Lecture Notes in Computer Science 3750

James S. Duncan   Guido Gerig (Eds.)

Medical Image Computing and Computer-Assisted Intervention – MICCAI 2005

8th International Conference
Palm Springs, CA, USA, October 26-29, 2005
Proceedings, Part II

Springer

Volume Editors

James S. Duncan
Yale University
Departments of Biomedical Engineering and Diagnostic Radiology
333 Cedar Street, P.O. Box 208042, New Haven, CT 06520-8042, USA
E-mail: james.duncan@yale.edu

Guido Gerig
University of North Carolina
Department of Computer Science
CB# 3175, 219 Sitterson Hall, Chapel Hill, NC 27599-3175, USA
E-mail: gerig@cs.unc.edu

Library of Congress Control Number: 2005933259

CR Subject Classification (1998): I.5, I.4, I.3.5-8, I.2.9-10, J.3, J.6

ISSN 0302-9743
ISBN-10 3-540-29326-4 Springer Berlin Heidelberg New York
ISBN-13 978-3-540-29326-2 Springer Berlin Heidelberg New York

Springer is a part of Springer Science+Business Media

springeronline.com

Printed in Germany

Typesetting: Camera-ready by author, data conversion by Scientific Publishing Services, Chennai, India
Printed on acid-free paper SPIN: 11566489 06/3142 5 4 3 2 1 0

Preface

The 8th International Conference on Medical Imaging and Computer Assisted Intervention, MICCAI 2005, was held in Palm Springs, California, USA, at the Riviera Resort, October 26–29, 2005.

MICCAI has become a premier international conference with in-depth papers on the multidisciplinary fields of medical image computing, computer-assisted intervention and medical robotics. The conference brings together clinicians, biological scientists, computer scientists, engineers, physicists and other researchers and offers them a forum to exchange ideas in these exciting and rapidly growing fields.

The impact of MICCAI increases each year and the quality and quantity of submitted papers this year was very impressive. We received a record 632 full submissions (8 pages in length), an increase of 22% from 2004, from 36 different countries and 5 continents (see fig. 2). Based on a decision of the MICCAI board, this year's conference employed a double-blind review procedure on a trial basis. Our Program Committee was made up of 11 area chairs, each of whom supervised the review of almost 60 papers. Four reviews were generated for each paper from 262 reviewers and the area chairs. A final paper selection meeting took place during two days in early June 2005 in Chapel Hill, North Carolina. We are especially grateful to Elizabeth Bullitt, Polina Golland, David Haynor, Rasmus Larsen, Greg Hager and Daniel Rückert, who attended this meeting and helped us make the final selections. Martin Styner provided valuable help with information management and the Web-site, and James Stewart is acknowledged for reliable and timely support of the Web-based reviewing system. We are grateful to everyone who participated in the review process; they donated a large amount of time and effort to make these volumes possible and insure a high level of quality. Because of the overall quality of the submissions and because of the limited number of slots available for presentation, paper selection was especially challenging. The MICCAI 2005 Program Committee finally accepted 236 full papers. The normal mode of presentation at MICCAI 2005 was as a poster; in addition, 46 papers were chosen for oral presentation. All of the full papers accepted are included in these proceedings in 8-page format. We also accepted 34 short communications (2 pages) which were presented as posters but not included in the proceedings.

The first figure below shows the distribution of the 236 full paper contributions by topic; the topics are defined by the primary keyword of the submission. The second figure illustrates the distribution of full paper submissions (a total of 632) by region.

We note that this year's program included some new features, including a session on Celullar and Molecular Imaging and Analysis. We hope that all who attended the 2005 meeting felt as we do that the program was both strong and diverse, within the range of topics covered by MICCAI.

It was our pleasure to welcome this year's MICCAI 2005 attendees to Palm Springs. Sitting in lush farming land, Palm Springs does not conform to any typical image of the desert, embodying a mix of Spanish Colonial and mid-twentieth century modern styling. Ever since Hollywood stars first came here in the 1930s, laying claim to ranch-style estates, holing up in elite hotels, and enjoying the clean dry air and sunshine, Palm Springs has been a special place to visit. We hope that the attendees, in addition to visiting the conference, took the opportunity to enjoy the hospitality and amenities of the Riviera Resort, and to explore the city, the desert region, and other parts of Southern California. For those unable to attend, we trust that these volumes will provide a valuable record of the state of the art in the MICCAI disciplines.

We also want to thank both our sponsors who are listed below and our two keynote speakers, Profs. Scott Fraser from Caltech and Arthur Toga from UCLA for excellent and stimulating lectures.

Finally, we note that this year a landmark event occurred in the life of MICCAI, namely the formation of the Medical Image Computing and Computer-Assisted Intervention Society (the MICCAI Society) which was officially announced on December 9, 2004. The main focus of the society is our annual international conference series (www.miccai.org) which has become the premier conference in the field of medical image computing and computer-assisted interventions, including biomedical imaging and robotics. The society is governed and administered by the MICCAI Board of Directors. The society will continue to publish the proceedings of the annual MICCAI conference in a prestigious scientific series. Having a paper accepted for publication in this series is highly meritorious and on a par with publication in highly regarded peer-reviewed journals in the field. The society is negotiating with three journals in the field of MICCAI themes, each to become "an affiliated MICCAI journal". These journals will offer significant benefits to members, including sharply discounted rates for paper subscriptions and access to on-line content. The society will continue to develop, enrich, and maintain a dynamic website with exclusive content for members (www.miccai.org).

We look forward to welcoming you to MICCAI 2006, to be held October 2–4, 2006 in Copenhagen, Denmark, and chaired by Mads Nielsen.

October 2005 James Duncan and Guido Gerig

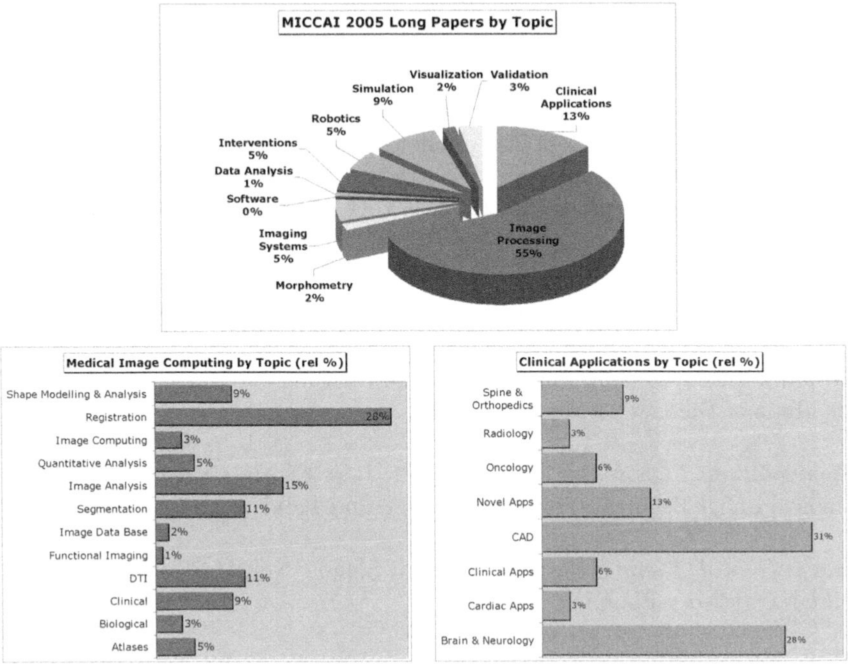

Fig. 1. View at a glance of MICCAI 2005 full paper contributions based on the declared primary keyword. A total of 236 full papers were presented

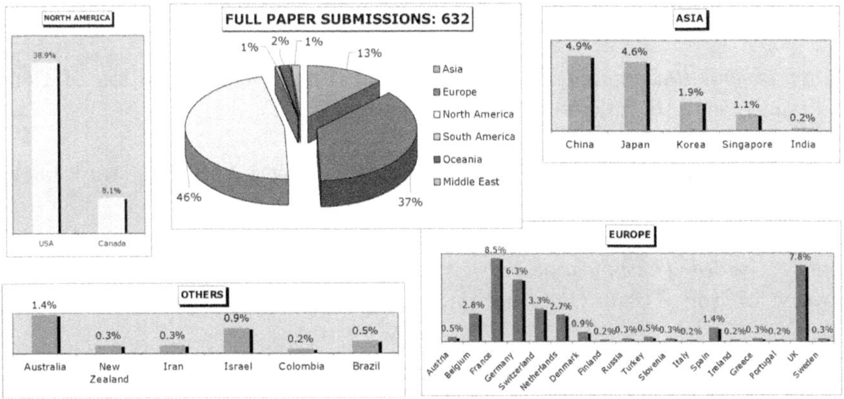

Fig. 2. Distribution of MICCAI 2005 full paper submissions (632 in total) by region

MICCAI Student Awards

Every year MICCAI awards outstanding work written and presented by students. Both oral and poster presentations are eligible for the awards, and the awards are presented to the winners in a public ceremony. Student awards at MICCAI 2003 and 2004 were sponsored by Northern Digital Incorporation (NDI), and NDI will also be the sponsor for the MICCAI 2005 awards.

MICCAI 2003 Student Awards

Robotics: Hashimoto, Ryuji: A Transurethral Prostate Resection Manipulator for Minimal Damage to Mucous Membrane

Segmentation: Pichon, Eric: A Statistically Based Surface Evolution Method for Medical Image Segmentation: Presentation and Validation

Image Guided Therapy Surgery: DiMaio, Simon: Needle Steering and Model-Based Trajectory Planning

Medical Image Analysis: Fillard, Pierre: Quantitative Analysis of White Matter Fiber Properties Along Geodesic Paths

Medical Image Processing and Visualization: Arsigny, Vincent: Polyrigid and Polyaffine Transformations: A New Class of Diffeomorphisms

MICCAI 2004 Student Awards

Image Segmentation and Processing: Dikici, Engin: Quantification of Delayed Enhancement MR Images

Image Registration and Analysis: Perperidis, Dimitrios: Spatio-temporal Free-Form Registration of Cardiac MR Image Sequences

Image Guided Therapy and Robotics: Stoyanov, Danail: Dense 3D Depth Recovery for Soft Tissue Deformation During Robotically Assisted Laparoscopic Surgery

Image Simulation and Display: Valtorta, Davide: Dynamic Measurements of Soft Tissue Viscoelastic Properties with a Torsional Resonator Device

Organization

Executive Committee

James Duncan (General Chair), New Haven, USA
Guido Gerig (Program Chair), Chapel Hill, USA
Christian Barillot, Rennes, France
Mads Nielsen, Copenhagen, Denmark
Terry Peters, London, Canada

Program Committee

Nicholas Ayache, Sophia-Antipolis, France
Elizabeth Bullitt, Chapel Hill, USA
Christos Davatzikos, Philadelphia, USA
Polina Golland, Boston, USA
Gregory D. Hager, Baltimore, USA
David Haynor, Seattle, USA
Leo Joskowicz, Jerusalem, Israel
Rasmus Larsen, Copenhagen, Denmark
Keith Paulsen, Hanover, USA
Daniel Rückert, London, UK
Ross Whitaker, Salt Lake City, USA

MICCAI Board

Alan Colchester (General Chair), Canterbury, UK
Nicholas Ayache, Sophia Antipolis, France
Christian Barillot, Rennes, France
Takeyoshi Dohi, Tokyo, Japan
James Duncan, New Haven, USA
Karl Heinz Höhne, Hamburg, Germany
Anthony Maeder, Brisbane, Queensland, Australia
Mads Nielsen, Copenhagen, Denmark
Terry Peters, London, Ontario, Canada
Richard Robb, Rochester, USA
Max Viergever, Utrecht, The Netherlands

MICCAI Society

Society Officers

President and Chair	Alan Colchester, Canterbury, UK
Executive Director	Richard Robb, Rochester, USA
Vice Chair (2005)	Christian Barillot, Rennes, France
Executive Secretary	Nicholas Ayache, Sophia Antipolis, France
Treasurer	Terry Peters, London, Ontario, Canada

Society Staff

Membership Coordinator	Gabor Székely, Zurich, Switzerland
Publications Coordinator	Nobuhiko Hata, Boston, USA

Tutorial Chair

Larry Staib, New Haven, CT, USA

Information Management and Web Administration

Martin Styner, Chapel Hill, NC, USA

Poster Coordination

Isabelle Corouge, Chapel Hill, WA, USA

Sponsors and Exhibits Coordination

Tina Kapur, Seattle, USA

Student Awards Coordination

Karl Heinz Höhne, Hamburg, Germany

Local Conference Management/Secretariat

Carolyn Meloling, New Haven, CT, USA
Delphine Bull, Chapel Hill, NC, USA

Sponsors

We are grateful to the following organizations for their generous financial support of MICCAI 2005:

- Northern Digital Inc. of Waterloo, Ontario
- Springer Lecture Notes in Computer Science (LNCS)
- GE Healthcare
- Medtronics Navigation
- Siemens Corporate Research
- NIBIB

Furthermore, the following organizations put up financial support: Claron Technology, Ascension Technology Corporation, BrainLAB and Elsevier.

Reviewers

Alberola-López, Carlos
Archip, Neculai
Asano, Takehide
Ashburner, John
Audette, Michel
Ayache, Nicholas
Aylward, Stephen
Azar, Fred S.
Bardinet, Eric
Barillot, Christian
Barratt, Dean
Bello, Fernando
Berger, Marie-Odile
Bhotika, Rahul
Boctor, Emad
Bouix, Sylvain
Bucholz, Richard
Bullitt, Elizabeth
Burghart, Catherina R.
Cahill, Nathan
Camara-Rey, Oscar
Castro, Alfonso
Castro-Pareja, Carlos
Cen, Feng
Chang, Hsun-Hsien
Chang, Sukmoon
Chen, Jian
Cheng, Lishui
Christensen, Gary
Chung, Moo
Colchester, Alan
Collins, D. Louis
Colliot, Olivier
Comaniciu, Dorin
Corouge, Isabelle
Coulon, Olivier
Crouch, Jessica
Dam, Erik
Davatzikos, Christos
Davis, Brad
Dawant, Benoit
de Bruijne, Marleen
Delingette, Hervé
Descoteaux, Maxime
Desvignes, Michel
Dillenseger, Jean-Louis
DiMaio, Simon
Duchesne, Simon
Duncan, James S.
El-Baz, Ayman
Ellis, Randy
Falcão, Alexandre
Fan, Yong
Faugeras, Olivier

Fenster, Aaron
Fichtinger, Gabor
Forest, Clément
Frangi, Alejandro
Friedman, Allan
Friman, Ola
Gan, Rui
Gee, James
Gerig, Guido
Gering, David
Gerritsen, Frans
Gibaud, Bernard
Golland, Polina
Gonzalez Ballester, Miguel Angel
Gooding, Mark
Grau, Vicente
Grimson, Eric
Haber, Eldad
Hager, Gregory D
Hahn, Horst
Haidar, Haissam
Haigron, Pascal
Hamarneh, Ghassan
Harders, Matthias
Hashizume, Makoto
Hassouna, Mohamed
Hastenteufel, Mark
Hastreiter, Peter
Hata, Nobuhiko
Hawkes, David
Haynor, David
He, Ying
Hedjidemetriou, Efstathios
Hellier, Pierre
Heng, Pheng Ann
Hibbard, Lyn
Holmes, David
Höhne, Karl Heinz
Hong, Byung-Woo
Hong, Helen
Hornegger, Joachim
Howe, Robert
Huang, Heng
Iseki, Hiroshi
Jannin, Pierre
Jaramaz, Branislav
Jomier, Julien
Joshi, Sarang
Joskowicz, Leo
Kang, MyungJin
Karron, DB
Kaus, Michael
Keeve, Erwin
Kerrien, Erwan
Khamene, Ali
Kikinis, Ron
Kim, Sun I.
Kissi, Adelaide
Kronreif, Gernot
Kruggel, Frithjof
Lötjönen, Jyrki
Lange, Thomas
Lapeer, Rudy
Larsen, Rasmus
Leahy, Richard
Lee, Sang-Chul
Li, Rongxin
Li, Shuo
Liang, Jianming
Liao, Hongen
Liao, Rui
Lienard, Jean
Linguraru, Marius George
Liu, Alan
Liu, Huafeng
Liu, Jundong
Liu, Tianming
Loog, Marco
Lorensen, William
Lorenzen, Peter
Macq, Benoit
Madabhushi, Anant
Maddah, Mahnaz
Maeder, Anthony
Maes, Frederik
Makram-Ebeid, Sherif
Malandain, Gregoire
Mancas, Matei
Mangin, Jean-Francois
Martin-Fernandez, Marcos

Mattes, Julian
Maurer, Calvin
McInerney, Tim
Metaxas, Dimitris
Meyer, Chuck
Miga, Michael I.
Mori, Kensaku
Muragaki, Yoshihiro
Navab, Nassir
Nicolau, Stephane
Niessen, Wiro
Noble, Alison
Nolte, Lutz
O'Donnell, Thomas
Okada, Kazunori
Olabarriaga, Silvia
Olsen, Ole Fogh
Ordas, Sebastian
Ortmaier, Tobias
Ourselin, Sebastien
Palm, Christoph
Papademetris, Xenophon
Paragios, Nikos
Patriciu, Alexandru
Paulsen, Keith
Peitgen, Heinz-Otto
Pelegrini-Issac, Mélanie
Pennec, Xavier
Peters, Terry M.
Pham, Dzung
Pichon, Eric
Pizer, Stephen
Pluim, Josien
Pommert, Andreas
Prager, Richard
Prastawa, Marcel
Prima, Sylvain
Prince, Jerry L.
Pujol, Sonia
Robb, Richard A.
Rohlfing, Torsten
Rohling, Robert
Rohr, Karl
Rosenthal, Michael
Rosiene, Joel
Rueckert, Daniel
Ruiz-Alzola, Juan
Russakoff, Daniel
Sato, Yoshinobu
Sauer, Frank
Schnabel, Julia
Shen, Dinggang
Shi, Pengcheng
Shimizu, Akinobu
Skrinjar, Oskar
Sonka, Milan
Stewart, James
Stokking, Rik
Studholme, Colin
Styner, Martin
Subramanian, Navneeth
Suetens, Paul
Sun, Hai
Syeda-Mahmood, Tanveer
Székely, Gabor
Tannenbaum, Allen
Tao, Xiaodong
Tasdizen, Tolga
Taylor, Chris
Taylor, Russell
Tek, Huseyin
ter Haar Romeny, Bart M.
Terzopoulos, Demetri
Thiran, Jean-Philippe
Thirion, Bertrand
Tohka, Jussi
Tosun, Duygu
Troccaz, Jocelyne
Vaillant, Regis
van Assen, Hans
van Ginneken, Bram
Van Leemput, Koen
Vandermeulen, Dirk
Vermeer, Koen
Vetsa, Yethiraja Sampath K.
Vos, Frans
Vosburgh, Kirby
Vossepoel, Albert
Wai, Lionel C.C.
Wang, Jianzhe

Wang, Yalin
Wang, Yongmei Michelle
Wang, Yuanquan
Warfield, Simon
Westin, Carl-Fredrik
Whitaker, Ross
Wildermuth, Simon
Williams, James
Wong, Wilbur C.K.
Wu, Chia-Hsiang
Wu, John Jue
Wu, Ziji
Wyatt, Chris
Xu, Xiaoyin
Xue, Zhong
Yan, Pingkun
Yang, Guang-Zhong
Yang, Jing
Yaniv, Ziv
Yoo, Terry
Yuan, Xiaohui
Yushkevich, Paul
Zeng, Jianchao
Zhao, Zheen
Zheng, Guoyan
Zhu, Chaozhe
Zou, Kelly
Zrimec, Tatjana

Table of Contents – Part II

Robotics, Image-Guided Surgery and Interventions

Sensor Guided Ablation Procedure of Left Atrial Endocardium
Hua Zhong, Takeo Kanade, David Schwartzman 1

A Method to Evaluate Human Spatial Coordination Interfaces for Computer-Assisted Surgery
M.A. Cardin, J.X. Wang, D.B. Plewes 9

3D TRUS Guided Robot Assisted Prostate Brachytherapy
Zhouping Wei, Mingyue Ding, Donal Downey, Aaron Fenster 17

Invisible Shadow for Navigation and Planning in Minimal Invasive Surgery
Marios Nicolaou, Adam James, Benny P.L. Lo, Ara Darzi, Guang-Zhong Yang 25

A Navigation System for Minimally Invasive CT-Guided Interventions
Markus Nagel, Gerd Schmidt, Ralf Petzold, Willi A. Kalender 33

Passive Markers for Ultrasound Tracking of Surgical Instruments
Jeffrey Stoll, Pierre Dupont 41

Optimal Trajectories Computation Within Regions of Interest for Hepatic RFA Planning
Caroline Villard, Claire Baegert, Pascal Schreck, Luc Soler, Afshin Gangi 49

Effects of Latency on Telesurgery: An Experimental Study
Reiza Rayman, Serguei Primak, Rajni Patel, Merhdad Moallem, Roya Morady, Mahdi Tavakoli, Vanja Subotic, Natalie Galbraith, Aimee van Wynsberghe, Kris Croome 57

A Novel Phantom-Less Spatial and Temporal Ultrasound Calibration Method
Ali Khamene, Frank Sauer 65

Electromagnetic Tracker Measurement Error Simulation and Tool Design
Gregory S. Fischer, Russell H. Taylor 73

Compact Forceps Manipulator Using Friction Wheel Mechanism and Gimbals Mechanism for Laparoscopic Surgery
Takashi Suzuki, Youichi Katayama, Etsuko Kobayashi, Ichiro Sakuma 81

Spatial Motion Constraints for Robot Assisted Suturing Using Virtual Fixtures
Ankur Kapoor, Ming Li, Russell H. Taylor 89

Contact Force Measurement of Instruments for Force-Feedback on a Surgical Robot: Acceleration Force Cancellations Based on Acceleration Sensor Readings
Shigeyuki Shimachi, Fumie Kameyama, Yoshihide Hakozaki, Yasunori Fujiwara 97

Development of the Needle Insertion Robot for Percutaneous Vertebroplasty
S. Onogi, K. Morimoto, I. Sakuma, Y. Nakajima, T. Koyama, N. Sugano, Y. Tamura, S. Yonenobu, Y. Momoi 105

Laparoscope Self-calibration for Robotic Assisted Minimally Invasive Surgery
Danail Stoyanov, Ara Darzi, Guang Zhong Yang 114

A Hand-Eye Robotic Model for Total Knee Replacement Surgery
Fanhuai Shi, Jing Zhang, Yuncai Liu, Zijian Zhao 122

Robot-Assisted Image-Guided Targeting for Minimally Invasive Neurosurgery: Planning, Registration, and In-vitro Experiment
R. Shamir, M. Freiman, L. Joskowicz, M. Shoham, E. Zehavi, Y. Shoshan 131

Soft-Tissue Motion Tracking and Structure Estimation for Robotic Assisted MIS Procedures
Danail Stoyanov, George P. Mylonas, Fani Deligianni, Ara Darzi, Guang-Zhong Yang 139

Image Registration II

Mass Preserving Registration for Heart MR Images
Lei Zhu, Steven Haker, Allen Tannenbaum 147

Liver Registration for the Follow-Up of Hepatic Tumors
Arnaud Charnoz, Vincent Agnus, Grégoire Malandain, Clément Forest, Mohamed Tajine, Luc Soler 155

Maximum a Posteriori Local Histogram Estimation for Image Registration
Matthew Toews, D. Louis Collins, Tal Arbel 163

Dynamic 3D Ultrasound and MR Image Registration of the Beating Heart
Xishi Huang, Nicholas A. Hill, Jing Ren, Gerard Guiraudon, Derek Boughner, Terry M. Peters 171

Learning Best Features for Deformable Registration of MR Brains
Guorong Wu, Feihu Qi, Dinggang Shen 179

Stochastic Inverse Consistency in Medical Image Registration
Sai Kit Yeung, Pengcheng Shi 188

A Novel Incremental Technique for Ultrasound to CT Bone Surface Registration Using Unscented Kalman Filtering
Mehdi Hedjazi Moghari, Purang Abolmaesumi 197

Automatic 4-D Registration in Dynamic MR Renography Based on Over-Complete Dyadic Wavelet and Fourier Transforms
Ting Song, Vivian S. Lee, Henry Rusinek, Manmeen Kaur, Andrew F. Laine 205

Model of a Vascular C-Arm for 3D Augmented Fluoroscopy in Interventional Radiology
S. Gorges, E. Kerrien, M-O. Berger, Y. Trousset, J. Pescatore, R. Anxionnat, L. Picard 214

2D/3D Deformable Registration Using a Hybrid Atlas
Thomas S.Y. Tang, Randy E. Ellis 223

Reconstruction-Based 3D/2D Image Registration
Dejan Tomaževič, Boštjan Likar, Franjo Pernuš 231

Comparison of Simultaneous and Sequential Two-View Registration for 3D/2D Registration of Vascular Images
Chetna Pathak, Mark Van Horn, Susan Weeks, Elizabeth Bullitt 239

Interpolation Artefacts in Non-rigid Registration
P. Aljabar, J.V. Hajnal, R.G. Boyes, D. Rueckert 247

Learning Based Non-rigid Multi-modal Image Registration Using Kullback-Leibler Divergence
Christoph Guetter, Chenyang Xu, Frank Sauer, Joachim Hornegger 255

Deformable Registration of Brain Tumor Images Via a Statistical Model of Tumor-Induced Deformation
Ashraf Mohamed, Dinggang Shen, Christos Davatzikos 263

Myocardial Motion Estimation in Tagged MR Sequences by Using αMI-Based Non Rigid Registration
E. Oubel, C. Tobon-Gomez, A.O. Hero, A.F. Frangi 271

Iterative 3D Point-Set Registration Based on Hierarchical Vertex Signature (HVS)
Jun Feng, Horace H.S. Ip 279

Automatic Patient Registration for Port Placement in Minimally Invasive Endoscopic Surgery
Marco Feuerstein, Stephen M. Wildhirt, Robert Bauernschmitt, Nassir Navab 287

Hybrid Formulation of the Model-Based Non-rigid Registration Problem to Improve Accuracy and Robustness
Olivier Clatz, Hervé Delingette, Ion-Florin Talos, Alexandra J. Golby, Ron Kikinis, Ferenc A. Jolesz, Nicholas Ayache, Simon K. Warfield 295

Automatic Registration and Fusion of Ultrasound with CT for Radiotherapy
Wolfgang Wein, Barbara Röper, Nassir Navab 303

Medical Image Computing - Atlases - Shape I

Lung Deformation Estimation and Four-Dimensional CT Lung Reconstruction
Sheng Xu, Russell H. Taylor, Gabor Fichtinger, Kevin Cleary 312

Automatic Parameter Optimization for De-noising MR Data
Joaquín Castellanos, Karl Rohr, Thomas Tolxdorff, Gudrun Wagenknecht 320

Towards a Dynamic Model of Pulmonary Parenchymal Deformation: Evaluation of Methods for Temporal Reparameterization of Lung Data
Tessa A. Sundaram, Brian B. Avants, James C. Gee 328

4D MR Imaging Using Internal Respiratory Gating
M. von Siebenthal, Ph. Cattin, U. Gamper, A. Lomax, G. Székely 336

Anatomically Constrained Surface Parameterization for Cortical Localization
C. Clouchoux, O. Coulon, D. Rivière, A. Cachia, J.-F. Mangin, J. Régis 344

Multiresolution Parametric Estimation of Transparent Motions and Denoising of Fluoroscopic Images
Vincent Auvray, Jean Liénard, Patrick Bouthemy 352

Plaque and Stent Artifact Reduction in Subtraction CT Angiography Using Nonrigid Registration and a Volume Penalty
Dirk Loeckx, Stylianos Drisis, Frederik Maes, Dirk Vandermeulen, Guy Marchal, Paul Suetens 361

Respiratory Motion Correction in Emission Tomography Image Reconstruction
Mauricio Reyes, Grégoire Malandain, Pierre Malick Koulibaly, Miguel A. González Ballester, Jacques Darcourt 369

Optimal Embedding for Shape Indexing in Medical Image Databases
Xiaoning Qian, Hemant D. Tagare 377

Retrospective Cross-Evaluation of an Histological and Deformable 3D Atlas of the Basal Ganglia on Series of Parkinsonian Patients Treated by Deep Brain Stimulation
Eric Bardinet, Didier Dormont, Grégoire Malandain, Manik Bhattacharjee, Bernard Pidoux, Christian Saleh, Philippe Cornu, Nicholas Ayache, Yves Agid, Jérôme Yelnik 385

Anatomical and Electrophysiological Validation of an Atlas for Neurosurgical Planning
M. Mallar Chakravarty, Abbas F. Sadikot, Jurgen Germann, Gilles Bertrand, D. Louis Collins 394

Construction of a 4D Statistical Atlas of the Cardiac Anatomy and Its Use in Classification
Dimitrios Perperidis, Raad Mohiaddin, Daniel Rueckert 402

Unbiased Atlas Formation Via Large Deformations Metric Mapping
Peter Lorenzen, Brad Davis, Sarang Joshi 411

Least Biased Target Selection in Probabilistic Atlas Construction
Hyunjin Park, Peyton H. Bland, Alfred O. Hero III, Charles R. Meyer 419

Automatic Selection of DBS Target Points Using Multiple Electrophysiological Atlases
Pierre-Francois D'Haese, Srivatsan Pallavaram, Ken Niermann, John Spooner, Chris Kao, Peter E. Konrad, Benoit M. Dawant 427

Nonrigid Shape Correspondence Using Landmark Sliding, Insertion and Deletion
Theodor Richardson, Song Wang 435

Statistical Face Models for the Prediction of Soft-Tissue Deformations After Orthognathic Osteotomies
Sebastian Meller, Emeka Nkenke, Willi A. Kalender 443

Fully Automatic Shape Modelling Using Growing Cell Neural Networks
Luca Ferrarini, Hans Olofsen, Mark A. van Buchem, Johan H.C. Reiber, Faiza Admiraal-Behloul 451

Multiscale 3D Shape Analysis Using Spherical Wavelets
Delphine Nain, Steven Haker, Aaron Bobick, Allen R. Tannenbaum 459

Structural and Functional Brain Analysis

Discriminative Analysis of Brain Function at Resting-State for Attention-Deficit/Hyperactivity Disorder
C.Z. Zhu, Y.F. Zang, M. Liang, L.X. Tian, Y. He, X.B. Li, M.Q. Sui, Y.F. Wang, T.Z. Jiang 468

Finding Landmarks in the Functional Brain: Detection and Use for Group Characterization
Bertrand Thirion, Philippe Pinel, Jean-Baptiste Poline 476

Topology Correction Using Fast Marching Methods and Its Application to Brain Segmentation
Pierre-Louis Bazin, Dzung L. Pham 484

New Ratios for the Detection and Classification of CJD in Multisequence MRI of the Brain
Marius George Linguraru, Nicholas Ayache, Miguel Ángel González Ballester, Eric Bardinet, Damien Galanaud, Stéphane Haïk, Baptiste Faucheux, Patrick Cozzone, Didier Dormont, Jean-Philippe Brandel 492

Model-Based Image Analysis

Statistical Representation and Simulation of High-Dimensional Deformations: Application to Synthesizing Brain Deformations
Zhong Xue, Dinggang Shen, Bilge Karacali, Christos Davatzikos 500

Model-Based Parameter Recovery from Uncalibrated Optical Images
S.J. Preece, I.B. Styles, S.D. Cotton, E. Claridge, A. Calcagni 509

MRI Tissue Classification with Neighborhood Statistics: A Nonparametric, Entropy-Minimizing Approach
Tolga Tasdizen, Suyash P. Awate, Ross T. Whitaker, Norman L. Foster 517

Image-Guided Intervention: Simulation, Modeling and Display

Robotic Assisted Radio-Frequency Ablation of Liver Tumors – Randomized Patient Study
A. Patriciu, M. Awad, S.B. Solomon, M. Choti, D. Mazilu, L. Kavoussi, D. Stoianovici 526

New Approaches to Catheter Navigation for Interventional Radiology Simulation
S. Cotin, C. Duriez, J. Lenoir, P. Neumann, S. Dawson 534

Hybrid Bronchoscope Tracking Using a Magnetic Tracking Sensor and Image Registration
Kensaku Mori, Daisuke Deguchi, Kenta Akiyama, Takayuki Kitasaka, Calvin R. Maurer Jr., Yasuhito Suenaga, Hirotsugu Takabatake, Masaki Mori, Hiroshi Natori 543

Toward Robotized Beating Heart TECABG: Assessment of the Heart Dynamics Using High-Speed Vision
Loïc Cuvillon, Jacques Gangloff, Michel de Mathelin, Antonello Forgione 551

Data-Fusion Display System with Volume Rendering of Intraoperatively Scanned CT Images
Mitsuhiro Hayashibe, Naoki Suzuki, Asaki Hattori, Yoshito Otake, Shigeyuki Suzuki, Norio Nakata 559

Simulation and Modeling II

A Hybrid Cutting Approach for Hysteroscopy Simulation
M. Harders, D. Steinemann, M. Gross, G. Székely 567

Hydrometra Simulation for VR-Based Hysteroscopy Training
R. Sierra, J. Zátonyi, M. Bajka, G. Székely, M. Harders 575

Brain Shift Computation Using a Fully Nonlinear Biomechanical Model
Adam Wittek, Ron Kikinis, Simon K. Warfield, Karol Miller 583

Finite Element Model of Cornea Deformation
Jessica R. Crouch, John C. Merriam, Earl R. Crouch III 591

Characterization of Viscoelastic Soft Tissue Properties from *In vivo* Animal Experiments and Inverse FE Parameter Estimation
Jung Kim, Mandayam A. Srinivasan 599

A Fast-Marching Approach to Cardiac Electrophysiology Simulation for XMR Interventional Imaging
M. Sermesant, Y. Coudière, V. Moreau-Villéger, K.S. Rhode, D.L.G. Hill, R.S. Razavi 607

An Inverse Problem Approach to the Estimation of Volume Change
Martin Schweiger, Oscar Camara-Rey, William R. Crum, Emma Lewis, Julia Schnabel, Simon R. Arridge, Derek L.G. Hill, Nick Fox 616

A Velocity-Dependent Model for Needle Insertion in Soft Tissue
Jessica R. Crouch, Chad M. Schneider, Josh Wainer, Allison M. Okamura 624

Material Properties Estimation of Layered Soft Tissue Based on MR Observation and Iterative FE Simulation
Mitsunori Tada, Noritaka Nagai, Takashi Maeno 633

Simulating Vascular Systems in Arbitrary Anatomies
Dominik Szczerba, Gábor Székely 641

Medical Image Computing - Shape II

Physiological System Identification with the Kalman Filter in Diffuse Optical Tomography
Solomon Gilbert Diamond, Theodore J. Huppert, Ville Kolehmainen, Maria Angela Franceschini, Jari P. Kaipio, Simon R. Arridge, David A. Boas 649

Brain Surface Parameterization Using Riemann Surface Structure
Yalin Wang, Xianfeng Gu, Kiralee M. Hayashi, Tony F. Chan, Paul M. Thompson, Shing-Tung Yau 657

Automated Surface Matching Using Mutual Information Applied to Riemann Surface Structures
Yalin Wang, Ming-Chang Chiang, Paul M. Thompson 666

Optimization of Brain Conformal Mapping with Landmarks
Yalin Wang, Lok Ming Lui, Tony F. Chan, Paul M. Thompson 675

A New Method for SPECT Quantification of Targeted Radiotracers Uptake in the Myocardium
Shimin Li, Lawrence W. Dobrucki, Albert J. Sinusas, Yi-Hwa Liu 684

Tracking and Analysis of Cine-Delayed Enhancement MR
Thomas O'Donnell, Engin Dikici, Randolph Setser, Richard D. White 692

Characterizing Vascular Connectivity from microCT Images
Marcel Jackowski, Xenophon Papademetris, Lawrence W. Dobrucki, Albert J. Sinusas, Lawrence H. Staib 701

Shape Modeling Using Automatic Landmarking
Jun Xie, Pheng-Ann Heng 709

A Computer-Aided Design System for Revision of Segmentation Errors
Marcel Jackowski, Ardeshir Goshtasby 717

Statistical Modeling of Shape and Appearance Using the Continuous Medial Representation
Paul A. Yushkevich, Hui Zhang, James C. Gee 725

Vertebral Shape: Automatic Measurement with Dynamically Sequenced Active Appearance Models
M.G. Roberts, T.F. Cootes, J.E. Adams 733

Geodesic Active Contours with Adaptive Neighboring Influence
Huafeng Liu, Yunmei Chen, Hon Pong Ho, Pengcheng Shi 741

A Construction of an Averaged Representation of Human Cortical Gyri Using Non-linear Principal Component Analysis
G. Lohmann, D.Y. von Cramon, A.C.F. Colchester 749

Efficient Kernel Density Estimation of Shape and Intensity Priors for Level Set Segmentation
Mikael Rousson, Daniel Cremers 757

Corpus Callosum Subdivision Based on a Probabilistic Model of Inter-hemispheric Connectivity
Martin A. Styner, Ipek Oguz, Rachel Gimpel Smith, Carissa Cascio, Matthieu Jomier 765

Image Segmentation and Analysis II

Random Walks for Interactive Organ Segmentation in Two and Three Dimensions: Implementation and Validation
Leo Grady, Thomas Schiwietz, Shmuel Aharon, Rüdiger Westermann 773

Robust Pulmonary Nodule Segmentation in CT: Improving Performance for Juxtapleural Cases
K. Okada, V. Ramesh, A. Krishnan, M. Singh, U. Akdemir 781

Tissue Classification of Noisy MR Brain Images Using Constrained GMM
Amit Ruf, Hayit Greenspan, Jacob Goldberger 790

Automatic Left Atrium Segmentation by Cutting the Blood Pool at Narrowings
Matthias John, Norbert Rahn 798

Automatic Vascular Tree Formation Using the Mahalanobis Distance
Julien Jomier, Vincent LeDigarcher, Stephen R. Aylward 806

The Use of Unwrapped Phase in MR Image Segmentation: A Preliminary Study
Pierrick Bourgeat, Jurgen Fripp, Andrew Janke, Graham Galloway, Stuart Crozier, Sébastien Ourselin 813

2D and 3D Shape Based Segmentation Using Deformable Models
Ayman El-Baz, Seniha E. Yuksel, Hongjian Shi, Aly A. Farag, Mohamed A. El-Ghar, Tarek Eldiasty, Mohamed A. Ghoneim 821

CT Hepatic Venography: 3D Vascular Segmentation for Preoperative Evaluation
Catalin Fetita, Olivier Lucidarme, Françoise Prêteux, Philippe Grenier 830

Shape-Based Averaging for Combination of Multiple Segmentations
T. Rohlfing, C.R. Maurer, Jr. 838

Automatic Initialization Algorithm for Carotid Artery Segmentation in CTA Images
Martijn Sanderse, Henk A. Marquering, Emile A. Hendriks, Aad van der Lugt, Johan H.C. Reiber 846

Automated Nomenclature of Bronchial Branches Extracted from CT Images and Its Application to Biopsy Path Planning in Virtual Bronchoscopy
Kensaku Mori, Sinya Ema, Takayuki Kitasaka, Yoshito Mekada, Ichiro Ide, Hiroshi Murase, Yasuhito Suenaga, Hirotsugu Takabatake, Masaki Mori, Hiroshi Natori 854

Spectral Clustering Algorithms for Ultrasound Image Segmentation
Neculai Archip, Robert Rohling, Peter Cooperberg, Hamid Tahmasebpour, Simon K. Warfield 862

Using the Fast Marching Method to Extract Curves with Given Global Properties
Xiaodong Tao, Christos Davatzikos, Jerry L. Prince 870

Robust Tissue Boundary Detection for Cerebral Cortical Thickness Estimation
Marietta L.J. Scott, Neil A. Thacker 878

Statistical Analysis of Pharmacokinetic Models in Dynamic Contrast-Enhanced Magnetic Resonance Imaging
Volker J. Schmid, Brandon J. Whitcher, Guang-Zhong Yang, N. Jane Taylor, Anwar R. Padhani 886

Image Registration III

Inter-breath-hold Registration for the Production of High Resolution Cardiac MR Volumes
Nicholas M.I. Noble, Redha Boubertakh, Reza S. Razavi, Derek L.G. Hill 894

Consistent Estimation of Cardiac Motions by 4D Image Registration
Dinggang Shen, Hari Sundar, Zhong Xue, Yong Fan, Harold Litt 902

Multispectral MR to X-Ray Registration of Vertebral Bodies by Generating CT-Like Data
Everine B. van de Kraats, Graeme P. Penney, Theo van Walsum, Wiro J. Niessen 911

Articulated Rigid Registration for Serial Lower-Limb Mouse Imaging
Xenophon Papademetris, Donald P. Dione, Lawrence W. Dobrucki, Lawrence H. Staib, Albert J. Sinusas 919

Incorporating Statistical Measures of Anatomical Variability in Atlas-to-Subject Registration for Conformal Brain Radiotherapy
Olivier Commowick, Radu Stefanescu, Pierre Fillard, Vincent Arsigny, Nicholas Ayache, Xavier Pennec, Grégoire Malandain 927

Accurate Image Registration for Quadrature Tomographic Microscopy
Chia-Ling Tsai, William Warger II, Charles DiMarzio 935

Riemannian Elasticity: A Statistical Regularization Framework for Non-linear Registration
X. Pennec, R. Stefanescu, V. Arsigny, P. Fillard, N. Ayache 943

3D Model-Based Approach to Lung Registration and Prediction of Respiratory Cardiac Motion
Mikhail G. Danilouchkine, Jos J.M. Westenberg, Hans C. van Assen, Johan H.C. van Reiber, Boudewijn P.F. Lelieveldt 951

Fast DRR Generation for 2D/3D Registration
W. Birkfellner, R. Seemann, M. Figl, J. Hummel, C. Ede, P. Homolka, X. Yang, P. Niederer, H. Bergmann 960

Validation of PET Imaging by Alignment to Histology Slices
Philip J. Edwards, Ayman D. Nijmeh, Mark McGurk, Edward Odell, Michael R. Fenlon, Paul K. Marsden, David J. Hawkes 968

Adaptive Subdivision for Hierarchical Non-rigid Registration of Multi-modal Images Using Mutual Information
Adrian Andronache, Philippe Cattin, Gábor Székely 976

3-D Diffeomorphic Shape Registration on Hippocampal Data Sets
Hongyu Guo, Anand Rangarajan, Sarang C. Joshi 984

Two-Stage Registration for Real-Time Deformable Compensation Using an Electromagnetic Tracking Device
Hui Zhang, Filip Banovac, Neil Glossop, Kevin Cleary 992

Cadaver Validation of Intensity-Based Ultrasound to CT Registration
Graeme P. Penney, Dean C. Barratt, Carolyn S.K. Chan, Mike Slomczykowski, Timothy J. Carter, Phillip J. Edwards, David J.Hawkes 1000

Author Index 1009

Table of Contents – Part I

Image Analysis and Validation

Classification of Structural Images via High-Dimensional Image Warping, Robust Feature Extraction, and SVM
Yong Fan, Dinggang Shen, Christos Davatzikos 1

Bone Enhancement Filtering: Application to Sinus Bone Segmentation and Simulation of Pituitary Surgery
Maxime Descoteaux, Michel Audette, Kiyoyuki Chinzei, Kaleem Siddiqi 9

Simultaneous Registration and Segmentation of Anatomical Structures from Brain MRI
Fei Wang, Baba C. Vemuri 17

Synthetic Ground Truth for Validation of Brain Tumor MRI Segmentation
Marcel Prastawa, Elizabeth Bullitt, Guido Gerig 26

Vascular Image Segmentation

Automatic Cerebrovascular Segmentation by Accurate Probabilistic Modeling of TOF-MRA Images
Ayman El-Baz, Aly A. Farag, Georgy Gimel'farb, Stephen G. Hushek 34

A Segmentation and Reconstruction Technique for 3D Vascular Structures
Vincent Luboz, Xunlei Wu, Karl Krissian, Carl-Fredrik Westin, Ron Kikinis, Stéphane Cotin, Steve Dawson 43

MRA Image Segmentation with Capillary Active Contour
Pingkun Yan, Ashraf A. Kassim 51

Spatial Graphs for Intra-cranial Vascular Network Characterization, Generation, and Discrimination
Stephen R. Aylward, Julien Jomier, Christelle Vivert, Vincent LeDigarcher, Elizabeth Bullitt 59

Image Registration I

Surface Alignment of 3D Spherical Harmonic Models: Application to Cardiac MRI Analysis
Heng Huang, Li Shen, Rong Zhang, Fillia Makedon, Bruce Hettleman, Justin Pearlman 67

Unified Point Selection and Surface-Based Registration Using a Particle Filter
Burton Ma, Randy E. Ellis 75

Elastic Registration of 3D Ultrasound Images
Pezhman Foroughi, Purang Abolmaesumi 83

Tracer Kinetic Model-Driven Registration for Dynamic Contrast Enhanced MRI Time Series
Giovanni A. Buonaccorsi, Caleb Roberts, Sue Cheung, Yvonne Watson, Karen Davies, Alan Jackson, Gordon C. Jayson, Geoff J.M. Parker 91

Generalised Overlap Measures for Assessment of Pairwise and Groupwise Image Registration and Segmentation
William R. Crum, Oscar Camara, Daniel Rueckert, Kanwal K. Bhatia, Mark Jenkinson, Derek L.G. Hill 99

Diffusion Tensor Image Analysis

Uncertainty in White Matter Fiber Tractography
Ola Friman, Carl-Fredrik Westin 107

Fast and Simple Calculus on Tensors in the Log-Euclidean Framework
Vincent Arsigny, Pierre Fillard, Xavier Pennec, Nicholas Ayache 115

3D Curve Inference for Diffusion MRI Regularization
Peter Savadjiev, Jennifer S.W. Campbell, G. Bruce Pike, Kaleem Siddiqi 123

Fiber Tract-Oriented Statistics for Quantitative Diffusion Tensor MRI Analysis
Isabelle Corouge, P. Thomas Fletcher, Sarang Joshi, John H. Gilmore, Guido Gerig 131

White Matter Tract Clustering and Correspondence in Populations
Lauren O'Donnell, Carl-Fredrik Westin 140

76-Space Analysis of Grey Matter Diffusivity: Methods and Applications
Tianming Liu, Geoffrey Young, Ling Huang, Nan-Kuei Chen, Stephen TC Wong 148

Fast Orientation Mapping from HARDI
Evren Özarslan, Timothy M. Shepherd, Baba C. Vemuri, Stephen J. Blackband, Thomas H. Mareci 156

An Automated Approach to Connectivity-Based Partitioning of Brain Structures
P.A. Cook, H. Zhang, B.B. Avants, P. Yushkevich, D.C. Alexander, J.C. Gee, O. Ciccarelli, A.J. Thompson 164

Deformable Registration of Diffusion Tensor MR Images with Explicit Orientation Optimization
Hui Zhang, Paul A. Yushkevich, James C. Gee 172

A Hamilton-Jacobi-Bellman Approach to High Angular Resolution Diffusion Tractography
Eric Pichon, Carl-Fredrik Westin, Allen R. Tannenbaum 180

Automated Atlas-Based Clustering of White Matter Fiber Tracts from DTMRI
Mahnaz Maddah, Andrea U.J. Mewes, Steven Haker, W. Eric L. Grimson, Simon K. Warfield 188

MR Diffusion-Based Inference of a Fiber Bundle Model from a Population of Subjects
V. El Kouby, Y. Cointepas, C. Poupon, D. Rivière, N. Golestani, J.-B. Poline, D. Le Bihan, J.-F. Mangin 196

Knowledge-Based Classification of Neuronal Fibers in Entire Brain
Yan Xia, And U. Turken, Susan L. Whitfield-Gabrieli, John D. Gabrieli 205

A Physical Model for DT-MRI Based Connectivity Map Computation
Erdem Yörük, Burak Acar, Roland Bammer 213

Image Segmentation and Analysis I

A Novel 3D Partitioned Active Shape Model for Segmentation of Brain MR Images
Zheen Zhao, Stephen R. Aylward, Eam Khwang Teoh 221

Cross Entropy: A New Solver for Markov Random Field Modeling and Applications to Medical Image Segmentation
Jue Wu, Albert C.S. Chung 229

Semi-automated Basal Ganglia Segmentation Using Large Deformation Diffeomorphic Metric Mapping
Ali Khan, Elizabeth Aylward, Patrick Barta, Michael Miller, M. Faisal Beg 238

Particle Filters, a Quasi-Monte Carlo Solution for Segmentation of Coronaries
Charles Florin, Nikos Paragios, Jim Williams 246

Hybrid Segmentation Framework for Tissue Images Containing Gene Expression Data
Musodiq Bello, Tao Ju, Joe Warren, James Carson, Wah Chiu, Christina Thaller, Gregor Eichele, Ioannis A. Kakadiaris 254

Fully Automatic Kidneys Detection in 2D CT Images: A Statistical Approach
Wala Touhami, Djamal Boukerroui, Jean-Pierre Cocquerez 262

Segmentation of Neighboring Organs in Medical Image with Model Competition
Pingkun Yan, Weijia Shen, Ashraf A. Kassim, Mubarak Shah 270

Point-Based Geometric Deformable Models for Medical Image Segmentation
Hon Pong Ho, Yunmei Chen, Huafeng Liu, Pengcheng Shi 278

A Variational PDE Based Level Set Method for a Simultaneous Segmentation and Non-rigid Registration
Jung-ha An, Yunmei Chen, Feng Huang, David Wilson, Edward Geiser 286

A Tracking Approach to Parcellation of the Cerebral Cortex
Chris Adamson, Leigh Johnston, Terrie Inder, Sandra Rees, Iven Mareels, Gary Egan 294

Cell Segmentation, Tracking, and Mitosis Detection Using Temporal Context
Fuxing Yang, Michael A. Mackey, Fiorenza Ianzini, Greg Gallardo, Milan Sonka 302

A Unifying Approach to Registration, Segmentation, and Intensity Correction
Kilian M. Pohl, John Fisher, James J. Levitt, Martha E. Shenton, Ron Kikinis, W. Eric L. Grimson, William M. Wells ... 310

Automatic 3D Segmentation of Intravascular Ultrasound Images Using Region and Contour Information
Marie-Hélène Roy Cardinal, Jean Meunier, Gilles Soulez, Roch L. Maurice, Éric Thérasse, Guy Cloutier ... 319

Automatic Segmentation of the Articular Cartilage in Knee MRI Using a Hierarchical Multi-class Classification Scheme
Jenny Folkesson, Erik Dam, Ole Fogh Olsen, Paola Pettersen, Claus Christiansen ... 327

Automatic Segmentation of the Left Ventricle in 3D SPECT Data by Registration with a Dynamic Anatomic Model
Lars Dornheim, Klaus D. Tönnies, Kat Dixon ... 335

Intravascular Ultrasound-Based Imaging of Vasa Vasorum for the Detection of Vulnerable Atherosclerotic Plaque
Sean M. O'Malley, Manolis Vavuranakis, Morteza Naghavi, Ioannis A. Kakadiaris ... 343

Parametric Response Surface Models for Analysis of Multi-site fMRI Data
Seyoung Kim, Padhraic Smyth, Hal Stern, Jessica Turner ... 352

Clinical Applications – Validation

Subject Specific Finite Element Modelling of the Levator Ani
Su-Lin Lee, Ara Darzi, Guang-Zhong Yang ... 360

Robust Visualization of the Dental Occlusion by a Double Scan Procedure
Filip Schutyser, Gwen Swennen, Paul Suetens ... 368

Segmentation of Focal Cortical Dysplasia Lesions Using a Feature-Based Level Set
O. Colliot, T. Mansi, N. Bernasconi, V. Naessens, D. Klironomos, A. Bernasconi ... 375

Effects of Healthy Aging Measured By Intracranial Compartment Volumes Using a Designed MR Brain Database
Bénédicte Mortamet, Donglin Zeng, Guido Gerig, Marcel Prastawa, Elizabeth Bullitt 383

Predicting Clinical Variable from MRI Features: Application to MMSE in MCI
S. Duchesne, A. Caroli, C. Geroldi, G.B. Frisoni, D. Louis Collins 392

Finite Element Modeling of Brain Tumor Mass-Effect from 3D Medical Images
Ashraf Mohamed, Christos Davatzikos 400

STREM: A Robust Multidimensional Parametric Method to Segment MS Lesions in MRI
L.S. Aït-Ali, S. Prima, P. Hellier, B. Carsin, G. Edan, C. Barillot 409

Cross Validation of Experts Versus Registration Methods for Target Localization in Deep Brain Stimulation
F. Javier Sánchez Castro, Claudio Pollo, Reto Meuli, Philippe Maeder, Meritxell Bach Cuadra, Olivier Cuisenaire, Jean-Guy Villemure, Jean-Philippe Thiran 417

Localization of Abnormal Conduction Pathways for Tachyarrhythmia Treatment Using Tagged MRI
G.I. Sanchez-Ortiz, M. Sermesant, K.S. Rhode, R. Chandrashekara, R. Razavi, D.L.G. Hill, D. Rueckert 425

Automatic Mammary Duct Detection in 3D Ultrasound
Mark J. Gooding, Matthew Mellor, Jacqueline A. Shipley, Kathy A. Broadbent, Dorothy A. Goddard 434

Automatic Segmentation of Intra-treatment CT Images for Adaptive Radiation Therapy of the Prostate
B.C. Davis, M. Foskey, J. Rosenman, L. Goyal, S. Chang, S. Joshi 442

Inter-Operator Variability in Perfusion Assessment of Tumors in MRI Using Automated AIF Detection
Edward Ashton, Teresa McShane, Jeffrey Evelhoch 451

Computer–Assisted Deformity Correction Using the Ilizarov Method
A.L. Simpson, B. Ma, D.P. Borschneck, R.E. Ellis 459

Real-Time Interactive Viewing of 4D Kinematic MR Joint Studies
Heinrich Schulz, Kirsten Meetz, Clemens Bos, Daniel Bystrov, Thomas Netsch 467

Computer-Assisted Ankle Joint Arthroplasty Using Bio-engineered Autografts
R. Sidler, W. Köstler, T. Bardyn, M.A. Styner, N. Südkamp, L. Nolte, M.Á. González Ballester 474

Prospective Head Motion Compensation for MRI by Updating the Gradients and Radio Frequency During Data Acquisition
Christian Dold, Maxim Zaitsev, Oliver Speck, Evelyn A. Firle, Jürgen Hennig, Georgios Sakas 482

Harmonic Skeleton Guided Evaluation of Stenoses in Human Coronary Arteries
Yan Yang, Lei Zhu, Steven Haker, Allen R. Tannenbaum, Don P. Giddens 490

Acquisition-Related Limitations in MRI Based Morphometry
Arne Littmann, Jens Guehring, Christian Buechel, Hans-Siegfried Stiehl 498

Combining Classifiers Using Their Receiver Operating Characteristics and Maximum Likelihood Estimation
Steven Haker, William M. Wells III, Simon K. Warfield, Ion-Florin Talos, Jui G. Bhagwat, Daniel Goldberg-Zimring, Asim Mian, Lucila Ohno-Machado, Kelly H. Zou 506

Two Methods for Validating Brain Tissue Classifiers
Marcos Martin-Fernandez, Sylvain Bouix, Lida Ungar, Robert W. McCarley, Martha E. Shenton 515

Comparison of Vessel Segmentations Using STAPLE
Julien Jomier, Vincent LeDigarcher, Stephen R. Aylward 523

Validation Framework of the Finite Element Modeling of Liver Tissue
Hongjian Shi, Rachid Fahmi, Aly A. Farag 531

A Complete Augmented Reality Guidance System for Liver Punctures: First Clinical Evaluation
S.A. Nicolau, X. Pennec, L. Soler, N. Ayache 539

Imaging Systems – Visualization

A Novel Approach to High Resolution Fetal Brain MR Imaging
F. Rousseau, O. Glenn, B. Iordanova, C. Rodriguez-Carranza, D. Vigneron, J. Barkovich, C. Studholme 548

Respiratory Signal Extraction for 4D CT Imaging of the Thorax from Cone-Beam CT Projections
Simon Rit, David Sarrut, Chantal Ginestet 556

Registering Liver Pathological Images with Prior In Vivo CT/MRI Data
Huadong Wu, Alyssa M. Krasinskas, Mitchell E. Tublin, Brian E. Chapman 564

Support Vector Clustering for Brain Activation Detection
Defeng Wang, Lin Shi, Daniel S. Yeung, Pheng-Ann Heng, Tien-Tsin Wong, Eric C.C. Tsang 572

Inter-frame Motion Correction for MR Thermometry
S. Suprijanto, M.W. Vogel, F.M. Vos, H.A. Vrooman, A.M. Vossepoel 580

Adaptive Multiscale Ultrasound Compounding Using Phase Information
Vicente Grau, J. Alison Noble 589

3D Freehand Ultrasound Reconstruction Based on Probe Trajectory
Pierrick Coupé, Pierre Hellier, Noura Azzabou, Christian Barillot 597

Self-Calibrating Ultrasound-to-CT Bone Registration
Dean C. Barratt, Graeme Penney, Carolyn S.K. Chan, Mike Slomczykowski, Timothy J. Carter, Philip J. Edwards, David J. Hawkes 605

A Hand-Held Probe for Vibro-Elastography
Hassan Rivaz, Robert Rohling 613

Real-Time Quality Control of Tracked Ultrasound
Emad M. Boctor, Iulian Iordachita, Gabor Fichtinger, Gregory D. Hager 621

Fully Truncated Cone-Beam Reconstruction on Pi Lines Using Prior CT
Krishnakumar Ramamurthi, Norbert Strobel, Rebecca Fahrig, Jerry L. Prince 631

C-arm Calibration - Is it Really Necessary?
Ameet Jain, Ryan Kon, Yu Zhou, Gabor Fichtinger 639

Laser Needle Guide for the Sonic Flashlight
David Wang, Bing Wu, George Stetten 647

Differential Fly-Throughs (DFT): A General Framework for Computing Flight Paths
M. Sabry Hassouna, Aly A. Farag, Robert Falk 654

Panoramic Views for Virtual Endoscopy
Bernhard Geiger, Christophe Chefd'hotel, Sandra Sudarsky 662

Computer Assisted Diagnosis

Toward Automatic Computer Aided Dental X-ray Analysis Using Level Set Method
Shuo Li, Thomas Fevens, Adam Krzyżak, Chao Jin, Song Li 670

Exploiting Temporal Information in Functional Magnetic Resonance Imaging Brain Data
Lei Zhang, Dimitris Samaras, Dardo Tomasi, Nelly Alia-Klein, Lisa Cottone, Andreana Leskovjan, Nora Volkow, Rita Goldstein 679

Model-Based Analysis of Local Shape for Lesion Detection in CT Scans
Paulo R.S. Mendonça, Rahul Bhotika, Saad A. Sirohey, Wesley D. Turner, James V. Miller, Ricardo S. Avila 688

Development of a Navigation-Based CAD System for Colon
Masahiro Oda, Takayuki Kitasaka, Yuichiro Hayashi, Kensaku Mori, Yasuhito Suenaga, Jun-ichiro Toriwaki 696

A Prediction Framework for Cardiac Resynchronization Therapy Via 4D Cardiac Motion Analysis
Heng Huang, Li Shen, Rong Zhang, Fillia Makedon, Bruce Hettleman, Justin Pearlman 704

Segmentation and Size Measurement of Polyps in CT Colonography
J.J. Dijkers, C. van Wijk, F.M. Vos, J. Florie, Y.C. Nio, H.W. Venema, R. Truyen, L.J. van Vliet 712

Quantitative Nodule Detection in Low Dose Chest CT Scans: New Template Modeling and Evaluation for CAD System Design
Aly A. Farag, Ayman El-Baz, Georgy Gimel'farb, Mohamed Abou El-Ghar, Tarek Eldiasty 720

Graph Embedding to Improve Supervised Classification and Novel Class Detection: Application to Prostate Cancer
Anant Madabhushi, Jianbo Shi, Mark Rosen, John E. Tomaszeweski, Michael D. Feldman 729

Quantification of Emphysema Severity by Histogram Analysis of CT Scans
Paulo R.S. Mendonça, Dirk R. Padfield, James C. Ross, James V. Miller, Sandeep Dutta, Sardar Mal Gautham 738

Cellular and Molecular Image Analysis

Efficient Learning by Combining Confidence-Rated Classifiers to Incorporate Unlabeled Medical Data
Weijun He, Xiaolei Huang, Dimitris Metaxas, Xiaoyou Ying 745

Mosaicing of Confocal Microscopic *In Vivo* Soft Tissue Video Sequences
Tom Vercauteren, Aymeric Perchant, Xavier Pennec, Nicholas Ayache 753

Segmentation and 3D Reconstruction of Microtubules in Total Internal Reflection Fluorescence Microscopy (TIRFM)
Stathis Hadjidemetriou, Derek Toomre, James S. Duncan 761

Physically-Based Modeling

Ligament Strains Predict Knee Motion After Total Joint Replacement – A Kinematic Analysis of The Sigma Knee
Elvis C.S. Chen, Joel L. Lanovaz, Randy E. Ellis 770

A Boundary Element-Based Approach to Analysis of LV Deformation
Ping Yan, Ning Lin, Albert J. Sinusas, James S. Duncan 778

Reconstruction of Cerebrospinal Fluid Flow in the Third Ventricle Based on MRI Data
Vartan Kurtcuoglu, Michaela Soellinger, Paul Summers, Kevin Boomsma, Dimos Poulikakos, Peter Boesiger, Yiannis Ventikos 786

Schwarz Meets Schwann: Design and Fabrication of Biomorphic Tissue Engineering Scaffolds
Srinivasan Rajagopalan, Richard A. Robb 794

Robotics and Intervention I

Automatic Detection and Segmentation of Robot-Assisted Surgical Motions
Henry C. Lin, Izhak Shafran, Todd E. Murphy, Allison M. Okamura, David D. Yuh, Gregory D. Hager 802

DaVinci Canvas: A Telerobotic Surgical System with Integrated, Robot-Assisted, Laparoscopic Ultrasound Capability
Joshua Leven, Darius Burschka, Rajesh Kumar, Gary Zhang, Steve Blumenkranz, Xiangtian (Donald) Dai, Mike Awad, Gregory D. Hager, Mike Marohn, Mike Choti, Chris Hasser, Russell H. Taylor 811

Design and Control of In-Vivo Magnetic Microrobots
K. Berk Yesin, Philipp Exner, Karl Vollmers, Bradley J. Nelson 819

3D Needle-Tissue Interaction Simulation for Prostate Brachytherapy
Orcun Goksel, Septimiu E. Salcudean, Simon P. DiMaio, Robert Rohling, James Morris 827

Development and Application of Functional Databases for Planning Deep-Brain Neurosurgical Procedures
Ting Guo, Kirk W. Finnis, Andrew G. Parrent, Terry M. Peters 835

Medical Image Computing for Clinical Applications

Gaze-Contingent Soft Tissue Deformation Tracking for Minimally Invasive Robotic Surgery
George P. Mylonas, Danail Stoyanov, Fani Deligianni, Ara Darzi, Guang-Zhong Yang 843

Registration and Integration for Fluoroscopy Device Enhancement
James C. Ross, David Langan, Ravi Manjeshwar, John Kaufhold, Joseph Manak, David Wilson 851

Computer Aided Detection for Low-Dose CT Colonography
Gabriel Kiss, Johan Van Cleynenbreugel, Stylianos Drisis, Didier Bielen, Guy Marchal, Paul Suetens 859

Photo-Realistic Tissue Reflectance Modelling for Minimally Invasive Surgical Simulation
Mohamed A. ElHelw, Stella Atkins, Marios Nicolaou, Adrian Chung, Guang-Zhong Yang 868

Biological Imaging - Simulation and Modeling I

Motion Tracking and Intensity Surface Recovery in Microscopic Nuclear Images
Lopamudra Mukherjee, Mingen Lin, Jinhui Xu, Ronald Berezney 876

Towards Automated Cellular Image Segmentation for RNAi Genome-Wide Screening
Xiaobo Zhou, K.-Y. Liu, P. Bradley, N. Perrimon, Stephen TC Wong 885

Adaptive Spatio-Temporal Restoration for 4D Fluorescence Microscopic Imaging
Jérôme Boulanger, Charles Kervrann, Patrick Bouthemy 893

Kinematic Geometry of Osteotomies
Erin J. Smith, J. Tim Bryant, Randy E. Ellis 902

Predictive Camera Tracking for Bronchoscope Simulation with CONDensation
Fani Deligianni, Adrian Chung, Guang-Zhong Yang 910

Experimental Validation of a 3D Dynamic Finite-Element Model of a Total Knee Replacement
Joel L. Lanovaz, Randy E. Ellis 917

An In Vitro Patient-Tailored Model of Human Cerebral Artery for Simulating Endovascular Intervention
Seiichi Ikeda, Fumihito Arai, Toshio Fukuda, Makoto Negoro, Keiko Irie, Ikuo Takahashi 925

Author Index 933

Sensor Guided Ablation Procedure of Left Atrial Endocardium

Hua Zhong[1], Takeo Kanade[1], and David Schwartzman[2]

[1] Computer Science Department, Carnegie Mellon University, USA
[2] University of Pittsburgh Medical Center, USA

Abstract. In this paper, we present a sensor guided ablation procedure of highly motile left atrium. It uses a system which automatically registers the 4D heart model with the position sensor on the catheter, and visualizes the heart model and the position of the catheter together in real time. With this system clinicians can easily map the motile left atrium shape and see where the catheter is inside it, therefore greatly improve the efficiency of the ablation operation.

1 Introduction

Recent years have witnessed an expanding need for percutaneous, endocardium-based cardiac interventions, including ablation, injection, and device deployment. These interventions are generally not focal, but rather involve a broad region of endocardial anatomy. This anatomy is complex topographically, as well as motile. Current modalities for real-time intraoperative endocardial imaging and navigation are highly inaccurate, which has been the cause of procedure inefficacy and complications. In the present paper, we will focus on catheter ablation of left atrial endocardium. This procedure is performed in an attempt to cure atrial fibrillation, a common heart rhythm disorder. The left atrium has the attributes noted above - complex topography and motility. At present, the ablation procedure is performed by attempting to "register" preoperative four-dimensional imaging data (derived from computed tomography) with two-dimensional intraoperative imaging data (derived from intracardiac echocardiography and fluoroscopy) using the mind's eye. This is laborious, highly operator-dependent (which prohibits dissemination) and inaccurate. To the clinician, the optimal situation would be one in he/she were "injected" into the operative environment with automatic registration, such that endocardial intervention would be akin to painting a wall (left atrial endocardium) with a brush (ablation catheter). When painting a wall, complex topographical hurdles (eg. molding on the wall, windows, light switches) are not a problem, because of real-time feedback provided by direct visualization of the paint target. Motion of the room could be easily overcome by registering the motion of the room with that of the painter.

To realize such a goal, the system should be able to visualize the dynamic shape of left atrium and together with real time updated catheter position. Currently GE's Litespeed CT scanner can provide up to 10 3D CT scan of

J. Duncan and G. Gerig (Eds.): MICCAI 2005, LNCS 3750, pp. 1–8, 2005.

heart during one cardiac cycle. Assuming the changes in shape of left atrium repeat from one cardiac cycle to another, this one cycle heart scan is sufficient to capture the dynamic shape of left atrium. With such CT scan (3D + time), we can reconstruct a 4D heart shape model. Besides, currently available magnetic tracking systems (CARTO and NOGA from Biosense) can track position of catheter tip in real time synchronized with ECG signals. However the heart model and magnetic tracking systems are working independently now. Our task is to automatically register the magnetic tracking system with the 4D heart model, and visualize the result to facilitate the ablation procedure.

In [1] a registration system (HipNav) of position sensors and CT/MRI scans for bones has been introduced. In [2] 3D MRI models are built to navigate in hearts. In our case we have to use a 4D model to represent motile heart shape. Our registration problem then becomes 4D as well. [3] introduced a 4D registration method for two MR image sequences. Our problem is also a 4D registration but for 4D points and 4D surface models. In section 2 we will show how to do a space time registration and in section 3 we will show experiment results which validate our system's correctness. Also we will discuss how we can take advantage of this 4D property of both model and points to make the registration even easier and more robust than 3D shape registration.

2 Sensor Guided Ablation Procedure

To register the heart model with the magnetic position sensor, we first need to collect some points which are on the inner heart wall of left atrium with magnetic tracking system. We call these points "*constraint point set*". Then our system will find a transformation function F which aligns these points to the 4D heart model so that all the points are on the inner heart wall of the model. We also need to align the time axis. Next we will describe our method step by step.

2.1 4D Heart Model Reconstruction from CT

CT scan is proceeded one day before the operation assuming the heart shape won't change within one day. We use GE's CT scanner which can generate a 3D heart scan at every 10% of a cardiac cycle, and totally 10 3D CT scans for one cardiac cycle. Left atrium is then segmented out manually. We extract the surface model from the segmented CT data using Marching Cube(MC) algorithm. The extracted surface should represent the inner heart wall. We remove the small floating parts by discarding all triangles except those in the largest connecting group of the model. Then we smooth the model based on geometry cues with an implicit integration method [4].

Each 3D surface model extracted from CT data corresponds to a time $t \in [0, 1)$ (suppose $t = 0$ is at the beginning of a cardiac cycle and $t = 1$ is at the end of a cardiac cycle) in a cardiac cycle when the CT was scanned. In the rest of the paper, we use $C = \{C_0, C_1, ..., C_{n-1}\}$ to represent the 4D heart model, n is the number of 3D models for one cardiac cycle. In our example we capture a 3D CT scan at every 10% of a cardiac cycle, we can extract $n = 10$ surface

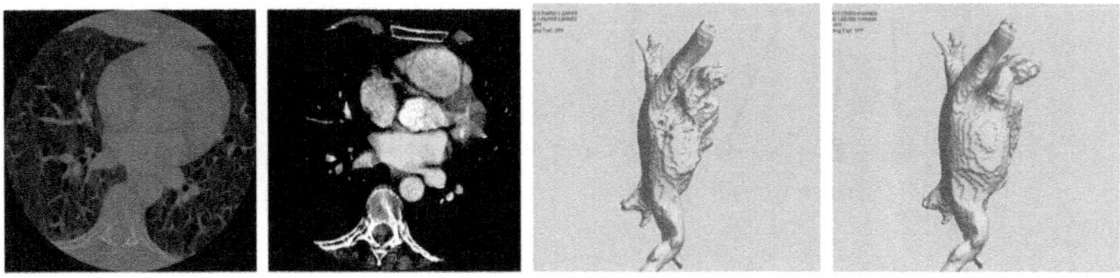

(a) CT scan (b) Segmented CT (c) Model t = 0.0 (d) sModel t = 0.5

Fig. 1. CT scan and 4D Heart Model of a patient. It contains 10 3D models for one cardiac cycle.

models $C = \{C_0, C_1, ..., C_9\}$ where each model C_i represents the heart shape at time $t = i/10, i = 0, 1, ...9$. This process is shown in Figure 1.

2.2 Constraint Point Set Collection

At the beginning of the operation, the clinician needs to capture 20-30 points spread on the inner heart wall with magnetic position sensor (Figure 2(b)). During this step, another catheter with intracardiac echocardiography sensor, which can generate 2D ultrasound images as shown in Figure 2(a) in real time, is used to verify the touching of ablation catheter tip on the inner heart wall. The magnetic tracking system can be setup to capture points at 10 evenly distributed time spots within a cardiac cycle as the CT scan, so each captured point will have a time coordinate of $t = 0, 0.1, ..., 0.9$. We group those points with same time coordinates together (though they may be captured in different cardiac cycles). Then all the recorded points can be organized into 10 groups: $P = \{P_0, P_1, ..., P_9\}$. P can be thought as a 4D point set.

2.3 Registration

Initial Registration. Space initial registration can be done in a coarse-to-fine scheme. First a rough alignment can be found based on the orientation of

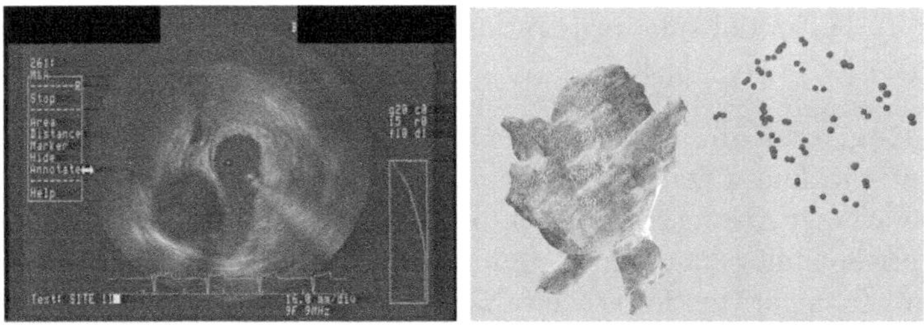

(a) Ultrasound Image (b) Captured Point Set

Fig. 2. Constraint Point Set. (a) Ultrasound image with the ablation catheter tip visible in it. Clinicians can verify if the ablation catheter tip is touching the heart wall. (b) A set of captured points (blue dots) at $t = 0.0$. They are not aligned with the heart model yet.

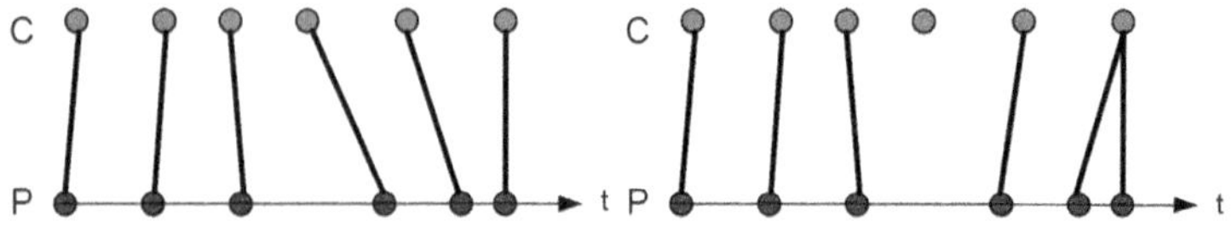

Fig. 3. Time Alignment. Upper row represents models, lower row represents point sets. x axis represents time. (a) Initial time alignment, we assume it's simple one-on-one correspondence. (b) The best correspondence scheme will be found after time alignment.

the patient on the bed. This rough alignment can be further refined by some points captured on some designated regions of the heart. These regions should be easy to locate solely from ultrasound images, such as the entrance region of pulmonary veins. Then we find an alignment so that these points are near the same regions in the heart model as where we know they are captured. Other information such as where the catheter enter the left atrium and some inside points can also help to eliminate global alignment ambiguities. If we define the registration error as the average distance from the real positions of constraint points from their calculated positions, the initial alignment should be able to reduce this error to approximate 10-20mm.

Time registration equals to a correspondence scheme S which tells for any point set P_i in P which C_j in C is its correspondence according to time. We know that we captured heart model $C = \{C_0, C_1, ..., C_9\}$ and points $P = \{P_0, P_1, ..., P_9\}$ both at $t = 0, 0.1, ..., 0.9$. Ideally the time registration should be P_i corresponds to C_i for any i. In reality, the heart model is synchronized to ECG signal one day before the operation during CT scan, while the magnetic tracking system is synchronized to ECG signal during the operation, and under the operation conditions, sometimes the patient's heart beat rate is not stable, then this one-on-one correspondence of C_i with P_i may not be true. This problem will be more noticeable if we have more CT scans in one cardiac cycle in the future, for example 100 3D models instead of 10. So time alignment is necessary (Figure 3). For initial time registration, we just use the correspondence scheme of P_i to C_i for any $i \in [0, 9]$.

Space Registration. Under a given correspondence scheme S, the space registration is to find a transform function F (rotation and translation) for P so that the average distance from each point in each transformed point set $F(P_i)$ to its corresponding model C_j is minimized. We use a modified Iterative Closest Points [5] algorithm for space registration. Different from original ICP, here during each iteration, when we try to find each constraint point's nearest point on the model, for any P_i, we only find nearest points from its corresponding model C_j, called P_{i_near}. And then we use $P = \bigcup_i P_i$ and its nearest point sets $P_{near} = \bigcup_i P_{i\_near}$ to find the transformation function for that iteration.

To accelerate, we use K-D tree structure for nearest neighbor searching. And we add random perturbation of the registration result use it as a new initialization and run the ICP again for multiple times to avoid local minimum. To reduce side effects of outlier points, we use a trimmed ICP with 95% of the points [6].

Space Time Registration. Under a given space registration F, the correspondence scheme can be decided by: for any P_i, C_j which has the least average distance from all the points in $F(P_i)$ to C_j is its corresponding model. But now we fall into a dilemma: to register time, we need to know the space registration; to register space, we need to know time registration (correspondence scheme).

To solve this problem, an EM algorithm is proposed assuming errors have a gaussian distribution. We take the correspondence scheme S as a hidden variable. The EM algorithm finds a space transformation function F and a time correspondence scheme S that maximize the expectation of log likelihood of $p(F(P)|S,C)$. The probability $p(F(P)|S,C)$ can be defined as

$$p(F(P)|S,C) = \prod_i p(F(P_i)|C_{si}) = \prod_i (exp(-||F(P_i), C_{si}||)) \quad (1)$$

Here C_{si} is the corresponding model for P_i defined by scheme S. Each $p(F(P_i)|C_{si})$ can be defined as an exponential function of the average distance from every point in $F(P_i)$ to model C_{si}, which is written as $||F(P_i), C_{si}||$. With this definition, the EM algorithm is:

Initial Alignment: We first use simple correspondence scheme of P_i to C_i, and calculate a space registration based on this initial time registration (with the help of other initial registration methods described before). This is our initial space registration F^0.

E step: At iteration k, given the spatial registration of iteration $k-1$: F^{k-1}, the probability of each possible correspondence scheme S can be calculated using the following formula:

$$p(S|F^{k-1}) = a^{-1} p(F^{k-1}(P)|S,C) prior(S) \quad (2)$$

where a^{-1} is a normalization constant. $p(F^{k-1}(P)|S,C)$ is similar as the probability in Equation 1. $prior(S)$ is the prior probability of each scheme S. We set $prior(S)$ to be very low or zero for schemes S that map P_i to a C_j where $||i-j||$ is large. From now we use term $p(S)$ to represent the probability in Equation 2.

M step: With $p(S)$ known, we can find a F^k that maximizes the expectation of log likelihood:

$$\arg\max_{F^k} \sum_S p(F^k(P)|C,S)p(S) \quad (3)$$

Maximizing Equation 3 equals to minimizing a weighted distance function

$$\arg\min_{F^k} \sum_S \sum_{i=1}^{m=10} ||F^k(P_i) - C_{si}|| p(S).$$

This distance function can be minimized similarly with our modified ICP algorithm. Only difference is here we need to combine the P and its nearest point set P_{near} under different correspondence scheme S with weight $p(S)$.

EM stops: when the registration improvement from F^k to F^{k-1} is less than a given threshold or a certain number of iterations has been reached whichever becomes true first. Time registration S is then computed based on the final space registration F^k.

2.4 Visualization of Ablation Procedure

After registration, the heart model and catheter position can be displayed together in real time: input catheter position in magnetic tracking system coordinate (x, y, z, t) will be transformed to model's coordinate $(F(x, y, z), S(t))$. The "beating" rate of the heart model is also synchronized with ECG signal from patient. Clinicians can setup a virtual camera anywhere in the space to monitor the whole ablation procedure. The procedure therefore is like a simple "painting the room" job (Figure 4).

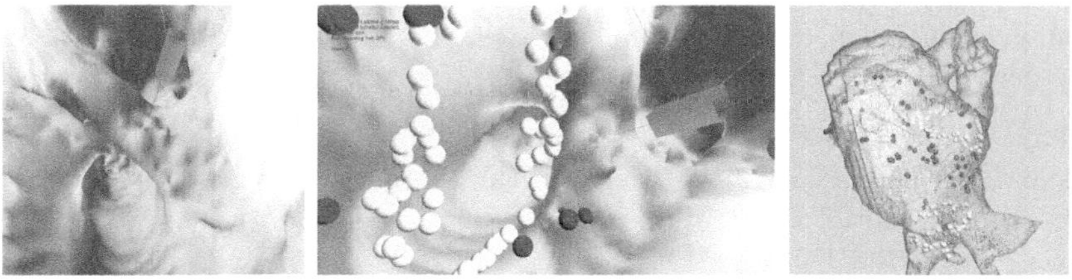

(a) (b) (c)

Fig. 4. Visualization (a) view of the catheter from inside left atrium. (b) view of ablation sites(yellow) together with constraint points(blue). (c) view from outside the left atrium.

3 Results and Discussion

3.1 Patient Data Test

To validate our system, we test it with a real patient's data. The CT scan's resolution is $512 \times 512 \times 116 \times 10$ (X×Y×Z×time). Voxel size is X: 0.48mm per voxel, Y: 0.48mm per voxel, Z: 0.625mm (or 1.25mm) per voxel, time: 10% of a cardiac cycle(Figure 1). We use CARTO system by Biosense to track the catheter position (1mm average error). CARTO can capture position at the beginning of each cardia cycle. So here the points we have is $P = P_0$(Figure 2(b)). We collect 76 constraint points to do the registration: for every location, we recorded two points both at $t = 0$. Then the clinician proceeded the ablation procedure *without* our system's help and recorded all the ablation sites. Our system then mapped where those ablation sites are based on registration. The correctness of registration is verified by the clinician who knows where those

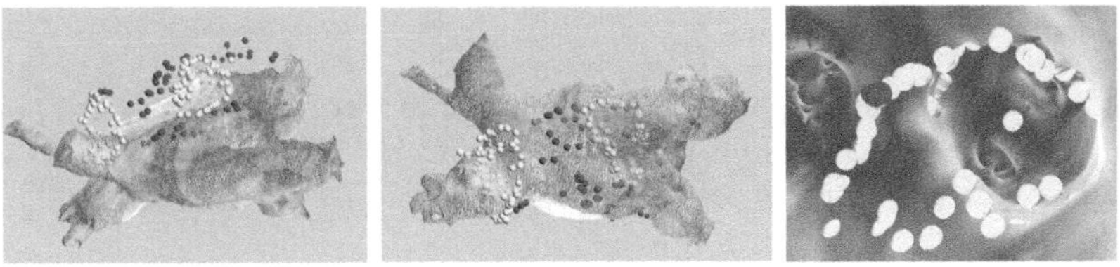

(a) (b) (c)

Fig. 5. Patient data test (a) Initial alignment (intensionally deteriorated to test robustness). (b) Outside view of the registration result. Yellow points are ablation sites. They are correctly mapped to the pulmonary veins entrance regions. (c) Inside view, these points are right on the surface.

ablation sites should be mapped to. The registration error is: 1.6347mm. This result may vary from case to case because of different heart shape and CT scan quality. Results are shown in Figure 5.

3.2 4D Registration Versus 3D Registration

To fully exploit the information of a 4D heart model, we record constraint points in such a way: we move the catheter to touch the heart wall, stay on the wall for a cardiac cycle, and record all 10 positions $p = \{p_0, ..., p_9\}$ at time $t = 0, 0.1, ..., 0.9$, generally $p_i \neq p_j$ if $i \neq j$ because the heart is beating. We can call p a 4D point. After we record one 4D point, we actually add one 3D point to each point set P_i, $i = 1$ to 10. No extra efforts are necessary to capture one 4D point than a 3D point. To demonstrate how 4D points can improve registration performance, we did the following experiments. For a 4D heart model of a patient, we simulate the collection of constraint points, both 4D points and 3D points (3D points are all recorded on model C_0). And we use a random transformation F_r to transform the points away from the heart model. F_r has $0-30$ degree of rotation and $0-20$mm of translation. Then we use our algorithm to find registration transformation F which maps points back to the surface model. We define the error as the average of $||v - F(F_r(v))||$ for every vertex v of the heart model. The result is shown in Figure 6. As we can see, 4D point registration achieves same registration accuracy with fewer constraint points than 3D point registration in our test. The spatial distribution of constraint point set is random but same for 3D and 4D points.

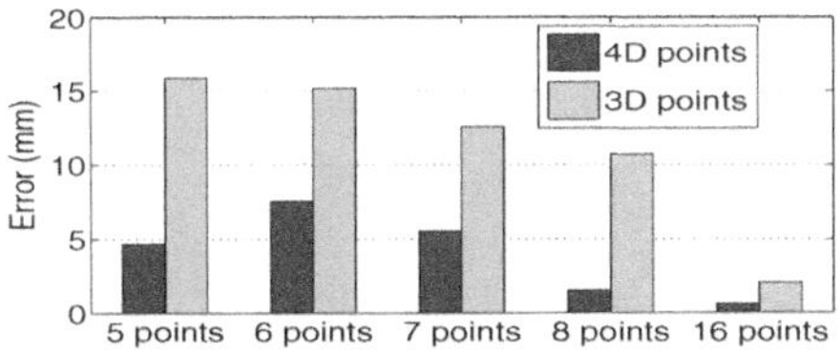

Fig. 6. Constraint point number vs registration error. For each item, we run the registration test for several times and the average error is shown here.

3.3 Speed Performance

Usually 15-30 seconds are needed for clinicians to record one constraint point, 2 minutes or less are needed for registration. With the automatic registration and visualization system, the whole procedure time can be greatly reduced.

4 Conclusion

In this paper, we described a new left atrial endocardium ablation procedure with automatic 4D registration and visualization. Registration for static objects (bones) can be thought as a subset of our registration problem. Promising results have been shown. Although the registration problem is far from totally solved, we believe 4D registration is the way we should go. In the future, we will focus on more lab animal tests to further verify and quantify the accuracy of 4D registration. Then more real patient tests will be done.

References

1. Gioia, D., etc.: Hipnav: Pre-operative planning and intra-operative navigational guidance for acetabular implant placement in total hip replacement surgery. In: Computer Assisted Orthopaedic Surgery Symposium. (1995)
2. Lardo, A., etc.: Mr guided radiofrequency ablation: Creation and visualization of atrial lesions. In: presented at International Society for Magnetic Resonance in Medicine, Sixth Scientific Meeting. (1998)
3. Dimitrios Perperidis, R.M., Rueckert, D.: Spatio-temporal free-form registration of cardiac mr image sequences. In: MICCAI. (2004)
4. Desbrun, M., Meyer, M., Schröder, P., Barr, A.H.: Implicit fairing of irregular meshes using diffusion and curvature flow. Computer Graphics **33** (1999) 317–324
5. Besl, P.J., McKay, N.D.: A method for registration of 3-d shapes. In: IEEE Trans. Pattern Analysis and Machine Intelligence. (1992) 14:239–256
6. Chetverikov, D., Stepanov, D.: Robust euclidean alignment of 3d point sets. In: First Hungarian Conference on Computer Graphics and Geometry. (2002) 70–75

A Method to Evaluate Human Spatial Coordination Interfaces for Computer-Assisted Surgery

M.A. Cardin, J.X. Wang, and D.B. Plewes

Department of Imaging Research,
Sunnybrook and Women's College Health Sciences Centre,
2075 Bayview Avenue, Toronto, Ontario, Canada
{ma.cardin, jxwang, don.plewes}@swri.ca
http://www.swri.ca/groups/dbp

Abstract. Computer assistance for breast conserving surgery requires a guidance method to assist a surgeon in locating tumor margin accurately. A wide array of guidance methods can be considered ranging from various pictorial representations, symbolic graphical interfaces as well as those based on other sensory cues such as sound. In this study, we present an experimental framework for testing candidate guidance methods in isolation or in combination. A total of 22 guidance approaches, based on stereographic, non-stereographic, symbolic and auditory cues were tested in a simulation of breast conserving surgery. Observers were asked to circumscribe a virtual tumor with a magnetically tracked scalpel while measuring the spatial accuracy, time and the frequency with which the tumor margin was intersected. A total of 110 studies were performed with 5 volunteers. Based on these findings, we demonstrated that a single view of the tumor with a stereo presentation in conjunction with an auditory guidance cue provided the best balance of accuracy, speed and surgical integrity. This study demonstrates a practical and helpful framework for testing guidance methods in a context dependent manner.

1 Introduction

Increasing interest in alternatives to conventional surgery for cancer applications has prompted a wide array of potential solutions, ranging from remote surgery under image driven, laparoscopic or robotic manipulation [1], direct real-time image guidance integrated into a more traditional surgical setting and the use of pre-operative imagery to track surgical maneuvers based on some model of tumor geometry [2][3]. Regardless of the approach, the need to integrate spatial information into a surgical decision making framework poses significant challenges to the engineer and the surgeon alike. This is particularly challenging when the surgeon attempts to integrate virtual data seamlessly into their appreciation of the surgical field. Ideally, one hopes to deliver the maximum amount of spatial information to the surgeon without inducing fatigue or being overwhelmed by

J. Duncan and G. Gerig (Eds.): MICCAI 2005, LNCS 3750, pp. 9–16, 2005.

excessive data. As each surgical task poses differing challenges, this balance will depend on the surgical context.

We have been exploring one such task which aims to integrate MRI information for the purpose of breast conserving surgery (BCS). Our approach is based on a segmented model of a breast tumor for resection which is coordinated to the patient's actual tumor location and geometry during surgery. The surgical task of BCS is to ensure complete removal of all cancerous tissue while sparing normal tissue. In this paper, we consider the challenge of creating a surgeon-computer interface that achieves the desired goal of guiding the surgical maneuvers while not burdening the surgeon with excessive and potentially distracting information.

Choices for surgical interfaces range from purely visual to those which attempt to integrate other perceptual cues. In addition to the inclusion of stereo presentation of visual data, other synthetic options include the use of tactile and auditory cues along with symbolic directives which aim to lead the surgeon in their task. These have the advantage of being used in isolation or in hybrid combination with virtual imagery with the hope of improving information transfer. However, it is often unclear which interface method or combination thereof is most effective. In this work, we attempt to address this question and demonstrate a surgical interface simulator which measures the efficacy of differing interfaces in isolation or in hybrid combinations.

2 Method

A surgical platform was constructed which allowed reproducible positioning of a tracking system (Figure 1(a)) in which a magnetic system was used to dynam-

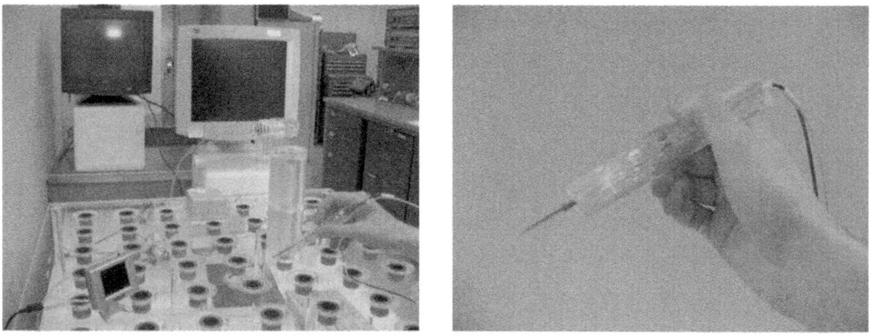

(a) (b)

Fig. 1. a) Experimental setup showing the positioning table offering precise 6 DOF positioning and orientation of the magnetic sensor. The mini-viewer seen on the left is used in some of the various interface combinations, together with the LCD and CRT monitors at the back. The modified scalpel containing another magnetic sensor is shown on the bottom-right. b) Modified radio frequency scalpel that contains the magnetic sensor.

ically locate a scalpel with respect to the boundaries of a virtual "tumor". The object of the experiment was to move the tip of the scalpel in a well-defined trajectory to simulate tissue cutting while recording the scalpel position. To achieve this, a 2 mm catheter-based, 6 DOF magnetic tracking probe (Ascension Technology) was embedded in a modified scalpel (Figure 1(b)). The desired trajectory was defined and fixed in space with another channel of the magnetic tracking system. The specific task was to trace out a circular path of radius of 200 mm while measuring the time taken to perform the task as well as the differences in the actual scalpel path relative to the desired path (i.e. the virtual tumor boundary). The operator was shown the "tumor" shape in various orientations as defined by the surgical platform.

In this experiment, we studied a number of visual and synthetic interface approaches. In the next, section we describe each of these approaches and the rationale behind their choice.

2.1 Interface Options

There were a total of 6 interface options we considered for this study. While many are possible, we chose these on the basis of our own experience and evidence from previous literature.

Interface 1 - Visual model of the scalpel and the desired task are viewed from a single viewport on a LCD monitor. This is shown in Figure 2(a) and represents the simplest visual presentation of the combined tracking task and the scalpel together. Motion of the scalpel is reflected by motion of the virtual scalpel in this presentation.

Interface 2 - Visual model of the scalpel and the desired task are shown from three orthogonal viewports together with a perspective rendering on the LCD monitor. This is shown in Figure 2(b) and provides complete three-dimensional presentation of the tracking task and the scalpel motions from three orthogonal points of view and a single perspective viewpoint. This was the most complex visual model we tested.

Interface 3 - A stereo presentation of the task on a CRT monitor with the observer wearing optical shutter glasses (Stereographics) as shown in Figure 2(c). By this means, the observer perceived a clear three dimensional perception of the tracking task and the scalpel.

Interface 4 - In this case, we provided the observer with an auditory cue in which the amplitude of a tone with constant frequency increased as the probe approaches the tumor boundary. Another element of this sound guidance interface is noted by a change in frequency when the scalpel was moved to a position inside the tumor, indicating an error in resection. This interface is shown in Figure 2(d).

Interface 5 - In this case, we generated a small, "navigation compass" viewport which was presented on the LCD monitor. The compass operates to dynamically point in a direction that the scalpel should move to approach the desired position

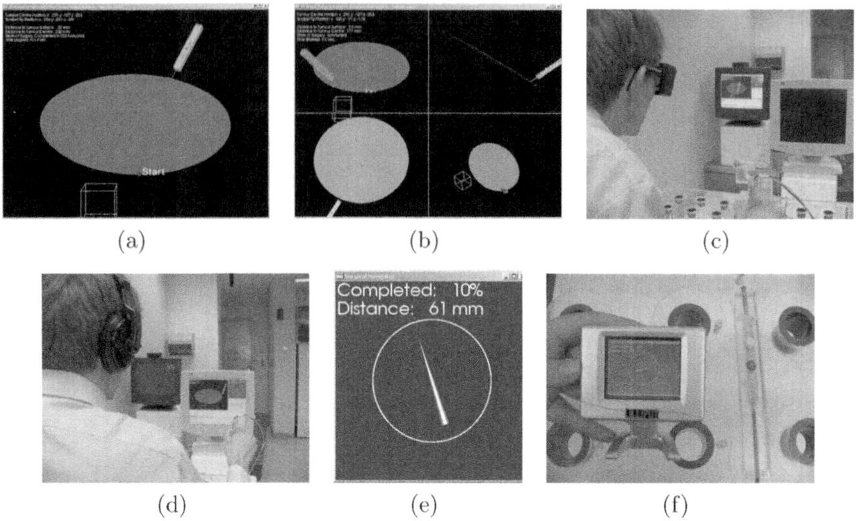

Fig. 2. a) Interface 1: one viewport with axial view and virtual scalpel. b) Interface 2: four viewports with axial, sagittal, coronal and a perspective view. c) Interface 3: stereo visualization on CRT monitor. d) Interface 4: Sound guidance and other visualization combination. e) Interface 5: Navigation compass. f) Interface 6: Navigation compass on mini-viewer and modified scalpel.

in a plane corresponding to the plane of trajectory. If the tip of the scalpel was found to be "above" the desired plane, the needle would increase in length. Likewise if it was below the desired level, the needle would shrink. The interface is shown in Figure 2(e). This was an attempt at a symbolic interface that was not pictorial but still provided all directional information for surgical guidance.

Interface 6 - In this interface, we explored the effect of "perceptual discontinuity" where the observer must constantly redirect their attention toward a monitor to gather perceptual information and away from the surgical area. To overcome this effect, we used a "mini-viewer" which shows the compass of interface 5, but placed immediately beside the surgical field so that the user does not need to look away from the surgical field when using it. This is shown in Figure 2(f).

2.2 Volunteer Studies

These six interfaces were studied in isolation and in combination. Table 1 shows the combinations of interfaces applied in this study. A total of 22 experiments were performed with varying combinations thought to provide interesting combinations of guidance methods. Each of the 22 experiments was performed with differing orientations of the virtual tumor, thus providing a diverse set of surgical trajectories. The volunteers were asked to move the scalpel around the virtual tumor boundary as accurately as possible. They were also informed not to move the scalpel to a point "inside" the tumor, as this would reflect a surgical error corresponding to degrading the tumor margin for histology. They were also told to complete the task as quickly as possible and that they were being timed. The balance between speed and accuracy was left to the volunteer. This experiment was repeated for five volunteers who were asked to complete all the experiments in a single sitting. The order of experiments was determined randomly and a total of 110 experiments were completed.

Each volunteer was asked to move the scalpel around the desired path assisted by the interface combination for that experiment. The positional error, the total time to encompass the path and the frequency with which the scalpel was found to "cut into" the tumor were all measured.

2.3 Measures of Surgical Efficiency

For each experiment, the distance between the surgical path and the actual tumor boundary was measured at all times with the magnetic trackers. The positional error was evaluated as the closest distance between the tip of the virtual scalpel and the virtual tumor boundary. From this data a root-mean-square (RMS) distance error was determined. The time taken to complete the task was also measured by providing a target on the virtual tumor boundary to keep track of the state of progression of the virtual surgery. This target point would advance on the circular path each time the closest point to the scalpel tip would cross the previously determined target point, thus simulating a virtual "cutting" of the tumor. The task was completed when the target point had swept over all point locations on the circular path. We also recorded the fraction of distance measurements that were positioned inside the virtual tumor. This error was recorded whenever a part of the virtual scalpel was touching the virtual tumor from the inside. It was recorded as a negative distance measurement to the scalpel tip, as seen on Figures 3(a) and 3(b).

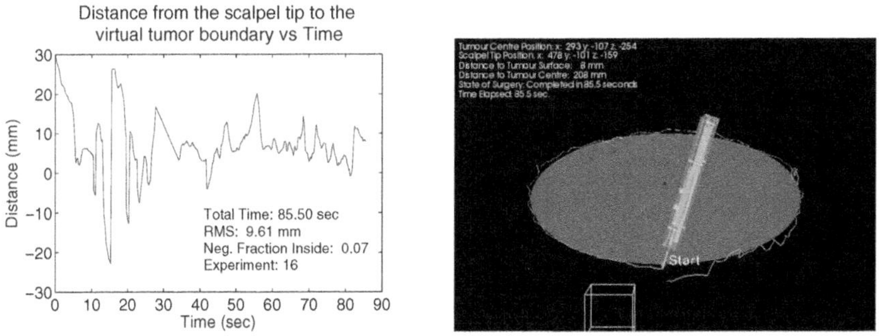

(a) (b)

Fig. 3. a) Typical positional error as a function of time for completion of experiment 16. The total time in seconds to complete the surgical task, RMS distance and fraction of distance measurements taken inside the tumor are also shown. b) Surgical path traced out by one volunteer in experiment 16.

3 Results

For all experiments described in Table 1, the average RMS distance was calculated across all 5 volunteers for each experiment. In addition, the average time to completion and the average percentage of distance measurements recorded inside the tumor were also considered (Figure 4). We can see from these data considerable variation in these parameters across each experiment. In general, we see a slight advantage for experiment number 16 in which the mean value is

Table 1. The combination of interface studies in the virtual surgical task

Method of Guidance	Experiment Number																					
	1	2	3	4	5	6	7	8	9	10	11	12	13	14	15	16	17	18	19	20	21	22
Single Viewport on LCD	X		X		X		X		X		X		X	X	X	X	X	X				
Four Viewports on LCD		X		X		X		X		X		X										
Stereo on LCD													X	X	X	X	X	X				
Sound Guidance							X	X	X	X	X	X				X	X	X			X	X
Compass on LCD			X	X					X	X				X			X			X		X
Compass on “Mini-viewer”					X	X					X	X			X			X	X		X	

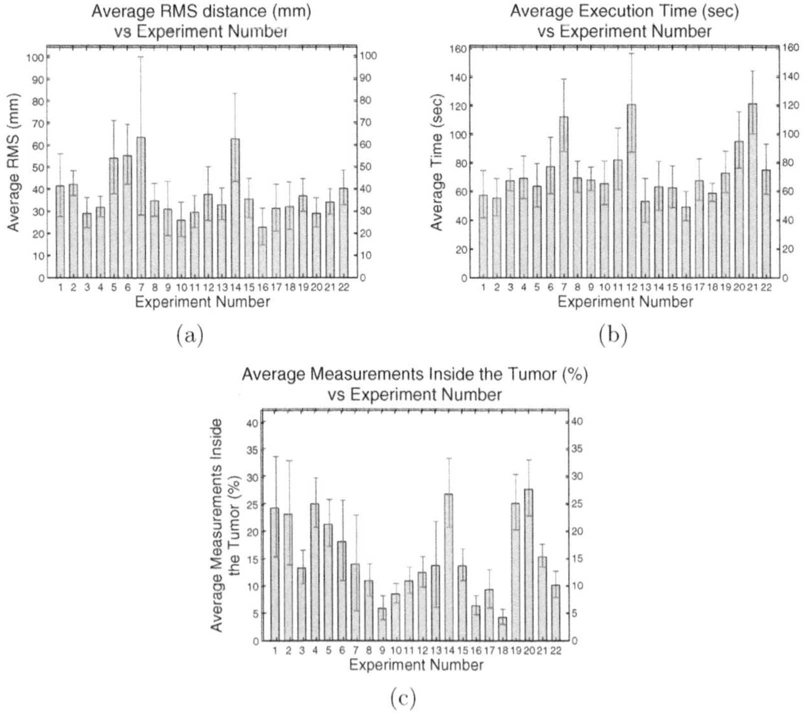

Fig. 4. The RMS error (a), the time to complete the task (b) and the frequency with which the scalpel cut into the tumor (c) versus the guidance method (see Table 1). The variation is the standard error of each parameter for the five observers.

minimized for RMS error and time. In addition, this same method also shows a low value for the frequency with which the scalpel ventured inside the tumor. However, in this latter case, experiments 9 and 18 also performed well. However, methods 9 and 18 did not perform as well with regard to spatial error and time.

On the basis of these pilot data, we determined that the guidance method tested in experiment 16 was the most successful approach. This guidance method involved the combination of a one viewport with the additional support of 3D stereography and auditory guidance. It is noteworthy that when the compass was provided in the mini-viewer, there appeared to be no significant advantage with regard to error and time but showed a slight benefit in terms of cutting into the tumor.

4 Discussion

These studies demonstrate that there is an optimum combination of guidance approaches for the guidance tasks presented in this paper. We note that providing as much imaging information does not necessarily increase the ability of the user to use this information. Furthermore, the use of stereo visualization was not always seen to be helpful. Rather, we found that the use of stereo data needed to be done in conjunction with other approaches to have a significant effect on its overall utility. Another interesting finding is that the use of the navigation compass did not contribute efficiently in improving the results. Furthermore, the degradation from "perceptual discontinuity" was not evident in these data as indicated by the use of the mini-viewer for the compass guidance as compared to the compass presented on the monitor. This does not mean that the notion of perceptual discontinuity was not operational in this study, but may reflect that use of a compass guidance approach did not appear to offer much advantage. In contrast, the use of an auditory cue was found to be of value when offered in conjunction with visual cues.

These general observations are corroborated by the comments received from volunteers while performing the experiments. They outlined that four viewports generally added on the complexity of the task while not providing additional support to improve performance. Volunteers would still resort to one or two viewports to complete the task. In addition, the results reflect a general appreciation of the sound guidance system, mainly for the evaluation of depth in performing the task. Volunteers also mentioned the difficulty in using the navigation compass, which is also reflected by it not having a large impact on the accuracy data.

5 Conclusion

This experimental method has been developed to test the efficacy of varying guidance methods for computer-assisted surgery. We tested a range of guidance methods which have been chosen to represent appropriate and potentially useful candidates for virtual surgical guidance. Our goal was to study the effect of combining guidance cues in a quantitative and controlled setting with the objective of seeking approaches which maximized the accuracy and speed of an intervention without burdening the user. We found, considerable variation in the utility of these approaches and that stereo and auditory guidance appeared to be a fruitful option. Clearly, other methods could have been chosen and this same experimental platform can be used to evaluate these. In the future, we will be using this approach to test other guidance methods with increased degree of complexity as we move toward developing a computer assisted surgical methods for breast conserving surgery.

References

1. Riva, G.: Applications of virtual environments in medicine. Methods of Information in Medicine **42(5)** (2003) 524–534
2. Shuhaiber, J.: Augmented reality in surgery. Archives of Surgery **139** (2004) 170–174
3. Tamaki, Y., et al.: Intraoperative navigation for breast cancer surgery using 3d ultrasound images. Computer Aided Surgery **4** (1999) 37–44

3D TRUS Guided Robot Assisted Prostate Brachytherapy

Zhouping Wei, Mingyue Ding, Donal Downey, and Aaron Fenster

Imaging Research Laboratories, Robarts Research Institute,
100 Perth Drive, London, ON N6A 5K8, Canada
{zwei, mding, ddowney, afenster}@imaging.robarts.ca

Abstract. This paper describes a system for dynamic intraoperative prostate brachytherapy using 3D ultrasound guidance with robot assistance. The system consists of 3D transrectal ultrasound (TRUS) imaging, a robot and software for prostate segmentation, 3D dose planning, oblique needle segmentation and tracking, seed segmentation, and dynamic re-planning and verification. The needle targeting accuracy of the system was 0.79 mm ± 0.32 mm in a phantom study.

1 Introduction

Transperineal prostate brachytherapy provides an improved alternative for minimal-invasive treatment of prostate cancer [1]. Current prostate brachytherapy involves placing about 80 to 100 radioactive seeds (e.g. ^{125}I or ^{103}Pd) into the prostate based on a predetermined plan (pre-plan). A template with a rectilinear pattern of holes is used to guide the implantation needles, loaded with radioactive seeds, to be inserted into the prostate according to the pre-plan. The needle insertion into the prostate is carried out under two-dimensional (2D) transrectal ultrasound (TRUS) guidance [2]. With accurate placement of the seeds, the high dose of radiation is expected to be confined, essentially, to the prostate, dramatically limiting treatment-related complications by minimizing radiation to nearby organs, such as the bladder and rectum.

However, it has been widely recognized that current prostate brachytherapy is still susceptible to variability. A dynamic intraoperative procedure, in which all steps are performed in one session, including planning, monitoring of prostate changes, dynamic re-planning, optimal needle insertion including oblique trajectories and automatic seed localization in US images, will help to solve some of the problems with current prostate brachytherapy [3].

To achieve dynamic intraoperative prostate brachytherapy, we developed a 3D TRUS guided and robot assisted system with new software. In this paper, we describe the development of the system and the related algorithms, and report on the targeting accuracy and variability achievable with the system.

2 Methods

2.1 System Description

Our prototype system (see Fig. 1) consists of a commercial robot, and a 3D TRUS imaging system including a B&K 2102 Hawk US system (B&K, Denmark) with a side-firing 7.5*MHz* TRUS transducer coupled to a rotational mover for 3D imaging [4]. The

J. Duncan and G. Gerig (Eds.): MICCAI 2005, LNCS 3750, pp. 17 – 24, 2005.

mover rotates the transducer about its long axis, while 2D US images are digitized and reconstructed into a 3D image while the images are acquired. A one-hole needle guide is attached to the robot arm, so that the position and orientation of the needle targeting can be changed as the robot moves. The robot and 3D TRUS coordinate systems are integrated with robot and image calibrations of the coordinate systems [5]. As a result, the robot can be controlled to target any point in 3D TRUS images, along any trajectory including oblique to avoid pubic arch interference (PAI).

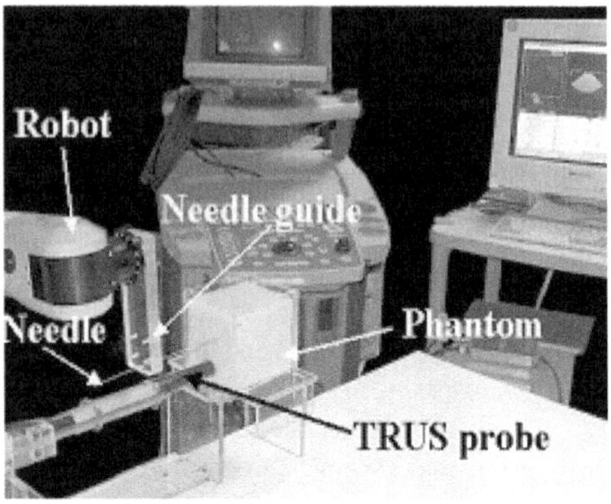

Fig. 1. 3D TRUS guided and robotic assisted prostate brachytherapy system

The software tools included in the system provide following functions:

1. Semiautomatic prostate segmentation in 3D TRUS images: We used the Discrete Dynamic Contour (DDC) method for semi-automatic prostate segmentation in 3D TRUS images [6]. First, the 3D TRUS image of the prostate is re-sampled into slices using a rotational re-slicing method (Fig. 2(a)). Then, in an initial slice, four or more points are chosen on the boundary of the prostate to obtain an initial contour using a cardinal-spline (Fig. 2(b)). In the next step, the initial contour is refined using the DDC method to obtain a prostate-fitted contour in the initial slice (Fig. 2(c)). The refined prostate contour in the initial slice is then propagated to adjacent slices and refined until the prostate boundaries in all slices have been segmented.

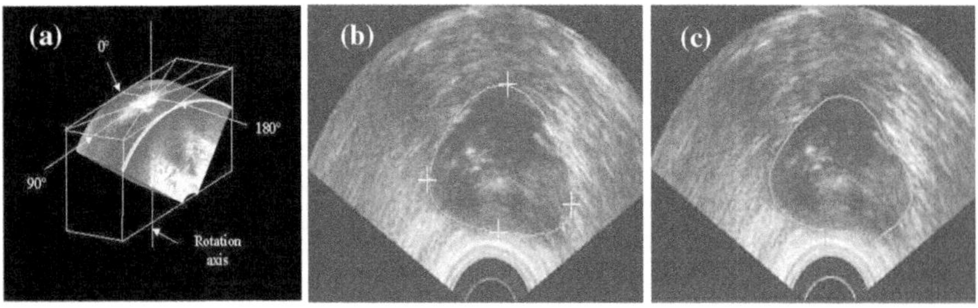

Fig. 2. Prostate segmentation. (a) Rotational re-slicing. (b) Initial slicing. (c) Refine the contour.

2. 3D prostate dose planning: Real time dose calculation is performed using TG43 formalism. Geometric optimization followed by simulated annealing is used to obtain the optimal dose distribution for pre-planning. The dose distribution is evaluated using dose volume histograms (DVH) for the delineated organs, as well as for the implant volume. The plan can be performed and displayed in 3D volume view, orthogonal planes view, transverse view, and needle rendered view. The user can switch on and off the contours, isodose curves, needles, etc., in order to view each separately, and obtain the dose at any point by simply clicking the mouse on the transverse image or by typing the coordinates. Dose volume histograms for different plans from the same patient or different DVH from the same plan can also be displayed for comparison.

3. Oblique needle segmentation and tracking: The aim of oblique needle segmentation is to determine needle's position and orientation, so that rapid dynamic re-planning could be performed, based on the actual needle trajectory and seed locations to obtain an optimum 3D dose distribution within the prostate. The oblique needle segmentation algorithm includes six steps [7]: 1) pre-scan to obtain the image prior to the insertion of the needle; 2) live-scans to obtain the images as the needle is being inserted; 3) image subtraction to obtain a difference images between the pre-scan and live-scans; 4) thresholding to remove background noise (Fig. 3(a)); 5) further removal of spurious needle voxels to obtain the needle candidate voxels (Fig. 3(b)); 6) linear regression of needle candidate voxels to obtain the needle vector in 3D TRUS image coordinate system (Fig. 3(c)).

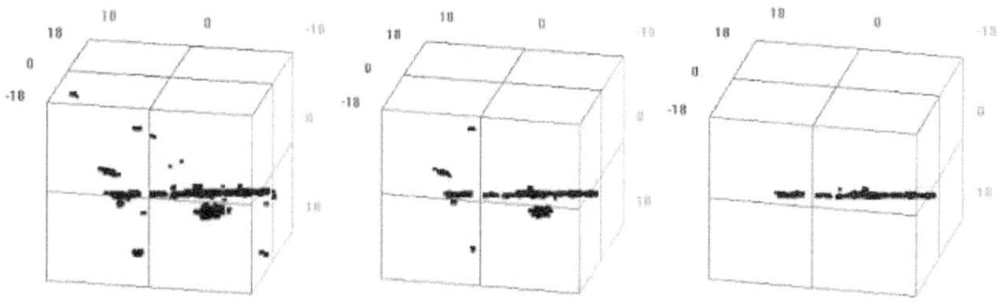

(a) (b) (c)

Fig. 3. Oblique needle segmentation procedure. (a) 3D difference map after the thresholding processing; (b) 3D difference map after the spurious needle voxels have been removed; (c) 3D difference map ready for final linear regression. Black regions are the needle candidate clusters.

4. Automatic seed localization in 3D TRUS images: Automated seed localization is important for intraoperative evaluation of dose delivery, which permits the identification of under-dosed regions, need for remedial seed placement, and ensures that the entire prostate receives the prescribed dose. The automatic seed segmentation algorithm is composed of following five steps: 1) 3D needle segmentation to obtain the needle position when implanting the seeds; 2) reducing the search space by volume cropping along the detected needle, as the implanted seeds are close to the needle; 3) non-seed structure removal based on model of orthogonal projections of the needle; 4) seed candidate recognition using 3D line segment detection; and 5) localization of seed positions using a peak detection algorithm described in [8] to localize the center of the seeds.

2.2 System Evaluation

To assess the performance of the 3D TRUS guided and robotic assisted system, we used tissue-mimicking prostate phantoms made from agar and contained in a Plexiglas box. A hole in the side allowed insertion of the TRUS transducer into the phantom, simulating the rectum (Fig. 4). Each phantom contained of two rows of 0.8mm diameter stainless steel beads. The bead configurations formed a $4 \times 4 \times 4$ cm polyhedron to simulate the approximate size of a prostate. These beads were scanned using the 3D TRUS system, and the positions of these seeds were determined manually in 3D TRUS image coordinate system. Then, these positions were transferred into the robot coordinate system, and the robot was controlled to guide the needle to target these beads. The displacements between the preinsertion bead position and the needle tip after the needle has been inserted into the phantom were used to analyze the needle insertion accuracy. A 3D principal component analysis (PCA) was performed to analyze needle targeting accuracy. The elements in the covariance matrix used for PCA analysis are defined as:

$$S_{ij} = \frac{\sum_{k=1}^{8} (x_{ik} - \overline{x}_i)(x_{jk} - \overline{x}_j)}{(n-1)} \qquad (i, j = 1, 2, 3) \tag{1}$$

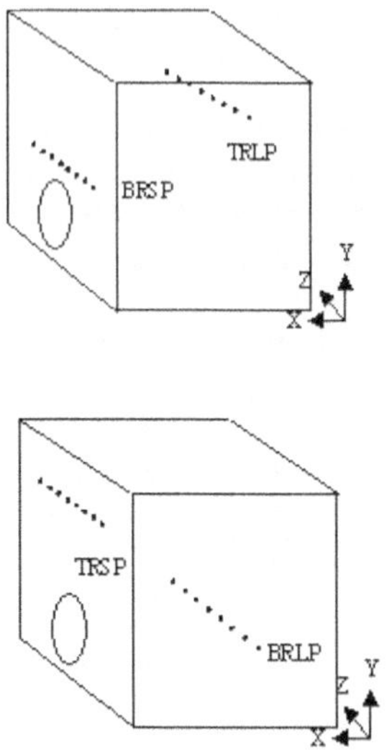

Fig. 4. The two different prostate phantom types with four different bead configurations were used for the needle targeting accuracy experiment. The needle entered from left-hand side, parallel to the x-axis, in each case.

where, x_{ik} is the displacement between the middle of the pre-insertion bead and the needle tip. i and j represent the direction component (*i.e.*, x, y or z), k is the target index (k = 1, 2, … , 8, i.e., for each bead, 8 targeting trials were performed) in each of four bead configurations as shown in Fig. 4. $\overline{x}_i = \frac{1}{8}\sum_{k=1}^{8} x_{ik}$ is the mean displacement in the ith component, and $n = 8$. Solving the determinant equation:

$$| \boldsymbol{S} - \lambda \boldsymbol{I} | = 0 \tag{2}$$

where $\boldsymbol{I}$ is the identity matrix. $\boldsymbol{S}$ is the covariance matrix, whose elements have been determined using Eq. (1). Eqs. (1) and (2) produce a third degree polynomial equation, with roots that are the eigenvalues of $\boldsymbol{S}$, λ_i (i = 1, 2, 3), and the corresponding normalized eigenvectors $\boldsymbol{u}_i$ (i = 1, 2, 3). The eigenvalues give us the variance along the corresponding eigenvectors, with maximum variance occurring along the principal axis. The two other axes, orthogonal to the first and each other, account for the remaining variance, which is calculated as the corresponding eigenvalues of the covariance matrix. The principal components, *i.e.*, the orthonormal eigenvectors, u_i, are not necessarily parallel to the image coordinate axes.

Three-dimensional 95% confidence intervals were calculated for the eight bead locations for each bead configuration. We assumed that the needle targeted the origin of the coordinate system, and plotted the 95% confidence interval as an ellipsoid about the average needle position. The orientation and length of the ellipsoid axis were given by the eigenvectors and eigenvalues from the PCA. Because the variance is the square of the STD, the length of the 95% confidence interval in one direction along each of the principal axes, $\boldsymbol{u}_i$ (i = 1, 2, 3), is given by:

$$a_i = 2\sqrt{\lambda_i} \qquad (i = 1, 2, 3) \qquad (3)$$

where λ_i is the eigenvalue of the covariance matrix. The equation of the resulting ellipsoid is then given by:

$$\sum_i \frac{(u_i)^2}{a_i^2} = 1 \qquad (i = 1, 2, 3) \qquad (4)$$

The ellipsoid equation was transformed back to the image coordinate system, and translated so that its center was at the average needle position relative to the preinsertion bead position. The displacements of the measured positions of the needle tip relative to the preinsertion bead positions at the origin were plotted for all eight targeting attempts for each bead configuration along with the 95% ellipsoid intervals. The volume of 95% ellipsoid was calculated by:

$$V = \frac{4\pi}{3}\prod_{i=1}^{3} a_i \qquad (5)$$

a_i ($i = 1, 2, 3$) are the ellipsoid axis lengths determined by Eq. (3). Projections through the ellipsoid and needle data were also plotted.

To assess the performance of the prostate segmentation algorithm, we compared the algorithm segmented prostate with manual segmentation. Due to the robot's high positioning and angulation accuracy, we used the robot as a "gold standard" to assess the performance of the needle segmentation algorithm. We compared the results of algorithm segmentation to the values measured by the robot.

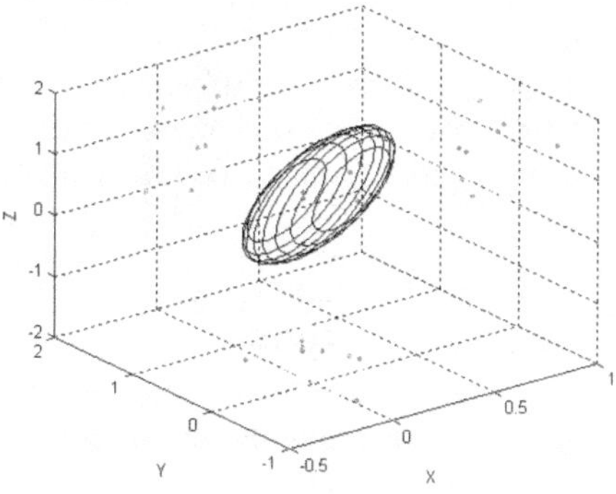

Fig. 5. An ellipsoid representing 95% confidence interval for needle targeting. The target locates at the origin of the coordinate system. The small dots are the real needle tip positions.

3 Results

Evaluation of the system showed that needle can be used to target positions in agar phantoms with a mean error of 0.79mm±0.32mm. The 3D 95% confidence ellipsoids (see Fig. 5) were found to have total volumes ranging from 0.54mm^3 to 1.92mm^3, depending on the location of the targets with respect to the ultrasound probe and insertion distance. The size of the ellipsoid, representing the 95% confidence interval, describes the random errors of the needle targeting. The random error results from poorer resolution in the 3D scanning direction (Z_i) due to insufficient sampling of 2D images and the poorer elevational resolution of the transducer. This image "blurring" would be exacerbated for the points farther away from the TRUS transducer, resulting the larger volumes for the targeting of the beads in the top row. Table 1 lists the widths of the 95% confidence intervals along the primary, secondary and tertiary axis for four different bead configurations.

The distance between the intersection of a radial line with the algorithm segmented surface, and the intersection of the same radial line with the manually outlined surface, was used as the measure of the algorithm's performance. Error analysis showed that the average difference between manual and the prostate segmentation algorithm boundaries was -0.20±0.28mm, the average absolute difference was 1.19±0.14mm, the average maximum difference was 7.01±1.04mm, and the average volume difference was 7.16%±3.45%. Figure 6 is an example of a segmented prostate in a 3D TRUS image. Figure 7 is an example of the 3D prostate dose planning tool showing a surface rendered view of a pre-plan with delineated organs and oblique needle targeting.

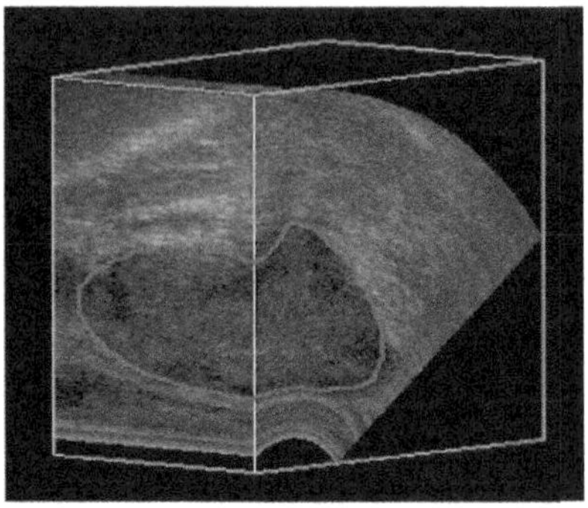

Fig. 6. Segmented prostate in 3D TRUS image

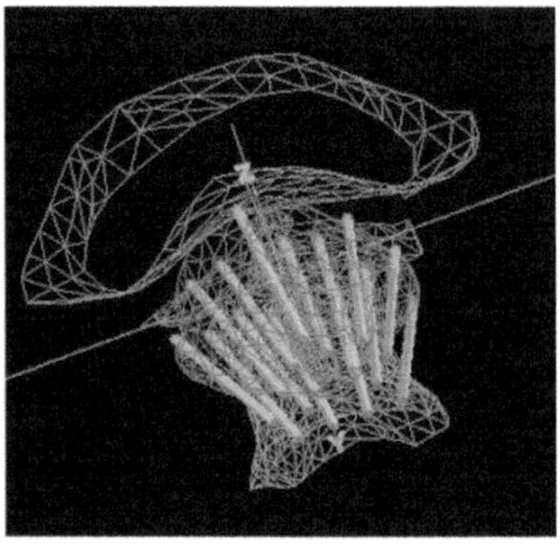

Fig. 7. Surface rendered view of the pre-plan with delineated organs

The error for the needle segmentation algorithm in determining the needle tip position was 0.8mm when the insertion distance was greater than 15mm. The mean error in determining the needle orientation in the *yaw* and *pitch* orientations was 0.20° and 0.03° respectively. Figure 8 shows the result of the needle segmentation algorithm in a patient image obtained during a prostate cryotherapy procedure.

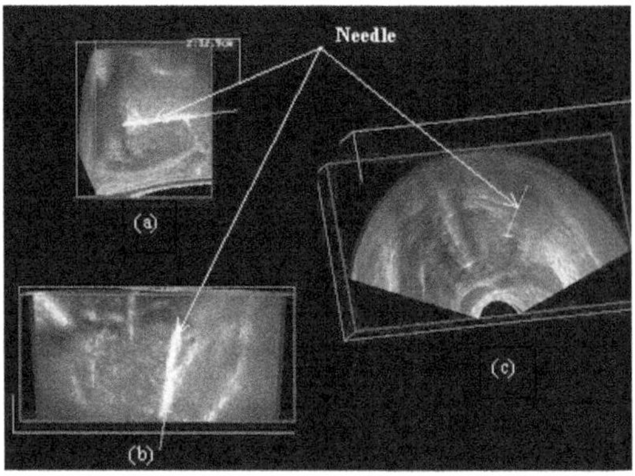

Fig. 8. Segmented needle. (a) Oblique sagittal view; (b) oblique coronal plane; (c) transverse view with a graphical 3D display of the needle targeting superposed on the view.

The true-positive rate for the seed segmentation algorithm was 100% for agar and 93% for chicken phantoms. This is acceptable, because according to Lindsay et al [9], variation in D90 (the lower bound on the minimum dose delivered to any

90% of the target volume) due to inability to localize 5% of the seeds is negligible. The average distance to the manually segmented seeds was 1.0 mm for agar and 1.7mm for chicken phantoms. The preliminary result for the segmentation time on a PC computer with dual AMD Athlon 1.8GHz processor was 280 seconds for 14 seeds. This is too long for routine brachytherapy, and we are improving the seed segmentation method so that the segmentation time is limited to less than 1 minute. Figure 9 is an example of the result of the seed segmentation algorithm for localization of the seeds in the 3D TRUS image.

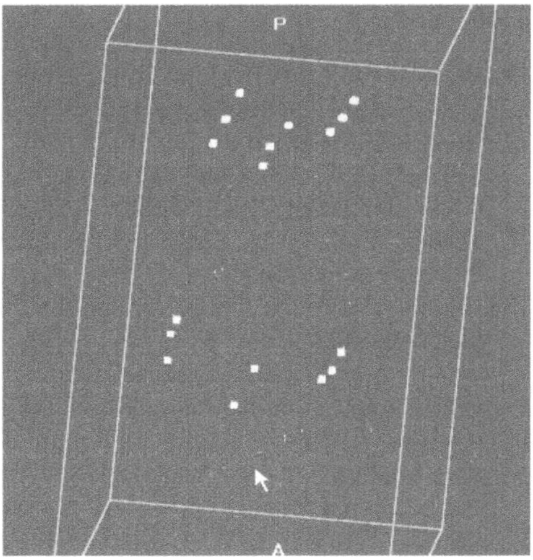

Fig. 9. Localized seeds in 3D TRUS image

4 Conclusion

Nath et al. has pointed out that the maximum difference between the needle tip and its planned target allowed in prostate brachytherapy is 5 mm [10]. Compared with our results from the phantom study, we concluded that with robotic assistance, the brachytherapy needle could be guided to accurately and consistently target any point identified in the 3D TRUS image along various trajectories including oblique. In addition, the software developed in this project provides various functions such as oblique needle segmentation and tracking, 3D dose planning, radioactive seed segmentation in 3D TRUS images, and dynamic re-planning, which are important for an intraoperative procedure. In the future, we will test our system *in vivo*, which will include realistic tissue deformation and mobility. We expect that the result of this work can provide a tool to achieve dynamic intraoperative prostate brachytherapy using 3D TRUS imaging and robotic assistance together with efficient segmentation software.

Table 1. A description of the 95% uncertainty intervals for brachytherapy needle insertion

Bead configuration	**Width of the 95% uncertainty interval (mm)**			**Center of confidence interval (mm)**	**Ellipsoid volume (mm^3)**
	Primary axis	Secondary axis	Tertiary axis		
Top row, long penetration (TRLP)	1.95	1.02	0.23	(-0.46,0.57,-0.98)	1.92
Bottom row, short penetration (BRSP)	1.06	0.55	0.22	(0.38,-0.22,-0.44)	0.54
Top row, short penetration (TRSP)	1.77	0.94	0.24	(0.03,0.49,-0.04)	1.68
Bottom row, long penetration (BRLP)	1.38	0.60	0.19	(0.17,0.39,0.68)	0.66

References

1. Blasko J.C., Ragde H., Luse R.W., Sylvester J.E., Cavanagh W., Grimm P.D.: Should brachytherapy be considered a therapeutic option in localized prostate cancer? Urol Clin North Am 23 (1996) 633-650
2. Rifkin M.D.: Ultrasound of the prostate: imaging in the diagnosis and therapy of prostatic disease. Lippincott-Raven Publishers, Philadelphia, New York (1997)
3. Todor D.A., Zaider M., Cohen G.N., Worman M.F., Zelefsky M.J.: Intraoperative dynamic dosimetry for prostate implants. Phys. Med. Biol. 48 (2003) 1153-1171.
4. Fenster A., Downey D.B., Cardinal H.N.: Three-dimensional ultrasound imaging. Phys Med Biol 46 (2001) R67-R99
5. Wei Z., Wan G., Gardi L., Mills G., Downey D.B., Fenster A.: Robot-assisted 3D-TRUS guided prostate brachytherapy: System integration and validation. Med Phys, 31 (2004), 539-548
6. Ding M., Chen C., Wang Y., Gyacskov I., Fenster A.: *Prostate segmentation in 3D US images using the cardinal-spline-based discrete dynamic contour.* In: Proc. SPIE Medical Imaging 2003 Vol. 5029: Visualization, Image-guided procedures, and display, San Diego, CA, USA, February 16-18, 2003, pp. 69-76
7. Wei Z., Gardi L., Downey D.B., Fenster A.: *Oblique needle segmentation for 3D TRUS-guided robot aided transperineal prostate brachytherapy.* In: Proc. IEEE International Symposium in Biomedical Imaging (ISBI'04), Arlington, VA, USA, April 15-18, 2004
8. Ding M., Wei Z., Downey D.B., Fenster A.: *Automated seed localization for intraoperative prostate brachytherapy based on 3D line segment patterns.* In: Proc. SPIE Medical Imaging 2005 Vol. 5744: Visualization, Image-guided procedures, and display, San Diego, CA, USA, February 13-15, 2005, pp. 417-424
9. Lindsay P.E., Van Dyk J., Battista, J.J: A systematic study of imaging uncertainties and their impact on ^{125}I prostate brachytherapy dose evaluation. Med Phys, 30 (2003), 1897-1907
10. Nath S, Chen Z, Yue N, Trumpore S, Peschel S. Dosimetric effects of needle divergence in prostate seed implant using ^{125}I and ^{103}Pd radioactive seeds. Med Phys, 27 (2000), 1058-1066

Invisible Shadow for Navigation and Planning in Minimal Invasive Surgery

Marios Nicolaou, Adam James, Benny P.L. Lo, Ara Darzi, and Guang-Zhong Yang

Royal Society/Wolfson Medical Image Computing Laboratory & Department of Surgical Oncology and Technology, Imperial College London, London, United Kingdom
{m.nicolaou, a.james, a.darzi, g.z.yang}@imperial.ac.uk

Abstract. Depth estimation is one of the most fundamental challenges for performing minimally invasive surgical (MIS) procedures. The requirement of accurate 3D instrument navigation using limited visual depth cues makes such tasks even more difficult. With the constant expectation of improving safety for MIS, there is a growing requirement for overcoming such constraints during MIS. We present in this paper a method of improving the surgeon's perception of depth by introducing an "invisible shadow" in the operative field cast by an endoscopic instrument. Although, the shadow is invisible to human perception, it can be digitally detected, enhanced and re-displayed. Initial results from our study suggest that this method improves depth perception especially when the endoscopic instrument is in close proximity to the surface. Experiment results have shown that the method could potentially be used as an instrument navigation aid allowing accurate maneuvering of the instruments whilst minimizing tissue trauma.

1 Introduction

Over the last decade, minimally invasive surgery (MIS) has attained great popularity and acceptance among surgeons and patients alike due to its improved cosmetic appearance, shorter rehabilitation, less pain and decreased hospital costs. However, MIS requires a higher degree of competency from the surgeon due to the presence of a number of constraints. Among them, vision is the primary element. The surgeon is required to reconstruct the 3D operative field and perform instrument navigation through the narrow monoscopic two-dimensional (2D) field of view provided by the endoscope. The perceptual cues that a surgeon uses to navigate are complex, and it is well understood and documented in *cue theory* that a variety of cues are utilized in order to estimate depth. The visual system typically infers depth based on information relating to the posture of the eyes as well as visual patterns projected onto the retina [1]. The particular cues that foster the perception of depth have been widely investigated [2,3] and are often classified as *primary* (physiological) cues, such as binocular disparity, convergence, and accommodation, and *secondary* (pictorial) cues, such as linear perspective, elevation, shading and shadow, texture and texture gradients, and reference frames [1]. It is not well understood, however, how these cues are assimilated in MIS. This is because the majority of cues are subtle and difficult to detect in the operative environment presented to the surgeon. Furthermore,

J. Duncan and G. Gerig (Eds.): MICCAI 2005, LNCS 3750, pp. 25 – 32, 2005.

there is a direct reduction in perceptual information that is available at any moment in time due to an ever-evolving surgical scene as a result of laparoscope translations and anatomical deformations. Ultimately, the monoscopic field-of-view provided by the laparoscope limits the 3D perception by presenting a scene onto 2D planes. It has been observed that surgeons tend to compensate for the lack of depth perception by developing new strategies such as groping forward and backward with instruments to gauge the relative depths of organs by touching them (Figure 1). The combined visual and haptic feedback helps to confirm the instrument position and orientation. This navigation approach, however, is not ideal particularly when undertaking delicate surgical maneuvers that require subtle control of instruments which must be performed slowly enough to avoid damaging the tissues in contact [4].

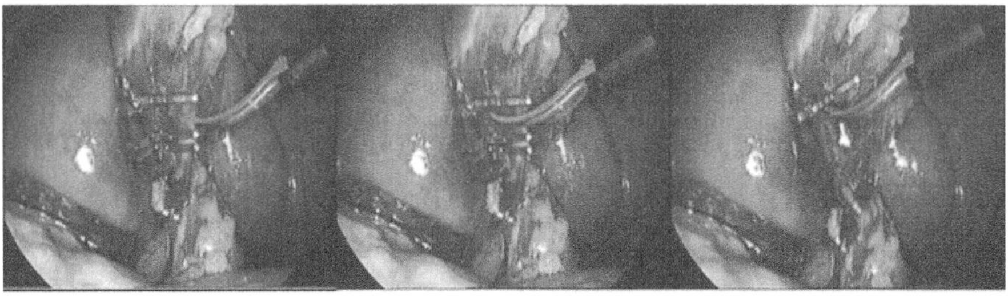

Fig. 1. Operative stills representing a collision sequence during MIS. In this sequence, the surgeon advances the instrument into the vessel to establish position before straddling the vessel instrument to transect it.

Currently, there is a constant requirement for surgery to become safer, particularly in the current climate of clinical governance. Practically, safety can be achieved by better training as well as by reducing the constraints set by the nature of MIS. Improving 3D visualization and ultimately facilitating instrument navigation and maneuvering should be a priority. Although advances in stereoscopic surgery aim to improve 3D perception, such systems have practical limitations with respect to their practical use as they tend to be extremely expensive and not widely available. For these reasons, it is useful to investigate other alternatives for conveying depth information and enhancing existing monocular visual cues. One of the primary cues that the visual system utilizes to infer depth is shadow [5]. Shadow can provide useful information about object shapes, relative 3D position, and surface characteristics within a scene [6,7,8,9]. Unfortunately, this visual cue is unavailable with MIS due to the coaxial alignment of the lens and light bundle of traditional rigid endoscopes. Under this setup, the operative field is generally shadowless [10]. It has been shown that inducing shadow by the introduction of a secondary light source within the surgical field improves endoscopic task performance [11]. The purpose of this paper is to introduce a new framework for improving depth perception for MIS by introducing a secondary light source. The unique feature of the proposed method is that it only casts a weak shadow of the laparoscopic instrument that is almost invisible under normal viewing conditions. During instrument maneuver, this "invisible shadow" is dynamically enhanced which introduces a strong depth cue from which the distance between the instrument and tissue can be accurately determined. This naturally avoids the use of the instrument to "crash" on the tissue surface to gauge the 3D relative position of tissue-instrument whilst maintaining normal laparoscope viewing condition when instrument depth cuing is not required.

2 Materials and Methods

To emulate the laparoscopic environment, a laparoscopic box trainer was used, within which a silicon based tissue surface model was placed. The surface was coated with silicone rubber mixed with acrylic to give it a specular finish that looks similar to wet tissue. The scene was illuminated primarily from the endoscope itself and a secondary light source was placed directly above the surface but away from the endoscope. The intensity of this source was carefully adjusted so as to cast a near invisible shadow to the surface to avoid any interference to the normal viewing condition. A laparoscopic instrument was held over the surface in different positions and the vertical distance from the tip to the surface was measured to the nearest half centimeter. A video stream of the instrument assuming each position was obtained from a camera within the endoscope and digitally stored for subsequent processing. Figure 1 outlines the main components used for dynamically enhancing the "invisible shadow" during instrument maneuver.

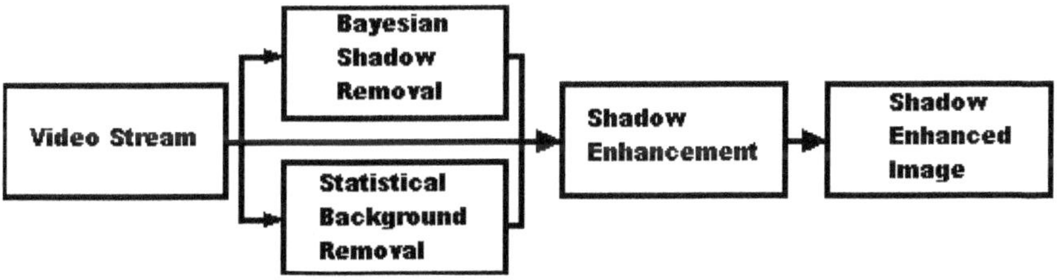

Fig. 2. A schematic illustration of the shadow enhancement filter design to generate the computer enhanced shadow

With this work, the shadow removal algorithm was based on the following four low level visual cues: intensity difference, intensity gain, angle between RGB vectors and color difference. Intensity difference is the absolute difference between the current image and the statistical background image B(x,y) calculated from the peak PDF of each pixel, $D(x,y)=|I(x,y)-B(x,y)|$ where $D(x,y)$ is the filter output. The use of intensity difference is biased towards the extraction of shadows in bright regions. For shadows in darker regions, however, one has to rely on the relative intensity attenuation between $I(x,y)$ and $B(x,y)$, given by $G(x,y)= | I(x,y)/B(x,y) |$. Based on the property of shadow color invariance, two color filters working in the RGB space have also been adopted:

$$R(x,y)=\frac{\langle \bar{I}\bullet\bar{B}\rangle}{\|\bar{I}\|\|\bar{B}\|}$$

where $\overline{I}$ and $\overline{B}$ are the RGB vectors of the background images. The final filter uses a color invariant model and addresses the limited color quantization steps:

$$c_1 = \arctan\left(\frac{R_i}{\max(G_i, B_i)}\right) \qquad b_1 = \arctan\left(\frac{R_b}{\max(G_b, B_b)}\right)$$

$$c_2 = \arctan\left(\frac{G_i}{\max(R_i, B_i)}\right) \qquad b_2 = \arctan\left(\frac{G_b}{\max(R_b, B_b)}\right)$$

$$c_3 = \arctan\left(\frac{B_i}{\max(R_i, G_i)}\right) \qquad b_3 = \arctan\left(\frac{B_b}{\max(R_b, G_b)}\right)$$

$$V(x, y) = (c_1 - b_1)^2 + (c_2 - b_2)^2 + (c_3 - b_3)^2$$

where (R_i,G_i,B_i) and (R_b,G_b,B_b) are the RGB components of a given pixel of the current background [12].

In order to evaluate the effect of shadow enhancement as an aid to depth perception, an experiment was devised comparing shadow enhanced to shadow unenhanced images. Ten volunteers with experiences in surgical imaging were recruited for this study. They were blinded to the aims of this study and asked to serially assess 36 images taken from the experimental setup described above on a 2D display. Each image showed part of laparoscopic instrument over a surface and the subjects were asked to estimate to the nearest half centimeter the vertical distance

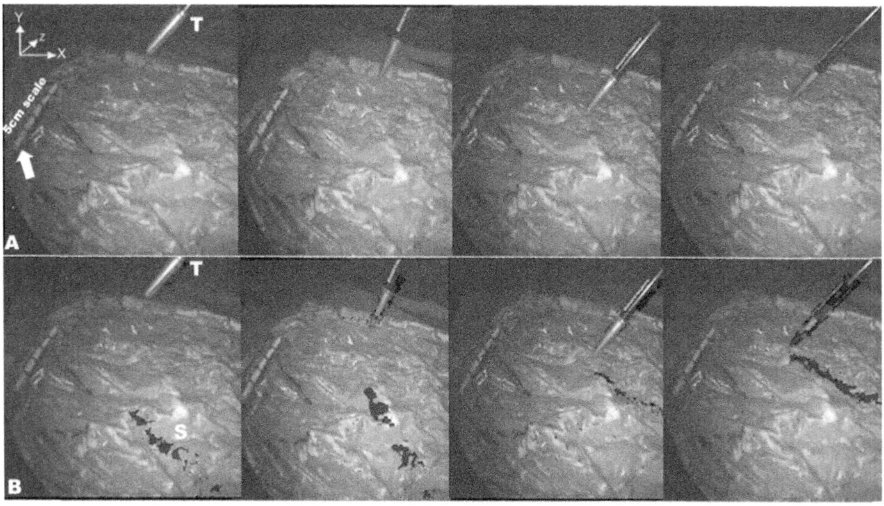

Fig. 3. (**A**) A series of raw images showing a laparoscopic instrument tip (T) as it approaches the silicon surface. (**B**) The same images following shadow (S) enhancement. Note the 5cm scaling aid to the left of each image (arrow).

from the tip of the instrument to the surface, with their answers recorded. The first 18 images were raw images (similar to those shown in Figure 3A) taken from the endoscope, whereas the remainder images were obtained by applying the described shadow enhancement algorithm (Figure 3B). For a better appreciation of the scaling and perspective, a 5cm marker with 1cm graduations was placed directly onto the surface in line with the z-axis.

To elucidate the underlying visual behavior of the users under normal and shadow enhanced viewing environments, gaze tracking was performed on all subjects performing the above task using a Tobii ET 1750 eye tracker. This is an infra-red video-based binocular eye-tracking system recording the position of gaze in the work plane (screen) at up to 38 samples per second with an accuracy of 1 degree across the work plane [13]. In this study the eye gaze data was analyzed qualitatively using the Clearview software (Tobii technology).

3 Results

To determine the perceptual accuracy, the absolute difference of the perceived distance of the tool-tip from the surface from the mean measured distance for all images for each subject was calculated. The mean difference for all subjects was 1.36cm for raw and 1.02cm for shadow enhanced images indicating an improvement in depth perception after shadow enhancement. This difference, however, was not statistically significant (t-test $p = 0.115$). The results indicate that the users are able to gauge large relative instrument distance to the surface when there are secondary visual cues. When the instrument is close to the tissue surface, however, the visual cues appreciable by the user are diminished if dynamic shadow enhancement is not applied. For this study, when the distance between the instrument and tissue surface is within 1cm (see Figure 4) (a situation that is most critical for relying on

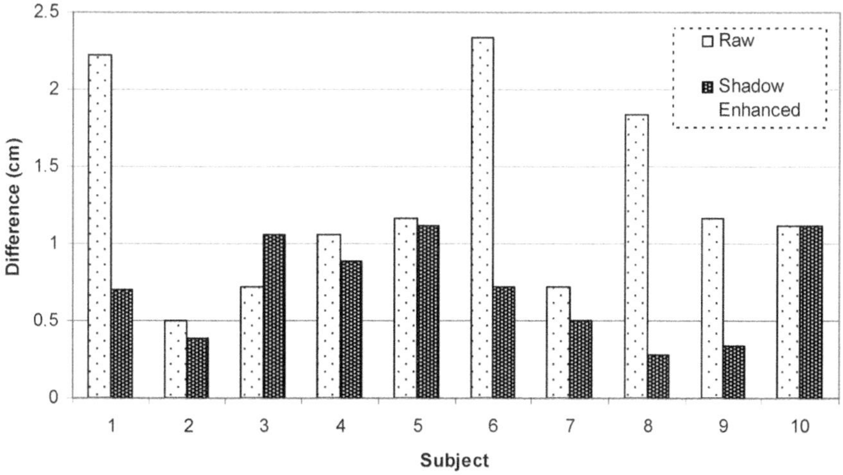

Fig. 4. Bar charts comparing the mean distance difference from reality perceived for raw and shadow enhanced images for each subject when the distance between the tool tip and tissue surface was set within 1cm

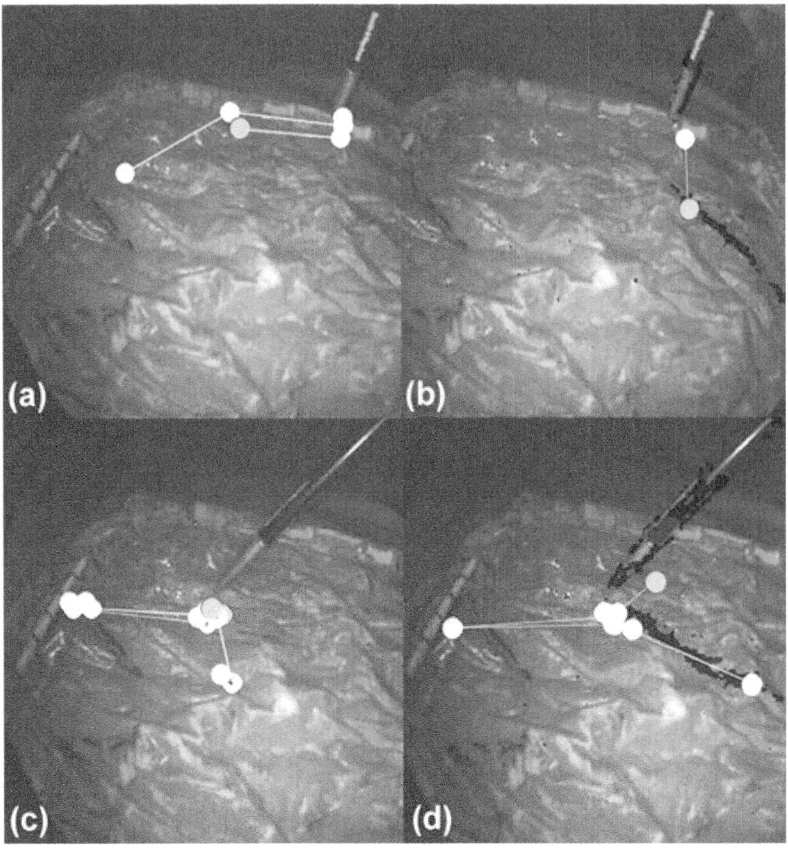

Fig. 5. An eye-gaze path demonstrating the fixations (white circles = fixations, yellow circle = first fixation, and white lines = saccades) recorded during the experiment. The effect of the "invisible shadow" enhancement to the accuracy of perceived tissue-instrument distance can be clearly demonstrated. In (a) and (b), the actual distance of the instrument tip from the tissue is 2cm and the subject whilst underestimating this to be 1cm in the raw image was able to estimate the exact distance correctly after shadow enhancement. In images (c) and (d) without shadow enhancement, the perceived distance was 2.5cm whereas by the use of shadow enhancement the perceived distance was 0.5cm, which is much closer to the ground truth.

tactile distance ranging), the mean errors for this group of observers were 1.283 and 0.709 (standard deviation 0.64 and 0.32) for raw and shadow enhanced images respectively (t-test p=0.020). This result was statistically significant. In addition, overall subjects were able to estimate depth faster from shadow enhanced images compared to raw images (5.8s versus 7.9s).

Verbal assessment of the participants has shown that all of them admitted that the enhanced "invisible" shadow had significantly facilitated their perception of depth. When a shadow was not present, most subjects based their answer on the scale of the instrument tip to estimate its position in space.

Figure 5 demonstrates the effect of the enhanced "invisible shadow" on general visual behavior revealed through eye tracking. It is evident that in Figures 5(a) and (b), the apex of the shadow provides direct cuing for depth perception with the subject drawing a visual line between the apex and tool tip. The real distance in this image is 2cm and the subject whilst underestimating to 1cm in the raw image was able to estimate the exact distance correctly after shadow enhancement. Figures 5(c) and (d), show a pair of images without and with "invisible shadow" enhancement when the instrument is in fact touching the surface. Without shadow enhancement, the perceived distance was 2.5 cm whereas by the use of shadow enhancement the perceived distance was 0.5cm, which is much closer to the ground truth.

4 Discussions and Conclusions

In this paper, we have demonstrated the effect of shadow on the accuracy of perceived tissue-instrument distance. One important feature of the algorithm is to cast an "invisible shadow" through the careful use of a secondary light source in a simulated laparoscopic environment. During instrument maneuver, this "invisible shadow" is dynamically enhanced which introduces a strong depth cue from which the distance between the instrument and tissue can be accurately determined. From a practical point of view, a faint shadow can theoretically be easily created by the introduction of a secondary light source through one of the accessory laparoscopic ports inserted during the procedure. The method naturally avoids the use of instrument to "crash" on the tissue surface, which is undesirable under delicate surgical maneuvers that require subtle control of the instruments to avoid damaging the tissues in contact. From both the objective and subjective assessment results of the study, it is evident that artificial shadow enhancement can be a useful aid for the perception of depth from 2D cues. Furthermore, the digital enhancement approach proved to be most effective when the instrument is in close proximity to a surface, which is the most critical time for enhanced instrument maneuver as *in vivo* mal-navigation at this level may lead to accidental injury to sensitive tissues.

Acknowledgements. We would like to thank our colleagues: Danail Stoyanov, George Mylonas and Xiao-Peng Hu from the Royal Society/Wolfson Medical Image Computing Lab for their support and contribution to the study. We would also like to thank Smith & Nephew for supplying the laparoscopic equipment used in this study.

References

1. Hubona GS, Shirah GW, Jennings DK. The effects of cast shadows and stereopsis on performing computer-generated spatial tasks *Systems, Man and Cybernetics, Part A, IEEE Transactions on* 2004; 34(4): 483-493.
2. Gibson JJ. Perception of the visual world. ed. Westport, Conn: Greenwood Press; 1974: pp. 235.
3. Kelsey C. Detection of visual information. In: The Perception of Visual Information, W. Hendee and P. Wells, Eds. New York: Springer-Verlag, 1993; 30-51.

4. Tendick F, Jennings R., Stark L, Tharp G. Sensing and Manipulation Problems in Endoscopic Surgery: Experiment, Analysis, and Observation. 1993; *Presence*, 2(1), 66-81.
5. Wanger L, Ferwanda J, Greenberg D. Perceiving spatial relationships in computer-generated images. *Computer Graphics and Applications, IEEE* 1992; 12(3): 44-58.
6. Huertas A, Nevatia R. Detecting Buildings in Aerial Images. *Comput. Vision Graphics and Image Processing.* 1988; 41: 131-152.
7. Irvin R B, NcKeown D.M. Methods for exploiting the relationship between building and their shadows in aerial imagery. *IEEE Tran. On System, Man and Cybernetics*, 1989; 19 (6): 1564-1575.
8. Liow Y, Pavlidis T. Use of shadows for extracting buildings in aerial images. *Computer Vision, Graphics and Image Processing*. 1990; 49: 242-277.
9. Thompson B W, Checky M T, Kaemmerer W F. Shadow stereo-locating object boundaries using shadows. *National Conf. on Art. Intel.* 1987; 761-766.
10. Mishra RK, Hanna GB, Brown SI and Cuschieri A. Optimum shadow-casting illumination for endoscopic task performance. *Arch Surg*, 2004; 139: 889-892.
11. Hanna GB, Cresswell AB, Cuschieri A. Shadow depth cues and endoscopic task performance. *Arch Surg* 2002; 137(10): 1166-1169.
12. Lo BPL and Yang GZ. Neuro-fuzzy shadow filter. *Lecture Notes In Computer Science:* Proceedings of the 7th European Conference on Computer Vision, 2002; 2352: 381-392.
13. Tobii technology. User Manual, 2003, http://www.tobii.se.

A Navigation System for Minimally Invasive CT-Guided Interventions

Markus Nagel[1], Gerd Schmidt[2], Ralf Petzold[3], and Willi A. Kalender[1]

[1] Institute of Medical Physics, University of Erlangen-Nürnberg, Germany
markus.nagel@imp.uni-erlangen.de
[2] Siemens Medical Solutions, Erlangen, Germany
[3] CAS innovations AG, Erlangen, Germany

Abstract. The purpose of our project was to develop a novel navigation system for interventional radiology. Fields of application are minimally invasive percutaneous interventions performed under local anaesthesia. In order to reduce unintentional patient movements we used a patient vacuum immobilization device. Together with the vacuum fixation and a newly developed reference frame we achieved a fully automatic patient-to-image registration independent from the tracking system. The combination of the software and a novel designed needle holder allows for an adjustment of the needle within a few seconds. The complete system is adapted to the requirements of the radiologist and to the clinical workflow. For evaluation of the navigation system we performed a phantom study with a perspex phantom and achieved an average needle positioning accuracy of less than 0.7 mm.

1 Introduction

CT-guided minimally invasive interventions on human subjects are today an established radiological procedure. Such interventions include percutaneous punctures, biopsies, vertebroplasties and radio frequency ablations, as well as therapies requiring the percutaneous advancing of a needle to a definite anatomical position in the patient. CT-guided interventions allow the radiologist to work rapidly with the greatest care and interest of the patient.

The exact placement of the needle in the patient requires a great deal of experience and considerable skills. A limiting factor is the time required to exactly position a needle at the required anatomical site in the patient. Particularly with interventions requiring a high degree of precision, where the incorrect positioning of the needle can lead to life-threatening complications, it is necessary to repeatedly control and correct the position of the advancing needle within the patient using CT control scans. This not only lengthens the entire intervention, but also increases radiation exposure for the patient.

In practice, a number of different auxiliary needle positioning devices are employed. For example, laser targeting devices attached to the gantry or targeting devices which can be fixed directly to the patient [1,2]. However, none

J. Duncan and G. Gerig (Eds.): MICCAI 2005, LNCS 3750, pp. 33–40, 2005.

of these auxiliary devices permits simultaneous real-time control of the needle, tremble-free needle advancement, and assistance for the implementation of an access path as planned in the patient data. Since the early 1990s, computer and robot-assisted navigation systems have been increasingly used as intervention aids, leading the way for applications in neurosurgery and orthopedics. Applications in the area of interventional radiology are, on the other hand, very rare. The Tirat Hacarmel company utilizes an electromagnetic localization system (UltraGuide1000). This system has already been successfully employed for hepatic and renal punctures, as well as for radio frequency ablations [3]. Bale et al. have employed an optical localization system for punctures and radio frequency ablations [4]. Medical research shows a continuously growing interest in navigation systems for interventional radiology, as seen by the ever increasing number of groups working on prototypes for needle positioning systems and robotic systems [5,6,7,8].

With CT-guided navigation systems, it is first necessary to register the patient according to the images acquired. For this purpose, a fixed reference point, defined by a Dynamic Reference Frame (DRF), is rigidly attached to the patient. For navigation systems used in orthopedics, the DRF is firmly attached to the bones by using surgical screws. For neurosurgical applications, stereotactic frames are attached to the head to allow for the registration of the patient. With minimally invasive interventions such as punctures and biopsies, the rigid attachment of a DRF to the patient represents a problem due to the absence of firm anatomic structures. One solution is to use skin markers which can be positioned in combination with DRFs either directly on the patient's skin, or nearby. However, in this case patient movement would impair the precision of registration or even render the registration useless. Since most minimally invasive interventions are performed under local anesthesia, patient movement is highly probable. A further difficulty with navigation systems is the guidance of the physician during the 3D orientation of the instruments such as the puncture needle along a planned access path. The orientation process must be fast, precise and simple. In order not to lengthen the entire interventional procedure, the workflow of the navigation system needs to be adapted to the clinical procedure.

We will introduce a new navigation system to solve the problem of patient movement and registration, at the same time enabling the fast, simple and precise orientation of the needle along a planned trajectory. Additionally, the navigation system is ideally matched to the clinical requirements and the clinical workflow.

2 Materials and Methods

2.1 System Overview and Architecture

The navigation system consists of an optical tracking system (Polaris, NDI, Canada), a standard PC with touch screen as user interface and dedicated navigation software (CAPPA IRad, CAS innovations, Germany), a needle holder, a patient fixation vacuum device (BodyFix™, Medical Intelligence, Germany) and a reference frame (RF) developed in this work. The RF is attached with

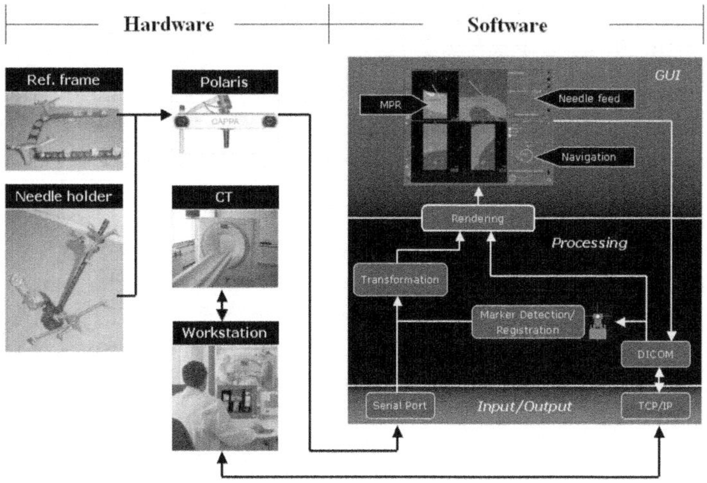

Fig. 1. Overview of the system architecture: CAPPA IRad (Input/Output, Processing, GUI) and hardware (reference frame, needle holder, polaris, CT with workstation)

markers that can be detected automatically in CT images as well as with reflective markers detectable by optical tracking. For image acquisition the navigation system is connected to a CT scanner (Sensation 64, Siemens Medical Solutions, Germany). The system architecture and interface between the components used are illustrated in Fig. 1.

The tracking system is used to localize the position of the reference frame and the needle holder in the operating room. For this purpose, reflecting spheres are fixed with a known geometry on both the reference frame and the needle holder. The position of the needle holder is measured by the tracking system relative to the reference frame in physical space. All necessary 3D coordinates are transmitted from the Polaris to the PC by using the serial port. For the communication of the CAPPA IRad System with the CT scanner we implemented a DICOM network application providing verification, storage and query/retrieve services to enable image transfer using a TCP/IP connection. The DICOM network application is implemented as a background process and set up to receive images as soon as CAPPA IRad is running. After receiving the images, these can be visualized in multi planar reconstruction (MPR) views. We also used the connection to send DICOM images back to the scanner for documentation of performed steps.

2.2 Description of the System Components and Steps

Needle holder: The needle holder was constructed such that any medical tool like biopsy syringes or needle hulls can be quickly attached and unmounted. The needle holder itself is mounted at the end of a hydraulic arm. By moving the hydraulic arm (6 DoF) which is mounted on the CT table, the needle holder can be positioned near the patient. Two independent pivot joints on the needle holder enable the precise and fast alignment of the needle holder with the planned surgical path, illustrated in Fig. 2.

Reference frame (RF) and image-to-patient registration: In order to visualize medical instruments like the needle in the CT images of the patient, an image-to-patient registration is necessary. For that the RF is positioned in proximity to the planned entry point prior to the first CT scan. In addition to the tracking markers, which are used as reference DRF to define the coordinate system of the tracking system, we also placed CT markers in a known geometry on the RF. During image acquisition, all CT markers at the frame must be inside the field of view. After sending the images to the CAPPA IRad system, an integrated marker detection algorithm in the navigation software finds the CT markers in the patient's data set and determines the marker centroids with sub-voxel accuracy. The coordinates of the CT markers in the patient coordinate system and the coordinates of the CT markers in the tracking system are used to derive the registration matrix. After this step, the relation between the images and the patient are fixed.

Patient fixation: We used the BodyFix™to fixate the patient to reduce any patient movements relative to the positioned RF. The BodyFix™is a double fixation device which consists of a vacuum bag, cushions and a pump. The patient is fitted to the vacuum bag and the cushions are placed on the patient. The air in the bag and in the cushions are exhausted by the pump. In that way the patient is fixed securely to the bag. The fixation device is used successfully in both radiation therapy for the reproducible positioning of the patient for beam delivery [9] and for medical navigation and robotic systems [4].

Calibration of the needle: We implemented and evaluated two kinds of needle navigation possibilities. The first method restricts the adjustment of the needle holder according to the prior planned trajectory without visualizing the length of the needle in the patient's data set. The adjustment of the needle outside the patient is visualized and the software only guides the radiologist to adjust the needle holder. During the needle feed, graduated marks on the needle can be used for depth information.

The second method requires a calibration of the needle to obtain the exact needle length. For that, the radiologist holds the needle tip on a calibration point on the RF. The 3D coordinates of the calibration point are known by the system. A second DRF (needle DRF) is fixed above the needle and calibrated in a way that the origin of the DRF is on top of the needle, as illustrated in Fig. 2. The needle length is defined as the length of the vector between the calibration point and the origin of the needle DRF. During the needle feed, the needle DRF is moved with the needle. The exact position of the needle, especially the tip of the needle, is visible in the patient's data set on the screen.

Software and graphical user interface (GUI): The GUI is designed to allow for an intuitive use of the navigation software. Transfer and loading of the images from CT and registration work fully automatically: The planning module is kept as simple as possible but contains comfortable planning features like oblique

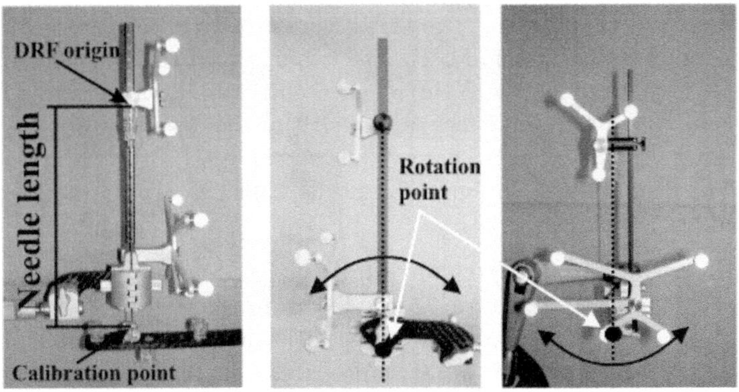

Fig. 2. Left: Calibration step. The length of the needle is calculated from the needle DRF to the calibration point located at the frame. Middle, Right: The needle holder with the two possible movements.

MPRs and accurate planning of trajectories with sub-voxel accuracy. It is also possible to plan arbitrary oblique trajectories. The planning can be performed with the mouse or by touch screen. The combination of the dedicated navigation software and the needle holder allows for an accurate adjustment of the needle according to the planned trajectory within a few seconds. For documentation, screenshots containing information about the final needle position are created, converted to DICOM images and finally sent to the PACS. After the intervention, all images and patient data are removed from the CAPPA IRad system since the local PACS is responsible for archiving and managing the image data.

2.3 Clinical Workflow

We analyzed the established clinical workflow of CT-guided, minimally invasive interventions. Based on our investigations we were able to derive the navigation workflow which consists of the following steps:

Preparation of the patient: The patient is placed on the CT bed and immobilized with the BodyFix^{TM}system. The RF is positioned close to the prospective entry point. A field of view is determined to ensure that all CT markers are inside the scanning area.

Importation of scanned images: After scanning, the images are sent from the CT system to the navigation system. All images are internally checked by the software to ensure consistency of patient data before visualization. Additionally, the images are verified by the radiologist and stored on the system to allow for a quick review during the intervention.

Preparation of trajectories: The radiologist defines a trajectory by setting a target and an entry point using the touch screen or the mouse.

Calibration of the needle (optional): The radiologist calibrates the needle used to obtain its length.

Adjustment of the needle: The adjustment process of the needle with respect to the planned trajectory is divided into two steps. First, the radiologist moves the needle holder in vicinity to the planned entry point, assisted by the navigation system. The next step is the adjustment of the needle holder to adapt the needle axis to the planned trajectory. The software gives the radiologist important information on how to move the needle holder at the two joints to adjust it within a few seconds.

Navigation of needle feed (optional): If the needle was calibrated, the actual position of the needle tip is visible within the CT images of the patient during the needle feed. By extracting information about the location of the needle within the CT coordinates, the system proposes a small region for a control scan in longitudinal direction.

Initiation of control scan: During the needle feed the radiologist is able to initiate control scans and load the images into the navigation system. It is also possible to continue the navigation in the images delivered by the control scan or switch back to the images of the preparation scan.

Documentation: After the needle is at the final position, screenshots can be taken and sent back to the PACS for documentation.

3 Phantom Test and Results

To evaluate the navigation system's accuracy we designed a perspex phantom with a base plate including 7 rods with tips, Fig. 3. The phantom was placed at the CT table and the RF was positioned above the phantom with a distance of 15 cm from the base plate to the RF. After scanning the phantom we selected the tips of the rods as targets in the planning step of the navigation software and planned trajectories with lengths of 120 mm and 180 mm.

A standard biopsy needle (18G) was calibrated and adjusted so that the needle tip was exactly on the top of the tips of the rods and the needle was adjusted according to the planned trajectory. The navigation system calculates the vector $\boldsymbol{v}$ between the current needle tip measured by the system and the planned target point and the perpendicular $\boldsymbol{l}$ of the needle path to the target point. The distance $\varepsilon = |\boldsymbol{v}|$ and the perpendicular $\kappa = |\boldsymbol{l}|$ were used to denote the error of the misadjustment. The error includes the error of construction (needle holder and RF), the image-to-patient registration error and the error caused by the tracking system.

For every rod we measured 30 values respectively 15 for both planned trajectory lengths (120 cm and 180 cm).

The resulting error ε of 105 measurements on 7 targets with a trajectory length of 120 mm was 0.635 mm rms with 0.228 mm standard deviation. The length of the perpendicular κ at this length was 0.481 mm with a standard deviation of 0.211 mm. The 105 measurements at the same 7 targets but with a trajectory length of 180 mm showed nearly the same results. The resulting error ε was 0.604 mm rms with 0.217 mm standard deviation and the perpendicular

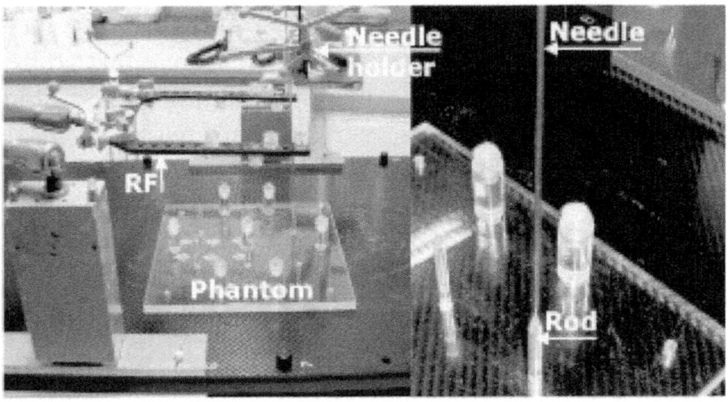

Fig. 3. Perspex phantom study: The needle is exactly adjusted to the planned target (tip of rod) and the needle deviation denoted by the software is used as system adjustment error

Table 1. Results of the phantom study

path length	n	rms (ε)	rms (κ)
120 mm	105	0.635 mm ± 0.228 mm	0,481 mm ± 0.211 mm
180 mm	105	0.604 mm ± 0.217 mm	0,489 mm ± 0.204 mm

κ was 0.489 mm with a standard deviation of 0.204 mm. All measured values are summarized in Table 1. The maximum measured deviation was 1.2 mm at a path length of 120 mm.

4 Discussion

We presented a new navigation system to be used for minimally invasive percutaneous procedures in interventional radiology. The main focus of the system was to support the radiologist during interventions and to provide a system which is at the same time fully integrated into the clinical workflow. The TCP/IP network connection of the navigation system with the CT scanner and the DICOM protocol enables a manufacturer independent and comfortable image transfer in both directions. By using the developed RF, a fully automatic, tracking system independent patient-to-image registration was achieved. Unpredicted patient movements relative to the RF which could influence the image-to-patient registration are minimized by the fixation. In that way risk related to patient movements was minimal. The calibration allows any needle to be used regardless of the manufacturer. Biopsy syringes or needle hulls can be easily integrated into the system during the intervention. With the combination of software and needle holder it was possible to adjust the needle holder in accordance with a prior planned trajectory. This process was fast and accurate. The needle feed is visualized in the patient's data set to verify the needle placement. This reduces the number of control scans which would otherwise be necessary. In contrast to conventional navigation systems or help devices, our navigation system was adapted to the requirements of the radiologist and therefore serves as an ideal tool for various CT-guided percutaneous interventional procedures.

The first accuracy studies with a perspex phantom illustrated a repetitious accuracy of less than 0.7 mm for two different path lengths (120 mm and 180 mm). The next step will involve a cadaver study prior to clinical evaluation which has already been approved by an ethics commission.

Acknowledgements. This work was supported by CAS innovations (Erlangen, Germany). The authors are grateful to S. Kurz and S. Wahl for their support during implementation of the complete software. Special thanks go to R. Bale et al. (Sib-Lab, University of Innsbruck, Austria) for helping during the complete development and W. Bautz and M. Uder (Department of Radiology, University of Erlangen-Nürnberg, Germany) for the clinical feedback.

References

1. Buecker, A., et al.: In: Circular spirit level guidance system for CT- and MR-guided punctures. In Journal of Computer Assisted Tomography **23** (1999) 552–554
2. Frederick, P., et al.: A light-guidance system to be used for CT-guided biopsy. In: Radiology **154** (1985) 535–536
3. Wood, B., et al.: Percutaneous radiofrequency ablation with three-dimensional position sensor guidance. In: Cardiovasc Intervent Radiol (2001) –
4. Bale, R., et al.: A novel vacuum immobilization device and a novel targeting device for computer assisted interventional procedures. In: Proc. of 16th International Congress on "Computer Aided Radiology and Surgery" (2002) 92–97
5. Ra, J., et al.: Spine needle biopsy simulator using visual and force feedback. In: Computer Aided Surgery **7** (2002) 353–363
6. Banovac, F., et al.: Liver tumor biopsy in a respiring phantom with the assistance of a novel electromagnetic navigation device. In: Proc. of Medical Image Computing and Computer-Assisted Intervention, MICCAI (2002) 200–208
7. Cleary, K., et al.: CT-directed robotic biopsy testbed: User interface and coordinate transformations. In: Proc of 15th International Congress on "Computer Aided Radiology and Surgery" (2001) 27–30
8. Megali, G., et al.: A computer-assisted robotic ultrasound-guided biopsy system for video-assisted surgery. In: Proc. of Medical Image Computing and Computer-Assisted Intervention, MICCAI (2003) 343–350
9. Fuss, M., et al.: Repositioning accuracy of a commercially available double-vacuum whole body immobilization system for stereotactic body radiation therapy. In: Technology in Cancer Research and Treatment (2004) 59–68

Passive Markers for Ultrasound Tracking of Surgical Instruments

Jeffrey Stoll and Pierre Dupont

Boston University, Aerospace and Mechanical Engineering Department,
Boston, MA
{jstoll, pierre}@bu.edu

Abstract. A family of passive markers is presented by which the position and orientation of a surgical instrument can be computed from its ultrasound image using simple image processing. These markers address the problem of imaging instruments and tissue simultaneously in ultrasound-guided interventions. Marker-based estimates of instrument location can be used in augmented reality displays or for image-based servoing. Marker design, measurement techniques and error analysis are presented. Experimentally determined in-vitro measurement errors of 0.22 mm in position and 0.089 rad in orientation were obtained using a standard ultrasound imaging system.

1 Introduction

While ultrasound imaging has traditionally been employed for diagnostic procedures, its use in minimally invasive interventions is growing. The advent of real-time 3D ultrasound is also likely to facilitate these procedures. For example, in cardiac surgery, ultrasound imaging can be used for beating-heart repair of internal defects [1].

A challenge arises, however, due to the substantial difference in both impedance and absorption of biological tissues and instruments. Imaging systems designed to differentiate tissue types based on small changes in impedance are not well suited to imaging metal instruments. As a result, instruments produce image artifacts due to specular reflection and scattering, which obscure both the location and geometric details of the instrument. The instrument markers presented here address this problem by providing a means to easily estimate an instrument's body coordinate frame from a single ultrasound image. Such estimates can be used to augment ultrasound images with precise instrument location or to register instruments with respect to a manipulating robot for image-based servoing.

Alternate solutions to the instrument imaging problem include instrument modification, image processing techniques and the use of active markers. In instrument modification, several researchers have focused on altering instruments' reflection characteristics to make them more visible [2]. This approach can involve the application of coatings or surface modifications to the instruments, which can add cost while not necessarily eliminating image artifacts. Image processing methods apply search techniques based on either actual instrument geometry or the geometry produced under ultrasound imaging [3]. This approach shows promise although the amount of processing involved may be tied to the complexity of the geometry. Other

J. Duncan and G. Gerig (Eds.): MICCAI 2005, LNCS 3750, pp. 41 – 48, 2005.

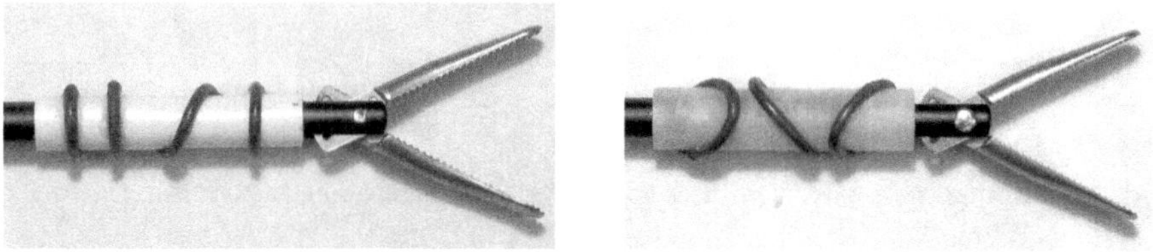

(a) (b)

Fig. 1. Two possible marker designs attached to a surgical grasping instrument

work has focused on actively tracking instruments and ultrasound transducers using electromagnetic and optical sensors. Lindseth et al. report measurement accuracy of 0.6 mm with optical tracking of the ultrasound scan head [4], and Leotta reported accuracy of 0.35 mm with electromagnetic tracking [5]. Merdes and Wolf reported a method for tracking an active ultrasound receiver mounted on a cardiac catheter [6]. They achieved a mean accuracy between 0.22±0.11 and 0.47±0.47 mm, depending on the distance between the catheter and the ultrasound transducer. Active tracking devices are more costly than passive ones. They also can require more complex calibration and can be more difficult to integrate with existing medical instruments.

The solution presented here consists of passive markers which can be easily added to existing surgical instruments and require minimal calibration. The markers are constructed to possess two properties: (1) they appear clearly when imaged along with tissue regardless of instrument appearance, and (2) they are shaped such that their positions and orientations can be determined from a single image using simple image processing.

In this paper, we assume that the instruments possess a cylindrical shaft over which the marker can be attached as shown in Figure 1. The cylindrical portion of the marker is used to determine the four degrees of freedom associated with the instrument shaft axis. The marker pattern is designed to indicate the location of the marker along the instrument shaft and the rotation of the marker about the shaft's axis. The proposed markers are applicable to both 2D and 3D ultrasound. For simplicity of presentation, only the 2D case is considered here.

These markers are similar to devices known as stereotactic frames, which have been studied extensively for imaging modalities such as CT and MRI [7][8]. A stereotactic frame consists of a shape that appears uniquely when imaged at various positions and orientations and is constructed of material easily seen in a particular imaging modality.

The next section describes the proposed family of markers – their design, image processing and error analysis. The subsequent section presents an experimental evaluation of one possible marker shape and the paper concludes with a discussion of the results.

2 Implementation

The markers consist of two parts, a cylindrical sleeve that can be fit over the shaft of a surgical instrument and ridges of constant height and width fixed to the outer surface of the sleeve, as shown in Figure 1. The cylindrical shape allows the markers to fit through access ports used in minimally invasive surgery. The ridges trace out prescribed paths on the sleeve's surface, which, when imaged, indicate the marker's position along and orientation about the cylinder's axis. The family of markers is characterized by a variable number of ridges and a variety of ridge paths. These are together referred to as the marker pattern.

The marker pattern must satisfy three constraints. First, each position along and rotation about the cylinder's axis must correspond to a unique ultrasound image of marker pattern. Second, the error in position and orientation should be small. Third, the length of the marker pattern should be small since ultrasound imaging systems typically have a small field of view. Note that the marker body can extend beyond the marker pattern in order to make the instrument shaft visible.

2.1 Marker Analysis

If the relative position and orientation of the instrument and marker are known, the rigid body transformation, T_I^M, relating the marker coordinate frame to the image-based coordinate frame defines the instrument's position and orientation relative to the ultrasound image. This transformation can be decomposed into two elements,

$$T_I^M = T_I^A T_A^M . \tag{1}$$

As shown in Figure 2, transformation T_I^A relates an intermediate frame, A, located on the instrument shaft's axis, with the image frame. This frame, determined in an initial processing step, serves to locate the axis of the instrument shaft in the image. The second transformation, $T_A^M(\theta,t)$, defines the marker frame with respect to the shaft axis frame in terms of θ and t, the rotation about, and the translation along, the shaft axis x_A. The entire length of the marker body can be used to estimate the shaft axis frame while the marker pattern is used to estimate θ and t.

Assuming the instrument shaft lies in the plane of the 2D ultrasound image, the marker body appears as a line of high pixel intensity. This line represents a thin strip along the surface of the marker facing the ultrasound transducer. The marker pattern appears as a sequence of bumps along the bright line produced by the body.

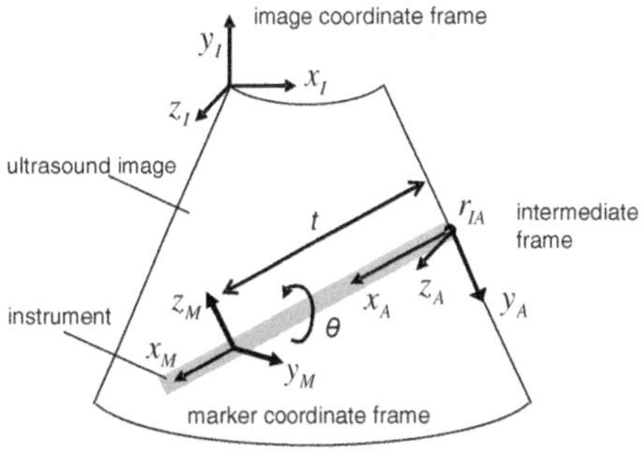

Fig. 2. Ultrasound image plane and coordinate systems

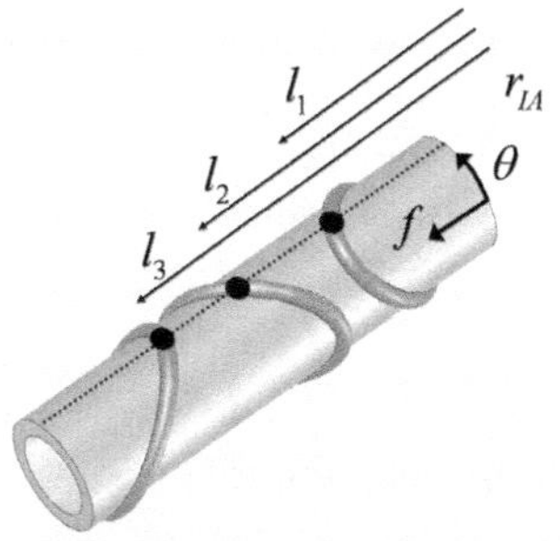

Fig. 3. Marker pattern

The transformation T_I^A is estimated by fitting a line to the high intensity marker body image and selecting as the frame's origin, r_{IA}, one of the two points where this line intersects the image boundary. The frame's *x*-axis, x_A is selected to lie along the instrument's shaft axis and its *z*-axis, z_A is taken to coincide with z_I, orthogonal to the image plane. Note that the axis x_A is offset from the image line in the $\pm y_A$ direction by the known radius of the marker body.

Transformation T_A^M is estimated from the bump locations associated with the imaged marker pattern. As shown in Figure 3, the x_A coordinates of the n bumps are combined in a vector $l = [l_1, l_2, \ldots, l_n]^T$. This vector is related to the marker pattern through θ and t by

$$\begin{bmatrix} l_1(\theta,t) \\ l_2(\theta,t) \\ \vdots \\ l_n(\theta,t) \end{bmatrix} = \begin{bmatrix} f_1(\theta) \\ f_2(\theta) \\ \vdots \\ f_n(\theta) \end{bmatrix} + tu, \qquad u = \begin{bmatrix} 1 \\ 1 \\ \vdots \\ 1 \end{bmatrix}, \tag{2}$$

in which the components of the vector $f(\theta)$ are functions describing the x_M coordinates of the marker ridges as functions of rotation angle θ about x_M . In this equation, t is seen to be the magnitude of r_{AM}, the vector describing the origin of marker frame M with respect to shaft axis frame A, measured along x_A.

In terms of the vector l, the constraint that each position along, and rotation about, the cylinder's axis corresponds to a unique ultrasound image of marker pattern can be expressed as

$$l(\theta_1,t_1) - l(\theta_2,t_2) = 0 \Leftrightarrow (\theta_1,t_1) = (\theta_2,t_2) \quad \forall \theta \in [0 \ldots 2\pi), t \in \Re . \tag{3}$$

Combining (2) and (3) gives the constraint in terms of $f(\theta)$,

$$f(\theta_1) - f(\theta_2) \neq au \quad \forall a \in \Re . \tag{4}$$

By (2), a marker pattern must possess at least two ridges ($n \geq 2$) to provide a unique solution for θ and t. By (4), the curves describing these two ridges must differ. For markers with more than two ridges, (2) is overdetermined providing the means to reduce measurement error. For marker patterns satisfying (4), solutions for θ and t can be found by the following procedure. First note that t can be expressed explicitly in terms of θ by

$$t = u^T (l - f(\theta)) / n . \tag{5}$$

The error vector $l - f(\theta) - tu$ can be expressed solely in terms of θ using (5) and its minimum norm solution corresponds to θ,

$$\theta = \arg \min_{0 \leq \alpha < 2\pi} \left\| l - f(\alpha) - \frac{u^T (l - f(\alpha))}{n} u \right\| . \tag{6}$$

2.2 Error Analysis

The resolution of the marker depends fundamentally on the error in measuring the individual components of l. This error arises from four sources: random noise, finite image resolution, marker manufacturing defects, and misalignment between the image plane and instrument shaft. Since noise and image resolution involve the imaging system, they are assumed to affect all elements of l equally and are treated as one error source. While manufacturing defects can cause unevenly distributed error, for simplicity they are treated here as noise affecting all elements equally. Distortion of l caused by misalignment of the instrument in the image plane is assumed to be small, due to both the length of the instrument shaft and the narrow width of the ultrasound image.

Error estimates in t and θ based on measuring the components of l can be obtained by first linearizing (2) about a nominal angle, θ_0.

$$l = \left(\frac{\partial f}{\partial \theta}\right)_{\theta_0} \theta + tu + \left(f(\theta_0) - \left(\frac{\partial f}{\partial \theta}\right)_{\theta_0} \theta_0\right) = \begin{bmatrix} f'(\theta_0) & u \end{bmatrix} \begin{bmatrix} \theta \\ t \end{bmatrix} + \gamma(\theta_0). \quad (7)$$

Least squares solutions for t and θ are given by the pseudoinverse of $\begin{bmatrix} f'(\theta_0) & u \end{bmatrix}$ as

$$t = \frac{b^T}{b^T u}(l - \gamma), \quad b = \left(u - \left(\frac{f'^T u}{f'^T f'}\right) f'\right) \quad (8)$$

$$\theta = \frac{c^T}{c^T f'}(l - \gamma), \quad c = \left(f' - \left(\frac{f'^T u}{u^T u}\right) u\right) \quad (9)$$

The linearized error estimate for t and θ is given by multiplying the error factors $\left\| b / b^T u \right\|$ and $\left\| c / c^T f' \right\|$, respectively, by the standard deviation of the error in the components of l. The error factors are functions of the nominal angle θ_0.

Marker pattern length corresponds to the total range of values in $f(\theta)$. As can be seen in (8) and (9), design changes, such as increasing the number of ridges (ie. increasing $\|u\|$) or increasing the ridge slope, f', can reduce the error factors. Such changes, however, also increase the marker pattern length. As a result, there exists a tradeoff in marker design between the stated design constraints of minimizing measurement error and minimizing pattern length.

3 Example

Figure 4 depicts one possible marker pattern (also shown in Figures 1b and 3) consisting of three ridges described by sine waves of equal amplitude, but with phase lags of $2\pi/3$ and displacement offsets of β,

$$f(\theta) = \left[\alpha \sin(\theta) + \alpha, \quad \alpha \sin\left(\theta + \frac{2\pi}{3}\right) + \beta + \alpha, \quad \alpha \sin\left(\theta + \frac{4\pi}{3}\right) + 2\beta + \alpha\right]^T. \quad (10)$$

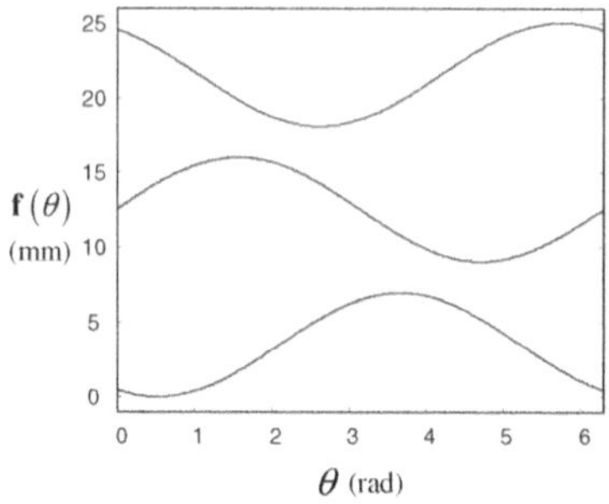

Fig. 4. Plot of $\mathbf{f}\left(\theta\right)$ versus θ for the example marker

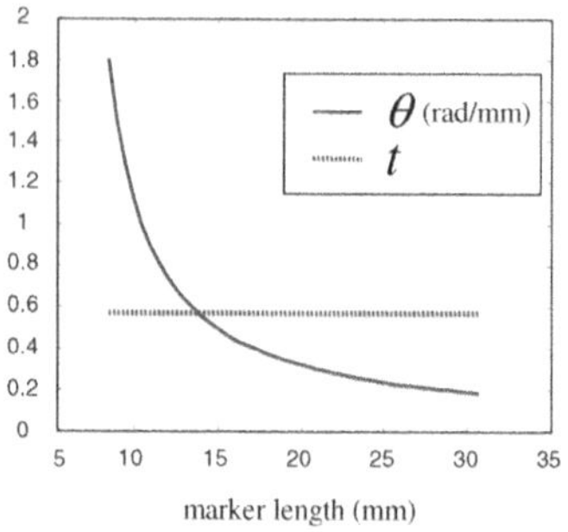

Fig. 5. Error factor versus length for the example marker

This choice of $f(\theta)$ is such that $u^T f(\theta) = 3(\alpha + \beta)$ for all θ. Consequently, the dependence of t on θ in (5) is eliminated yielding the explicit solution,

$$t = \left(u^T l - 3(\alpha - \beta)\right)/n \tag{11}$$

and the expression for θ simplifies to

$$\theta = \arg \min_{0 \le \alpha < 2\pi} \left\| l - f(\alpha) - tu \right\|. \tag{12}$$

The pattern parameters are $\alpha = 3.48$ mm and $\beta = 9.02$ mm resulting in a pattern length of 25 mm. Here, β is selected to ensure minimum separation of the ridges.

Using (8) and (9), the error factors for t and θ are 0.58 and 0.23 rad/mm, respectively. A plot of theoretical error factors for a variety of other lengths, obtained by varying α, is shown in figure 5.

The marker's cylindrical body is constructed with plastic by a rapid prototyping process. This enables shallow grooves to be located precisely on the outer surface, in which 1 mm diameter hollow plastic tubing is glued to form the ridges. Marker dimensions are as follows: body inner diameter 5mm, body outer diameter 7 mm, and overall marker diameter 8mm.

3.1 Experimental Evaluation

Two imaging experiments were performed to determine the example marker's accuracy and verify its predicted error factor. Images were generated using a 3.5 MHz 2D ultrasound probe (Analogic, Peabody, MA). The scan head was mounted to a linear micrometer stage over a tank filled with degassed water. A rotational micrometer was fixed to the side of the tank, and a 5mm diameter stainless steel rod, simulating the shaft of a surgical instrument, was attached such that it extended into the imaging plane and could rotate about its axis. The markers were then placed on the rod for imaging. The complete test apparatus is shown in figure 6.

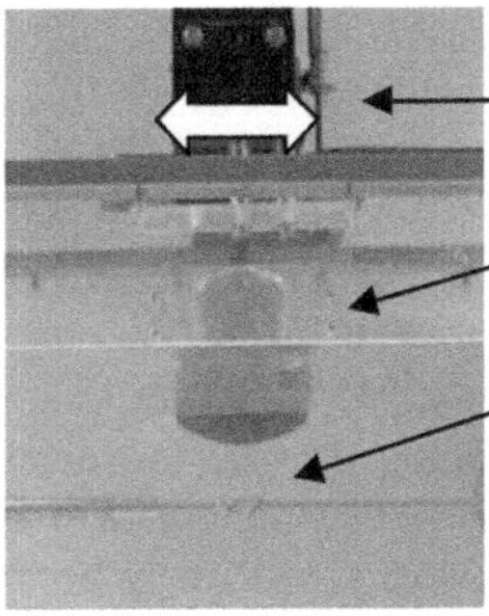

Fig. 6. Test apparatus

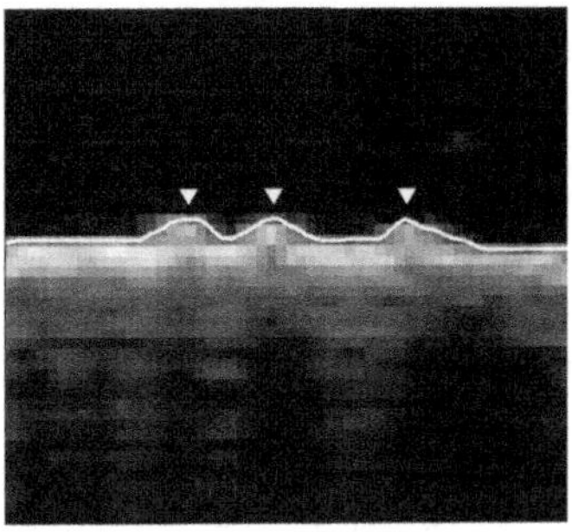

Fig. 7. Ultrasound image of a marker showing surface contour (line) and bump locations (arrows)

In all experiments, ultrasound images were analyzed offline in Matlab (Mathworks, Natick, MA). Images were initially filtered with a Gaussian kernel to remove high frequency noise. Surface contours were then obtained via threshold edge detection, super-sampled by cubic interpolation, and filtered to smooth the bumps. An example surface contour is shown in Figure 7. Analysis required an average of 0.047 sec. per image (21 Hz) on a Pentium 4, 3.5 Ghz desktop.

The first experiment established the error in the components of l at a variety of image regions. At each region, the scanhead was translated randomly 20 times within a 15 mm range along the marker's axis while the marker rotation angle was held constant. The locations of bumps in image coordinates were compared to the corresponding scan head positions recorded by micrometer. A line was fit to the data to determine the image resolution in pixels/mm, and the standard deviation from this line was taken as the error in components of l. At depths of 20 to 80 mm and ±40mm horizontally from center, error in the components of l ranged from ±0.20 to ±0.40 mm, increasing with distance from the transducer focal depth of ~60 mm.

The second experiment determined the marker's accuracy. Images were taken of the marker at a random set of 100 angles ($0 - 2\pi$ rad) and positions across the width of the image (~80 mm). Actual marker angle and scan head position were recorded by micrometer. The errors in t and θ were taken as the standard deviation of the difference between measured values and actual values. Finally, actual errors in t and θ were compared with predictions based on the error in the components of l and the marker's error factors defined by (8)-(9).

Error in the components of l was found to be ±0.33 mm at a depth of 70 mm. At this depth, the marker showed measurement errors in t and θ of ±0.22 mm and ±0.089 rad. Based on the marker error factors, predicted measurement errors are ±0.19 mm and ±0.077 rad.

4 Discussion

The experimental results show that the example markers have comparable accuracy to other methods of tracking instruments. They also confirm the marker error analysis by showing a small difference between actual and predicted measurement errors. Higher image resolutions and higher probe frequencies will likely lower the error in the components of l and thereby increase marker accuracy.

The results also verify that marker analysis can be accomplished with simple image processing. More sophisticated approaches, such as physics-based techniques, may produce further reductions in error.

The family of markers proposed in this paper is also amenable to 3D ultrasound imaging. In particular, it removes the constraint of 2D imaging that the instrument shaft be aligned with the image plane. Since the 3D analysis will be comparable to the 2D approach, the marker accuracy demonstrated with 2D images will likely be the same for 3D images which possess the same error in the components of l .

In conclusion, the markers presented have been shown to be a simple, cost-effective, and accurate approach to image-based instrument guidance.

Acknowledgment. This research was funded by the NIH, grant #R01 HL073647.

References

1. Cannon, J et al.: Application of Robotics in Congenital Cardiac Surgery, Seminars in Thoracic and Cardiovascular Surgery: Pediatric Cardiac Surgery Annual. 6(1):72-83, 2003.
2. Nichols, K. et al.: Changes in ultrasonographic echogenicity and visibility of needles with changes in angles of insonation. J Vasc Interv Radiol. 14(12):1553-7 Dec. 2003.
3. Novotny, P., J. Cannon, and R. Howe: Tool Localization in 3D Ultrasound Images. MICCAI, 2003.
4. Lindseth F. et al.: Probe Calibration for Freehand 3-D Ultrasound. Ultrasound in Med. & Biol. 29(11):1607-1623, 2003.
5. Leotta D.: An Efficient Calibration Method for Freehand 3-D Ultrasound Imaging Systems. Ultrasound in Med. & Biol. 30(7):999-1008, 2004.
6. Merdes, C. and P. Wolf: Locating a Catheter Transducer in a Three-Dimensional Ultrasound Imaging Field. IEEE trans Biomed Eng Dec. 2001.
7. Galloway, R. et al.: The accuracies of four stereotactic frame systems: an independent assessment. Biomed Instrum Technol 25(6):457-60 Nov-Dec 1991.
8. Fichtinger, G. et al.: Robotically Assisted Percutaneous Local Therapy and Biopsy. ICAR 2001.

Optimal Trajectories Computation Within Regions of Interest for Hepatic RFA Planning

Caroline Villard[1], Claire Baegert[1], Pascal Schreck[1], Luc Soler[2], and Afshin Gangi[3]

[1] LSIIT, Pôle API, F67400 Illkirch, France
{villard, baegert, schreck}@lsiit.u-strasbg.fr
[2] IRCAD, 1 place de l'Hôpital, F67091 Strasbourg, France
[3] Hôpital Civil, Radiologie B, 1 place de l'Hôpital, F67091 Strasbourg, France

Abstract. Percutaneous radiofrequency ablation has become a frequently used technique for the treatment of liver cancers, but still remains very difficult to plan. In this paper, we propose a robust method to delineate on the skin of a 3D reconstructed patient the zones that are candidate for an insertion, because they allow a safe access to the tumor without meeting any organ, and to compute automatically within these zones an optimal trajectory minimizing the volume of necrosis covering the tumor.

1 Introduction

Radiofrequency ablation (RFA) of liver tumors is a relatively recent technique, that has been increasingly used in the past few years. The percutaneous procedure has proved its effectiveness, relative safety and predictability. It has the advantage to be minimally invasive, that means lighter operations and shorter hospital stays, becoming a good option for unresectable cases or small tumors.

This approach consists in inserting a probe through the skin towards the tumor, and causing coagulative necrosis of the tumor by heating the tissues surrounding the probe's tip above 60°C thanks to an ionic agitation due to the principle of microwave. The success of such an operation closely depends on the choice of an optimal strategy for the insertion of the RF probe through the skin, even though this choice remains very difficult for a physician, who can only rely on 2D slices acquired from CT scan or MRI.

Our long term objective is to elaborate a complete tool for patient-specific treatment planning, surgeons training, and even robotically assisted interventions, including all steps from the 3D reconstruction of the acquired images to simulation and assistance, including image analysis, 3D modeling, 3D interaction, haptics and virtual reality, augmented reality, automatic planification, and robotics. In this paper, we will only focus on one part of this work, currently in progress, concerning the automatic planification of an appropriate strategy for needle placement, and detail our first encouraging results.

After a brief state of the art in Section 2, we will expose our new method in Sections 3 and 4. Then we will discuss the results, report the few remaining problems of our approach, and give perspectives for our future works.

J. Duncan and G. Gerig (Eds.): MICCAI 2005, LNCS 3750, pp. 49–56, 2005.

2 Previous Works

2.1 General

First of all, our work is based on an abundant literature about RFA, explaining widely the profile of candidate patients, the principle and the effects of the process, existing devices and usual treatment strategies, the nature of possible complications, the reasons why complications or failure may occur and the occurring rates, and the procedures that improve the treatment, for hepatic or other tumors, and for percutaneous, open, or laparoscopic procedures [1,2,3,4].

In addition to a need from radiologists, our project also takes its motivations from works proving how an important part of the success of an intervention was played by the training and experience of the surgeons [5]. That is why a realistic training simulator can be very useful in the formation of novices. Moreover, it has been underlined that an volumic view improved the success rates [6], so we think that helping the radiologists in having a better visualization, and even providing him an assistance for the treatment planning can be of valuable help.

In computer science, many works have been focused on simulations of cancer treatments, a few ones concerning RFA, or cryotherapy that has a lot of common points. Most of the developments use finite elements methods, reproducing the thermic exchanges within the teated area [7,8]. However, this approach has the drawback to be quite slow, whereas one of our objectives is to have a low-cost and transportable solution, working on a common laptop. Treatment planning has been less studied for RFA, but there are close works in neurosurgery, where we find comparable objectives: destroying tumors and damaging as less surrouding tissue as possible, even if the constraints are not the same [9].

2.2 Basis of Our Works

The tool we are developping is based on works, presented a few years ago, about automatic 3D reconstruction of slices from enhanced spiral CT scans with 2 mm cuts acquired from patients with liver metastases [10]. The software detects, delineates and reconstructs automatically their liver, pathologies, and surrounding organs. It produces realistic and manipulable 3D scenes representing the anatomy of the patients.

Then, we added the possibility to perform simulations of RFA [11], based upon the characteristics of the Berchtold HITT needle. A user of the simulator can add virtual probes into the 3D scene of the patient's organs, and then freely manipulate them. During a simulation, the lesion zone is estimated and simulated as a simple mesh representing the 60 °C isosurface, most of the time approximated as being a simple spheroid, that is deformed when necessary to simulate the heat-sink effect caused by large vessels.

First attempts were also leaded to perform an automatic treatment planning for RFA [12]. We proposed an algorithm able to find automatically a secure trajectory for the needle, covering the whole tumor plus an additional security margin while minimizing the damages on healthy cells and avoiding other organs. The first part of this algorithm finds the minimal spheroid containing the tumor given a fixed trajectory for the needle, and computes its volume. The second part is based on a classic minimization method, the Downhill Simplex algorithm [13], and tries to find the smallest minimal spheroid by varying a set of parameters corresponding to the needle's position and orientation. To avoid organs, we simply return a penalty volume for candidate trajectories that would meet an organ, in order to eliminate this candidate. With this method, we managed to obtain satisfying results in terms of volume, with acceptable computation times.

However, a few problems still remained. The major of them was that we observed that this approach was quite dependent on the initial position from which the process was launched. Two phenomena were involved. The first one was due to the Downhill Simplex method we use, that is known to be sensitive to local minima. The second one was due to the way we avoid organs: it leads the minimization process to be bounded into a zone delimited by the surrounding presence of organs. Then, if the initial position was located within such an area, the minimization process was not able to cross the virtual boundary, and was limited to the minimum of the considered area. Due to these problems, the planning could not be really considered as being fully automatic, as it depended on the initial data determined by the user. As we wanted it to be fully automatic, we tried to find ways to solve these problems. That is the main purpose of this paper, and we describe in next section the solutions we propose.

3 Determination of the Candidate Zones for Needle Insertion

The algorithm we propose acts in 3 phases. The first one is the delimitation of the zones of the skin where a needle can be inserted and reach the target without meeting an organ. Let us describe this phase more in detail.

3.1 Simplified Algorithm

If we consider the tumor as a visualization point, we have to solve a visibility problem. All the points that are visible from the tumor point of view without being hidden by any organ are candidates. Of course, the tumor cannot be considered as a single point of view, because it has a volume, but we'll explain later how we can extend the proposed algorithm. For simplicity and computing efficiency, we do not consider all the points of the surface of the skin, but only the triangles of the mesh. One triangle is considered as visible if every point in this triangle is visible, hidden otherwise. That means that if one triangle belongs to the accessibility zone, any needle insertion in this triangle that reaches the tumor (tumor considered as a point) will not collide any organ. Then we only have to determine the visibility of each skin's triangle from the tumor. To do this, we place a camera at the point of view, and compute 6 views of the scene, each one corresponding to one face of an imaginary projection cube around the tumor. If one triangle is hidden by an organ (except liver), there will be at least one view in which it will be detected. Triangles not detected as hidden are visible.

3.2 Algorithm Taking into Account Tumor's Volume

Let's now consider the whole tumor volume. We will say that a triangle is visible from the tumor if it is visible from at least $p\%$ of its voxels. In practice, we will only consider triangles that have a 100% visibility, in order to ensure that the whole tumor is reachable from the zone without any obstructing organ. To compute the 100% visible triangles, we could launch the previous algorithm from each tumor's voxel, considering it as the projection cube. In order to optimize the algorithm, we only examine external voxels of the tumor. Among them, we only compute the views corresponding to faces adjacent to other external voxels. On Fig.1 the considered faces in the tumor are drawn in thick. For each view, if a triangle is hidden we eliminate it from the list of candidates, that will be called the 100% zone. An example of the 100% zone is shown on left of Fig.2.

The time taken to determine the 100% zone mainly depends on the number of tumor's external voxels, as seen in Table 1, but it is not the only influencing factor, as can be seen comparing cases 2 and 3, and cases 4 and 5, where the number of tumor's external voxels are quite the same but times are different. The complexity of the scene and the skin's mesh have a reduced but not insignificant influence on the execution time. We can see for instance in cases 1 and 2 that,

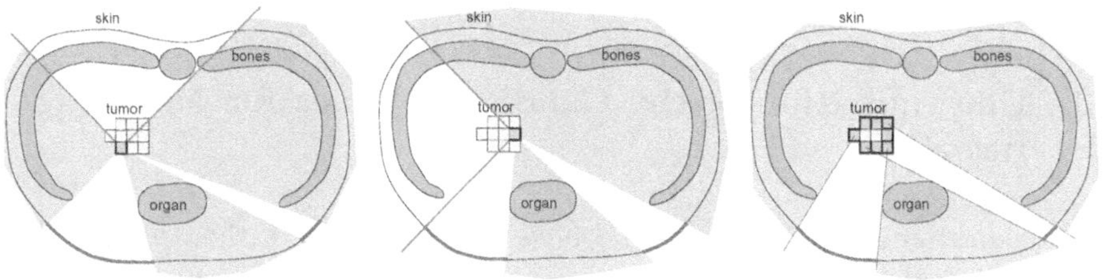

Fig. 1. Computation of the candidate zones on the skin

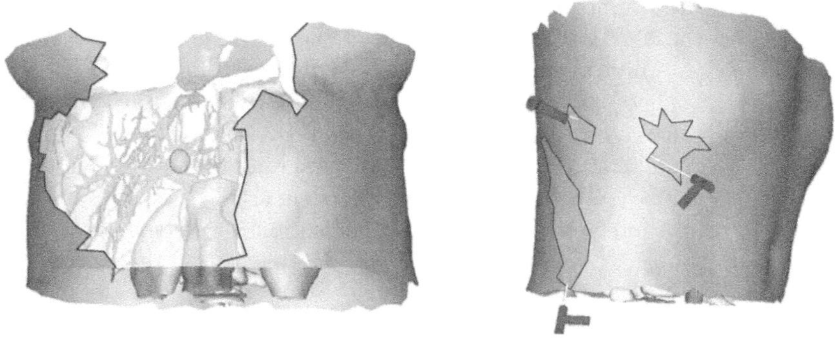

Fig. 2. Left: example of a computed 100% zone (in transparent with a thick border, 1 c.c.); Right: example of computed optimal trajectories for each of the 3 c.c. of the 100% zone (here in opaque with a thick border)

Table 1. Execution times for the computation of candidate zones in 5 cases. The number and surfaces of the obtained zones can be found on Table 2.

case #	nb. of tumor's external voxels	nb. of skin's triangles	nb. of other organs triangles	execution time (s)
1	220	2106	207257	43
2	401	2055	150187	63
3	417	2062	185509	74
4	1198	2074	141285	186
5	1120	1953	171401	175

the execution time is barely the same, showing that a large number of triangles compensates for a small number of voxels. In cases 4 and 5, the number of skin's triangles seems to make the difference and to lengthen the process. Times are computed with a Pentium 4 with 1,5 GHz and 768 Mo RAM and a Radeon 8500.

4 Candidate Optimal Trajectory for Each Zone

After the computation of each connected component, the goal is to launch the minimization algorithm in each component in order to compare the respective minima and choose the best one. In previous works, we used to choose randomly an initial position of the needle, and launch the minimization process. When a candidate trajectory collided an organ, the volume of the lesion was artificially increased. Here, for the second phase, we will use a quite similar approach.

On a first idea, we tried to launch the minimization from a randomly chosen triangle of the connected component. The results were satisfying for small, convex zones. But in larger zones, the algorithm often fell into local minima. We decided to add an initialization phase, to bring the initial position closer to the minimum. We make a quick estimation of the burnt volume for the barycentre of each candidate triangle, with the tip of the needle placed in the centre of the tumor's bounding box (not axis-aligned). Then we compare the obtained volumes and initialize the needle in the position of the smallest one. If the initial position corresponds to the good valley, the needle will reach the good minimum.

On Table 2 we can see the difference between the obtained minima, with or without initialization phase. In this table, we only mentioned connected components containing more than one triangle, because we consider zones with only one triangle as being too risky (too closely surrounded by organs). We can see on Fig.2 the result of this process for the three 100% zones obtained in case #4.

We observe that the initialization phase is more or less efficient according to the size of the region. The bigger the region is, the more the minimization with initialization can improve the result: we notice that we obtain an average gain of -0.213 mL for zones larger than 10 cm^2, whereas we obtain no gain (or infinitesimal) for smaller zones. This is probably because in large regions there are more local minima in which the process could fall, and starting the process in the appropriate valley prevents more often from a wrong convergence. When the zone is small, the method provides approximately the same result in volume.

Table 2. Results of the minimization for each candidate zone, for 5 patient cases, with and without initialization. Last column: objective to reach.

case #	connected component #	size of the component (cm^2)	without init. min. vol. (mL)	without init. time (s)	with init. min. vol. (mL)	with init. time (s)	theor. min. vol (mL)
1	1	234,4	3,588	12	3,067	13	2,730
2	1	1,1	7,227	18	7,222	16	
	2	1,6	7,180	12	7,180	12	
	3	2,2	6,888	13	6,859	13	6,830
	4	2,3	7,532	8	7,534	8	
	5	12,0	7,698	12	7,596	12	
	6	92,0	7,070	15	7,073	13	
3	1	3,2	5,823	11	5,837	7	
	2	5,0	5,846	10	5,827	8	
	3	5,2	5,740	12	5,739	12	
	4	150,6	3,858	26	3,831	14	3,059
4	1	4,3	13,707	16	13,751	11	
	2	10,8	12,270	15	11,960	13	
	3	28,1	10,610	16	10,618	14	8,876
5	1	12,0	13,698	20	13,678	13	
	2	79,0	11,841	19	11,805	13	
	3	162,9	10,216	18	9,301	20	9,304

Concerning execution time, we noticed that the minimization process itself converges faster when the needle is previously positioned. If we add initialization and minimization times the total time sometimes increases, but in most cases does not exceed the time witout initialization. We even have an average gain of -2.41s. In conclusion, we think that the initialisation is always useful: for large regions it allows to provide a sizeable better volume, in other cases it speeds up the process.

On this table, we also mentioned in the last column the theoretical minimal covering volume that could be reached if the surrounding organs were not taken into account, that can be seen as a goal: for each case, this volume is written in front of the best candidate trajectory. This value is computed thanks to an exhaustive sampling method. Most of the time, this theoretical minimal volume doesn't correspond to a possible needle insertion point, but we can see that we manage to find a very close result within authorized areas, with an average of only +0.57 mL, *i.e.* +11.52% of the theoretical values, that is encouraging.

5 Discussion

Until now, we always considered the optimal trajectory as being the one providing a minimal volume of burnt tissue, that was the aim of this work. However, we have to notice that a radiologist would not always make the same choice.

First of all, we did not take into account some additional constraints, such as the length of the needle, or the level of risk. Sometimes, the trajectory is good, but impossible to reproduce in practice. To solve these problems, we plan to eliminate triangles being too far from the tumor, and to add an extra margin around organs, except bones that can usually be safely approached by the needle, in order to eliminate unfeasible insertion points from candidates. An other solution would be to compute a "risk level" for every candidate triangle, and to give triangles with a high risk level a penalty when performing the minimization. The strength of the penalty could be chosen by the radiologist, from 0 to 100% penalty, the latter leading to a total elimination of the risky insertion points.

Another criterion that could be taken into account is the distance between the chosen entry point and the tumor, as in some cases a radiologist may prefer a more direct insertion. But in some other cases, if the tumor is located close to the capsule, the radiologist would choose a trajectory including a portion of healthy liver tissue instead of a direct access to avoid a possible hemorrhage. Many other criteria like these ones can be cited, and the planning process would benefit if they were included in the process. That is why we plan to work on the integration of these numerous and not always quantifiable constraints.

We also plan to find ways to include those various informations into the interface, in order to help the radiologist if he wants to choose himself among the possible trajectories or even among the proposed insertion zones. The major problem is the amount of necessary information that would be added to the visualization area. To avoid an overload of the visual information, that is very rich yet with the view of the volumic data, we are currently studying the approach of using haptic interfaces for the materialization of extra information.

Finally, we would also like to try to speed up the process. At first, we considered the idea to eliminate very small regions, for instance $< 5cm^2$, that would sometimes reduce significantly the computation time. But we decided to keep them because for some cases a very optimal solution could be found in one of those very small regions, and according to radiologists the small size of a region is not really a problem to reproduce. Moreover, as we plan to couple our method with a robot [14], trajectories in these zones can easily be reproduced.

6 Conclusion

In this paper, we presented an algorithm that automatically computes an optimal needle trajectory, for the planning of a RFA intervention. This algorithm first selects the possible entry zones on the skin, *i.e.* the zones from which we can reach the tumor without meeting any organ, then computes for each zone the trajectory minimizing the volume of the necrosis zone covering the whole target.

In the future, we plan to improve the algorithm by integrating other criteria in the planning process, as the minimization of the volume is sometimes not the only factor that is taken into account by radiologists to consider a trajectory as optimal, always keeping in mind the reproducibility of the proposed trajectory.

References

1. McGahan, J., Dodd III, G.: Radiofrequency ablation of the liver: Current status. American Journal of Roentgenology **176** (2001) 3–16
2. Cady, B., Jenkins, R., Steele Jr, G., et al.: Surgical margin in hepatic resection for colorectal metastasis: a critical and improvable determinant of outcome. Annals of Surgery **227** (1998) 566–571
3. De Baere, T., Denys, A., Wood, B., Lassau, N., Kardache, M., Vilgrain, V., Menu, Y., Roche, A.: Radiofrequency liver ablation: Experimental comparative study of water-cooled versus expandable systems. American Journal of Roentgenology **176** (2001) 187–192
4. Rossi, S., Garbagnati, F., Lencinoni, R.: Unresectable hepatocellular carcinoma: percutaneous radiofrequency thermal ablation after occlusion of tumor blood supply. Radiology **217** (2000) 119–126
5. Poon, R., Ng, K., Lam, C., Ai, V., Yuen, J., Fan, S., Wong, J.: Learning curve for radiofrequency ablation of liver tumors: Prospective analysis of initial 100 patients in a tertiary institution. Annals of Surgery **239** (2004) 441–449
6. Antoch, G., Kuehl, H., Vogt, F., Debatin, J., Stattaus, J.: Value of ct volume imaging for optimal placement of radiofrequency ablation probes in liver lesions. Journal of Vascular and Interventional Radiology **13** (2002) 1155–1161
7. Butz, T., Warfield, S., Tuncali, K., Silverman, S., van Sonnenberg, E., Jolesz, F., Kikinis, R.: Pre- and intra-operative planning and simulation of percutaneous tumor ablation. In: Medical Image Computing and Computer-Assisted Intervention, LNCS 1935. (2000) 317–326
8. Tungjitkusolmun, S., Staelin, S., Haemmerich, D., Cao, H., Tsai, J.Z., Cao, H., Webster, J., Lee, F., Mahvi, D., Vorperian, V.: Three-dimensional finite element analyses for radio-frequency hepatic tumor ablation. IEEE Trans. Biomed. Eng. **49** (2002) 3–9
9. Tombropoulos, R., Adler, J., Latombe, J.: Carabeamer: A treatment planner for a robotic radiosurgical system with general kinematics. Medical Image Analysis **3** (1999) 237–264
10. Soler, L., Delingette, H., Malandain, G., Montagnat, J., Ayache, N., Koehl, C., Dourthe, O., Malassagne, B., Smith, M., Mutter, D., Marescaux, J.: Fully automatic anatomical, pathological, and functional segmentation from ct scans for hepatic surgery. Computer Aided Surgery **6** (2001) 131–142
11. Villard, C., Soler, L., Papier, N., Agnus, V., Thery, S., Gangi, A., Mutter, D., Marescaux, J.: Virtual radiofrequency ablation of liver tumors. In: International Symposium on Surgery Simulation and Soft Tissue Modeling (IS4TM), LNCS 2673. (2003) 366–374
12. Villard, C., Soler, L., Gangi, A., Mutter, D., Marescaux, J.: Towards realistic radiofrequency ablation of hepatic tumors 3d simulation and planning. In: Medical Imaging 2004 : Visualization, Image-Guided Procedures, and Display, SPIE 5367. (2004) 586–595
13. Press, W., Teukolsky, S., Vetterling, W., Flannery, B.: Numerical Recipes in C++: The Art of Scientific Computing (Second Edition). (2002)
14. Maurin, B., Gangloff, J., Bayle, B., de Mathelin, M., Piccin, O., Zanne, P., C., D., Soler, L., Gangi, A.: A parallel robotic system with force sensors for percutaneous procedures under ct-guidance. In: Medical Image Computing and Computer-Assisted Intervention MICCAI 2004, LNCS 3217. (2004) 176–183

Effects of Latency on Telesurgery: An Experimental Study

Reiza Rayman[1], Serguei Primak[2], Rajni Patel[2], Merhdad Moallem[2], Roya Morady[1], Mahdi Tavakoli[2], Vanja Subotic[2], Natalie Galbraith[2], Aimee van Wynsberghe[1], and Kris Croome[1]

[1] Canadian Surgical Technologies & Advanced Robotics (CSTAR), 339 Windermere Road, London, Ontario, N6A 5A5, Canada
[2] CSTAR & Department of Electrical and Computer Engineering, The University of Western Ontario, London, Ontario, N6A 5B9, Canada

Abstract. The paper is concerned with determining the feasibility of performing telesurgery over long communication links. It describes an experimental testbed for telesurgery that is currently available in our laboratory. The tesbed is capable of supporting both wired and satellite connections as well as simulated network environments. The feasibility of performing telesurgery over a satellite link with approximately 600 ms delay is shown through a number of dry and wet lab experiments. Quantative results of these experiments are also discussed.

1 Introduction

The use of minimally invasive surgical systems for performing remote surgery (telesurgery) has the potential to significantly improve healthcare in remote communities and provide cost effective services. While robot-assisted on-site minimally invasive surgery (MIS) has became a routine procedure, there has been very little experience gained so far in remote teleoperations of robotic MIS systems [1]-[5]. Our aboratory is currently developing and testing new infrastracture to investigate the feasibility of telesurgery over wired and satellite communication links. This work concentrates on the following issues: 1) development of an appropriate testbed; 2) dry lab experiments to evaluate the effects of communication latency; 3) determination of tasks that are appropriate for telesurgery; 4) wet lab experiments in the presence of different amounts of latency; 5) determination of the type and amount of training required for telesurgery.

It is well known that delays and disturbances in communication links can severely degrade the quality of teleoperation. However even approximate limits on such operations are currently not known. The experiments conducted in our Telesurgery Research Laboratory at CSTAR are aimed at addressing some of the issues related to telesurgery over large distances. In this paper, we present results that provide a quantitative evaluation of the effect of latency on the performance of telesurgery using both dry lab and wet lab (animal) experiments.

J. Duncan and G. Gerig (Eds.): MICCAI 2005, LNCS 3750, pp. 57–64, 2005.

2 Experimental Setup

The experimental setup consists of the following two major units: a teleoperation capable ZEUS^{TM} robotic MIS system [1] with both the surgeon's console and the surgical robot located in our laboratory and a communication network with its monitoring equipment.

A redundant dedicated communication link consisting of three different modalities has been established with the help of Bell Canada and Telesat Canada. These include a wired link via Halifax with a roundtrip delay of 64 ms, a satellite link with a roundtrip delay of 580 ms, and a software simulated delay link through a local switch. The network design provides considerable flexibility for expansion and redeployment, sufficient redundancy and graceful degradation in case of communication failures. The setup has been found to be suitable for both dry and wet lab experiments as described below.

2.1 Telesurgery Unit

The ZEUS^{TM} robotic MIS system has been designed using a master-slave philosophy as described in [1] with the master (surgeon's console) and the slave (surgical robot located in the operating room) comprising completely separate units that are both IP capable. The surgical robot at the patient side contains three robotic arms, two of which are used to manipulate laparoscopic surgical intruments while the third holds an endoscopic camera. The latter provides a 2D view of the surgical area inside the patient. All three arms are controlled from the surgeon's console. The arms are controlled remotely through a sequence of packet-oriented digital commands from the surgeon's console, and are delivered through a standard 100 base T ethernet network connection. The surgeon's console has two 5 degrees-of-freedom "arms" that are used by the surgeon to manipulate the two robotic arms at the patient side that are connected to laparoscopic surgical tools. The endoscopic camera unit at the patient side is controlled from the surgeon's console. The surgeon also has a view of a video stream provided by a color video camera located at the patient side.

An additional unit described in [1] allows the telesurgery system to operate in UDP/IP mode thus avoiding time-outs due to large delays. The unit is designed to lock the operation of the robot if the packet loss in the communication network becomes unacceptably high.

The video signal from the endoscopic camera in compressed by an encoder to preserve bandwidth. The encoder introduces a 100 ms processing delay. The image is restored into the original video format at the surgeon side by means of a decoder. An additional function of the encoder/decoder is to enable one to vary the effective transmission bandwidth utilized by the system. This is because most of the bandwidth resource is consumed by the videotraffic. Two sets of encoders and coders are used to provide redundancy. Both the surgeon and the patient sides are equipped with IP compatible Polycom ViewStations allowing lower quality video and audio interaction between the two sides. This link is also used to convey instructions from the surgeon to the remote side (such as turn on/off ultrasound scalpel, *etc.*).

2.2 Networking

The general network configuration is shown in Fig. 1. All individual devices are connected to each other using a standard IP interface. This enables the system to be easily deployed, be readjusted or be augmented by new tools. Signals from all devices are collected and multiplexed by aswitch, creating a single data stream directed by a router. The networking hardware is fully redundant on both sides. The system automatically chooses between switches to obtain the most reliable link. The total bandwidth provided by Bell amounts to 10 Mbps which is sufficient for transmitting all of the necessary signals with a high level of priority. Routers on each side can be connected in different ways to emulate different modalities of the deployment. The first possibility it to connect through a dedicated computer equipped with the NetDisturb software [2]. This modality can be used for the purpose of training and testing of the system under a great variety of simulated conditions. The software allows one to isolate particular network parameters to study their influence on the setup performance. The second option includes a wired high quality, low latency (approximately 65 ms round trip)connection which loops from London to Halifax and back. Coupled with the delay in the codecs, this is roughly equivalent to a 200 ms round trip delay. Finally, a Telesat satellite link can also be included in the loop, providing a link with a variable time delay of approximately 600 ms round trip with some jitter and packet losses. Inclusion of such a segment is a substantial contribution since no such experiments have been reported in the literature. A protocol of switching between the wired and satellite loops has been agreed upon between the involved parties and the switching itself has been routinely used during actual experimentation.

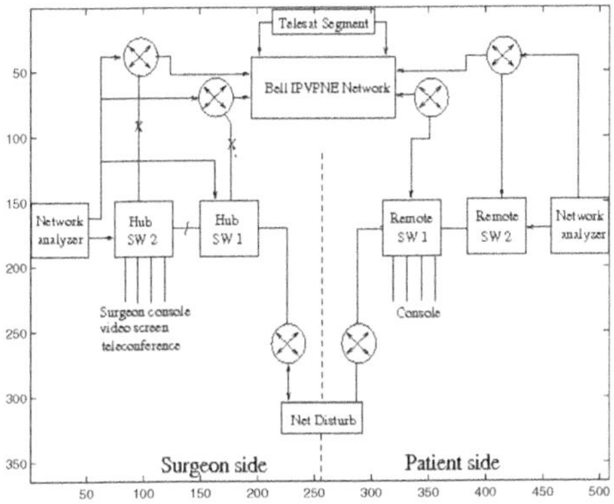

Fig. 1. Network configuration

2.3 Experiments

We have conducted numerous experiments to evaluate the performance of the system. In contrast to previously reported feasibility experiments [1],[3]-[6], we have conducted a number of trials that provide more quantative information about such important parameters as completion time and quality of surgery. In this paper, we focus our attention on the dry lab experiments while briefly reporting the results of the wet lab experiments which are still ongoing and will be reported in detail at another time.

2.4 Dry Lab Experiments

The robotic exercises were designed to simulate typical surgical maneuvers. These involved object grasping and precise placement, object steering, and curved needle manipulation using the laparoscopic tools manipulated by the robot arms. We did not simulate more complex tasks such as knot tying or precise suture placement. Due to the technical limitations of the ZEUS robotic system, such complex tasks are quite difficult to complete even without any latency thus resulting in a very 'noisy' data set. The following exercises were evaluated:

1. Pick up a cone with the left hand. Place in a circle. Return the cone to its original position with the right hand. Pass it back and forth six times. Repeat this procedure four times for one data set.
2. Pick up a 6-0 suturing needle with the left hand. Maneuver the needle to enter at the left dot and exit from right dot. Retrieve the exiting needle with the right hand. Hand over the needle to the left hand and repeat six times. Repeat this procedure four times for one data set.
3. Pick up a ring with the left hand, grasping the ring at the black line. Maneuver the ring with both hands so that the right hand only holds it at the black line. Do not drop or let the ring touch the surface during the maneuver. Pass the ring back and forth four times. Repeat this procedure eight times for one data set.
4. Pick up a rod with the left hand. Pass the rod through three hoops without touching the hoops. Pass it back and forth through the hoops four times. Repeat this procedure three times for one data set;

Four test subjects with no previus experience (students with science backgrounds) were assigned to complete the surgical exercises. These subjects had dayly access to the robotic system and has performed the exercises five days per week over a period of four months. Therefore, they were continuously exposed to the system and had the opportunity to learn and adapt to the system.

The group performed the surgical exercises at latencies from 0 to 1 s, in increments of 100 ms. At each latency, each subject completed four data sets for each exercise. Additionally, the subjects performed the exercises with random delays between 0 to 1 s at the end of the training period. Task completion times and error rate were recorded for all exercises.

The delay in the network was controlled by the NetDisturb software. For each delay, the completion time and a number tally of errors for the maneuver were recorderd and later plotted as a function of delay. It was observed that a relatively small number of repetitions of the same maneuver led to a reduction of task completion times due to learning. It was also found that the effect of delay is not pronounced until the round trip time exceeds 400 ms.

2.5 Wet Lab Experiments

The wet lab experiments were designed to conduct an internal mammary artery (IMA) takedown on a pig using the ZEUS^{TM} Telesurgical System. The procedure was divided into two 45 *min.* segments each using a different C-STAR network asset. The first segment used the Halifax loop (64 *ms* roundtrip delay) and the second used the satellite (537 *ms* round trip delay). Following each segment, the length of the IMA dissected was measured and the surgeon's skills were assessed according to the "Objective Structured Assessment of Technical Skills" sliding scale. During the first segment, 3.5 *cm* of the IMA was dissected, and in the second segment, 4.5 *cm* of the IMA was dissected. The surgeon was able to perform at both latencies with fluid instrument movements, maximum efficiency and no inadvertent damage to the tissue.

3 Experimental Results

A few representative results of the dry lab experiments described above are shown in Fig. 2. It shows the completion time for different experiments as a function of the delay. The experiments were conducted by a group of inexperienced users who were asked to repeatedly conduct the experiments starting from a negligible delay and then with delay increasing by 100 *ms* for each new set of runs. Solid lines in Fig. 2 illustrates the effect that we call long-term learning. This type of learning has to do with improving performance through repeating a task a number of times. The effect of long term learning remains with the participant over the whole period of experiments (just over three months). The gradual decline in completion time upto about 300 *ms* delay can thus be explained by this long-time learning. This figure also indicates that the minimum amount of training needed to properly perform simple tasks can be achieved over relatively short periods of time, equivalent to 3-4 weeks of one hour a day, three times a week training period.

This point can be further verified by comparing the results with incremental and random delay distribution. The latter was performed under random delays that were unknown to the users. The experiments were conducted after all the users had gained significant experience in manipulating the robot thereby reducing the effect of any long-time learning. The curves clearly show that delays of upto 300 *ms* do not have any significant impact on the performance of teleoperation tasks. Further increase in the delay gradually degrades the performance. However, one can conclude that it is possible to perform simple tasks with delays as high as 800 *ms* with a high level of accuracy. Overall it can be concluded that it is possible to perform basic surgical tasks in a simulated environment with delays as large as 800 *ms* with moderate training.

The results shown in Fig. 3 illustrate the effect we refer to as short-term learning. This phenomenon was observed experiments with random delays that are unknown to the operator. Each task was performed a number of times and it can be seen from the figure that the perfomance improved significantly at the second attempt. This indicates that the operator adapted to a particular delay

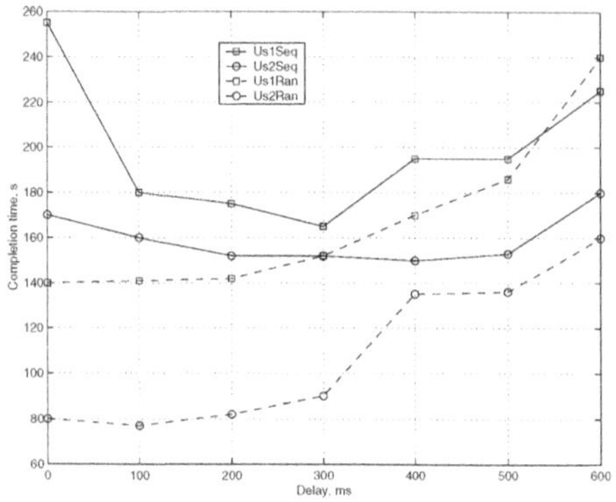

Fig. 2. Dependence of the completion time on the delay. The delay was gradually increased from 0 ms to 600 ms with 100 ms increments solid lines, or chosen at random, dashed lines.

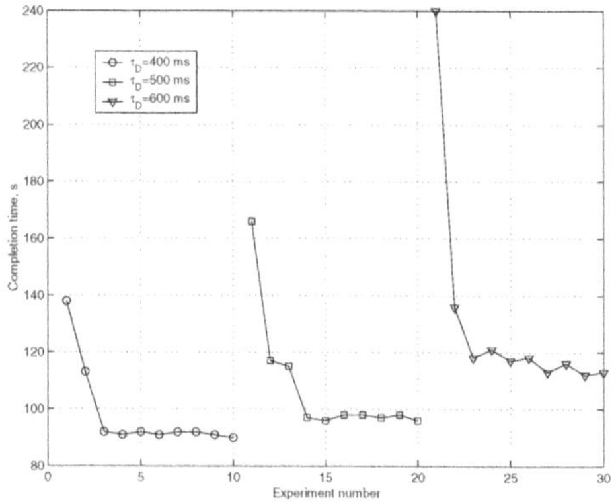

Fig. 3. Short term adaptation to a random delay

and his/her performance is optimized for this delay. However, once the delay changes, the skills acquired are no longer applicable and the operator has to adapt to a new delay. The skills acquired are therefore helpful only for a short period of time.

4 Heuristic Mathematical Model

While one cannot expect that a simple and accurate mathematical description of telesurgery can be developed, it is reasonable to explore the applicability of some basic models, based on Fitts' law [9] or feedback control.

The crossover model [7]-[8] with one pole the open loop transfer function: $G(s) = \omega_c/s \exp(-s\tau_D)$ and the unity feedback is widely accepted as a model for a human operated control system. In essence, this is the simplest possible model which reflects the following fundamental properties of a human operator:

Decision is based on some sort of information feedback; the human operator is able to react only to relatively slow changes in stimuli limited by the so-called crossover frequency ω_c, and there is some delay τ_D between an observation and the reaction of the motor system.

In the absence of the delay $\tau_D = 0$, the model gives a simple estimate of the task completion time for moving an object over a distance A and placing it onto a target of width W: $T_c = 1/\omega_c \ln(2A/W)$ if the task can be considered complete when the position of the target is in the range $A \pm 0.5W$. This result agrees with Fitts' law [9]. In the presence of a delay, one can distinguish three different regimes of operation: for relatively small delays, the exponential approach to the target remains, albeit the time of completion may be reduced ; for intermediate delays the system maintains stability; however, the approach to the target becomes oscillatory which, in turn, increases the completion time. For large delays the system becomes unstable or even chaotic [10].

While the model is simple and describes the main features concerning the human operator, it does not reflect such features as learning due to repeated practicing and adaptation to the delay during a single run of an experiment. We suggest the following generalization. The open-loop network is a series connection of a time-varying gain $K_D(t, \tau_D)$, a time-varying crossover frequency gain $1/\tau_h(t, \tau_D)$, and the delay term. The variable gain represents short-term learning: decreasing the gain is equivalent to slowing the operation. It is assumed that at the initial stage of the movement, the human operator estimates the delay τ_D and adjusts the gain to avoid oscillatory movement. We suggest simple models of the dynamics of time delay estimation and gain adjustment as follows:

$$\tau_D = \tau_{D0} + (\tau_D^* - \tau_{D0}) \exp\left(-\frac{t}{\tau_a}\right), \quad K_D = K_{D0} + (K_D^* - K_{D0}) \exp\left(-\frac{t}{\tau_a}\right) \quad (1)$$

This model reflects the fact that it takes a certain amount of time τ_a to acquire the necessary information about the delay, possible errors in the delay estimation, $\tau_D^* \neq \tau_D$, and that there is some initial guess about the delay in the network.

The variation in the parameter $\tau_h\,(\tau_D, N)$ reflects the long-term learning (i.e. learning over a number N of repetitions of the same maneuver). During one run of the experiment, it remains constant but from run to run it may change due to a training process. It is reasonable to assume that the time needed to complete a task decreases from some level τ_{h0} to a level of the best possible performance τ_h^*. It is suggested that the task completion time decreases according to a power law $N^{-\alpha}$ [7].

5 Concluding Remarks

Preliminary results of the experiments indicate that telesurgery over long communication links is possible. It has been found that the maximum tolerable delay is approximately 600 ms. This allows operations to be performed over wired links that cover most of continental Canada as well as through a one hop satellite link which allows for a much wider coverage. While there was some degradation in task completion times, it was shown experimentally that this was within tolerable limits. It was shown that the completion time complies with the basic Fitts' law. The results also show that significant improvement in performance can be achieved with proper training. However, additional work is required to quantify the effect of learning and to determine the maximum tolerable delay. Furthermore, an investigation of the quality of the communication channel on performance also needs to be performed.

Acknowledgements

The Authors would like to thank the Government of the Province of Ontario, Canada, Natural Sciences and Engineering Research Council of Canada, Canadian Foundation for Innovation, Bell Canada, Telesat Canada, Intuitive Surgical Inc, CA, USA for financial and technical support of this project.

References

1. S. E. Butner and M. Ghodoussi, "Transforming a surgical robot for human telesurgery", *IEEE Trans. Robotics & Automation*, Vol. 19, No. 5, pp. 818-824, Oct. 2003.
2. ZTI-Telecom NetDisturb *http://www.zti-telecom.com/fr/pages/netdisturb.htm*
3. J. C. Rosser, N. Gabriel, B. Herman and M. Murayama, "Telementoring and teleproctoring", *World J. Surg.*, Vol.25, pp. 1438–1448, 2001.
4. R. E. Link, P. G. Schulam and L. R. Kavoussi, "Telesurgery, Remote monitoring and assistance during laparoscopy", *Urol. Clin. North Am* , Vol. 28, pp. 177–188, 2001.
5. B. R. Lee, D. J. Png, L. Liew et al., "Laparoscopic telesurgery between the United States and Singapore," *Ann Acad. Med. Singapore*, Vol. 29, pp. 665–668, 2000.
6. W. K. Cheah, B. Lee, J.E. Lenzi, P. M. Goh, "Telesurgical laparoscopic cholecystectomy between two countries," *Surg. Endosc.*, Vol. 14, pp. 1085, 2000.
7. D. McRuer, D. Graham, E. Krendel, and W. Reisener, "Human Pilot Dynamics in Compensatory Systems - Theory, Models, and Experiments with Controlled Elements and Forcing Function variations," *AFFDL-TR-65-15*, July, 1965.
8. D. McRuer, and D. Graham, "Manual Control of Single Loop Systems: Part I," *J. Franklin Institute*, Vol. 283, pp. 1-29, 1967.
9. P. Fitts, "The information capacity of the human motor system in controlling the amplitude of movement," *J. of Experimental Psychology*, vol. 47, 1954, pp. 381-391.
10. P. Tass, J. Kurths, M.G. Rosenblum, G. Guasti, and H. Hefter, "Non-linear tracking Systems with Delay," *Physical Review E*, Vol. 54, pp. R2224-R2227, 1996.
11. A. McFoulkes, and C. Miall, "Adaptation to Visual Feedback Delays in a Human manual Tracking Task," *Experimental Brain Research*, Vol. 131, pp. 101-110, 2000.

A Novel Phantom-Less Spatial and Temporal Ultrasound Calibration Method

Ali Khamene and Frank Sauer

Imaging and Visualization Dept.,
Siemens Corporate Research,
755 College Road East, Princeton NJ 08540, USA
<first name>.<last name>@scr.siemens.com

Abstract. This paper introduces a novel method for ultrasound calibration for both spatial and temporal parameters. The main advantage of this method is that it does not require a phantom, which is usually expensive to fabricate. Furthermore, the method does not require extensive image processing. For spatial calibration, we solve an optimization problem established by a set of equations that relate the orientations of a line (i.e., calibration pointer) to the intersection points appearing in the ultrasound image. The line orientation is provided through calibration of both ends of the calibration pointer. Temporal calibration is achieved by processing of the captured pointer orientations and the corresponding image positions of intersection along with the timing information. The effectiveness of the unified method for both spatial and temporal calibration is apparent from the quality of the 3D reconstructions of a known object.

1 Introduction and Background

Ultrasound imaging systems are being widely used in many interventional and radiation therapy applications. In these applications, ultrasound probe is usually instrumented with a tracking sensor (either magnetic or optical) or an articulated arm providing the estimates of position and orientation (i.e., pose) of the probe at all times. A calibration process has to establish the transformation from an anatomical location appearing in the ultrasound image to the coordinate system established by the external tracking device. This is referred to as spatial calibration. Furthermore, the exact timing at which the ultrasound image is captured has to be synchronized to the positional information read from the external tracking system. This is referred to as temporal calibration. The cumulative accuracy of tracking system and calibration parameters dictates the fidelity of the overall system to quantify anatomical locations in the desired coordinate system. A tracked ultrasound imaging system can be used to bring anatomical location and surgical instruments or the iso-center of a radiation beam into the same coordinate system [2,4]. Another application is to compound 3D ultrasound volumes for visualization and quantification [8].

J. Duncan and G. Gerig (Eds.): MICCAI 2005, LNCS 3750, pp. 65–72, 2005.

Ultrasound spatial calibration methods have widely been investigated in the literature. There are varieties of geometrical phantoms proposed in the literature mainly to facilitate the calibration procedure. Phantoms with sparse set of wires are proposed in [1,3]. In these procedures, intersection points of the wires are being imaged and are related to the known 3D position of the same point in the phantom. In [9], the proposed phantom has a special shape with known control points, which is then used to relate the local coordinate system of the phantom to that of the tracking system. In [2], a Z-shaped based phantom is used reduce the scan time and to facilitate the process of establishing correspondences between features in the ultrasound image and that in the phantom. In [6], a more sophisticated phantom is used, which combines strings and fiducials.

The main problem in using a phantom is that first the manufacturing of an accurate phantom is expensive and second no matter how accurate the phantom is, its position (or local coordinate system) has to be determined in the tracking system either by attaching another sensor to the phantom at the some exact position or to use control points on the phantom as beacons for registration. In either case the accuracy of the phantom is bound to the accuracy of the tracking system. In [7], authors propose a single-wall phantom that is very easy to use and does not require establishing any correspondences. The equation of the wall has to be determined in the tracking device coordinate system. Furthermore, a special holder has to be used for scanning procedure. The number of images required for this calibration process is rather high. In [5], authors propose a calibration method that does not require a phantom. A calibrated pointer tip is placed into the ultrasound beam. The traces of the pointer tip in the image and the three-dimensional locations acquired with the tracking system are collected and used to compute calibration parameters. The drawback of this approach is that it is very hard to pinpoint the exact position at which the pointer enters the plane. This is mostly because of the beam width of the ultrasound imaging system. This effect makes the whole process inaccurate in determining the calibration parameters, specifically regarding translation in the direction perpendicular to the ultrasound plane.

Our proposed method is inspired by the method described in [5]. However, we address the shortcomings of the previous method. Furthermore, we add an essential piece for estimating the temporal lead/lag between tracking information and ultrasound frame. In contrast to [5], we use a line pointer instead of a "point pointer". I.e., we formulate the problem, in a way that we only require the direction of a tracked pointer in 3D and not the location of pointer tip. Therefore, as long as the pointer intersects the ultrasound plane, we are acquiring valid information for the calibration process.

2 Ultrasound Calibration

Conventional ultrasound imaging systems provide real-time two dimensional array of pixels (i.e., $I(u, v)$) refreshed at the frequency of f_{us}. Real-time optical, magnetic, or mechanical tracking devices are used to map ultrasound images taken from various positions into a global coordinate system. Let us denote the world coordinate system of the tracking device as $\mathbf{W}$, and the coordinate system of the sensor i as $\mathbf{S}_i$. Tracking device provides homogenous transformation matrices ${}^{W}\mathbf{T}_{S_i}$ relating the sensor coordinate $\mathbf{S}_i$ to the world coordinate system $\mathbf{W}$ with certain refresh frequency of f_{tr}. Spatial calibration parameters can be presented as the combination of a homogenous scaling matrix $\mathbf{T}_s$ and a transformation matrix $\mathbf{T}_c$. In order to map any point in the ultrasound image plane (i.e., $P_u = [u, v, 0, 1]^\top$) to the world coordinate system the following matrix multiplication chain has to be computed:

$$P_w^t = {}^{W}\mathbf{T}_{S_0}^t \mathbf{T}_c \mathbf{T}_s P_u^t, \tag{1}$$

where the scaling factors in horizontal and vertical directions are built into $\mathbf{T}_s = diag(s_x, s_y, 0, 1)$, and it is assumed that the ultrasound probe is instrumented with the tracking sensor number 0. Furthermore, time dependency is denoted by t. Sampling interval is usually dictated by $\delta t = \frac{1}{f_{us}}$. Temporal calibration (synchronization) process is to infer $\mathbf{T}_{S_0}$ at time $n\delta t$ (n is an integer) from the samples available at the time intervals of $\frac{1}{f_{tr}}$. The synchronization is dominated by inherent delays, which exist in both ultrasound image formation and tracking. Therefore, the temporal calibration parameter is a single number τ representing the delay, which is usually much larger than the sampling interval of either ultrasound or tracker. For the case where the sampling frequency is identical (i.e., $f_{us} = f_{tr}$) perfect synchronization can be achieved. However, in the case where the sampling frequencies are not identical, the time discrepancy varies in the range of $\tau \pm min(\frac{1}{f_{us}}, \frac{1}{f_{tr}})$.

2.1 Phantom-Less Calibration

A calibration procedure that does not require a phantom is proposed in [5]. In this approach, a secondary tracked coordinate system (i.e., $\mathbf{S}_1$) is considered. The pointer is in fact a known fixed coordinate P_p within such a coordinate system. By carefully placing the pointer tip into the ultrasound beam and recording both the trace of the point in the image P_u^i and the coordinate transformation of the sensor attached to the pointer, one can establish the following relationship:

$${}^{W}\mathbf{T}_{S_1}^i P_p = {}^{W}\mathbf{T}_{S_0}^i \mathbf{T}_c \mathbf{T}_s P_u^i, \tag{2}$$

Therefore, the spatial calibration procedure can be thought of as an optimization process finding eight parameters (i.e., six for translation and rotation and two for the scaling) lumped into matrices $\mathbf{T}_c$ and $\mathbf{T}_s$, as follows:

$$\{\widetilde{\mathbf{T}_c}, \widetilde{\mathbf{T}_s}\} = \arg \min_{[\mathbf{T}_c, \mathbf{T}_s]} \sum_i \left|\left|[{}^{W}\mathbf{T}_{S_1}^i P_p - {}^{W}\mathbf{T}_{S_0}^i \mathbf{T}_c \mathbf{T}_s P_u^i]_3\right|\right|^2 \tag{3}$$

where operator $[.]_3$ converts homogenous to Euclidian coordinates by dropping the fourth element, and $||.||$ represents Euclidian norm. The main problem with this approach is that it is very hard to make sure that the pointer tip is exactly in the ultrasound plane. The trace of the pointer observed within the ultrasound

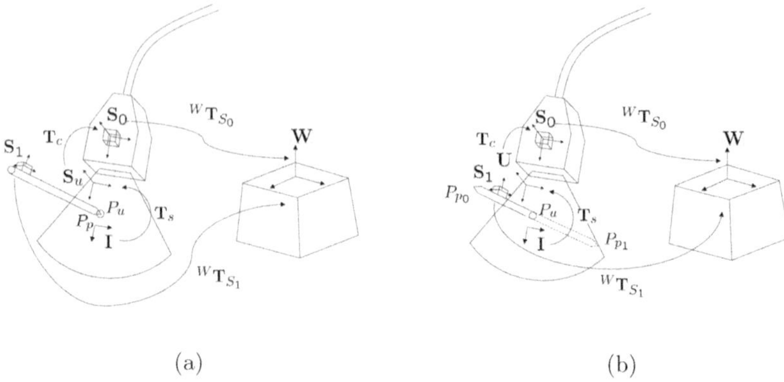

Fig. 1. (a) depicts the calibration method, which requires exact placement of the pointer tip in the ultrasonic plane. (b) shows our new method that only requires intersection anywhere along the pointer.

image is poorly resolved. Furthermore, the width (elevational thickness) of the ultrasound beam is not infinitesimally small, the lower bound of the error in determining the position of the pointer tip is half of the beam width.

2.2 Proposed Phantom-Less Calibration Method

The proposed phantom-less calibration method addresses the problem of the method discussed in section 2.1. Two or more points on the calibration stylus (pointer) are assumed to be known. In this way, the orientation of the calibration pointer is known. We denote the coordinates of these points as P_{p_0} and P_{p_1} in the coordinate system of the tracker sensor $\mathbf{S}_1$ attached to the pointer. If we position the stylus in a way that it intersects the ultrasound beam, we have the following equation:

$$ {}^W\mathbf{T}_{S_1}\left(P_{p_0} + \lambda \frac{P_{p_1} - P_{p_0}}{|P_{p_1} - P_{p_0}|}\right) = {}^W\mathbf{T}_{S_0}\mathbf{T}_c\mathbf{T}_s P_u, \tag{4} $$

where λ is an unknown real number with in $[0\ 1]$. In order to omit the unknown factor λ, equation 4 can e re-written as follows:

$$ [L_{01}]_x \left[{}^W\mathbf{T}_{S_0}\mathbf{T}_c\mathbf{T}_s P_u - {}^W\mathbf{T}_{S_1} P_{p_0}\right]_3 = \mathbf{0}_{3\times 1}, \tag{5} $$

where the operator $[.]_x$ converts a vector to a skew symmetric matrix, and $\mathbf{0}_{3\times 1}$ represents a null point. Furthermore, L_{01} is the normalized vector within the world coordinate system, which is connecting the points P_{p_0} and P_{p_1} with $L_{01} = \frac{{}^W\mathbf{R}_{S_1}[P_{p_1}]_3 - {}^W\mathbf{R}_{S_1}[P_{p_0}]_3}{||[P_{p_1} - P_{p_0}]_3||}$. ${}^W\mathbf{R}_{S_1}$ is the 3×3 rotation matrix imbedded in ${}^W\mathbf{T}_{S_1}$. Finally if the measurements are done for various points i, a similar relationship as in equation (3) can be established to solve for calibration parameters:

$$\{\widetilde{\mathbf{T}_c}, \widetilde{\mathbf{T}_s}\} = \arg \min_{[\mathbf{T}_c, \mathbf{T}_s]} \sum_i \left|\left|[L^i_{01}]_x \left[{}^W\mathbf{T}^i_{S_0}\mathbf{T}_c\mathbf{T}_s P^i_u - {}^W\mathbf{T}_{S_1} P_{p_0}\right]_3\right|\right|^2 \quad (6)$$

The difference between equations (3) and (6) is the matrix $[L^i_{01}]_x$, which specifies the direction of the pointer and relaxes the constraint of exact intersection of the pointer tip with the ultrasound plane.

2.3 Calibration Workflow

The calibration can be divided into three processes. First is the pointer calibration, during which the coordinates of two points along the stylus have to be determined accurately within the coordinate system of the sensor attached to the stylus. In the second step, the spatial calibration acquisition is done. The pointer is placed into multiple positions within the ultrasonic beam, preferably using a grid guide that is well spread over the ultrasound image plane. The 6DOF sensor readings along with the 2D coordinates of the intersection points on the image is recorded and used for recovering the spatial calibration parameters. The third process is for temporal calibration. During this step, we continuously move the pointer while keeping it intersecting the ultrasound plane. We record 2D coordinates of the pointer trace within the ultrasound image, 6DOF coordinates of the pointer sensor,and the corresponding time stamps. These recordings are then used to recover the (semi) constant delay between the magnetic pose and the ultrasound image acquisition.

Pointer Calibration. Pointer tip calibration can be performed by fixing the tip of the pointer and rotating the pointer about the fixed point. For two distinctive poses of the pointer (e.g., ${}^W\mathbf{T}^0_{S_1}$ and ${}^W\mathbf{T}^1_{S_1}$), we have ${}^W\mathbf{T}^0_{S_1} P_p = {}^W\mathbf{T}^1_{S_1} P_p$. Therefore, the pointer tip is simply:

$$[P_p]_3 = ({}^W\mathbf{R}^0_{S_1} - {}^W\mathbf{R}^1_{S_1})^{-1}({}^W\mathbf{t}^0_{S_1} - {}^W\mathbf{t}^1_{S_1}). \quad (7)$$

where $\mathbf{R}$ is the rotation matrix and $\mathbf{t}$ is the translation vector embedded in homogenous transformation matrix $\mathbf{T}$. For more robust and accurate solution and to avoid degeneracy in equation 7 more than two poses (e.g., n) should be used. In this case, we select any combination pair of points, and solve a least squares problem using matrix manipulations, as follows:

$$[P_p]_3 = (\mathbf{RR}^\top\mathbf{RR})^{-1}\mathbf{RR}^\top\mathbf{tt} \quad (8)$$

where $\mathbf{RR} = [\ldots |{}^W\mathbf{R}^i_{S_1} - {}^W\mathbf{R}^j_{S_1} | \ldots]$, and $\mathbf{tt} = [\ldots |{}^W\mathbf{t}^i_{S_1} - {}^W\mathbf{t}^j_{S_1} | \ldots]$, and (i, j) is a combination pair from $[1, n]$.

Spatial Calibration. For the spatial calibration, we first overlay an equidistant grid of points onto the ultrasound image plane. The user's task is to intersect the pointer with the ultrasound plane in a way that the grid points are lined up with the trace of the pointer in the image. In order to avoid degeneracy in the solution of equation (6), it is required the user change the orientation of the pointer from one grid point to another. At each grid point, the coordinates

Table 1. (a) Pointer calibration results, (b) extracted spatial calibration parameters

Point	x	y	z
P_{p_0} (mm)	-58.644	-1.1899	-11.371
P_{p_1} (mm)	34.800	6.6530	-9.1214

(a)

Calib.	x	y	z
Trans. (mm)	27.891	21.967	-62.082
Rot. (deg)	-47.038	-70.526	-44.386
Scale	0.187	0.196	-

(b)

of the grid and the pose of the sensors attached to the pointer and ultrasound probe are saved. It is desirable that the user performs the acquisition in the vicinity of the workspace, where the final measurements are done specially in the case, where magnetic trackers are used. This ensures that magnetic tracker readings are as consistent as possible. Furthermore, it is better to change the pose of the ultrasound probe as the user select different grid point to account for possible variations in magnetic readings and minimize the bias in the results by perturbing the measurement error.

Temporal Calibration. We assume that tracker and ultrasound acquisition frequencies are known. What remains unknown is the inherent delay that exists between the two processes. In order to measure this delay, the user holds the pointer intersecting the ultrasound plane in a perpendicular fashion. The user should periodically move the pointer in horizontal or vertical direction back and forth, while the ultrasound probe is steady. During the motion, both the ultrasound images and the pose of the pointer sensor are recorded together with the time stamps. We then process the recorded images and extract the bright points (in pixels) representing the pointer intersections. The dominant direction of the point in the image (in pixels) and dominant translation parameter of the sensor (in millimeters) are then used to recover the delay. Let us assume the dominant direction of image point movement is in horizontal direction (i.e. $r(t)$, where t is time) and the dominate translation is in x direction (i.e., $x(t)$). The delay can be computed using the following equation:

$$\tau = \arg\ \max \left(\mathbf{F}^{-1} \left\{ \frac{\mathbf{F}\{r(t)\}\mathbf{F}^{*}\{x(t)\}}{|\mathbf{F}\{r(t)\}\mathbf{F}^{*}\{x(t)\}|} \right\} \right) \tag{9}$$

where $\mathbf{F}$ and $\mathbf{F}^{-1}$ represent Fourier and inverse Fourier transforms, respectively, and $(*)$ denotes the complex conjugate operation.

3 Experimental Results

We performed a series of tests in order to verify the performance of the proposed calibration process. Performance measures are considered to be the amount of residual error in the optimization process for the calibration parameters and the quality of three dimensional compounding of the tracked B-plane images. In this experiments , we used images acquired by a SONOLINE Elegra ultrasound (Siemens Medical Solutions, Issaquah, WA) with a 50HDPL40 probe. As tracking device, we used a MicroBird magnetic tracking system (Ascension,

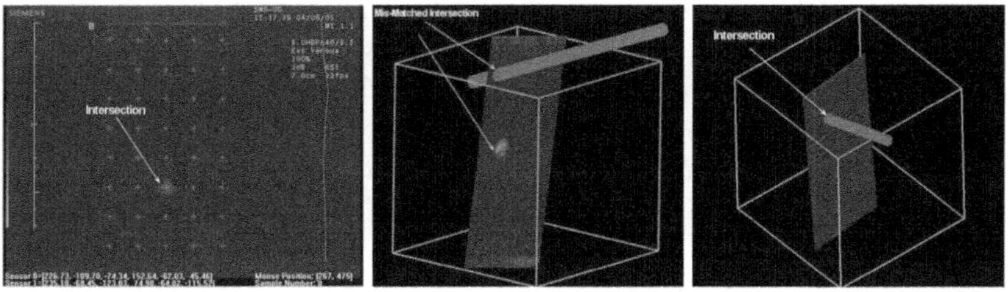

(a) (b) (c)

Fig. 2. (a) depicts the ultrasound image with projected grid pattern, (b) shows the discrepancy between the pointer intersection according to the tracking system and its trace in the image, (c) the discrepancy is minimized after the calibration process.

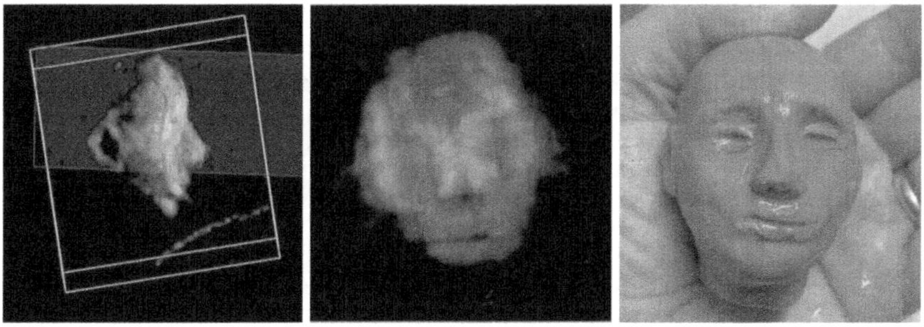

(a) (b) (c)

Fig. 3. (a) depicts the compounded volume with overlaid B-plane, (b) shows the volume from another view and (c) is the photograph of the actual clay model.

Burlington, VT). We prepared a 10cm stainless steel rod as the pointer. We attached a magnetic sensor to the middle of the rod ,sharpened and calibrated both ends using the method described in section 2.3. The standard deviations of the end points in the world coordinate system were 0.9501mm and 0.6068mm. The estimated coordinates of the end points are listed in Table 1(a). We acquired calibration data as explained in section 2.3. By assuming nominal scaling for the ultrasound image, and relaxing the orthonormality constraints of the rotation matrix, we found an estimate of the calibration parameters in a closed-form fashion using various measurements through equation (5). The results were then used as initial values for the optimization in equation (6). We used Levenberg-Marquardt method to solve the non-linear optimization problem. The residual error of the optimization process was 0.8913 mm. Figure 2 (b) shows the intersection of the virtual pointer and the ultrasound plane with arbitrary calibration parameters.There is a clear discrepancy between the virtual and real intersections. Figure 2 (c) shows a good match after computing the correct calibration parameters. The temporal calibration delay was computed to be about 96 milliseconds. The refresh rates of the magnetic tracker and ultrasound device were 60 and 30 Hz, respectively. Since the frequencies were not synchronized up to 16 millisecond variable time discrepancy exists between image and tracked pose. Figures 3 (a) and (b) show reconstruction of the clay head, depicted in Figure 3 (c), using the real-time compounding method described in [4]. The reconstruction is performed by sweeping the B-plane axially from head to neck. Figure 3 (a) shows the reconstruction overlaid by a B-plane in sagittal orientation. Matching outlines in B-plane and reconstruction confirm the fidelity of the calibration parameters.

4 Summary and Conclusion

Calibration is essential for a tracked ultrasound system. In this paper, we propose a robust phantom-less calibration approach. With this method, one can extract both spatial and temporal calibration parameters in a unified way. During spatial calibration, no image processing is needed. Some image processing is required for temporal calibration. Main advantage of the method is minimizing the user dependency during the acquisition of the data for spatial calibration. The new approach relies on the orientation of the tracked pointer instead of the exact tip position. Reconstruction of clay model illustrates the quality of the calibration.

References

1. Barry, C. D., Allot, C. P., John, N. W., Mellor, P. M., Arundel, P. A., Thomson, D. S. and Waterton, J., Three-dimensional freehand ultrasound: image reconstruction and volume analysis. Ultrasound in Med. and Biol. 23(8), 1997, 1209-1224.
2. Bouchet, L. G., Meeks, S. L., Goodchild, G., Bova, F. J., Buatti, J. M., and Friedman W. A., Calibration of three-dimensional ultrasound images for image guided radiation therapy, Physics in Med. and Biol., 46, 2001, 559-577.
3. Detmer, P. R., Bashin, G., Hodges, T., Beach K. W., Filter, E. P., Burns, D. H., Strandness Jr., D. E., 3D Ultrasound image feature localization based on magnetic scanhead tracking: in vitro calibration and validation, Ultrasound in Med. and Biol., 20(9), 1994, 923-936.
4. —
5. Muratore, D. M. , and Galloway, Jr, R. L.,Beam calibration without a phantom for creating a 3D free-hand ultrasound system, Ultrasound in Med. and Biol., 27(11), 2001, 1557-1566.
6. Pagoulatos, N, Haynor, D. R., and Kim, Y.,A Fast calibration method for 3D tracking of ultrasound images using a spatial localizer, Ultrasound in Med. and Biol., 27(9), 2001, 1219-1229.
7. Prager, R.W., Rohling, R. N., Gee, A. N., Berman, L., Rapid calibration for 3-D freehand ultrasound, Ultrasound in Med. and Biol. 24(6),1998, 855-869.
8. Prager, R.W., Gee, A. N., Berman, L., StradX: Real-time acquisition and visulization of freehand three-dimensional ultrasound, Med. Image Anal. 3(2),1999, 129-140.
9. Sato, Y., Nakamoto, M., Tamaki, Y., Sasama, T., Sakita, I., Nakajima, Y., Monden, M., Tamura, S., Image guidance of breast cancer surgery using 3-D ultrasound images and augmented reality visualization, IEEE Trans. on Med. Imag. 17(5), 1998, 681-693.

Electromagnetic Tracker Measurement Error Simulation and Tool Design

Gregory S. Fischer and Russell H. Taylor

Johns Hopkins University, CISST ERC, Baltimore, Maryland, USA
{gfisch, rht}@jhu.edu
http://www.cisst.org

Abstract. Developing electromagnetically (EM) tracked tools can be very time consuming. Tool design traditionally takes many iterations, each of which requires construction of a physical tool and performing lengthy experiments. We propose a simulator that allows tools to be virtually designed and tested before ever being physically built. Both tool rigid body (RB) configurations and reference RB configurations are configured; the reference RB can be located anywhere in the field, and the tool is virtually moved around the reference in user-specified pattern. Sensor measurements of both RBs are artificially distorted according to a previously acquired error field mapping, and the 6-DOF frames of the Tool and Reference are refit to the distorted sensors. It is possible to predict the tool tip registration error for a particular tool and coordinate reference frame (CRF) in a particular scenario before ever even building the tools.

1 Introduction

Optimal design of new electromagnetically (EM) tracked tools requires determining the quantity, relative position, and pose of sensors on tools and the corresponding coordinate reference frames (CRFs). Design is a tedious and time consuming process; to optimize a tool experimentally it takes many design iterations; for each it is necessary to build the tool, collect data, and perform error analysis. We propose a simulator that allows arbitrary tool rigid body (RB) configurations and arbitrary CRF configurations of any number of sensors to be virtually positioned in user-specified patterns and distorted according to a model of a previously acquired measurement distortion error map. This predicts the tool tip registration error for a particular tool with respect to a patient-mounted CRF in a particular scenario before ever building the physical tools.

This work spans two distinct fields related to Image Guided Surgery (IGS). First is tool design and optimization. There appears to be no analytical work directly related to EM tool design, but there has been in depth analysis of optically tracked tool design. The primary work in this field is presented in a series of papers by Fitzpatrick, West, and Maurer, the most recent of which being [1] and [2]. The second key field is EM tracker characterization and calibration, where there has been much work so this summary is far from exhaustive. Tracker characterization involves measurement of the tracking errors with respect to a ground truth reference; recent work describing this can be found in [3] and [4]. Calibration, which takes characterization information to make a model of the measurement distortion has been presented in many papers, including [5] and [6]. In this work, we adapted the formulation of [7], which specifically modeled Aurora tracker's distortion.

J. Duncan and G. Gerig (Eds.): MICCAI 2005, LNCS 3750, pp. 73 – 80, 2005.

2 Measurement Error Modeling

It is important to be able to map the measurement error in a distorted measurement field of an EM tracker; such a mapping is essential for understanding how error is affected by the environment and for modeling the distortion and further error analysis.

2.1 Measurement Error Assessment

Sensor measurement distortion is assessed by collecting a large quantity of measurements from the EM tracker along with corresponding reference measures from a ground truth. In our trials, the NDI Optotrak optical tracking system (OTS) is used as a reference for the NDI Aurora EM tracking system (EMTS); the Optotrak has an accuracy that is about one order of magnitude better than that of the Aurora and is effectively immune to field distortion. The EM sensors are moved throughout the working volume of the Aurora and simultaneously tracked with the EMTS and OTS. By registering the EM sensors to this OTS RB and optically tracking Aurora, it is possible to know the ground truth position and orientation (pose) of each sensor. Reference measurements are then compared to EMTS measurements for the same time step to obtain the measurement error's position and orientation components. Position error is simply the translation required to align the ideal reference position to the distorted EMTS position. Orientation error is defined as a Rodriguez vector that corresponds to the magnitude, θ, and axis of rotation, $\vec{\omega}$, required to align the OTS reference to the EMTS measurement. The errors are mathematically represented as

$$\vec{e}_{pos} = \vec{p}_{measured} - \vec{p}_{ideal} \in \mathbb{R}^3 \quad \text{and} \quad \vec{e}_{ori} = \vec{\omega}\theta \in \mathbb{R}^3 \; . \tag{1}$$

2.2 Polynomial Modeling of Measurement Error

The detailed error mapping is used to generate a model that estimates a sensor's measurement error at a given position and orientation in the workspace of the characterized environment. Bernstein polynomials are used as the basis for these distortion models. In general, n^{th} order Bernstein polynomials are defined for $0 \le i \le n$ by

$$B_i^n(x) = \binom{n}{i} x^i (1-x)^{n-i} \, , \text{ where } \binom{n}{i} = \frac{n!}{i!(n-i)!} \; . \tag{2}$$

Extending Bernstein polynomial models for measurement error in 3D measurement space where the six error values from (1) are interpolated, for each value we have

$$e(x,y,z) = \sum_{i=0}^{n} \sum_{j=0}^{n} \sum_{k=0}^{n} c_{i,j,k}^{b} B_i^n(x) B_j^n(y) B_k^n(z) \in \mathbb{R}^6 \; . \tag{3}$$

The model in (3) is sufficient if the measurement error of the EM system being modeled is independent of the orientation of the sensors. However, this is not a valid assumption for many tracking system; in particular, this is not valid for the Aurora system and the sensor orientation must be accounted for. The following algorithm accounts for both position-related and orientation-related measurement error:

- Choose a set of basis orientations vectors for which the polynomials in (3) will be generated. They should be evenly distributed as the example shown in Fig. 1.

Basis orientation vectors (14):

1	0	0
0	1	0
0	0	1
0.57735	0.57735	0.57735
-0.57735	0.57735	0.57735
0.57735	-0.57735	0.57735
-0.57735	-0.57735	0.57735
-1	0	0
0	-1	0
0	0	-1
-0.57735	-0.57735	-0.57735
0.57735	-0.57735	-0.57735
-0.57735	0.57735	-0.57735
0.57735	0.57735	-0.57735

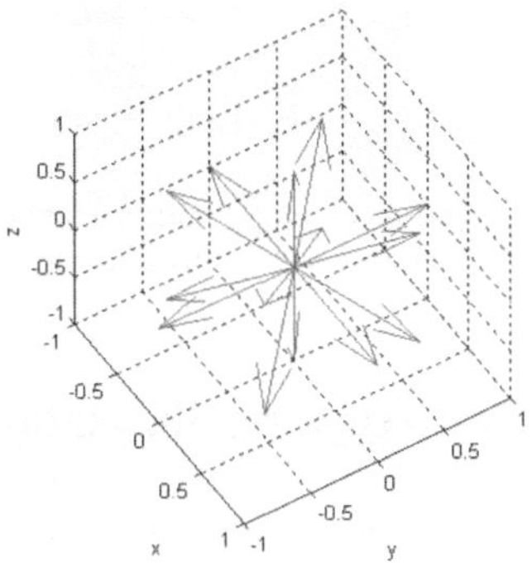

Fig. 1. Basis orientations along which distortion models are created when using 14 basis vectors. Measurements are interpolated between these to determine relative contributions of each.

- For each measurement, determine the closest three base orientation vectors that enclose the z-axis of the measured sensor reading, $\vec{n}_i$, inside of a spherical triangle defined by $\vec{b}_1, \vec{b}_2$, and $\vec{b}_3$ as shown in Fig. 2. Determine the corresponding areas of each of the three spherical triangles; these that are directly proportional to the weighting of a particular base vector's contribution, $w_{i,b}$, to the error.
- Calculate the Bernstein coefficients. For each base orientation, there are six sets of coefficients in (4) to solve for: X, Y, Z, Rx, Ry, Rz.
  - Normalize the measured positions to fit inside a unit cube.
  - Build the six sets of equations in $A\vec{x} \approx \vec{b}$ form to solve in the least squares (LS) sense for each base vector and dimension being interpolated,

$$\begin{bmatrix} w_{1,b}e_x^1 \\ \vdots \\ w_{i,b}e_x^i \end{bmatrix} \approx \beta \begin{bmatrix} w_{1,b}c_{x_{0,0,0}} \\ \vdots \\ w_{i,b}c_{x_{n,n,n}} \end{bmatrix} \quad , \ldots , \quad \begin{bmatrix} w_{1,b}e_{Rz}^1 \\ \vdots \\ w_{i,b}e_{Rz}^i \end{bmatrix} \approx \beta \begin{bmatrix} w_{1,b}c_{Rz_{0,0,0}} \\ \vdots \\ w_{i,b}c_{Rz_{n,n,n}} \end{bmatrix} . \tag{4}$$

Where, $w_{i,b}$ is the weight of the ith data point for the bth basis vector and

$$\beta = \begin{bmatrix} B_0^n(x_1)B_0^n(y_1)B_0^n(z_1) & \cdots & B_n^n(x_1)B_n^n(y_1)B_n^n(z_1) \\ \vdots & & \vdots \\ B_0^n(x_i)B_0^n(y_i)B_0^n(z_i) & \cdots & B_n^n(x_i)B_n^n(y_i)B_n^n(z_i) \end{bmatrix}_{i,(n+1)^3} . \tag{5}$$

  - Solve for $6m*(n+1)^3$ coefficients in the LS sense using singular value decomposition (SVD), where m is the number of basis orientations.

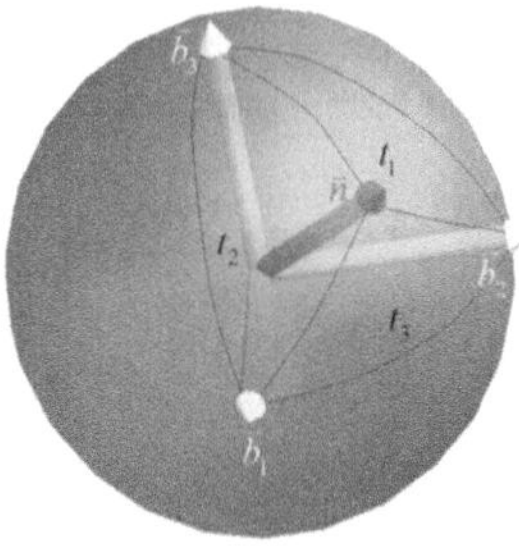

$\vec{n}$	Measured orientation (z-axis of sensor)
$\vec{b}_1, \vec{b}_2, \vec{b}_3$	Enclosing three base orientation vectors
t_1, t_2, t_3	Areas of corresponding spherical triangles (normalized to sum to 1)

Fig. 2. Spherical interpolation techniques determine the relative contributions of the three closest orientations to a sensor's measurement error (and vice versa for model generation)

3 Tool Tracking Simulation

Contrary to the more traditional application of modeling field distortion so that measurements can be compensated in real-time (which is also a feature of our software), we are focused on simplifying tool design by removing the necessity to construct and test each physical tool in each environment of interest. The method is similar to compensation methods, but sensor measurements are artificially distorted rather than corrected.

3.1 Calculating Measurement Distortion

For a given position and orientation error at a given simulated sensor pose we have the distorted sensor position and orientation as

$$\vec{p}_{distorted} = \vec{p}_{actual} + \vec{e}_{pos} \quad \text{and} \tag{6}$$

$$R_{distorted} = R_{error}^{-1} R_{actual}, \quad \text{where} \quad R_{error} = e^{-\hat{\omega}\theta} \in SO(3). \tag{7}$$

Where, $\hat{\omega}\theta = skew(\vec{\omega}\theta) \in so(3)$ and $\vec{e}_{ori} = \vec{\omega}\theta$ is the Rodriguez vector representing the axis and angle of the estimated orientation error.

The above equations require the estimated measurement distortion for a given sensor pose, $\vec{e}_{pos}$ and $\vec{e}_{ori}$. The process for determining the error is very similar to that of generating the distortion model; the error is calculated as

$$\vec{e}(x,y,z) = \sum_{b=1}^{3} w_b \left(\sum_{i=0}^{n} \sum_{j=0}^{n} \sum_{k=0}^{n} \vec{c}_{i,j,k}^{\,b} B_i^n(x) B_j^n(y) B_k^n(z) \right) = \begin{bmatrix} \vec{e}_{pos} \\ \vec{e}_{ori} \end{bmatrix} \in \mathbb{R}^6. \tag{8}$$

Where, the values for b correspond to one of the three closest basis orientations as described earlier and w_b corresponds to the contribution of each basis orientation.

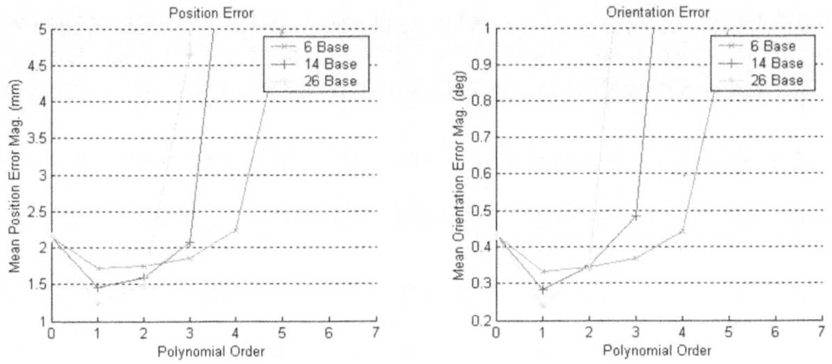

Fig. 3. Residual error for 1025 sensor measurements compensated for with a model generated an using independent data set of 1025 sensors as a function of polynomial order and angular resolution. An order of zero represents the original measurement error with no compensation.

3.2 6-DOF Frame Fitting

The frames $\{F_1, F_2, \cdots, F_n\}$ represent the known position and orientation of n sensors with respect to the given RB frame of reference (i.e. a frame centered at a tool tip and aligned with a pointer shaft). Since sensor frames for the Aurora are only specified in 5 DOF, they can be represented as $F_i = (\vec{n}_i, \vec{p}_i)$.

De-meaned values of sensor positions are necessary to compute the optimal rotational alignment of an RB configuration to the corresponding measurements. These values are the measurements in the RB frame with the position of the center of gravity (CG) in the RB frame subtracted off. The best rigid point cloud to point cloud rotation that aligns the sensor RB configuration to the measurements is found in the LS sense.

Weighted orientations are treated the same way as the demeaned points; the weighting factor, w, keeps the position and orientation contributions balanced. The method is a modified version of that presented in [8], with the modification being the addition of orientations as just mentioned. Two variables are defined in (9); X represents the configuration of the rigid body's sensors with respect to its own frame (denoted by subscript RB), and Y represents the corresponding positions and orientations for the actual sensor measurements (denoted by subscript $Meas$).

$$X = \begin{bmatrix} (\vec{p}_{RB_1} - \bar{p}_{RB})^T \\ \vdots \\ (\vec{p}_{RB_n} - \bar{p}_{RB})^T \\ \hline w \begin{pmatrix} \vec{n}_{RB_1}{}^T \\ \vdots \\ \vec{n}_{RB_n}{}^T \end{pmatrix} \end{bmatrix} \qquad Y = \begin{bmatrix} (\vec{p}_{Meas_1} - \bar{p}_{Meas})^T \\ \vdots \\ (\vec{p}_{Meas_n} - \bar{p}_{Meas})^T \\ \hline w \begin{pmatrix} \vec{n}_{Meas_1}{}^T \\ \vdots \\ \vec{n}_{Meas_n}{}^T \end{pmatrix} \end{bmatrix} \tag{9}$$

Where, n represents the number of sensors, $\bar{p}$ represents the mean position of the measurement set, $\vec{n}_i$ represents the unit vector pointing along the z-axis of the given sensor, w represents the weighting of the orientation measurements relative to the position measurements. This weight was analytically determined and experimentally confirmed to be a function of the relative position and orientation accuracy of the tracker. In the environment present in our lab, a weight of w=100 is satisfactory.

Using the notation in [8], two variables are defined as

$$q_i = X(i,1:3)^T \quad \text{and} \quad q_i' = Y(i,1:3)^T \quad \text{for} \quad i=\{1,\ldots,2n\}\,. \tag{10}$$

Using the variables in (10), the matrix H is calculated as

$$H = \sum_{i=1}^{n} q_i q_i'^T\,. \tag{11}$$

The best rigid rotation in the LS sense that aligns the tool configuration to the measurements is determined by taking the SVD of H and calculating R where,

$$H = U \Lambda V^T \quad \text{and} \quad R = VU^T\,. \tag{12}$$

The optimal translation that aligns the RB with the measurements is then given by

$$\bar{v} = \bar{p}_{Meas} - R * \bar{p}_{RB}\,. \tag{13}$$

3.3 Tool Tracking

The primary contribution of this method is that it allows for simulated tracking of a tool with respect to a reference body and determining the relative tracking error. The frame transformations of interest are detailed in Fig. 4, the '^' and the dotted lines indicate approximate, measured transformations.

The important transformation from Fig. 4 is that of the tool with respect to the patient-fixed reference frame. It is defined as

$$\hat{F}_{CRF}^{Tool} = \left(\hat{F}_{CRF}\right)^{-1} \hat{F}_{Tool}\,. \tag{14}$$

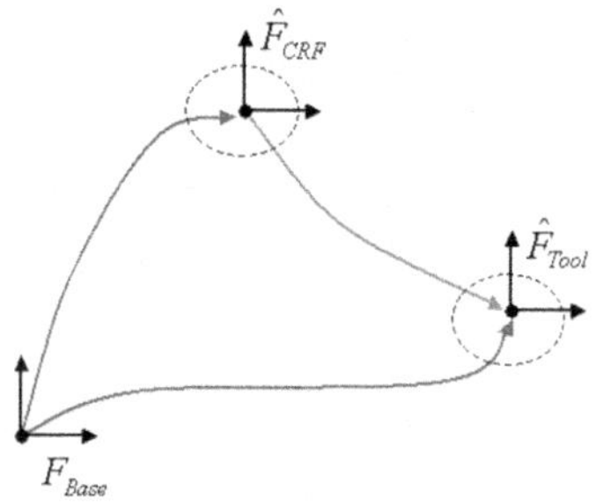

Fig. 4. Tool tracking scenario of where a tool is measured with respect to a coordinate reference frame (CRF). This is critical for IGS applications where a surgical tool is tracked with respect to a patient-fixed reference.

4 Simulation Software

The above algorithms have been incorporated into a single program that allows for data collection, frame fitting, real-time measurement compensation, and tool simulation; Fig. 5 displays the GUI for the simulator. The software takes a tool configuration and reference configuration from user-specified files or native NDI SROM formats. The reference is virtually placed at its commanded pose and the tool is placed with respect to the reference. Sensor locations in the base frame of the EM tracker are determined based on the RB configuration and are distorted based upon the polynomial model of the error for the chosen environment from (8). Tool RBs are refit to the distorted sensor readings as in (12) and (13); tracking error is the relative change in frame transformation between the reference and the tool.

The software can be run in three modes. The first mode, ‘Single Point’ mode, places the two RBs at the specified poses and outputs the relative tracking error. In ‘Range of Motion’ mode, the reference is fixed in a pose selected by the user, and the tool is moved in the specified range of positions and orientations with respect to the reference. This represents a tool being moved about a patient-fixed CRF. Finally, in ‘Input Data’ mode, the program accepts a text file with arbitrarily specified positions and orientations for both the tool and the reference. For all modes, summary statistics are displayed on the screen and results from each trial can be logged to file.

4.1 Tool Design Using Simulator

The simulator proves to be a very helpful tool for design of EM tracked instruments because a tool’s performance can be gauged without ever even building it; this allows for a very large quantity of trials. In general, the tool design procedure is as follows:

1. Generate a CRF design (skip this step if one is already available)
2. Simulate the CRF design in the appropriate environment with respect to the EMTS base. Many different environments can be used for the experiments.
3. Analyze the results and decide if design satisfies requirements. If Yes, continue; if No, return to step 1.
4. Generate a Tool design and simulate with respect to the CRF.
5. Analyze the results and decide if design satisfies requirements. If Yes, continue; if No, return to step 4.
6. Build the reference and tool and compare the results.

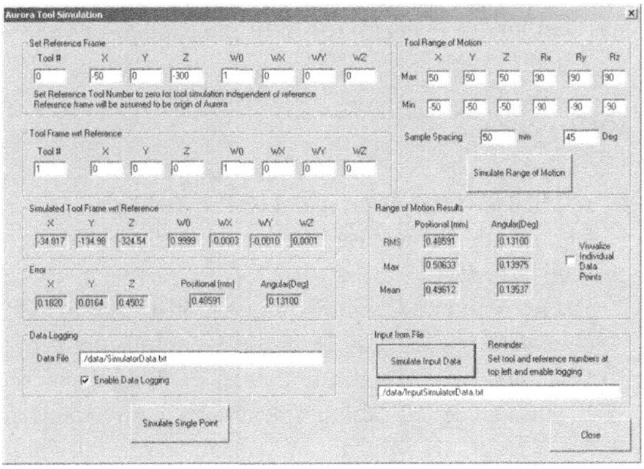

Fig. 5. GUI front end for simulation software. Allows for simulated tracking of pre-defined tools with respect to pre-defined references in a given characterized environment.

5 Discussion

A new tool for design of electromagnetically tracked instruments is presented here. It allows for rapid prototyping and design of EM tracked tools without the necessity to physically build and experiment with many different designs. This allows for the prospect of faster design of higher quality tracked instruments. Initial experiments show that the polynomial model, when used for measurement compensation, produces a very accurate representation of the data. The RMS residual error for a mildly disturbed data set that began with RMS errors of 2.30mm and 0.45° was below 0.20mm and 0.05° for a 6th order model with 14 basis orientations.

To get a better idea of how representative the measurement distortion model really is, it was applied to an independent set of sensor measurements with know reference measurements; the results are shown in Fig. 3. Realistically, it appears that we can expect the model to decrease the residual error by a factor of about two. Fortunately, the minimum residual error occurs at a lower order model (1st or 2nd order), so the quantity of data required for generation of the model can be reduced to make collection reasonable for a given practical environment such as an operating room. The compensation results are quite good, and therefore, we can expect the simulator to produce realistic distortions since it based off of the same model. Thus far, the procedure has been used successfully to help design instruments and references for ENT surgery including a head-mounted CRF, endoscope, pointer, and tissue shaver. Further results and more detail of these methods are available in [9].

Acknowledgements

Funding for this work was provided by Northern Digital Inc., Waterloo, Canada. General infrastructure support was provided by the CISST ERC under agreement EEC-9731478. We would also like to thank Paul MacDonald, Jeff Stanly, Saibal Chakraburtty, John Niemenan, Stefan Kirsch, Gouthami Chintalapani, Xiaofeng Liu, and Katherin Peperzak for their assistance in various aspects of this work.

References

1. J. Michael Fitzpatrick and Jay B. West. The Distribution of Target Registration Error in Rigid-Body Point-Based Registration. IEEE Trans. on Med. Imaging. Vol. 20. No. 9. Sept. 2001: 917-927.
2. Jay B. West and Calvin R. Maurer, Jr. Designing Optically Tracked Instruments for Image-Guided Surgery. IEEE Trans. on Med. Imaging, Vol. 23. No. 5. May 2004: 533-545.
3. J. Hummel, M. Figl, C. Kollmann, H. Bergmann, W. Birkfellner. Evaluation of a Miniature Electromagnetic Position Tracker. Med. Physics. Oct. 2002. Vol. 29, No. 10: 2205-2212.
4. A. Wagner, K. Schicho, W. Birkfellner et. al. Quantitative Analysis of Factors Affecting Intraoperative Precision and Stability of Optoelectronic and Electromagnetic Tracking Systems. Medical Physics. May 2002. Vol. 29, No. 5: 905-912.
5. A.J. Chung, P.J. Edwards, F. Deligianni, and G. Yang. Freehand Cocalibration of Optical and Electromagnetic Trackers for Navigated Bronchoscopy. MIAR 2004. Aug. 2004, Springer LNCS 3150: 320-328.
6. K. Kanada, et. al. A Rapid Method for Magnetic Tracker Calibration Using a Magneto-Optical Hybrid Tracker. MICCAI 2003. Nov. 2003. Springer LNCS 2879: 285-293.
7. Xiaohui Wu and Russell Taylor. A Direction Space Interpolation Technique for Calibration of Electromagnetic Surgical Navigation Systems. MICCAI 2003. Nov. 2003. Springer LNCS 2879: 215-222.
8. K.S. Arun, T.S. Huang, and S.D. Blostein. Least-Squares Fitting of Two 3-D Point Sets. IEEE PAMI. Vol. 9. No. 5. Sept. 1987: 698-700.
9. Gregory S. Fischer. Electromagnetic Tracker Characterization and Optimal Tool Design - With Applications to ENT Surgery. Masters thesis, Johns Hopkins University, Baltimore, MD, USA. May 2005. (http://www.cisst.org/~gfischer)

Compact Forceps Manipulator Using Friction Wheel Mechanism and Gimbals Mechanism for Laparoscopic Surgery

Takashi Suzuki, Youichi Katayama, Etsuko Kobayashi, and Ichiro Sakuma

Institute of Environmental Studies, Graduate School of Frontier Sciences,
The University of Tokyo, 7-3-1, Hongo, Bunkyo-ku, Tokyo 113-8656, Japan
{t-suzuki, katayama, etsuko, sakuma}@miki.pe.u-tokyo.ac.jp
http://bme.pe.u-tokyo.ac.jp/index_e.html

Abstract. This paper reports evaluation of compact forceps manipulator designed for assisting laparoscopic surgery. The manipulator consists of two miniaturized parts; friction wheel mechanism which rotates and translates forceps ($62\times52\times150[mm^3]$, 0.6[kg]), and gimbals mechanism which provides pivoting motion of forceps around incision hole on the abdomen ($135\times165\times300[mm^3]$, 1.1[kg]). The four-DOF motion of forceps around the incision hole on the abdomen in laparoscopic surgery is realized. By integration with robotized forceps or a needle insertion robot, it will work as a compact robotic arm in a master-slave system. It can also work under numerical control based on the computerized surgical planning. This table-mounted miniaturized manipulator contributes to the coexistence of clinical staffs and manipulators in the today's crowded operating room. As the results of mechanical performance evaluation with load of 4 [N], positioning accuracy was less than 1.2 [deg] in pivoting motion, less than 4 [deg] in rotation of forceps, less than 1.2 [mm] in longitudinal translation of forceps. As future works, we will modify mechanism for sterilization and safety improvement, and also integrate this manipulator with robotized forceps to build a surgery assisting robotic system.

1 Introduction

Today, as a means of minimally invasive surgery, laparoscopic surgery is widely performed. Surgeons cut small holes on the abdomen to insert laparoscope and forceps, and conduct all operations inside the abdominal cavity. Small incisions damage patients much less than conventional laparotomy, and patients can get relief from postoperative pain or medication. This patient-friendly technique, however, is rather difficult and cannot be applied to all cases, mainly because the limited degrees of freedom (DOF) of forceps eliminate the dexterity of surgeons (Fig.1(a)). Surgeons must take special training for laparoscopic surgery.

Responding to these issues, surgery-assisting robotic manipulators are developed. Some of them are clinically applied and show their availability [1,2]. Those new systems have provided surgeons with technologically advanced hand skills,

J. Duncan and G. Gerig (Eds.): MICCAI 2005, LNCS 3750, pp. 81–88, 2005.

and enabled higher-quality and more precise operation, that could not be realized in the conventional laparoscopic surgery. Meanwhile, the large size of them caused problems. Some robotic systems require larger room and are difficult to install into conventional crowded operating theater. As the operation space above the patient's abdomen is occupied by the manipulator arms, clinical staffs have troubles to observe the patient and have danger of collision with manipulators. Thus, a new compact surgery-assisting robotic system is required [3].

We have developed a compact forceps manipulator using "friction wheel mechanism" (FWM) [4] and gimbals mechanism (Fig. 1(b)). In the former study, a prototype was manufactured, and feasibility was shown as a forceps manipulator [5]. At the same time, some problems emerged. The rotational speed of ultrasonicmotor varied depending on various factors, that is, the motor we adopted for actuation was unstable, being affected by temperature and load, so that the motion of forceps was also unstable under the open-loop controlling system [6]. In the recent presentation [7], we reported mechanical implementation of miniaturized ultrasonic motors with rotary encoder into the mechanically-modified prototype, and reported evaluation of basic performance using feedback control system. Positioning accuracy of the gimbals mechanism was less than 0.6 [deg], and that of friction wheel mechanism was less than 0.2 [mm] in translation and 1 [deg] in rotation.

In the former studies, the accuracy was measured as a static positioning device without load. Thus, in this study, we measured and evaluated static position accuracy with load of 4 [N]. In section 2, we introduce the configuration and mechanism of our compact forceps manipulator. Experimental apparatus and evaluation results are shown in section 3. We discuss the results of performance evaluation in section 4. Conclusions are presented in section 5.

2 System Configuration

We adopted following two mechanisms to realize four-DOF motion of forceps required in laparoscopic surgery(Fig.1(a)); "Friction wheel mechanism" (FWM) provides the rotation around the forceps shaft and translation along the shaft (number (1) and (2) in Fig.1(b)). Gimbals mechanism realizes the pivoting motion to determine the direction of the forceps (number (3) and (4) in Fig.1(b)). The dimension of the FWM is $62\times52\times150[mm^3]$ and the weight was 0.6[kg]. Those of gimbals mechanism are $135\times165\times300[mm^3]$ and 1.1[kg]. We mount this manipulator near the incision hole using multiple joint arm (ex. Iron intern$^{(R)}$ [8] or Point setter [9]). This is because mechanisms and actuators should be mounted near the operating field so that they require less torque or force [3].

Friction wheel mechanism (FWM) consists of three titled idle rollers and outer case (Fig. 2(a)). Three idle rollers around the forceps shaft travel spirally on the surface of shaft when outer case rotates (Fig. 2(b)) [10]. A couple of FWMs with opposite tilting angle (like right-handed screw and left-handed one) hold the forceps shaft(Fig. 2(c)). When they rotate in the same direction, the shaft held statically by rollers rotates around its longitudinal axis (Fig. 3(a)).

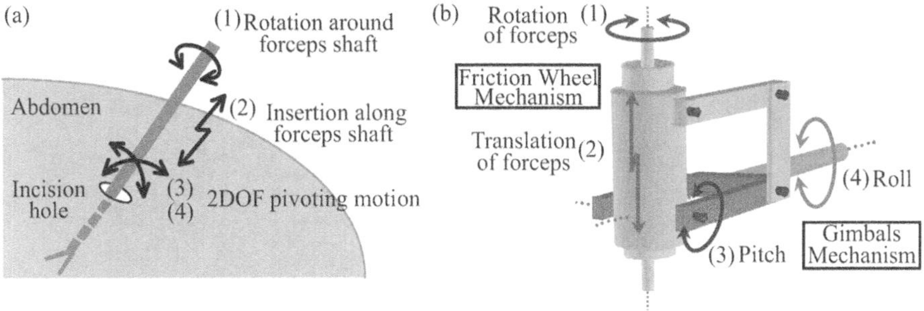

Fig. 1. System configuration, (a) In laparoscopic surgery, forceps have only four degrees of freedom; two for rotation(1) and insertion(2) of forceps, two for pivoting motion(3)(4) around the incision hole. (b) Friction Wheel Mechanism provides two motions of (1) and (2). Gimbals mechanism realizes the rotational motions of (3) and (4).

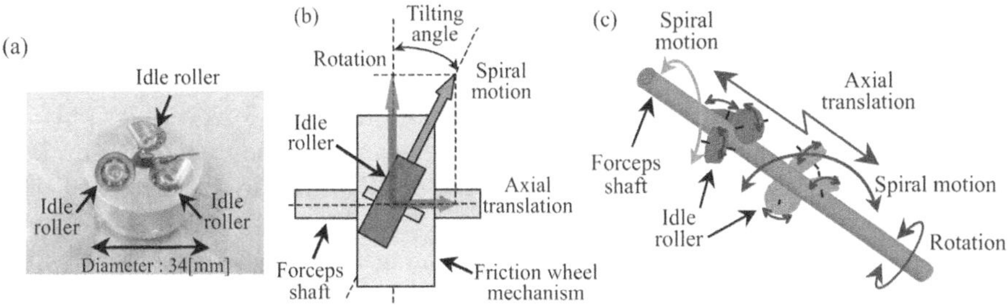

Fig. 2. Friction wheel mechanism, (a) a FWM has three rollers (arrow). (b) Rollers travel spirally on the surface of shaft. That motion can be divided into axial translation along the shaft and rotation around the shaft. (c) We combine two different spiral motions to realize rotation and translation.

Alternatively, when they rotate in the opposite direction, rollers travel on the shaft spirally and rotational motion is cancelled by rotational component of each spiral motion, so that forceps moves along its axis (Fig. 3(b)). The tilting angle was set at 30 [deg] in this study. We used hollow-shaft ultrasonic motors with rotary encoder (custom order, Fukoku, Japan) to drive the outer case of FWM for miniaturization of the system. The resolution of the rotary encoder was 0.2 [deg/pulse].

Gimbals mechanism provides pivoting motion, two rotational motions around the mutually-perpendicular axes. It is to be noted that pivot center of this manipulator is not located at the incision hole, but at the intersectional point of two axes. As for a surgery assisting robot for laparoscopic surgery, "remote center of motion (RCM)" mechanism should be mounted to bind the rotational center of manipulator at the incision hole (ex,[11,12]). However, as we reported in [5], it is not always necessary. This was because abdominal muscle under anesthesia gets flaccid and manipulator does not damage the abdominal wall by driving the

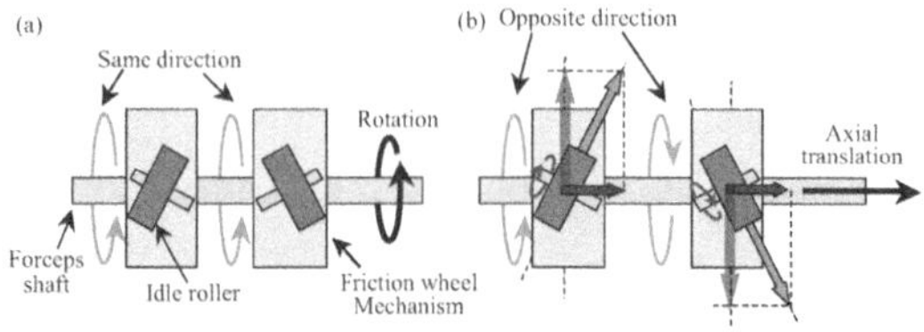

Fig. 3. Driving mechanism of forceps, (a) Rotation, (b) Translation

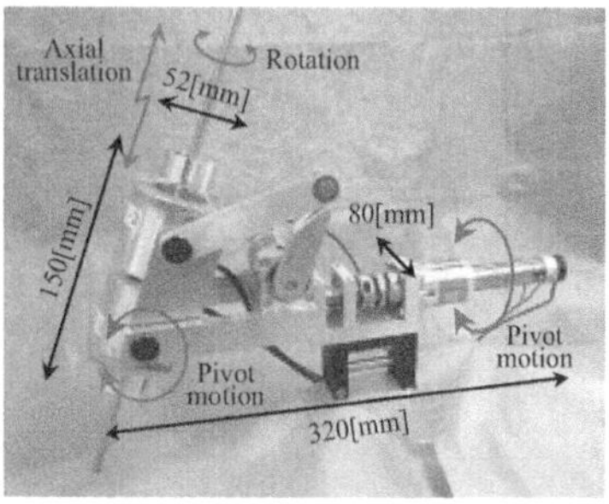

Fig. 4. New prototype

forceps. We used geared DC servomotors (ENC-185801, Chiba Precision Co.,Ltd, Japan) for actuation. The reduction gear ratio was 1/576. The resolution of the rotary encoder was 0.36[deg/pulse]. The prototype is shown in Fig. 4.

3 Evaluation Experiments

We conducted mechanical performance evaluation of our forceps manipulator. In the former studies, we conducted performance evaluation without any load [5,6,7]. Thus, in this study, we applied a load of 4[N], that was equivalent to the one third weight of Japanese male liver.

We measured working range and positioning accuracy of each axis (pitch and roll motions in gimbals mechanism, rotation and longitudinal translation of forceps in FWM) with load. Motion of manipulator was recorded using digital microscope (VH-7000C, KEYENCE, Japan), and working range and positioning

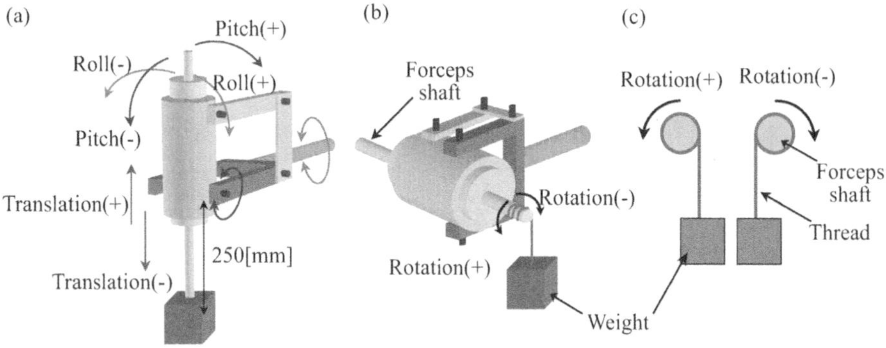

Fig. 5. Experimental setup, (a) Forceps were initially set in the vertical position to measure the motion of gimbals mechanism and the translation. Input direction is defined as shown here. (b) In the evaluation of rotation, forceps were set horizontally. (c) We measured the rotational positioning accuracy of forceps when forceps were pulling up the weight.

accuracy were measured by its accompanying utility software. Each measurement was repeated for twelve times. In order to reduce the measuring error, maximum and minimum values were eliminated, and the average and standard deviation of other ten values were calculated. Positive value in positioning error means that manipulator overruns beyond the input command, and negative means that it does not reach the goal. The definition of +/- input direction is shown in Fig. 5. As the initial setting, the forceps were set vertically in the evaluation of gimbals mechanism and translation of forceps (Fig. 5(a)), and horizontally in rotation (Fig. 5(b)). The distance between the weight and the center of gimbals mechanism was 250 [mm].

3.1 Gimbals Mechanism

Working range of gimbals mechanism was measured. No decrease of working range was shown (Table. 1). Positioning accuracy of the gimbals mechanism was measured at every 5 [deg] from −30 [deg] to +30[deg]. Measurement results are shown in Fig.6, comparing the results of evaluation without load [7]. Accuracy was less than 1.2 [deg] in pitch and roll motions.

3.2 Friction Wheel Mechanism (FWM)

As for the working range, FWM has no mechanical limitation, and the load did not limit the working range (Table. 1).

Before measuring the positioning accuracy, we evaluated the separation of rotation and translation. Because rotation and translation of forceps are generated by combining a couple of spiral motions, if each spiral motion differs from each other because of machining error, rotational error occurs in translation and translational error occurs in rotation [7,13]. Thus we measured the motion error beforehand and added compensation factor. When 45 [mm] translation command (that corresponds to 5 revolutions or 1800[deg] rotation of friction wheel) was input, forceps rotated 14.3 [deg]. This means that the difference of rotational traveling distance between FWMs is 14.3 [deg]. Thus we applied two coefficients; 1 - (14.3 / 1800) to longer traveling one, and 1 + (14.3 / 1800) to shorter traveling one.

Positioning accuracy of FWM was measured at every 45 [deg] from −180 [deg] to +180[deg] in rotation, and at every 20[mm] from −80 [mm] to +80[mm]

Table 1. Results of Working Range Evaluation

	Working Range	
	with load	w/o load
Pitch [deg]	−35.0 – +37.0	−35.0 – +37.0
Roll [deg]	± 180.0	± 180.0
Rotation [deg]	no limitation	no limitation
Translation [mm]	no limitation	no limitation

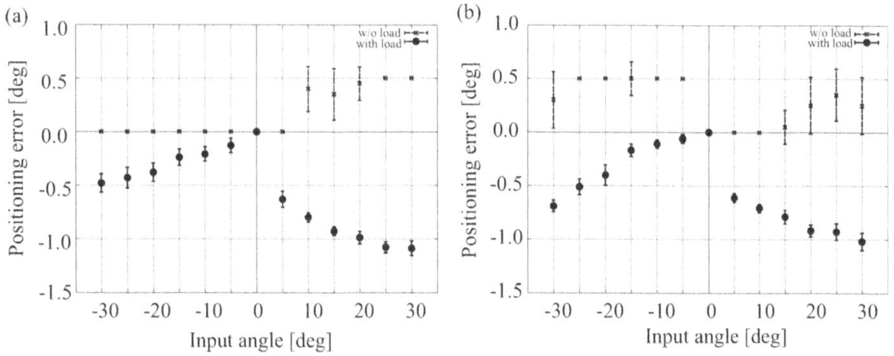

Fig. 6. Positioning accuracy of gimbals mechanism, (a) Pitch, (b)Roll

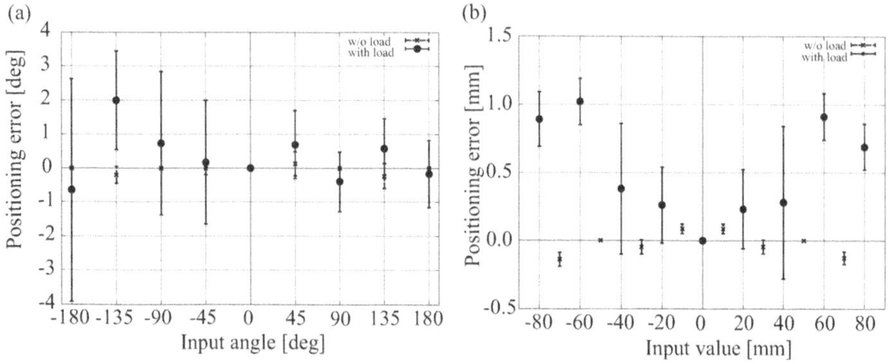

Fig. 7. Positioning accuracy of friction wheel mechanism, (a) Rotation, (b) Translation

in translation. The diameter of the forceps was 5 [mm], thus the torque applied by the weight was 10 [mNm]. Results are shown in Fig. 7. The accuracy was less than 4 [deg] in rotation of forceps, less than 1.2 [mm] in longitudinal translation.

4 Discussion

4.1 Working Range and Positioning Accuracy

Working range of gimbals mechanism and FWM did not affected by the load of 4 [N]. As for the roll motion of gimbals mechanism and rotation and translation of FWM, they have no mechanical limitation to realize wide range of motion. However, we can think mechanical limitation is desirable to ensure the safety in the case of malfunction. Some kind of safety mechanism should be implemented without wasting the advantages of gimbals mechanism and FWM.

As for the positioning accuracy of gimbals mechanism, it decreased as the input value increased. However, results showed the relative small standard deviation and high repeatability, thus high positioning accuracy will be realized by adding offset into input command depending on the load.

Positioning accuracy of FWM also decreased, especially in the rotation of forceps. This would be because the friction force between idle roller and forceps shaft to hold the forceps is smaller than external force by the load. Though we used stainless steel for idle rollers and shaft from the viewpoint of future washing and sterilization in the current prototype, we have to consider other materials to strengthen the friction force.

4.2 Future Works

We have following plans as near-term future works.

1. We will measure the dynamic response characteristics with/without load. The dynamic characteristics must be known to drive this manipulator smoothly as a slave robotic arm in a master-slave system.

2. As a related work, we evaluated the tilting angle of idle rollers in FWM [15]. In that study, FWM with rollers of 45 [degree] tilting angle showed higher speed, torque and force, and did not show any decrease in the positioning accuracy, comparing with those of 30 [degree], those were used in this study. Thus we will replace the FWMs with new ones.

3. Sterilization-compatible mechanism should be implemented for the clinical application. We will use "separation method" that separates sterilized and non-sterilized part via transmission part [14].

5 Conclusion

In this study, we evaluated the compact forceps manipulator using gimbals mechanism and FWM. As the results of experiments applying 4[N] load, positioning accuracy of the gimbals mechanism was less than 1.2 [deg], and that of friction wheel mechanism was less than 4 [deg] in rotation and 1.2 [mm] in translation.

This manipulator can work as a compact robotic arm to manipulate various kinds of forceps, ex. wire-driven bending forceps [16], bending forceps using linkage mechanism [17], and laser surgical tool [18], or rigid laparoscope can be manipulated with this system. In other words, this manipulator can be a common platform for robotized forceps. Thus we are going to integrate various surgical instruments with this manipulator to use robotized sophisticated surgical equipments.

Acknowledgement

This work is partially supported by "Research for the Future Program (JSPS-RFTF 99I00904)" funded by Japan Society for the Promotion of Science, Electro-Mechanic Technology Advancing Foundation, "Research and Development of the Compact Surgical Robot System for Future Medical Care" funded by New Energy and Industrial Technology Development Organization (NEDO), and "Research on medical devices for analyzing, supporting and substituting the function of human body" funded by Ministry of Health, Labour and Welfare.

References

1. M.Hashizume, et al. Robotic Surgery and Cancer: the Present State, Problems and Future Vision. *Jpn.J.Clin.Oncol.*, 34(5):227–237, 2004.
2. A.R.Lanfranco, et al. Robotic Surgery: A Current Perspective. *Annals of Surgery*, 239(1):14–21, 2004.
3. Y.Kobayashi, et al. Small Occupancy Robotic Mechanisms for Endoscopic Surgery. In *Proc. of MICCAI2002*, pages 75–82, 2002.
4. M.Vollenweider, et al. Surgery Simulator with Force Feedback. In *Proc. of* 4th *International Conference on Motion and Vibration Control (MOVIC98)*, 1998.
5. T.Suzuki, et al. A new compact robot for manipulation forceps using friction wheel and gimbals mechanism. In *Proc. of CARS2002*, pages 314–319, 2002.
6. Y.Katayama, T.Suzuki, et al. New compact robot for manipulating forceps using friction wheel and gimbals mechanism. In *Proc. of JSPE*, 2004, (in Japanese).
7. T.Suzuki, et al. Compact Forceps Manipulator for Laparoscopic Surgery. In *Proc. of IEEE/RSJ IROS2005*, page accepted, 2005.
8. http://www.ironintern.com/amp/.
9. http://www.mitakakohki.co.jp/english/med_index.html.
10. http://www.zero-max.com/products/rohlix/rohlixmain.asp.
11. R.H.Taylor, et al. A Telerobotic Assistant for Laparoscopic Surgery. *IEEE Engineering in Medicine and Biology*, 14(3):279–288, MayJune 1995.
12. A.J.Madhani, et al. The Black Falcon : A Teleoperated Surgical Instrument for Minimally Invasive Surgery. In *Proc. of IEEE/RSJ IROS'98*, pages 936–944, 1998.
13. K.Ikuta et al. Virtual Endoscope System with Force Sensation. In *Proc. of MICCAI98*, pages 293–304, 1998.
14. J.L.Hefti, et al. Robotic Three-Dimensional Positioning of a Stimulation Electrode in the Brain. *Journal of Computer Aided Surgery*, 3(1):1–10, 1998.
15. T.Suzuki, et al. Improvement of compact forceps manipulator using friction wheel mechanism. In *The* 1st *Asian symposium on computer aided surgery*, page OR1, 2005.
16. R.Nakamura, et al. Multi-DOF Forceps Manipulator System for Laparoscopic Surgery - Mechanism miniaturized & Evaluation of New Interface -. In *Proc. of MICCAI2001*, pages 606–613, 2001.
17. H.Yamashita, et al. Handheld Laparoscopic Forceps Manipulator Using Multi-slider Linkage Mechanisms. In *Proc. of MICCAI 2004*, pages 121–128, 2004.
18. T.Suzuki, et al. Development of a Robotic Laser Surgical Tool with an Integrated Video Endoscope. In *Proc. of MICCAI2004*, pages 25–32, 2004.

Spatial Motion Constraints for Robot Assisted Suturing Using Virtual Fixtures

Ankur Kapoor, Ming Li, and Russell H. Taylor

Dept. of Computer Science, Johns Hopkins University

Abstract. We address the problem of the stitching task in endoscopic surgery using a circular needle under robotic assistance. Our main focus is to present an algorithm for suturing using guidance virtual fixtures (VF) that assist the surgeon to move towards a desired goal. A weighted multi-objective, constraint optimization framework is used to compute the joint motions required for the tasks. We show that with the help of VF, suturing can be performed at awkward angles without multiple trials, thus avoiding damage to tissue. In this preliminary study we show the feasibility of our approach and demonstrate the promise of cooperative assistance in complex tasks such as suturing.

1 Introduction

The benefits of Minimally Invasive Surgery (MIS) over conventional open surgery are well known, however, the surgeon faces the challenge of limited and constrained motion as well as loss of direct visualization. These factors make the simple act of suturing probably the most difficult and time consuming of all MIS tasks. For these reasons, robotic assisted MIS has gained increasing popularity during the last decade. As shown in [1] by Ruurda *et al.* there is a significant improvement in time needed per stitch with robotic assistance even for experienced surgeons. Hubens [2] reaches a similar conclusion for standardized surgical tasks performed by inexperienced surgeons. To further augment the surgeon's ability to manipulate the surgical instruments using robotic system in a confined environment, various techniques have been proposed in literature. In [3] the surgeon's view is enhanced by 3D vision. Kitagawa *et al.* [4] provide force feedback through sensory substitution to achieve suture results that are closer to ideal conditions. It is important to note that in the various surgical systems described above the surgical procedures are still performed by surgeon; the robotic device merely follows the human commands. Estimation of distances and angles with a "key hole" view provided by endoscopic cameras becomes difficult and time consuming for surgeons. Consequently, the suturing motion is often realized by multiple trials that extend the operating time as pointed out by Ruurda *et al.* [1]. This indicates that a robotic assistant system that uses surgeon's intelligence for high level cognition tasks and at the same time fills the gap in sensory perception by providing motion guidance will be useful.

Different techniques [5,6,7,8] have been proposed to provide interaction modes in which the surgeon shares the control of the robot with the computer process.

J. Duncan and G. Gerig (Eds.): MICCAI 2005, LNCS 3750, pp. 89–96, 2005.

The goal of the computer process is to provide anisotropic motion behavior to the surgeon's motion command besides filtering out tremor and disturbance to enhance precision and stability. Li and Taylor [9] extended Funda's work [10] to generate virtual fixtures (VF) to assist the surgeon to manipulate surgical tools in a complex work space environment, in which anatomical constraints are automatically generated from 3D medical images.

The suturing task was observed and analyzed as performed in training videos. This task involves the following steps 1) *(Select)* Determine a suitable entry and exit point for the suture needle leaving sufficient room from the edge to be approximated. 2) *(Align)* Grasp the needle, move and orient it such that the tip is aligned with the entry point. 3) *(Bite)* Entry and exit "bites" are made such that the needle passes from one tissue to be approximated to the other. 4) *(Loop)* Create a suture loop to tie a knot. 5) *(Knot)* Secure the knot under proper tension. Previous works have focuses on steps 4 and 5 and used a shuttle device to address the issue of manipulation of curved needle. Kang and Wen [11] and Nagy *et al.* [12] have focused on the knot tying aspects of suturing. Both of them use tele-manipulation with haptic feedback to perform these tasks. Nageotte *et al.* [13] have presented a kinematic analysis of the entrance and exit bites involved in stitching task. In this work we describe our recent approach to VF that can combine guidance with forbidden regions relative to features on the target and its application to the task of stitching.

2 Methods

In this work we address the align and bite steps of the suturing process described above, where the primary challenges are manipulation of curved needle under non-ideal haptic using a robot with complex kinematics. In the align step, the goal is to move the robot to align the position and orientation of the suture needle such that it pierces the tissue correctly, at the same time minimizing extraneous motion of the needle and robot. The goal of the bite step is to move the needle tip from entry point to the exit point with minimum damage to the tissue through which the needle passes.

2.1 Constrained Control Algorithm Overview

For this work, we assume that the robot is holding the needle and the needle tip and target have been registered in the robot coordinate system. The outline of the algorithm is as follows: 1) Obtain the incremental motion desired by the user through force sensor, joystick or master 2) Formulate a set of linear constraints based on current robot state and specified task 3) Use the robot and task instantaneous kinematics to generate a quadratic program with linear constraints. The general form of the program is

$$\begin{array}{l} \arg\min_{\Delta q} \|W(\Delta \boldsymbol{x} - \Delta \boldsymbol{x}^d)\|, \\ s.t. \quad H\Delta \boldsymbol{x} \geq \boldsymbol{h}, \qquad \Delta \boldsymbol{x} = J\Delta \boldsymbol{q} \end{array} \tag{1}$$

where $\Delta \boldsymbol{q}$ is the desired incremental motions of the joint variables, $\Delta \boldsymbol{x}^d$, $\Delta \boldsymbol{x}$ are the desired and the computed incremental motions of the task variables in Cartesian space, respectively. J is the Jacobian matrix relating task space to joint space. W is a diagonal matrix for weights selected so that the errors of critical motion elements are close to zero, while errors in other non-critical motions simply stay as low as possible within tolerances allowed by the constraint set. 4) Solve the quadratic program for the incremental joint motion, which is used to move the robot. We would like to note that the constraints of step 3 might not be linear such as the distance function. In such cases we use a linear approximation, which allows us to utilize the structure of least squares problem with linear constraints, and solve the quadratic program in time frames suitable for robot control. We have used the Lawson and Hanson's algorithm as presented in [14].

2.2 Modeling of Task

We assume that the entry and exit points are known in the robot coordinate frame. These could be specified by surgeon using an optical marker tool to indicate points in space or by using a computer vision system to determine suitable points on the surface based on distance from the edge to be approximated and transferred to the robot coordinate frame (Reader is refered to [15] for a general purpose toolkit for computer vision).For the purpose of this work we use a point based registration method using Optotrak. We shall denote $\boldsymbol{p}_i$ as the position of the origin of frame $\{i\}$ with respect to world coordinates, where $\{i\}$ is any one of the frames shown in Figure 1.

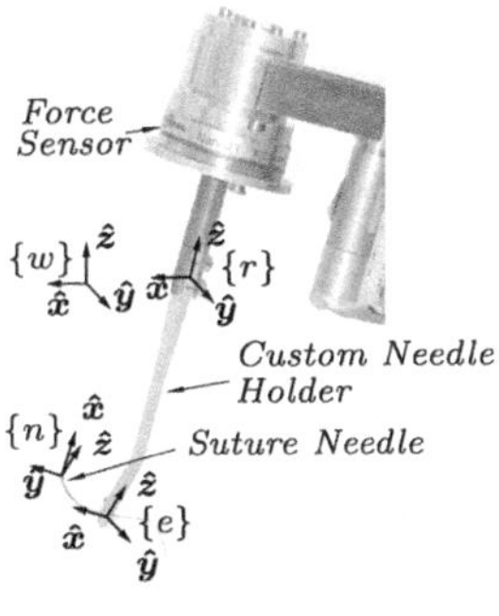

Fig. 1. Custom needle holder, needle and assigned frames

Align Step. We now present a strategy that could be used for the align step with the following substeps. *(Substep 1)* First the needle tip is allowed to move in a straight line such that the needle tip coincides with the desired entry point; at the same time its orientation is allowed to change only about an axis such that this motion will result in the tangent at needle tip being coincident with the normal to the surface at the entry point. *(Substep 2)* In the next substep the orientation of the normal to the needle plane is allowed to change, such that the needle plane coincides with line joining entry and exit points. Assistance is provided by not allowing any motion of needle tip or the tangent at the needle tip. *(Substep 3)* Once the desired orientations are reached we allow the surgeon to penetrate the tissue by a small distance, *(Substep 4)* followed by motion constraints that would let the surgeon bring the tangent at needle tip to coincide with the desired entry direction without changing the plane normal and tip position. The align step is completed once the desired orientation is reached, which is computed using the entry and exit points specified by the surgeon and the needle radius. In all these substeps only those motions that bring the needle closer to the desired position and orientation are allowed.

The above sequence of substeps ensures that the needle tip (cutting point) is normal to the tissue surface at the time of piercing the tissue. This is particularly favorable for hard tissue such as muscle as it makes the optimal use of the cutting point of needle. In case of soft tissue, the surgical needles used do not have a sharp cutting point. Thus in order to reduce the number of substeps and hence the time, an alternate strategy in which the substeps are to align needle tip directly with desired direction instead of surface normal and skiping the last two substeps could be used. For the remainder of this paper, we shall focus on the former approach. For our algorithm, the later approach can be considered as a special case of former.

Moreover, for the current work we ignore the deformation in the tissue. For the future we want to extend this approach by regarding the deformation and updating the targets accordingly.

Bite Step. *(Substep 5)* Once the entry and exit points are determined, and the radius of needle is known, it easy to see that the trajectory of the needle tip that would cause minimum damage to the tissue lie on a circle with entry and exit points as points on a chord and with radius equal to needle radius. To ensure sufficient depth of penetration in the tissue we ensure that the needle plane is parallel to the line joining entry and exit points and the surface normal at entry point. In this step our constraint motion algorithm permits only those motions that satisfy these constraints.

2.3 Algorithm Implementation

In our approach the required VF constraints for each substep are analyzed and broken into a combination of one or more of basic constraints. We make use of the common structure between the different substeps and construct generalized constraints that take desired target into consideration. Furthermore we utilize the sequential nature of the task to switch between different substeps. The switch could be triggered when the error between the current value and target decreases below a threshold. We now describe a method to compute H and $\boldsymbol{h}$ in the inequality subject function of (1) corresponding to one of basic constraints, then we show how we can combine then together to form the desired VF behavior. We use MOVE (and ROTATE) for the constraint of moving along a desired direction (or rotate about a desired direction). We use the name STAY (and MAINTAIN) for a VF designed to maintain a desired position (or orientation). We denote signed error for target by $\boldsymbol{\delta}$, its translational part by $\boldsymbol{\delta}_p$ and the rotation component by a Rodriguez vector $\boldsymbol{\delta}_r$. Since the angles are small, we can approximate the Rodriguez vector by Euler angles.

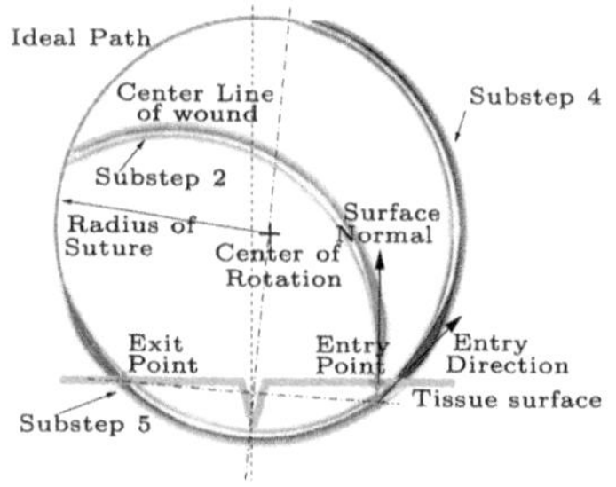

Fig. 2. Ideal path of needle tip for minimal tissue tear is a circle with the same radius as the suture needle and centered at needle center

STAY Constraint. We are given a desired target point $\boldsymbol{p}_i^d$ in some frame $\{i\}$. This gives signed error as $\boldsymbol{\delta} = [\boldsymbol{p}_i - \boldsymbol{p}_i^d, 0]^t$. We require that after incremental motion due to input, the position be as close as possible to the target point. This requires that $\|\boldsymbol{\delta}_p + \Delta\boldsymbol{p}_i\| \leq \epsilon_1$ where ϵ_1 is a small positive number that defines the size of the range that can be considered as the target. To gain computational efficiency we would like to solve a quadratic program with linear constraints. Thus, we linearize the above constraint by considering projections of $\boldsymbol{\delta}_p + \Delta\boldsymbol{p}_i$ on a finite set of lines through target point. These can be written as

$$\left[c_{\alpha i}c_{\beta j},\ c_{\alpha i}s_{\beta j},\ s_{\alpha i},\ 0,\ 0,\ 0 \right]^t (\boldsymbol{\delta}+\Delta\boldsymbol{x}) \leq \epsilon_1; \quad i=1,\cdots,n;\ j=1,\cdots,m. \quad \text{where} \quad c_{\alpha i}=\cos\tfrac{2\pi i}{n};\ c_{\beta j}=\cos\tfrac{2\pi j}{m};\ s_{\alpha i}=\sin\tfrac{2\pi i}{n};\ s_{\beta j}=\sin\tfrac{2\pi j}{m} \tag{2}$$

Then we set $H \in \Re^{6\times mn}$ and $\boldsymbol{h} \in \Re^{mn}$ as

$$H = \begin{bmatrix} -c_{\alpha 1}c_{\beta 1}, & -c_{\alpha 1}s_{\beta 1}, & -s_{\alpha 1}, & 0, & 0, & 0 \\ & \cdots & & & & \\ -c_{\alpha 1}c_{\beta m}, & -c_{\alpha 1}s_{\beta m}, & -s_{\alpha 1}, & 0, & 0, & 0 \\ & \cdots & & & & \\ -c_{\alpha n}c_{\beta 1}, & -c_{\alpha n}s_{\beta 1}, & -s_{\alpha n}, & 0, & 0, & 0 \\ & \cdots & & & & \\ -c_{\alpha n}c_{\beta m}, & -c_{\alpha n}s_{\beta m}, & -s_{\alpha n}, & 0, & 0, & 0 \end{bmatrix}, \quad \boldsymbol{h} = \begin{bmatrix} -\epsilon_1 \\ \vdots \\ -\epsilon_1 \end{bmatrix} - H\boldsymbol{\delta} \tag{3}$$

MOVE Constraint. We are given a desired line $L(s) = \boldsymbol{L}_0 + \hat{\boldsymbol{l}} \cdot s$ in some frame $\{i\}$. We require that the position after incremental motion due to input be as close to the line as possible. If $\boldsymbol{p}_i^c$ is the closest point on the line to the current position, then the signed error is $\boldsymbol{\delta} = [\boldsymbol{p}_i - \boldsymbol{p}_i^c, 0]^t$. We define $\boldsymbol{u_i}$ as the projection of $\boldsymbol{p}_i - \boldsymbol{p}_i^c$ on a plane Π that is perpendicular to the line. Our requirement is that $\|\boldsymbol{u}_i\|$ be close to zero. If R denotes a rotation matrix that would transform a vector in plane Π to world coordinates, then any unit vector in plane Π with O (Figure 3) as origin can be written in world coordinate frame as $R\left[\cos\gamma, \sin\gamma, 0\right]^t$.

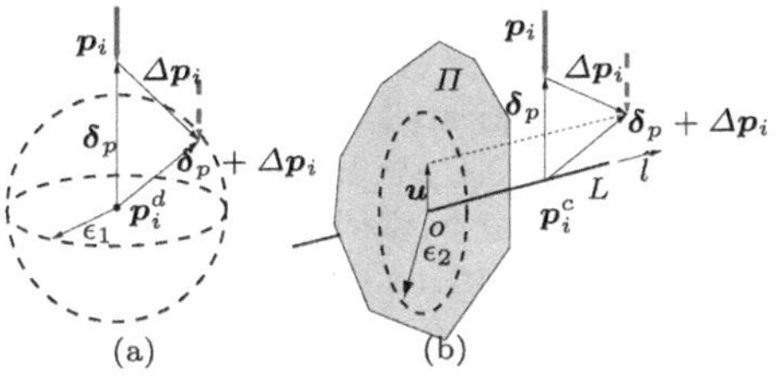

Fig. 3. Geometric relation for (a) STAY and (b) MOVE

Like before we approximate by considering only a finite set of vectors, and our constraint can be written as

$$\left[\left[R\left[c_{\gamma i},\ s_{\gamma i},\ 0 \right]^t \right]^t,\ 0,\ 0,\ 0 \right]^t (\boldsymbol{\delta}+\Delta\boldsymbol{x}) \leq \epsilon_2; \quad c_{\gamma i}=\cos\tfrac{2\pi i}{k};\ s_{\gamma i}=\sin\tfrac{2\pi i}{k};\ i=1,\cdots,k \tag{4}$$

We can set $H \in \Re^{6\times k}$ and $\boldsymbol{h} \in \Re^{k}$ as,

$$H = \begin{bmatrix} -\left[R\left[c_{\gamma 1},\ s_{\gamma 1},\ 0\right]^t\right]^t, & 0, & 0, & 0 \\ \cdots & & & \\ -\left[R\left[c_{\gamma k},\ s_{\gamma k},\ 0\right]^t\right]^t, & 0, & 0, & 0 \end{bmatrix}, \quad \boldsymbol{h} = \begin{bmatrix} -\epsilon_2 \\ \cdots \\ -\epsilon_2 \end{bmatrix} - H\boldsymbol{\delta} \tag{5}$$

The construction of H and $\boldsymbol{h}$ for MAINTAIN and ROTATE follow the same lines, and uses the later three columns of matrix H corresponding to three rotational components in $\Delta \boldsymbol{x}$. We refer the reader to [16] for further details on contruction of matrix H for different constraints. A combined constraint can be applied to a same frame or to different frames. For the case of different frames we consider Jacobian corresponding to each frame and the inequality subject function is of the form (6a) where $J_i(q)$ is the Jacobian matrix that maps Cartesian velocities of frame $\{i\}$ to joint space. For the case of same frame the inequality subject function of (1) is of the form (6b) where subscript p and r denotes the translational and rotational constraints respectively.

$$\begin{bmatrix} H_1 & & 0 \\ & \ddots & \\ 0 & & H_k \end{bmatrix} \begin{bmatrix} J_1(q) \\ \vdots \\ J_k(q) \end{bmatrix} \Delta \boldsymbol{q} \geq \begin{bmatrix} \boldsymbol{h}_1 \\ \vdots \\ \boldsymbol{h}_k \end{bmatrix} \quad \text{(6a)} \qquad \begin{bmatrix} H_p \\ H_r \end{bmatrix} J(q) \Delta \boldsymbol{q} \geq \begin{bmatrix} \boldsymbol{h}_p \\ \boldsymbol{h}_r \end{bmatrix} \quad \text{(6b)}$$

3 Materials

As a preliminary test bed (Figure 4) we have used a Johns Hopkins University Steady-Hand robot [17], which is equipped with a custom needle holder and a 6-DoF force-torque sensor (ATI Nano43 F/T transducer) mounted on the tool handle. For these experiments we have selected a 3/8 circle $30mm$ cutting needle from Ethicon (needle diameter $1mm$). The Optotrak (Northern Digital Inc, Waterloo, CA) infrared optical position tracking system was used for robot calibration.Our control algorithm is independent of manipulator type and input form a joystick or a master robot can easily replace the force input to the controller. The phantom to mimic the tissue is contructed by dissolving 4% by weight of agar in distilled water, maintaing this solution at $90 \deg C$ for one hour and solidifying the solution by rapidly cooling it to $-20 \deg C$.

4 Experiments

We performed three sets of experiments; The first set was computer simulation to check the feasiblity of motion given the constraints and robot kinematics. The second set was experiments with the robot. We recoreded the encoder reading of the robot joints and used direct kinematics of the robot to verify our algorithm by measuring the errors between the ideal target path and that followed by the robot. Figure 5 show the errors between actual and ideal robot motion as

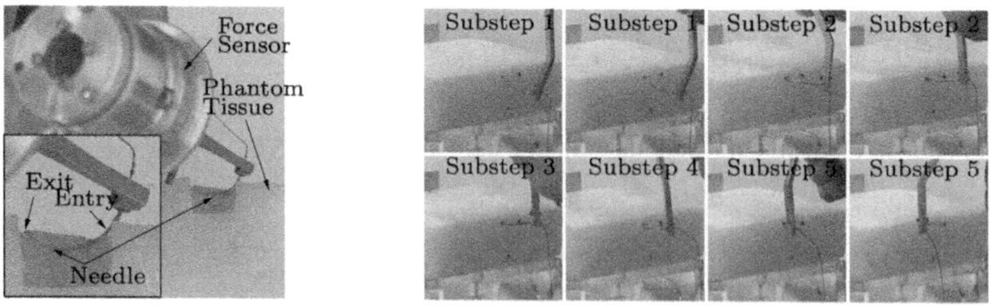

Fig. 4. (left) Experimental Setup, Insert: Path of needle (right) Phantom being sutured

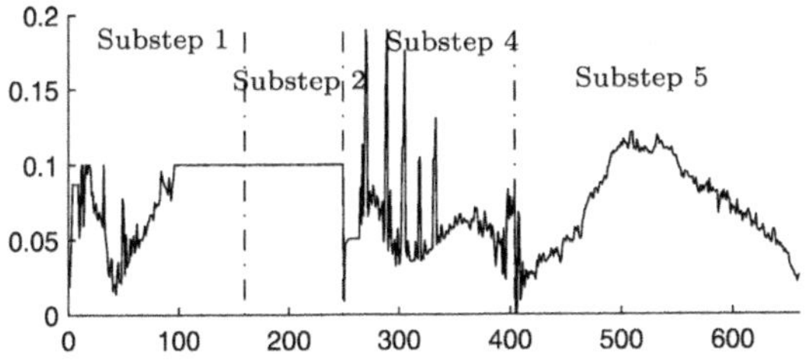

Fig. 5. The magnitude of error in needle tip with respect to ideal path as measured by robot encoders

Table 1. The error in ideal and actual points as measured by OptoTrak

	Entry	Exit
Robot	0.6375	0.7742
Manual	-	2.1

measured with robot encoders and kinematics for different substeps. The values (ϵ_i in equations 3 and 5) for positional and angular tolerance were selected as $0.5mm$ and 0.25 deg. The diameter of the needle was $1mm$. The last set of experiments were a demonstration of our algorithm using a phantom tissue. Since the phantom is opaque, the measurements available are the entry and exit points of the needle. Table 1 presents the differences between the user specified targets and the actual ones as measured by an optical tool. As expected the errors measured by Optotrak are higher than measured by encoders alone, because this represents the overall accuracy of the system, which also includes errors arising from calibration of the needle and accuracy of Optotrak ($0.1mm$). The residual calibration errors are appear as errors in the entry point errors in Table 1 above. Average errors for free hand suturing as performed by four users (5 trials each), using the same needle holder and without robot assistance, are presented in Table 1. We believe that robot assistance can improve accuracy especially in constrained environment such as that of endoscopic surgery. Moreover, robot assisted motions did not require multiple trials and large undesirable movements of tissue, which is often the case in free hand suturing. Figure 4 shows the progression of different substeps for one of the trials. The insert in Figure 4 shows the phantom with a portion cut out so that the actual path taken by the needle is visible; the entry and exit points are $13.5mm$ apart. As seen in the Figure 4 we have selected an angle that places limits on performing the suture manually, to emphasize the ability of our algorithm to assist in non-favorable orientations.

5 Conclusion

Endoscopic surgery presents a constrained working environment for surgeons, and the surgeons must deal with the realities of long instruments and awkward angles. In this paper we have implemented the constrained control for performing "align" and "bite" steps, given a surface, entry and exit points. Using guidance virtual fixtures we provide assistance to the surgeon allowing only those motions of the needle that are feasible and move the needle towards the desired goal. This helps realize the stitching motion without multiple trials and large undesirable movements of tissues involved. This formulation can be extended to include additional constraints such as collision avoidance and anatomy-based constraints

[9]. We plan to extend these results by integrating vision to take into account deformation and also add force feedback. We are also working on implementing this algorithm for control of a high dexterity snake-like robot [18] geared towards long and slender anatomy such as throat.

Acknowledgements

We thank Iulian Iordachita for his assistance with the robot and the needle holder. This work was partially funded by the National Science Foundation (NSF) under Engineering Research Center grant #EEC9731478, NSF grant #IIS9801684, and by the Johns Hopkins University internal funds.

References

1. Ruurda, J.P., et al: Manual robot assisted endoscopic suturing: Time-action analysis in an experimental model. Surg. End. **18** (2004) 1249–1252
2. Hubens, G., et al: A performance study comparing manual and robotically assisted laparoscopic surgery using the da vinci system. Surg. End. **17** (2003) 1595–1599
3. Guthart, G., Salisbury, K.: The intuitive TM telesurgery system: Overview and application. In: ICRA. (2000) 618–621
4. Kitagawa, M., et al: Effect of sensory substitution on suture-manipulation forces for robotic surgical systems. J Thorac Cardiovasc Surg **129** (2005) 151–158
5. Kazanzides, P., et al: Force sensing and control of a surgical robot. In: Trans. Robot. Automat. (1992)
6. Rosenberg, L.B.: Virtual fixtures: Perceptual tools for telerobotic manipulation. In: IEEE Virtual Reality Annual International Symposium. (1993) 76–82
7. Davies, B.L., et al: Active compliance in robotic surgerythe use of force control as a dynamic constraint. Proc Inst Mech Eng [H]. **211** (1997) 285–292
8. Dewan, M., et al: Vision-based assistance for ophthalmic micro-surgery. In: MICCAI. (2004)
9. Li, M., Taylor, R.H.: Spatial motion constraints in medical robot using virtual fixtures generated by anatomy. In: ICRA. (2004) 1270–1275
10. Funda, J., et al: Constrained cartesian motion control for teleoperated surgical robots. Trans. Robot. Automat. **12** (1996) 453–465
11. Kang, H., Wen, J.T.: Endobot: a robotic assistant in minimally invasive surgeries. In: ICRA. (2001) 2031–2036
12. Nagy, I., et al: Endo[PA]R: An open evaluation system for minimally invasive robotic surgery. In: Mechatronics and Robotics. (2004)
13. Nageotte, F., et al: Computer-aided suturing in laparoscopic surgery. In: CARS. (2004) 781–786
14. Lawson, C.L., Hanson, R.J.: Solving Least Squares Problems. Prentice-Hall, Inc. (1974)
15. Hager, G., Toyama, K.: The xvision system: A general-purpose substrate for portable real-time vision applications. CVIU **69** (1998) 23–37
16. Li, M., Kapoor, A., Taylor, R.: A constrained optimization approach to virtual fixtures. In: ICRA. (2005) Submitted for review Submitted for review.
17. Taylor, R.H., et al: A steady-hand robotic system for microsurgical augmentation. IJRR **18** (1999) 1201–1210
18. Simaan, N., et al: High dexterity snake-like robotic slaves for minimally invasive telesurgery of the upper airway. In: MICCAI. (2004)

Contact Force Measurement of Instruments for Force-Feedback on a Surgical Robot: Acceleration Force Cancellations Based on Acceleration Sensor Readings

Shigeyuki Shimachi[1], Fumie Kameyama[1], Yoshihide Hakozaki[1], and Yasunori Fujiwara[2]

[1] Iwate University, 4-3-5 Ueda, Morioka, Japan, 020-8551
shimachi@iwate-u.ac.jp
[2] Ichinoseki National College of Technology, Hagisho, Ichinoseki, Japan, 021-8551

Abstract. For delicate operations conducted using surgical robot systems, surgeons need to receive information regarding the contact forces on the tips of surgical instruments. For the detection of this contact force, one of the authors previously proposed a new method, called the overcoat method, in which the instrument is supported by sensors positioned on the overcoat pipe. This method requires cancellation of the acceleration forces of the instrument/holder attached to the overcoat sensor. In the present report, the authors attempt to use acceleration sensors to obtain the acceleration forces of the instrument/holder. The new cancellation method provides a force-detection accuracy of approximately 0.05-0.1 N for a dynamic response range of up to approximately 20 Hz, compared to approximately 1 Hz, which was achieved by using acceleration forces based on the theoretical robot motion.

1 Introduction

In laparoscopic surgery, a surgeon operates using specially designed instruments through ports formed in the patient's abdomen. This technique reduces surgical damages to the patient's body and results in a shortened recovery period. However, the surgeon is significantly constrained with respect to the loss of direct visual information and manual operations. Surgical robot systems such as the da Vinci system and the Zeus system have substantially reduced these constraints. However, at present, haptic feedback is not provided by these systems. Although surgeons are able to view tissue deformation as a measure of external force, this type of visual compensation is limited to elastic materials and is not suitable for bone structure or suture materials.

A great number of studies have been conducted, though the references are omitted here, in order to investigate 1) the tactile force, 2) the grasping force of the forceps, and 3) the tip end force of the instrument, in combination with a) the effect of force feedback on the surgeon's skills as well as the development of b) force sensors, c) a man-machine interface and d) bilateral controls. The present report concerns the development of b) force sensor equipment for use on a slave robot for sensing the 3) tip end force of the instrument.

Taylor [1] pointed out that the friction force between the instrument and the trocar may limit sensitivity of the external force detection. Madhani [2] reported a vital

J. Duncan and G. Gerig (Eds.): MICCAI 2005, LNCS 3750, pp. 97 – 104, 2005.

method for estimating the tip force from the motor torques that drive a multiple-degree-of-freedom forceps. Although this system was tested on a master slave system, the force feedback was reported to give the operator annoyance. Seibold [3] installed a six-axis force sensor to the end of a forceps, but reported that precise sensing is difficult with respect to forces in the direction of the shaft, which include the pulling force for the gripping jaws of the forceps.

One of authors [4] proposed a new method, called the overcoat method, in which the instrument is supported by force sensors that are located on the inner face of the overcoat pipe, as shown in Fig.1. The overcoat sensing system accepts most types of instruments. In addition, this system allows measurement of the external force acting on the tip of the surgical instrument attached to the slave robot in laparoscopic robotic surgery and is free from the frictional forces generated on the trocar.

The main concern regarding the overcoat method is the construction of the force sensors. In our first attempt [4], three-axis force sensors were placed on the outside of the abdomen and were driven at semi-static speed. This structure provided only a short sensing range of force magnitude. In our second stage attempts [5],[6], in order to provide higher speed of the instrument motion, the acceleration force derived from the instrument mass was compensated with the acceleration force due to the robot motion. However, the obtained dynamic response was only up to approximately 1 Hz. This poor response is a result of the robot arm motion. Robot has inherently character frequency. Main character frequency of industrial robot is around from several Hz to 20 Hz. The robot used as test equipment has the character frequency of approximately 7 Hz. Low-pass filtering of 2Hz yields a measuring system response of around 1 Hz.

For detecting delicate changes of contact force and for applying the overcoat method to a robot that has such rigidity as that of industrial robot, we have to improve the dynamic response of the force measurement system.

Recently, small acceleration sensors have become available. The present report describes an attempt to improve the response characteristic of the measurement system by means of direct measurement of the acceleration of the instrument mass for compensating the acceleration force.

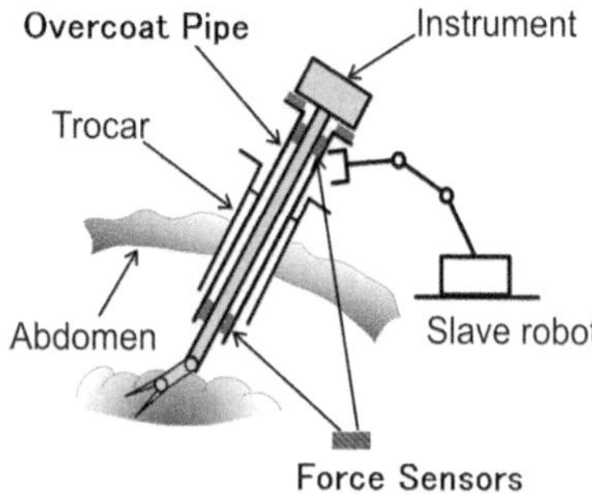

Fig. 1. Basic principle of overcoat method. Force sensors support instrument.

2 Theory of Force Measurement

Feedback Force Components. The goal of the present study is to provide force feedback to the fingertips of the surgeon. So, three orthogonal force components acting on the tip end of the instrument are measured herein.

Outline of the Overcoat Method. Fig.1 shows the basic principle of the overcoat method. A number of sensors that are installed inside the overcoat pipe support the instrument/holder that contains the instrument, the driving mechanisms and the holders for the instrument. The overcoat pipe is inserted into a trocar and is handled by a slave robot hand. In actual construction, the instrument shaft is inserted into an inner pipe and the force sensors are arranged between the inner pipe and the overcoat pipe. The mass of the instrument/holder and its acceleration make up the acceleration force. If the acceleration force can be subtracted from the force measured by the overcoat force sensors, then the force acting on the tip end of the instrument can be detected.

Coordinate System and Force Balance. Fig.2 shows the shaft of the instrument and the X, Y, Z coordinate system fixed on the ground. As shown in Fig.2, in the present report, the shaft direction of the instrument will be oscillated. For the expression of forces, let us introduce new coordinate axes and fix them to the instrument so as that the z axis coincides with the shaft of the instrument, the x axis is set parallel to the ground plane at the starting position of the instrument and the x, y and z coordinates form an orthogonal coordinate system, as shown in Fig.5.

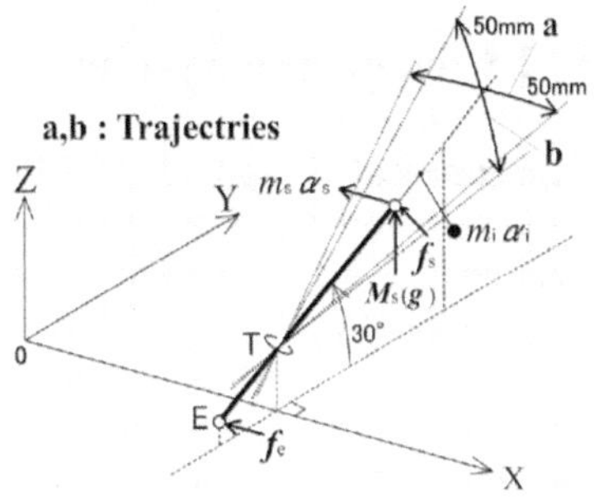

Fig. 2. Test trajectories for point "R"

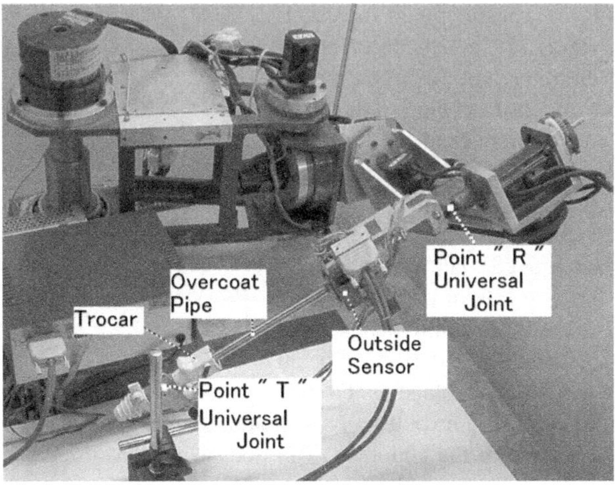

Fig. 3. Test setup of the overcoat sensing system

Let us define the following: $\boldsymbol{f}_e$ (f_x, f_y, f_z) is the detected force that acts on the tip end of the instrument, $\boldsymbol{f}_s(f_{sx}, f_{sy}, f_{sz})$ is the force sensed by the overcoat sensors, m_i is the mass of the instrument/holder, $\boldsymbol{a}_i$ is the motional acceleration of the center of gravity of the instrument/holder, m_s is the mass of the overcoat sensor frame, $\boldsymbol{a}_s$ is the motional acceleration of the gravity center of the overcoat sensor frame, and $\boldsymbol{g}$ is the gravitational acceleration. The force balance of the instrument/holder is as follows:

$$f_e + f_s + m_i\ (a_i + g)\ + m_s\ (a_s + g)\ = 0,$$
$$a_i = a_i + g\ ,\ a_s = a_s + g. \tag{1}$$

Here, the accelerations $a_i(a_{ix}, a_{iy}, a_{iz})$ and $a_s\ (a_{sx}, a_{sy}, a_{sz})$ are to be measured directly using acceleration sensors.

3 Experimental System

Experimental System. Fig.3 shows anoverview of the experimental system. The system is composed of a six-axis slave robot, the overcoat sensor, an instrument/holder and a trocar (commercial item) supported by a universal joint mechanism. The base frame of the overcoat sensor is attached to the robot hand through a universal joint for adjusting miss-alignment between the overcoat sensor pipe axis and the robot hand rotational axis.

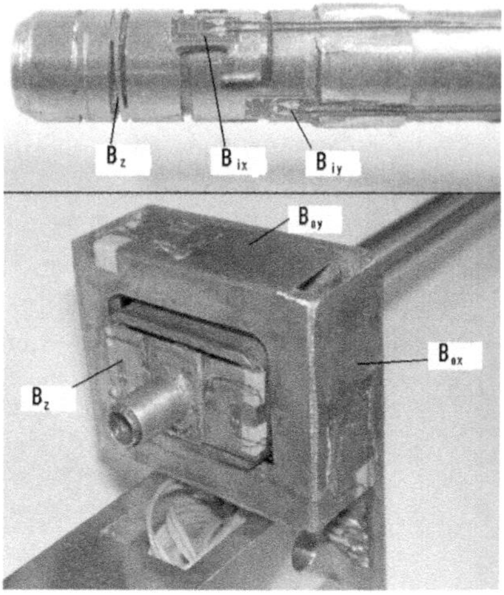

Fig. 4. Overcoat sensor. (top); inner part that is set on the inside B_Z: bending beams for x, y and z forces, of abdomen, B_{ix}, B_{iy}, B_Z: bending beams for x, y and z directional forces, (bottom); outer part, B_{ox}, B_{oy}, bending beams for x, y and z forces.

Overcoat Sensor. The overcoat sensor consists of three stainless pipes: an inner pipe, through which the instrument is inserted, a force sensor pipe, to which deflectable beams are attached for strain gauges, and an outer pipe (overcoat pipe), which covers the sensor pipe. The inner pipe has an inner diameter of 5.5 mm, and the outer pipe has an outer diameter of 10 mm. Fig.4 (top photograph) shows the inner part of the sensor pipe. Here, the outer pipe is removed. The 0.5-mm-thick sensor pipe has two sets of parallel deflection beams for the force component f_{sxi} and that for the f_{syi}, as well as a deflection beam structure for allowing displacement by f_{sz} in the shaft direction. Fig.3 (bottom photograph) shows the outside sensor part that is placed on the outside of the abdomen. This sensor part has three sensor components. Each sensor component has a set of two parallel bending plates for sensing each force component. The three sensor components for the f_{sxo}, f_{syo} and f_{sz} directional forces are stacked one-by-one inside the sensor in a box shape.

The overcoat sensor has five outputs f_{sxi}, f_{syi}, f_{sxo}, f_{syo} and f_{sz}. The x and y components are summed as $f_{sx} = f_{sxi} + f_{sxo}$ and $f_{sy} = f_{syi} + f_{syo}$ using a computer. The masses of the outer sensor frames, onto which parallel bending plates are fixed, are 120.4 g for f_{sx}, 85.7 g for f_{sy}, and 10.7 g for f_{sz}, respectively. The sensors have the linearity approximately 5% for 10 N and the resolution smaller than around 0.02N, as low pass filtered signals.

Trocar and Instrument/Holder. A commercially available trocar for an instrument shaft diameter of 10 mm was attached to a universal joint mechanism. The design of instrument/holder mechanisms is one of the future subjects. To test the overcoat method, we have to assume the instrument/holder mass. So, the authors made a simple holder in which a commercial and hand operate forceps is installed and the open-close motion of the jaws of forceps is driven by a geared motor (back side of the plate) that has larger power than the required one, as shown in Fig.5. The total weight of the trial instrument/holder is approximately 350g. So, the authors attached a model weight (400g ≅ 350g) to the inner pipe, as shown in Fig. 6. Authors expect now that the weight of instrument/holder may have around 500g. In this case, $\boldsymbol{a}_s$ and $\boldsymbol{a}_i$ become equal (, and it will be expressed as $\boldsymbol{a}_s$ (a_{sx}, a_{sy}, a_{sz})).

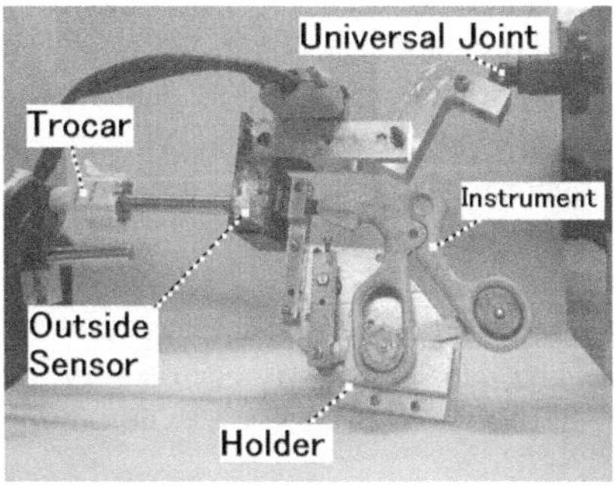

Fig. 5. An example of the instrument/holder setup

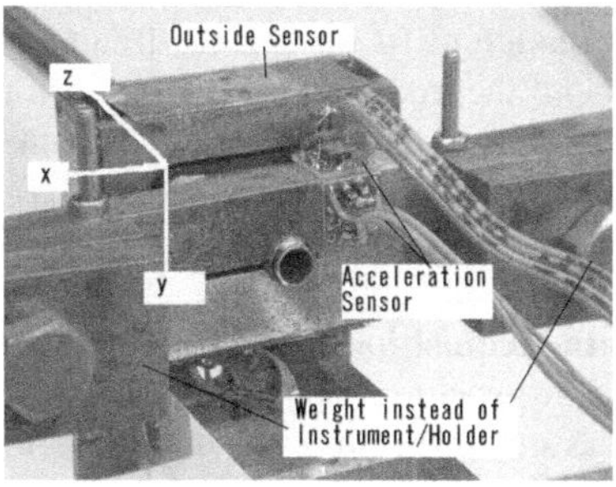

Fig. 6. Acceleration sensors and weight that represents the instrument/holder

Acceleration Sensor and Low Pass Filters. A two-directional acceleration sensor ADXL202E (Analog Devices Co.) was used as an acceleration sensor. The sensor has the outer dimensions of approximately 5mm×5mm×2mm and a cross-axis sensitivity of approximately 2%. For three-directional sensing, two sensors are arranged as shown in Fig.6.

The sensor outputs were passed through Low-Pass Filter (LPF) system, as shown in Fig. 7. The LPF generally gives a phase sift to the signal. Calculation must be performed for several output signals. So, we used filters that have almost the same characteristic for each of the signal passes. The acceleration sensor has two types of output signal; analog type and pulse width modulation (PWM) type. PWM type was selected in consideration of noise mixing in signal transmission. In order to obtain a smooth analog signal, a 2nd-order Butterworth LPF (approximately 50 Hz) was used, as shown in Fig. 7. The LPF for the outputs of the force sensors were adjusted to those of the acceleration sensors, in

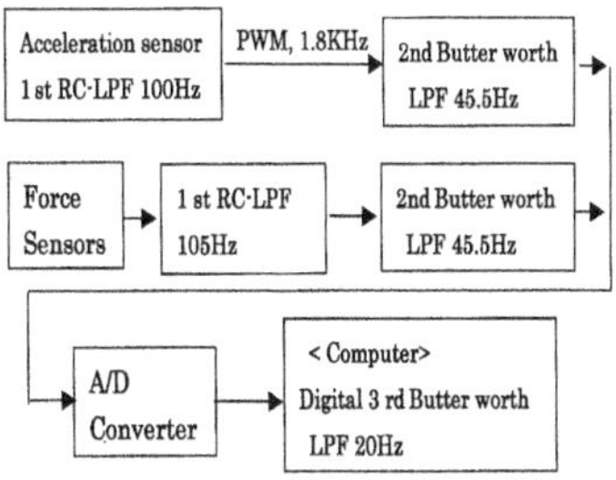

Fig. 7. Low-pass filter system

order to obtain almost the same characteristic. The above-mentioned values depend on the nominal values of the R C electric parts, and so have the same accuracy.

Slave Robot. The slave robot is a type of six-axis serial linkage. The rotation rigidity around the first axis of the robot arm is low, and its character frequency is approximately 7-8 Hz which is in the character frequency range of typical industrial robot.

4 Experimental Results

Experimental Trajectories of the Robot Hand. The robot hand point "R" was driven sinusoidally in two trajectories "a" and "b", as shown in Fig.2. The starting position of the instrument shaft is inclined 30° from X-Y plane and is parallel to the Z-Y plane. Trajectory "a" exists on a plane parallel to the Z-Y plane and has an oscillation of (u sin($2\pi ft$), f: frequency) for an amplitude (u = 50 mm in circular arc) around the trocar point "T". Trajectory "b" has the same oscillation as that of trajectory "a", but the swing axis exists on a plane parallel to the Z-Y plane. We can easily observe the motional acceleration effect in trajectory "a" and the gravitational acceleration effect in the trajectory "b".

Data Acquisition and Procession. All of the input signals were reset to zero at the starting position of the trajectories. The force and acceleration by each sensor were measured three times for both trajectories "a" and "b" at a speed 0.5 Hz without loading the tip end of the instrument, i.e., $f_x = f_y = f_z = 0$.

In canceling the acceleration forces, we have to consider the cross-axis sensitivity of the acceleration sensor. Therefore, the overcoat force sensor outputs f_{sx}, f_{sy}, and f_{sz} were cancelled through the following expression:

$$(f_x, f_y, f_z)^{\mathrm{T}} = (f_{sx}, f_{sy}, f_{sz})^{\mathrm{T}} - \mathrm{K}((a_x, a_y, a_z)^{\mathrm{T}} - \mathrm{c}^{\mathrm{T}}),$$

$$\mathrm{K}=\begin{pmatrix} -0.6360 & 0.0626 & -0.0182 \\ 0.0242 & -0.4120 & 0.0249 \\ 0.0081 & 0.0651 & -0.4504 \end{pmatrix}, \quad \mathrm{c}=(0.0021,-0.0166,0.0035). \tag{2}$$

Here, the diagonal coefficients of the matrix "K" correspond to the masses of each directional sensor, and the other values show the effects of the cross-axis sensitivity. The constant "c" corresponds to the offset of the acceleration sensor outputs.

The constants "K" and "c" are calculated using a regression for each force direction x, y and z, for each data corresponding to the three measurements for both trajectories "a" and "b", under the condition $f_x = f_y = f_z = 0$. The 18 sets of constants are averaged to obtain the constants shown in Eq. (2).

The diagonal constant referring to the x direction on the matrix "K" shows that the mass in the x direction is approximately 0.636 Kg. This value differs from the measured mass, i.e., (0.400 + 0.120 = 0.520 Kg/0.636 Kg), and the same method yields 0.486 Kg/0.412 Kg for y and 0.411Kg/0.450Kg for z, respectively. These values exceed the expected accuracy, which is smaller than 10%. Poor accuracy with regard to the x directional data, will also be shown later.

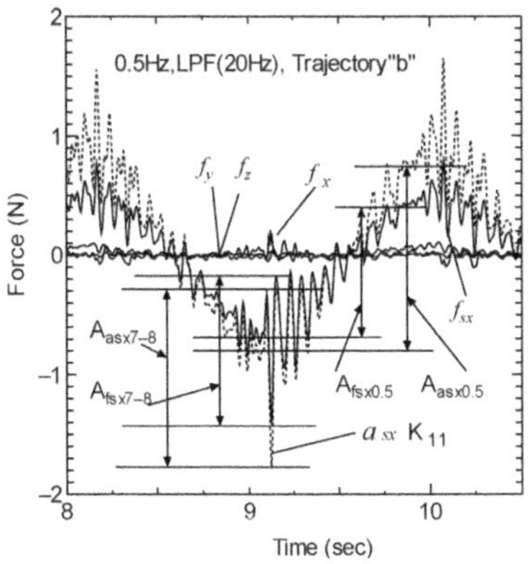

Fig. 8. Example of force cancellation on trajectory "b". f_{sx}; force sensor output, a_{sx}; acceleration sensor output, f_x, f_y, f_z; detected forces, A_{fsx},A_{asx}: amplitude of f_{sx}, a_{sx} for frequency $_{\text{subscript } 7\text{-}8}$:7-8Hz, $_{\text{subscript } 0.5}$:0.5Hz, K_{11}:11 component of matrix K.

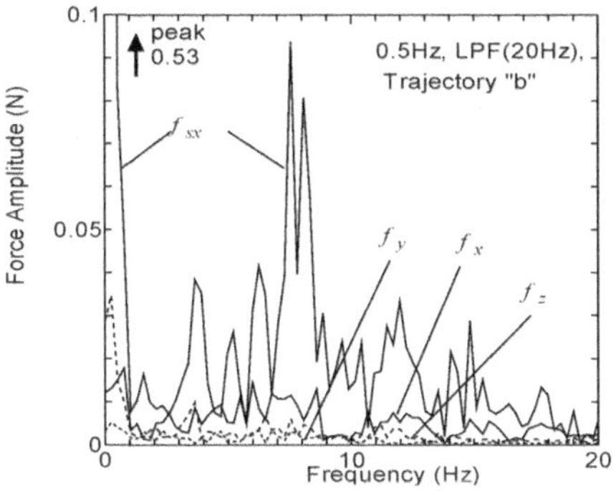

Fig. 9. Force amplitude/frequency analysis by FFT for the data shown in Fig.8

Measurement Errors. As the worst case, which shows the largest error in the detected forces, Fig.8 shows the force component f_{sx} for trajectory "b" and the detected forces f_x, f_y, and f_z that should be zero. Fig.9 shows the results of FFT analysis for the same data of the forces f_{sx}, f_x, f_y and f_z. Fig.9 shows that the amplitude of the signal f_{sx} in the frequency ranges of up to approximately 20 Hz is almost canceled by the acceleration forces.

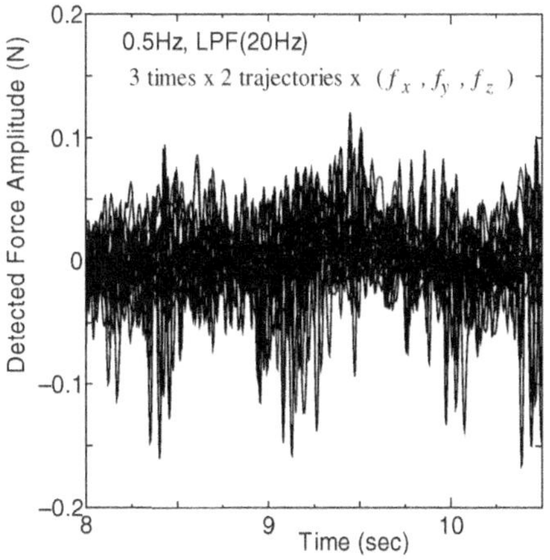

Fig. 10. Detected force amplitude for hand starts oscillating severely no-contact condition, i.e. measurement error

As shown in Fig.8, the accelerationsensor output a_{sx} follows the force f_{sx} without phase lag of the signal, even though the robot and with large amplitude after approximately 9 seconds. However, the large amplitude of the resonance frequency of 7-8 Hz gives the largest error for the detected force f_x. In Fig. 8, the four arrows indicate two types of amplitude A_{fsx}, A_{asx} for the force f_{sx} and the acceleration a_{sx}, and for frequency 0.5 Hz and 7-8 Hz, respectively. The ratio (amplitude $A_{fsx7\text{-}8}$ of the force f_x at a frequency 7-8 Hz) /(amplitude $A_{fsx0.5}$ of the force f_x at a frequency of 0.5 Hz) is approximately 1.3 times of that ($A_{asx7\text{-}8}$ /$A_{asx0.5}$) of the acceleration a_{sx}. This makes the detected force errors large. This is a future problem that must be solved in order to improve fine force detection.

Fig.10 shows the detected forces f_x, f_y, and f_z for trajectories "a" and "b", and for three measurements. The amplitude of the detected force for no-contact condition corresponds to the measurement error of the system. The amplitude of the force is in the range of approximately 0.05-0.1 N, for every kind of the forces.

5 Conclusion

In order to feed back the contact force of a surgical instrument to the surgeon in a laparoscopic surgical robot system, the overcoat method has been previously proposed by one of authors. This method requires cancellation of the acceleration force of the instrument/holder. In the present study, the authors attempted to use acceleration sensors to estimate the acceleration forces of the instrument/holder, and the following results were obtained. The cancellations performed using the acceleration sensors can provide a force-detection accuracy of approximately 0.05-0.1 N for a dynamic range of up to approximately 20 Hz.

The cancellation method examined herein improved the dynamic response range to 20 Hz from 1 Hz by using robot motion for calculating the acceleration of the instrument/holder.

References

1. R. H. Taylor, J. Funda, B. Eldridge, S. Gomory, K. Gruben, D. LaRose, M. Talamini, L. Kavoussi, and J. Anderson:A Telerobotic Assistant for Laparoscopic Surgery,IEEE Engineering in Medicine and Biology, Vol. 14, No. 3, pp. 279-288 (1995).
2. A. J. Madhani, G. Niemeyer and J. K. Salisbury Jr.,The Black Falcon: A Teleoperated Surgical Instrument for Minimally Invasive Surgery, Proc. IEEE Int. Conf. Intelligent Robots and Systems, pp.936-944 , 1998.
3. Ulrich Seibold, Gerd Hirzinger, A 6-Axis Force/Torque Sensor Design for Haptic feedback in minimally invasive robotic surgery, Proc. of the 2nd VDE World Microtechnologies Congress, October, 2003
4. S.Shimachi, A. Oguni, and A. Hashimoto:Assist Robot System for Laparoscopic Surgery (Feedback Performance on the Forceps Load), Proc. 36th JSME Spring Annual Meeting at Tohoku Branch, pp. 88-89 (2001) (in Japanese).
5. S.Shimachi,Y.Hakkozaki,T.Tada,Y.Fujiwara, Measurement of force acting on surgical instrument for force-feedback to master robot console, CARS2003 (Elsevier), pp538-546
6. S.Shimachi, Y.Fujiwara, Y.Hakkozaki, New sensing method of force acting on instrument for laparoscopic robot surgery, CARS2004 (Elsevier), pp775-780

Development of the Needle Insertion Robot for Percutaneous Vertebroplasty

S. Onogi[1], K. Morimoto[1], I. Sakuma[1], Y. Nakajima[2], T. Koyama[3], N. Sugano[3], Y. Tamura[4], S. Yonenobu[4], and Y. Momoi[5]

[1] Graduate School of Frontier Sciences, The University of Tokyo, Japan
[2] Intelligent Modeling Laboratory, the Univeristy of Tokyo, Japan
[3] Graduate School of Medicine, Osaka University, Japan
[4] Osaka Minami Medical Center, Japan
[5] Hitachi Ltd

Abstract. Percutaneous Vertebroplasty (PVP) is an effective and less invasive medical treatment for vertebral osteoporotic compression fractures. However, this operative procedure is quite difficult because an arcus vertebra, which is narrow, is needled with accuracy, and an operator's hand is exposed to X-ray continuously. We have developed a needle insertion robot for Percutaneous Vertebroplasty. Its experimental evaluation on the basic performance of the system and needle insertion accuracy are presented. A needle insertion robot is developed for PVP. This robot can puncture with accuracy and an operator does not need to be exposed to X-ray. The mechanism of the robot is compact in size (350 mm $\times$ D 400 mm $\times$ H270 mm, weight: 15 kg) so that the robot system can be inserted in the space between C-arm and the patient on the operating table. The robot system is controlled by the surgical navigation system where the appropriate needle trajectory is planned based on pre-operative three-dimensional CT images. The needle holding part of the robot is X-ray lucent so that the needle insertion process can be monitored by fluoroscopy. The position of the needle during insertion process can be continuously monitored. In vitro evaluation of the system showed that average position and orientation errors were less than 1.0 mm and 1.0 degree respectively. Experimental results showed that the safety mechanism called mechanical fuse released the needle holding disk properly when excessive force was applied to the needle. These experimental results demonstrated that the developed system has the satisfactory basic performance as needle insertion robot for PVP.

1 Introduction

Percutaneous Vertebroplasty(PVP) is an effective treatment for vertebral osteoporotic compression fractures (Figure 1). In this technique, the surgeon inserts one or two bone biopsy needles into fractured vertebral body, and injects semi-liquid plastic cement called bone cement into the vertebral body through the needle. After injection the bone cement hardens, the vertebra is stabilized. In

J. Duncan and G. Gerig (Eds.): MICCAI 2005, LNCS 3750, pp. 105–113, 2005.

this treatment technique, it is one of the most important procedure that the surgeon inserts needle into vertebra precisely. Because the spinal cord and nerves exist through the vertebra, if the surgeon injures nerves by the needle, it will cause critical accidents such as a partial paralysis of the patients. The surgeon must insert needles along appropriate trajectory that locates in a narrow space of pedicle of arch of vertebra. Thus, surgeons must have considerably high skill and experiences in order to control the position of needle. When the needle is inserted percutaneously, the surgeon uses X-ray fluoroscopy to confirm the position of needle resulting in continuous exposure of surgeon's hand to X-ray. A new engineering assistance is required to improve the reliability, accuracy, and safety of this procedure.

In order to improve the above-mentioned subject, we have developed a needle insertion robot for PVP (Figure 2)[1]. Cleary et al. developed needle insertion robot for nerve and facet blocks under X-ray fluoroscopy[2]. Compared with robot for nerve and facet blocks, the robot for PVP must generate larger insertion force to make the needle penetrate cortical bone of vertbra. On the other hand, the size of the robot must be compact. In this report, design of the developed needle insertion robot for percutaneous vertebroplasty, its experimental evaluation on the basic performance of the system and needle insertion accuracy are presented. The positioning accuracy of the robot itself was evaluated and the safety mechanism in case of excessive applied force was also tested. Finally, accuracy of needle insertion of the robot under image guidance was evaluated using a vertebra model.

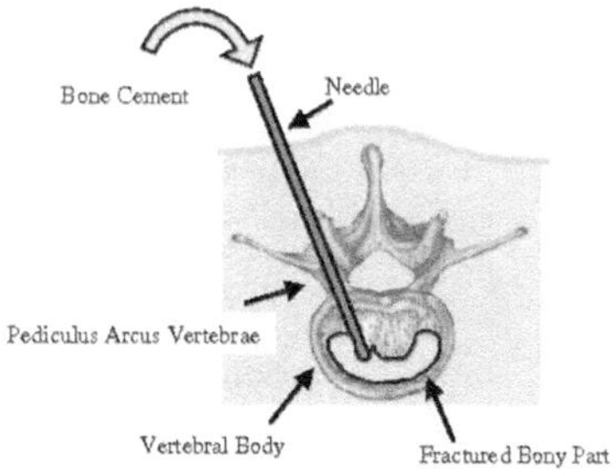

Fig. 1. Percutaneous Vertebroplasty

2 Materials and Methods

Design of the Needle Insertion Robot

The developed robot has the following features:

1. The robot is rigid enough to generate required needle insertion force.
2. The robot is compact so that the robot system (needle positioning mechanism, needle insertion and rotation mechanism) can be inserted in the space between C-arm and the patient on the operating table. We have also developed an X-ray lucent operating table made of carbon reinforced fiber materials (Mizuho Ltd., Japan).
3. The needle holding part of the robot is X-ray lucent so that the needle insertion process can be monitored by fluoroscopy (Figure 3).
4. The position and orientation of the needle can be adjusted with five degrees of freedom in three-dimensional space.

5. The robot system is controlled by the surgical navigation system where the appropriate needle trajectory is planned based on pre-operative three dimensional CT images.
6. The safety mechanism that avoid injury of the patient by the needle when excessive force is applied to the needle due to malfunction of the system.

The needle insertion robot is shown in Figure 2. The robot consists of three parts: 1) Rough positioning mechanism, 2) Accurate positioning mechanism, 3) Puncture mechanism. The rough positioning mechanism does not have any actuator. It has only electro-magnetic brake to fix two joints. (X, and Y in Figure 4). It positions the accurate positioning mechanism and puncture mechanism in two-dimensional plane parallel to the operation bed surface. One actuated translational positioning mechanism is used to position the mechanism in z direction shown in Figure 4.

The accurate positioning mechanism has four degrees of freedom for determination of orientation and position of the puncture mechanism: two DOF for to perpendicular translational motions (±10 mm in s[1] and s[2] direction shown in Figure 4) and two DOF for rotating motions around two axis intersecting with each other at right angle (±30 degrees in α and ±5 degrees in β shown in

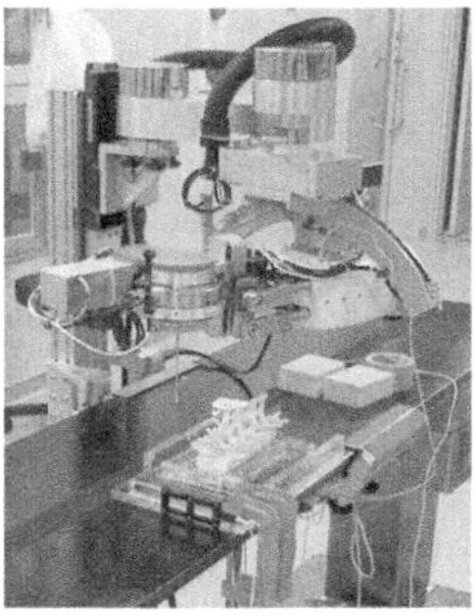

Fig. 2. Developed Needle Insertion Robot

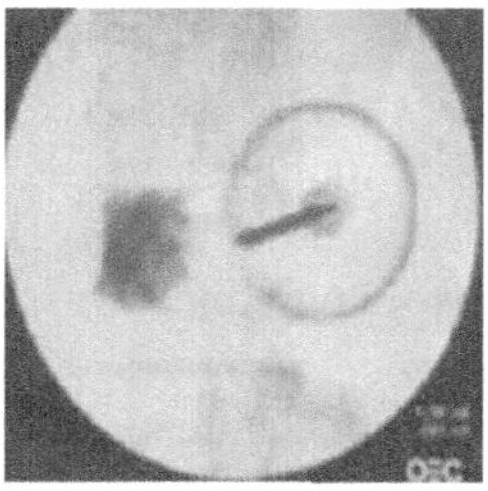

Fig. 3. C-arm X-ray image of the robot which has radiolucent

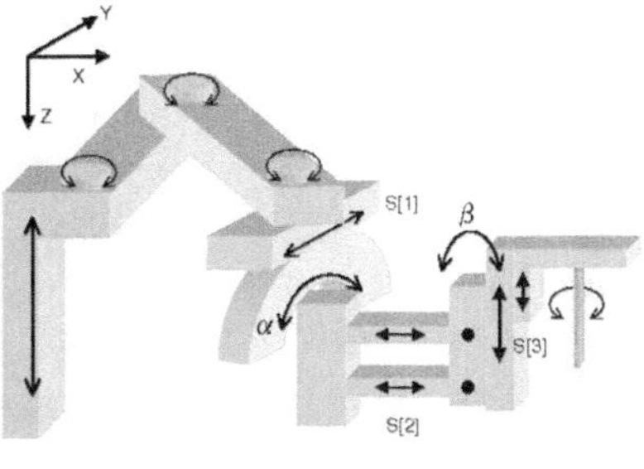

Fig. 4. Robot Mechanism

Figure 4). R-guide was used to realize the rotation for α axis, and remote center of motion mechanism consisting of two linear actuation mechanism was used to reduce the thickness of the mechanism[3].

The puncture mechanism inserts the needle into the patients (shown as s[3] in Figure 4) and rotates the needle in reciprocal manner with amplitude of 120 degrees. The stroke and resolution of the needle insertion mechanism are 110 mm and ± 0.2 mm respectively (Figure 4). The holder is a plastic disk fixed to cylindrical part made of stainless steel that is rotated by a DC motor. Inner diameter of the cylinder is 52 mm. We can observe the position of needle by intra operative X-ray fluoroscopy through the cylinder. Surgeon can monitor the position of the tip of the needle during needle insertion process. It also has a force/torque sensor to measure the force applied on the robot during needle insertion. It is reported that the axial force during needle insertion to human vertebra preserved under formalin fixation. And it is reported that the forces did not exceed 25 N when feed rate of the needle was 0.05-0.5 mm/s. We designed the needle insertion mechanism to generate up to 60 N of axial force.

This robot has safety mechanism, called "Mechanical Fuse" (Figure 5). The needle was fixed on the disk plate. The holder grasps the disk with four contacting parts supported by springs as shown in Figure 6. When unexpected excessive force is applied to a needle, the disk comes off from the holder to avoid possible damage to the patient.

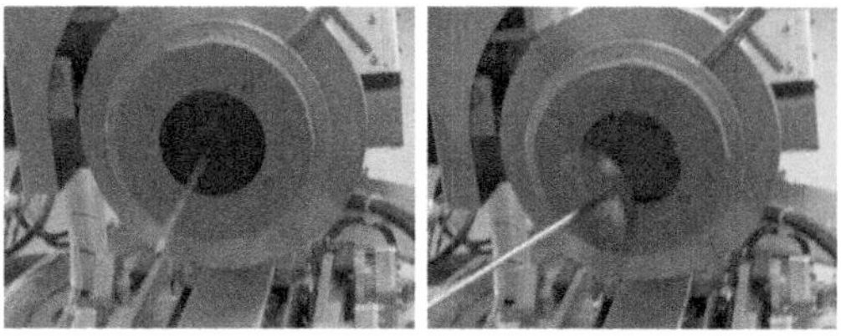

Fig. 5. Left: Normal setting, Right: Situation of Needle comes off by Mechanical Fuse

The entire mechanism was designed to be fixed to the operating table. The size of the entire mechanism was 350 mm $\times$ D 400 mm $\times$ H270 mm, and its weight was 15 kg. It can be inserted in the space between C-arm of the patient on the operating table as shown in Figure 7.

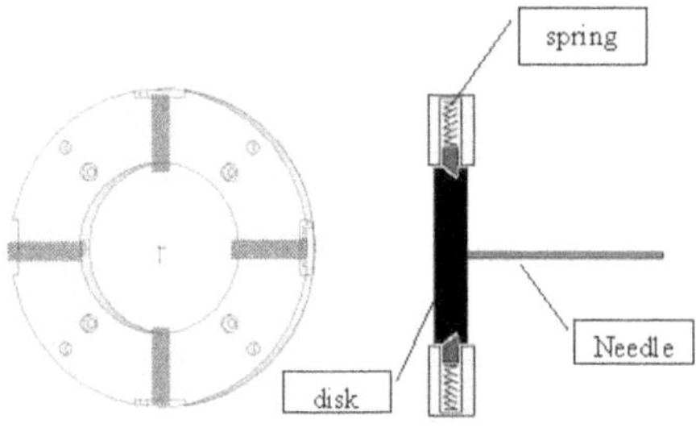

Fig. 6. Mechanism of the Mechanical Fuse

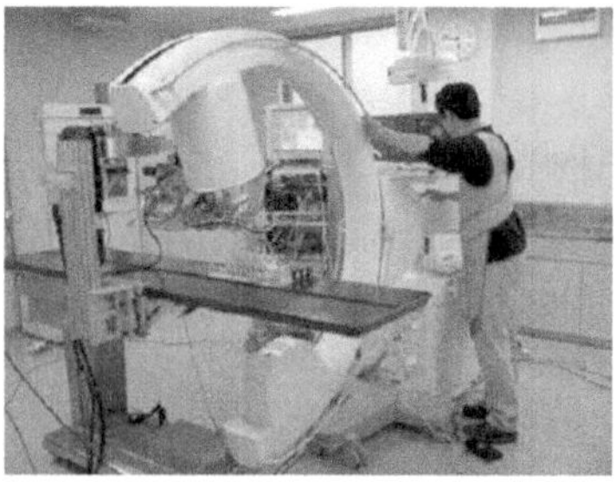

Fig. 7. The robot can be installed between a patient and C-Arm X-Ray Equipment

Description of Control System

Next, control system is shown in Figure 8. The system consists of the following three devices: 1) Needle Insertion Robot, 2) Navigation System([4]), 3) Optical Position Sensor (Optotrak, NDI, Canada). The robot is connected the navigation system by LAN cable (TCP/IP). And the navigation system is connected with an optical Position Sensor by serial cable (RS232C). The navigation system sends the position and orientation data to the robot. The robot drives the target position and orientation using this data by software.

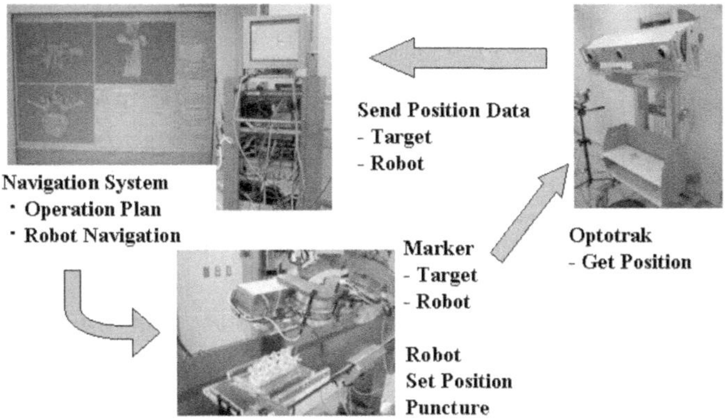

Fig. 8. Total System

Evaluation of Needle Positioning Accuracy

In this study, three experiments were conducted. First experiment is accuracy evaluation of the robot positioning ability. Target values in robot coordinate system were input to the robot and errors between target values and real values which were measured with a position sensor (Polaris, NDI, Canada) placed at the needle insertion mechanism. The errors were evaluated for various points and orientations in the range of motion of the robot.

Second experiment was evaluation of the Mechanical Fuse. The needle was hold by a material-testing instrument with force sensor. The force was applied along the needle and from the direction perpendicular to the needle. The force applied to the needle when the disk came off from the holder was recorded.

Third experiment is evaluation of needle insertion accuracy as a entire system including positioning errors due to needle insertion robot, surgical navigation system, and optical position sensor using a vertebra model (Sawbones, Pacific Research Laboratories, USA). (Figure 9). Three dimensional computer model of the vertebra model was obtained based on its

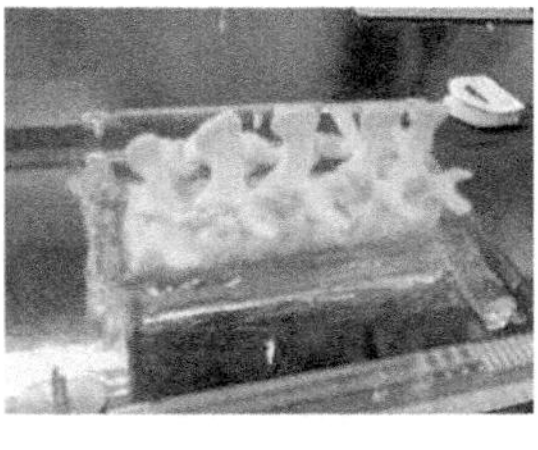

Fig. 9. Polyurethane Vertebra Phantom

CT data. The surface registration was used for surgical navigation [5,6,7,8]. The total errors between target values and determinate needle positions were measured by comparing the planned positions of the needle insertion mechanism and measured position data obtained by the optical position sensor. CT data after the needle insertion was also obtained to identify the difference between the actual needle trajectory and needle insertion plan for one case of the experiments.

The operation with this robot has three stages. At first stage, rough position is set manually. Second, accurate position is set automatically by interaction with the navigation system. Third, needle is inserted to a vertebra.

3 Results

Accuracy Evaluation of the Robot Positioning

Accuracy evaluation is performed on each axis. Result is shown in Table 1. All axes are satisfied requested specifications. However, errors of axis X and Z are somewhat large.

Next, target values in a robot coordinate system are inputted the robot. Result is shown in Table 2. In this case, all axes are satisfied requested specifications, too.

Evaluation of the Mechanical Fuse

Force along the insertion direction larger than 50 N made the disk came off the holder. Needle holding disk came off when force larger than 3 N was applied at the tip of the needle perpendicular to the needle direction. To simulate the possible situation in clinical setting, position of the vertebra model after initial needle insertion was shifted purposely by manual. The needle came off by mechanical fuse successfully. When a vertebra model is moved suddenly, the needle came off from the robot, too.

Evaluation of Puncture in a Vertebra Model

The target value is set by the navigation system with CT image of pre-operation. The position and orientation errors before and after contacting the model were shown in Table 3. The contact of the needle was detected by the force sensor signals from the system.

X-ray images of one vertebra model used in the experiments were obtained by CT to identify the position of holes created by the needle. The position and trajectory of the needle insertion was evaluated as the center of the respected

Table 1. Accuracy evaluation result of each axis (n=)

X (n=15)	Y (n=15)	Z (n=12)	α (n=36)	β (n=27)
0.54 mm	0.09 mm	0.80 mm	0.25 deg	0.41 deg

Table 2. Accuracy evaluation result of multiple axes

	Ave.	SD	Max. Err.
X[mm] (n=675)	-0.437	0.325	-1.197
Y[mm] (n=900)	-0.158	0.197	-0.675
Z[mm] (n=1428)	-0.540	0.361	-1.476
α[deg] (n=2448)	0.122	0.0448	0.230
β[deg] (n=279)	0.138	0.0661	0.364

Table 3. Result of Puncture Experiment

		Average Error ± SD	Maximum Error	Minimum Error
Pre-Puncture (n=10)	Position [mm]	0.80 ± 0.29	1.13	0.31
	Orientation [deg]	0.06 ± 0.08	0.21	0.00
Contact (n=8)	Position [mm]	0.81 ± 0.40	1.51	0.41
	Orientation [deg]	0.20 ± 0.26	0.80	0.03

volume due to needle insertion. The difference between the planned position and the entry point of the needle at the surface was 0.21 mm and the orientation error was 0.9 deg.

4 Discussion

The developed robot is compact enough to be set in the space between C-arm and operating table, while being able to generate required force for needle insertion to vertebra. It can insert 10 G needle into porcine vertebra sample with surrounding tissue and skin (data not shown.) Thus, it can generate enough force for PVP.

In accuracy evaluation, the robot is satisfied requested specifications (error less than 1 mm). The reason that errors of axis X and Z are somewhat large is mechanism of X-axis for small size. We used a remote center of motion mechanism consisting of two linear actuation mechanisms to reduce the thickness of the mechanism placed in the space between the C-arm of the fluoroscopy and operating table. This deteriorates positioning accuracy of the robot. However, since required positioning accuracy was satisfied as a whole. The system has enough positioning accuracy for PVP.

The Mechanical Fuse functioned as designed. For further validation of the mechanical fuse, experiments simulating possible disturbances observed in actual clinical situations to confirm the safety of the system. In addition to the mechanical safety measures, we have to develop the software to stop the system when the abnormal needle force is detected in the embedded force sensors in the system.

In total system error evaluation experiments, average of error is satisfied requested specifications (position error less than 1 mm and orientation error less than 1 deg). However, there was a case of the error exceeding required specification. We have to investigate the possible causes of errors to reduce the total positioning accuracy. Another possible factor not evaluated in the present study is the slip of the needle tip at the contact to the cortical bone. When the surface of the vertebra is inclined, the needle may slip from the appropriate insertion position. Thus the appropriate needle insertion plan must be designed to reduce the possibility of needle slip based on the geometrical information of the vertebra. Although the system can be inserted into the space between the C-arm and patient on the operating table, the system must be further miniaturized for ease of operation for easier setting and operation. We will analyze the cause of errors and optimize the mechanical design.

5 Conclusion

We have developed a needle insertion robot for Percutaneous Vertebroplasty. Its experimental evaluation on the basic performance of the system and needle insertion accuracy is presented. This robot can puncture with accurate and an operator does not need to be exposed to X-ray. The mechanism of the robot is compact in size (350 mm × D 400 mm × H270 mm, weight: 15 kg) so that the robot system can be inserted in the space between C-arm of the patient on the operating table. The position and orientation of the needle can be adjusted with five degrees of freedom in three-dimensional space. The robot system is controlled by the surgical navigation system where the appropriate needle trajectory is planned based on pre-operative three-dimensional CT images. The needle holding part of the robot is X-ray lucent so that the needle insertion process can be monitored by fluoroscopy. The position of the needle during insertion process can be continuously monitored. In vitro evaluation of the system showed that average positioning and orientation errors were less than 1.0 mm and 1.0 degree respectively. Experimental results showed that the safety mechanism called mechanical fuse released the needle holding disk properly when excessive force was applied to the needle. These experimental results demonstrated that the developed system has the satisfactory basic performance as needle insertion robot for PVP.

Acknowledgement. This study was partly supported by "Research for the Future Program JSPS-RFTF 99I00904"

References

1. Matsumiya, K.: Proc. miccai 2003. Medical Image Computing and Computer-Assisted Intervention (2003) 271–278
2. Cleary, K., Stoianovici, D., Patriciu, A., Mazilu, D., Lindisch, D., Watson, V.: Robotically assisted nerve and facet blocks. Academic Radiology (2002) 821–825
3. Kim, D., Kobayashi, E., Dohi, T., Sakuma, I.: A new, compact mr-compatible surgical manipulator for minimally invasive liver surgery. Lecture Notes in Computer Science **2488** (2002) 99–106

4. Nakajima, Y., Yamamoto, H., Sato, Y., Sugano, N., Momoi, Y., Sasama, T., Koyama, T., Tamura, Y., Yonenobu, K., Sakuma, I., Yoshikawa, H., Ochi, T., Tamura, S.: Available range analysis of laser guidance system and its application to monolithic integration with optical tracker. CARS 2004, Chicago, USA (2004-06)
5. Besl, P.J., Mckay, N.D.: A method for registration of 3-d shapes. IEEE Trans. Pattern Anal. Machin. Intell. **14** (1992) 239–256
6. Simon, D., Hebert, M., Kanade, T.: Techniques for fast and accurate intrasurgical registration. The Journal of Image Guided Surgery **1** (1995) 17–29
7. C.R.Maurer, J.Maciunas, J.M.Fitzpatrick: Registration of head ct images to physical space using a weighted combination of points and surfaces. IEEE Trans. Med. Imag. **17** (1998) 753–761
8. R.Bächler, H.Bunke, L.P.Nolte: Restricted surface matching–numerical optimization and technical evaluation. Computer Aided Surgery **6** (2001) 143–152

Laparoscope Self-calibration for Robotic Assisted Minimally Invasive Surgery

Danail Stoyanov[1], Ara Darzi[2], and Guang-Zhong Yang[1,2]

[1] Royal Society/Wolfson Foundation Medical Image Computing Laboratory
[2] Department of Surgical Oncology and Technology
Imperial College of Science, Technology and Medicine, London SW7 2BZ, UK
{danail.stoyanov, a.darzi, g.z.yang}@imperial.ac.uk
http://vip.doc.ic.ac.uk

Abstract. For robotic assisted minimal access surgery, recovering 3D soft tissue deformation is important for intra-operative surgical guidance, motion compensation, and prescribing active constraints. We propose in this paper a method for determining varying focal lengths of stereo laparoscope cameras during robotic surgery. Laparoscopic images typically feature dynamic scenes of soft-tissue deformation and self-calibration is difficult with existing approaches due to the lack of rigid temporal constraints. The proposed method is based on the direct derivation of the focal lengths from the fundamental matrix of the stereo cameras with known extrinsic parameters. This solves a restricted self-calibration problem, and the introduction of the additional constraints improves the inherent accuracy of the algorithm. The practical value of the method is demonstrated with analysis of results from both synthetic and *in vivo* data sets.

1 Introduction

With the maturity of master-slave robotic manipulators, the clinical applications of minimally invasive surgery (MIS) are rapidly advancing. Robotic assistance provides enhanced instrumental control and intuitive 3D manipulation of the operating field, and advanced systems can include image guidance, motion compensation and active constraints. For MIS involving large soft tissue deformation, intraoperative guidance with patient specific anatomy presents a significant challenge and reliable 3D reconstruction of soft-tissue deformation *in situ* is essential [1]. The prerequisite of this for optical methods, however, is accurate and robust camera calibration. Existing research has shown that after calibration and feature correspondence, it is possible to perform real-time 3D reconstruction of soft tissue deformation with stereo laparoscope cameras [2].

Thus far, preoperative calibration for robotic assisted MIS is generally achieved with a calibration object [3] based on the assumption that during the operation the intrinsic parameters of the laparoscope remain fixed. This, however, is not true for complex procedures as for example in thoracoscopic surgery, where parameters such as the focal length may change in order to optimize the surgical field-of-view. In such cases, frequent recalibration of the laparoscope is not feasible and *in situ* self-calibration is the only practical way forward. Hitherto, self-calibration has received

J. Duncan and G. Gerig (Eds.): MICCAI 2005, LNCS 3750, pp. 114 – 121, 2005.

extensive interest in computer vision and most existing techniques assume a rigid world, which can be viewed from a number of different positions [4]. For continuously deforming scenes, however, such temporal constraints are invalid and only inter-stereo epipolar geometry can be used to derive camera parameters. Hartley [5] has shown that the focal lengths of the stereo camera can be extracted from the fundamental matrix by using Singular Value Decomposition (SVD) and a number of other techniques based on the same constraint have also been developed [6,7]. Brooks *et al.* [8] demonstrated that in a typical stereo configuration, the problem is degenerate for cameras with different focal lengths [9]. Strum [10] subsequently provided a detailed analysis for deriving matching focal lengths of the cameras based on epipolar geometry, and outlined the potential singularities when variable focal lengths were used [11].

It has been recognized that the above methods are susceptible to noise in the proximity of singularities. Frahm *et al* [12] proposed a method based on known rotations between views and using one epipole for embedding the unknown translations. Earlier work by Stein [13] and McLaughlin *et al* [14] also used partial knowledge of rotation to restrict the problem. These techniques, however, are not specifically designed for stereo camera setups and can result in complex formulations with additional degenerate configurations. Whilst for many vision systems critical motion can be avoided through appropriate setups, this is not the case for stereo laparoscopes where the camera arrangement is on a much smaller scale to assist the 3D perception of the surgeon. The purpose of this paper is to develop a parameterization scheme for the intrinsic parameters of the stereo laparoscope based on the epipolar constraint with known intrinsic parameters. This simplifies the traditional self-calibration to an over determined problem with respect to focal lengths. We demonstrate that the problem is solvable with a minimum of two correspondences and the stability of the algorithm to different noise levels can be further improved by using a robust estimator. The practical value of the technique is demonstrated with both numerical simulation and *in vivo* robotic assisted MIS data.

2 Methods

2.1 Stereoscopic Laparoscope Model

It is assumed in this study that the stereo laparoscope cameras follow the standard pinhole model, with which the mapping of a point $\mathbf{M} = [X \quad Y \quad Z \quad W]^T$ in projective 3D space onto the corresponding image point $\mathbf{m} = [x \quad y \quad w]^T$ can be described up to a scale by a matrix multiplication with homogeneous coordinates:

$$\mathbf{m} \sim \mathbf{PM} \tag{1}$$

where $\sim$ denotes equality up to scale. The matrix $\mathbf{P}$ is the camera's projection matrix and may be decomposed into the intrinsic and extrinsic camera parameters:

$$\mathbf{P} = \mathbf{K}[\mathbf{R} \mid -\mathbf{RC}] \tag{2}$$

The camera orientation and position with respect to a reference coordinate system are expressed by a rotation matrix $\mathbf{R}$ and a translation vector $\mathbf{t} = -\mathbf{RC}$, where $\mathbf{C}$ is the location of the optical center. The upper triangular matrix $\mathbf{K}$ encompasses the focal length, f, skew, s, aspect ratio, μ, and the image coordinates of the principal point, $[u, v]$:

$$\mathbf{K} = \begin{bmatrix} f & s & u \\ & \mu f & v \\ & & 1 \end{bmatrix} \tag{3}$$

Without a loss of generality, the camera matrices for the stereoscopic laparoscope can be represented with the following equation by taking the left camera as the reference coordinate system:

$$\mathbf{P} = \mathbf{K}[\mathbf{I} \mid \mathbf{0}] \ \textit{and} \ \mathbf{P}' = \mathbf{K}'[\mathbf{R} \mid \mathbf{t}] \tag{4}$$

The inherent relationship between the left and right camera frames is described by the epipolar geometry, which is algebraically encapsulated by the fundamental matrix, $\mathbf{F}$ [15]. The fundamental matrix is a rank two matrix, defined up to scale and thus it has seven degrees of freedom. Its dependency on the camera parameters can be expressed as:

$$\mathbf{F} \sim \mathbf{K}'^{-\mathrm{T}}\left([\mathbf{t}]_{\times} \mathbf{R}\right)\mathbf{K}^{-1} \sim \mathbf{K}'^{-\mathrm{T}}\mathbf{E}\mathbf{K}^{-1} \tag{5}$$

where $[.]_{\times}$ is used to denote a skew symmetric matrix and $\mathbf{E}$ is the essential matrix defined by the rotation and translation between the cameras [15]. For corresponding image points (points which are projections of the same 3D world point), $\mathbf{F}$ can be used to express the constraint:

$$\mathbf{m}'^{\mathrm{T}}\mathbf{F}\mathbf{m} = 0 \tag{6}$$

Given sufficient corresponding points (eight or more for a unique solution) the fundamental matrix can be determined from Eq. (6) and this is the basic knowledge about the camera geometry, which can be directly obtained from the images.

2.2 Self-calibration with Varying Focal Lengths

Without prior knowledge about the cameras, Eq. (5) is governed by 15 unknowns, and the seven degrees of freedom of the fundamental matrix are insufficient to provide a solution for the camera parameters from a single pair of stereo images. In robotically assisted MIS, however, it is feasible to calibrate the stereoscopic laparoscope before the procedure. Therefore, the knowledge about the initial extrinsic and intrinsic parameters of the cameras can be used to simplify Eq. (5) for deriving a solution for the varying focal length problem. By assuming all parameters except for the focal lengths are known, Eq. (5) can be written as:

$$\tilde{\mathbf{F}} \sim \mathit{diag}(1,1,f')\mathbf{E}\mathit{diag}(1,1,f) \sim \begin{bmatrix} e_{11} & e_{12} & e_{13}f \\ e_{21} & e_{21} & e_{13}f \\ e_{31}f' & e_{31}f' & e_{13}ff' \end{bmatrix} \tag{7}$$

For computing $\tilde{\mathbf{F}}$ based on Eq. (6), the coordinates of the corresponding image points are normalized by the known intrinsic parameters to $\tilde{\mathbf{m}}$ and $\tilde{\mathbf{m}}'$ [15]. Since the knowledge of the essential matrix is also available from the initial calibration, Eq. (7) yields a bilinear equation with respect to the focal length for each point correspondence:

$$\begin{aligned}&\left(xy'e_{21}+xw'e_{31}\right)f+\left(wx'e_{13}+wy'e_{23}\right)f'+ww'e_{33}ff'=\\&xx'e_{11}+xy'e_{21}+yx'e_{12}+yy'e_{22}\end{aligned} \tag{8}$$

It is evident that the above equation can be solved from a minimum of two correspondences. But in practice, the problem is likely to be over determined and may be solved in a least-squares sense. The minimum solution required is important, however, to robust estimation schemes such as the random sampling consensus (RANSAC) approach [15], which outperform linear methods in the presence of noise. We have therefore used an approach analogous to the RANSAC estimation of the fundamental matrix using the minimum solution obtained from Eq. (8). With the proposed technique, inliers are determined using the first-order approximation to the geometric re-projection error:

$$\sum_i \frac{\left(\tilde{\mathbf{m}}_i'^{T}\tilde{\mathbf{F}}\tilde{\mathbf{m}}_i\right)^2}{\left(\tilde{\mathbf{F}}\tilde{\mathbf{m}}_i\right)_1^2+\left(\tilde{\mathbf{F}}\tilde{\mathbf{m}}_i\right)_2^2+\left(\tilde{\mathbf{F}}^{\mathsf{T}}\tilde{\mathbf{m}}_i'\right)_1^2+\left(\tilde{\mathbf{F}}^{\mathsf{T}}\tilde{\mathbf{m}}_i'\right)_2^2} \tag{9}$$

The number of samples used in the robust estimation is determined adaptively and once the desired solution is determined, Eq. (9) is used as a cost function to refine the estimated focal lengths by using the Levenberg-Marquardt algorithm. With the proposed framework, incremental changes of the known extrinsic parameters, as well as shifts of the principal points, can also be incorporated in the minimization procedure.

It can be shown that the practical critical motion (extrinsic configuration of the stereo cameras for which the solution is degenerate) for the proposed method is when the optical axis are parallel. This configuration is a generic singularity for most existing methods, which results in a reduced version of the fundamental matrix so that Eq. (8) cannot be solved. In practice, however, the stereo laparoscope is always setup with a small vergence angle to assist stereoscopic fusion of the surgeon with the left and right visual channels. Although this naturally avoids the singularity problem, it is important to note that the cameras can be in proximity of the degeneracy.

2.3 Numerical Validation and *In vivo* Experiment

To assess the general performance of the proposed method, particularly in the vicinity of the singular configuration, a synthetic test data set was used. In this experiment, the left and right cameras started from a degenerate position with parallel image planes with optical axes as shown in **Fig. 1**. We varied the vergence angle, θ, from zero with increasing steps up to ten degrees. In this configuration, the problem can be unstable [8] as the e_{33} element of the essential matrix is zero, and therefore there is a single

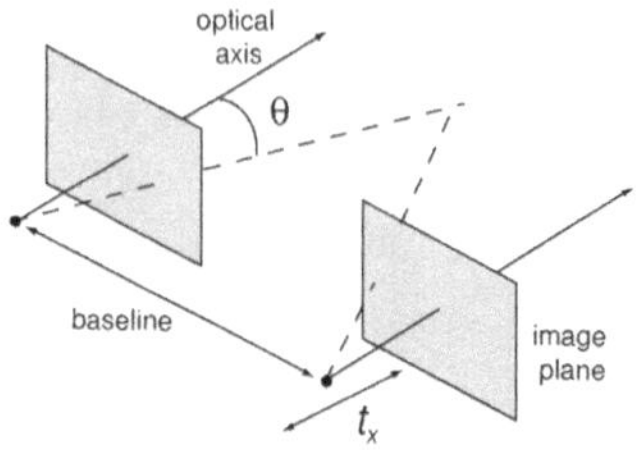

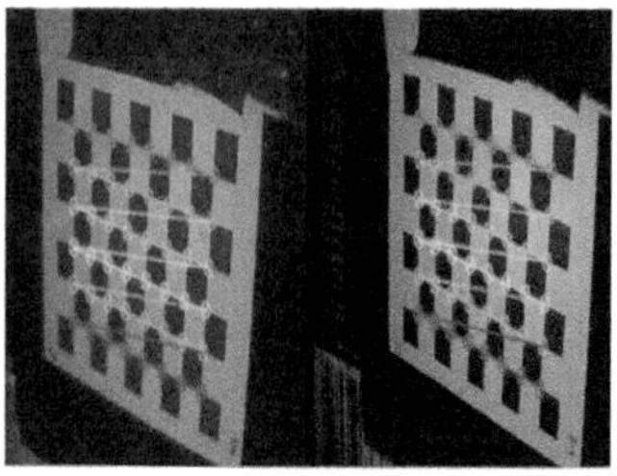

(a) (b)

Fig. 1. (a) A schematic illustration of the setup used for synthetic simulation. **(b)** An example stereo view of the calibration grid used for deriving the ground truth data.

linear solution for Eq. (8) when only two correspondences are available. For numerical validation, a total of 100 random 3D points in the viewing volume in front of the cameras were used, and the projection of each point in the image planes was corrupted by additive zero mean Gaussian noise with standard deviation varied from zero to two pixels. The effect of error with known extrinsic parameters was analyzed also by corrupting the known vergence angle and baseline with zero mean Gaussian noise with standard deviation varying from zero to two in units of degrees and millimeters, respectively. We performed a total of 100 trials for each noise level and the mean estimation was used for final analysis.

For *in vivo* validation of the proposed technique, a surgical procedure with the daVinci™ surgical robot was used. The ground truth of the calibration data was obtained by using a planar grid method [17] before the insertion of the laparoscope into the patient. The proposed algorithm was used to intraoperatively compute the focal length of the stereo system. Image correspondences were obtained by using a variant of the stereo feature matching algorithm described by Pilu [18]. With this experiment, the focal lengths of the cameras were altered during the procedure in order to validate the proposed method. The ground truth parameters were recalculated immediately after the change of parameters by removing the stereo laparoscope out of the patient for recalibration.

3 Results

In **Fig. 2,** we demonstrate the overall performance of the proposed method as the cameras rotate about their own vertical axis forming a vergence angle. **Fig. 2 (a)** shows the results of solving Eq. (8) by using a least-squares-method (LSM), whereas **Fig. 2 (b)** shows the corresponding results by using the robust algorithm. It is evident that in the presence of noise, the robust algorithm clearly out-performs LSM and it retains a good accuracy in the vicinity of degeneracy.

In **Fig. 3,** the effects of noise in the known extrinsic parameters are analyzed for the proposed calibration method by varying stereo vergence angle. It is evident that the algorithm performed well in the presence of significant errors in the baseline and rotation angles. Similarly to **Fig. 2**, the algorithm is also relatively robust in the neighborhood of the singular camera configuration.

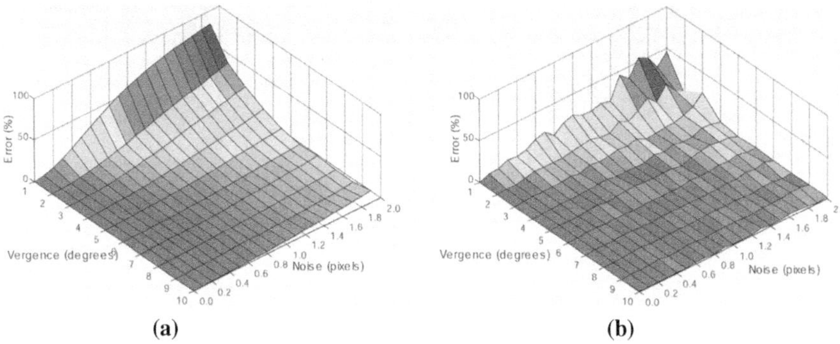

Fig. 2. Average percentage errors in focal length estimation by varying vergence angle near the singularity point with noise corrupted synthetic data. (**a**) Results with least-squares solution using SVD, and (**b**) results with the proposed robust algorithm.

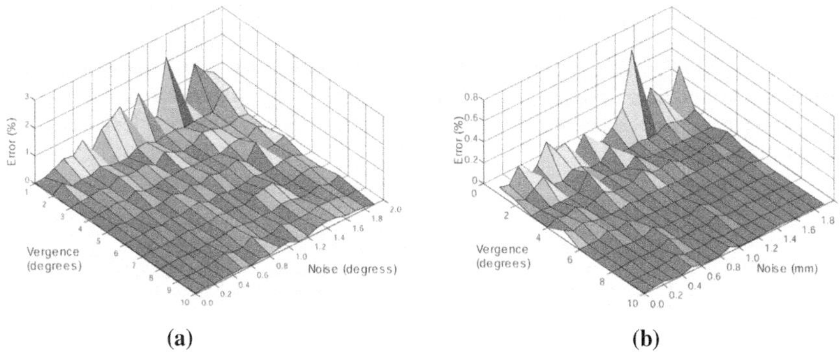

Fig. 3. Percentage errors in focal length estimation w.r.t. noise in the known extrinsic parameters of (**a**) vergence angle, (**b**) baseline

The results obtained from *in vivo* experiment are listed in **Fig. 4.** For the calculation of the ground truth calibration data, the intrinsic accuracy of the method had a pixel reprojection error of 0.12 pixels, and a reconstruction error of 0.78 mm. **Fig. 4 (b)** demonstrates the estimated focal lengths over the acquired video sequence, where the solid lines correspond to the ground truth data. It is clear from **Fig. 4** that after the change in camera focal length, the algorithm is able to reliably quantify the shift involved. For providing a detailed statistical analysis of data, **Fig. 5** illustrates the standard deviation of focal length estimation for the left laparoscope camera before and after the change in focal length. The shaded region outlines the standard deviation of the derived focal length value in every 0.4s window of the video sequence. The variance in the estimation is dominated by the accuracy of feature matching in the stereo pair, which can vary for images with many specular highlights or significant motion blurring from caused instrument or tissue movement.

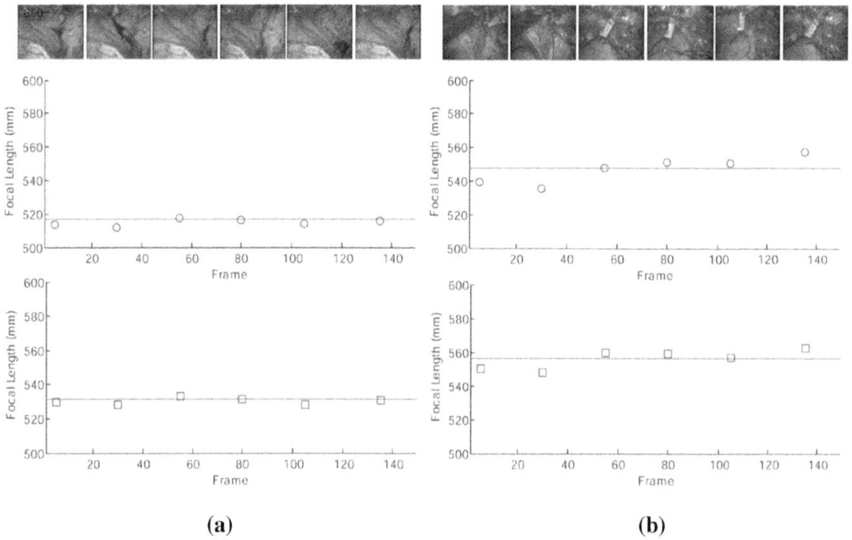

Fig. 4. *In situ* calibration results for a robotic assisted MIS video where the ground truth is shown as a solid red line. Columns **(a)** and **(b)** show the changes in focal length during the operation. The circular and square markers represent the estimations of the focal lengths of the left and right cameras, respectively.

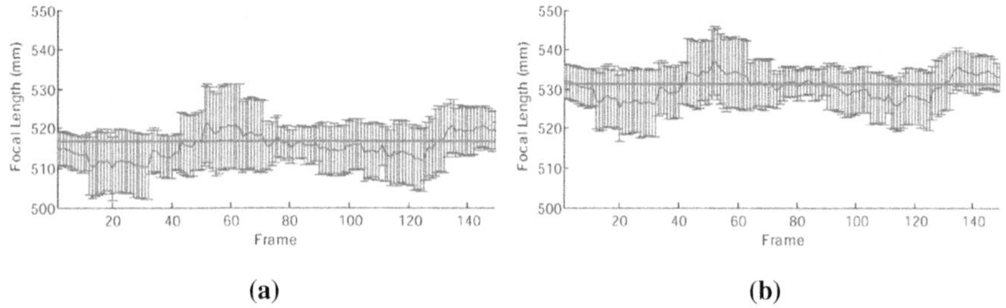

Fig. 5. The standard deviation of focal length estimation for the left stereo laparoscope camera before (a) and after (b) focal length change (the estimation window was set to be 0.4s)

4 Discussion and Conclusions

In this paper, we have proposed a practical method for intra-operatively determining the varying focal length of stereo laparoscopes. The validity of the method has been demonstrated on both synthetic and *in vivo* data. The results indicate the high accuracy obtained despite the near singular arrangement of the cameras. The performance of the algorithm against noise of the known extrinsic parameters, suggests that it may be possible to fully calibrate the system in different surgical procedures by using a prior estimate of the camera parameters. Thus far, approaches to self-calibration typically involve temporal constraints over rigid multi-view geometry. Due to extensive deformation of the soft tissue, constraints can only be enforced across two-view inter-stereo epipolar geometry for robotic MIS procedures. The proposed method represents a first step towards active calibration of changing camera parameters during surgery, and the results derived have shown the robustness of the technique in proximity of the generic degeneracy and against noise influence.

References

1. Taylor, R. H., Stoianovici, D.: Medical Robotics in Computer-Integrated Surgery. IEEE Transactions on Robotics and Automation, (19):765-781, 2003.
2. Stoyanov, D., Darzi, A., Yang, G-.Z.: Dense 3D Depth Recovery for Soft Tissue Deformation During Robotically Assisted Laparoscopic Surgery. In: Proc. MICCAI, 41-48, 2004.
3. Morgues, F., Coste-Manière, È.: Flexible calibration of actuated stereoscopic endoscope for overlay in robot assisted surgery. In: Proc. MICCAI, 2488, 24-34, 2002.
4. Pollefeys, M.: Self-Calibration and Metric 3D Reconstruction from Uncalibrated Image Sequences. PhD Thesis, Katholieke Universiteit Leuven, Belgium, 1999.
5. Hartley, R. I.: Estimation of Relative Camera Positions for Uncalibrated Cameras. In: Proc. ECCV, 579-587, 1992.
6. Bougnoux, S.: From Projective to Euclidean Space under Any Practical Situation, A Criticism of Self-Calibration. In: Proc. ICCV, 790-796, 1998.
7. Kanatani, K., Matsunaga, C.: Closed Form Expressions for Focal Lengths from the Fundamental Matrix. In: Proc. ACCV, 128-133, 2000.
8. Brooks, M.J., De Agapito, L., Huynh, D.Q., Baumela, L.: Towards Robust Metric Reconstruction Via A Dynamic Uncalibrated Stereo Head. Image and Vision Computing, (16):989-1002, 1998.
9. De Agapito, L., Huynh, D. Q., Brooks, M. J.: Self Calibrating a Stereo Head: An Error Analysis in The Neighbourhood of Degenerate Configurations. In: Proc. ICCV, 747-753, 1998
10. Sturm, P.: On Focal Length Calibration from Two Views. In: Proc. CVPR, 145-150, 2000.
11. Sturm, P.: Critical Motion Sequences for the Self-Calibration of Cameras and Stereo Systems with Variable Focal Length. Image and Vision Computing, (20):415-426, 2002.
12. Frahm, F., Koch, R.: Camera Calibration with known Rotation. In: Proc. ICCV, 1418-1425, 2003.
13. Stein, F.: Accurate Internal Camera Calibration Using Rotation with Analysis of Sources of Error. In: Proc. ICCV, 230 - 236, 1995.
14. McLauchlan, P. F., Murray, D. W.: Active camera calibration for a head-eye platform using the variable state-dimension filter. IEEE Transactions on Pattern Analysis and Machine Intelligence, (18):15-22, 1996.
15. Hartley, R., Zisserman, A.: Multiple view geometry in computer vision. Cambridge University Press. 2000.
16. Zhang, Z.: A flexible new technique for camera calibration. IEEE Transactions on Pattern Analysis and Machine Intelligence, (22):1330-1334, 2000.
17. Pilu, M.: A Direct Method for Stereo Correspondence based on Singular Value Decomposition. In: Proc. CVPR, 261-266, 1997.

A Hand-Eye Robotic Model for Total Knee Replacement Surgery

Fanhuai Shi[1], Jing Zhang[1], Yuncai Liu[1], and Zijian Zhao[2]

[1] Inst. Image Processing & Pattern Recognition,
Shanghai Jiao Tong University,
Shanghai 200030, P.R. China
{fhshi, zhjseraph, whomliu}@sjtu.edu.cn
[2] School of Information Science & Engineering, Shandong University,
Jinan 250100, P.R. China
zhaozijian@sdu.edu.cn

Abstract. This paper presents a hand-eye robotic model for total knee replacement (TKR) surgery. Unlike existent robot assisted TKR surgery, the proposed model is a surgical robot that combines with a movable hand-eye navigation system, which would use the full potential of both computer-assisted systems. Without using CT images and landmark pins in the patient's bones, it can directly measure the mechanical axis with high precision. This system provides a new approach of the minimally invasive surgery. Experiment results show that the proposed model is promising in the future application.

1 Introduction

Total knee replacement (TKR) surgery is a common orthopaedic procedure to replace damaged articular surfaces of the knee with prosthetic implants. To fit the prosthesis, each of the knee bones (tibia, femur and patella) should be cut to a specific shape to mate the mounting side of the corresponding prosthesis component. To ensure normal functionality of the knee, all components must be placed onto the bones with high precision. For this aim, we must consider both the bone axes and the mating surfaces between the bone and prosthesis [1].

During the operation, traditionally, a complex jig system composed of cutting blocks, alignment rods, etc., is used to help the surgeon to estimate the geometry of the bones and select the appropriate size and location of the components. The accuracy of this process relies on the surgeon's individual experience. Besides, the traditional jig-based systems also introduce several sources of inaccuracy in alignment of the prosthetic components [2]. The limitations of traditional knee surgery have prompted the research for a more accurate and repeatable system for TKR.

The rapid development of robotics provides a new approach to improve the surgery quality. Due to the rigid nature of bone, it is relatively easy to image in computed X-ray tomography (CT) and X-ray fluoroscopy [3]. So orthopaedics suits for robotic assistance. Moreover, robot assisted TKR can enhance the quality of the bone cuts and require less time for surgery [2].

J. Duncan and G. Gerig (Eds.): MICCAI 2005, LNCS 3750, pp. 122 – 130, 2005.

1.1 Related Work

There are already commercially available surgical robots for joint replacement surgery, such as ROBODOC [4] and CASPAR [5]. Both systems adapted industrial robots for surgical task and were initially aimed at hip replacement. Unfortunately, they still require additional surgery to preimplant fiducial markers. ROBODOC recently started using an anatomical registration procedure [6]. Researchers in Imperial College, London developed a "hands-on" robot, called Acrobot, for TKR surgery [1]. Intraoperatively, the surgeon guides the special-purpose robot, which is mounted on a gross positioning device. Acrobot uses active constraint control to constrain the motion of the cutter to a predefined region, and thus allows the surgeon to safely cut the knee bones with high precision. Nevertheless, all the above systems need to take plenty of CT images for registration.

The technology of knee replacement is evolving, changing, and improving. Laskin and Richard [7] described some new techniques and concepts in TKR, especially Minimally Invasive Surgery (MIS). A good approach for MIS is the use of a CT-free image-guided system, which usually based on optically tracked surgical tools with a visual display of the bone models to aid in the positioning and alignment of tools. Aesculap Inc. has developed Unveils OrthoPilot, which is the industry's first CT-free navigation system for orthopedic surgery and has been routinely used in orthopaedic surgery [8]. Other commercialized systems include BrainLab's (BrainLab, Germany), Stryker Leibinger's (Leibinger, Germany), and PiGalileo (PLUS Orthopedics USA, Inc.). These navigation systems, however, while helping to improve accuracy, should not be moved during the operation, which greatly constrains the field of view of the optic sensors. In brief, we call such system as static navigation system. More recently, DiGioia et al. provided rich review of these relevant technologies in [9].

1.2 Contributions of This Paper

In this paper, we propose a hand-eye robotic model for TKR surgery. In this model, both the optic sensors and the cutting tool are fixed on the end-effecter/gripper of a surgical robot, which can be moved freely to anywhere within the capability of the robot. Thus, we combine the surgical robot and navigation system together, which would use the full potential of both computer-assisted systems. As the navigation system can move while the robot gripper is moving, we call it a movable navigation system. The remainder of this paper decomposes as follows. Section 2 recalls the target problem in TKR surgery. Then the proposed model is presented in detail in section 3. Section 4 describes how to use the proposed model for TKR surgery. Some experiments on performance test are conducted in section 5.

2 Problem Formulation

Let's revisit the target problem in TKR surgery. Shown as Fig. 1(a), the normal mechanical axis of the leg is formed by a straight line starting from the center of the femoral head B, passing through the center of the knee joint O and ending at the center of the ankle C. The transverse axis passing through the joint is parallel to the floor when

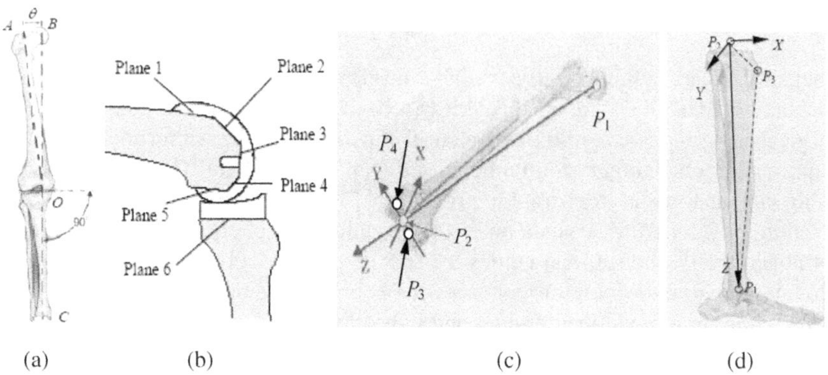

Fig. 1. Main task of TKR surgery. (a) Restoration of the mechanical axis. (b) Surface of the bone to be cut. (c) Femoral positioning and measure. (d) Tibia positioning and measure.

one stands. The angle θ between the normal mechanical axis *OB* and the axis of the femur canal *OA* is about 5°~ 9° [10]. The aim of TKR surgery is to restore the normal mechanical axis and create a joint plane, which is vertical to the mechanical axis, while sacrificing minimal bone stock and maximizing collateral ligament. Thus, shown in Fig. 1(b), five planes on the distal femur (plane 1-plane 5) and one plane on tibia (plane 6) must be cut to fit on prosthesis components. Therefore, there are mainly two tasks in the TKR surgery: one is the precise measurement of the mechanical axis and the other is the accurately milling of the fitting plane. The former task is especially dependent on the accuracy of the navigation system.

Unfortunately, the mechanical axis is not directly measurable by the surface of the femoral, tibia, or deforming joint. For example, present methods of measuring *OB* firstly figure out the axis of the femur canal *OA*, and then make a rotational alignment of 5°~ 9°. This kind of alignment heavily depends on the experience of the surgeons.

3 Techniques of the New Model

In this paper, we propose a flexible hand-eye robotic model, in which the navigation system can directly measure the mechanical axis without using CT images or other indirect ways. In contrast to previous navigation system for orthopaedic surgery, which uses static navigation system, a hand-eye, special-purpose robot, called WATO, has been built for a movable navigation and operation in TKR surgery. Besides, the cutting tool is fixed on the end-effecter of the robot, which would use the full potential of both computer-assisted systems.

3.1 System Configuration

The WATO is a 6-DOF industrial robot (MOTOMAN) with the cutting tool and a pair of CCD cameras attached on the end-effecter. After the stereo rig is precisely calibrated, we mount an infrared filter on each camera. Thus, we get an infrared stereovision system, see Fig. 2. In order to make precise measuring on the bone, some infrared positioning devices, such as infrared marker and infrared probe, are developed.

3.2 Positioning and Measuring in the Surgery

Positioning and measuring are the most important and difficult technology in TKR surgery. Traditional mechanical guidance relies heavily on an individual surgeon's experience with a given jig system. CT-based image-guidance system has greatly promoted the measure in robot assisted TKR surgery. However, early approach requires an additional surgery to implant several metal pins into the bone and the later developed noninvasive anatomical registration method is time-consuming.

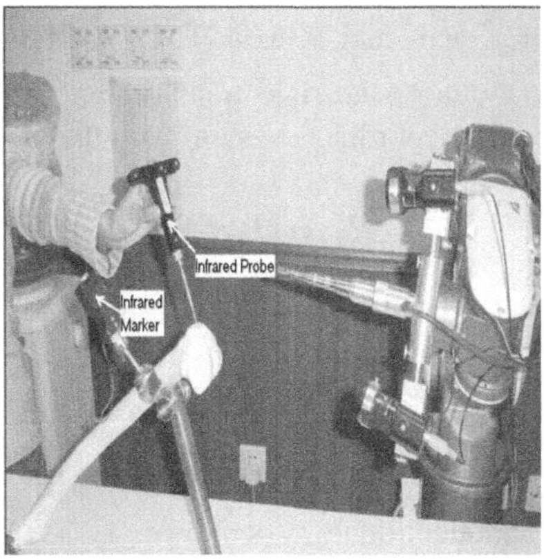

Fig. 2. WATO Experimental System

In WATO system, neither CT models nor metal markers on the patient's bone are needed. Instead, an infrared guide system is used which consists of a binocular vision system and its associated infrared marker/probe. Several special infrared emitters are embedded in the infrared probe, whose 3-D coordinates can be detected by the binocular vision system. After the infrared probe calibration, the position of the probe tip relative to those diodes can be obtained. Therefore, when the probe picks up a space point, the position of infrared diodes can be detected and then the position of the probe tip. To build femoral and tibia coordinate system, surgeons are requested to detect some physiological marks on patient's bone by probe. Fig. 2 shows a probe that was used in WATO system. Similar to infrared probe, the infrared marker also consists of some infrared emitters and is clamped on the distal femur or tibia. According to the relationship between the marker and the bone, the motion of the bone can be monitored by the vision system. We will explain it in detail in the following.

Femoral measure. Sufficient surgical exposure is needed to fix the infrared marker, surgeons instead of robot complete this procedure. After surgical exposure, we clamp an infrared marker on the distal femur, see Fig. 2.

In the jig-based surgery, see Fig. 1(a), a baseline axis AO is first measured by inserting a T-rod into the femoral canal. Then they can restore the mechanical axis BOC by adjust AO 5°~ 9°. In WATO system, however, the axis BOC can be acquired directly. Shown as Fig. 1(c), P_1 is the center of the femoral head, P_2 is the center of intercondylar fossa, P_3 is the epicondylus medialis, and P_4 is the epicondylus lateralis. With the infrared marker clamped on the femur, the surgeon manually flexes and abducts the entire leg (which is able to rotate only about the femoral head) through substantial arcs, while the hand-eye navigation system observing the position of the infrared marker. As the detected positions of the infrared emitters are on a sphere whose center is also the center of the femoral head, then we can obtain the coordinate of P_1. It is important that the surgeon must take special care during the pivot motion with the femur and not to move the pelvis, which would invalidate the pure rotation. This approach is inspired by the work of Kienzle et al. [2]. Meantime, the coordinates of P_2, P_3 and P_4 can be obtained by infrared probe. Straight line P_1P_2 is equivalent to the mechanical axis BOC in Fig. 1(a). Take the center of intercondylar fossa P_2 as the origin, $\overrightarrow{P_1P_2}$ as the direction of Z axis, the cross product of the vectors $\overrightarrow{P_3P_4}$ and $\overrightarrow{P_1P_2}$ as the direction of X axis. Then one can obtain the direction of Y axis by cross product of Z axis and X axis. Thus, the femoral coordinate system P_2 - XYZ is constructed. We denote the rigid transformation between the femoral coordinate system and the camera coordinate system with the couple (R_{fc}, t_{fc}), and then we have

$$R_{fc} = [\overrightarrow{P_3P_4} \times \overrightarrow{P_1P_2}, \overrightarrow{P_1P_2} \times (\overrightarrow{P_3P_4} \times \overrightarrow{P_1P_2}), \overrightarrow{P_1P_2}], t_{fc} = \overrightarrow{P_2} \tag{1}$$

The transformation from camera to gripper (R_{cg}, t_{cg}) can be obtained by hand-eye calibration [11] in advance and the transformation from gripper to robot base (R_{gr}, t_{gr}) can be computed from the recorded gripper pose. After constructing femoral coordinate system, we can obtain the relationship (R_{fr}, t_{fr}) between the femur and the robot coordinate system by

$$\begin{bmatrix} R_{fr} & t_{fr} \\ 0 & 1 \end{bmatrix} = \begin{bmatrix} R_{gr} & t_{gr} \\ 0 & 1 \end{bmatrix} \begin{bmatrix} R_{cg} & t_{cg} \\ 0 & 1 \end{bmatrix} \begin{bmatrix} R_{fc} & t_{fc} \\ 0 & 1 \end{bmatrix} \tag{2}$$

Therefore, any point $(x_f, y_f, z_f)^T$ in the femoral coordinate system can be transformed to the coordinate $(x_r, y_r, z_r)^T$ in robot base as

$$(x_r, y_r, z_r)^T = R_{fr} \cdot (x_f, y_f, z_f)^T + t_{fr} \tag{3}$$

In making surgical plans, a planning software is used to interactively decide prosthesis size according to the sampled data of individual patient's femur. Then the placement of the prosthesis and cutting quantity could be estimated automatically. All the data in femoral coordinate system are transformed to the data in robotic coordinate system, then the robot are controlled to perform bone resection with special designed cutting tool.

Tibia measure. Similar to femoral positioning, as shown in Fig. 1(d), surgical exposure of the tibia is made by surgeons in advance and then the infrared marker is clamped onto the distal tibia. Since the mechanical axis passes through the center of the knee joint and ends at the center of the ankle, tibia coordinate system must be constructed in accordance with this axis. Firstly, the positions of the physiology fiducial mark of malleolus medialis and malleolus lateralis are sampled by using infrared probe. We assume that the mid-point of the two points is the center of ankle joint. In the similar way, surgeons can obtain the position of 1/3 part on the tuberculum intercondylare mediale (P_2) and tuberositas tibiae (P_3). Define the plane $P_1P_2P_3$ formed by tuberculum intercondylare mediale, center of ankle and tuberositas tibiae. We define the direction of vector $\overrightarrow{P_2P_1}$ as the direction of Z axis. The line in plane

$P_1P_2P_3$ which is perpendicular to Z axis is defined as the direction of X axis. Then Y axis is the cross product of Z and X axis. So we have constructed tibia coordinate system. After constructing tibia coordinate system, we can obtain the relationship between the two coordinate systems of tibia and infrared marker. When the infrared marker is combined with the tibia, the pose monitoring and resection of it are similar to the way of femur.

3.3 Visual Servoing in the Surgery

In the surgery, the milling track of the cutting tool can be planned in advance. However, in conventional system, patient is not fixed completely during the whole operation. Consequently, when unwanted micro-movements of the leg occurs during robotic surgery, the surgical plan must be re-designed, which is time-consuming. In order to deal with this problem, the traditional method is trying to fix the patient's leg and an alarming device is mounted on the patient's leg. For example, in ROBODOC TKR system [6], bony spiculas are fitted into the femur and tibia to guarantee the patient's leg unmovable. However, in TKR surgery, it often requires a different flexion angle of the knee in order to find an optimal pose for operation. Once the patient's leg is fixed completely, the surgeons will have some trouble in operation especially in an emergency. All the above disadvantages constrain the applications of such systems.

The above problems have been solved in WATO system when we fix the infrared markers onto the bones. During the surgery, the passive markers are constantly monitored by the cameras, so does the associated femur or tibia coordinate system. In this way, a position-based visual servoing system [12] comes into being. In CASPAR system, the movement of the leg is also monitored by an infrared camera system [5], however, it is based on a static navigation system. When the navigation system keeps tracking the position and orientation of the infrared marker (or the bone), the movement of the bone will not affect the bone resection, which guarantee a safe operation. Besides, as the position-based visual servo in the system needs only simple stereo computation, it performs much faster than that of registration between CT model and the patient's bone. The refresh time of the visual servoing system is less than 0.2 second, which can fulfill the surgical requirement.

4 System Operation

To apply our model to TKR surgery, the basic steps are as follows.

Preoperative procedures

1. Mount two cameras and the cutting tool (a milling cutter) on the end-effector/gripper of the robot (see Fig. 2). Calibrate the stereo rig (camera calibration) and the transformation relationship between the robot gripper and the stereo rig (hand-eye calibration).
2. Mount an infrared filter on each camera. Calibrate the infrared probe using the stereo rig and find the 3-D position of the probe tip in the probe coordination system.
3. Carry out the sterilize process.

Surgical procedures

1. Immobilize the pelvis using specially designed fixtures and clamped the infrared markers onto the distal femur. Find the center of the femoral head using the method described in section 3.2.
2. Use the infrared probe to determine the coordinate of the physical fiducial marks on the distal femur in order to construct the femur coordinate system.
3. Use planning software to interactively decide the prosthesis size and placement.
4. Use the robot to guide the surgical cuts for placement of the femoral component.
5. Clamp the infrared marker on the tibia and use the similar method as that of femur to construct the tibia coordinate system.
6. Use the robot to guide the surgical cuts for placement of the tibia component.

5 Performance Test of the Navigation System

The hand-eye navigation system is the most distinctive part in the proposed model. In this section, we test the performance of the navigation system with two different measurement schemes. First, a fixed infrared marker was used to test the calibration accuracy of the stereo rig and the hand-eye relationship. In the second test, we use a calibrated infrared probe to sample the crossings of a chessboard, which will test the positioning accuracy of the infrared probe, see Fig. 4.

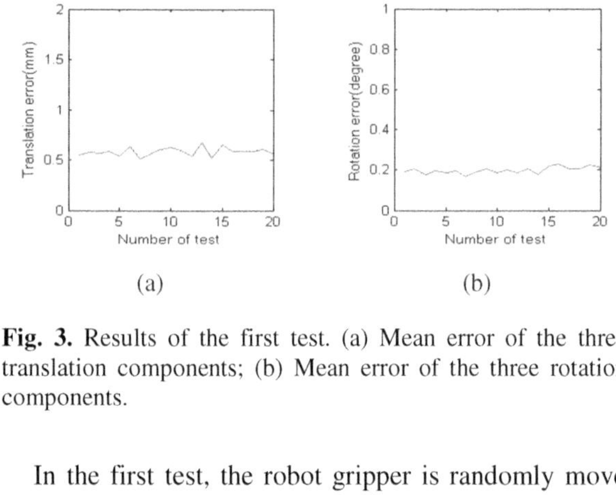

(a) (b)

Fig. 3. Results of the first test. (a) Mean error of the three translation components; (b) Mean error of the three rotation components.

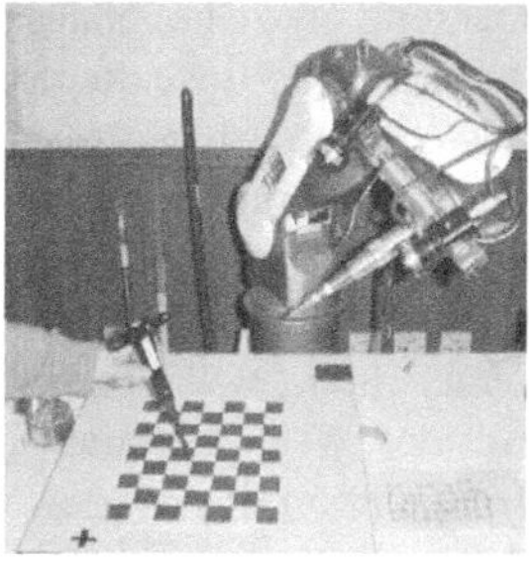

Fig. 4. Positioning test with the infrared probe

In the first test, the robot gripper is randomly moved to 30 different positions to observe a static infrared marker and each recorded gripper pose is denote as $P_i = (X_i, Y_i, Z_i, RX_i, RY_i, RZ_i)$, i=1,2,...,30; repeat the test for 20 times. X_i, Y_i, Z_i are the translation components and RX_i, RY_i, RZ_i are the three pose angles of robot gripper. Then camera motion B_j (j=1,2,...,29) between frame i and frame i+1 can be calculated according to pose of the infrared marker. Then, from the basic equation of robotic hand-eye relationship $A_j X_0 = X_0 B_j$ [11], where X_0 is the relation between robotic gripper and cameras, the gripper motion A_j can be obtained. Notice that $P_{i+1} = P_i A_j$, we can obtain a sequence of calculated robotic positions $\tilde{P}_{i+1}$. We compare the translation part and rotation angle of P_{i+1} with that of $\tilde{P}_{i+1}$ respectively. Shown as

Fig. 3, the mean error is illustrated in solid line, in which mean error of the translation part is 0. 58 mm, the standard deviation is 0.44 mm, while rotation angle is 0.19 degree and 0.17 degree respectively.

In another test, a calibrated infrared probe is used to sample the crossings of a chessboard, where the real distance *d* between crossings is known. The distance between crossings that calculated from the 3-D coordinates sampling by the probe is *d*'. Here, the coordinates sampled by the probe are all in the camera coordinate system. We randomly move the chessboard to 10 locations with different translation and orientation while keeping the cameras or the robot gripper static. In each location, 40 pairs of crossings are sampled. To qualify the results, we take RMS of the error $\|d-d'\|$. The mean error is 0.40 mm.

From the experimental results, we can see that a goal of less than 0.6 mm of translational error and less than 0.2 degree of rotational error is achievable, which means that WATO can fulfill the requirement of the TKR surgery.

6 Summary and Future Work

A new robot assisted surgical model (WATO) is proposed for TKR in this paper. Unlike existent solutions, WATO is a surgical robot that combines together with a movable, hand-eye navigation system. Without using CT images and landmark pins in the patient's bones, WATO can directly measure the mechanical axis with high precision, which affords a new approach for the development of the minimally invasive surgery. Experimental results show that WATO is promising in the future application.

However, there are still some places to be improved. The present infrared marker needs too much surgical exposure to fix on the femur, which increases the invasiveness of the procedure. So, we need to design more efficient clamps to fix the infrared marker. In addition, as the proximity of the camera to the cutting tool, some splash-guard and vibration control mechanism should be considered in the future.

References

[1] Jakopec M., Baena F. R. Y., Harris S. J., Gomes P., Cobb J., and Davies B. L.: The Hand-On Orthopaedic Robot 'Acrobot': Early Clinical Trials of Total Knee Replacement Surgery. IEEE Trans. Robot. Automat. 19(5):902-911,2003.

[2] Kienzle, T.C., III; Stulberg, S.D.; Peshkin, M.; Quaid, A.; Lea, J.; Goswani, A.; Wu, C.-h.: Total Knee Replacement. IEEE Engineering in Medicine and Biology Magazine, 14(3): 301-306, 1995.

[3] Taylor R. H. and Stoianovici D.: Medical Robotics in Computer- Integrated Surgery. IEEE Trans. Robot. Automat. 19(5):765-781, 2003.

[4] Taylor R. H., Paul H.A., Kazandzides P., Mittelstadt Hanson B. D.,W., Zuhars J. F., Williamson B., Musits B. L., Glassman E., and Bargar W. L.: An image-directed robotic system for precise orthopaedic surgery. IEEE Trans. Robot. Automat., vol. 10, pp. 261-275, Apr. 1994.

[5] Siebert W., Mai S., Kober R., Heeckt P.F.: Technique and first clinical results of robot-assisted total knee replacement. The Knee. 9(3): 173-180, 2002.

[6] Wiesel U., Lahmer A., Tenbusch M., and Borner M.: Total knee replacement using the ROBODOC system. in Proc. 1st Annu. Meeting CAOS Int., Davos, Switzerland, 2001, p. 88.
[7] Laskin, Richard S. MD.: Session IV, New Techniques and Concepts in Total Knee Replacement. Clinical Orthopaedics & Related Research. 1(416): 151-153, November 2003.
[8] Sundaraj, K.; Laugier, C.; Boux de Casson, F.: Intra-operative ct-free examination system for anterior cruciate ligament reconstruction. Proc. IEEE/RSJ International Conference on Intelligent Robots and Systems, Oct. 2003, Vol. 3, pp:2829-2834.
[9] DiGioia A. M., Jaramaz B., Picard F., and Nolte L. P.: Computer and Robotic Assisted Hip and Knee Surgery. Oxford University Press, 2004.
[10] Gray M. Ferguson, M.D., Richard J. Friedman, M.D. and FRCS(C): Foundation Knee System Primary Surgical Technique, Encore Orthopedics, Inc. 1999.
[11] Andreff N., Horaud R., and Espiau B.: Robot hand-eye calibration using structure from motion. Int. J. Robot. Res., 20(3):228-248, 2001.
[12] Hutchinson, S., Hager, G. D., and Corke, P. I.: A tutorial on visual servo control. IEEE Trans. Robot. Automat. 12(5):651-670, 1996.

Robot-Assisted Image-Guided Targeting for Minimally Invasive Neurosurgery: Planning, Registration, and In-vitro Experiment

R. Shamir[1], M. Freiman[1], L. Joskowicz[1], M. Shoham[2,3], E. Zehavi[3], and Y. Shoshan[4]

[1] School of Eng. and Computer Science, The Hebrew Univ. of Jerusalem, Israel
[2] Dept. of Mechanical Engineering, Technion, Haifa, Israel
[3] Mazor Surgical Technologies, Caesarea, Israel
[4] Dept. of Neurosurgery, School of Medicine, Hadassah University Hospital, Israel
josko@cs.huji.ac.il

Abstract. This paper present a novel image-guided system for precise automatic targeting in keyhole minimally invasive neurosurgery. The system consists of a miniature robot fitted with a mechanical guide for needle/probe insertion. Intraoperatively, the robot is directly affixed to a head clamp or to the patient skull. It automatically positions itself with respect to predefined targets in a preoperative CT/MRI image following an anatomical registration with a intraoperative 3D surface scan of the patient facial features. We describe the preoperative planning and registration modules, and an in-vitro registration experiment of the entire system which yields a target registration error of 1.7mm (std=0.7mm).

1 Introduction

Precise targeting of tumors, lesions, and anatomical structures with a probe or a needle inside the brain based on preoperative CT/MRI images is the standard of care in many keyhole neurosurgical procedures. The procedures include tumor biopsies, catheter insertion, deep brain stimulation, aspiration and evacuation of deep brain hematomas, and minimal access craniotomies. Additional procedures, such as tissue and tumor DNA analysis, and functional data acquisition, are rapidly gaining acceptance and also require precise targeting. These minimally invasive procedures are difficult to perform without the help of support systems that enhance the accuracy and steadiness of the surgical gestures.

Four types of support systems for keyhole neurosurgery are currently in use: 1. stereotactic frames; 2. interventional imaging systems; 3. navigation systems, and; 4. robotic systems. Stereotactic frames provide precise positioning with a manually adjustable frame rigidly attached to the patient skull. These extensively used frames provide rigid support for needle insertion, and are relatively accurate and inexpensive ($< 1mm$, USD 50K). However, they require preoperative implantation of frame screws, head immobilization, and manual adjustment during surgery. They cause patient discomfort and do not provide real-time validation. Interventional imaging systems produce images showing the actual needle

J. Duncan and G. Gerig (Eds.): MICCAI 2005, LNCS 3750, pp. 131–138, 2005.

position with respect to the predefined target [1,2,3]. Their key advantage is that they account for brain shift. A few experimental systems also incorporate optical real-time tracking and robotic positioning devices. However, their nominal and operational costs are high and their availability is very limited. Furthermore, brain shift is a secondary issue in keyhole neurosurgeries.

Navigation systems (e.g., Medtronic, USA and BrainLab, Germany) show in real time the location of hand-held tools on the preoperative image onto which targets have been defined [4,5,6]. Augmented with a manually positioned tracked passive arm (e.g., Phillips EasyTaxis^{TM}), they also provide mechanical guidance for targeting. While these systems are now in routine clinical use, they are costly (USD 250K), require head immobilization and maintenance of line-of-sight for tracking, and additional time for registration and manual arm positioning.

Robotic systems provide frameless stereotaxy with a robotic arm that automatically positions itself with respect to a target defined in the preoperative image [7,8,9,10]. Registration between the image and the intraoperative situation is done by direct contact or with video images. Two floor-standing commercial robots include NeuroMate^{TM} (Integrated Surgical Systems, USA) and PathFinder^{TM} (Armstrong HealthCare, UK). Their advantages are that they are rigid, accurate, and provide a frameless integrated solution. However, since they are bulky, cumbersome, and costly (US 300K), they are not commonly used.

2 System Overview and Protocol

We are developing a novel image-guided system for precise automatic targeting of structures inside the brain that aims at overcoming the limitations of existing solutions [11]. The system automatically positions a mechanical guide to support keyhole drilling and insertion of a needle or probe based on predefined entry point and target locations in a preoperative CT/MRI image. It incorporates the miniature MARS robot (Mazor Surgical Technologies) [12,14], originally developed for orthopaedics, mounted on the head immobilization clamp or directly on the patient skull via pins (Fig. 1). Our goal is a robust system for keyhole neurosurgical procedures which require clinical accuracy of 1–1.5mm.

The key idea is to establish a common reference frame between the preoperative CT/MRI image and the intraoperative patient head and robot locations with an intraoperative 3D surface scan of the patient's facial features. Once this registration has been performed, the transformation that aligns the planned and actual robot targeting guide location is computed. The robot is then automatically positioned and locked in place so that its targeting guide axis coincides with the entry point/target axis.

The system hardware consists of: 1) the MARS robot and its controller; 2) a custom robot mounting base, targeting guide, and registration jig; 3) an off-the-shelf 3D surface scanner, and; 4) a standard PC. MARS is a $5 \times 8\text{cm}^2$ cylinder, 250–gram six-degree-of-freedom parallel manipulator with workvolume of about 10cm^3 and accuracy of 0.1mm. It operates in semi-active mode; when locked, it is rigid and can withstand lateral forces of up to 10N [13]. The adjustable robot

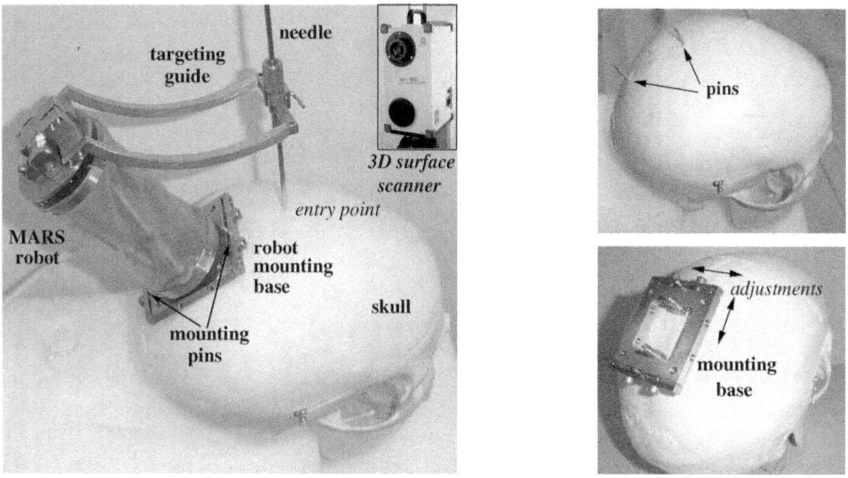

Fig. 1. The MARS robot mounted on the skull

mounting jig attaches the robot base to either the head immobilization frame or to skull-implanted pins. The system software modules are: 1) preoperative planning; 2) intraoperative execution; 3) surface scan processing; and 4) three-way registration. This paper describes the first and last modules.

The surgical protocol is as follows. A preoperative marker- and frame-less CT/MRI image of the patient is acquired. Next, with the preoperative planning module, the surgeon defines on the image the entry points and target locations, and determines the robot mounting type (head clamp or skull) and the desired robot location. Intraoperatively, guided by a video-based intraoperative module, the surgeon places the robot approximately in its planned location. When the robot is mounted on the head frame, the robot base is attached to an adjustable mechanical arm affixed to the head clamp. When mounted on the skull, two 4mm pins are screwed under local anesthesia on the skull and the robot mounting base is attached to them. Next, the registration jig is placed on the robot mounting base and a surface scan showing both the patient forehead and the registration jig is acquired. The registration jig is then replaced by the robot with the targeting guide on it, and the registration module automatically computes the offset between the actual and the desired targeting guide orientation. It then positions and locks the robot so that the actual targeting guide axis coincides with the planned needle insertion trajectory. On surgeon demand, the system automatically positions the robot for each of the predefined trajectories.

3 Preoperative Planning

The preoperative planning module inputs the CT/MRI image and geometric models of the robot, its workvolume, and the targeting guide. It automatically builds from the CT/MRI image the face surface and extracts four landmarks

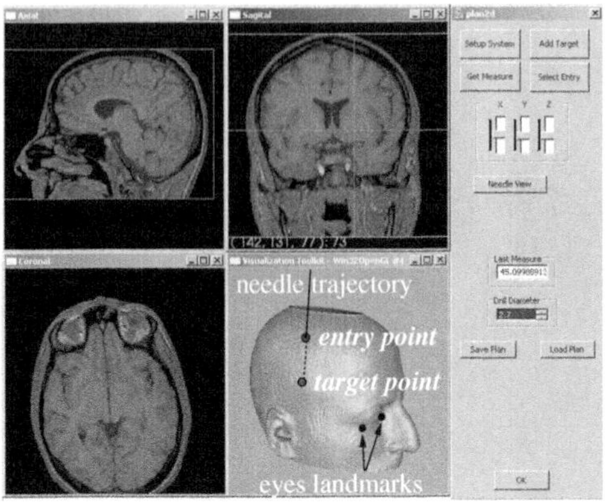

(a) entry and target point selection

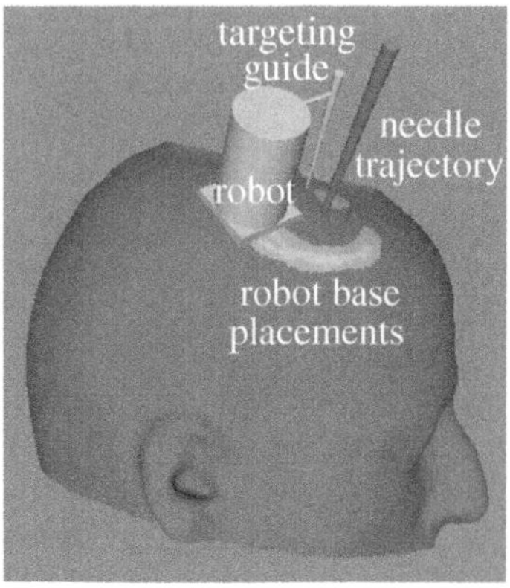

(b) robot base location and range

Fig. 2. Preoperative planning module screens

near the eyes to be used later for coarse registration. The module allows interactive visualization of the CT/MRI slices and the face surface, and enables the surgeon to define entry and target points and visualize the resulting needle trajectories (Fig 2a). Based on the surgeon-defined entry and target points, and the robot mounting mode (on the skull or on the head clamp), the module computes a suggested preferred approximate robot base placement and its range. The computed robot base placement is such that the needle trajectories are at the center of the robot work volume. Placements away from it are assigned a score based on how far they are from the robot work volume center. The results are graphically shown to the surgeon (Fig 2b), who can then select the approximate actual position to satisfy clinical criteria, such as avoiding placements near the cranial sinuses, temporal muscle, or emissary vein. The output includes the surgical plan (entry and target points), the approximate robot base placement, and the patient face surface mesh and landmarks.

The algorithm for computing and rating the robot placements proceeds as follows. A needle trajectory is associated with a coordinate frame whose z axis is aligned with the needle axis and points towards the target. For each point on a uniform $5 \times 5\text{mm}^2$ grid of possible robot base placements over the skull, the rigid transformation that aligns the targeting guide z axis, held by the robot in its home position, with the needle trajectory axis, is computed based on Horn's closed-form solution. The robot base location is then computed by composing the fixed transformation from the targeting guide to the robot top, and the transformation from the robot top to the robot base. The resulting robot transformation is scored against the robot home position based on their distance.

4 Registration

The three-way registration module computes the transformation that establishes a common reference frame between the preoperative CT/MRI, the robot mount-

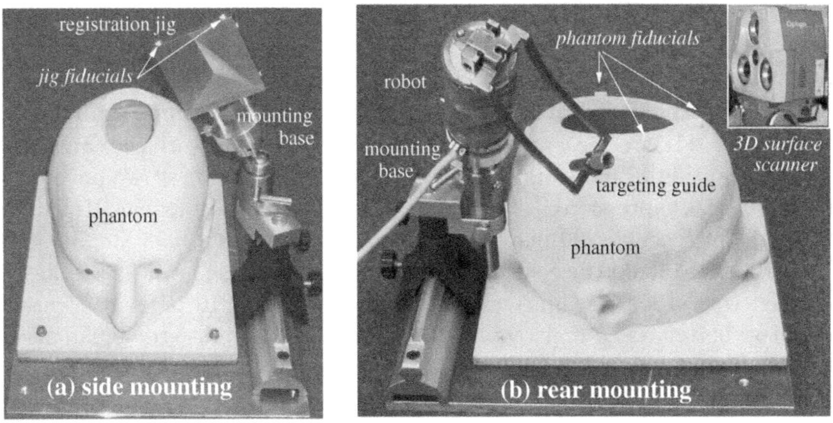

(a) front view, with registration jig (b) side view, with robot

Fig. 3. In-vitro experimental setup

ing base, and the intraoperative patient situation. Two transformations are computed to this end: CT/MRI to intraoperative patient face and robot mounting base to intraoperative patient face. The module inputs the intraoperative surface scans of the registration jig and of the patient's face, and four eye landmarks from the 3D surface scan processing module.

The transformation between the face surface scanner cloud of points and the corresponding CT/MRI surface is performed by first computing a coarse correspondence between them from the extracted landmark eye points in both datasets. This correspondence is then refined with robust Iterative Closest Point (ICP) registration [15], which is performed between a small (1,000–3,000) subset of the surface scan points and the CT/MRI points on the face/ear surface.

The transformation between the robot mounting base and the patient face is performed with a custom-designed registration jig. The registration jig is a $75 \times 75\text{mm}^2$ base with a wide-angled tetrahedron of 9mm height that is placed on the robot mounting base (Fig 3a). It is designed so that all four planes can be seen from a wide range of scanning viewpoints, with sufficient area for adequate scan sampling. To facilitate plane identification, all pairwise plane angles are different. The registration jig model is matched to the surface scanner data as follows. First, we compute a Delaunay triangulation of the registration jig scanner cloud of points. Next, the normals of each mesh triangle are computed and classified into five groups according to their value: four groups correspond to each one of the planes of the registration jig, and one to noise. A plane is then fitted to the points in each of the groups, and four points, corresponding to the intersection between any three planes, are computed. The affine transformation between these four points and the corresponding ones in the model is then computed. Finally, an ICP rigid registration on the plane points is computed to further reduce the error. The actual robot mounting base location with respect to the preoperative plan is determined from this transformation, and from it and the robot characteristics, the targeting guide location.

5 Experimental Results

We have implemented a complete hardware and software prototype of the proposed system and designed an in-vitro registration experiment to validate it. In earlier work [11], we measured the accuracy of the MRI/surface scan registration by acquiring 19 pairs of MRI/3D surface scans of the first two authors with different facial expressions – worried or relaxed, eyes open or closed. The MRI scans are $256 \times 256 \times 200$ pixels^3 with voxel size of $0.93 \times 0.93 \times 0.5\text{mm}^3$ from which 100,000-150,000 face surface points are extracted. The surface scans were obtained with a laser scanner (Konica Minolta Vivid 910, USA – accuracy of 0.1mm or better). The registration RMS error was 1.0mm (std=0.95mm) computed in 2 secs, which is adequate and compares favorably with [16].

In this in-vitro registration experiment of the entire system, we manufactured the registration jig, a positionable robot mounting base, and a precise stereolithographic phantom replica of the outer head surface of the second author from an MRI dataset (Fig 3). Both the phantom and the registration jigs include fiducials for contact-based registration. The phantom is attached to a base with a rail onto which slides a manually adjustable robot mounting base.

To verify the accuracy of the three-way registration algorithm, we used an optical tracking system (Polaris, Northern Digital, Canada – 0.3mm accuracy) to measure the relative locations of the phantom and the registration jig. Their spatial location was determined by touching with a calibrated tracked pointer the phantom and registration jig fiducials. The phantom and the registration jig were scanned with a video scanning system (Optigo200, CogniTens – 0.03mm accuracy). We then computed two registration chains (Fig 4), and measured the

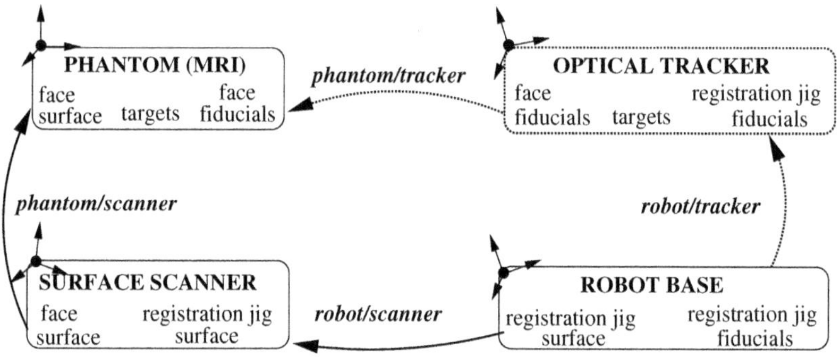

Fig. 4. Registration chains for in-vitro experiment. Each box corresponds to an independent coordinate system. The location of the phantom targets with respect to the robot base origin is computed once via the surface scanner (phantom/scanner and robot/scanner transformations) using the face and registration face surfaces, and once via the optical tracker (phantom tracker and robot/tracker transformations) using the registration jig and the face fiducials. By construction, the phantom and the MRI are in the same coordinate system.

Table 1. In-vitro registration results (in mm) of five experiments. The 2nd and 3rd are the surface scanner phantom and robot base surface registration errors. The 4th and 5th column are the fiducial tracker phantom and registration jig registration errors (both FRE – Fiducial Registration Error – and TRE – Target Registration Error for a target at about 150mm from the mounting base. The 6th column is the error between the target scanner and tracker fiducial locations.

Set	phantom/scan RMS (std)	robot/scan RMS (std)	phantom/tracker FRE (TRE)	robot/tracker FRE (TRE)	Error (std)
1.	0.45 (0.16)	0.31 (0.22)	0.50 (0.61)	0.71 (0.68)	2.71
2.	0.46 (0.17)	0.28 (0.20)	0.50(0.61)	0.71 (0.68)	1.85
3.	0.46 (0.17)	0.25 (0.13)	0.22 (0.53)	0.65 (0.69)	1.31
4.	0.46 (0.18)	0.34 (0.27)	0.22 (0.53)	0.65 (0.69)	1.09
5.	0.44 (0.14)	0.21 (0.08)	0.76 (0.79)	0.73 (0.73)	1.49
Avg.	0.46 (0.17)	0.28 (0.18)	0.44 (0.62)	0.67 (0.69)	1.69 (0.7)

location error of phantom targets with respect to the robot mounting base as computed by the surface scanner and the optical tracker.

Table 1 shows the results of five experiments. The Target Registration Error (TRE) is 1.7mm, which is close to the desired clinical goal. It includes the positional error tracked pointer tip, estimated at 0.5mm (this can be improved with a more accurate measuring system). In addition, we measured the accuracy of the registration between the real faces and the CogniTens scans, taken several months apart, as we did in the earlier experiment. The RMS error is 0.7mm (std=0.25mm), which shows that registration based on facial features is accurate and stable over time. We also measured the accuracy of the robot and registration jig mounting with the optical tracker by putting on and off 10 times the registration jig and measuring the fiducial offset location. The FRE is 0.36mm (std=0.12mm), which is within the measuring error of the optical tracker.

6 Conclusion

We have described a system for automatic precise targeting in minimally invasive keyhole neurosurgery that aims at overcoming the limitations of the existing solutions. The system, which incorporates the miniature parallel robot MARS, will eliminate the morbidity and head immobilization requirements associated with stereotactic frames, eliminate the line-of-sight and tracking requirements of navigation systems, and provide steady and rigid mechanical guidance without the bulk and cost of large robots. This paper presents the preoperative planning and registration modules, and the first results on an in-vitro registration experiment. It establishes viability of the surface scan concept and the accuracy of the location error of phantom targets with respect to the robot base to 1.7mm, which is close to the required 1–1.5mm clinical accuracy in many keyhole neurosurgical procedures.

Acknowledgments. This research is supported in part by a Magneton grant from the Israel Ministry of Industry and Trade. We thank Dr. Tamir Shalom and CogniTens for their generous assistance in acquiring the scans, ad Haim Yeffet for manufacturing the experimental setup platform.

References

1. Tseng, C-S. Chen, H-H. Wang, S-S, et al., "Image guided robotic navigation system for neurosurgery". *Journal of Robotic Systems* **17**(8), 2000, pp 439-447.
2. Chinzei, K. Miller. K. "MRI Guided Surgical Robot". *Australian Conf. on Robotics and Automation*, Sydney, 2001.
3. Kansy, K. Wikirchen, P. Behrens, U. et al. "LOCALITE - a frameless neuronavigation system for interventional magnetic resonance imaging". *Proc. of Medical Image Computing and Computer Assisted Intervention*, 2003, pp 832-841.
4. Kosugi, Y. Watanabe, E. Goto, J. et al. "An articulated neurosurgical navigation system using MRI and CT images". *IEEE Trans. on Biomedical Eng.* **35**(2), 1998.
5. Akatsuka, Y. Kawamata, T. Fujii, M. et al. "AR navigation system for neurosurgery". *Proc. of Medical Imaging and Computer-Aided Interventions*, 2000.
6. Grimson, E, Leventon, M. Ettinger, G. et al., "Clinical experience with a high precision image-guided neurosurgery system". *Proc. of Medical Imaging and Computer-Aided Interventions*, 1998, pp 63-72.
7. Chen, MD. Wang, T. Zhang, QX et al.,"A robotics system for stereotactic neurosurgery and its clinical application". *Proc. Conf. Robotics and Automation*, 1998.
8. Masamune, K. Ji, LH. Suzuki, M. et al., Takeyoshi Dohi, Hiroshi Iseki, "A newly developed stereotactic robot with detachable drive for neurosurgery". *Proc. of Medical Image Computing and Computer Aided Imaging*, 1998, pp. 215-222.
9. Davies, B. Starkie, B. Harris, S. et al. "Neurobot: a special-purpose robot for neurosurgery", *Proc. Int. Conf. and Robotics and Automation*, 2000, pp 410-414.
10. Hang, Q. Zamorano, L. Pandya, A. et al., "The application of the NeuroMate Robot: a quantitative comparison with frameless and frame-based surgical localization systems". *Computer Aided Surgery* **7**(2), 2002, pp 90-98.
11. Joskowicz, L. Shoham, M. Shamir, R. Freiman, M. Zehavi, E. and Shoshan, Y. "Miniature robot-based precise targeting system for keyhole neurosurgery: concept and preliminary results". *19th Int. Conf. on Computer-Assisted Radiology and Surgery*, CARS'2005, H.U. Lemke et. al. editors, Elsevier 2005, to appear,
12. Shoham, M. Burman, M. Zehavi, E. et al., "Bone-mounted miniature robot for surgical procedures: concept and clinical applications". *IEEE Trans. on Robotics and Automation* **19**(5), 2003, pp 893-901.
13. Wolf, A. Shoham, M. Schinder M. and Roffman, M. "Feasibility study of a mini robotic system for spinal operations: analysis and experiments", *European Spine Journal*, 2003.
14. Yaniv, Z. and Joskowicz, L. "Registration for robot-assisted distal locking of long bone intramedullary nails", *IEEE Trans. on Medical Imaging*, to appear, 2005.
15. Besl, P.J. and McKay, N.D. "A method for registration of 3D shapes", *IEEE Trans. on Pattern Analysis and Machine Intelligence*, **14(2)**, 1992.
16. Marmulla, R. Hassfeld, S. and Lueth, T. "Soft tissue scanning for patient registration in image-guided surgery", *Computer-Aided Surgery* **8**(2), 2003, pp70-81.

Soft-Tissue Motion Tracking and Structure Estimation for Robotic Assisted MIS Procedures

Danail Stoyanov[1], George P. Mylonas[1], Fani Deligianni[1], Ara Darzi[2], and Guang Zhong Yang[1,2]

[1] Royal Society/Wolfson Foundation Medical Image Computing Laboratory
[2] Department of Surgical Oncology and Technology,
Imperial College of Science, Technology and Medicine, London SW7 2BZ, UK
{danail.stoyanov, george.mylonas, fani.deligianni, a.darzi, g.z.yang}@imperial.ac.uk
http://vip.doc.ic.ac.uk

Abstract. In robotically assisted laparoscopic surgery, soft-tissue motion tracking and structure recovery are important for intraoperative surgical guidance, motion compensation and delivering active constraints. In this paper, we present a novel method for feature based motion tracking of deformable soft-tissue surfaces in totally endoscopic coronary artery bypass graft (TECAB) surgery. We combine two feature detectors to recover distinct regions on the epicardial surface for which the sparse 3D surface geometry may be computed using a pre-calibrated stereo laparoscope. The movement of the 3D points is then tracked in the stereo images with stereo-temporal constrains by using an iterative registration algorithm. The practical value of the technique is demonstrated on both a deformable phantom model with tomographically derived surface geometry and *in vivo* robotic assisted minimally invasive surgery (MIS) image sequences.

1 Introduction

Recent advances in robotic assisted Minimally Invasive Surgery (MIS) for performing micro-scale tasks using motion scaling and miniaturized mechanical wrists have made it possible to perform closed-chest cardiothoracic surgery on a beating heart. This approach minimizes patient trauma and avoids certain adverse effects associated with cardiopulmonary bypass. In practice, deformation of the epicardial surface due to cardiac and respiratory motion can impose significant challenges to delicate tasks such vessel anastomosis. The use of mechanical stabilizers can effectively remove most of the bulk motion, but residual tissue deformation remains significant in most cases. For intraoperative guidance and applying image guided active constraints to avoid critical anatomical structures such as nerves and blood vessels, it is necessary to develop complementary techniques for accurate 3D surface structure reconstruction and motion estimation *in situ* [1].

The determination of tissue deformation can be approached with a number of approaches that involve intraoperative imaging such as endoscopic ultrasound, or motion sensors such as mechanically or optically based accelerometers [2,3]. Marker based techniques have been proposed, but they involve suturing or projecting fiducals

J. Duncan and G. Gerig (Eds.): MICCAI 2005, LNCS 3750, pp. 139 – 146, 2005.

onto the heart surface [4,5]. Region based tracking of natural epicardial regions has also been investigated using monocular video sequences [6], but only for recovering 2D image motion. Since robotic assisted MIS procedures typically involve a pair of miniaturized stereo cameras, detailed 3D motion and structure recovery from the stereo laparoscope with image registration was recently proposed [7,8]. The major advantage of these methods is that they do not necessitate additional modification to the existing MIS hardware, but computationally they require complex computer vision algorithms inferring dense 3D correspondence which is often an ill-posed problem. Existing research has shown that sparse sets of well known feature correspondences can be used as ground control points to enforce additional constraints and increase the inherent accuracy and robustness of dense stereo techniques [9]. Furthermore, the integration of other visual cues such as shading and specular reflectance and their temporal characteristics in response to soft-tissue deformation can further improve the practical value of optically based methods.

The purpose of this paper is to introduce a method for inferring precise 3D structure and motion for a set of sparse salient features on the soft-tissue surfaces during robotic assisted MIS procedures. With a calibrated stereo laparoscope, a combination of landmarks is used to provide robust performance in the presence of specular reflections. The temporal behavior of each landmark is then derived by using constraints in the stereo video sequence. Detailed validation of the proposed method was performed on both a phantom model with known geometry and *in vivo* robotic assisted MIS data.

2 Methods

2.1 Salient Landmarks on the Epicardial Surface

Traditionally, the identification of salient landmarks is usually achieved with edge or corner features for sparse stereo matching and motion tracking. For robotically assisted MIS, these features can be unstable and prone to errors due to the homogeneity of surface texture and the presence of specular highlights, which can cause clustering of high frequency features on the specular boundary. In the context of wide-baseline stereo matching, Matas *et al.* [10] defined maximally stable extremal regions (MSER) based on thresholding the image intensity to create connected components with local minima. The use of MSER landmarks has a number of desirable properties as they are invariant to monotonic changes in illumination. Furthermore, if they are detected by starting from the lowest intensity (MSER-), they can implicitly avoid specular reflections. It can also be shown that on MIS cardiac surfaces, MSER- generally corresponds to physically meaningful texture details such as superficial blood vessels or small tissue bruising.

In this paper, a combination of MSER- regions and the traditional gradient based image features [11] is used for salient landmark selection. The use of different feature descriptors can provide added robustness [12], which is necessary in the presence of occlusions and specular highlights as encountered in cardiac MIS procedures. We associate a measurement region (MR) around each landmark for computing the dissimilarity metrics. The MR is a rectangular window for corner features and an ellipse that bounds the convex hull of the component for MSER- regions.

2.2 Stereo Feature Matching

To recover 3D measurements from a stereoscopic laparoscope, the correspondence of landmarks of the stereo pair needs to be determined. There are many algorithms for matching sparse feature sets, and in this work we used the method proposed by Pilu [13] for combining proximity and similarity measures to discriminate between potential matches. For each feature type, we build a cost matrix with row entries corresponding to features in the left image and columns for the right image. Each entry of the cost matrix depicts how well respective features correspond to each other by using the following dissimilarity measure:

$$Cost_{ij} = e^{-\frac{(C_{ij}-1)^2}{2\gamma^2}} e^{-\frac{r_{ij}^2}{2\mu^2}} \tag{1}$$

In Eq. (1), r is the Euclidian distance between features, γ and μ are sensitivity control parameters set to the values suggested in [13], and C_{ij} is the normalized cross correlation (NCC) between the measurement regions of features i and j. When matching MSER-, we used the largest MR for computing correlation. The algorithm makes use of the properties of Singular Value Decomposition (SVD) of the cost matrix to attenuate matrix values for poor matches. Once corresponding points are determined, 3D points on the epicardial surface can be inferred by using the centre of mass of the MSER- as a reference. By calibrating the camera before the MIS procedure, the epipolar constraint can be introduced to the proximity cost. Calibration is also important to the intrinsic accuracy of the proposed technique as otherwise the recovered 3D points will be ambiguous up to a projective transformation if just using the determined stereo correspondences for estimating the camera matrices.

2.3 Temporal Tracking Using Stereo Constraints

Once the stereo correspondence is established, we used temporal motion tracking of salient features to iteratively update their temporal positions in 3D space by using both stereo frames. This extends the Lucas-Kanade (LK) [15, 16] registration algorithm for incorporating the inter-stereo epipolar constraint. The goal of the LK tracker is to align a reference image template $T(\mathbf{x})$ with an image region subject to the squared pixel difference, given a warping function $W(\mathbf{x};\mathbf{p})$ of arbitrary complexity and $\mathbf{p}$ parameters. The algorithm starts with an initial estimate of the warping parameters $\mathbf{p}$ and iteratively computes an update term $\Delta\mathbf{p}$ until convergence below a predefined threshold $\Delta\mathbf{p} \leq \xi$. The error function e used for minimizing the modified stereo LK tracker is defined as:

$$\varepsilon = \sum_{\mathbf{x}} \left[\left[I\left(W\left(\mathbf{x};\mathbf{p}+\Delta\mathbf{p}\right)\right) - T(\mathbf{x}) \right]^2 + \left[J\left(W'\left(\mathbf{x}';\mathbf{p}+\Delta\mathbf{p}\right)\right) - T'(\mathbf{x}') \right]^2 \right] \tag{2}$$

where $I(W(\mathbf{x};\mathbf{p}))$ and $J(W'(\mathbf{x};\mathbf{p}))$ are the images transformed by the respective warping function. The error function can be linearized by taking the first order Taylor expansion about $\mathbf{p}$, such that the partial derivative with respect to $\Delta\mathbf{p}$ can be determined by using the chain rule. Setting the partial derivative to zero and solving for $\Delta\mathbf{p}$ yields a least-squares solution (constants are ignored), we have:

$$\Delta\mathbf{p} \approx H^{-1} \sum_{\mathbf{x}} \left[\left[\nabla I \frac{\partial W}{\partial \mathbf{p}} \right]^T \left[I(W(\mathbf{x};\mathbf{p})) - T(\mathbf{x}) \right]^2 + \left[\nabla J \frac{\partial W'}{\partial \mathbf{p}} \right]^T \left[J(W'(\mathbf{x}';\mathbf{p})) - T'(\mathbf{x}') \right]^2 \right] \tag{3}$$

Where ∇I and ∇J are the warped image gradients of each stereo channel, $\partial W / \partial \mathbf{p}$ is the *Jacobian* of each warping function and H^{-1} is the inverse of the *Hessian* matrix:

$$H = \sum_{\mathbf{x}} \left[\nabla I \frac{\partial W}{\partial \mathbf{p}} \right]^T \left[\nabla I \frac{\partial W}{\partial \mathbf{p}} \right] + \left[\nabla J \frac{\partial W'}{\partial \mathbf{p}} \right]^T \left[\nabla J \frac{\partial W'}{\partial \mathbf{p}} \right] \tag{4}$$

The motion parameterization used in this is study is based on a pure translation model for each feature, which incorporates terms for the vertical and horizontal motion in the reference image, and an additional term for disparity changes in the stereo pair. More complex models can readily be incorporated into the proposed framework (for further details consult the study by Baker *et al* [16]) but the increased search space may have an adverse effect on the actual system performance [6]. Furthermore, it has been demonstrated that for small inter-frame motion, the use of translation tracking alone can be sufficient [11].

2.4 Experimental Design

The proposed method was implemented in C++ on a standard desktop PC with a Pentium IV 2.4 GHz CPU and 512 Mb RAM, running the Windows XP operating system. In the current implementation, initialization took 0.5s (mostly for MSER detection) after which the algorithm processed 320×288 images at 11 frames per second (fps). With further optimization real-time performance can be achieved.

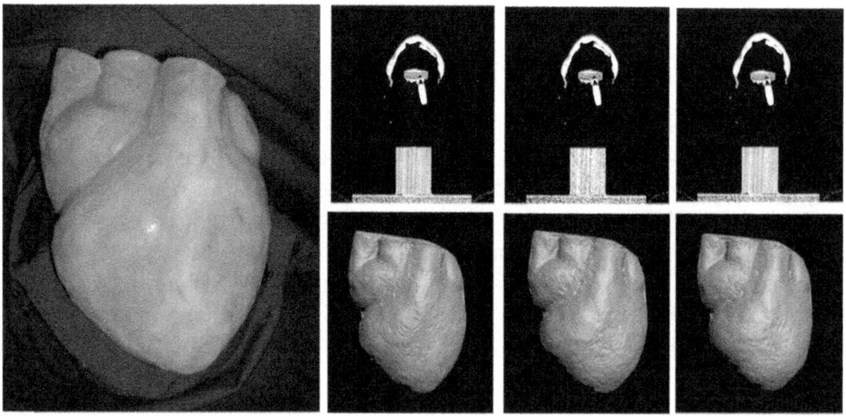

(a) (b)

Fig. 1. The cardiac phantom model used for validating the proposed technique **(a)** image of the heart model showing the visual and geometrical fidelity of the model and **(b)** CT slice for three levels of deformation and 3D renditions of reconstructions from the respective CT series

To validate the proposed method, a scaled simulation environment was created with a phantom heart model shown in **Fig. 1 (a)**. A stereo rig mounted on a Stäubli RX60 robotic arm with six degrees of freedom (DOF) and repeatability accuracy of ±0.02mm. The phantom model was created using thixotropic silicone mould rubber and pre-vulcanized natural rubber latex with rubber mask grease paint to achieve a specular appearance and high visual fidelity. The deformable silicone surface was mounted onto a piston mechanism with controllable injection levels to simulate the heart beat motion in a reproducible manner. The precise phantom model geometry was recovered at seven discrete heart beat simulation levels using a Siemens Somatom Sensation 64 CT scanner with slice thickness of 0.6mm, an example CT slice and 3D rendition of a reconstruction are shown in **Fig. 1 (b)**.

For *in vivo* analysis, data from robotic assisted cardiac surgery carried out with a daVinci™ surgical system (Intuitive Surgical, CA) was used. The cameras of the stereoscopic endoscope were hardware synchronized by using a proprietary FPGA device designed by this institution. The stereo cameras were calibrated before the procedure using a planar calibration object [17]. The proposed method was used to detect and then track landmarks on the epicardial surface after the positioning of a mechanical stabilizer. Since, ground truth data for the 3D structure and motion of the soft-tissue cannot be easily obtained for robotic procedures, we used the motion of landmarks on the epicardial surface to determine the respiratory and cardiac motion as a means of qualitative analysis.

3 Results

The phantom heart model described above was used to generate an image sequence of 50 frames, with each frame showing consecutive deformation of the heart associated with the CT data. The setup was devised so that the resultant inter-frame pixel motion

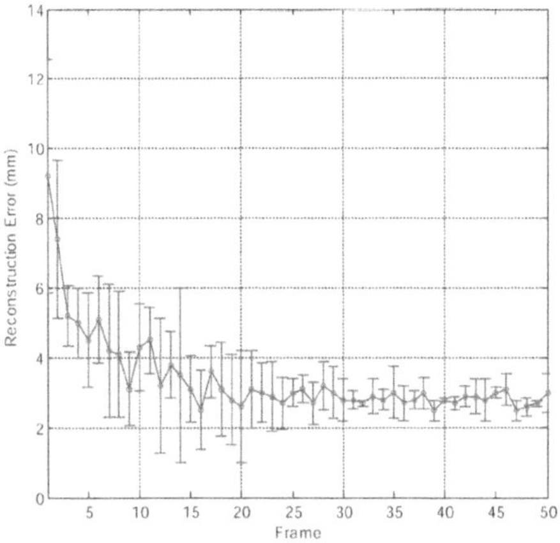

(a)

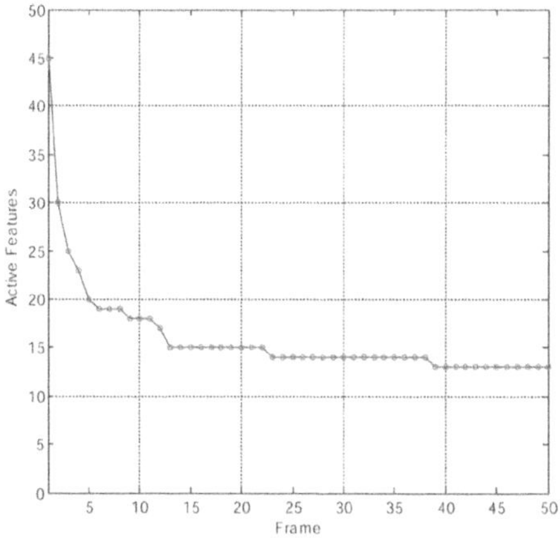

(b)

Fig. 2. Phantom model experiment for evaluating reconstruction accuracy of stereo feature tracking **(a)** the average and standard deviation of error in millimeters for feature correspondences in each experimental frame **(b)** the number of features actively tracked at each frame of the sequence

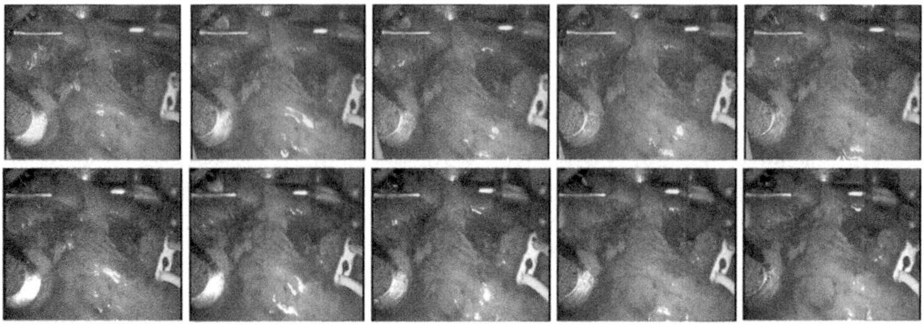

Fig. 3. Example stereoscopic image pairs of robotic assisted totally endoscopic coronary artery bypass surgery used for the *in vivo* analysis in this study

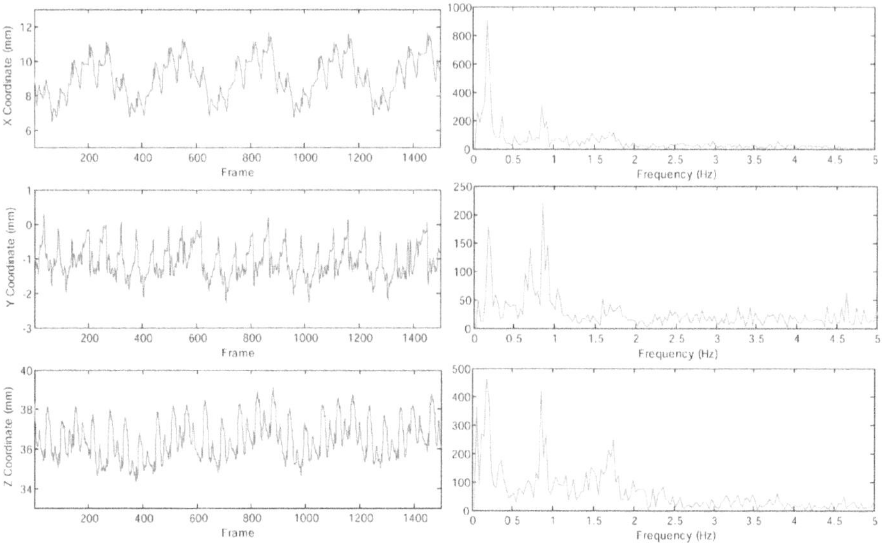

(a) **(b)**

Fig. 4. Results for *in vivo* robotic assisted MIS (**a**) the recovered 3D coordinates in the left camera reference system for a landmark tracked through 1500 video frames at 50 fps (**b**) power spectral analysis clearly identifies the heart beat and respiratory frequencies in the 3D motion

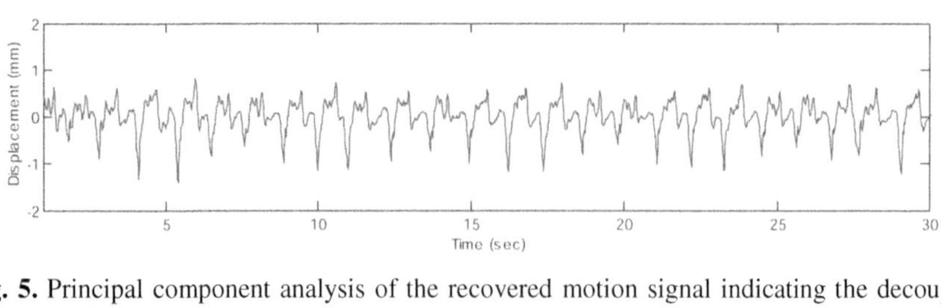

Fig. 5. Principal component analysis of the recovered motion signal indicating the decoupled cardiac motion component

did not exceed 15 pixels, which was consistent with observations from *in vivo* data for consecutive frames. Metric error was measured as the distance between the reconstructed 3D point and the point on the CT reconstructed surface along the ray back-projected from the left camera. In **Fig. 2**, we demonstrate the reconstruction accuracy of stereo correspondence obtained with the proposed technique. Not all features are suitable for temporal tracking, and initial outliers were rejected depending on the correlation threshold. This results in fewer features being tracked over the entire period but improves the overall accuracy by ensuring that only consistent landmarks are considered. With the proposed framework additional landmarks may be introduced at any stage.

The *in vivo* performance of the algorithm is assessed with a robotic assisted totally endoscopic coronary artery bypass graft (TECAB) as shown in **Fig. 3**. In **Fig. 4**, it is evident that the recovered motion clearly captures the coupled deformation of the epicardial surface due to cardiac as well as respiratory motion. It is worth noting that the graph shown in **Fig. 4** illustrates the surface motion as projected onto the x, y and z axes of the camera coordinate system. Within this figure, the power spectrum of each of the motion components is also provided, which illustrates the dominant frequencies derived from the proposed algorithm. In **Fig. 5**, we show the decoupled motion component indicating only the cardiac motion by using a localized principal component analysis (PCA) cardiac/respiratory decoupling technique.

4 Discussion and Conclusions

In this paper, we have proposed a practical method for determining soft-tissue deformation for robotic assisted MIS from a set of landmarks. We have used a combination of landmarks including MSER- regions and the traditional gradient-based image features for ensuring robust system performance. Results from the phantom model have demonstrated the accuracy of 3D reconstruction that can be achieved and analysis of *in vivo* robotic assisted MIS data has further demonstrated the clinical value of the proposed technique. With the current implementation, features occluded by the instruments or tissue effects such as bleeding are detected through correlation and epipolar geometry thresholds and set as outliers in the tracking process. The introduction of new features or labeling lost features as occluded and performing subsequent searches with statistical motion models can be used improve the tracking process.

Acknowledgements

The authors thank Eddy Kavanagh, Danny Sharpe and Bob Pullen for their valuable help and Roberto Casula for kindly providing the *in vivo* data used in this study.

References

1. Taylor, R. H., Stoianovici, D.: Medical Robotics in Computer-Integrated Surgery. IEEE Transactions on Robotics and Automation, (19):765-781, 2003.
2. Hoff, L.,Elle, O.J., Grimnes, M.J., Halvorsen, S., Alker, H.J., Fosse, E.: Measurements of heart motion using accelerometers. In: Proc. EMBC, 2049 – 2051, 2004.

3. Thrakal A, Wallace J, Tomlin D, Seth N, Thakor N. Surgical Motion Adaptive Robotic Technology (SMART): taking the motion out of physiological motion. In: Proc. MICCAI, 317-325, 2001.
4. Nakamura, Y., Kishi, K., Kawakami, H.: Heartbeat synchronization for robotic cardiac surgery. In: Proc. ICRA, 2014-2019, 2001.
5. Ginhoux, R., Gangloff, J. A., de Mathelin, M. F., Soler, L., Arenas Sanchez, M., Marescaux, J. : Beating Heart Tracking in Robotic Surgery Using 500 Hz Visual Servoing, Model Predictive Control and an Adaptive Observer. In: Proc. ICRA, 274-279, 2004.
6. Gröger, M., Ortmaier, T., Sepp, W., Hirzinger, G.: Tracking local motion on the beating heart. In: Proc. SPIE Medical Imaging Conference, 233-241, 2002.
7. Stoyanov, D., Darzi, A., Yang, G-.Z.: Dense 3D Depth Recovery for Soft Tissue Deformation During Robotically Assisted Laparoscopic Surgery. In: Proc. MICCAI, 41-48, 2004.
8. Lau, W., Ramey, N., Corso, J., Thakor, N., Hager, G.: Stereo-Based Endoscopic Tracking of Cardiac Surface Deformation. In: Proc. MICCAI, 494-501, 2004.
9. Bobick, A. F., Intille, S. S.: Large occlusion stereo. International Journal of Computer Vision, (33):181-200, 1999.
10. Matas, J., Chum, O., Martin, U., Pajdla, T.: Robust wide baseline stereo from maximally stable extremal regions. In: Proc. BMVC, 384-393, 2002.
11. Shi, J., Tomasi, C.: Good features to track, In: Proc. CVPR, 593 - 600, 1994.
12. Mikolajczyk, K., Tuytelaars, T., Schmid, C., Zisserman, A., Matas, J., Schaffalitzky, F., Kadir, F., Van Gool, L.: A comparison of affine region detectors. International Journal of Computer Vision, *in press*.
13. Pilu, M.: A Direct Method for Stereo Correspondence based on Singular Value Decomposition. In: Proc. CVPR, 261-266, 1997.
14. Hager, G. D., Belhumeur, P. N.: Efficient Region Tracking With Parametric Models of Geometry and Illumination. IEEE Transactions on Pattern Analysis and Machine Intelligence, (20):1-15, 1998.
15. Lucas, B. D., Kanade, T.: An Iterative Image Registration Technique with an Application to Stereo Vision. In: Proc. IJCAI, 674-679, 1981.
16. Baker, S., Matthews, I.: Lucas-Kanade 20 Years On: A Unifying Framework. International Journal of Computer Vision, (56):221-255, 2004.
17. Zhang, Z.: A flexible new technique for camera calibration. IEEE Transactions on Pattern Analysis and Machine Intelligence. (22):1330-1334, 2000.

Mass Preserving Registration for Heart MR Images

Lei Zhu[1], Steven Haker[2], and Allen Tannenbaum[1,⋆]

[1] School of Biomedical Engineering,
Georgia Institute of Technology, Atlanta, GA 30332
{zlzl, tannenba}@ece.gatech.edu
[2] Surgical Planning Lab, Brigham and Women's Hospital,
Harvard Medical School, Boston, MA 02115
haker@bwh.harvard.edu

Abstract. This paper presents a new algorithm for non-rigid registration between two doubly-connected regions. Our algorithm is based on harmonic analysis and the theory of optimal mass transport. It assumes an underlining continuum model, in which the total amount of mass is exactly preserved during the transformation of tissues. We use a finite element approach to numerically implement the algorithm.

1 Introduction

Image registration is the process of generating a common geometric frame of reference between two or more image datasets. This technique is especially useful in the context of medical image processing. A successful registration technique allows for the integration of pre-operative information with intra-operative imaging to improve image-guided surgery and therapy. For example, in brain surgery where craniotomy is performed, the ventricles in the brain may be compressed due to pressure changes. A surgical plan based on pre-surgical images must therefore be updated accordingly to reflect these shape deformations. There have been numerous algorithms proposed for non-rigid registration. See [9] for a detailed review and the references therein. Our method employs optimal mass transport, and therefore belongs to the category of warping algorithms based on continuum and fluid mechanics. The approach may be formulated as an energy minimization problem. We should point out that our methodology may not be suitable under circumstances where the mass preservation assumption is invalid, such as the matching of two different perspective projections of a spatial object.

⋆ Allen Tannenbaum is also with the School of Electrical and Computer Engineering. This work is part of the National Alliance for Medical Image Computing (NAMIC), funded by the National Institutes of Health through the NIH Roadmap for Medical Research, Grant U54 EB005149. This work was also supported by a grant from NIH (P41 RR-13218 NAC through Brigham and Women's Hospital). S. Haker's work is supported by NIH grants R01CA109246, R01LM007861, R01CA1029246 and P41RR019703.

J. Duncan and G. Gerig (Eds.): MICCAI 2005, LNCS 3750, pp. 147–154, 2005.

In the work of [5,11], an algorithm was presented for finding an optimal warping function between two simply-connected domains, or more specifically two rectangular regions. The assumption was that the mass is preserved at all points in the image domain. However, this is not always the case. Sometimes, the mass preserving (MP) assumption is valid only in parts of the two images. The specific example we have in mind concerns two magnetic resonance (MR) images of the heart taken at different times in the cardiac cycle, but corresponding to the same spatial position. Indeed, during the cycle, the MP assumption is valid in the myocardium, but not in the ventricles where the volume of blood varies from time point to time point. With this key example in mind, we will derive an algorithm for extending previous approaches to two doubly-connected domains, based on harmonic analysis and a Finite Element Method (FEM). Here, we treat image intensity as tissue mass density, due to the fact that in MR images intensity is related to proton density, thus related to mass density. After registration, image intensity (mass density) can change, but the total amount of mass (mass density times area or the integral of intensity) preserves.

We now outline the contents of this paper. In Section 2, we give a brief review of the optimal mass transport problem and a general gradient descent solution. In Section 3, we summarize the approach for finding an optimal MP mapping between two doubly-connected domains. In Section 4, we illustrate the proposed algorithm using a pair of heart MR images. Finally, in Section 5, we summarize the contribution of this paper and discuss some possible future research directions.

2 Background on Optimal Mass Transport

The Monge-Kantorovich Problem (MKP) is concerned with the optimal way of moving certain amount of mass from one domain into another. The total amount of mass remains constant in this process. It has been widely studied in various fields such as econometrics, fluid dynamics, transportation, and image retrieval [7]; see [6] and the references therein. In this paper, we will consider only 2D problems. Accordingly, let Ω_0 and Ω_1 be domains of $\mathbf{R^2}$, having smooth boundaries. On each domain Ω_i, we assume that there exists a positive mass density function $\mu_i, i = 0, 1$. It is further assumed that the same total amount of mass is associated with the two domains.

We will be considering a class of diffeomorphisms u from Ω_0 to Ω_1 which satisfy the "Jacobian equation" in the form of

$$\mu_0 = |Du| \mu_1 \circ u, \tag{1}$$

where $|Du|$ is the determinant of the Jacobian of u, and $\circ$ represents the composition of functions. Equation (1) is an infinitesimal form of the mass preservation (MP) constraint. We are interested in finding an MP mapping u which differs minimally from the identity. To this end, we introduce the L^2 Kantorovich–Wasserstein penalty functional on $u \in$ MP, defined as:

$$M[u] := \int_{\Omega_0} \|u(x) - x\|^2 \mu_0(x) dx \tag{2}$$

This functional places a penalty on the distance the map u moves each bit of material, weighted by the material's mass. The resulting distribution of material is constrained to be the given density μ_1. The "optimal" mapping $\tilde{u}$ is the one that minimizes functional (2), and is the "cheapest" way of transporting mass from one domain into the other. An energy term penalizing intensity change can also be added, please refer to [5].

Theoretical results [2,3] show that there is a unique minimizer $\tilde{u} \in \mathrm{MP}$, and that this minimizer is characterized as being the gradient of a convex function w, *i.e.*, $\tilde{u} = \nabla w$. There have been a number of algorithms proposed for solving this problem, *e.g.* linear programming [6], which is the most popular one. However, the linear programming approach has a high computational complexity. In the method presented here, we use a gradient descent approach to solve for the optimal transport problem, based on the equivalent problem of polar factorization. Here we will briefly describe the procedure; for mathematical details we refer the reader to [5].

The first step of the method is to construct an initial MP mapping. For two rectangular regions, the initial mapping can be found by solving a family of 1D problems unsing simple numerical integration. Assume the two domains have shapes of $\Omega_0 = [0, A_0] \times [0, B_0]$ and $\Omega_1 = [0, A_1] \times [0, B_1]$, respectively. Assume further that the initial mass preserving mapping has the form of $u^0(x, y) = (a(x), b(x, y))$. Since both μ_0 and μ_1 are positive everywhere, it is easy to solve $u^0 = (a(x), b(x, y))$ from the following equations:

$$\begin{aligned} \int_0^{a(x)} \int_0^{B_1} \mu_1(\eta, y) dy d\eta &= \int_0^{x} \int_0^{B_0} \mu_0(\eta, y) dy d\eta \\ a'(x) \int_0^{b(x,y)} \mu_1(a(x), \rho) d\rho &= \int_0^{y} \mu_0(x, \rho) d\rho. \end{aligned} \tag{3}$$

The second step is to find the minimizer $\tilde{u}$ of the energy functional (2), using an iterative approach. In [5], it is shown that the evolution of u should have the following form in order to satisfy the mass preserving constraint:

$$u_t = \frac{2}{\mu_0} Du \nabla^{\perp} \triangle^{-1} \mathrm{div} \left[(u - \underline{id})^{\perp} \right], \tag{4}$$

where $\perp$ rotates a vector by $\pi/2$ in the counterclockwise direction, $\triangle^{-1}$ denotes the inverse of Laplacian, and $\underline{id}$ stands for the identity map. It can be shown that the optimal mapping $\tilde{u}$ is a curl-free vector field [5].

3 Mass-Preserving Registration Between Two Doubly-Connected Domains

In the previous section, we briefly described the approach for solving the transport problem between two rectangular regions. However, this approach cannot be applied on doubly-connected regions (*i.e.* an annular region) without some modifications. The main difficulty comes from the construction of an initial MP mapping u^0 between two irregular doubly-connected domains. In this section, we present an algorithm which constructs such a mapping by using harmonic parametrization. In this approach, the two domains are first harmonically parameterized, then the initial MP mapping u^0 is constructed by solving a 1D transport problem along one harmonic coordinate, followed by a family of 1D transport problems along the other harmonic coordinate.

3.1 Harmonic Parametrization

Here we sketch the steps for constructing an analytic function $f^h = u^h + iv^h$ for the harmonic parametrization. Similar techniques have been applied for measuring tissue thickness [10], for colon surface visualization [4], and for parametrization of ventricular regions of the heart [8].

Assume we have a triangulated doubly-connected domain Σ, which has an inner boundary denoted by σ_0 and an outer boundary denoted by σ_1 as shown in Figure 1. First, we want to construct u^h, which is the real part of f. It is assumed that u^h satisfies

$$\begin{aligned} \triangle u^h &= 0 \\ \text{with } u^h(\sigma_0) = 0 &\text{ and } u^h(\sigma_1) = 1 \end{aligned} \tag{5}$$

The Laplace equation can be solved by using standard FEM techniques [4]. A cut C is then found from σ_0 to σ_1 by following the gradient of u^h from an arbitrary point $x_0 \in \sigma_0$ to another point $x_1 \in \sigma_1$. The cut C and two original boundaries σ_0 and σ_1 form a new closed and oriented boundary B for the domain,

$$B : x_0 \xrightarrow{\sigma_0} x_0 \xrightarrow{C} x_1 \xrightarrow{\sigma_1} x_1 \xrightarrow{-C} x_0$$

The boundary condition of the imaginary part v^h can be then prescribed by,

$$v^h(\zeta) = \int_{\zeta_0}^{\zeta} \frac{\partial v}{\partial s} ds = \int_{\zeta_0}^{\zeta} \frac{\partial u}{\partial n} ds$$

according to the Cauchy-Riemann equations. Inside the cut surface, v^h is found as the solution of Laplace's equation $\triangle v^h = 0$.

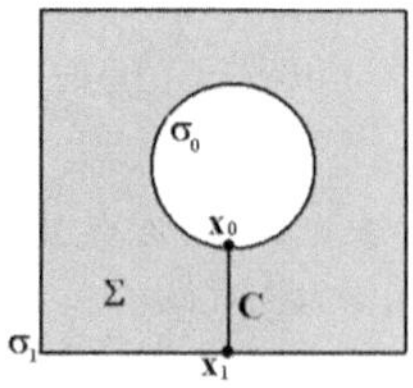

Fig. 1. A doubly-connected domain Σ with two boundaries

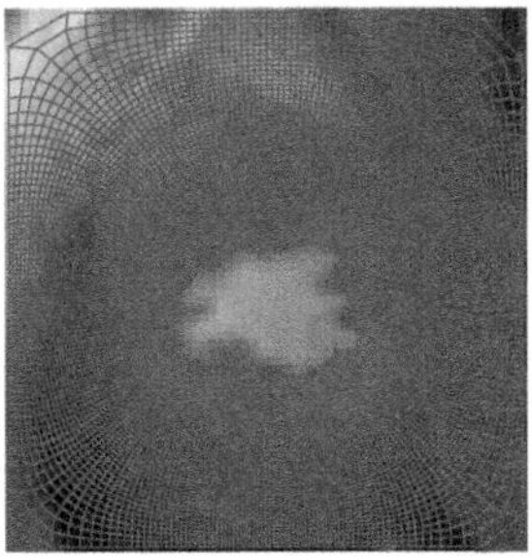

Fig. 2. Harmonic parametrization of a heart image

Once the analytic function $f^h = u^h + iv^h$ is constructed, a curvilinear harmonic polar coordinate system is defined by taking u^h as one coordinate axis and v^h as the other. The coordinate u^h can be thought of as a curvilinear "radius" and v^h as the "angle". By scaling u^h and v^h by a constant, v^h can be made to run from 0 to 2π. Figure 2 shows such a parametrization on a heart MR image without involving the ventricle area.

3.2 Finding the Initial Mapping u^0

By performing harmonic parametrization, the first doubly-connected domain (Ω_0, μ_0) is cut and mapped onto a rectangular region (Ω_0^h, μ_0^h) via a harmonic (conformal) mapping $f_0^h = u_0^h + iv_0^h$. If we *define* the mass density μ_0^h by

$$\mu_0^h = |Df_0^h|^{-1}\mu_0, \tag{6}$$

then the mapping from Ω_0 to Ω_0^h is mass-preserving. Similarly, the second doubly-connected domain (Ω_1, μ_1) is mapped onto another rectangular region (Ω_1^h, μ_1^h) via $f_1^h = u_1^h + iv_1^h$. Here, μ_1^h is taken to be

$$\mu_1^h = |Df_1^h|^{-1}\mu_1. \tag{7}$$

The remaining task is to find an MP mapping from (Ω_0^h, μ_0^h) to (Ω_1^h, μ_1^h). Since Ω_0 and Ω_1 are now rectangular regions, we can use the algorithm presented in Section 2 to find an initial MP mapping u_{init} between them. This process can be illustrated by the following diagram.

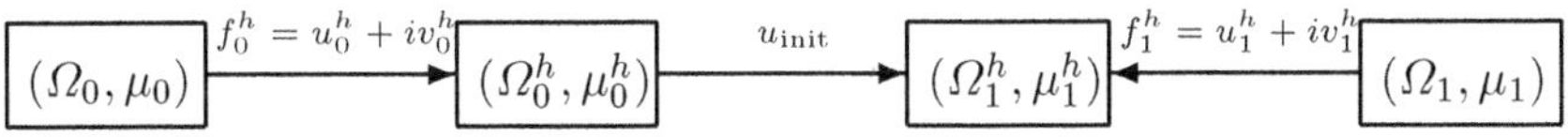

The resulting initial mapping u^0 is the composition of f_0^h, u_{init} and $(f_1^h)^{-1}$, so that

$$u^0 = (f_1^h)^{-1} \circ u_{\text{init}} \circ f_0^h. \tag{8}$$

Compositions of MP mappings and inverses of MP mappings are also MP mappings. Thus u^0 is and MP mapping, since f_0^h, f_1^h and u_{init} are.

3.3 Finding the Minimizer $\tilde{u}$

The equation we use to evolve u is the same as for rectangular regions. The finite element method (FEM) is used to solve the Poisson equation (the $\triangle^{-1}$ part of equation (4)) on a triangulated irregular domain.

In the evolution equation of u (equation (4)), we use an upwinding scheme for computing Du. For all other derivatives, we use a Least Mean Square (LMS) method to numerically implement the spatial derivatives. For example, assume that a given point (x_0, y_0) has N neighbors $(x_i, y_i), i = 1...N$, and a function Φ is defined such that $\Phi(x_i, y_i) = \Phi_i$ for $i = 0...N$. It is easy to show that the derivatives of Φ should satisfy

$$\begin{pmatrix} \Phi_x \\ \Phi_y \end{pmatrix} = (A^T A)^{-1} A^T \begin{pmatrix} \Phi_1 - \Phi_0 \\ \cdots \\ \Phi_N - \Phi_0 \end{pmatrix}, \tag{9}$$

where A is the position difference matrix given by

$$A = \begin{pmatrix} x_1 - x_0, \; y_1 - y_0 \\ \cdots \\ x_N - x_0, \; y_N - y_0 \end{pmatrix}. \tag{10}$$

A time step was chosen as in [5] to make the algorithm stable.

4 Example

We illustrate the procedure outlined above on two 256×256 MR images of the heart acquired on a GE scanner. Referring to Figure 3, we show the diastolic (Figure 3(a)) and systolic (Figure 3(b)) time points of the cardiac cycle.

The black regions in Figure 3 (c) and (d) are two multi-connected domains, corresponding to the heart muscle and other tissues in which we use image intensity as the mass density. Uniform mass densities could also be used, in which case mass preservation becomes a simple area preservation constraint. These regions were chosen as natural candidates to apply an MP deformation (in contrast to the left ventricle in which the change is too drastic to sensibly apply the procedure). Harmonic parametrization is first done on each domain (as shown in Figure 2 for the diastolic image), and an FEM-based L^2 MKP is

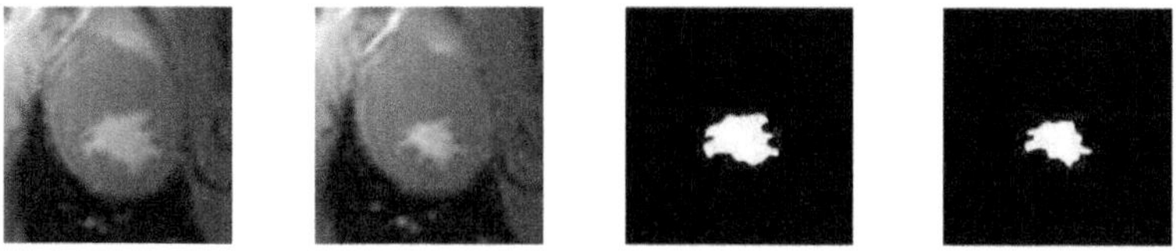

(a) diastolic phase (b) systolic phase (c) the mask of (a) (d) the mask of (b)

Fig. 3. Two heart MR images and their segmentation results

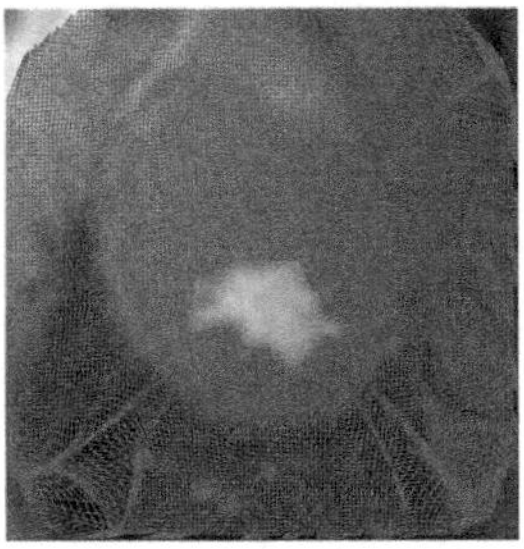

Fig. 4. The deformed grid on the systolic heart image

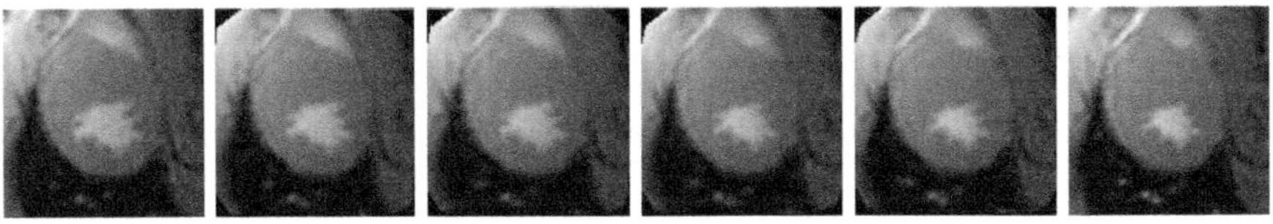

Fig. 5. Morphing movie for two heart images in Figure 3

then solved between the two domains to find the correspondence. Figure 4 shows the deformed grid. We can also create a morphing video to show the deformation of the first image into the second. Figure 5 shows some key frames in the video.

5 Conclusions

In this note, we extended the methodology for applying MP registration [5] to a pair of doubly-connected domains. For an L^2 version of the problem, a gradient descent algorithm is proposed to solve the problem iteratively. Harmonic analysis is employed in this approach for constructing an initial MP mapping. If the radius of the inner boundary is small enough, the inner boundary can be considered as a single landmark. In this sense, we have solved for MP registration on two domains with a pair of corresponding landmarks. This technique can also be extended into multi-connected domains (corresponding to multiple landmarks).

In the present work, the pure L^2 Kantorovich-Wasserstein functional is proposed as the similarity measure. A modified energy functional penalizing the intensity change can also be implemented [12]. Other types of distance measures, *e.g.* minimizers of the Dirichlet energy integral, can also be combined with a mass preservation constraint [1]. We plan to implement these ideas in some future work.

References

1. S. Angenent, S. Haker, and A. Tannenbaum. Minimizing flows for the Monge-Kantorovich problem. *SIAM J. Math. Analysis*, 35(1):61–97, 2003.
2. Y. Brenier. Polar factorization and monotone rearrangement of vector-valued functions. *Com. Pure Appl. Math.*, 64:375–417, 1991.

3. W. Gangbo and R. McCann. The geometry of optimal transportation. *Acta Math.*, 177:113–161, 1996.
4. S. Haker, S. Angenent, A. Tannenbaum, and R. Kikinis. Nondistorting flattening maps and the 3D visualization of colon CT images. *IEEE Trans. on Medical Imaging*, 19:665–670, 2000.
5. S. Haker, L. Zhu, A. Tannenbaum, and S. Angenent. Optimal mass transport for registration and warping. *International Journal on Computer Vision*, 60(3):225–240, 2004.
6. S. Rachev and L. Ruschendorf. *Mass transportation problems*, volume Volumes I and II: Probability and Its Applications. Springer, New York, 1998.
7. Y. Rubner, C. Tomasi, and J. Guibas. The earth mover's distance as a metric for image retrieval. Technical Report STAN-CS-TN-98-86, Department of Computer Science, Stanford University, September 1998.
8. H. Tagare. Deformable 2-d template matching using orthogonal curves. *IEEE Trans. Med. Imaging*, 16(1):108–117, 1997.
9. A. Toga. *Brain Warping.* Academic Press, San Diego, 1999.
10. A. Yezzi and J. Prince. An Eulerian PDE approach for computing tissue thickness. *IEEE Trans. on Medical Imaging*, 22(10):1332–1339, 2003.
11. L. Zhu and A. Tannenbaum. Image interpolation based on optimal mass preserving mappings. In *Proc. of International Symposium on Biomedical Imaging (ISBI'04)*, pages 21–24, 2004.
12. L. Zhu, Y. Yang, A. Tannenbaum, and S. Haker. Image morphing based on mutual information and optimal mass transport. In *Proc. of Int. Conf. on Image Processing 2004 (ICIP2004)*, pages 1675–1678, 2004.

Liver Registration for the Follow-Up of Hepatic Tumors

Arnaud Charnoz[1,3], Vincent Agnus[1], Grégoire Malandain[2], Clément Forest[1], Mohamed Tajine[3], and Luc Soler[1]

[1] IRCAD R&D, Strasbourg, France
[2] Epidaure Research group, INRIA, Sophia Antipolis, France
[3] LSIIT, CNRS/ULP, Strasbourg, France

Abstract. In this paper we propose a new two step method to register the liver from two acquisitions. This registration helps experts to make an intra-patient follow-up for hepatic tumors.

Firstly, an original and efficient tree matching is applied on different segmentations of the vascular system of a single patient [1]. These vascular systems are segmented from CT-scan images acquired (every six months) during disease treatement, and then modeled as trees. Our method matches common bifurcations and vessels. Secondly, an estimation of liver deformation is computed from the results of the first step.

This approach is validated on a large synthetic database containing cases with various deformation and segmentation problems. In each case, after the registration process, the liver recovery is very accurate (around 95%) and the mean localization error for 3D landmarks in liver is small (around 4mm).

1 Introduction

Motivations: Liver Tumors Follow-Up: The main purpose of our work is to make an intra-patient follow-up of tumors (see our previous work [2]). This task is difficult since the liver is a highly deformable organ. Thus, tumor matching relies on the liver deformation. To estimate this deformation, we propose to compute a deformation field from reliable landmarks and then extrapolate it to a dense field. It is a well-known result that the most reliable landmarks to estimate deformations sustained by the liver are provided by its vascular network [3,4,5,6,7]. We use our iterative tree matching algorithm on the vascular system, to match common bifurcations and edges (see [1] for more details). Thus, each match provides a displacement vector. From this sparse data a dense deformation field is built.

Proposal: The remainder of this paper is organized as follows. We briefly recall related methods to solve the problematics of our approach to compare and to justify our approach. Then, we summarize our iterative oriented tree matching (detailed in [1]). The next part describes the registration algorithm. The last section deals with the validation protocol and demonstrates the efficiency of this global approach (localization error reduced from 20mm to 4mm).

J. Duncan and G. Gerig (Eds.): MICCAI 2005, LNCS 3750, pp. 155–162, 2005.

2 Related Works

Matching: Related works propose algorithms to match and/or register vascular systems (brain, liver and, in a similar manner, lung airways). Generally, veins are modeled as graphs computed from segmented images and skeletons [8]. Some authors use tree structure notions in their algorithms to register a tree with an image [3] or two trees [4]. Other approaches match structures (nodes and vessels), but use general graph matching methods [5,6,9] or specific methods like subtree isomorphism [7] which do not take segmentation problems into account.

The oriented tree matching problem is more specific than graph matching because the structure is oriented and the path that connects two nodes is unique. Moreover, it cannot be considered as an oriented subtree isomorphism problem because of the segmentation errors. Indeed, the segmentation process can miss some vessels (edges). This implies a (virtual) pruning on both trees (for example an edge in a tree could be represented by several successive edges on the other tree) and thus the tree topology differs between acquisitions.

In our previous work [1], vascular systems are modeled as trees. Then, tree vertices are matched using a cost function that takes possible segmentation errors into account. Our algorithm does not focus on the best solution (given two edge sets to match) but on the most likely solutions which are updated during the process.

Vector Field Interpolation: Several methods exist to produce a deformation vector field from sparse displacements : the method in [10] is based on the computation of the optical flow. Another approach uses krigging [11] or considers the deformation field as a derivate of a potential scalar map modeled by Green's function [12]. A generalization of scalar splines to vector interpolation is proposed in [13] to estimate displacements.

Our first time method is simpler and less computive consuming than previously cited ones. Indeed liver deformations are less complicated than generalized flow fields (no vortex for instance). Our method is decribed in section 4 and its efficiency which is encouraging is discussed in section 5.

3 Iterative Tree Matching Technique

This section describes how we build correspondences among common structures in the vascular system. Skeletons computed from segmented vascular systems can be represented as oriented trees. The orientation symbolizes blood circulation flow. Nodes represent bifurcations and edges correspond to vessels between two bifurcations. Furthermore in our algorithm, some geometric attributes are added to the vessels (3D positions, radius, path).

Vascular trees segmented for a patient follow-up represent the same vascular system and our goal is to find common bifurcations and to register them. However, their topology and 3D positions may differ due to segmentation errors and deformations applied to them. The main challenge consists in using tree topology

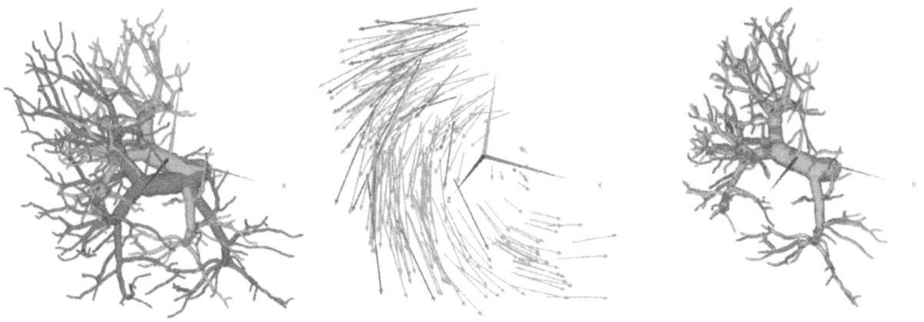

Fig. 1. **[Left]** A large deformation case is pruned at 20% (% of branch area randomly removed in both trees). **[Center]** The figure shows the result of our oriented tree matching, good matches are represented by light gray arrows and represent 91% of all nodes and wrong matches by dark gray arrows. **[Right]** The figure shows the tree registration after the process.

to detect deformations, and in parallel, geometric information to detect topology problems.

The idea of our algorithm [1] is to search for the best tree matching starting from roots (vascular system entrance). Since possibilities are numerous, we propose to generate and select the most relevant solutions. The algorithm starts by studying the root match and updates selected solutions while it explores and finds other possible matches in both trees. This means that some solutions selected at a given process step can be eliminated later if they become less relevant. The relevance of the solutions is evaluated at each step using a quality match criteria. We show in [1] that this algorithm matches 90% of common nodes on standard deformation and pruning. An example is shown in Fig. 1 and other results are shown on Tab. 2. For more information on this topic, please refer to our previous paper [1] in which this method is described and validated.

4 Registration

The previous step provides us with a match set which represents a deformation vector field. We explain here how we extrapolate it to a dense field in order to predict the liver deformation.

The matching provides us with a vector deformation $\boldsymbol{T_i} = P_i' - P_i$ in each correspondence point (bifurcation) (P_i',P_i). Our method extrapolates this vector flow to yield deformation vectors in each point inside the liver. To compute the deformation $\boldsymbol{T_M}$, we use Voronoi cells $V_i = \{P \in \mathcal{R}^3 : \|P - P_i\| \leq \|P - P_j\|, \forall j \neq i\}$. The extrapolated deformation $\boldsymbol{T_M}$ in a point $M \neq P_i$ is defined by :

$$\boldsymbol{T_M} = \frac{1}{volume(S_M)} \times \sum_i volume(V_i \cap S_M) \times \boldsymbol{T_i} \tag{1}$$

where S_M is a sphere centered on M and of radius $d = \min_i \|M - P_i\|$. This deformation is a linear combination of surrounding bifurcation displacements. The impact of each displacement is correlated with its influence zone $(V_i \cap S_M)$.

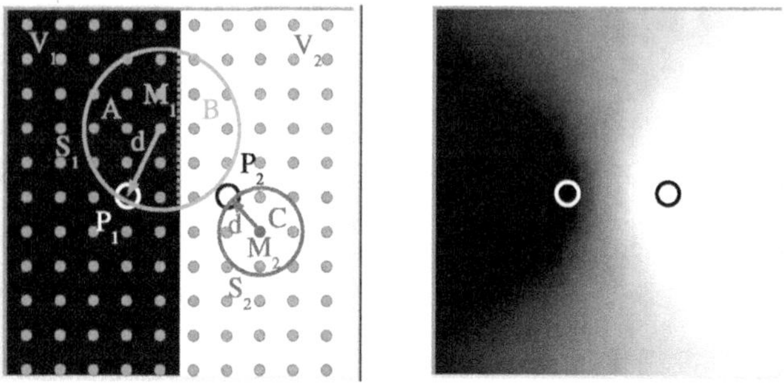

Fig. 2. [**Left**] The figure shows two color points P_1 (black) and P_2 (white), their associated Voronoi cell V_1 and V_2. The circles S_i are defined using the distance d from M_i to the closest point P_i. [**Right**] The figure shows the result of our color interpolation.

To speed up the process,the displacement field is computed on a regular subsampled liver. Then, we use a trilinear interpolation to extend the results to whole liver. A 2D example with color interpolation of two points (white and black) is illustrated on Fig. 2.

5 Experiments and Validation

To validate this registration algorithm, it is necessary to have a large patient database. However, we lack multi-acquisitions of the same patient mostly because the time between two acquisitions is long as it is imposed by the disease treatment (around 6 months). This is why our real patient database is not sufficient to provide a clinical validation of our method. However, a real case is studied at the end of this paper and results are encouraging for the future.

At the moment, we have tested our algorithm on a large synthetic database. Even if synthetic cases differ slightly from real cases (deformations and segmentation problems are simulated), working with a synthetic database has some advantages. It allows to test many configurations and to have a gold standard, so that we can estimate the algorithm efficiency. In this section, we present how we build this database and obtain our results.

5.1 Creating Virtual Patient

To test and validate our algorithm, we worked on synthetic deformation applied on a liver and its hepatic vascular system. The liver model has been extracted from the Visible Man image which voxel resolution is $0.33 \times 0.33 \times 1$mm (cf. The Visible Human Project of NLM) with a segmentation that provides us an accurate quality model.

To simulate deformations, we use the minimally invasive hepatic surgery simulator prototype developed at INRIA [14]. This simulator provides a realistic deformation model for the liver and its vascular system. It uses complex biomechanical models, based on linear elasticity and finite element theory, including

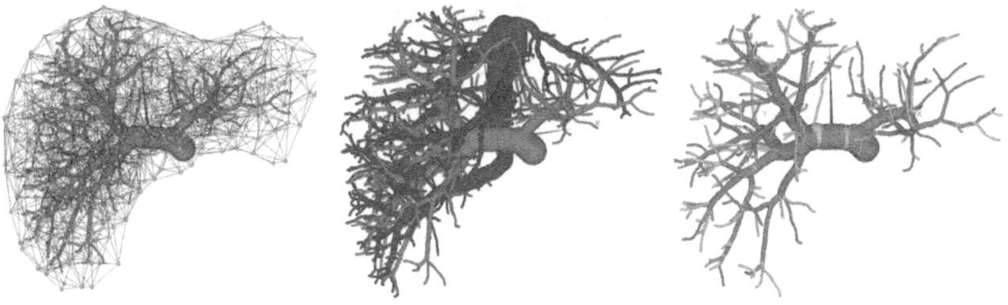

Fig. 3. The EPIDAURE surgery simulator is used to simulate liver and vascular system deformations. **[Left]** Volumetric model with the portal vascular system. **[Center]** Portal and sus-hepatic vascular system of Visible Man **[Right]** Portal vascular system is randomly pruned to lose approximately 40% of its branches. Lost branches appear in light gray.

anisotropic deformations. Thanks to a discussion with surgeons, we try to render realistic deformations by simulating pressure applied on the liver (breathing, patient positions, etc). The left of Fig.5 shows an example of an applied deformation.

To simulate segmentation errors, we have pruned random tree branches. Since segmentation errors are mostly observed on small vessels, the probability to lose small vessels is greater than to lose large ones. A database of 600 patient follow-up cases has been generated from 5 types of deformations and 5 pruning steps (0,10,20,30,40 %) with, on each step, 20 randomly generated prunings.

5.2 Results on a Virtual Patient

Matching: In our previous paper [1], we have demonstrated the efficiency and robustness of our matching algorithm on standard deformations. An average of 90% of all possible matches was found in the 600 different cases, even with large pruning. The process is fast and matches 380 nodes in 10 minutes on a 1GHz PC. Fig. 1 shows an example of a matching process where we obtain an efficiency of 91% for a standard deformation case.

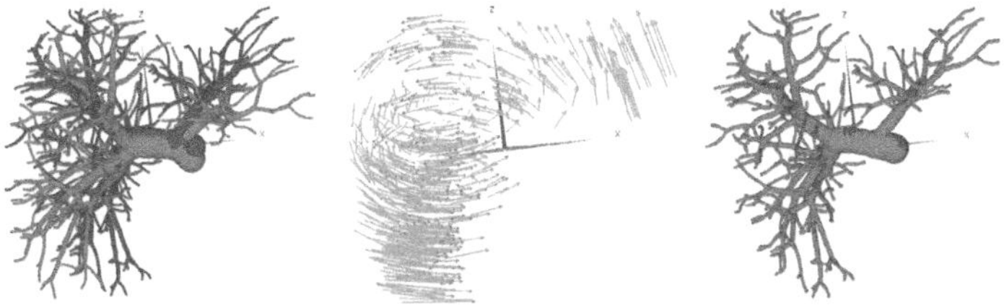

Fig. 4. **[Left]** Portal vascular system before the deformation estimation. **[Center]** Perfect match between both portal trees. **[Right]** Portal vascular system after the registration.

Table 1. Deformation results on deformation n 5 : All distances are in millimeters. The liver similarity is $\frac{vol(L_1 \cap L_2)}{vol(L_1 \cup L_2)}$ with L_i the liver area. Before the registration, the liver similarity is **72.3%** and the mean displacement distance between livers is **22.7 ± 10.3** . With a perfect registration, these distances (errors) should be equal to 0 and liver similarity to 100%.

% pruning	portal system		portal & sus-hepatic system	
	error	similarity	error	similarity
0-0	3.0 ± 2.0	95.4	2.3 ± 1.8	96.4
10-10	3.2 ± 2.1	94.9	2.5 ± 1.9	96.0
20-20	**3.9 ± 2.6**	**93.9**	2.8 ± 2.0	95.6
30-30	4.6 ± 3.1	92.4	3.3 ± 2.6	94.4
40-40	5.0 ± 3.3	92.5	3.8 ± 2.8	94.0
50-50	5.6 ± 3.5	91.3	4.5 ± 3.1	92.7

Table 2. Matching and deformation results: Each vascular system of these five configurations has been pruned at 20%. The sensitivity (S) is the number of correct found matches among the number of perfect solution matches (here 165 nodes). The efficiency (E) is the number of correct found matches among the number of found matches (correct and incorrect). The average distance between same points in the liver are shown before registration (references), after the deformation estimated from our matching and after a deformation estimated from a perfect matching.

cases	S	E	references		found matches		perfect matches	
			error	similarity	error	similarity	error	similarity
def1	98.8	90.4	9.9 ± 4.2	84.1	1.5 ± 1.3	97.0	1.3 ± 1.2	97.3
def2	95.5	87.1	28.9 ± 13.6	73.3	4.9 ± 4.2	94.2	4.4 ± 3.4	94.2
def3	98.2	86.9	22.9 ± 11.8	67.8	3.2 ± 2.0	96.0	3.3 ± 2.2	95.6
def4	96.0	87.1	19.7 ± 9.8	75.9	3.5 ± 2.5	95.3	3.3 ± 2.3	95.5
def5	96.1	87.1	**22.7 ± 10.3**	72.3	4.2 ± 3.0	93.6	**3.9 ± 2.6**	**93.9**

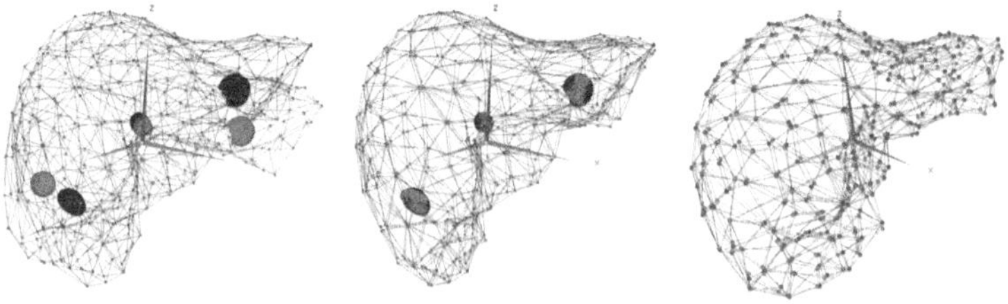

Fig. 5. **[Left]** Liver and its tumors before the deformation estimation. **[Center]** Liver and its tumors after the registration. **[Right]** Details on liver superimposition after the registration.

Deformation Field: Here, we test the registration robustness only. Thus, the estimation is computed from a perfect matching. Firstly, we study the registration estimated from portal vascular system matches with different level of pruning. Secondly, we improve the estimation by adding the sus-hepatic vascular system analysis. Table 1 shows the results of these experiments. The synthetic deformation on the volumetric mesh gives us the true displacement inside the liver. Thus we compare this displacement with the one estimated from the deformation field by studying the distance between matching 3D landmarks. We compute a mean and a standard deviation on the distance between the corresponding points. According to surgeons, results are sufficient to permit a tumor follow-up: the mean error to localize a 3D point in the liver is 5.6 mm in the worst case and our registration estimation is robust against the pruning of data. Results are better when the sus-hepatic analysis is added to the process. However, the gain (about 1 mm) appears small compared to the 10 additional minutes necessary to match the vascular system. Fig. 4 shows the vascular system registrations estimated from a perfect matching on the case number 5 with a 20% pruning.

6 Conclusion

The purpose of this paper was to present a new robust method to register the liver between two CT/MRI acquisitions using the segmented vascular systems. This registration provides us a powerful tool for the follow-up of hepatic tumors. It is easier to match tumors after this registration despite the disease evolution. Thanks to the synthetic database automatically generated by the INRIA simulator, we have tested numerous configurations. These different cases allow us to gain in robustness.

Currently, we are improving the liver deformation by testing another vector flow extrapolation. Moreover we are taking the liver surface into account to better estimate the deformation close to the surface (generally far from the vascular system). In parallel, we have started tests on a real patient database with very encouraging results (Fig. 6) and we plan to provide surgeons with a new tool for automatic diagnosis of liver tumor evolution.

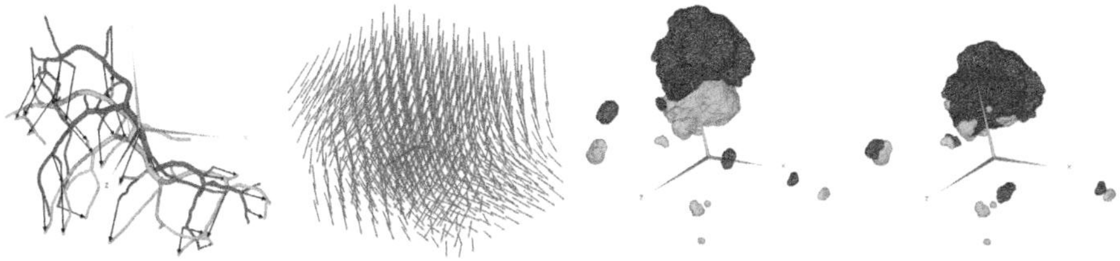

Fig. 6. [**a**]Real patient where the vascular system has been matched whose vertex matches are represented by black arrows. [**b**]Deformation field computed from matches. [**c,d**]Tumors before and after registration.

Acknowledgments. We wish to thank the Strasbourg hospital and their surgeons for providing images as well as for their advice on "standard" deformations applied to the liver. This work has benefited from the segmentation program of the vascular system developed by the IRCAD R&D team. The realistic liver deformations are provided by the INRIA simulator from the Epidaure project. Many thanks to Clément Forest for his assistance during the use of the simulator.

References

1. Charnoz, A., Agnus, V., Malandain, G., Nicolau, S., Tajine, M., Soler, L.: Design of robust vascular tree matching: validation on liver. In: IPMI. Volume 3565 of LNCS., Glenwood Springs, Colorado, USA, Springer Verlag (2005) 443–455
2. Charnoz, A., Agnus, V., Soler, L.: Portal vein registration for the follow-up of hepatic tumours. In: MICCAI. Volume 3216 of LNCS., Saint-Malo, France, Springer Verlag (2004) 878–886
3. Aylward, S., Jomier, J., Weeks, S., Bullitt, E.: Registration and analysis of vascular images. IJCV **55** (2003) 123–138
4. Lange, T., Eulenstein, S., Hunerbein, M., Lamecker, H., Schlag, P.M.: Augmenting intraoperative 3D ultrasound with preoperative models for navigation in liver surgery. In: MICCAI. Volume 3217 of LNCS., Saint-Malo, France, Springer Verlag (2004) 534–541
5. Tschirren, J., Palágyi, K., Reinhardt, J., Hoffman, E., Sonka, M.: Segmentation, Skeletonization, and Branchpoint Matching - A Fully Automated Quantitative Evaluation of Human Intrathoracic Airway Trees. In: MICCAI. Volume 2489 of LNCS., Springer-Verlag (2002) 12–19
6. Park, Y.: Registration of linear structures in 3D medical images. PhD thesis, Osaka University, Japan. Departement of informatics and Mathematical Science (2002)
7. Pisupati, C., Wolff, L., Mitzner, W., Zerhouni, E.: Tracking 3D pulmonary tree structures. In: MMBIA, IEEE Computer Society (1996) 160
8. Soler, L., Delingette, H., Malandain, G., Montagnat, J., Ayache, N., Clément, J.M., Koehl, C., Dourthe, O., Mutter, D., Marescaux, J.: A fully automatic anatomical, pathological and fonctionnal segmentation from CT-scans for hepatic surgery. In: Medical Imaging. SPIE proceedings, San Diego (2000) 246–255
9. Pelillo, M., Siddiqi, K., Zucker, S.: Matching hierarchical structures using association graphs. PAMI **21** (1999) 1105–1120
10. Gibson, D., Spann, M.: Robust optical flow estimation based on a sparse motion trajectory set. IEEE Transactions on Image Processing (2003)
11. Cressie, N.: Statistics for Spatial Data (Revised Edition). Wiley: New York (1993)
12. Mussa-Ivaldi: From basis functions to basis fields: Vector field approximation from sparse data. In: Biological Cybernetics. Volume 67. (1992) 479–489
13. Cachier, P., Ayache, N.: Isotropic energies, filters and splines for vector field regularization. Journal of Mathematical Imaging and Vision archive **20** (2004) 147–167
14. Picinbono, G., Lombardo, J.C., Delingette, H., Ayache, N.: Improving realism of a surgery simulator: linear anisotropic elasticity, complex interactions and force extrapolation. JVCA **13** (2002) 147–167

Maximum a Posteriori Local Histogram Estimation for Image Registration

Matthew Toews[1], D. Louis Collins[2], and Tal Arbel[1]

[1] Center for Intelligent Machines, McGill University, Montréal, Canada
{mtoews, arbel}@cim.mcgill.ca
[2] McConnell Brain Imaging Center, Montreal Neurological Institute,
McGill University, Montréal, Canada
louis@bic.mni.mcgill.ca

Abstract. Image similarity measures for registration can be considered within the general context of joint intensity histograms, which consist of bin count parameters estimated from image intensity samples. Many approaches to estimation are ML (maximum likelihood), which tends to be unstable in the presence sparse data, resulting in registration that is driven by spurious noisy matches instead of valid intensity relationships. We propose instead a method of MAP (maximum a posteriori) estimation, which is well-defined for sparse data, or even in the absence of data. This estimator can incorporate a variety of prior assumptions, such as global histogram characteristics, or use a maximum entropy prior when no such assumptions exist. We apply our estimation method to deformable registration of MR (magnetic resonance) and US (ultrasound) images for an IGNS (image-guided guided neurosurgery) application, where our MAP estimation method results in more stable and accurate registration than a traditional ML approach.

1 Introduction

The evaluation of intensity similarity between two images for the task of image registration can be framed in the general context of joint intensity histograms, for a wide variety of similarity measures including correlation, correlation ratio, mutual information and others [12]. In this context, the task of similarity evaluation is to calculate the relevant similarity measure based on *an estimate* of the joint intensity histogram. Thus, the quality of image similarity evaluation is dependent on the quality of joint histogram estimation.

Histogram estimation can be considered in the context of statistical parameter estimation, where the parameters to be estimated are the bin counts of the joint histogram. A variety of estimation techniques have been presented in the literature, the majority of which are variants of ML (maximum likelihood) estimation [6]. The hallmark of ML estimators is that they become unstable in the presence of sparse image data, and are undefined in the absence of image data. As such, ML estimators perform poorly in the presence of sparse data, tending to latch onto spurious, noisy matches despite the variety of techniques designed to improve their performance such as Parzen windowing, partial volume interpolation, robust ML estimation, etc.

J. Duncan and G. Gerig (Eds.): MICCAI 2005, LNCS 3750, pp. 163–170, 2005.

In this article, we present a method of joint histogram estimation based on MAP (maximum a posteriori) parameter estimation. In contrast to ML estimation, MAP histogram estimates are well-defined in sparse data or even in the complete absence of data by a prior distribution over histogram bins. As such, MAP histogram estimates are not subject to instability as are ML estimates. Furthermore, MAP estimation provides a principled way incorporating prior information in terms of the number of samples required to obtain a valid histogram estimate. As a result, one can bias histogram estimates such that if the number of samples is insufficient, the MAP estimate will favor a benign prior unlikely to lead to spurious matches.[1]

In practical terms, our method involves pre-populating joint histogram bin counts before the arrival of data, according to an estimate of number of samples M required for valid joint histogram estimation. This pre-population constitutes our prior belief as to the joint histogram, which is gradually outweighed as data samples are added. This general approach is known to stabilize probability estimates of infrequently observed events [10], but it is not commonly used to stabilizing image similarity estimates for registration.

Our MAP estimation method was developed for the purpose of on-line nonlinear registration of MR (magnetic resonance) and US (ultrasound) imagery in the context of an IGNS (image-guided neurosurgery) application. This is a demanding registration task for the following reason: the joint intensity relationship between MR and US imagery is noisy, multi-modal and highly non-stationary (i.e. varying with spatial location), thus computing image similarity for registration requires a sophisticated similarity measure such as MI (mutual information) with a high degree of parameterization. At the same time, precise nonlinear registration requires evaluating similarity within small local image windows, meaning a relatively large number of histogram parameters must be estimated from a relatively small number of intensity samples. A principled method of histogram estimation is therefore needed to overcome the problem of sparsity. Preliminary results based on stereotactic ground truth are promising, indicating a greater degree of registration stability and accuracy when based on MAP as opposed to ML histogram estimation.

2 Methods for Dealing with Sparsity

Sparsity in histogram estimation is a problem touched on by many authors, although rarely in the framework of statistical parameter estimation. Here we present some common approaches histogram estimation, particularly for the purpose of dealing with data sparsity:

Parzen windowing: Parzen windowing [15], involves smoothing histograms with a Parzen window kernel, often a Gaussian. Parzen windowing has the drawback of populating histogram estimates with fictitious samples, and does not generally converge to the true histogram estimate with increased sample size. To

[1] We stress here that we refer not to MAP estimation for registration, but the estimation of the joint histogram used to evaluate similarity given a fixed image alignment.

see this, consider the case in which the joint intensity histogram is completely contained in a single histogram bin. Using Parzen windowing, this histogram will always contain a smoothed peak, regardless of the amount of image data.

Coarse histogram binning: Coarse histogram binning reduces the number of parameters to be estimated from a limited amount of data [16]. Coarse histogram binning in itself is not sufficient to deal with sparsity, however, as the coarser the histogram quantization, the more impoverished the histograms become for the purpose of registration. In addition, even highly quantized histograms can suffer from undersampling given small local window sizes. Finally, the question of an optimal quantization scheme is difficult and task dependent.

Probabilistic Segmentation of Before Registration: A new approach which serves to reduce problems with sparse intensity histogram estimation is to compute histograms based on probabilistically labeled images [2]. Here, histograms are based on low-dimensional probability distributions, resulting in bins that are non-zero. Although seemingly well suited to it's purpose, such an approach requires the extra step of probabilistic data segmentation, which in our experience tends to blur out local structures in favor of global segmentation.

Weighting Local Histograms with Global Intensity Relationships: Weighting local histograms with global intensity relationships has been touched on by several authors [9,7,4,8,14], suggesting agreement that a means of dealing with sparsity is to populate histograms based on other sources of relevant information. The drawback with considering global histograms is that they do not generally reflect local intensity relationships, as in the case of MR and US modalities (See Figure 1), and can result in inappropriately biased estimates. That being said, our method of MAP estimation can be used to bias local histogram estimates using a variety of prior information within the principled context of statistical parameter estimation, allowing incorporation of global histogram information when relevant and providing other options when it is not.

3 MAP Histogram Estimation

The majority of techniques have difficulty with local histogram estimation because they are based on ML estimation, which becomes increasingly unstable in the presence of sparse data. In practical terms, this results in registration that tends latch onto spurious incorrect matches as data sparsity increases. To deal with this instability, we propose MAP estimation with a maximum entropy prior, which tends to produce strong matches only when justified by sufficient intensity samples.

3.1 Maximum Likelihood vs. Maximum a Posteriori

The task of estimating a local histogram for the purpose of registration is one of estimating a set of K discrete bin frequency counts $\theta = \{\theta^1, \ldots, \theta^K\}$. The goal in histogram estimation is to determine the values of θ that maximize $p(\theta|I)$, the conditional probability of θ given the image data I. By Bayes rule, the following equality holds:

$$p(\theta|I) = \frac{p(I|\theta)p(\theta)}{p(I)}. \tag{1}$$

For the purpose of statistical parameter estimation, $p(I)$ is constant as image data I is constant, $p(I|\theta)$ naturally takes the form of a multinomial distribution, and $p(\theta)$ and $p(\theta|I)$ are Dirichlet distributions [6].

There are two significantly different methods of estimating $p(\theta|I)$: ML and MAP. We advocate the MAP strategy, as it provides a principled mechanism for explicitly incorporating prior information in the form of the number of intensity samples M required for valid estimation.

ML Estimation: ML estimation is based on the assumption that $p(\theta)$ is constant. Under this assumption, we seek an estimate θ_{ML} such that:

$$\theta_{ML} = \underset{\theta}{\text{argmax}} \{ p(I|\theta) \}. \tag{2}$$

Here, to maximize $p(\theta|I)$, it suffices to maximize the term $p(I|\theta)$, which is known as the *likelihood*, hence the name maximum likelihood estimation. In ML estimation, histogram bin counts θ are simply set to counts of intensity data I, optionally processed with Parzen windowing, etc.

MAP Estimation: MAP estimation does not treat all histograms as equally probable, and $p(\theta)$ is not constant. In particular, certain histograms are more probable than others, based on prior assumptions we may have regarding θ, and we seek an estimate θ_{MAP} such that:

$$\theta_{MAP} = \underset{\theta}{\text{argmax}} \{ p(I|\theta)p(\theta) \}. \tag{3}$$

It can be shown that as the number of intensity samples I approaches infinity, both ML and MAP estimation converge to the same optimal histogram estimate of θ [6]. In intuitive terms, this is because the prior distribution $p(\theta)$ of the MAP approach becomes swamped by $p(\theta|I)$. Being swamped with intensity data is hardly a problem in histogram estimation however, particularly when attempting to calculate similarity for the purpose of localized deformation [11]. It is precisely in the case of sparse data samples I that the difference between ML and MAP estimation is most telling. MAP estimation allows the incorporation of a prior distribution $p(\theta)$ as to the value of θ in the absence of data I. In the presence of sparse data, i.e. an image window I with insufficient samples to estimate the histogram, we would like estimation to default to our expectation as to the true histogram values, or at least a benign histogram θ that is not likely to result in spurious, noise-driven matches.

In general, $p(\theta)$ could be based on a variety of prior assumptions, i.e. the global histogram approach, although the global histogram may not be representative of local intensity relationships, as in the case of MR/US registration. In the absence of constraints, we follow the rule of maximum entropy [5] and suggest a uniform prior - in the case of undersampling, the uniformly-weighted histogram is adverse to making a strong decision regarding registration, and the effect of spatial neighborhood constraints will dominate. In the case where the number of intensity sam-

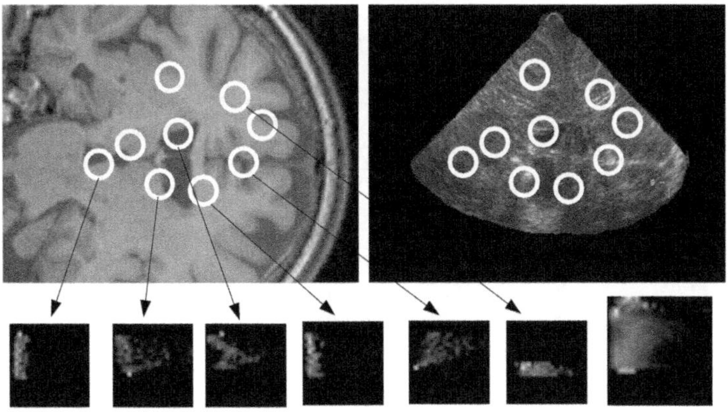

Fig. 1. The image intensity relationship between MR and US image modalities is multi-modal and non-stationary, i.e. varying spatial position. The upper left image is a 2D slice from T1-weighted MRI brain volume, and the upper right image is a corresponding US image slice. Correspondence was determined via a stereotactic positioning of the US probe relative to the volume coordinate system. The white circles overlaying the image indicate local regions within which local likelihood histograms $p(US|MR)$ are calculated. The smaller images along the bottom are likelihood histograms, where the vertical axis is MR intensity and the horizontal axis is US intensity. The histograms corresponding to local regions are indicated by arrows, and the larger histogram in the bottom right is the global histogram. It can be seen that the statistical likelihood pixel relationship is non-stationary, as it varies significantly with spatial location. In addition, local likelihood relationships are significantly different from the global likelihood.

ples is significant, the uniform prior will be outweighed by evidence and valid registration will occur. The intuition is that M should be set according to the number intensity samples required to obtain a valid histogram estimate, which is related to a number of factors such as noise, the number of histogram bins to be estimated, etc. Our MAP estimation approach can be summarized as follows:

MAP Histogram Estimation:

1) Generate an estimate as to the number of intensity samples M required to obtain a valid estimate of the histogram bins.

2) Pre-populate histogram counts according to M, either uniformly or according to other sources of prior information.

4 Deformable MR to US Registration

We developed our MAP estimation method for the purpose of deformable registration of MR and US imagery in the context of an IGNS application, where the goal is to update a detailed pre-operative 3D MR volume of the brain used in intervention planning with real-time US gathered inter-operatively, in order to reflect brain shift that occurs once the dura lining has been entered. With

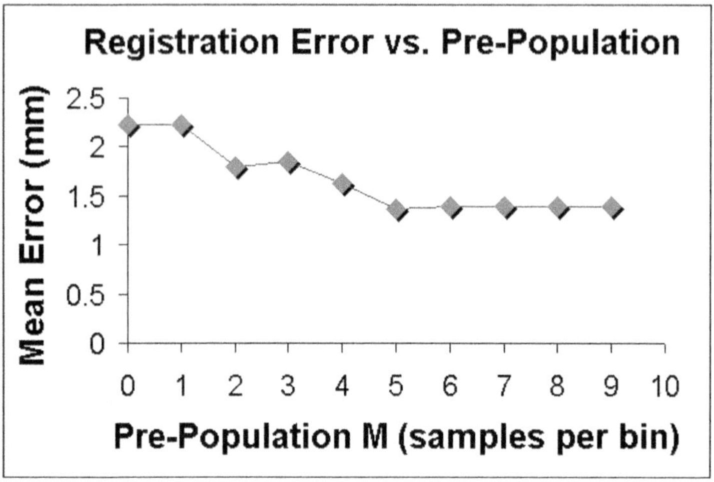

Fig. 2. A plot of mean displacement vector registration error vs. the degree of uniform prior incorporated MAP estimation. The error for a 9-point displacement field drops by a factor of 1.6 as the joint histogram pre-population is increased from M=0 to M=5 samples per bin. Note that when M=0, MAP and ML estimation are equivalent. The error is high for low M, as the posterior is dominated by spurious local MI maxima. Error reaches a minimum at $M = 5$ samples per histogram bin, after which point it rises slightly as the elastic prior begins to dominate the posterior.

both the US probe and the patient's head registered rigidly via a stereotactic tracking apparatus, the task becomes one of updating the 3D MR volume based on non-linear registration with 2D US slices.

For the purpose of validation, we have compiled a database of US slices taken inter-operatively. To test registration, we focus on recapturing the deformation relative to stereotactic ground truth. US image structure is due to the reflection of acoustic waves at the boundaries of structures of differing density, and is an inherently noisy and difficult image modality to work with, due to speckle noise, signal attenuation artifacts such as acoustic shadows, etc. Figure 1 illustrates how the joint intensity relationship between MR and US varies to a large degree with spatial position.

In order to model nonlinear brain shift, we are interested in recovering a field of displacement vectors $\mathbf{T} = \{\mathbf{t_i}\}$ mapping fixed points in the MR image to their displacements in the US image. Adopting a Bayesian strategy as in [3], we formulate registration as a posterior probability over $\mathbf{T}$ given the images to be matched:

$$p(\mathbf{T}|US, MR) \propto p(US|\mathbf{T}, MR)p(\mathbf{T}). \tag{4}$$

The Bayesian formulation requires specification of the terms $p(US|\mathbf{T}, MR)$ and $p(\mathbf{T})$ which are referred to as the likelihood and prior, respectively. In registration, the likelihood is the data term serving to evaluate similarity between images US and MR given $\mathbf{T}$, and the prior serves to incorporate regularization constraints on $\mathbf{T}$ independent of image information, such smoothness, elasticity, etc. The strength of Bayesian registration is that the likelihood and prior terms can be be changed to suit the registration task at hand without altering the overall formulation.

For our purposes, we choose to model $p(US|\mathbf{T}, MR)$ using the MI (mutual information) of intensities. The MI is a widely-used measure of statistical intensity similarity based on information theory [15,1]. Many excellent references exist regarding the details of MI calculation [11]. Alternatively, we could have adopted the correlation ratio approach of [13] based on intensity and gradient images or a learning based similarity measure as in [7]. In order to model nonlinear deformation, we choose to model $p(\mathbf{T})$ using an elastic prior between pairs of neighboring deformation vectors in $\mathbf{T}$. The final Bayesian posterior is of the form:

$$p(\mathbf{T}|US, MR) \propto exp\{\alpha \sum_{i}^{N}(MI(US|\mathbf{t_i}, MR) - MI_{max}) - \beta \sum_{i,j}^{N,N} d(\mathbf{t_i}, \mathbf{t_j})\}, \quad (5)$$

where MI_{max} is the maximum MI achievable using a 25x25 bin joint histogram, N is the number of vectors in $\mathbf{T}$, $d(\mathbf{t_i}, \mathbf{t_j})$ represents an elastic prior energy between $\mathbf{t_i}$ and $\mathbf{t_j}$, and $\alpha = 5$ and $\beta = 2$ are empirically determined parameters that balance the relative strengths of the likelihood and prior terms.

For experimentation, we attempt to recover the known transform $\mathbf{T}$ between US and MR image pairs. Given a fixed local window size, we compare the result of registration $\mathbf{T}$ using ML and MAP estimation. The number of joint histogram bins used is 25x25=625 and the local window size is 43x43=1849 pixels. Optimization of the posterior in (5) was achieved via gradient ascent from 100 random seeds, and the best solution, i.e. the deformation field maximizing equation (5) was used in the result analysis. Random seeds were generated by perturbing vectors $\mathbf{t_i}$ to random displacements within a 25 pixel radius of the known transform. The resolution of registration was 1mm per pixel.

Figure 2 shows the impact of MAP estimation on registration error, as the degree of prior pre-population in the joint histogram is increased. Here we see that with little or no histogram pre-population, i.e. ML estimation, poor histogram estimates result in unstable, inaccurate registration.

5 Conclusion

In this article, we presented a principled means of estimating joint intensity histograms for the purpose of similarity calculation in the presence of sparse image data. Given the number of intensity samples M required to reliably estimate intensity histograms, we proposed a MAP estimation method based on a uniform prior histogram. The advantage of this method is that histogram estimates only result in strong matches when sufficient evidence exists to justify them, i.e. when the number of intensity samples is sufficiently high. In the case of undersampling, histogram estimates will default to a benign prior histogram that is unlikely to result in strong false matches. Traditional ML estimation, on the other hand, tends to produce strong false matches in the case of undersampling, which can throw off registration. Practically, our method is simple to implement, where histogram bin counts are pre-populated by M uniformly distributed samples prior to estimation, representing the prior assumption of MAP estimation. We expect that MAP histogram estimation will result in improved registration in other methods of similarity calculation based on histograms, such as correlation, correlation ratio, etc. Future work will involve further clinical validation, testing with other similarity measures, and determining of an optimal degree of prior information M to incorporate given the images to be registered.

References

1. A. Collignon, *Multi-modality medical image registration by maximization of mutual information*, Ph.D. thesis, Catholic University of Leuven, Leuven, Belgum, 1998.
2. Emiliano D'Agostino, Frederik Maes, Dirk Vandermeulen, and Paul Suetens, *An information theoretic approach for non-rigid image registration using voxel class probabilities*, MICCAI2003, 2003, pp. 812–820.
3. J.C. Gee, L. LeBriquer, and C. Barillot, *Probabilistic matching of brain images*, IPMI95, Kluwer, July 1995.
4. A. Guimond, A. Roche, N. Ayache, and J. Meunier, *Three-dimensional multimodal brain warping using the demons algorithm and adaptive intensity corrections*, IEEE Transactions on Medical Imaging **20** (2001), no. 1, 58–69.
5. E.T. Jaynes, *Prior probabilities*, I.E.E.E Transactions of systems,science, and cybernetics **SSC-4** (1968), no. 3, 227–241.
6. Michael I. Jordan, *An introduction to probabilistic graphical models*, In preparation, 2003.
7. Michael E. Leventon and W. Eric L. Grimson, *Multi-modal volume registration using joint intensity distributions*, Lecture Notes in Computer Science **1496** (1998), 1057–1066.
8. B. Likar and F. Pernus, *A heirarchical approach to elastic registration based on mutual information*, Image and Vision Computing **19** (2001), no. 1-2, 33–44.
9. J.B.A. Maintz, H.W. Meijering, and M.A. Viergever, *General multimodal elastic registration based on mutual information*, Medical Imaging (1998), 144–154.
10. Alon Orlitsky, Narayana P. Santhanam, and Junan Zhang, *Always good turing: Asymptotically optimal probability estimation*, Science **302** (2003), 427–431.
11. J.P.W. Pluim, J.B.A. Maintz, and M.A. Viergever, *Mutual-information-based registration of medical images: a survey*, MedImg **22** (2003), no. 8, 986–1004.
12. A. Roche, N. Malandain, Ayache, and S. Prima, *Toward a better comprehension of similarity measures used in medical image registration*, MICCAI99, 1999, pp. 555–566.
13. A. Roche, X. Pennec, G. Malandain, and N. Ayache, *Rigid registration of 3D ultrasound with MR images: a new approach combining intensity and gradient information*, IEEE Transactions on Medical Imaging **20** (2001), no. 10, 1038–1049.
14. P. Rogelj, S. Kovacic, and J. C. Gee, *Point similarity measures for non-rigid registration of multi-modal data.*, Computer Vision and Image Understanding **92** (2003), no. 1, 112–140.
15. P.A. Viola and W.M. Wells, III, *Alignment by maximization of mutual information*, International Journal of Computer Vision **24** (1997), no. 2, 137–154.
16. L. Zollei, W.E.L. Grimson, A. Norbash, and W.M. Wells, III, *2d-3d rigid registration of x-ray fluoroscopy and ct images using mutual information and sparsely sampled histogram estimators*, CVPR01, 2001, pp. II:696–703.

Dynamic 3D Ultrasound and MR Image Registration of the Beating Heart

Xishi Huang[1,6], Nicholas A. Hill[2,6], Jing Ren[3], Gerard Guiraudon[4,6], Derek Boughner[5,6], and Terry M. Peters[1,2,6]

[1] Department of Biomedical Engineering
[2] Department of Medical Biophysics
[3] Department of Electrical and Computer Engineering, The University of Western Ontario
[4] Canadian Surgical Technology and Advanced Robotics (CSTAR)
[5] London Health Sciences Centre
[6] Imaging Research Labs, Robarts Research Institute, London, ON, Canada N6A 5K8
{xhuang, nhill, tpeters}@imaging.robarts.ca
{jren2, gguiraud}@uwo.ca
derek.boughner@lhsc.on.ca

Abstract. Real-time three-dimensional ultrasound (RT3D US) is an ideal imaging modality for the diagnosis of cardiac disease. RT3D US is a flexible, inexpensive, non-invasive tool that provides important diagnostic information related to cardiac function. Unfortunately, RT3D US suffers from inherent shortcomings, such as low signal-to-noise ratio and limited field of view, producing images that are difficult to interpret. Multi-modal dynamic cardiac image registration is a well-recognized approach that compensates for these deficiencies while retaining the advantages of RT3D US imaging. The clinical application of multi-modal image registration methods is difficult, and there are a number of implementation issues to be resolved. In this work, we present a method for the rapid registration of RT3D US images of the beating heart to high-resolution magnetic resonance (MR) images. This method was validated using a volunteer image set. Validation results demonstrate that this approach can achieve rapid registration of images of the beating heart with fiducial landmark and registration errors of 1.25 ± 0.63 and 1.76 mm respectively. This technique can potentially be used to improve the diagnosis of cardiac disease by augmenting RT3D US images with high-resolution MR images and to facilitate intra-operative image fusion for minimally invasive cardio-thoracic surgical navigation.

1 Introduction

Cardiovascular disease is the most frequent cause of death by disease in North America and accounts for the death of more Canadians than any other disease. Early diagnosis of heart failure is essential for successfully addressing the underlying diseases and/or causes, and the prevention of further myocardial dysfunction and clinical deterioration.

J. Duncan and G. Gerig (Eds.): MICCAI 2005, LNCS 3750, pp. 171 – 178, 2005.

The ability of MRI to be employed in a dynamic mode allows cardiologists to acquire high quality images of cardiac anatomy that assist diagnosis, yet it is an expensive procedure that may not yield all of the relevant diagnostic information. Echocardiography, also used to diagnose cardiac disease, is a flexible, inexpensive, non-invasive tool. However, the cardiac images produced are of lower quality and the small field of view (FOV) makes it difficult for the cardiologist to mentally place abnormal cardiac structures and congenital defects in the proper clinical context, which increases the risk of misdiagnosis. While both real time echocardiography and dynamic MRI are routinely used in the diagnosis of cardiac disease, there is no mechanism to easily integrate information from both image sets in order to take maximum advantage of both modalities. Techniques currently used to examine the heart provide valuable information, but do not represent the complete picture of cardiac health. It is therefore important for the cardiologist to dynamically relate the images generated from US studies to dynamic MR images from the same patient. We believe that ability to correlate real time echocardiography images with previously acquired dynamic 3D MR images would be a significant contribution to the diagnosis of cardio-vascular abnormalities and to interventional and minimally-invasive cardiac surgery.

While existing literature outlines procedures and methods for multi-modal image registration [1, 2, 3], these approaches have mainly been used in neurosurgical applications [4, 5] and abdominal interventions [6]. These methods show promising results, however these techniques are insufficient to meet the demands of real time cardiac image registration. To account for the periodic motion of the beating heart, image registration must be performed very rapidly. The lower quality of the US images of the heart makes the realization of a fast, robust US-MR image registration technique difficult.

In this paper, we present a method for the rapid registration of RT3D US images with dynamic 3D MR images. This method integrates electrocardiogram (ECG) signals and a spatial tracking system with a commercially available US machine. Compared to the existing methods for fusing RT3D US with dynamic 3D MR images, our technique is the first to simultaneously address the issues of image acquisition, image processing timing constraints, and the motion of the beating heart.

2 Methods

In medical image registration one approach for modeling the beating heart is to represent the heart as a deformable model [7]. A major concern relating to this approach for real time 3D US-MR image registration is the associated computation time. For the method to operate in real time, the entire process (image acquisition, processing and visualization) must be completed at least 20 times per second. Accounting for time lag due to image acquisition and visualization, for real time image integration to be possible, image registration must be completed in 20-50 ms. If a deformable model is used, then the integration process requires substantially more computation time, because additional registration parameters need to be adjusted and optimized [8]. Therefore, the use of a deformable model to represent the heart is not a suitable choice in this case. To meet these strict time constraints we propose a registration method that employs a rigid-body transformation between US and MR images.

2.1 Rigid-Body Representation

During cardiac diagnosis and surgery planning the heart remains relatively fixed with respect to the thoracic cage between dynamic 3D MRI and RT3D US examinations. Breath-holding is employed during both MRI and US acquisitions to ensure that organ motion is due solely to the beating heart, and not a combination of the beating heart and patient respiration. Although the shape and size of the heart differs at different phases in the cardiac cycle, it is reasonable to assume that the overall pattern of shape and size variation does not change beat-to-beat. This assumption is especially true in the case of diagnosis where there is no significant change in heart rate or blood pressure. We further observe that if we subdivide the cardiac cycle into discrete cardiac phases, the US and MR images acquired at the same moment in the cardiac cycle represent the same physical heart features. Given these observations, it is straightforward to represent the registration for each pair of the US and MR frames of the same cardiac phase with a rigid-body transformation.

Furthermore, if we consider any two pairs of US and MR images in different phases, the non-rigid transformation between the two MRI frames is the same as that for the two US frames, because they represent the same physical heart deformation between the two cardiac phases. Aligning any pair of MRI and US frames automatically aligns the other sets of frames.

These observations imply that a single rigid-body transformation between the MR images and US images can be used to rapidly register the image sets.

2.2 Registration Method

To register RT3D US images with 4D MR images we track the US probe using a Polaris optical tracking system (OTS) (NDI, Waterloo, Canada) while simultaneously recording ECG signals. One major advantage of using US imaging systems lies in the flexibility of image acquisition. During a cardiac examination, the operator has the freedom to position/orientate the US probe in any manner to obtain the necessary views of the heart. Since the position and orientation of US probe is continuously tracked with the Polaris OTS, the tracking information can be used to register the US images to the world coordinate system (WCS).

ECG signals are employed to temporally align the US and MRI frames. Dynamic 3D MRI frames are often acquired with a fixed sampling rate, whereas the sampling rates for US systems vary with any on-the-fly adjustments made to the FOV by the operator. This difference in sampling rates implies that the US and MRI frames will not in general be temporally synchronized. To overcome this difficulty, we utilize ECG signals to phase-stamp the US images with timing information derived from the ECG signals. The MR images are temporally interpolated, and using this phase data, US and MR images with coincident cardiac phases are identified. The US images are transformed into the WCS and the US and MR images are registered together. Recognizing that there will be sampling errors in the ECG signal, the tracking system, and variations in the heart rate between MRI and US acquisitions, it is necessary to perform a final 'fine-tuning' of the registration to ensure optimal spatial and temporal alignment.

In order to fine-tune the registration result, the transformation matrix generated by the registration procedure is used as the starting position/orientation for a mutual information (MI) registration method [9], which further optimizes the registration with respect to seven parameters: translations (x, y, z), rotations (θ_x, θ_y, θ_z) and time (t).

2.3 Registration Procedure

Based on the above considerations and the analysis of cardiac diagnostic and planning problems, we outline the following procedures for real time image registration. Our approach involves two steps: 1) a pre-registration step and 2) a real-time registration step (Figure 1). The steps for the registration procedure are as follows:

Step 1. Pre-registration before procedure (diagnosis/planning):
Pre-operative
1. acquire dynamic 3D MR images (gradient echo T1-weighted imaging sequence with a voxel size of 1.5 mm^3 [10]) at different phases over one cardiac cycle

Immediately prior to procedure
2. acquire a 3D US image (denoted US_1) recording the US probe's tracking information ($T_{WCS \leftarrow US_1}$) and the ECG signal at some cardiac phase
3. the MR images are temporally interpolated and based on the ECG information ($\hat{t}_1$) the MR image with the closest cardiac phase is identified (denoted mr_1)
4. the two image sets are manually registered together, generating a temporary transformation matrix, $T_{mr_1 \leftarrow US_1}$
5. using $T_{mr_1 \leftarrow US_1}$ as the starting point, the two image sets are registered together using a MI registration method, optimizing the positional, rotational and temporal variables (x, y, z, θ_x, θ_y, θ_z, t) to obtain $T_{MR_1 \leftarrow US_1}$. We use the notation MR_1 to denote the optimal aligned MR image corresponding to US_1
6. finally, using the following relation, the pre-registration transformation $T_{MR \leftarrow WCS}$ is calculated

$$T_{MR \leftarrow WCS} = T_{MR_1 \leftarrow US_1} \left(T_{WCS \leftarrow US_1} \right)^{-1} \tag{1}$$

Step 2: Real-time registration during procedure:
1. acquire an intra-operative RT3D US image (denoted US_2), recording the probe tracking information ($T_{WCS \leftarrow US_2}$) and ECG signal
2. use the ECG signal to estimate the cardiac phase, $\hat{t}_2$, corresponding to US_2
3. derive a 'near-optimal' transformation, $T_{mr_2 \leftarrow US_2}$, using the following equation

$$T_{mr_2 \leftarrow US_2} = T_{MR \leftarrow WCS} T_{WCS \leftarrow US_2} \tag{2}$$

   where $T_{MR \leftarrow WCS}$ is the initial position/orientation estimated from the pre-registration procedure, and $T_{WCS \leftarrow US_2}$ is the US to WCS calibration transformation for US_2 and mr_2 denotes the MR image interpolated based on the ECG information ($\hat{t}_2$)

4. using $\hat{t}_2$ as the cardiac phase and $T_{mr_2 \leftarrow US_2}$ as the starting position/orientation, register the two image sets together using a MI registration method and generate the final transformation, $T_{MR_2 \leftarrow US_2}$, where MR_2 denotes the optimal interpolated MR image corresponding to US_2.

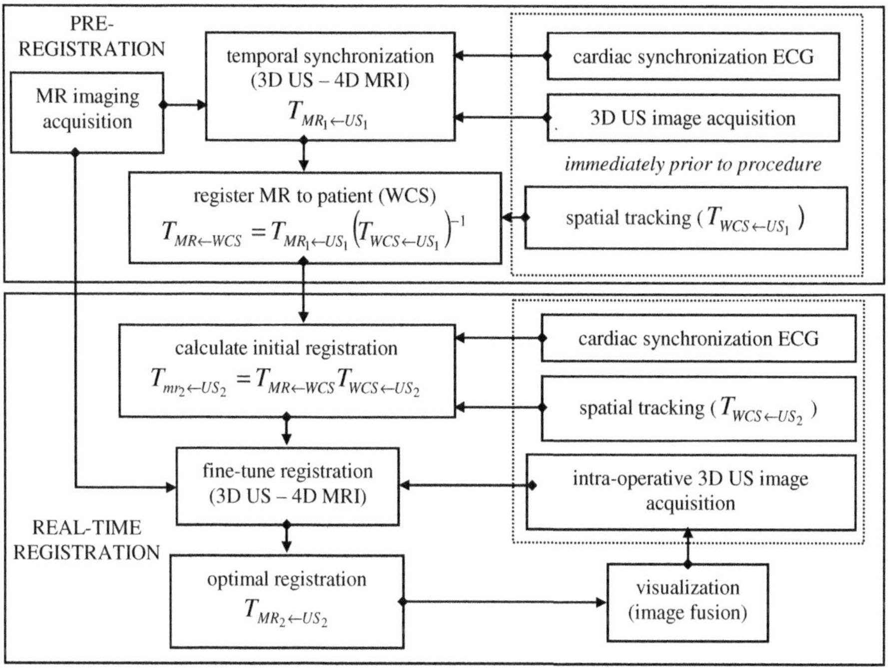

Fig. 1. The proposed method is a two-step registration procedure. The first step, *pre-registration*, involves registering pre-operative dynamic 3D MR images to RT3D US images at an arbitrary point in the cardiac cycle. This step is performed while the patient is on the OR/examination table. The second step, *real-time registration*, is performed during the procedure and involves acquiring RT3D US images augmented with both ECG signals and spatial tracking information. A series of these 'augmented' RT3D US images are continuously acquired and registered with the pre-operative dynamic 3D MR images to provide accurate, real time image registration.

3 Experimental Results

In this experiment, 20 dynamic 3D MR images of one cardiac cycle, acquired on a 1.5T GE CVi scanner (GE Medical systems, Milwaukee) and 14 RT3D US images, acquired on a Phillips SONOS 7500 real time US machine, from the same volunteer were registered together. The image sets were temporally aligned, and then spatially registered using a MI registration algorithm. This method was able to achieve image registration within 1 second.

The registration was visually satisfactory in all image pairs (see Figure 2), but it is not a trivial task to perform a quantitative validation, since the ground truth is unknown. We discuss below two methods used to evaluate the registration accuracy: 1) a landmark-based method, and 2) an average transformation method.

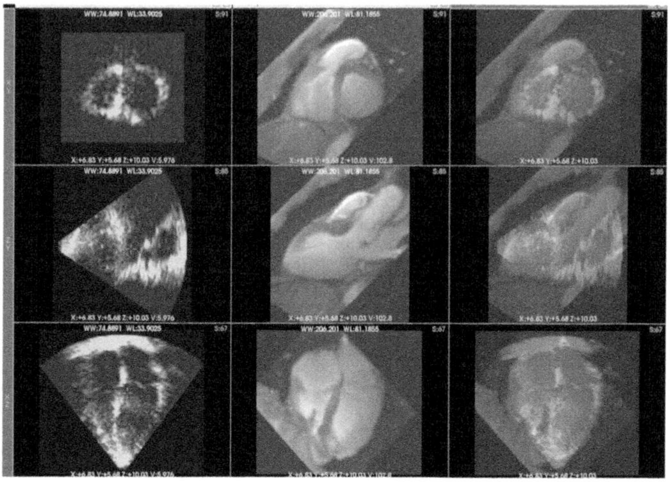

Fig. 2. Registration between RT3D US and dynamic 3D MR images. (a) orthogonal slices of the US volume of the beating heart; (b) the MRI volume of the beating heart; (c) the overlay of the two image sets after registration.

3.1 Landmark Based Validation

Anatomical landmarks within the heart were used to evaluate the registration accuracy. Five such landmarks, the mitral annular septal site (MASS), mitral valve (MV), anterior tricuspid valve (ATV), septal tricuspid valve (STV) and the coronary sinus (CS), were identified in both the US and MR images by six observers and the landmark (or fiducial) localization error (FLE) and fiducial registration error (FRE) were determined. The FLE is defined as the error in locating the landmarks (i.e. the distance of the localized landmark from the "forever unknown" actual landmark location) [11] and is approximated by the average of the landmark locations for the six observers. The FRE is defined as the root mean square (RMS) distance between landmarks in the US image after registration and the corresponding homologous landmarks in the MR image. In this experiment the FLE and the FRE were 1.25 ± 0.63 and 1.76 mm respectively.

3.2 Average Transformation Based Validation

Since the heart beats periodically there should be little variation between the resultant registration transformations of all cardiac phases. Using this assumption it is reasonable to approximate the average transformation over all cardiac phases as the "ground truth" transformation. We evaluate the registration accuracy by using the average distance error, which is defined as the average of displacement error at the eight vertices of a hypothetical cube centered with the bounding box of a data volume [8]. The side of the cube is 100 mm. We compute the average distance error from the average transformation for each registration of the paired images at the same cardiac phase. Compared to the average transformation of all cardiac phases, the average distance error is 0.86 ± 0.40 mm (mean ± SD). While this result is smaller than the values represented in the landmark-based method, it is nevertheless reasonable considering the FLE previously reported.

4 Discussion and Conclusion

In this paper we presented a method for the rapid registration of RT3D US and dynamic 3D MR images of the beating heart. This technique will improve the ease and accuracy of cardiac disease diagnosis, as well as aid in surgical planning and guidance.

We employed image data of a volunteer's beating heart to validate the proposed method with encouraging results. In the future we plan to investigate more effective approaches to preprocessing US images and develop a more robust registration method to improve the registration accuracy and speed.

This method can also be employed to register real-time dynamic 2D US images with dynamic 3D pre-operative CT/MR images and other multi-modal dynamic images, and has the potential to be used in other clinical applications such as liver and lung surgeries, where the organs are subject to approximately periodic respiratory motion.

This method was validated using volunteer data to yield a registration accuracy of 1.76 mm. This method will provide real-time high quality image guidance for cardiac disease diagnosis and surgical planning by improving interpretation of images of the beating heart. We also expect this work to lead to the development of a novel cardiac diagnostic US device that can output real-time high quality cardiac images, fused with high-resolution anatomical information. This device will retain all the merits of conventional US system, and will also have applicability for the guidance of intra-cardiac interventions by improving interpretation of images acquired from various cardiac US modalities (trans-thoracic, trans-esophageal and intra-cardiac echo techniques).

Acknowledgements

The authors thank Dr. Xiaping Yuan for her help in data acquisition and image processing. We also acknowledge the financial support from the Canadian Institute of Health Research (CIHR), Natural Sciences and Engineering Research Council of Canada (NSERC), the Ontario Research & Development Challenge Fund (ORDCF), the Canada Foundation for Innovation (CFI), and the Ontario Innovation Trust (OIT).

References

1. Makela, T., Clarysse, P., Sipila, O., Pauna, N., Pham, Q.C., Katila, T., Magnin, I.E., A review of cardiac image registration methods, IEEE trans. on Med. Imag., 21(9):1011-1021, 2002.

2. Hill, D.L.G., Batchelor, P.G., Holden, M., Hawkes, D.J., Medical image registration, Phys. Med. Biol., 46:R1-R45, 2001.
3. Maintz, J.B., Viergever, M.A., A survey of medical image registration, Med. Image Anal., 2: 1-36, 1998.
4. Gobbi, D.G., Comeau, R.M., Peters, T.M., Ultrasound/MRI overlay with image warping for neurosurgery. MICCAI 2000, LNCS 1935, 106–114, 2000.
5. Lindseth, F., Kaspersen, J.H., Ommedal, S., Langø, T., Unsgaard, G., Hernes, T.A.N., Multimodal image fusion in ultrasound-based neuronavigation: improving overview and interpretation by integrating preoperative MRI with intraoperative 3D ultrasound, submitted to Computer Aided Surgery, 2002.
6. Kaspersen, J.H., Sjølie, E., Wesche, J., Asland, J., Lundbom, J., Odegard, A., Lindseth, F., Three-dimensional ultrasound-based navigation combined with preoperative CT during abdominal interventions: a feasibility study, Cardiovasc Intervent Radiol, 26:347-356, 2003.
7. Wierzbicki M., Drangova M., Guiraudon G., Peters T., Validation of dynamic heart models obtained using non-linear registration for virtual reality training, planning, and guidance of minimally invasive cardiac surgeries, Medical Image Analysis 8:387-401, 2004.
8. Shekhar, R., Zagrodsky, V., Mutual Information-based rigid and nonrigid registration of ultrasound volumes, IEEE Trans. on Medical Imaging, 21(1):9-22, 2002.
9. Mattes, D., Haynor, D.R., Vesselle, H., Lewellen, T.K., Eubank, W., PET-CT image registration in the chest using free-form deformations, IEEE Transactions on Medical Imaging, 22(1): 120 - 128, 2003.
10. Moore, J., Drangova, M., Wierzbicki, M., Barron, J., Peters, T., A high resolution dynamic heart model based on averaged MRI data, MICCAI 2003, LNCS 2878, 549-555, 2003.
11. Fitzpatrick, J.M., West, J.B., Maurer, Jr. C.R., Predicting error in rigid-body point-based registration, IEEE Trans. Med. Imaging, 17:694-702, 1998.

Learning Best Features for Deformable Registration of MR Brains*

Guorong Wu[1], Feihu Qi[1], and Dinggang Shen[2]

[1] Department of Computer Science and Engineering,
Shanghai Jiao Tong University, Shanghai 200030, China
{grwu, fhqi}@cs.sjtu.edu.cn
[2] Section of Biomedical Image Analysis, Department of Radiology,
University of Pennsylvania, Philadelphia, PA 19104
Dinggang.Shen@uphs.upenn.edu

Abstract. This paper presents a learning method to select best geometric features for deformable brain registration. Best geometric features are selected for each brain location, and used to reduce the ambiguity in image matching during the deformable registration. Best geometric features are obtained by solving an energy minimization problem that requires the features of corresponding points in the training samples to be similar, and the features of a point to be different from those of nearby points. By incorporating those learned best features into the framework of HAMMER registration algorithm, we achieved about 10% improvement of accuracy in estimating the simulated deformation fields, compared to that obtained by HAMMER. Also, on real MR brain images, we found visible improvement of registration in cortical regions.

1 Introduction

Deformable registration is very important for medical image analysis. So far, various methods have been proposed [1-7], either based on feature matching or intensity similarity. HAMMER registration algorithm [8] uses an attribute vector, instead of only intensity, as a signature of each point, for reducing the ambiguity in correspondence matching during the image registration procedure. Each attribute vector includes image intensity, edge type and a number of geometric moment invariants (GMIs) calculated in certain neighborhoods for reflecting the anatomy around that point. However, GMIs are calculated from the fixed sizes of neighborhood around each point at each resolution, regardless of whether this point is localizing in the complicated cortical regions or in the simple uniform regions. Thereby, it might be difficult to obtain the distinctive GMIs for every image point, by using *identical* neighborhood size for the whole image.

Recently, in computer vision area, Kadir and Brady [9] studied the implicit relationship between scale and saliency, and found that scale is intimately related to the problem of determining saliency and extracting relevant descriptions. They also proposed an effective method to detect the most salient regions in image, by considering the entropy of local image regions over a range of scales, in order to select regions with highest local saliency in both spatial and scale spaces. Based on [9], Huang *et al*

* This work is supported by NSFC (National Science Foundation of China) 60271033.

J. Duncan and G. Gerig (Eds.): MICCAI 2005, LNCS 3750, pp. 179 – 187, 2005.

[10] proposed to align images under arbitrary poses, by finding the correspondences between salient region features. Although best features have been studied for active shape models [11, 12], however, to our knowledge, it seems that no previous non-rigid registration method considered the relationship between scale and saliency and used this relationship to guide image matching and correspondence detection during the deformable registration procedure.

This paper presents a learning-based method to compute GMIs from the best scales, for significantly reducing the ambiguity in image registration. Each image location will have its own best scale to calculate its GMIs, and simultaneously best scales are made smooth spatially. It is required that, for each point, its GMIs computed from its best-scale neighbor be *similar* across the corresponding points in the training samples, and also be *different* from GMIs of nearby points in all training samples. Entropy used in [9] is adopted here to measure this requirement, and the best scales are obtained by solving an energy minimization problem. Finally, by incorporating those best-scale GMIs into the original HAMMER algorithm, we achieved about 10% improvement in estimating the simulated deformation fields, compared to that obtained by HAMMER.

2 Method

2.1 Attribute Vector with Best Scales

Attribute vector is defined for each point $\mathbf{x}$ in the image I, and it is designed as distinctive as possible, in order to distinguish this point from others in its neighborhood, $N_\mathbf{x}$. In HAMMER registration algorithm [8], each attribute vector includes edge type, image intensity, and GMIs. GMIs are computed from a spherical neighborhood around point $\mathbf{x}$, with radius of $S_\mathbf{x}$ that is identical at all image locations. Images, i.e., brain MR images, are usually spatially complicated, thus different regions usually need features computed from its best scale $S_\mathbf{x}$ [9], to distinguish itself from others. For example, for brain MR images, the point $\mathbf{x}$ in cortical regions requires a different best scale $S_\mathbf{x}$ to compute the distinctive GMIs $\vec{G}(S_\mathbf{x})$, compared to the points in uniform regions. Therefore, it is significant to obtain a best scale $S_\mathbf{x}$ for each image point $\mathbf{x}$, based on particular image content around that point.

A machine learning based method is proposed to select best scales in the template space, in order to capture the distinctive attributes for robustly establishing correspondences. Three criteria are used to select best scales. *First*, the GMIs of a point $\mathbf{x}$, computed from the best-scale neighborhood, should be different from the GMIs of the nearby points in its neighborhood $R_\mathbf{x}$, thereby this point $\mathbf{x}$ can be easily recognized. *Second*, the resulted GMIs of a point $\mathbf{x}$ should be statistically similar to the GMIs of its corresponding points in training samples, if a set of training samples is available. *Third*, the selected best scales should be spatially smooth.

Entropy of GMIs is used to measure the above requirements, by following an idea of using entropy for salient region detection [9]. Thus, the *first* criterion requires that the entropy of GMIs in the neighborhood $R_\mathbf{x}$, $E_1(\mathbf{x},S_\mathbf{x})$, be maximized, and the *second* criterion requires that the entropy of GMIs over the corresponding points in training samples, $E_2(\mathbf{x},S_\mathbf{x})$, be minimized. Entropy can be computed from the histograms of GMIs [9]. The *third* criterion requires that the differences between $S_\mathbf{x}$ and scales $S_\mathbf{y}$ of its small neighborhood $r_{\mathbf{x}}$, $E_3(\mathbf{x}, S_{\mathbf{x}}) = \sum_{\mathbf{y} \in r_{\mathbf{x}}} (S_{\mathbf{x}} - S_{\mathbf{y}})^2$, be minimized. Therefore, we can obtain best scales for all image points, by using a gradient-based algorithm to minimize the following cost function:

$$E = \sum_{\mathbf{x}} \left(-E_1(\mathbf{x}, S_{\mathbf{x}}) + \alpha E_2(\mathbf{x}, S_{\mathbf{x}}) + \beta E_3(\mathbf{x}, S_{\mathbf{x}})\right) \quad (1)$$

where α and β are two weights. Notably, if there is no training samples available, then we just use the best scale selection method [9], with spatial smoothness constraint, to compute the best scales based on the template image itself.

A learning-based method for selecting the best scale $S_{\mathbf{x}}$ can be summarized next:

- Select a set of brain samples, such as 18 brains we used.
- Use a linear registration algorithm [13] to linearly align those samples to a selected template, thereby obtaining the linearly aligned brain samples.
- Use HAMMER algorithm [8] to register template with each linearly aligned brain sample, thereby obtaining the correspondences of each template point in any brain samples.
- For each template point $\mathbf{x}$ and their corresponding points in training samples, compute their GMIs of different scales $S_{\mathbf{x}}$, from the linearly aligned brains.
- Determine best scales for all template points jointly, by minimizing the cost function in equation (1).

For increasing the robustness of registration, the registration algorithms are usually implemented in a multi-resolution fashion [8]. Thus, we need to select best scales separately for each resolution, by performing the same best-scale selection method at each resolution.

Smooth maps of best scales are obtained, from fine to low resolutions, as shown in Fig 1 with the smallest scale (radius) 4 and the largest scale 24. The resulted best scales are actually adaptive to the brain anatomy, such as small scales selected in rich edge regions like cortex, and scales increased gradually from exterior to interior brain regions with the largest best scales selected for the uniform regions like white matter (WM) region. Notably, in low resolution, even a small best scale on cortex will capture a large region in the fine resolution (Fig 2), thereby providing the possibility of distinguishing between precentral and postcentral gyri. Also, since the registration algorithm is implemented in a multi-resolution fashion, the registration results from low and middle resolutions will make the two images approximately aligned, thereby local features, based on small best scales selected for cortex, can be used to refine the registration in cortex during the high-resolution registration stage. Fig 2 shows the best scales selected for seven points on ventricular corners, sulcal roots, gyral crowns, and putamen boundary, in three different resolutions, respectively. For convenience, both low and middle resolution images have been upsampled to the same size of high resolution image. The size of circle denotes the value of the best scale. Also, best scales ranged from 4 to 8 are displayed by solid circles, best scales ranged from 8 to 15 displayed by densely-dashed circles, and best scales over 15 displayed by sparsely-dashed circles.

Advantages of using best-scale GMIs. By employing a learning-based best scale selection method described above, we can use adaptive scale to compute GMIs for each point, thus making it distinctive among its neighboring points as well as similar to its correspondences in other brains. For example, for a template point on sulcal root in Fig 3(a), as indicated by the cross, it is similar to its true correspondence indicated by the asterisk and the false correspondence indicated by the dot in subject (Fig 3(b)), if local image content is compared. Therefore, by measuring the similarities of this template point with all points in the subject image (Fig 3(b)) by the attribute vectors computed from neighborhoods of fixed scale (or size) such as S_x=3,4,7 used for low, middle, and high resolution images in HAMMER algorithm, it is not easy to establish correct correspondences, since multiple peaks are existing in the similarity map, as color-coded and shown in Fig 3(c). Red represents the most similar points, which include the false correspondence indicated by the dot in Fig 3(b). *Importantly*, by using our learning-based best scale selection method, we can determine the best scales for this template point at different image resolutions (i.e., S_x=7,14,8, respectively for low, middle and high resolutions), and further obtain for this template point all GMIs computed from different resolution images using the selected best scales. The best scales selected in low and middle resolutions (7x4=28, 14x2=28) actually correspond

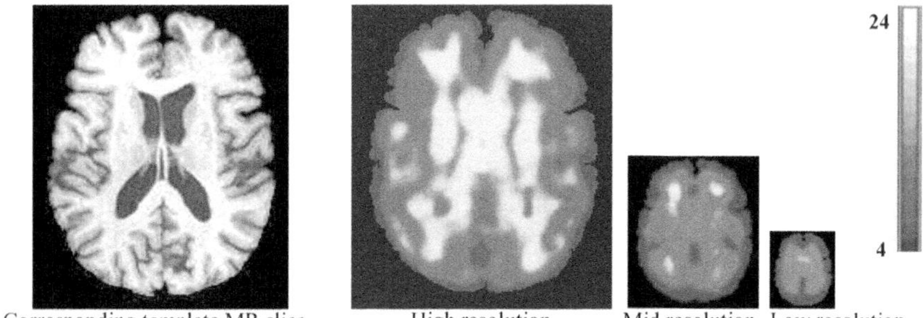

Fig. 1. Best scales selected for the image at three different resolutions, and further color-coded according to the color bar on the right. *This figure is best viewed with color.*

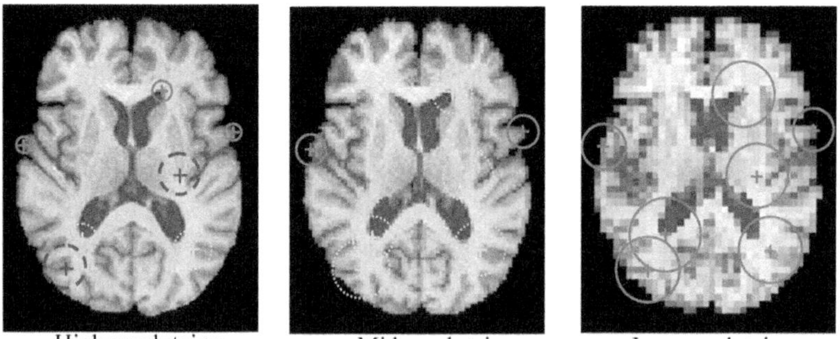

Fig. 2. Best scales of seven selected points in three different resolutions. For convenience, the low and middle resolution images (b,c) were zoomed to the same size of the original image. Here, best scales ranged from 4 to 8 are displayed by solid circles, best scales ranged from 8 to 15 displayed by densely-dashed circles, and best scales over 15 displayed by sparsely-dashed circles. *This figure is best viewed with color.*

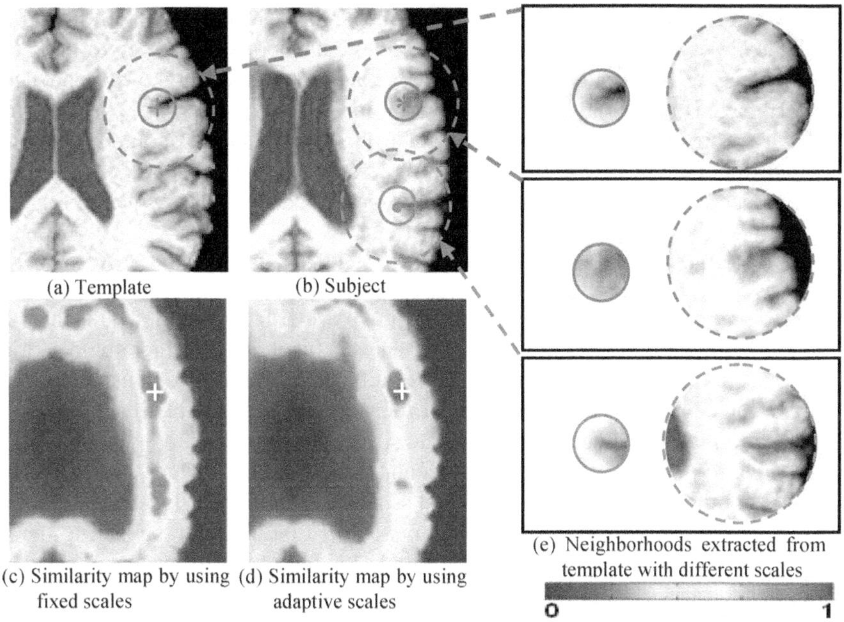

Fig. 3. Advantages of using adaptive scales to compute GMIs for correspondence detection. The similarity of a template point indicated by the cross in (a), is compared to any point in the subject (b), by respectively using GMIs with fixed scales (c) and with learned adaptive scales (d). The color-coded similarity map in (d) indicates distinctive correspondences, compared to the similarity map in (c) which has multiple peaks, with one peak corresponds to the false correspondence which is indicated by the dot in (b). *This figure is best viewed with color.*

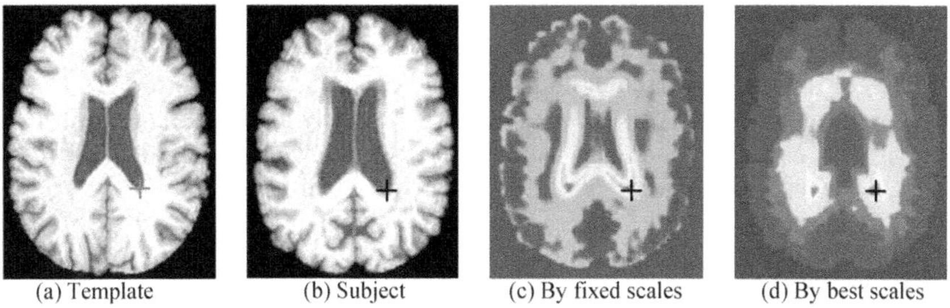

Fig. 4. Similar performances of using fixed scales and learned best scales for distinguishing some brain points, such as ventricular corners. The point in (b), as indicated by black cross, is a detected correspondence of the point in (a), by comparing the GMIs of either fixed scales or learned best scales. The red denotes similar, and blue denotes different. *This figure is best viewed with color.*

to big regions around this template point in the fine resolution, such as big circled images in the right panel of Fig 3. Thus, by using new attribute vectors, we can easily distinguish this template point from two candidate points in Fig 3(b), which has been clearly demonstrated by a color-coded similarity map in Fig 3(d).

Although it is possible to distinguish correspondences for many brain points even using the GMIs with a fixed scale, it may be less distinctive, compared to the method of using learned best scales. Fig 4 shows an example of detecting correspondences in subject image (Fig 4(b)), for a template point in Fig 4(a). According to a color-coded similarity map in Fig 4(c), the method of using fixed scales to compute GMIs can distinguish corresponding points, while it is less distinctive, compared to our method of using learned best scales, as indicated by a color-coded similarity map in Fig 4(d).

2.2 Image Registration by Matching Best-Scale Attributes

All image registration strategies developed in HAMMER algorithm [8], such as definitions of attribute vector similarity and energy function, and hierarchical driving point selection, are adopted by our registration algorithm, except using best-scale GMIs to replace the fixed-scale GMIs for image matching. Notably, the best scale for each location is determined in the template space, thus it is easy to compute GMIs for each *template* point by using the pre-calculated best scale. However, for *subject* image, it is not direct to use appropriate best scales to compute GMIs, since subject is in its own space. To overcome this problem, we will first align the subject to the template space by a linear registration algorithm [13], and then compute in advance the GMIs of all scales (used in the template space) for each subject point. When matching two template and subject points during the deformable registration procedure, we use the particular GMIs included in the attribute vector of the template point as standard and take the corresponding GMIs from the subject point, to measure their similarity. For saving time to compute GMIs of all possible best scales for each subject point, we limit the number of scales used as best scales, such as selecting best scales from a small set of scales $\{i| \, i=4*j, j=1,2,3,\ldots,6\}$.

HAMMER algorithm selects the initial driving points at sulcal roots, crown gyri, and certain areas of strong boundary, and then gradually adds more driving points according to a simple criterion. Here, we adopt the saliency definition in [9], and similarly define the salient measure for each brain point as follows. Given the best scale $S_{\mathbf{x}}$ for a point $\mathbf{x}$, its salient measure can be defined by the entropy of GMI vectors in its neighborhood $N_{\mathbf{x}}$, i.e. $E_1(\mathbf{x},S_{\mathbf{x}})$, multiplied by a weight that penalizes self-similarity of $E_1(\mathbf{x},S_{\mathbf{x}})$ around the best scale $S_{\mathbf{x}}$ [9]. Notably, the definition of $E_1(\mathbf{x},S_{\mathbf{x}})$ is the same as that in equation (1).

3 Results

The proposed method has been evaluated by both real and simulated MR brain images with comparison of HAMMER algorithm [8]. All experiments are performed in PC (Pentium 4, 3.0GHz), by using the same set of parameters.

3.1 Experiment on Real MR Brain Images

The proposed registration algorithm has been used to register 18 brain images, and the results by our method are further compared with those by HAMMER algorithm. The average brain produced from 18 normalized brains by our method is visually very similar to that obtained by HAMMER algorithm. However, when we further check individual registration results, we find the visual improvement by our method in the areas such as cortical regions, although two methods perform equally well on most parts of brain regions. Fig 5 shows two examples, which compare the template with the results obtained by both methods, indicating that our method can align cortical regions more accurately.

3.2 Experiment on Simulated Brain Images

Simulated data is used to quantitatively evaluate the performance of our method. Our simulated data is created by using an elastic warping method [14] to warp a selected brain to be similar to five real brains, respectively, thereby obtaining five simulated brains that are actually five deformed versions of the selected brain. Besides, the regions of precentral gyrus and superior temporal gyrus have been manually labeled in this selected brain, thereby the labels of these two regions can be warped together by the same deformation fields during the simulation procedure. Thus, by using our proposed registration method, we can estimate deformations between the selected brain and each of its deformed brains, and further bring two labeled regions in the simulated brains to the original space of the selected brain. Then, we can measure the overlay degree of the labeled regions. Our method achieves average overlay percentage 88.29%, which is very close to that by HAMMER algorithm on the same dataset (88.48%). The average volume error by our method is 5.18%, while it is 6.67% by HAMMER; this indicates *28.8% of volume error reduction* by our method. Moreover, we compare the deformations estimated by our method with those simulated, thus obtaining a histogram of estimation errors as shown by red bars in Fig 6. This result is compared with that obtained by HAMMER algorithm, whose histogram of estimation errors is shown as blue bars in Fig 6. Obviously, the result obtained by our method is

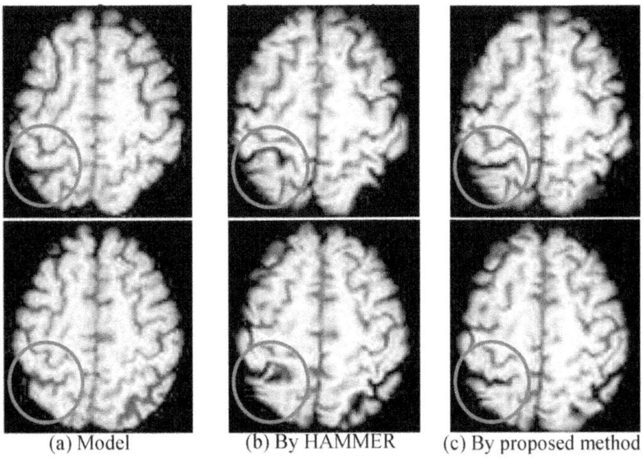

Fig. 5. Visual improvement in registering some brain images by the proposed method, particularly in the cortical regions circled.

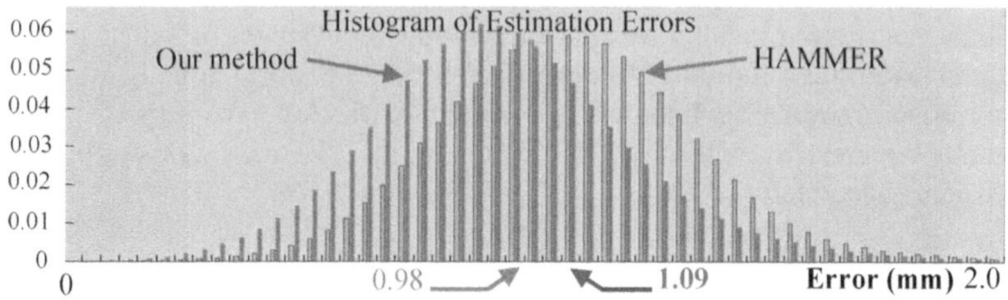

Fig. 6. Performances of estimating simulated deformations by our method (red) and by HAMMER algorithm (blue). The average error is 0.98 mm by our method, and 1.09 mm by HAMMER algorithm, which indicates 10.1% of improvement by our method.

much better, since its histogram is shifted to left, i.e., small errors. The average deformation error is 0.98mm by our method, and 1.09mm by HAMMER, indicating 10.1% of improvement by our method.

4 Conclusion

We have presented a learning based method to adaptively select best-scale GMIs for different image locations, thereby achieving higher registration accuracy by incorporating the selected best-scale GMIs into the HAMMER registration framework. Our learning method requires simultaneously the similarity of corresponding points in the training samples and the difference of a point to its nearby points, in terms of GMIs. It further requires the spatial smoothness of best-scale map. All of these requirements are formulated by a single entropy-based energy function, thereby solved by an energy optimization method. Importantly, our learning method can also be used to learn best features from others, i.e., wavelet-based features [15].

References

1. Y. Wang and L. H. Staib, "Elastic model-based non-rigid registration incorporating statistical shape information," *MICCAI'98*, vol. 1496, pp. 1162-1173, 1999.
2. J. C. Gee, M. Reivich, and R. Bajcsy, "Elastically deforming 3D atlas to match anatomical brain images," *Journal of Computer Assisted Tomography*, vol. 17, pp. 225-236, 1993.
3. G. E. Christensen and H. J. Johnson, "Consistent Image Registration," *IEEE Trans on Med. Imaging*, vol. 20, pp. 568-582, 2001.
4. B. M. Dawant, S. L. Hartmann, and S. Gadamsetty, "Brain Atlas Deformation in the Presence of Large Space-occupying Tumours," *MICCAI'99*, vol. 1679, pp. 589-596, 1999.
5. P. Thompson and A. W. Toga, "A surface-based technique for warping three-dimensional images of the brain," *IEEE Trans on Med. Imaging*, vol. 15, pp. 402-417, 1996.
6. I. Wells, William M., P. Viola, H. Atsumi, S. Nakajima, and R. Kikinis, "Multi-modal volume registration by maximization of mutual information," *Medical Image Analysis*, vol. 1, pp. 35-51, 1996.
7. Studholme C, Hill DLG, and H. DJ, "Multiresolution voxel similarity measures for MR-PET registration," *Proc. IPMI, Ile de Berder, France.*, pp. 287-298, 1995.

8. D. Shen and C. Davatzikos, "HAMMER: Hierarchical attribute matching mechanism for elastic registration," *IEEE Trans on Med. Imaging*, vol. 21, pp. 1421-1439, 2002.
9. T. Kadir and M. Brady, "Saliency, scale and image description," *International Journal of Compter Vision*, vol. 45(2), pp. 83-105, 2001.
10. X. Huang, Y. Sun, D. Metaxas, F. Sauer, and C. Xu, "Hybrid image registration based on configural matching of scale-invariant salient region features," *IEEE Workshop on Image and Video Registration, Washington D.C.,*, July, 2004.
11. B. v. Ginneken, A. F. Frangi, J. J. Staal, B. M. t. H. Romeny, and M. A. Viergever, "Active Shape Model Segmentation With Optimal Features," *IEEE Trans. on Medical Imaging*, vol. 21, pp. 924-933, 2002.
12. S. Li, L. Zhu, and T. Jiang, "Active Shape Model Segmentation Using Local Edge Structures and AdaBoost," *MIAR*, pp. 121-128, 2004.
13. M. Jenkinson, P.R. Bannister, J.M. Brady, and S. M. Smith, "Improved optimisation for the robust and accurate linear registration and motion correction of brain images," *NeuroImage*, vol. 17, pp. 825-841, 2002.
14. C. Davatzikos, "Spatial transformation and registration of brain images using elastically deformable models," *Comp. Vision and Image Understanding*, vol. 66, pp. 207-222, 1997.
15. S. Mallat, "A theory for multiresolution signal decomposition: The wavelet representation," *IEEE Trans. on PAMI*, vol. 11, pp. 674--693, July 1989.

Stochastic Inverse Consistency in Medical Image Registration

Sai Kit Yeung[1] and Pengcheng Shi[2]

[1] Bioengineering Program
[2] Department of Electrical and Electronic Engineering,
Hong Kong University of Science and Technology,
Clear Water Bay, Kowloon, Hong Kong
{beysk, eeship}@ust.hk

Abstract. An essential goal in medical image registration is, the forward and reverse mapping matrices should be inverse to each other, i.e., inverse consistency. Conventional approaches enforce consistency in deterministic fashions, through incorporation of sub-objective cost function to impose source-destination symmetric property during the registration process. Assuming that the initial forward and reverse matching matrices have been computed and used as the inputs to our system, this paper presents a stochastic framework which yields perfect inverse consistency with the simultaneous considerations of the errors underneath the registration matrices and the imperfectness of the consistent constraint. An iterative generalized total least square (GTLS) strategy has been developed such that the inverse consistency is optimally imposed.

1 Introduction

One of the most desirable properties for registration is inverse consistency or source-destination symmetry in which the correspondence is one-to-one and also unambiguous. Consistent transformations maintain the topology of the registering pair. This is important in medical image registration for generating biologically meaningful results [1]. The inverse consistent constraint has been enforced with other information such as image intensity and geometric characteristics to become part of the optimization criterion in medical image registration [1] or to act as a sub-objective cost function in point set matching [3]. Since the inverse consistency in the latter case is only part of the metric which needs to be minimized, the resulting transformation matrices are, in general, not perfectly inverse consistent. Furthermore, all the above approaches solve the transformations in a deterministic nature, meaning that the stochastic properties of these matrices are not considered.

We propose a stochastic framework for registration problems which generates perfect source-destination symmetric mapping between the data sets. Instead of imposing inverse consistency in a *deterministic* and *imperfect* sense, we enforce the inverse consistent property optimally with the systematic considerations of the stochastic uncertainties of the input forward and reverse transformation matrices to achieve *perfect* source-destination symmetry. The adoption of the

J. Duncan and G. Gerig (Eds.): MICCAI 2005, LNCS 3750, pp. 188–196, 2005.

Generalized Total Least Square(GTLS) technique [6] allows simultaneous considerations of the errors in the input transformation matrices and the inverse consistent constraint during a post-registration fitting process to solve a set of new forward and reverse transformations iteratively until they are *perfectly inverse to* each other. This framework can be used with any registration algorithms which have already shown their validity in establishing forward/reverse mappings for different matching problems.

2 Inverse Consistency in Medical Image Registration

2.1 Discrete Nature of the Information Sources

Due to the discrete nature of data, either the point representation or the digital medical image of the biological objects and the discrete optimization process, correspondences extracted from conventional registration algorithms are always ambiguous, i.e., the forward and reverse mapping is not consistent. Fig.1(g) and (j) show 2 simple 1D examples to illustrate the point: A_n and B_n are discrete version of the original continuous signals A and B which B is shifted to right by 0.5s from A=sin(x). A_c and B_c are the reconstructed signals for registration. Notice that A_c and B_c on the above examples are unable to represent the original signals perfectly due to the inadequate sampling rate of A_n and B_n. Conventional optimization processes initialize one way to start climbing the hill (the matching criteria curve), e.g. from left to right. In Fig.1(h), the possible forward and reverse registration results would be an ambiguous pair (-1.1,-0.5) instead of the ground truth pair (-0.5,0.5). In Fig.1(k), the matching criteria curves give a consistent pair (-1,1), however, it is not the ground truth transformation[1].

2.2 Deterministic Inverse Consistent Constraint

One typical scheme to incorporate inverse consistency for registration is to assign a cost metric E_{Cons} for the inverse consistent property as part of the matching cost function E, i.e., $E = E_{Sim} + E_{Cons}$ where E_{Sim} measures the similarity (i.e. image intensity and geometrical properties) between the data sets. Since the consistency is only part of the overall cost function, the optimal solution to Equ. 1 in general would not produce the perfect source-destination symmetry one desires.

Moreover, this type of formulation didn't consider the underlying stochastic uncertainties such that the forward transformation T_{12} and the reverse transformation T_{21} are solved in *deterministic* nature in order to get a one-to-one consistent mapping (consistent correspondence), i.e.,

$$T_{12} * T_{21} = I. \tag{1}$$

[1] It should be noticed that inverse consistency can always be automatically achieved if the registering pair is continuous (Fig.1(a),(b)) or the digital signal is sampled under very high sampling rate such that the original continuous signal can be perfectly reconstructed (Fig.1(d),(e)).

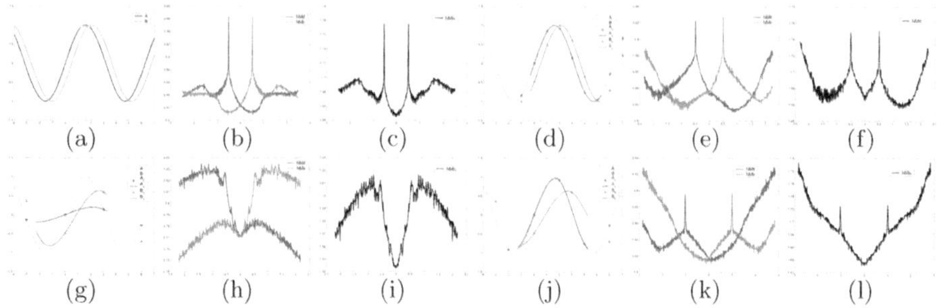

Fig. 1. Column 1 and 4: A_c and B_c are the registering pair reconstructed from A_n and B_n which are the sampled version of A and B respectively (in (a): A_c=A, B_c=B). Column 2 and 5: the blue curve (NMIf) shows the forward matching criteria (registering B_c to A_c) while the red one (NMIr) for registering A_c to B_c. Column 3 and 6: The combined matching criteria curve (NMIc) from the forward and reverse registration process, here the combination is simple addition. NMI is the normalized mutual information [5].

2.3 Role of Inverse Consistency in Registration

In one dimensional, imposing inverse consistency deterministically means the hill climbing process should be in pairwise nature: (1,-1)...(8,-8) for the testing signal over the reference signal. Equivalently, there would be a new matching criteria curve that is a combination of the forward and reverse matching criteria curve. The simplest way is to have a non-weighted linear combination [4], which is equivalently a simple addition, as shown column 3 and 6 in Fig.1. Here, a critical rule for combining the forward and reverse matching criteria curves under a deterministic sense is that they should be combined in the corresponding transformation position, i.e. the NMIf value at 0.5 translation have to combine with the NMIr value at 0.5 translation also. In fact, deterministic consistency will only give better registration results if a new peak closer to the ground truth is formed as shown in Fig.1(i), which the transformation pair corresponding to optimum will be around (-0.8,0.8) instead of (-1.1,-0.5) and also closer to the ground truth (-0.5,0.5).

3 Stochastic Inverse Consistency in Medical Image Registration

3.1 Stochastic Inverse Consistent Constraint

As we have stated above, the discrete nature of the information source makes the matching criteria drive to incorrect maximum, simply combine them deterministically will not be an optimal way to utilize the information from the forward and reverse process. In this paper, we are arguing that one should model inverse consistency stochastically with the simultaneous consideration of the underlying stochastic uncertainties within the forward and reverse transformation matrices and hence the imperfectness of the inverse consistent constraint, i.e,

$$(T_{12} + E_{T_{12}}) * (T_{21} + E_{T_{21}}) = I + R_i \tag{2}$$

$$E_{T_{12}} = |T_{12} - T_{21}^{-1}| \qquad E_{T_{12}^{-1}} = |T_{21} - T_{12}^{-1}| \tag{3}$$

We adopt a simple absolute difference approach for $E_{T_{12}}$ and $E_{T_{21}}$ ($E_{T_{21}}$ is obtained from $E_{T_{12}^{-1}}$, which will be explained later) to model the stochastic error properties of the transformation matrix T_{12} and T_{21} [2] respectively since the forward and inverse of the reverse transformation has already set up a loose upper bound of the error. R_i is the error imposed on the imperfectness of the inverse consistent constraint[3]. Under this formulation, we can provide more flexibility on imposing source-destination symmetry between the forward and reverse registration processes, without compromising accuracy.

To further simplify our current error model, we assume all the elements in the error matrices have zero mean and are independent to each other. These matrices will be involved in building the error equilibration matrices for the Generalized Total Least Solvers in the following section.

3.2 GTLS Formulation

As the stochastic property are not the same for every entry and some of the entries are error free, in order to solve the problem while considering all the errors simultaneously, a Generalized Total Least Square (GTLS) [6] approach is adopted. Consider a overdetermined system of linear equations

$$AX \approx B \qquad A \in R^{m\times n}, B \in R^{m\times d} \text{ and } X \in R^{n\times d},\ m \geqslant n + d \tag{4}$$

If the first n_1 column in A is error free, A can be partitioned into $[A_1, A_2]$ where $A_1 \in R^{m\times n_1}$, $A_2 \in R^{m\times n_2}$ and n $= n_1 + n_2$. A GTLS solution of (4) is any solution of the set $\widehat{A}X = A_1X_1 + \widehat{A_2}X_2 = \widehat{B}$. $\widehat{A} = [A_1, \widehat{A_2}]$ and $\widehat{B}$ are determined such that Range($\widehat{B}$) $\subseteq$ Range($\widehat{A}$) and $\| R_D^{-T}[\triangle\widehat{A_2}, \triangle\widehat{B}]R_C^{-1} \|_F = \| R_D^{-T}[A_2 - \widehat{A_2}, B_2 - \widehat{B}]R_C^{-1} \|_F$ is minimal where $R_D \in R^{m\times m}$ and $R_C \in R^{(n_2+d)\times(n_2+d)}$ are the given equilibration matrices such that the errors on $R_D^{-T}[A_2, B]R_C^{-1}$ are equilibrated, i.e. uncorrelated with zero mean and same variance.

Our objective is to solve the fitting transformation matrices under the consideration of the errors in the transformation matrices and the source-destination symmetric constraint simultaneously by making use of the GTLS property. Notice that the last row of the affine transformation matrix is actually error free. By making use of this property, the transformation matrices can be first transposed and permuted to fit the GTLS formulation:

$$Q_{12} = T_{12}^T * P \qquad Q_{21} = T_{21}^T * P \tag{5}$$

$$invQ_{12} = (T_{12}^{-1})^T * P \qquad invQ_{21} = (T_{21}^{-1})^T * P \tag{6}$$

---

[2] In this paper we test on the 4-by-4 affine transformation matrices, in theory, we can also enforce the stochastic relationship on non-rigid deformation. Notice that we didn't apply our model on rigid transformation due to the orthonormality issue.

[3] We simply assume all the entries in R_i have the same stochastic uncertainty and set it as $\triangle_r$, i.e., $R_i \in R^{4\times 4}$ with all the entries equal to $\triangle_r$.

$$P = P_{14} * P_{24} * P_{34}, \; P_{14} = \begin{pmatrix} 0\,0\,0\,1 \\ 0\,1\,0\,0 \\ 0\,0\,1\,0 \\ 1\,0\,0\,0 \end{pmatrix} \; P_{24} = \begin{pmatrix} 1\,0\,0\,0 \\ 0\,0\,0\,1 \\ 0\,0\,1\,0 \\ 0\,1\,0\,0 \end{pmatrix} \; P_{34} = \begin{pmatrix} 1\,0\,0\,0 \\ 0\,1\,0\,0 \\ 0\,0\,0\,1 \\ 0\,0\,1\,0 \end{pmatrix} \tag{7}$$

Q_{12} will be a 4-by-4 matrix with the form:

$$Q_{12} = \begin{pmatrix} 0 & T_{12}(1,1) & \cdots & T_{12}(3,1) \\ 0 & T_{12}(1,2) & & \vdots \\ 0 & \vdots & \ddots & \vdots \\ 1 & \vdots & \cdots & T_{12}(3,4) \end{pmatrix} \qquad Q_{21} = \begin{pmatrix} 0 & T_{21}(1,1) & \cdots & T_{21}(3,1) \\ 0 & T_{21}(1,2) & & \vdots \\ 0 & \vdots & \ddots & \vdots \\ 1 & \vdots & \cdots & T_{21}(3,4) \end{pmatrix} \tag{8}$$

So the first column of Q_{12} and Q_{21} is error free and suit the form of the GTLS approach stated before. Hence the GTLS formulation of our stochastic inverse consistent model becomes:

$$\begin{bmatrix} Q_{12} \\ invQ_{21} \end{bmatrix} X \approx \begin{bmatrix} I \\ I \end{bmatrix} \qquad \begin{bmatrix} invQ_{12} \\ Q_{21} \end{bmatrix} Y \approx \begin{bmatrix} I \\ I \end{bmatrix} \tag{9}$$

The optimal forward and reverse transformation T^*_{12} and T^*_{21} are obtained by performing the permutation and transpose on the GTLS solutions X and Y:

$$T^*_{21} = (P * X)^T \qquad T^*_{12} = (P * Y)^T \tag{10}$$

Apart from the input transformation matrices, the error properties are also necessary to specify the GTLS formulation. The error matrices $E_{Q_{12}}$, $E_{invQ_{12}}$ for Q_{12}, $invQ_{12}$ are derived as the same in Equ.(3) i.e.,

$$E_{Q_{12}} = |Q_{12} - invQ_{21}| \quad E_{invQ_{12}} = |Q_{21} - invQ_{12}| \tag{11}$$

and the first column is dropped as the first column of Q_{12} is error free. The error matrices $E_{invQ_{21}}$ and $E_{Q_{21}}$ transformation matrix are formed respectively by:

$$E_{invQ_{21}} = \frac{(1-\alpha)}{\alpha} * E_{Q_{12}} \quad E_{Q_{21}} = \frac{(1-\alpha)}{\alpha} * E_{invQ_{12}} \tag{12}$$

where α is the weighting on the error of the forward transformation matrix T_{12}:

$$\alpha = \frac{\text{voxel size of } I_1}{\text{voxel size of } I_2} \quad \text{or} \quad \alpha = \frac{\text{\# of points in point set 2}}{\text{\# of points in point set 1}} \tag{13}$$

So by imposing the above relationship, the registration result with a higher resolution testing image or point matching result with more points in the testing point set will be trusted more. While in this paper we use this simple assumption to model the weighting function between the error on forward and reverse registration results from two images under different resolutions. More complicated way can be investigated and would be one possibility of our future work.

The error equilibration matrices R_C and R_D are obtained from the Cholesky decomposition of the error covariance matrices C and D, where $C = \Delta^T \Delta$, $D = \Delta \Delta^T$, $\Delta = \begin{bmatrix} E_{Q_{12}} & R_i \\ E_{invQ_{21}} & R_i \end{bmatrix}$. Δ represents the stochastic property of the error in solving X in Equ.(9), while Δ matrix in solving Y is $\begin{bmatrix} E_{invQ_{12}} & R_i \\ E_{Q_{21}} & R_i \end{bmatrix}$.

3.3 Inverse Consistency by Iterative GTLS Solution

After defining the GTLS model for fitting the transformation matrix based on our stochastic source-destination symmetric model, we set up the whole iterative process from the registration results T_{12} and T_{21} in order to extract both the forward transformation matrix T_{12}^* and the reverse transformation matrix T_{21}^* which are inverse of each other. The input for the iteration process is Q_{12}, Q_{21}, $invQ_{12}$, $invQ_{21}$ in Equ.(5) and (6).

$$\begin{bmatrix} Q_{12}^{(0)} \\ invQ_{21}^{(0)} \end{bmatrix} X^{(0)} \approx \begin{bmatrix} I \\ I \end{bmatrix} \quad \begin{bmatrix} invQ_{12}^{(0)} \\ Q_{21}^{(0)} \end{bmatrix} Y^{(0)} \approx \begin{bmatrix} I \\ I \end{bmatrix} \tag{14}$$

with the corresponding stochastic property in the noise data:

$$\begin{bmatrix} E_{Q_{12}}^{(0)} & R_i \\ E_{invQ_{21}}^{(0)} & R_i \end{bmatrix} \quad \text{and} \quad \begin{bmatrix} E_{invQ_{12}}^{(0)} & R_i \\ E_{Q_{21}}^{(0)} & R_i \end{bmatrix} \tag{15}$$

the '0' in the brackets is the number of iteration and the solved $X^{(0)}$ and $Y^{(0)}$ are:

$$X^{(0)} = P^{-1} * (T_{21}^{(1)})^T \qquad Y^{(0)} = P^{-1} * (T_{12}^{(1)})^T \tag{16}$$

$$\text{so} \quad (X^{(0)})^{-1} = invQ_{21}^{(1)} \quad \text{and} \quad P * (X^{(0)}) * P = Q_{21}^{(1)} \tag{17}$$

$$(Y^{(0)})^{-1} = invQ_{12}^{(1)} \quad \text{and} \quad P * (Y^{(0)}) * P = Q_{12}^{(1)} \tag{18}$$

The corresponding error matrices for the transformation matrices are also updated during the iteration, i.e., getting $E_{Q_{12}}^{(1)}, E_{Q_{21}}^{(1)}, E_{invQ_{12}}^{(1)}, E_{invQ_{21}}^{(1)}$ by Equ.(11) and (12) to fit the input matrices of the GTLS solvers as the transformation errors should be smaller during the iteration (closer to the ground truth) while the error matrix R_i for the source-destination symmetric constraint is fixed as the initial input stochastic consistent model is kept unchanged. So all the components for the GTLS solvers are updated and the process can be repeated until

$$||(P * X^{(n)})^T * (P * Y^{(n)})^T - I||_F < \text{threshold} \tag{19}$$

and the GTLS solution matrices will be:

$$T_{21}^* = (P * X^{(n)})^T \qquad T_{12}^* = (P * Y^{(n)})^T \tag{20}$$

4 Experiments and Discussion

We have applied our stochastic inverse consistent model on registration of point sets which representing the human brain in Fig.2. Feature points are selected from the brain image to act as the testing point set, then a non-rigid mapping, Gaussian radial basis functions was applied on it to form the reference point set. Different degree of gaussian noise and different proportion of outliers are added to both point sets in the experiment. The Robust point matching algorithm

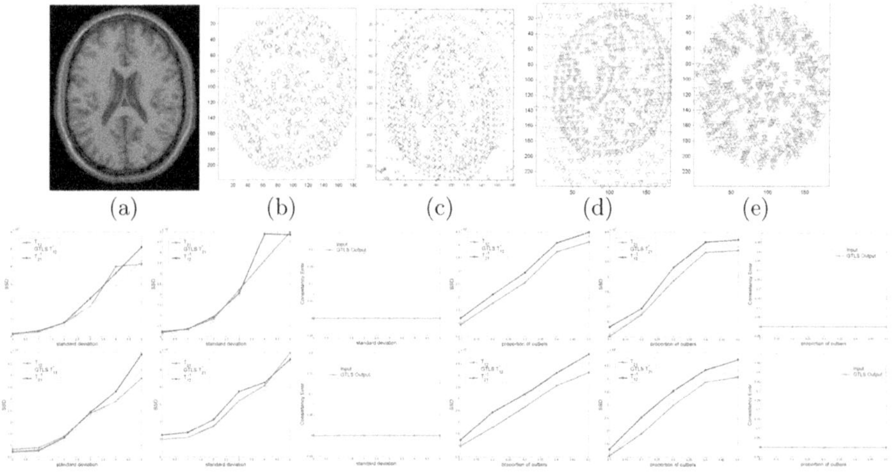

Fig. 2. (a):Brain image with the extracted point set (the testing point set). (b),(c): Testing point sets (blue circle) and the reference point sets (black cross). (b) small deformation, noise level = 2SD. (c) large deformation, outlier proportion = 0.5. (d):Forward wrapping results: small deformation, outlier proportion = 0.1. (e):Reverse wrapping results: large deformation, noise level = 4SD. Color convention for all the results shown in the figure: forward process - red:T_{12}, green:T_{12}^*, blue:T_{21}^{-1}, reverse process - red:T_{21}, green:T_{21}^*, blue:T_{12}^{-1}. The 2nd and 3rd row are the results for small deformation and large deformation respectively. Column 1 to 3 are the results for different noise level, column 4 to 6 are for different proportion of outliers. Column 1 and 4 are the errors computed as sum of squared distance (SSD) between the points in the warped testing point set and the reference point set for forward process while column 2 and 5 are for reverse process. Column 3 and 6 are the consistency error computed as $\| T_{12} * T_{21} - I \|_F$ for the input and $\| T_{12}^* * T_{21}^* - I \|_F$ for the GTLS output.

RPM [2] is run on the pair of point sets to obtain the forward and reverse transformation matrices for our system. The position error of the points is computed as the sum of squared distance (SSD) between the points in the warped testing point set and the reference point set for the evaluation of the transformations obtained. We also compare the error on consistency by $\| T_{12} * T_{21} - I \|_F$. As it is expected, our stochastic inverse consistent model generates a perfect source-destination symmetric registration results from the input forward and reverse transformation matrices which are inconsistent in nature.

Moreover, our GTLS solutions will produce results those will always better than the worst and sometimes be the best as shown in column 1 and 2 in Fig.2. Actually proper modelling of individual element of the error matrices, their relationship within the matrix and also the interrelation among the error matrices will be the potential mean to improve the registration results through consistency so that the GTLS solutions always yield the best results. This modelling is depended on the actual data and also the corresponding matching criteria

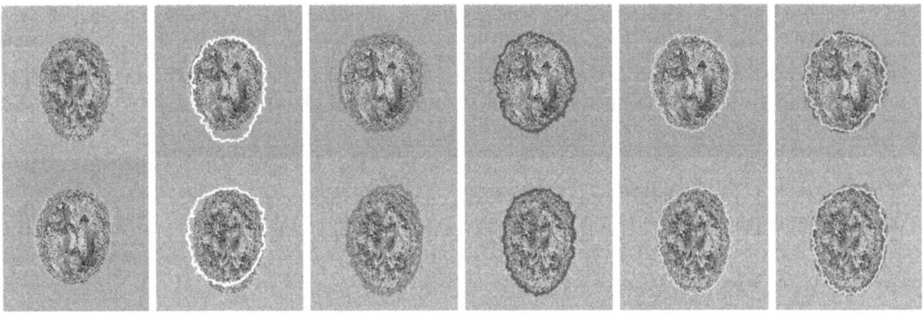

Fig. 3. Column 1: two different PD-weighted MRIs. Row 1 and 2 are the forward and reverse registration results. Forward results - red:T_{12}, green:T^*_{12}, blue:T^{-1}_{21}, reverse results - red:T_{21}, green:T^*_{21}, blue:T^{-1}_{12}. White: contour of the unregistered testing image overlay the reference image.

which is very complicated and will be investigated in our future work. In real registration problem, ground truth is not available and the complicated input image or point data make it very difficult to determine the forward or reverse transformation is superior than the other. Hence our stochastic inverse consistent model can always produce better result in terms of robustness. Fig.3 shows the registration results for 2 PD-weighted MRIs. The inconsistency of the forward and reverse process is shown in the figures by the red and blue contours. T^*_{12} and T^*_{21} is in-between their inputs and also perfectly inverse to each other. In addition, the observable registration errors in T_{12} and T_{21} from the red contours are not appeared in our GTLS solutions which show that the stochastic model produce better registrations.

5 Conclusion

We presented a novel framework for modelling inverse consistency stochastically, by simultaneously considering the stochastic uncertainties on both of the transformation matrices and the source-destination symmetric constraint through the Generalized Total Least square fitting from the transformation matrices obtained after the registration process. With our stochastic inverse consistent model, source-destination symmetry can be enforced perfectly with the consideration of any other similarity constraints. This work is supported by HKRGC CERG Grant HKUST6151/03E.

References

1. Gary E. Christensen and Hans J. Johnson. Consistent image registration. *IEEE Trans. Med. Imaging*, 20(7):568–582, 2001.
2. Haili Chui and Anand Rangarajan. A new algorithm for non-rigid point matching. In *CVPR*, pages 2044–2051, 2000.

3. Hongyu Guo, Anand Rangarajan, S. Joshi, and Laurent Younes. Non-rigid registration of shapes via diffeomorphic point matching. In *ISBI*, pages 924–927, 2004.
4. Oskar M. Skrinjar and Hemant Tagare. Symmetric, transitive, geometric deformation and intensity variation invariant nonrigid image registration. In *ISBI*, pages 920–923, 2004.
5. Colin Studholme, Derek L. G. Hill, and David J. Hawkes. An overlap invariant entropy measure of 3d medical image alignment. *Pattern Recognition*, 32(1):71–86, 1999.
6. S. Van Huffel and J. Vandewalle. Analysis and properties of the generalized total least squares problem $AX \approx B$ when some or all columns in A are subject to error. *SIAM J. Matrix. Anal. Appl.*, 10:294–315, 1989.

A Novel Incremental Technique for Ultrasound to CT Bone Surface Registration Using Unscented Kalman Filtering

Mehdi Hedjazi Moghari[1] and Purang Abolmaesumi[1,2]

[1] Department of Electrical and Computer Engineering, Queen's University, Canada
[2] School of Computing, Queen's University, Canada
{purang, hedjazi}@cs.queensu.ca

Abstract. We propose a novel incremental surface-based registration technique that employs the Unscented Kalman Filter (UKF) to register two different data sets. The method not only reports the variance of the registration parameters but also has significantly more accurate results in comparison to the Iterative Closest Points (ICP) algorithm. Furthermore, it is shown that the proposed incremental registration algorithm is less sensitive to the initial alignment of the data sets than the ICP algorithm. We have validated the method by registering bone surfaces extracted from a set of 3D ultrasound images to the corresponding surface points gathered from the Computed Tomography (CT) data.

1 Introduction

Registration is a crucial step in applications of medical imaging in computer-assisted surgery. Two general methods for registration are intensity-based and feature-based approaches [1]. The former uses the intensity of two images or volumes of the targeted anatomy to calculate the registration parameters by using a variety of similarity measures, such as the mutual-information or normalized correlation. The latter, extracts corresponding geometric features in order to perform the registration. In the feature-based registration technique, if corresponding points between two data sets are available, then one could easily find the registration parameters by employing the closed-form solution provided by Horn [2]. However, the problem becomes more challenging when the corresponding points between the two cloud of points are unknown. In this case the most widely used registration method is the Iterative Closest Points (ICP) algorithm [3]. But the ICP algorithm is very sensitive to the initial alignment of data sets and easily gets trapped in a local minimum. Recently, Ma [4] has proposed a novel approach for estimating the registration parameters and visualizing the error distribution by using the Unscented Particle Filter (UPF). While excellent registration results are reported for a small size of data set (24 points), the algorithm converges very slowly due to the employment of 5000 particles. The need to employ a large number of particles makes this algorithm practically impossible to run for large data sets. The Particle Filtering is a powerful method when

J. Duncan and G. Gerig (Eds.): MICCAI 2005, LNCS 3750, pp. 197–204, 2005.

one is dealing with a nonlinear process or model corrupted by a non-Gaussian random noise. In the case of the Gaussian distribution assumption for the noise distribution, one could significantly reduce the computation time by using the Unscented Kalman Filtering (UKF), while achieving similar registration performance. Due to the significantly small computational requirements of the UKF algorithm in comparison to the UPF algorithm, it is possible to apply the UKF technique to large data sets.

In this paper, we propose a novel incremental registration algorithm based on the Unscented Kalman Filtering. It is shown that the proposed registration algorithm is less sensitive to the initial alignment and is more accurate than the ICP method. Finally, the robustness and accuracy of the proposed technique is examined by registering a 3D ultrasound data set of a Scaphoid bone surface to the corresponding 3D Computed Tomography (CT) data.

2 Method

2.1 Unscented Kalman Filter Registration

In 1960, R. E. Kalman published his famous paper describing a recursive and incremental solution to the discrete data linear filtering problem [5]. Since that time the Kalman Filtering (KF) has been the subject of research with several applications, specifically in the navigation and target tracking area [6]. The KF addresses the state vector estimation, $\mathbf{x} \in \Re^n$, of a discrete time control process model governed by a linear equation:

$$\mathbf{x}_k = \mathbf{A}\mathbf{x}_{k-1} + \mathbf{w}_{k-1}, \tag{1}$$

from the observation model which is a linear function as well:

$$\mathbf{z}_k = \mathbf{C}\mathbf{x}_k + \mathbf{v}_k, \tag{2}$$

where $\mathbf{A}$ and $\mathbf{C}$ are defined by the system dynamics, $\mathbf{z}_k \in \Re^m$ is the observation vector at time k, $\mathbf{w}_k$ and $\mathbf{v}_k$ represent the process and the observation noise at time k, respectively, and are independent Gaussian random vectors with distributions $\mathcal{N}(0, \mathcal{W})$ and $\mathcal{N}(0, \mathcal{V})$ respectively. The KF algorithm estimates the state vector by minimizing the mean square error. This estimation is optimum if the process and the observation models are defined by linear equations, and the process and the observation noises are independent Gaussian random variables. However, in a general case, the process and the observation models can be governed by non-linear equations:

$$\mathbf{x}_k = \mathbf{F}(\mathbf{x}_{k-1}, \mathbf{w}_{k-1}), \tag{3}$$

$$\mathbf{z}_k = \mathbf{H}(\mathbf{x}_k, \mathbf{v}_k). \tag{4}$$

In this case the KF estimation of the state vector is not optimum anymore. There are two well known solutions for dealing with nonlinearities in the process or the observation model. As a first solution, the non-linear function in the observation or process model can be linearized around a good initial guess, using the first order Taylor approximation, and then the KF algorithm is used to estimate the state vector. This method is called Extended Kalman Filtering (EKF) [6]. However, to use the EKF, one needs to have the first derivative of the nonlinear functions (Jacobian Matrix) for linearization. Finding the Jacobian matrix is usually cumbersome and makes the algorithm complicated.

As a second approach, one could use the true non-linear models and approximate the distribution of the state random variable rather than approximating the non-linear process or observation model. This method, called the Unscented Kalman Filtering (UKF) [7], uses the true non-linear models to approximate the distribution of the state or observation vector with the Gaussian distribution by using a set of deterministically chosen sample points. These sample points completely capture the true mean and covariance of the Gaussian random variables, and when propagated through the true non-linear system, accurately capture the posterior mean and covariance to the third-order of Taylor series expansion for any nonlinearity. The EKF algorithm, in contrast, only achieves first-order of Taylor series expansion accuracy, with the same order of complexity as that of the UKF algorithm [8]. Once distributions of the state and the observation vectors are estimated, one could easily estimate the state vector by using the KF technique.

The problem of estimating the state vector becomes more challenging by assuming that the observation and the process noise have non-Gaussian distributions. In this situation, where one is dealing with the system governed by nonlinearity functions and distorted by a non-Gaussian noise, the Particle Filter algorithm is used to estimate the state vector [9].

2.2 Incremental Registration Algorithm Based on UKF

Since we would like to estimate rigid transformation parameters which register a cloud of data set (register data set) to the desired data set (model data set), the state vector contains three rotational (θ_x, θ_y, θ_z) and three translational (t_x, t_y, t_z) parameters. We assume that the scale factors between two data sets are known. Therefore, the state space model can be defined as follows:

$$\mathbf{x}_k = \mathbf{x}_{k-1} + \mathcal{N}(0, \mathcal{W}_k), \tag{5}$$

where, $\mathbf{x}_k = [t_x, t_y, t_z, \theta_x, \theta_y, \theta_z]^T \in \Re^6$ and $\mathcal{W}_k$ is the covariance matrix of the zero-mean Gaussian random vector. This covariance matrix allows the algorithm to move from a poor initial estimate to the successively better ones. However, the process noise variances should be small values, since the state vector (transformation parameters) is time invariant.

The observation model is defined as follows:

$$\mathbf{y}_{1:k} = \mathbf{R}_{[\theta_x,\theta_y,\theta_z]}(\mathbf{t}_{[t_x,t_y,t_z]} + \mathbf{u}_{1:k}) + \mathcal{N}(0, \mathcal{V}_k), \tag{6}$$

where $\mathbf{R}$ is an Euler rotation matrix about $\mathbf{x}$, $\mathbf{y}$ and $\mathbf{z}$ axes, respectively, and $\mathbf{t}$ is a translation matrix along $\mathbf{x}$, $\mathbf{y}$ and $\mathbf{z}$ coordinates. Furthermore, $\mathbf{u}_k$ is the

k_{th} registering point in the register data set and $\mathbf{y}_k$ is its corresponding point in the model data set; However, these correspondence points are unknown and we have used the well-known nearest-neighbor approximation method proposed by Besl and Mckay [3] for finding the correspondences. Finally, it is assumed that the observations are stimulated by a zero-mean Gaussian random vector with the covariance matrix of $\mathcal{V}_k$. This assumption can be verified by the following argument: Since the data sets' points are not accurately extracted because of the calibration and segmentation errors, it is logical to assume that they are degraded by a zero-mean uniformly distributed and independent random vector noise with a specific variance in each dimension. In the sequel, for simplicity, it is assumed that the variance of the noise is the same in each dimension; however in the reality they might be different. Also, different modality data sets have different uniformly distributed random noise vector characteristics. Hence, by assuming that the registration parameters (rotation matrix and translation vector) between two data sets are known, one can write:

$$\mathbf{y} + \mathbf{n}_y = \mathbf{R}(\mathbf{t} + \mathbf{u} + \mathbf{n}_u), \tag{7}$$

where $\mathbf{n}_y = [n_{1y}, n_{2y}, n_{3y}]^T$ and $\mathbf{n}_u = [n_{1u}, n_{2u}, n_{3u}]^T$ are zero-mean independent uniformly distributed random vectors in the two data sets with covariance matrices of $\sigma_y^2\mathbf{I}$ and $\sigma_u^2\mathbf{I}$ ($\mathbf{I}_{3\times3}$ is the identity matrix), respectively. $\mathbf{y} + \mathbf{n}_y$ is the selected point in the model data set and $\mathbf{u} + \mathbf{n}_u$ is its correspondence in the register data set. Equation (7) can be simplified as:

$$\mathbf{y} = \mathbf{R}(\mathbf{t} + \mathbf{u}) + \mathbf{R}\mathbf{n}_u - \mathbf{n}_y = \mathbf{R}(\mathbf{t} + \mathbf{u}) + \mathbf{n}, \tag{8}$$

where $\mathbf{n} = \mathbf{R}\mathbf{n}_u - \mathbf{n}_y$, is a random vector with three components. The first element of $\mathbf{n}$ can be written as:

$$n_1 = r_{11}n_{1u} + r_{12}n_{2u} + r_{13}n_{3u} + n_{1y}, \tag{9}$$

where r_{11}, r_{12} and r_{13} are the first row components of the rotation matrix $\mathbf{R}$. Using central limit theorem, it is easy to show that, with a good approximation, n_1 has a Gaussian distribution with the mean of zero and the variance of:

$$\sigma_{n_1}^2 = r_{11}^2\sigma_u^2 + r_{12}^2\sigma_u^2 + r_{13}^3\sigma_u^2 + \sigma_y^2 = \sigma_u^2 + \sigma_y^2. \tag{10}$$

In the same way, it can be verified that the two other components of $\mathbf{n}$ have the variance of $\sigma_u^2 + \sigma_y^2$ as well. Considering that the components of $\mathbf{n}$ are statistically independent, by a good approximation, $\mathbf{n}$ can be considered as a zero-mean independent Gaussian random vector with the covariance matrix of $(\sigma_u^2 + \sigma_y^2)\mathbf{I}$. Since the defined observation model is governed by a non-linear function distorted by a Gaussian observation noise, we have employed the UKF algorithm for estimating the registration parameters as follows:

In the first iteration, the state vector is initialized to zero, and only one random point is selected from the register data set. Next, the state vector is used to transfer the selected point to the model data set. Then the closest point in the model data set to the transferred selected point is transferred back to the register data set using the inverse of the transformation matrix represented by the state vector. The distance between this point and the original selected point is used to update the state vector and its covariance by using the UKF algorithm. The procedure is iteratively repeated by incrementally adding more points from the register data set to the algorithm in the next iterations.

3 Results

Two sets of experiments are performed to validate the accuracy of the proposed registration method. In addition, the registration results of the proposed method are compared to the well-known ICP algorithm. In the first experiment, a set of known random transformations are applied to a cloud of points and the proposed algorithm is employed to register the original point cloud to the transformed one. This experiment shows the performance of the proposed algorithm where there is no ultrasound calibration or segmentation error involved. In the second experiment, the point cloud representing the bone surface extracted from 3D ultrasound data is registered to its corresponding surface points extracted from the mesh data generated by segmenting CT images. This experiment shows the degradation of the registration parameters caused by segmentation and calibration errors.

3.1 Two Point Clouds Registration

By using the ultrasound calibration and segmentation methods proposed in [10], the 2D ultrasound images of a phantom Scaphoid bone surface are transferred to the 3D real-world coordinates. Then a set of random transformations are applied to the 3D ultrasound point cloud, and for each transformation, registration parameters are estimated between the original point cloud and the transferred one. For constructing the 3D ultrasound data set, 280 points of the bone surface

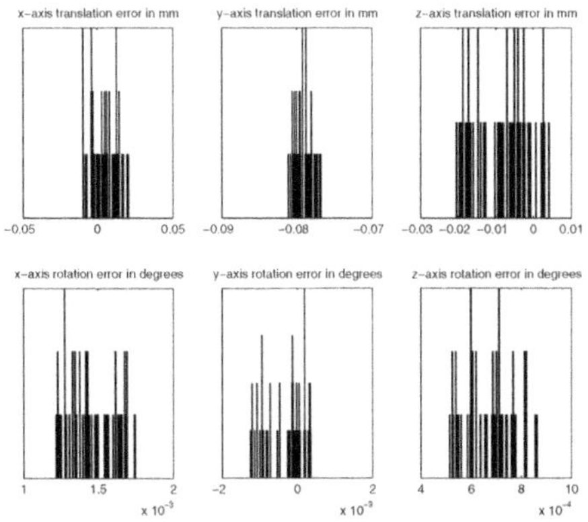

Fig. 1. Error distributions for 50 UKF registrations; standard deviations are $2.6° \times 10^{-8}$, $2.7° \times 10^{-7}$ and $9.5° \times 10^{-9}$ for **x**, **y** and **z** axis rotation errors, and 6.8×10^{-5}mm, 1.4×10^{-6}mm and 5.3×10^{-5}mm for the **x**, **y** and **z** axis translation errors, respectively.

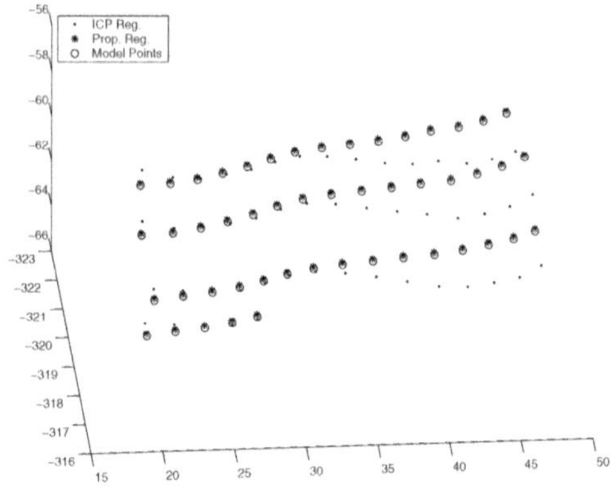

Fig. 2. Registration of model and registered data sets using ICP and our proposed method with the same initial conditions (units are in millimeters)

from 14 ultrasound images are selected. By drawing from the uniform distribution $\mathcal{U}(\pm 10mm, \pm 10mm, \pm 10mm, \pm 10°, \pm 10°, \pm 10°)$, 50 random transformations are generated and each transformation is applied to the 3D ultrasound point cloud to construct the model data set. Next, the proposed registration method is used to register the original data set (register data set) to the model data set. The distribution of the rotation and translation errors are shown in Figure 1. As expected, the variance and the mean of errors are very small (almost zero), since there is no calibration or segmentation errors in the data sets. For the same set of data and initial conditions, the registration results for the ICP algorithm and our proposed registration method are compared as well. The same uniform distribution mentioned above is used to generate the initial conditions. Figure 2 shows the registration result for the ICP algorithm and the proposed registration method for one of the simulations. It is seen that the proposed method's performance is significantly higher than that of the ICP algorithm. On average, the maximum distance error using the ICP registration algorithm is 1.5mm, whereas this error reduces to 0.8mm using the proposed registration method.

3.2 CT to Ultrasound Registration

In this experiment the constructed 3D ultrasound cloud is registered to the bone mesh surface, extracted from the CT data. Here, the two data sets have different number of points and are extracted from different imaging modalities, therefore containing different inherent calibration and segmentation errors. At first the 3D ultrasound data is manually aligned to the CT mesh using the fiducial points mounted on the Scaphoid bone. We were able to align two data sets manually within the range of 2mm fiducial registration error. Then a set of random transformations are applied to the 3D ultrasound point cloud, and for each transformation, registration parameters are estimated between the CT mesh data and the transferred 3D ultrasound points. The 3D ultrasound data set is constructed by selecting 450 points from the bone surface within 30 ultrasound images. Obviously, due to the uncertainty caused by the thickness of the bone response in each ultrasound image, these points are just approximations to the location of the bone within these images. As before, 45 random transformations are produced by drawing from the uniform distribution $\mathcal{U}(\pm 10mm, \pm 10mm, \pm 10mm, \pm 10^\circ, \pm 10^\circ, \pm 10^\circ)$ and each transformation is applied to the randomly selected 3D ultrasound points. Then the proposed registration method is employed to register the transformed 3D ultrasound point cloud to the CT mesh data set. The distribution of the rotation and translation error of the estimated transformation parameters are shown in Figure 3. For the similar data sets and the same initial conditions, the registration result for the ICP algorithm and the proposed registration method is compared in Figure 4. As shown, the proposed method registers the two data sets much

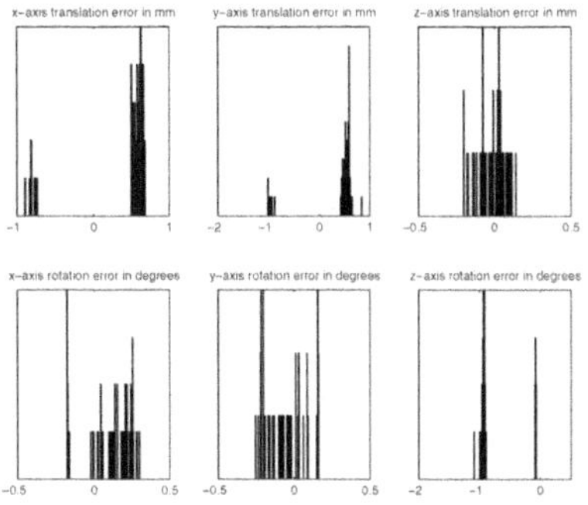

Fig. 3. Error distributions for 45 UKF registrations; standard deviations are 0.022°, 0.018° and 0.1° for **x**, **y** and **z** axes rotation errors, and 0.26mm, 0.32mm and 0.008mm for the **x**, **y** and **z** axes translation errors, respectively.

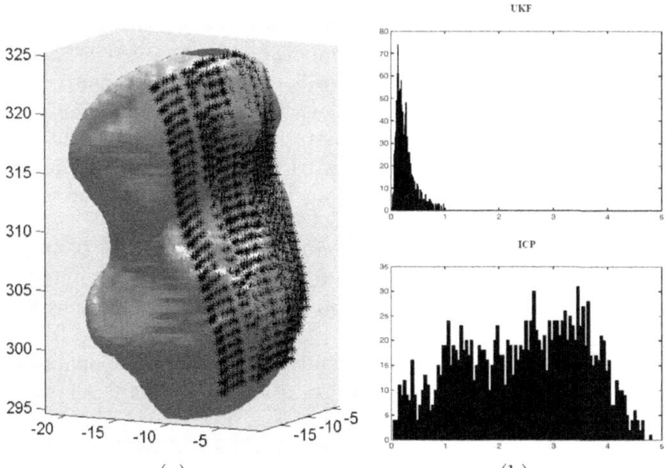

(a) (b)

Fig. 4. Comparison of the proposed method to ICP: a) The black star points represent the bone surface extracted from the ultrasound images, overlaid on the 3D surface mesh extracted from CT using UKF; b) Surface registration error (units are in mm).

more accurately than the ICP algorithm which is trapped in a local minimum. Figure 4(b) shows the distance error histogram between the 3D ultrasound points cloud and the corresponding CT data set after registration. The maximum and the root mean square distance errors using the ICP algorithm are 6mm and 3.7mm, respectively, whereas these errors reduce to 1.4mm and 0.31mm using the UKF method.

4 Discussion and Conclusions

A novel incremental surface-based registration technique based on the UKF is proposed. It is shown that the proposed method accurately registers the bone surface points extracted from the 3D ultrasound images to the ones from CT images. This method offers notable advantages to the other approaches such as the ICP and UPF algorithms. The proposed registration method not only is less sensitive to the initial guess or alignment, but also is significantly more accurate than the ICP algorithm as shown in Section 2. Moreover, against the UPF algorithm, the proposed registration method has less limitation on the size of the registration points due to the significantly less computational complexity. On the average, the complexity of the proposed method is $\mathcal{O}(N^2)$, N is the number of points in the register data set, while the complexity of the ICP algorithm and the UPF registration method with P particles, in the best case, are $\mathcal{O}(N \log N)$ and $\mathcal{O}(PN^2)$, respectively. In the future, further simulations and experiments will be performed to validate the UKF algorithm and its capture range under different measurement noise conditions.

References

1. Hill, D., Batchelor, P., Holden, M., Hawkes, D.J.: Medical image registration. Physics in Medicine and Biology **46** (2001) R1–R45
2. Horn, B., Hilden, H., Negahdaripour, S.: Closed-form solution of absolute orientation using orthonormal matrices. J. Opt. Soc. Am. **5** (1988) 1127–1135
3. Besl, P., McKay, H.: A method for registration of 3-d shapes. IEEE Trans. on Patterns Analysis and Machine Intelligence **14** (1992) 239–256
4. Ma, B., Ellis, R.: Surface-based registration with a particle filter. In: Medical Image Computing and Computer Assisted Interventions. (2004) 566–573
5. Kalman, R.E.: A new approach to linear filtering and prediction problems. Trans. of ASME. J. of Basic Eng. **82** (1960) 35–45
6. Welch, G., Bishop, G.: An introduction to kalman filter. TR 95-041, Department of Computer Science, University of Noth Carolina, Chapel Hill (1995)
7. Julier, S.J., Uhlmann, J.K.: Unscented filtering and nonlinear estimation. Proc. IEEE **92** (2004)
8. Wan, E.A., Merwe, R.V.D.: The unscented kalman filter for nonlinear estimation. In: Adapt. Syst. Signal Proc. Comm. Control Symp. (2000) 153–158
9. van der Merwe, R., Freitas, N.D., Doucet, A., Wan, E.A.: The unscented particle filter. In: Adv. Neural Inform. Proc. Syst. Volume 13., MIT Press (2000)
10. Peters, C., Abolmaesumi, P., Chen, T., Pichora, D., Sellens, R.: A novel interface for ultrasound guided percutaneous pinning of fractured scaphoids,. In: Computer-assisted Orthopaedic Surgery (CAOS) Conference, Helsinki, Finland (2005)

Automatic 4-D Registration in Dynamic MR Renography Based on Over-Complete Dyadic Wavelet and Fourier Transforms

Ting Song[1], Vivian S. Lee[2], Henry Rusinek[2], Manmeen Kaur[2], and Andrew F. Laine[1]

[1] Department of Biomedical Engineering, Columbia University, New York, NY, U.S.A
{ts2060, laine}@columbia.edu
[2] Department of Radiology, New York University School of Medicine, New York, NY, U.S.A
{Vivian.Lee, manmeen.kaur}@med.nyu.edu, hr18@nyu.edu

Abstract. Dynamic contrast-enhanced 4-D MR renography has the potential for broad clinical applications, but suffers from respiratory motion that limits analysis and interpretation. Since each examination yields at least over 10-20 serial 3-D images of the abdomen, manual registration is prohibitively labor-intensive. Besides in-plane motion and translation, out-of-plane motion and rotation are observed in the image series. In this paper, a novel robust and automated technique for removing out-of-plane translation and rotation with sub-voxel accuracy in 4-D dynamic MR images is presented. The method was evaluated on simulated motion data derived directly from a clinical patient's data. The method was also tested on 24 clinical patient kidney data sets. Registration results were compared with a mutual information method, in which differences between manually co-registered time-intensity curves and tested time-intensity curves were compared. Evaluation results showed that our method agreed well with these ground truth data.

1 Introduction

Single kidney glomerular filtration rate and split renal function can be measured by gadolinium-enhanced MR renography. Despite the fact that the kidney is a 3-D organ, most previous animal and clinical studies have been restricted to serial 2-D MRI data [1]. With three-dimensional magnetic resonance renography [2, 3], 3-D MR acquisitions are recorded repeatedly for at least 4 minutes after intravenous injection of a low dose of gadopentetate dimeglumine. In this context, image analysis of perfusion images aims to construct representative time-intensity curves from specified regions of interest such as the renal cortex, medulla, and collecting system. When patients cannot hold their breath reproducibly during perfusion data acquisition, accurate computation of time-intensity curves becomes complicated because of image misalignment over time. In an earlier study [2], three-dimensional registration and segmentation of all images were performed separately for each kidney by two investigators. For each case, manual registration and segmentation required

J. Duncan and G. Gerig (Eds.): MICCAI 2005, LNCS 3750, pp. 205 – 213, 2005.

approximately 2-3 hours at the workstation. For clinical applications, this workload is prohibitively time- and labor-intensive. Therefore, automated and semi-automated image registration techniques to correct respiration motion are of great clinical interest. There has been little work related to the registration of dynamic renal perfusion MRI data in which registration in time series is restricted in 2-D plus time and in-plane motion only [1, 4, 5]. Automated full 3-D serial image registration remains an unsolved problem especially in the context of internal organs [6-9]. We propose a novel fully automated four-dimensional (3-D plus time) MRI renography registration framework based on wavelet and Fourier transforms (WTFT). First, a preprocessing of denoising is employed using edge-preserving anisotropic diffusion; secondly, an edge detection is implemented using a 3-D overcomplete dyadic wavelet expansion; thirdly, based on the previous edge images, a 3-D registration is applied using the Fourier transform; then an existing sub-voxel registration scheme, which was extended to 3-D, is used to refine the registration results. Our method was quantitatively evaluated by phantom studies as well as on 24 clinical data sets compared with manually registered ground truth. WTFT was also compared with an existing 3-D mutual information based registration method.

2 Methodology

2.1 Anisotropic Diffusion

If edge detection is applied directly on the original serial 3-D images, the edges caused by noise prevent the registration process from achieving accuracy. Therefore, we needed to apply a denoising process before edge detection. Here, we have applied a computationally efficient denoising filter based on anisotropic diffusion previous developed by Duan et al. [10].

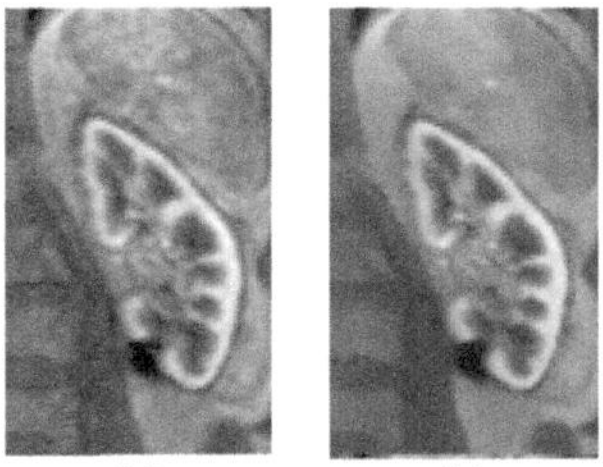

(a) (b)

Fig. 1. The effect of anisotropic diffusion comparison (coronal view): (a) original image; (b) processed image

2.2 Wavelet Edge Detection

Due to the gadopentetate dimeglumine perfusion process, intensities of serial images change with time, therefore, it is unreliable to use intensity images directly. Instead, we can use edge information which is preserved fairly well in the serial 3-D image volumes. Compared with gradient and 3-D Sobel edge detection, wavelet transforms, which can also be used for edge detection, provide smooth and strong edge detection results. One way of implementing a multi-dimensional discrete dyadic transform is to use a filter bank scheme with separable wavelet bases [11]. Since the research in this paper focuses on three-dimensional processing, we used a three-dimensional discrete dyadic transform. We selected the modulus at level 2 for registration. A comparison of the three different edge detection methods is shown in Figure 2.

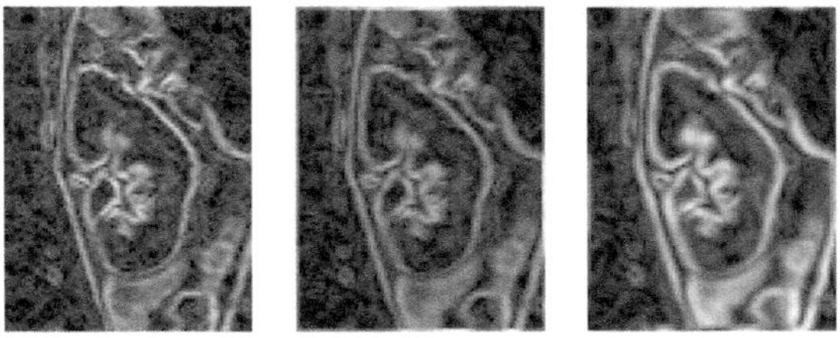

(a) (b) (c)

Fig. 2. A sample slice (coronal view) to compare different edge-detection methods: (a) gradient; (b) 3-D Sobel; (c) 3-D over-complete dyadic wavelet transform modulus

2.3 Fourier Based Registration

Using edge images acquired from previous step, a 4-D registration framework was accomplished by considering the first frame the reference as a 3-D object; the following 3-D frames were registered to the first one. Our work utilized a 3-D motion correction method based on the Fourier transform. The procedure can lead to an unsupervised 3-D rigid body registration method. One of the benefits of the method is that it makes use of all available information instead of limited features from the images. This makes the procedure very robust. Let $f(x,y,z)$ be a 3-D volume data, and let $g(x,y,z)$ be a translated and rotated version of $f(x,y,z)$, then

$$g(x,y,z) = f(Rx+t) \tag{1}$$

where $t \in R^3$ is a translation vector, and $R \in SO(3)$ is a rotation matrix.

The three-dimensional Fourier transform is defined as:

$$\mathfrak{F}[f(x,y,z)] = \int_{-\infty}^{\infty}\int_{-\infty}^{\infty}\int_{-\infty}^{\infty} f(x,y,z) e^{-j2\pi[w_x x + w_y y + w_z z]} dxdydz\,. \tag{2}$$

According to the property of the Fourier transform,

$$\mathfrak{F}[g](w_x,w_y,w_z) = R\mathfrak{F}[f](w_x,w_y,w_z) e^{j2\pi[w_x x + w_y y + w_z z]Rt} \tag{3}$$

and

$$\left|\mathfrak{F}[g](w_x,w_y,w_z)\right| = \left|R\mathfrak{F}[f](w_x,w_y,w_z)\right|. \tag{4}$$

From above equations, we can see that the estimation of rotation has been decoupled from the estimation of translation. Thus the first estimation of R should be implemented before the estimation of t. In three dimensional spaces, the rotation cannot be expressed in polar or spherical coordinates, in which case it would be reduced to a translation and be estimated by phase-correlation [8] as in the 2-D case. In other words, whereas rotation in 2-D space can be completely expressed by one angle, in order to represent a rotation in 3-D space, three angles are needed (Euler's rotation theorem). Rodrigues' rotation formula is adopted, which gives an efficient method for computing the rotation matrix $R \in SO(3)$ ($SO(3) = \{R \in \mathbb{R}^{3\times3}, R^{-1} = R^T, \det(R) = 1\}$ is a group of the 3-D special orthogonal matrices) corresponding to a rotation by an angle $\psi \in \mathbf{R}$ about a rotation axis specified by the unit vector $\tilde{\omega} = (\omega_x, \omega_y, \omega_z) \in \mathbb{R}^3$. Then R is given by

$$R = \begin{bmatrix} \cos\psi + \omega_x^2(1-\cos\psi) & \omega_x\omega_y(1-\cos\psi) - \omega_z\sin\psi & \omega_y\sin\psi + \omega_x\omega_z(1-\cos\psi) \\ \omega_z\sin\psi + \omega_x\omega_y(1-\cos\psi) & \cos\psi + \omega_y^2(1-\cos\psi) & -\omega_x\sin\psi + \omega_y\omega_z(1-\cos\psi) \\ -\omega_y\sin\psi + \omega_x\omega_z(1-\cos\psi) & \omega_x\sin\psi + \omega_y\omega_z(1-\cos\psi) & \cos\psi + \omega_z^2(1-\cos\psi) \end{bmatrix} \quad (5)$$

Since any unit vector in 3-D space can be expressed by two angles (θ, ϕ), the rotation axis unit vector can be calculated by three angles (θ, ϕ, ψ):

$$\omega_x = \cos\theta\cos\phi, \quad \omega_y = \sin\theta\cos\phi, \quad \omega_z = \sin\phi. \quad (6)$$

Since the kidney is a fairly symmetric object in 3-D, if we use the same method in Lucchese's work [7], which is mainly designed for binary images, the solution of the rotation axis is not unique because the intensity projection from different directions may be equal to the projection on the rotation axis. Furthermore, projection loses the information in the spatial domain, where the intensity profile along a fixed direction would provide extra information to find the rotation axis. Instead of three steps, in this context, only two steps were applied: rotation matrix, R, estimation and translation vector, t, estimation.

Step1. Recovering the rotation matrix

By using the relationship between the Fourier transform magnitudes in equation(4) and to avoid the effects of aliasing introduced by rotation to the energy minimization procedure, we use the energy term as

$$E = \iiint \left(\mathfrak{F}[g](w_x, w_y, w_z) - \mathfrak{F}[Rf](w_x, w_y, w_z)\right)^2 dw_x dw_y dw_z \quad (7)$$

and the optimum rotation axis and rotation angle can be recovered by

$$\left(\hat{\theta}, \hat{\phi}, \hat{\psi}\right) = \arg\min_{\theta,\phi,\psi} E \quad (8)$$

The minimization problem in equation (8) can be efficiently solved by the Quasi-Newton Method [12].

Step2. Recover translation vector.

After the rotation estimation, the rotational version of *f*, *Rf*, is calculated. Thus, the translation vector can be easily recovered by a phase-correlation technique:

$$\widehat{corr} = \frac{\mathfrak{F}[g](w_x, w_y, w_z)\mathfrak{F}^*[Rf](w_x, w_y, w_z)}{|\mathfrak{F}[g](w_x, w_y, w_z)||\mathfrak{F}[Rf](w_x, w_y, w_z)|} = e^{j[w_x \ w_y \ w_z]\bullet t} \quad (9)$$

where * denotes complex conjugate and • denotes vector dot product. The inverse Fourier transform of the right-hand side of equation (9) is the Dirac impulse function. So the translation vector can be trivially found by finding the position of that impulse function. According to the rotation and translation estimation, an aligned image from $g(x,y,z)$ to $f(x,y,z)$ can be denoted as $\widetilde{g}(x,y,z)$ and $\widetilde{f}(x,y,z)$, whose spectrum are $\widetilde{F}(w_x,w_y,w_z)$ and $\widetilde{G}(w_x,w_y,w_z)$.

2.4 Subvoxel Refinement in Frequency Domain

Based on the integer voxel translation estimation and correction, a subvoxel refining process can be used to make more accurate registration results. A 2-D subpixel registration method put forward by Stone et al. [9] was extended to a 3-D framework in this article for the first time. The method requires integer voxel accuracy because it can only correct subvoxel misalignment.

From the property of the Fourier transform,

$$\widetilde{G} = \Im[f(x+x_0, y+y_0, z+z_0)] = \widetilde{F}e^{-j(2\pi/N)(w_x x_0 + w_y y_0 + w_z z_0)} \tag{10}$$

i.e.

$$\widetilde{F}/\widetilde{G} = e^{j(2\pi/N)(w_x x_0 + w_y y_0 + w_z z_0)}. \tag{11}$$

In other words, the phase of $\widetilde{F}/\widetilde{G}$ should be a plane in the (w_x, w_y, w_z) space. Therefore, the subvoxel registration problem can be converted into a 3-D plane fitting problem, which can be solved by least square fitting. For any voxel in the (w_x, w_y, w_z) space, in theory, the following equation holds:

$$phase(\widetilde{F}/\widetilde{G}) = (2\pi/N)(w_x x_0 + w_y y_0 + w_z z_0). \tag{12}$$

Using matrix representation, the above equation is equivalent to

$$\frac{2\pi}{N}\begin{bmatrix} w_x & w_y & w_z \end{bmatrix}\begin{bmatrix} x_0 & y_0 & z_0 \end{bmatrix}^T = \begin{bmatrix} phase(\widetilde{F}/\widetilde{G}) \end{bmatrix}. \tag{13}$$

Equation (13) can be solved by pseudo inverse methods or singular value decomposition for the subvoxel translation vector $[x_0, y_0, z_0]^T$.

In both Fourier registration and subvoxel refinement process, a 3-D window is applied, which is recognized for eliminating the spurious introduction of high-frequency spectral energy due to the boundary effects [9]. We tried Blackman, Hann, and Tukey windows (r=0.5, which is r is the ratio of taper to constant sections), and we found that Blackman window worked the best for this dynamic renal data. Although in some time frames, when contrast agent intake is maximum and kidney boundaries are not clear, inner structures and outside edges surround the kidney, such as part of liver edges, will help the registration process.

3 Experiments and Results

3.1 Simulated Clinical Study

Based on a manually registered 4-D MR renography data set, a simulated data set with dimension [77 97 40 20] and voxel resolution 1.66mm x 1.66mm x 2.5 mm was generated by translating and rotating the kidney. Simulated motions included head to feet (HF) translation, left to right (LR) translation, anterior to posterior (AP) translation and rotation (Rot) with respect to three different axes, represented in terms of (θ, ϕ, ψ), where (θ, ϕ) defined the axis of rotation; ψ the angle of the rotation along that axis (Table 1).

The estimated errors in translation and rotation are shown in Figure 3. Translation estimation errors were lower than 1.4 voxels in all the directions with mean value 0.53± 0.47, 0.51±0.46, and 0.60±0.41 in x, y, and z direction respectively; for rotation, except for one case, the errors in the two angles representing the rotation axis were less than 0.5 degrees, and the errors in rotation angle were less than 2.5 degrees with mean value 0.003±0.003, 0.07±0.26, and 1.14±0.72 degrees in (θ, ϕ, ψ).

Table 1. Simulated Motion for Each Time Frame (T)

T	Motion	T	Motion	T	Motion
1	Baseline	8	LR(-1.66mm)+(90,0,5)	15	HF(3.32mm)
2	AP(-2.5mm)+(0,90,-9)	9	AP(2.5mm)	16	AP(5.0mm)
3	LR(3.32mm)+(90,0,-2)	10	Baseline	17	Baseline
4	HF(6.64mm)	11	HF(1.66mm)	18	HF(-4.98mm)
5	(0,0,-4)	12	HF(-1.66mm)	19	Baseline
6	HF(-6.64mm)	13	Baseline	20	LR(-4.98mm)
7	Baseline	14	LR(6.64mm)		

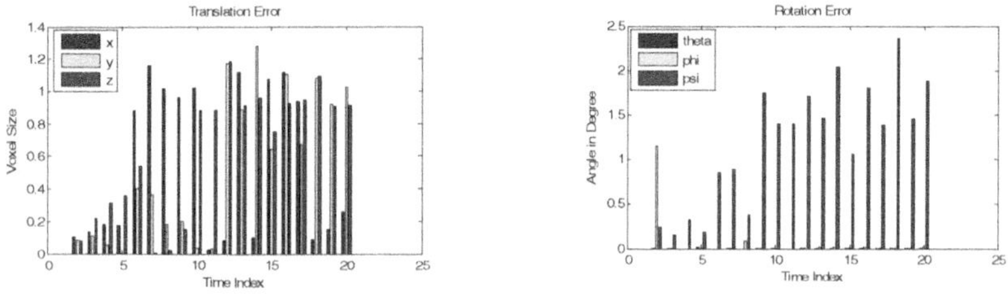

(a) (b)

Fig. 3. Clinical phantom study results: (a) translation error; (b) rotation error

3.2 Clinical Evaluation

In order to evaluate the performance of our algorithm (WTFT) clinically, our algorithm was applied to 12 clinical patient datasets (24 kidneys in total), with manual registration and segmentation as ground truth. All datasets consisted of at least 41 3-D acquisitions, where each 3-D dataset comprised 40 interpolated partitions of 2.5 mm thickness, with inplane matrix of 256 and inplane voxel size 1.66 x 1.66 mm. After registration, the cortex, medulla, and collecting system were differentiated by applying manual segmentation labels on the first frame, assuming following frames were been correctly registered. The time-intensity curves of cortex, medulla, and collecting systems were calculated based on manual registration treated as ground

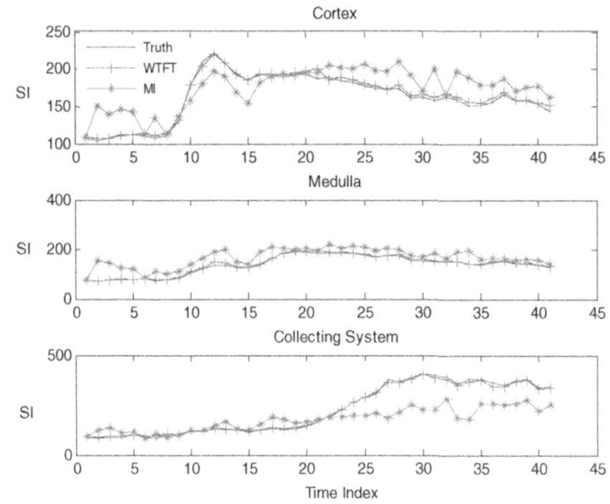

Fig. 4. Average intensity curves for one of the data sets using manual registration, WTFT, and mutual information registration

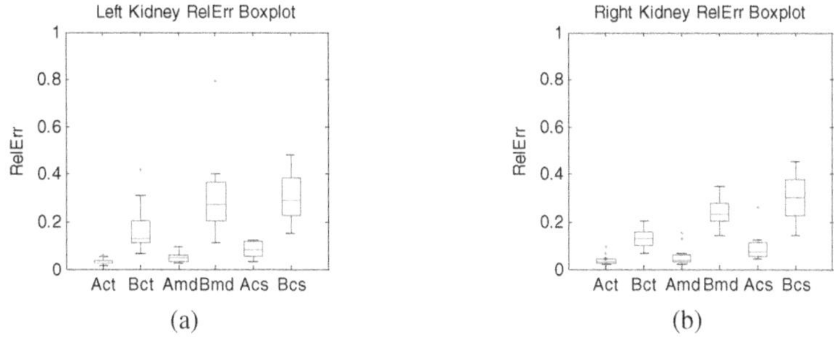

Fig. 5. Boxplot for RMS evaluation of the time-intensity curves generated from WTFT (A) and MI (B) methods. 'ct' stands for cortex; 'md' stands for medulla; 'cs'stands for collecting system. (a) left kidneys, (b) right kidneys.

Table 2. Significance values for Left and Right cortex, medulla and collecting systems for pairs of two methods

P	Left Kidney			Right Kidney		
	Cortex	Medulla	CollSys	Cortex	Medulla	CollSys
WTFT/MI	<0.0005	<0.0005	<0.0005	<0.0005	<0.0005	<0.0005

truth and our automatic registration method. As a comparison, the time-intensity curves based on Viola-Wells Mutual Information (MI) [13, 14] were also calculated. In Figure 4, results from the three registration methods are shown for each kidney structure. Qualitatively, time-intensity curves based on WTFT registration are much closer to the ground truth than MI. To quantitatively evaluate the performance, root mean squared (RMS) relative errors of time-intensity curves between automatic registration methods, WTFT or MI, and ground truth were calculated and are shown in Figure 5. From the box-plot, the relative errors based on our WTFT method are much smaller than the MI methods in terms of average and standard deviation of RMS measurements. However, we note that both automated registration methods performed best for cortex but lower agreement for the collecting systems. The average errors for cortex, medulla and collecting systems in WTFT method were 3.24%±1.41%, 5.31%±2.19%, and 8.23%±3.35% respectively for the left and 3.99%±2.23%, 5.67%±4.13%, and 9.26%±5.94% for the right. Evaluation of the statistical differences of results from the two registration methods was performed at the significance level 0.05 with a Wilcoxon signed rank test for paired data. Significance values for the three tissue types for each pair of registration methods are reported in Table 2. Small p values (below 0.0005) indicate a significant statistical difference between the methods. From box plot, we can see WTFT had lower mean and smaller standard deviation compared with MI, so WTFT statistically performed better than MI.

4 Conclusion

In this paper, we proposed a novel fully automated four-dimensional MRI renography registration framework based on over complete dyadic wavelet and Fourier transform (WTFT), which was tested in terms of automation, robustness, and accuracy. Simulated motion studies and clinical evaluation studies were used to evaluate the new method. Comparison between different edge detection methods and comparison between WTFT and mutual information (MI) were performed to illustrate the effectiveness of the proposed scheme. An edge-preserving anisotropic diffusion operator was also introduced as a denoising method. Experimental results showed accurate registration results when compared to manual registration, by expert radiologists.

References

[1] Y. Sun, M.-P. Jolly, and J. M. F. Moura, "Integrated Registration of Dynamic Renal Perfusion MR Images," presented at IEEE International Symposium on Image Processing, ICIP'04, Singapore, 2004.

[2] V. S. Lee, H. Rusinek, M. E. Noz, P. Lee, M. Raghavan, and E. L. Kramer, "Dynamic Three-dimensional MR Renography for the Measurement of Single Kidney Function: Initial Experience," *Radiology*, vol. 227, pp. 289-294, 2003.

[3] J. Sajous, Y. Boykov, C. Chefdhotel, H. Rusinek, and V. Lee, "Performance of semi-automatic registration and segmentation on 4D contrast-enhanced magnetic resonance renography," presented at Radiological Society of North America 2003, 2003.

[4] G. Gerig, R. kikinis, W. Kuoni, G. K. v. Schulthess, and O. Kubler, "Semiautomated ROI Analysis in Dynamic MRI-Studies: PartI: Image Analysis Tools for Automatic Correction of Organ Displacement," *IEEE Transaction on Image Processing*, vol. 11, pp. 221-232, 1992.

[5] E. L. W. Giele, J. A. dePriester, J. A. Blom, J. A. d. Boer, J. M. S. v. Engelshoven, A. Hasman, and M. Geerlings, "Movement Correction of the Kidney in Dynamic MRI Scans Using FFT Phase Difference Movement Detection," *Journal of Magnetic Resonance Imaging*, vol. 14, pp. 741-749, 2001.

[6] J. B. A. Maintz, "Retrospective Registration of Tomographic Brain Images." Utrecht, the Netherlands: Utrecht University, 1996, pp. 17.
[7] L. Lucchese, G. Doretto, and G. M. Cortelazzo, "A Frequency Domain Technique for Range Data Registration," *IEEE Transaction on Pattern Analysis and Machine Intelligence*, vol. 24, pp. 1468-1484, 2002.
[8] Y. Keller, A. Averbuch, and M. Israeli, "Pseudopolar-Based Estimation of Large Translations, Rotations, and Scalings in Images," *IEEE Transaction on Image Processing*, vol. 14, pp. 12-22, 2005.
[9] H. S. Stone, M. T. Orchard, E.-C. Chang, and S. A. Martucci, "A Fast Direct Fourier-Based Algorithm for Subpixel Registration of Images," *IEEE Transaction on Geoscience and Remote Sensing*, vol. 39, pp. 2235-2243, 2001.
[10] Q. Duan, E. D. Angelini, and A. Laine, "Assessment of visual quality and spatial accuracy of fast anisotropic diffusion and scan conversion algorithms for real-time three-dimensional spherical ultrasound," presented at Proceedings of SPIE, Medical Imaging 2004: Ultrasonic Imaging and Signal Processing, 2004.
[11] Y. Jin, "Multi-Scale Processing of Tomographic Images Using Dyadic Wavelet Expansions," in *Biomedical Engineering*. New York: Columbia University, 2004, pp. 1-221.
[12] D. F. Shanno, "Conditioning of Quasi-Newton Methods for Function Minimization," *Matheamtics of Computing*, vol. 24, pp. 647-656, 1970.
[13] ITK, *www.itk.org*.
[14] W. M. Well, P. Viola, and R. Kikinis, "Multimodal volume registration by maximzation of mutual information," presented at Proc. Med. Robot. Comp. Assist. Surg., Baltimore, 1995.

Model of a Vascular C-Arm for 3D Augmented Fluoroscopy in Interventional Radiology

S. Gorges[1,2], E. Kerrien[1], M-O. Berger[1], Y. Trousset[2], J. Pescatore[2], R. Anxionnat[1,3], and L. Picard[3]

[1] LORIA-INRIA Lorraine, France
[2] GE Healthcare, Buc, France
[3] Diagnostic and Therapeutic Neuroradiology Dept, Univ Hosp of Nancy, France
Sebastien.Gorges@loria.fr

Abstract. This paper deals with the modeling of a vascular C-arm to generate 3D augmented fluoroscopic images in an interventional radiology context. A methodology based on the use of a multi-image calibration is proposed to assess the physical behavior of the C-arm. From the knowledge of the main characteristics of the C-arm, realistic models of the acquisition geometry are proposed. Their accuracy was evaluated and experiments showed that the C-arm geometry can be predicted with a mean 2D reprojection error of 0.5 mm. The interest of 3D augmented fluoroscopy is also assessed on a clinical case.

1 Introduction

In order to guide tools during the procedure, the interventional radiologist uses a vascular C-arm to acquire 2D fluoroscopy images in real time. Today, 3D X-ray angiography (3DXA) is widely available on modern vascular C-arms. Such 3D images are recognized as being of a daily clinical usefulness for the planning and follow-up of the treatment of cerebral pathologies [1]. One next step is to leverage the high-resolution volumetric information provided by 3DXA to complement fluoroscopy images and ease the tool guidance. This requires registering 3DXA with fluoroscopy images, for any orientation of the C-arm.

Image-based registration [2] was investigated to match MRA with Digital Subtracted Angiography (DSA) images. Though providing accurate registration, such methods require the injection of contrast agent for the reference 2D image. Furthermore, their computation time together with the manual interaction necessary to initiate the registration [3] still hampers their wide integration in an ever tighter medical workflow.

Using 3DXA, both images to register are acquired on the same machine. Registration can be deduced from a model of the C-arm, based on the information provided in real-time by the system sensors, such as the C-arm angles. The *a priori* model in [4] does not accurately fit the acquisition geometry, due to slight mechanical deformations undergone by the C-arm. More sophisticated models have been proposed in [5,6]. Though encouraging with regards to the precision of the registration, these works proved that the *a priori* model was not accurate enough to render the effective mechanical behavior of the C-arm.

J. Duncan and G. Gerig (Eds.): MICCAI 2005, LNCS 3750, pp. 214–222, 2005.

In this paper, an *a posteriori* model of the C-arm motion is built through a series of measurements relying on vision-based methods. The aim is twofold: on one hand improve the quality of the registration and on a second hand effectively render the mechanical behavior of the C-arm, including mechanical deformations.

2 The Vascular C-Arm

2.1 The C-Arm and Its Sensors

During a clinical procedure, the C-arm can be oriented in any incidence that the physician reckons as the best suitable for the treatment (Fig. 1). The orientation is classically described by two anatomical angles: α = cranio-caudal (CC) and β = right/left anterior orientation (RAO/LAO). Furthermore, the imager can be translated to adjust its distance to the X-ray tube (Source to Image Distance, or SID). The SID and the α and β angles are measured in real time by sensors.

2.2 The Acquisition Geometry

The C-arm can be modeled as a pinhole camera by a projection matrix $\mathbf{M}$, relating any 3D point X to its corresponding projection q in the acquired image:

$$q = \mathbf{M}X \quad \text{with} \quad \mathbf{M} = \mathbf{IE} = \begin{bmatrix} f & 0 & u_0 \\ 0 & f & v_0 \\ 0 & 0 & 1 \end{bmatrix} [\mathbf{R}|\mathbf{T}]$$

The *intrinsic parameters* $\mathbf{I}$ describe the projection parameters from the X-ray tube to the 2D view: (u_0, v_0) is the principal point and f is the focal length in pixels (square pixels); the *extrinsic parameters* $\mathbf{E}$ define the orientation $\mathbf{R}$ and position $\mathbf{T}$ of the acquisition system in a world coordinate system.

2.3 The Predictive C-Arm Model

Model-based approaches [4,5,6] all aim at estimating the intrinsic and extrinsic parameters, thus building up the $\mathbf{M}$ matrix. The intrinsic parameters (u_0, v_0) are assumed constant while f directly depends on the SID.

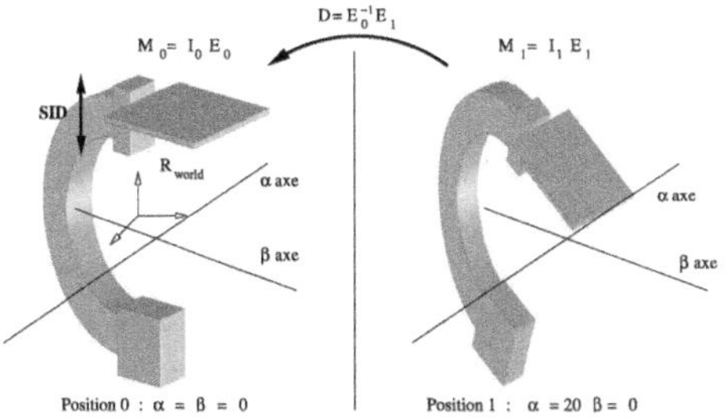

Fig. 1. The vascular C-arm in two different orientations. The change in the acquisition geometry $\mathbf{M}$ is given by the rigid motion $\mathbf{D}$, expressed in the world coordinate frame.

The extrinsic parameters are assumed to be known in a reference position, which is straightforward. To compute them in a different orientation, the rigid motion $\mathbf{D}$ of the C-arm is modeled as a function of the α and β angles (Fig. 1). Dumay [4] modeled $\mathbf{D}$ as made of two independent rotations around the α and β axes respectively. Both axes were assumed to be orthogonal and to intersect. Kerrien [5] showed that this does not exactly hold and proposed to calibrate the axes. Cañero [6] compared 4 models with growing complexity, starting from Dumay's model, that significantly improved the accuracy of the registration.

Still, the C-arm bears slight mechanical bendings that impair the accuracy of the previous models. Reliable and independent measurements of intrinsic and extrinsic parameters should help understand these deformations. Next section describes how such measurements can be made.

3 Robust Estimation of the Acquisition Geometry

3.1 Classical Geometric Calibration

The projection matrix $\mathbf{M}$ is classically estimated through the minimization of the reprojection error $\mathcal{E}_r$ on a set of 3D markers (X_i):

$$\mathcal{E}_r(\mathbf{M}) = \frac{1}{n}\sum_{i=0}^{n} ||\mathbf{M}X_i - q_i||^2$$

where n is the number of detected markers (q_i) in the image. In practice, we use a phantom called "helix phantom" which is made of a hollow Lucite cylinder in which lead markers are inserted according to an helicoidal pattern. Although the estimated projection matrix is known with a sub-pixel reprojection error, its decomposition into intrinsic and extrinsic parameters is known to be unstable.The statistical noise affecting this measurement prevents us from computing independent and reliable intrinsic and extrinsic parameters.

3.2 Multi-image Calibration

To reduce the statistical noise, calibration can be repeated with varying extrinsic parameters and fixed intrinsic parameters. Thereby, the inter-dependence between both sets of parameters is reduced, so that reliable intrinsic parameters are estimated. In [7], the camera is moved around the calibration target. In our case, there is no valid reason to believe the intrinsic parameters do not depend on the C-arm orientation. As a result, for a given C-arm orientation, N images of the helix phantom are taken, with the phantom being moved in both rotation and translation between each image acquisition. This step is called *multi-image calibration.* The common intrinsic parameters $\mathbf{I}$ and N extrinsic parameters $(\mathbf{E}_i)$ are then estimated simultaneously by minimizing the residual reprojection error $\mathcal{R}_m$ on the N images, using Levenberg-Marquardt algorithm:

$$\mathcal{R}_m = \frac{1}{N}\sum_{i=0}^{N} \mathcal{E}_r(\mathbf{M}_i) \quad \text{with} \quad \mathbf{M}_i = \mathbf{I}\mathbf{E}_i \tag{1}$$

3.3 Per-Axis Analysis

Our medical institution is equipped with a vascular C-arm mounted with the latest generation of flat panel detectors (INNOVA 4100 – GE Healthcare, Buc, France), thus bearing no geometrical distortions. The pixel size is 0.2 mm.

Experimental values showed that 30 images were enough to obtain a stable estimation of the intrinsic parameters. More, bootstrap techniques showed that the precision of the intrinsic parameters was always better than 2.5 pixels.

The Intrinsic Parameters. The multi-image calibration was used to study how the intrinsic parameters varied when the C-arm was rotated around either the α axis or the β axis, with a fixed SID (1180mm). For each axis, 5 orientations were chosen: $\mathcal{P}_\alpha = \{(\alpha,\beta)\,|\,\beta = 0\,\&\,\alpha \in [-40°, -20°, 0°, 10°, 20°]\}$ and $\mathcal{P}_\beta = \{(\alpha,\beta)\,|\,\alpha = 0\,\&\,\beta \in [-90°, -40°, 0°, 40°, 90°]\}$. For each orientation, a multi-image calibration was performed using $N = 30$ images.

The focal length remained almost constant whatever the orientation of the C-arm. Figure 2.a shows the measurements made on (u_0, v_0), the shorter lines being related to the α rotation. Given the 2.5 pixels precision of the method, no definite change of the intrinsic parameters could be observed except for u_0 which clearly presents a smooth variation during a rotation around the β axis. This imprecision also explains why the curves do not intersect for $\alpha = \beta = 0$.

The Extrinsic Parameters. The multi-image calibrations also provide N extrinsic matrices $\mathbf{E}$ for each orientation in the $\mathcal{P}_\alpha$ and $\mathcal{P}_\beta$ sets (see eq. 1). These parameters are stable, since estimated with stable intrinsic parameters. A subset of images, one per orientation, was taken with a common helix phantom position, thereby providing a subset of extrinsic matrices, one per orientation, expressed in the same coordinate system.

The orientation common to both sets was chosen as the reference position $(\alpha = \beta = 0)$. Following [5], the rigid motion $\mathbf{D}$ of the C-arm was computed by

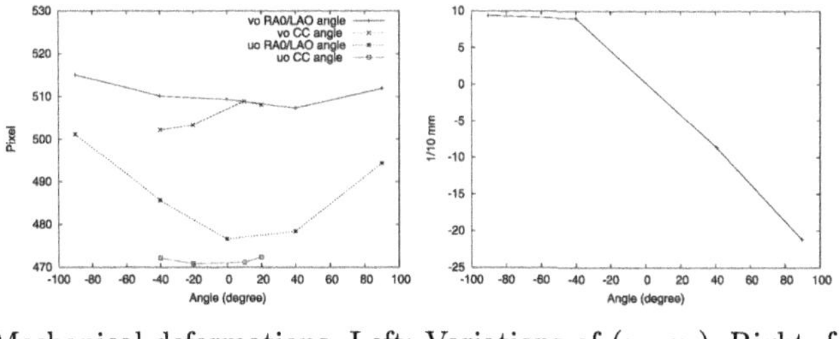

Fig. 2. Mechanical deformations. Left: Variations of (u_0, v_0). Right: factor λ.

Table 1. Per-axis rotation parameters

	α		β		
	C [x,y,z] (mm)	ϕ (°)	C [x,y,z] (mm)	ϕ (°)	θ_{err}(°)
mean	[1.75 0.53 -29.04]	0.48	[0.72 4.86 -0.04]	0.06	0.26
std	[0.33 0.17 1.20]	0.30	[0.90 0.67 0.003]	0.02	0.18

compositing extrinsic parameters (see also Fig. 1). For analysis purpose, $\mathbf{D}$ was expressed as:

$$\mathbf{D} = [\mathbf{R}_\theta \,|\, T] = [\mathbf{R}_\theta \,|\, (\mathbf{Id} - \mathbf{R}_\theta)C + \Delta T] \tag{2}$$

where $\mathbf{R}_\theta$ is a rotation of angle θ and axis ν, C is the closest point to the origin on the axis of rotation, and ΔT is a residual translation, proportional to ν: $\Delta T = \lambda\nu$.

A per-axis basis analysis of the rigid motions $\mathbf{D}$ is reported in table 3.3: the stability of the rotation axis is verified through statistics on the position of C and by computing the angular deviation ϕ of ν with respect to its average value. The difference θ_{err} observed between the computed θ and the sensor data is also very small. The norm of ΔT is below 0.2 mm for the α axis. On the opposite, it cannot be neglected for the β axis: provided that $\Delta T = \lambda\nu$, figure 2 displays the variation of λ according to the angle β. As a conclusion, the rotation model is valid for the C-arm motion around the α axis, but not for β which requires a further translation parallel to the rotation axis.

3.4 Conclusion

The multi-image calibration is an accurate method to determine reliable intrinsic and extrinsic parameters. A per-axis analysis unveiled a variation of the u_0 intrinsic parameter and an important residual translation during a β rotation. These may be interpreted as respectively a physical change of the relative position between the X-ray tube and the flat panel, and a global mechanical bending of the C-arm under its own weight in lateral positions. Such effects are taken into account in two models described in the next section.

4 Predictive Models of the C-Arm Acquisition Geometry

4.1 Description

The aim in modeling the C-arm acquisition geometry is to be able to predict, for any orientation (α, β) of the C-arm, the acquisition geometry:

$$\mathbf{M}_{\alpha,\beta} = \mathbf{I}_{\alpha,\beta}\mathbf{E}_{\alpha,\beta}$$

The extrinsic parameters $\mathbf{E}_{\alpha,\beta}$ are recovered by modeling the rigid motion imparted to the C-arm to move from a reference orientation ($\alpha = \beta = 0$) to (α, β). Under the hypothesis that the α and β motions are independent, this rigid motion is a composition of two rigid motions: $\mathbf{D}_\alpha$ around the α axis, and $\mathbf{D}_\beta$ around the β axis:

$$\mathbf{E}_{\alpha,\beta} = \mathbf{E}_0\mathbf{D}_\alpha\mathbf{D}_\beta$$

where $\mathbf{E}_0 = [\mathbf{R}_0|T_0]$ are the extrinsic parameters in the reference orientation.

According to the above measurements, $\mathbf{D}_\alpha$ is a rotation of angle α, read on the sensor, and parameterized by an axis vector ν_a and a fixed point C_a. $\mathbf{D}_\beta$ is a rotation of angle β, read on the sensor, and parameterized by an axis

Table 2. Reprojection error in pixels for the matrices predicted by both models. The mean error for model $\mathcal{M}_f$ was 2.37 pixels (std=1.48). The mean error for model $\mathcal{M}_m$ was 2.31 pixels (std=1.31). The pixel size is 0.2 mm.

α (°)	-28.8	-28.8	-28.8	-8.8	-8.8	-8.8	-8.8	-8.8	-0.3	-0.3	-0.3	-0.3	-0.3	19.1	19.1
β (°)	-40.4	1.3	40	-90.4	-39.1	0.1	41.1	79.8	-90.4	-39.6	0.4	41.2	80.3	-19.3	0.1
$\mathcal{M}_f$	5.81	3.43	5.61	1.93	1.90	2.24	2.59	2.24	1.20	1.27	1.28	1.38	1.60	1.83	1.25
$\mathcal{M}_m$	3.63	3.44	6.10	1.47	1.72	2.25	2.26	3.20	1.59	1.39	1.28	1.26	1.66	2.19	1.25

vector ν_b and a fixed point C_b associated to a translation along ν_b of amplitude λ. Provided the general function shape in figure 2.b, second- and third-order polynomials were tested to model the parameter λ as a function of β. The latter gave better results: $\lambda = \sum_{i=0}^{3} \lambda_i \beta^i$.

The intrinsic parameter v_0 is constant, and the focal length f only depends on the SID. The models are described considering a fixed SID, allowing the assumption that f is also constant. According to the above experiments, u_0 varies as a function of β. Figure 2.a suggests the shape of a low-order polynomial. Again third-order polynomial proved best: $u_0 = \sum_{i=0}^{3} \mu_i \beta^i$.

Thereby a model was built to render the mechanical properties of the C-arm. This model, denoted $\mathcal{M}_m$, is parameterized by the vector:

$$\phi_m = \{\mathbf{R}_0, T_0; \nu_a, C_a; \nu_b, C_b, (\lambda_i)_{i=0..3}; (\mu_i)_{i=0..3}, v_0, f\}$$

A second model was considered, only differing from $\mathcal{M}_m$ by considering u_0 is also constant, thereby assuming intrinsic parameters are constant. The model is denoted by $\mathcal{M}_f$ and is parameterized by:

$$\phi_f = \{\mathbf{R}_0, T_0; \nu_a, C_a; \nu_b, C_b, (\lambda_i)_{i=0..3}; u_0, v_0, f\}$$

4.2 Calibrating the Models

Model $\mathcal{M}_f$. Since intrinsic parameters are constant, a classical multi-image calibration can be performed, with a moving C-arm and a fixed helix phantom as in [7]. One image was acquired for every orientation in $\mathcal{P}_\alpha$ and $\mathcal{P}_\beta$. The only difference with section 3.2 is that the N extrinsic parameters are replaced by the components of ϕ_f modeling the extrinsic parameters. Images of the fixed helix phantom were also taken for C-arm orientations outside $\mathcal{P}_\alpha$ and $\mathcal{P}_\beta$ for validation purpose. The orientations of this test set are provided in table 2.

Model $\mathcal{M}_m$. Due to the varying intrinsic parameter u_0, one multi-image acquisition has to be made for each orientation in $\mathcal{P}_\alpha$ and $\mathcal{P}_\beta$. These come in addition to the same acquisition as for $\mathcal{M}_f$, necessary to manage the extrinsic parameters. This results in the same type of acquisition as made in section 3.3 to study the extrinsic parameters. Again, a global cost function could be designed and minimized but the relatively small influence of the intrinsic parameters compared to that of the extrinsic parameters leads to poorly optimized intrinsic parameters. As often in numerical optimization, we found the adequate cost function to be the weighted sum of two residuals:

$$\mathcal{R} = \mathcal{R}_f + \gamma \sum_{(\alpha,\beta)\in\mathcal{P}_\alpha\cup\mathcal{P}_\beta} \mathcal{R}_m(\mathbf{M}_{\alpha,\beta})$$

where $\mathcal{R}_f$ is the residual of the classical multi-image calibration as for the $\mathcal{M}_f$ model, and $\mathcal{R}_m$ is the residual of our multi-image calibration, as described in section 3.2. γ was fixed at 1000, to balance the influence of both terms on $\mathcal{R}$.

5 Validation – Application to 3D Augmented Fluoroscopy

The limitations of fluoroscopy are well known: contrast medium has to be injected repetitively to visualize the vessels, its image quality is reduced compared to DSA, and finally, it does not provide 3D information. The real-time superimposition of fluoroscopic images with pre-operative 3DXA images could potentially overcome some of these limitations. We call this clinical application "3D augmented fluoroscopy". The various validation studies that follow were targeted to such an application. As a result, the reprojection error was chosen as the figure of merit to evaluate our models.

5.1 Comparison of the Models

Both $\mathcal{M}_f$ and $\mathcal{M}_m$ models where calibrated as described above. For each orientation (α, β) in the test set, the matrix $\mathbf{M}_{\alpha,\beta}$ predicted by each model was built up and its reprojection error computed. Results are reported in table 2.

Each model presents a mean reprojection error of about 2.5 pixels which represents 0.5 mm of error in the image plane (pixel size=0.2 mm). In both cases, the error was below this average error in 84% of the test orientations. This precision is sufficient for many medical applications and in particular for 3D augmented fluoroscopy. No major differences could be noted between the models. Indeed, in $\mathcal{M}_f$, nothing prevents the coupling effect between intrinsic and extrinsic parameters from counteracting the error made when assuming u_0 is constant.

5.2 Evaluation of 3D Augmented Fluoroscopy

Phantom experiment. A silicon phantom of the cerebral vasculature was injected with a contrast medium and a 3DXA was acquired. Then, one fluoroscopy image was taken for each test orientation in table 2. 3D augmented views were

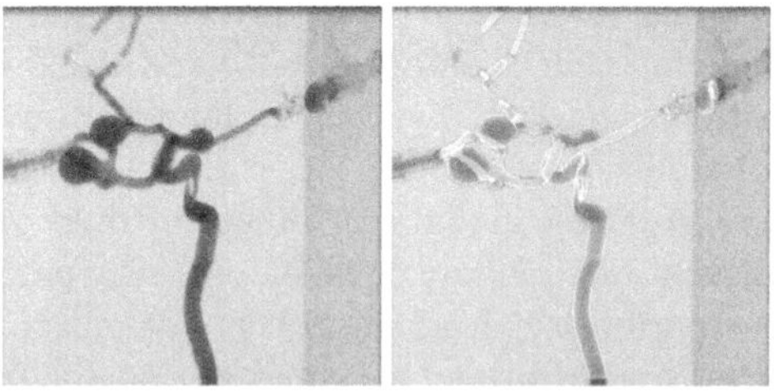

Fig. 3. 3D augmented fluoroscopy on phantom dataset. Left: fluoroscopic image of the phantom; right: superposition of the 3DXA onto the fluoroscopic image.

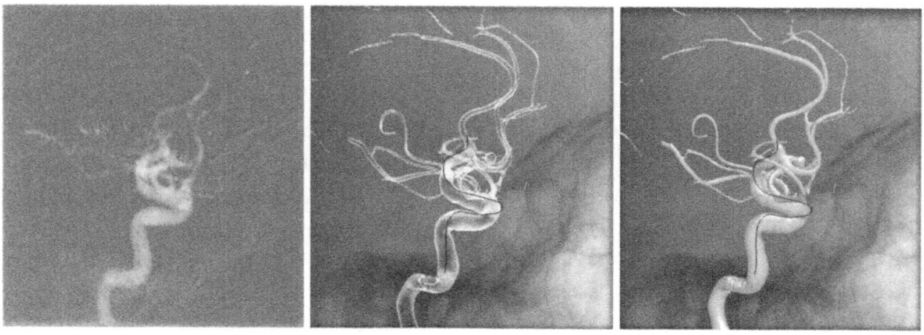

Fig. 4. 3D augmented fluoroscopy on a clinical case with model $\mathcal{M}_m$: Comparison of contrast-enhanced fluoroscopy (left) and 3D augmented fluoroscopy width blending (middle) and surface (right) views. Only the main vessels are shown and the guide wire was manually overlined in black.

generated, using model $\mathcal{M}_m$, to allow a visual assessment of the local reprojection error to complement the above global statistics. In Fig.5.2 an augmented image is shown for $\alpha = 8.8°$ and $\beta = 41.1°$. The precision of this position is 0.45 mm (see table.2) which, from a visual standpoint, corresponds to a perfect fit.

Patient Data. A patient underwent an endovascular treatment for an aneurysm. A 3DXA was acquired and fluoroscopy images were captured under an oblique orientation ($\alpha = 2°, \beta = -82°$) while the micro-catheter was moved up to the aneurysm. The SID (1070 mm) used during the procedure was different from the SID used to calibrate the models (1180 mm). Therefore, the focal length given by the models was updated as $f + (1070 - 1180)/s_p$ where $s_p = 0.2$mm is the pixel size.

Visual assessment of 3D augmented views indicated a very accurate match on the region of medical interest, i.e. around the aneurysm. Compared to fluoroscopic images (Fig.5.2 left), the augmented images (Fig.5.2 middle & right) present a higher image quality and ease the assessment of the tool position within the 3D vascular anatomy in real time. Furthermore, the surface view (Fig.5.2 right) allows to better analyze superimpositions of vascular structures and can dramatically help the radiologist to understand the vascular bifurcations. Thus, 3D augmented fluoroscopy can make micro-catheter navigation and tool deployment easier.

6 Conclusion

A robust calibration method for the intrinsic and extrinsic parameters of a vascular C-arm was proposed and evaluated. Thereby, some mechanical characteristics of the C-arm were assessed and realistic models were built, including slight deformations of the system. These models were evaluated as being able to predict the acquisition geometry for any C-arm orientation with a mean 2D reprojection error of 0.5 mm. This accuracy enables many medical applications such as 3D augmented fluoroscopy. A clinical case showed that 3D augmented fluoroscopy has the potential to facilitate the classical navigation of the radiologists.

References

1. R. Anxionnat, S. Bracard, X. Ducrocq, Y. Trousset, L. Launay, E. Kerrien, M. Braun, R. Vaillant, F. Scomazzoni, A. Lebedinsky and L. Picard. Intracranial Aneurysms : Clinical Value of 3D Digital Subtraction Angiography in the Therapeutic Decision and Endovascular Treatment. In *Radiology*, (218):799-808, 2001.
2. J.H. Hipwell, G.P. Penney, R.A. McLaughlin, K. Rhode, P. Summers, T.C. Cox, J.V. Byrne, A. Noble, and D.J. Hawkes. Intensity-based 2D-3D registration of cerebral angiograms. In *IEEE Trans. on Med. Imag.*, 22(11):1417-1426, 2003.
3. J.V. Byrne, C. Colominas, J.H. Hipwell, T.C. Cox, A. Noble, G.P. Penney, and D.J. Hawkes. Assessment of a technique for 2D-3D registration of cerebral intra-arterial angiography. In *The British Journal of Radiology*, 77:123-128, 2004.
4. A. Dumay, J. Reiber and J. Gerbrands. Determination of optimal angiographic viewing angles: Basic principles and evaluation study. In *IEEE Trans. on Med. Imag.*, 13(1):13-24, 1994.
5. E. Kerrien, R. Vaillant, L. Launay, M-O. Berger, and E. Maurincomme. Machine precision assessment for 3D/2D digital subtracted angiography images registration. In *SPIE Medical Imaging'98, San Diego, USA*, February 1998.
6. C. Cañero, E. Nofrerías, J. Mauri, and P. Radeva. Modelling the acquisition geometry of a C-arm angiography system for 3D reconstruction. In *Conferencia Catalana d'Inteligència Artificial - CCIA'2002*, 322-335, 2002.
7. J.M. Lavest, M. Viala and M. Dhome. Do we really need an accurate calibration pattern to achieve a reliable camera calibration. In *European Conference on Computer Vision - ECCV'98, Freiburg, Germany* ,Vol 1, 158-174, 1998.

2D/3D Deformable Registration Using a Hybrid Atlas

Thomas S.Y. Tang and Randy E. Ellis

School of Computing, Queen's University, Kingston, Canada K7L 3N6
{ttang, ellis}@cs.queensu.ca

Abstract. Statistical atlases built by point distribution models (PDMs) using a novel hybrid 3D shape model were used for surface reconstruction. The hybrid shape model removes the need for global scaling in aligning training examples and instance generation, thereby allowing the PDM to capture a wider range of variations. The atlases can be used to reconstruct, or deformably register, the surface model of an object from just two to four 2D x-ray projections of the object. The methods was tested using proximal and distal femurs. Results of simulated projections and fluoroscopic images of cadaver knees show that the new instances can be registered with an accuracy of about 2 mm.

1 Introduction

Variations of a shape in a population can be described using a statistical shape model (SSM). The point distribution model (PDM) proposed by Cootes *et al.* has been shown to be very successful in applications modeling anatomical objects.

In this paper, we propose a hybrid 3D shape model which can be used in a PDM framework. We show how to use the hybrid shape model and the resulting PDM to reconstruct the surface model of an object from a set of 2D x-ray projections using intensity-based registration techniques.

Methods for reconstructing 3D surfaces by a PDM usually use the PDM in a simple way, requiring a global scale factor to align the training examples and to correct the surface model generated by a PDM. The problem of global scaling is that, because the scaling changes the original shapes, so the PDM is actually constructed from altered shapes. The use of the hybrid shape model removes the need of global scaling, therefore the PDM can capture a wider range of variations. Nonetheless, traditional PDM still has good variability given enough training examples are used. Fleute *et al.* [4] used a PDM for the reconstruction using the segmented contours of the 2D projections. Yao [7] used a PDM with tetrahedral meshes with intensity-based registration. Benameur *et al.* [1] used an edge-based method for registering 2D projections with the surface model generated by a PDM.

2 Shape Modeling and Atlas Building

A shape model should be able to describe both global (overall) characteristics and local (detail) characteristics of a shape. The hybrid shape model used in the present work explicitly modeled both characteristics. The global characteristics were described by a set

J. Duncan and G. Gerig (Eds.): MICCAI 2005, LNCS 3750, pp. 223–230, 2005.

of connecting inscribed spheres – *in-spheres* – contained within the bounding surface of the shape. The local characteristics were described by parameterizing a surface with respect to each in-sphere.

2.1 Global Model

The global model here, as is the case for Blum's medial-axis description [2], uses in-spheres. One problem with medial-axis models, in general, is that a slight change in a shape can result in a very different set of medial axes. Instead of putting inscribed circles into a 2D shape (or in-spheres in 3D) that satisfy the medial constraints, one can instead fit in-spheres so that they take up the space inside the shape as much as possible. A crucial difference between the medial-axis description and the global model here is that spheres in the former may overlap, whereas in-spheres here serve as constraints on how subsequent in-spheres are positioned and sized. A given shape that is globally modeled by k in-spheres can be parameterized by k four-component tuples of the form $(\boldsymbol{c}_i, r_i)$, where $\boldsymbol{c}_i$ and r_i are respectively the center and radius of the ith in-sphere. Figure 1 shows the global model of a proximal and distal femur.

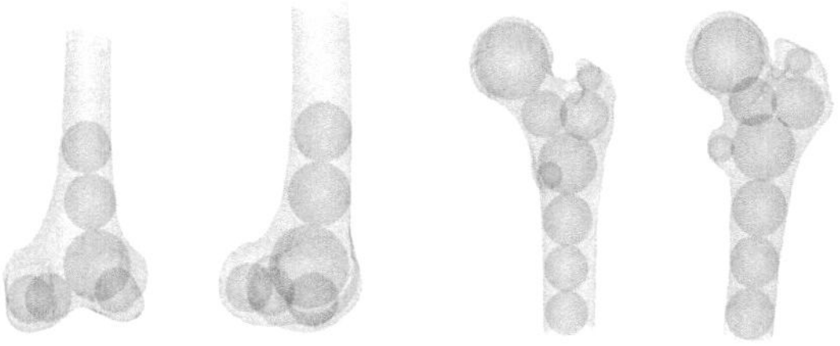

Fig. 1. Global model of the reference femur

2.2 Local Model

The local model parametrically represents the surface of a given shape around each in-sphere in the global model. In this work the parameterization was done by systematically shooting rays from the center of each sphere. Each ray had a parameter that represented the distance of the surface from the center of the sphere. Ideally the rays should be uniformly distributed on a sphere; this is only possible with the Platonic solids, but the rays would not be dense enough to capture the relevant details of the surface to be modeled. Nonetheless, approximation by a geodesic dome is sufficient. We used the octahedron and subdivided it such that it approximates a sphere with 1026 vertices and 2048 triangles. These vertices can then be used as directions of rays that emanate from the center.

Suppose that, for a given in-sphere, n rays are produced. The local model of the shape's surface is derived from the intersections of the rays with the surface. This is done in two stages; first, the length of the rays are found and then a polygon is constructed from the tips of the rays. A set $\mathcal{L}$ consisting of n distances suffice to parameterize the shape.

2.3 Merging the Global and Local Model

If a given shape is represented by k in-spheres, then it would be parameterized by k tuples of the form $(\boldsymbol{c}_i, r_i, \mathcal{L}_i)$, where $\boldsymbol{c}_i$ and r_i are the center and radius of the i-th sphere, and $\mathcal{L}_i$ is the n-dimensional set of ray lengths that describes the local shape. Each tuple can be used to reconstruct a mesh using the triangulation of the subdivided octahedron, in which the mesh describes part of the shape. The entire shape can be recovered by combining these meshes.

2.4 Building a Shape Atlas

Given a set of training examples, one of them, $\mathcal{M}_{ref}$ was selected as the reference example, and its shape parameter, $\boldsymbol{y}_{ref}$, was determined. For a new training example $\mathcal{M}_i$, an affine transformation was performed with the reference example, such that $\mathcal{M}_{ref} \approx T_{affine}(T_{rigid}(\mathcal{M}_i))$, where $T(\cdot)$ is a transformation. This affine transformation was used on the in-spheres locations of the reference example, so that they become the initial guess for the in-sphere location of the new training example. The in-sphere description is then determined in the same sequential order of the reference example. For the alignment, the only rigid part of the transformation is used. The local model of the new training example can be calculated after aligning it with the reference example, and the shape parameter $\boldsymbol{y}_i$ for $\mathcal{M}_i$ is now determined. Mathematically, $\mathcal{S}^{-1}(\boldsymbol{y}_{ref}) \approx T_{affine}(\mathcal{S}^{-1}(\boldsymbol{y}_i))$.

With the shape parameters of all the training examples known, a hybrid statistical shape atlas was generated using principal component analysis (PCA) [3]. PCA reduces the dimension of the shape parameter from thousands to $\hat{y}$, whose dimension has only a few values, such that $\hat{y} = C(\boldsymbol{y})$, and $\boldsymbol{y} \approx C^{-1}(\hat{y})$.

The hybrid shape model provides a method for parameterizing a shape, which can be denoted as functions $\mathcal{S}(\cdot)$ and $\mathcal{S}^{-1}(\cdot)$, such that for a given a shape $\mathcal{M}$ that is represented as a triangle mesh:

$$\boldsymbol{y} = [(\boldsymbol{c}_1, r_1, \mathcal{L}_1), \ldots, (\boldsymbol{c}_k, r_k, \mathcal{L}_k)]^T = \mathcal{S}(\mathcal{M}) \tag{1}$$

$$\mathcal{M}' = \mathcal{S}^{-1}(\boldsymbol{y}) \tag{2}$$

where $\mathcal{M}'$ is a retriangulated version of $\mathcal{M}$.

3 Shape Reconstruction

Given data from a surface that is not one of the training examples, the parameters can be optimized to best match the given data, such that a model for this surface is reconstructed. This process also includes registration, because the given data is under some coordinate system that is different from the coordinate system of the atlas. Therefore the reconstruction gives the shape parameter $\hat{y}$, a rotation R and translation $\boldsymbol{t}$, such that the mesh $\mathcal{S}(C^{-1}(\hat{y}))$ transformed by $T_{R,\boldsymbol{t}}(\cdot)$ is the best match to the given data.

The given data may be of various forms. The two most important forms for orthopedic applications are when the data are 3D points obtained from the surface of an anatomical object, and when the data are 2D projections of an anatomical object. As for

2D/3D rigid registration, a crucial component of reconstruction is the use of an appropriate similarity measure that can be used to compare the given data with an instance generated from the atlas. In other words, the reconstruction is essentially a minimization problem, that some error measure is minimized by using some values of $\hat{y}$ R, and $\boldsymbol{t}$. Here we address the reconstruction using a few 2D projections.

Given a set of calibrated 2D projections (i.e., the projection geometry for each projection, and the relative poses of the projections are known) the reconstruction was done in an iterative manner in two steps. First, starting with the mean shape ($\hat{y} = \mathbf{0}$) and an initial estimate of the pose, an intensity-based registration [6] was performed so that a similarity measure [5] between the digital reconstructed radiographs (DRRs) of the shape, and the given projections, was optimized. By fixing the resulting transformation, the similarity measure was further optimized using the dimension-reduced shape parameter, which was done using a non-gradient-based optimization technique. By repeating these steps, the shape of the given surface was determined. Because we focus on orthopedic application, we used gradient correlation as the similarity measure. For the optimization of the shape parameter, we used the downhill simplex method.

Note that the shape atlas only provides a surface mesh, not an image volume that is required for DRR generation. To simulate an image volume using the surface mesh, one can intersect the mesh with a set of parallel planes. The result would be a contour of the shape, represented by line segments. Guided by the local surface normals, these segments were "grown" inward to simulate the thickness of the cortical bone in a real CT slice.

4 Experiments

The shape model was tested using 20 dry human femurs. CT scans were acquired for each femur, using an (x, y) pixel size varying from 0.50 to 0.65 mm and a slice thickness of 1.25 mm. The resolution of the CT volumes was 512×512, comprised from 380 to 400 slices. Left femurs were mirrored to produce only right-femur shapes. The surface meshes were computed from the CT volumes. The proximal and the distal femurs were treated separately.

In building and testing the atlas a leave-one-out approach was used, i.e., 19 femurs were used for training the atlas and the remaining one was used for testing the atlas. The dimensions of the shape parameters were about 6620 and 5180 for the proximal and distal femur; after performing PCA they were reduced to 9 and 7, with a cumulative variance of $85.9 \pm 0.4\%$, and $86.1 \pm 0.5\%$, respectively.

RMS error was used for quantifying the error in the reconstruction of a surface $\mathcal{M}$, which can be defined as the sum of the distances between all the mesh vertices of $\mathcal{M}$, and the reconstructed shape:

$$RMS\ Error(\hat{y}, R, \boldsymbol{t}) = \sqrt{\sum_{\boldsymbol{m} \in \mathcal{M}} \|\boldsymbol{m} - closest(\boldsymbol{m}, T_{R,\boldsymbol{t}}(\mathcal{S}(C^{-1}(\hat{y})))\|^2 / |\mathcal{M}|} \quad (3)$$

where $|\mathcal{M}|$ is the number of mesh vertices in $\mathcal{M}$. Note that a rigid transformation has already been performed for $\mathcal{M}$ in the simulation, so the RMS error contains not only the error in the shape, but also the error in the registration.

Retrospective analyses show that the atlases were capable of describing the left-out femurs with mean RMS error±SD for the proximal and distal femur was 0.84 ± 0.17 mm and 0.70 ± 0.15 mm from 3D surface data.

4.1 Reconstruction from 2D Projections

Both simulated and cadaver data were used for testing.

For simulated data, reconstruction was done with two, three, and four images using all proximal and distal femurs. The view angle difference was approximately 15°, 60°, and 90° for reconstruction with two images, 15°, 30°, and 45° with three and four images. 2D projection images of the left-out femurs were simulated by DRRs with a resolution of 512×512. The mean initial pose error was normally distributed with zero mean and SD of 5° and 10 mm. Each set was done with and without calibration error. The calibration error included the error in finding the x-ray source location of the fluoroscope (in-plane SD = 0.25 mm, out-of-plane SD = 0.9 mm), and the relative orientation between projections (SD = 0.5°, 0.2 mm).

Two human cadaver knees with soft tissues intact were used in this study. The distal femurs were implanted with seven fiducial markers, such that they could be used to provide ground truth for the pose of the femur from the fluoroscopic images (OEC 9800, General Electric, USA). The knees were flexed in nine or ten positions, with three images of about 45° view angle difference for each position. CT scans with the same resolution of the dry bones were performed to determine the 3D models of the femurs, and the locations of the fiducial markers.

Table 1. Simulation of reconstruction using 2D projections for the proximal femur. All errors are in mm. Note that the histograms contain cases that were failed.

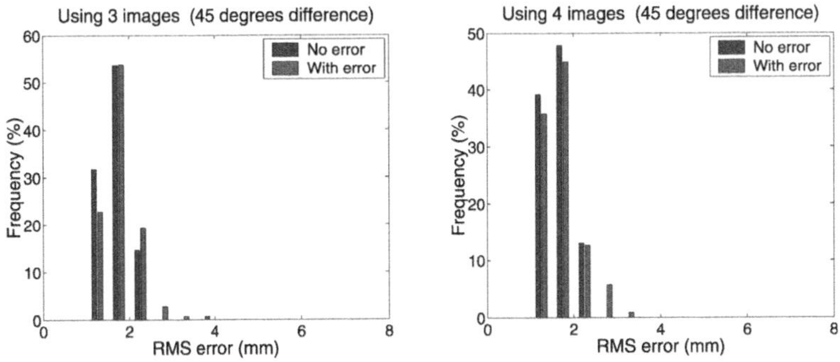

Proximal Femur	No Error			With Error			Number of cases
	Mean	SD	Failure	Mean	SD	Failure	
2 images (all)	1.80	0.45	0.9%	2.03	0.54	2.9%	490
3 images (all)	1.70	0.34	0.0%	1.89	0.45	0.5%	432
4 images (all)	1.66	0.34	0.0%	1.76	0.45	0.0%	512
2 images, 90°	1.73	0.37	0.0%	1.80	0.39	0.0%	152
3 images, 45°	1.66	0.32	0.0%	1.79	0.38	0.0%	145
4 images, 45°	1.61	0.34	0.0%	1.69	0.43	0.0%	229

Table 2. Simulation of reconstruction using 2D projections for the distal femur. All errors are in mm. Note that the histograms contain cases that were failed.

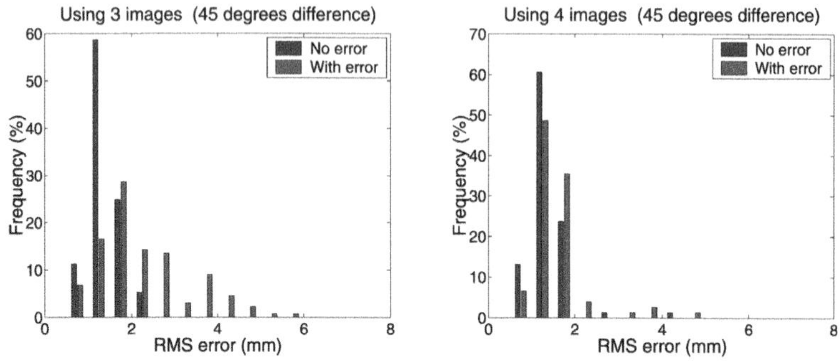

Distal Femur	No Error			With Error			Number
	Mean	SD	Failure	Mean	SD	Failure	of cases
2 images (all)	1.55	0.46	0.8%	2.34	0.82	40.4%	532
3 images (all)	1.46	0.40	0.2%	1.99	0.70	15.0%	513
4 images (all)	1.42	0.40	0.5%	1.70	0.56	5.8%	399
2 images, 90°	1.42	0.39	0.8%	2.20	0.82	44.4%	133
3 images, 45°	1.36	0.35	0.0%	2.09	0.82	8.3%	133
4 images, 45°	1.31	0.34	1.3%	1.57	0.50	1.3%	76

Table 3. Reconstruction from sets of three 2D projections of the distal femur of the two cadaver knees. Errors are in mm.

	Mean RMS Error	SD	n	Failure
Femur 1	1.95	0.55	171	6.9%
Femur 2	1.72	0.25	190	0%

The average time taken for reconstruction with two, three, and four images were 4.5, 6, and 8 minutes. Table 1 and 2 summarize the overall simulation results, and also the setting which produced the best results (4 images at 45°). A mean RMS error of over 4 mm was considered a failure. As a reference, reconstruction of a femur phantom using 60 surface points had an mean RMS error of 1.35 mm for the proximal femur, and 1.34 mm for the distal femur.

5 Discussion

The error of reconstruction using 2D images were about 2 mm, which is impressive because atlas-based reconstruction, or non-rigid registration, is a difficult problem. The use of more images significantly improved the accuracy. For both the proximal and distal femur, best results were obtained by using four images with view angles that were 45° apart. The cadaver results were better than the simulation with errors, which means that the actual calibration errors were likely not as high as we simulated.

Figures 2 and 3 show the average error for the proximal and distal femurs. In both cases, the error was extracted from a set of four test cases registered with four images at 45° apart. These particular sets were chosen as they had a relatively high error, so they better illustrate the most problematic cases. In the proximal femur, the femoral head is the most stable, with very small errors except around the fovea capitis. The greater trochanter, the lesser trochanter, and the medial/posterior side were not accurately reconstructed. In the distal femur, most error occurred around the intercondylar notch. An explanation for the higher error in these regions is that they can only be seen in one viewing angles, and for some parts like the tip of the greater trochanter and the intercondylar notch, they are hardly visible, so they could only be inferred indirectly from the atlas simultaneously with other regions.

Although the atlases were capable of generating left-out femurs with a mean error of under 1 mm, the error of the actual reconstruction was much higher. This does not imply that the deduced shape parameters are not optimal, as pose error is also included in the RMS error. Furthermore, the RMS errors reported here were only slightly higher than

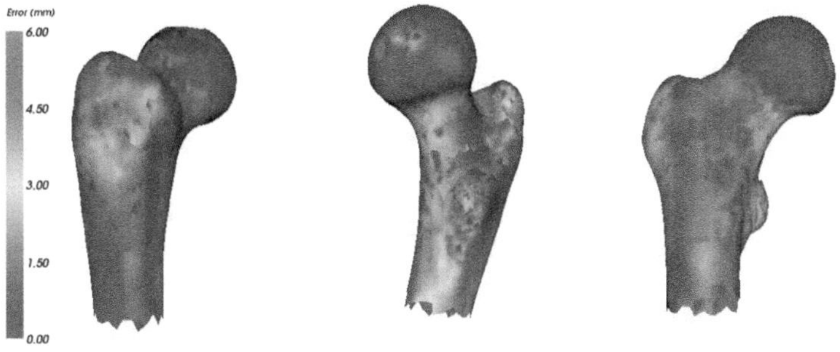

Fig. 2. Average error occurred in a proximal femur reconstructed by 2D images. The error was extracted from a set of four test cases registered with four images and 45° apart, and with calibration error.

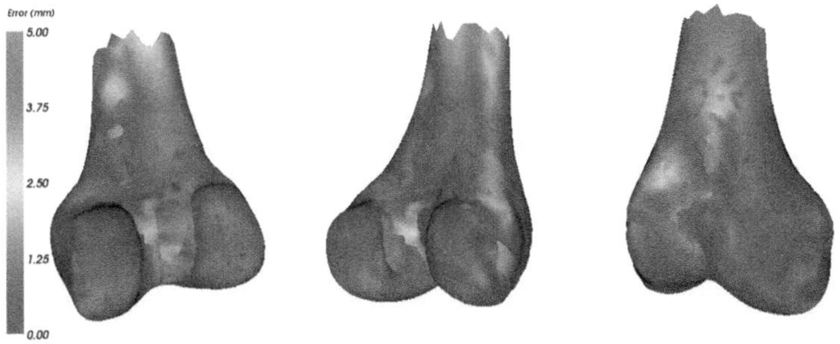

Fig. 3. Average error occurred in a distal femur reconstructed by 2D images. The error was extracted from a set of four test cases registered with four images and 45° apart, and with calibration error.

(if not comparable to) errors reported in the literature of intensity-based registration using the original CT scan.

In summary, we have shown that a PDM generated using our hybrid shape model can be used for registration using 2D x-ray projection with good accuracy, with the best results using four projections in 45° difference. The only human intervention needed in the process of the reconstruction was the specification of the initial pose estimate.

References

1. S. Benameur, M. Mignotte, S. Parent, H. Labelle, W. Skalli, and J. E. Guise. 3D/2D registration and segmentation of scoliotic vertebrae using statistical models. *Computerized Medical Imaging and Graphics*, 27(5):321–337, 2003.
2. H. Blum and R. N. Nagel. Shape description using weighted symmetric axis features. *Pattern Recognition*, 10:167–180, 1978.
3. T. F. Cootes, C. J. Taylor, D. H. Cooper, and J. Graham. Active shape models — their training and application. *Computer Vision and Image Understanding*, 61(1):38–59, 1995.
4. M. Fleute, S. Lavallée, and R. Julliard. Incorporating a statistically based shape model into a system for computer-assisted anterior cruciate ligament surgery. *Medical Image Analysis*, 3(3):209–222, 1999.
5. G. P. Penney, J. Weese, J. A. Little, P. Desmedt, D. L. G. Hill, and D. J. Hawkes. A comparision of similarity measures for use in 2-D–3-D medical image registration. *IEEE Transactions on Medical Imaging*, 17(4):586–595, 1998.
6. T. S. Y. Tang, N. J. MacIntyre, H. S. Gill, R. A. Fellows, N. A. Hill, D. R. Wilson, and R. E. Ellis. Hardware-assisted 2D/3D intensity-based registration for assessing patellar tracking. In *Medical Image Computing and Computer-Assisted Intervention - MICCAI 2004*, volume 2, pages 1095–1096, 2004.
7. J. Yao. *A Statistical Bone Density Atlas and Deformable Medical Image Registration.* PhD thesis, Johns Hopkins University, 2001.

Reconstruction-Based 3D/2D Image Registration

Dejan Tomaževič, Boštjan Likar, and Franjo Pernuš

University of Ljubljana, Faculty of Electrical Engineering,
Tržaška 25, 1000 Ljubljana, Slovenia
{dejan.tomazevic, bostjan.likar, franjo.pernus}@fe.uni-lj.si

Abstract. In this paper we present a novel 3D/2D registration method, where first, a 3D image is reconstructed from a few 2D X-ray images and next, the preoperative 3D image is brought into the best possible spatial correspondence with the reconstructed image by optimizing a similarity measure. Because the quality of the reconstructed image is generally low, we introduce a novel asymmetric mutual information similarity measure, which is able to cope with low image quality as well as with different imaging modalities. The novel 3D/2D registration method has been evaluated using standardized evaluation methodology and publicly available 3D CT, 3DRX, and MR and 2D X-ray images of two spine phantoms [1], for which gold standard registrations were known. In terms of robustness, reliability and capture range the proposed method outperformed the gradient-based method [2] and the method based on digitally reconstructed radiographs (DRRs).

1 Introduction

In image-guided therapy, preoperative three-dimensional (3D) computed tomography (CT) or magnetic resonance (MR) images and models of anatomical structures, obtained by image segmentation, serve for preoperative planning and simulation, and as "background" shown on the monitor in the treatment room onto which models of surgical instruments or of radiation beams are projected. The link between a preoperative 3D image and intraoperative physical space of the patient is established by registration of the preoperative image either directly to the patient or to intraoperative images of the patient. When two-dimensional (2D) images are acquired intraoperatively the pre- to intraoperative image registration is called 3D/2D registration. In the last decade, different 3D/2D image registration methods have been proposed. The segmentation-based 3D/2D registration methods [3-6] minimize the spatial distance between positions of corresponding geometrical features that have previously been extracted from pre- and intraoperative images. The drawback of these methods is that intraoperative segmentation errors propagate to errors in registration. Intensity-based 3D/2D registration methods [7-10] rely on image intensities or intensity gradients of pixels and voxels. The most popular intensity-based 3D/2D registration method optimizes the similarity measure calculated from overlapping CT-based digitally reconstructed radiographs (DRRs) and X-ray images [7-10]. Intensity-based 3D/2D registration methods are considered to be more accurate than segmentation-based methods but slower due to time consuming calculation of DRRs. Hybrid methods combine elements of segmentation- and intensity-based methods with the purpose to achieve

J. Duncan and G. Gerig (Eds.): MICCAI 2005, LNCS 3750, pp. 231 – 238, 2005.

the speed of segmentation-based methods and the accuracy of intensity-based methods [2, 11, 12]. From validation results provided by the authors of intensity-based and hybrid methods and from a recent comparison study of van de Kraats *et al.* [1], it is obvious that some of these methods are highly accurate when registering a CT image to two or more X-ray images. However, their capture ranges are rather small and they are not robust enough. Besides, 3D/2D registration of MR to X-ray images remains a challenging problem.

In this paper we propose a novel 3D/2D image registration method which first reconstructs a 3D image from a few 2D X-ray images and then matches this image to either a CT, MR, or 3DRX pre-operative image. The quality of a 3D image, reconstructed from a small number of 2D images will definitively be low. The similarity measure applied in such a registration should therefore be able to cope, among others, with low image quality of one image as well as with differences in imaging modalities. For this purpose we introduce a novel and powerful similarity measure, which we call asymmetric multi-feature mutual information measure. The measure is based on the multi-feature mutual information measure, recently proposed by Tomaževič at al. [13].

2 Asymmetric Multi-feature Mutual Information

Let the two images to be registered be denoted as floating image A and reference image B and represented by vector functions $\mathbf{z}_a(x)$ and $\mathbf{z}_b(x)$ of position x in image space, respectively. Each vector function $\mathbf{z}(x)$ is comprised of values of K image features, $\mathbf{z}(x)=(z_1(x),\ldots, z_K(x))$. Let, for a given spatial transformation T, SM denote the similarity measure between corresponding feature sets $\mathbf{z}_a(x)$ and $\mathbf{z}_b(T(x))$. Registration seeks the spatial transformation $\hat{T}$ that maximizes SM

$$\hat{T} = \arg\max_{T} SM(\mathbf{z}_a(x), \mathbf{z}_b(T(x))) . \tag{1}$$

Let the values of $\mathbf{z}_a(x)$ and $\mathbf{z}_b(x)$ be the observed values of vectors of random variables $\mathbf{Z}_a$ and $\mathbf{Z}_b$, respectively. In terms of entropy, multi-feature mutual information (MMI) [13], which represents a generalization of the widely used single-feature mutual information criteria [14, 15], is defined as

$$MMI(\mathbf{Z}_a, \mathbf{Z}_b) = H(\mathbf{Z}_a) + H(\mathbf{Z}_b) - H(\mathbf{Z}_a, \mathbf{Z}_b) \tag{2}$$

where $H(\mathbf{Z}_a)$, $H(\mathbf{Z}_b)$ and $H(\mathbf{Z}_a,\mathbf{Z}_b)$ are entropies of vectors of random variables $\mathbf{Z}_a=(Z_{a1},\ldots,Z_{aK})$, $\mathbf{Z}_b= (Z_{b1},\ldots,Z_{bK})$ and $(\mathbf{Z}_a,\mathbf{Z}_b)=(Z_{a1},\ldots, Z_{aK},Z_{b1},\ldots,Z_{bK})$, respectively. In general, entropy of a K-dimensional random variable $\mathbf{Z}$, $\mathbf{Z}=(Z_1,\ldots,Z_K)$ is defined as

$$H(\mathbf{Z}) = -\int p(\mathbf{z}) \log p(\mathbf{z}) d\mathbf{z} = -\int \ldots \int p(z_1,\ldots,z_K) \log p(z_1,\ldots,z_K)\, dz_1 \ldots dz_K . \tag{3}$$

In case $Z_1,\ldots,Z_K$ are discrete random variables, entropy $H(\mathbf{Z})$ is obtained as

$$H(\mathbf{Z}) = -\sum_{\mathbf{z}} p(\mathbf{z}) \log p(\mathbf{z}) = -\sum_{z_1} \ldots \sum_{z_K} p(z_1,\ldots,z_K) \log p(z_1,\ldots,z_K) . \tag{4}$$

As for single-feature mutual information, the multivariate probability distributions $p(\mathbf{z}_a)$, $p(\mathbf{z}_b)$ and $p(\mathbf{z}_a,\mathbf{z}_b)$ can be estimated from joint histograms [16]. Unfortunately, even in case of two features, the four-dimensional histogram $h(z_a,z_b)$, will probably be so sparse that a meaningful estimation of $p(\mathbf{z}_a,\mathbf{z}_b)$ will become practically impossible. For this reason, Tomaževič *et al.* [13] proposed to decompose the floating and the reference image features into a basic feature $i(x)$ and additional features $\mathbf{v}(x)$, i.e. $\mathbf{z}_a(x)=(i_a(x),\mathbf{v}_a(x))$ and $\mathbf{z}_b(x)=(i_b(x),\mathbf{v}_b(x))$. For the purpose of registering a preoperative image to a reconstructed image we propose that only one vector function, say $\mathbf{z}_a(x)$, is divided, resulting in $\mathbf{z}_a(x)=(i_a(x),\mathbf{v}_a(x))$. Using the known property of entropy [17] that

$$H(\mathbf{Z}) = H(Z_k) + H((Z_1,...,Z_{k-1},Z_{k+1},...,Z_K)|Z_k), \tag{5}$$

MMI is obtained as

$$\begin{aligned} MMI(\mathbf{Z}_a,\mathbf{Z}_b) &= H(\mathbf{Z}_a) + H(\mathbf{Z}_b) - H(\mathbf{Z}_a,\mathbf{Z}_b) = \\ &= H(I_a,\mathbf{V}_a) + H(\mathbf{Z}_b) - H(I_a,\mathbf{V}_a,\mathbf{Z}_b) = \\ &= H(I_a) + H(\mathbf{V}_a|I_a) + H(\mathbf{Z}_b) - H(I_a) - H(\mathbf{V}_a,\mathbf{Z}_b|I_a) = \\ &= H(\mathbf{Z}_b) + H(\mathbf{V}_a|I_a) - H(\mathbf{V}_a,\mathbf{Z}_b|I_a) \end{aligned} \tag{6}$$

where $H(\mathbf{Z}_b)$ is the entropy of $\mathbf{Z}_b$, and $H(\mathbf{V}_a|I_a)$ and $H(\mathbf{V}_a,\mathbf{Z}_b|I_a)$ are entropies of $\mathbf{V}_a$ and $\mathbf{V}_a\mathbf{Z}_b$ under the condition I_a, respectively. We call this similarity measure the asymmetric MMI (AMMI). Assuming that distributions of $\mathbf{Z}_b$, $\mathbf{V}_a|i_a$ and $\mathbf{V}_a\mathbf{Z}_b|i_a$ are normal, and knowing the distribution $p(i_a)$ and covariance matrices $\Sigma_{\mathbf{Z}b}$, $\Sigma_{\mathbf{V}a|ia}$ and $\Sigma_{\mathbf{V}a\mathbf{Z}b|ia}$, entropy $H(\mathbf{Z}_b)$ and conditional entropies $H(\mathbf{V}_a|I_a)$ and $H(\mathbf{V}_a,\mathbf{Z}_b|I_a)$ may be defined by

$$H(\mathbf{Y}\,|\,I) = \sum_i p(i)H(\mathbf{Y}\,|\,i), \tag{7}$$

$$H(\mathbf{Y}) = \frac{1}{2}\log\left|\Sigma_{\mathbf{y}}\right| + \frac{n}{2}\log(2\pi e) \tag{8}$$

Covariance matrices $\Sigma_{\mathbf{V}a|ia}$ and $\Sigma_{\mathbf{V}a\mathbf{Z}b|ia}$, are estimated for every feature value i_a. This approach requires much fewer samples than the estimation through high dimensional histograms. Moreover, in the case of AMMI, a one-dimensional histogram $h(i_a)$ is needed to estimate the probability distribution of the basic feature. With a one-dimensional histogram more samples become available for estimation of an individual covariance matrix. Entropies $H(\mathbf{Z}_b)$, $H(\mathbf{V}_a|I_a)$ and $H(\mathbf{V}_a,\mathbf{Z}_b|I_a)$, estimated by Eqs. 7 and 8 are monotonically increasing functions of variances of random variables $\mathbf{Z}_b$, $\mathbf{V}_a|i_a$ and $\mathbf{V}_a\mathbf{Z}_b|i_a$, respectively. The condition that random variable $\mathbf{Z}_b$, and conditional random variables $\mathbf{V}_a|i_a$ and $\mathbf{V}_a\mathbf{Z}_b|i_a$ are normally distributed will, generally, not be fulfilled in practice. Nevertheless, Eqs. 7 and 8 may be used to estimate entropies needed to calculate AMMI as long as the real, but unknown entropies are also monotonically increasing functions of variances of $\mathbf{Z}_b$, $\mathbf{V}_a|i_a$ and $\mathbf{V}_a\mathbf{Z}_b|i_a$.

3 Experiments

The proposed method has been evaluated and compared to the gradient-based method of Tomaževič at al. [2] using publicly available image data [1]. The image dataset comprised 2D fluoroscopic X-ray images and 3D 3DRX, CT and MR images of two defrosted segments of a vertebral column. The first vertebral column consisted of three thoracolumbar vertebrae bodies while the second segment comprised five thoracic vertebrae bodies. Some soft tissue was still present around both segments. The 2D fluoroscopic images were obtained with a clinical 3DRX system (Integris BV5000, Philiphs Medical System, Best, The Netherlands). A set of 100 X-ray images was acquired for each spinal segment in 8 seconds run of 180 degrees rotation around the imaged object. For each vertebral column, a 3DRX image was reconstructed from a set of 100 X-ray images using a filtered back-projection reconstruction technique [18]. The two CT-images were acquired with a clinical 16-detector-row multi-slice CT scanner (MSCT, Philips Medical System, Best, The Netherlands). The MR images were obtained with a clinical 1.5 Tesla MR scanner (Gyroscan NT, Philips Medical System, Best, The Netherlands) using a sagittal 3D turbo spin echo acquisition and turbo factor of 29, TR/TE of 1500 ms/90 ms. The MR images were corrected with the retrospective intensity inhomogeneity correction method based on information minimization [19]. The ground truth registration between 3DRX images and 2D projection images was established in the process of creating 3DRX images, while the gold-standard registration between CT and MR images with 2D fluoroscopic images was obtained by 3D/3D rigid registration of CT and MR images to corresponding 3DRX images using the mutual information maximization registration method [16]. Eight volumes of interest (VOIs), each containing a whole vertebra body and less than a quarter of neighboring vertebrae, were manually determined on 3DRX image volumes. VOIs in CT and MR images corresponding to 3DRX VOIs were defined by the gold standard registration. Examples of fluoroscopic, 3DRX, CT, and MR images of a VOI are shown in Fig. 1.

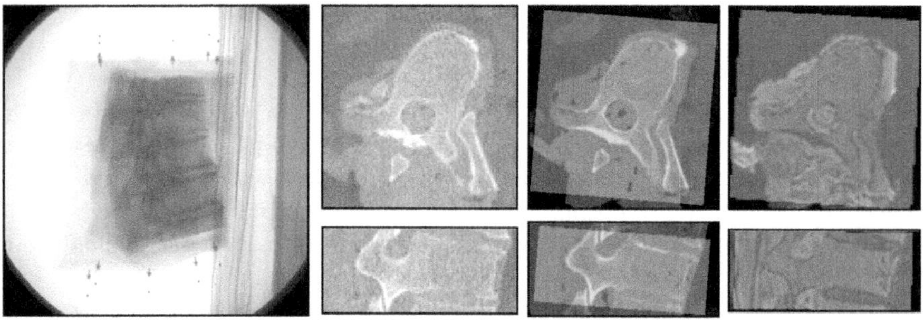

Fig. 1. Fluoroscopic (left) and transversal (top row) and lateral planes (bottom row) of corresponding VOIs taken from 3DRX (second column), CT (third column) and MR volumes (right column)

The gradient-based method was implemented as in [2]. The 2D X-ray images were blurred with a Gaussian kernel of 0.5 mm, the 3D images were isotropically resampled to 0.96 mm voxel sizes by linear interpolation, while the threshold to extract bone edges from VOIs was set to 18 for 3DRX and CT images and 15 for MR images. 3DRX and CT VOIs were registered to 3 X-ray images while MR VOIs were registered to 11 X-ray images because of the larger difference in modalities. The angle between each of the 3 (11) image views was approximately 60° (15°). For the novel method, the 3D image of a whole spinal segment was reconstructed from the same 3 and 11 X-ray images by the SART reconstruction method [20]. The sizes of reconstructed 3D images were 128x128x128 and 128x188x128 image elements for the first and second spinal segment, respectively, with isotropic spatial resolution of 0.63 mm. The preoperative 3D image was taken as the floating image A and the reconstructed image as the reference image B. Both feature sets $\mathbf{z}_a(x)$ and $\mathbf{z}_b(x)$, characterizing the preoperative and reconstructed image, respectively, consisted of image intensity $i(x)$ and image intensity gradient $\mathbf{v}(x)$ features, i.e. $\mathbf{z}_a(x)=(i_a(x),\mathbf{v}_a(x))$ and $\mathbf{z}_b(x)=(i_b(x),\mathbf{v}_b(x))$. To reduce sensitivity to image noise and non-isotropic image acquisition, the gradients of all 3D images were obtained after convolving 3D intensities with a Gaussian. Kernel scales of 0.5 mm and 0.35 mm were applied to the original 3D images and 3D reconstructed images, respectively. The AMMI similarity measure (Eq. 6) was used to measure the match between $\mathbf{z}_a(x)$ and $\mathbf{z}_b(T(x))$. Image intensity of the preoperative (floating) image $i_a(x)$ was the only feature whose probability distribution was estimated by using one-dimensional histogram $h(i_a)$ of intensity values. A histogram, having 64 bins was used to assure statistical power. Assuming normal distribution of $\mathbf{Z}_b$, $\mathbf{V}_a|i_a$ and $\mathbf{V}_a\mathbf{Z}_b|i_a$, the multivariate probability distribution $p(\mathbf{z}_b)$ was estimated through the covariance matrix $\Sigma_{\mathbf{z}b}$, while the distributions $p(\mathbf{v}_a|i_a)$ and $p(\mathbf{v}_a,\mathbf{z}_b|i_a)$ were estimated through conditional covariance matrices $\Sigma_{\mathbf{v}a|ia}$ and $\Sigma_{\mathbf{v}a\mathbf{z}b|ia}$, respectively, for every intensity value i_a. Powell's optimization method [21] was used in both methods to optimize the given similarity measure for six rigid-body transformation parameters (t_x, t_y, t_z, ω_x, ω_y, ω_z).

Both 3D/2D registration methods were evaluated using the standardized evaluation methodology of van de Kraats *et al.* [1]. The evaluation methodology uses the mean target registration error (mTRE) to measure the distance of a VOI position from the gold standard before and after registration. The positions of all image elements in a VOI were used as target points. For evaluating the capture range and robustness of a 3D/2D registration method, van de Kraats *et al.* [1] provided 200 starting positions for each VOI. The 200 starting position were randomly generated around the gold standard position in such a way that the distance from gold standard measured by mTRE was uniformly distributed in the interval of 0-20 mm. For each of 3DRX, CT or MR modalities 1600 registrations to X-ray images (reconstructed images) were thus performed, 200 per each of the 8 VOIs. Each registration was considered successful, if mTRE after registration was lower than 2 mm. The registration error was defined as mTRE of all successful registrations, while the capture range was defined as the distance from gold standard for which the registration had proved to be successful in at least 95% of all cases.

4 Results and Conclusion

The registration errors, capture ranges and percentages of successful registrations for both methods and different modalities are shown in Table1. The novel method is a little less accurate, has a somewhat larger capture range, especially for MR to X-ray registrations and is much more robust that the gradient-based method. Fig. 2 shows

Table 1. Mean TREs, capture ranges and percentage of successful registrations for the gradient-based (GBM) and reconstruction-based (RBM) methods

Modality	Views	mTRE (mm)		Capturing range (mm)		Successful registrations (%)	
		GBM	RBM	GBM	RBM	GBM	RBM
3DRX	**3**	0.19	0.33	7	9	68%	89%
CT	**3**	0.32	0.37	7	7	63%	78%
MR	**11**	0.50	0.67	2	7	23%	84%

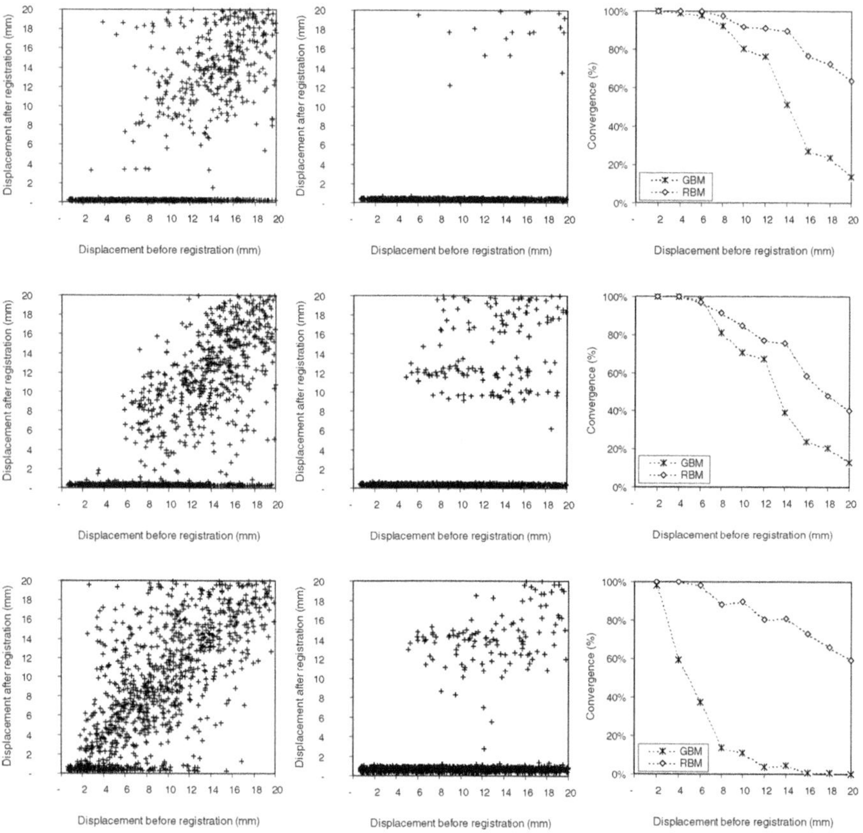

Fig. 2. Registration results of 3DRX (first row) and CT VOIs (second row) to 3 X-ray images and MR VOIs to 11 X-ray images (third rows). Scatter diagrams of displacements before and after registration for the gradient-based method (GBM) (left column) and the reconstruction based method (RBM) (middle column), and the proportions of correct registrations (right column).

the results in more detail. The results are in the form of scatter diagrams of displacements (mTRE) before and after registration and proportions of successful registrations (convergence) with respect to the initial displacement. For all modalities the proposed reconstruction-based method was successful in a significantly larger number of registrations than the gradient-based method. As expected, the proportion of successful registrations fell with the extent of initial displacement.

The proposed novel approach to 3D/2D registration based on 3D integration of 2D information is general and does not make any constraints on the modalities and anatomies involved in the registration. The experimental results show that the proposed method outperforms the gradient-based method with respect to capture range and proportion of correct registrations.

Acknowledgements

The authors would like to thank Dr. R.L.A.W. Bleys from the Anatomy department at the University Medical Center Utrecht for making the spinal segments available and E.B. van de Kraats from Image Sciences Institute, Utrecht, for acquiring and processing image data.

References

1. E. B. van de Kraats, G. P. Penney, D. Tomaževič, T. van Walsum, and W. J. Niessen, "Standardized Evaluation of 2D-3D Registration," in Lecture Notes in Computer Science, vol. 3216, *Medical Image Computing and Computer-Assisted Intervention - MICCAI 2004*, C. Barillot, D. R. Haynor, and P. Hellier, Eds., 2004, pp. 574-581.
2. D. Tomaževič, B. Likar, T. Slivnik, and F. Pernuš, "3-D/2-D registration of CT and MR to X-ray images," *IEEE Trans Med Imaging*, vol. 22, pp. 1407-16, 2003.
3. J. Feldmar, N. Ayache, and F. Betting, "3D-2D projective registration of free-form curves and surfaces," *Computer Vision and Image Understanding*, vol. 65, pp. 403-424, 1997.
4. A. Gueziec, P. Kazanzides, B. Williamson, and R. H. Taylor, "Anatomy-based registration of CT-scan and intraoperative X-ray images for guiding a surgical robot," *IEEE Trans Med Imaging*, vol. 17, pp. 715-728, 1998.
5. A. Gueziec, K. Wu, A. Kalvin, B. Williamson, P. Kazanzides, and R. Van Vorhis, "Providing visual information to validate 2-D to 3-D registration," *Med Image Anal*, vol. 4, pp. 357-74, 2000.
6. S. Lavallee and R. Szeliski, "Recovering the Position and Orientation of Free-Form Objects from Image Contours Using 3d Distance Maps," *IEEE Transactions on Pattern Analysis and Machine Intelligence*, vol. 17, pp. 378-390, 1995.
7. L. Lemieux, R. Jagoe, D. R. Fish, N. D. Kitchen, and D. G. Thomas, "A patient-to-computed-tomography image registration method based on digitally reconstructed radiographs," *Med Phys*, vol. 21, pp. 1749-60, 1994.
8. G. P. Penney, J. Weese, J. A. Little, P. Desmedt, D. L. Hill, and D. J. Hawkes, "A comparison of similarity measures for use in 2-D-3-D medical image registration," *IEEE Trans Med Imaging*, vol. 17, pp. 586-595, 1998.
9. J. H. Hipwell, G. P. Penney, R. A. McLaughlin, K. Rhode, P. Summers, T. C. Cox, J. V. Byrne, J. A. Noble, and D. J. Hawkes, "Intensity-based 2-D-3-D registration of cerebral angiograms," *IEEE Trans Med Imaging*, vol. 22, pp. 1417-26, 2003.

10. J. Weese, G. P. Penney, P. Desmedt, T. M. Buzug, D. L. Hill, and D. J. Hawkes, "Voxel-based 2-D/3-D registration of fluoroscopy images and CT scans for image-guided surgery," *IEEE Trans Inf Technol Biomed*, vol. 1, pp. 284-93, 1997.
11. K. G. Gilhuijs, P. J. van de Ven, and M. van Herk, "Automatic three-dimensional inspection of patient setup in radiation therapy using portal images, simulator images, and computed tomography data," *Med Phys*, vol. 23, pp. 389-99, 1996.
12. H. Livyatan, Z. Yaniv, and L. Joskowicz, "Gradient-based 2-D/3-D rigid registration of fluoroscopic X-ray to CT," *IEEE Trans Med Imaging*, vol. 22, pp. 1395-406, 2003.
13. D. Tomaževič, B. Likar, and F. Pernuš, "Multi-feature mutual information," in *Medical Imaging: Image Processing*, vol. 5370, J. M. Fitzpatrick and M. Sonka, Eds. Bellingham, WA: SPIE, 2004, pp. 143-154.
14. P. Viola and W. M. Wells, 3rd, "Alignment by maximization of mutual information," in *Proc. 5th Int. Conf. Computer Vision*. Boston, MA, 1995, pp. 16-23.
15. A. Collignon, F. Maes, D. Delaere, D. Vandermeulen, P. Suetens, and G. Marchal, "Automated multi-modality image registration based on information theory," in *Information Processing in Medical Imaging*. Norwell, MA: Kluwer, 1995, pp. 263-274.
16. F. Maes, A. Collignon, D. Vandermeulen, G. Marchal, and P. Suetens, "Multimodality image registration by maximization of mutual information," *IEEE Trans Med Imaging*, vol. 16, pp. 187-98, 1997.
17. T. M. Cover and J. A. Thomas, *Elements of Information Theory*. New York, USA: John Wiley & Sons, 1991.
18. M. Grass, R. Koppe, E. Klotz, R. Proksa, M. Kuhn, H. Aerst, and J. O. d. B. Beek, "Three-dimensional reconstruction of high contrast objects using C-arm image intensifier projection data," *Computerized Medical Imaging and Graphics*, vol. 23, pp. 311-321, 1999.
19. B. Likar, M. A. Viergever, and F. Pernuš, "Retrospective correction of MR intensity inhomogeneity by information minimization," *IEEE Trans Med Imaging*, vol. 20, pp. 1398-410, 2001.
20. A. H. Andersen and A. C. Kak, "Simultaneous algebraic reconstruction technique (SART): a superior implementation of the art algorithm," *Ultrason Imaging*, vol. 6, pp. 81-94, 1984.
21. W. H. Press, B. P. Flannery, S. A. Teukolosky, and W. T. Vetterling, *Numerical Recipes in C*, Second ed. Cambridge, UK: Cambridge University Press, 1992.

Comparison of Simultaneous and Sequential Two-View Registration for 3D/2D Registration of Vascular Images

Chetna Pathak[1], Mark Van Horn[1], Susan Weeks[2], and Elizabeth Bullitt[1]

[1] Department of Surgery, University of North Carolina, Chapel Hill, NC
http://casilab.med.unc.edu/
[2] Department of Radiology, University of North Carolina, Chapel Hill, NC
{cpathak, mark_vanhorn, sue_weeks, bullitt}@med.unc.edu

Abstract. Accurate 3D/2D vessel registration is complicated by issues of image quality, occlusion, and other problems. This study performs a quantitative comparison of 3D/2D vessel registration in which vessels segmented from preoperative CT or MR are registered with biplane x-ray angiograms by either a) simultaneous two-view registration with advance calculation of the relative pose of the two views, or b) sequential registration with each view. We conclude on the basis of phantom studies that, even in the absence of image errors, simultaneous two-view registration is more accurate than sequential registration. In more complex settings, including clinical conditions, the relative accuracy of simultaneous two-view registration is even greater.

1 Introduction

The objective of 3D/2D registration is to align spatial data to projective data. Given a 3D model and its 2D projection, 3D/2D registration determines the pose (orientation and position) of the model at which its 2D image was taken. This paper discusses the registration of 3D vessels, segmented preoperatively from computed tomographic (CT) or magnetic resonance (MR) images, to biplane, x-ray angiograms.

The driving clinical problem is the Transjugular Intrahepatic Portosystemic Shunt (TIPS) procedure, which creates a channel between the portal and hepatic veins [1]. We are currently developing an image-guided system for this procedure. One of the major challenges has been achieving accurate 3D/2D registration under conditions in which the x-ray angiograms are noisy and contain severe projection overlap (Fig. 1).

Several groups have described effective methods of 3D/2D vascular registration [2,3,4,5]. The purpose of the current paper is not to evaluate a specific registration metric, but rather to compare the efficacy of simultaneous, two-view registration with sequential registration. This issue has received little attention, although one paper notes in passing that simultaneous, two-view registration appears more effective than single-view registration [6]. However, no quantitative assessment or detailed analysis was provided.

This study uses phantom and clinical data to evaluate accuracy in registering a presegmented, 3D vessel model to biplane fluoroscopic images under two conditions. In the first, the relationship between cameras capturing the two views is determined in advance and the 3D model is registered simultaneously to the two views. In the second, the 3D model is registered sequentially and independently to each view.

J. Duncan and G. Gerig (Eds.): MICCAI 2005, LNCS 3750, pp. 239–246, 2005.

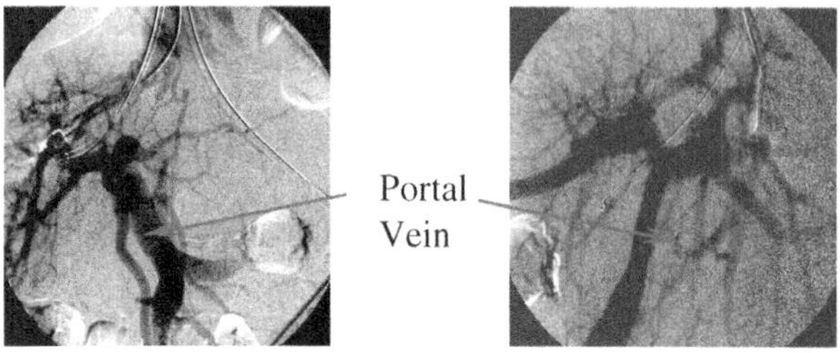

Fig. 1. Sample AP (left) and lateral (right) portograms used in the TIPS procedure. Note the thickness of the vessels and the projection overlap.

We conclude that the simultaneous approach is more accurate than the sequential approach even under ideal conditions. In the presence of image errors, the difference between the performance of the two methods increases. Although this report employs a particular registration metric [5], the findings in regard to sequential/simultaneous registration should be applicable to 3D/2D registration methods using other metrics.

2 Methods

2.1 Phantom Studies

The purpose of the phantom studies was to evaluate registration accuracy under conditions of known ground truth and varying image quality. All tests were performed in blinded fashion, with the individual performing the registration unaware of the 3D pose of the vessels until after study completion.

Simulated angiograms were created by generating projections of four different portal venous trees, each segmented from the CT or MR of a different patient, and each containing 7-15 vessels. The fields of view ranged from 9° to 16.5°, and the relative angle between the two views ranged from 80° to 90°, with arbitrary placement and rotation of the 3D model within the imaged field. Two sets of pseudoangiogram pairs were generated for each of the four vascular models, using different model poses and different combinations of camera intrinsics. For each 3D vessel point, a circle was projected upon the view-plane with radius calculated using the vessel radius and rules of projection geometry. Using a combination of buffers and summing image intensities, the generated images simulate angiograms with vessel overlap (Fig. 2).

For simultaneous registration, the operator was given the camera intrinsics and the relationship between the two views, and registration was performed on both views simultaneously, giving one set of registration matrices for each view. For sequential registration, the operator was given each view's camera intrinsics and registration was performed individually, also giving one set of registration matrices for each image. Single-view registrations are independent and the order in which they are carried out unimportant. Both AP and lateral views were registered in order to make a complete comparison with results of simultaneous registration. The initial estimate of 3D model pose was up to 16° off and up to 65 mm away from the actual position of the model.

3D/2D registration was performed using a metric that optimizes a view-plane based disparity measure based on the iterative closest point algorithm between the 3D vessel skeletons and the skeletons of the vessel projections seen on angiograms [5]. Three different phantom studies were performed:

1) Ideal case pseudoangiograms: Registrations of the 8 image pairs with their respective 3D models were evaluated under conditions of projection overlap, but without added noise and with perfect one-to-one correspondence between vessels of the 3D model and their projections on pseudoangiograms. Fig. 2 illustrates a perspective projection of the 3D model and its AP and lateral pseudoangiograms.

2) Noisy pseudoangiograms: This study was identical to the one above, but with Gaussian noise of standard deviation 2.5 added to the pseudoangiograms. The addition of noise both obscures smaller vessels and can confuse the determination of vessel skeletons (Fig. 3).

3) Noisy pseudoangiograms without one-to-one vessel correspondence: This study was identical to the two above, but with the deletion of 3-8 branches from the 3D model. This situation provides a partial simulation of the actual clinical condition, in which a noisy x-ray angiogram can show vessels that the 3D model does not. Similarly, the 3D model may contain vessels that are not visible in the angiogram.

Registration accuracy was measured by comparing the location of each point in the 3D model following registration with its known location during synthetic image

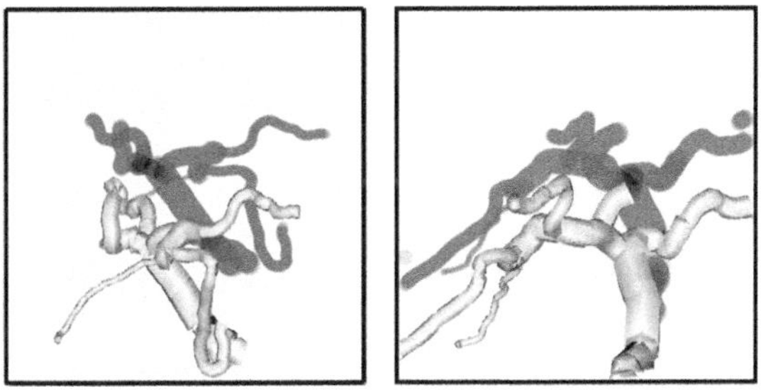

Fig. 2. An example of ideal-case simulated pseudoangiograms (gray), AP (left) and lateral (right). Also shown is a perspective projection of the 3D segmented vasculature (red).

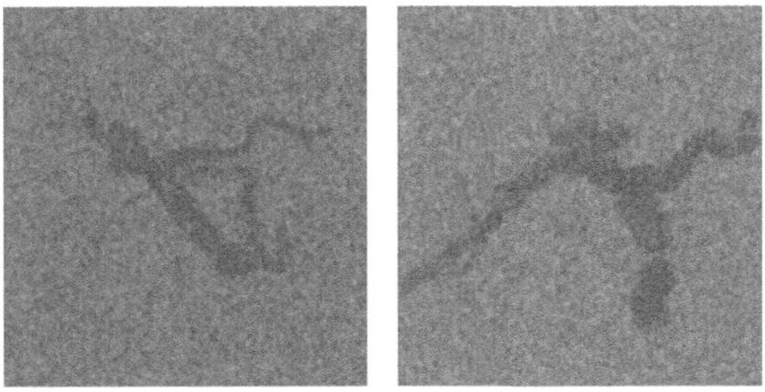

Fig. 3. Simulated angiograms with added noise. Vessels have the same pose as shown in Fig. 2

generation. Mean 3D point placement errors were calculated for each case during each study. One result was reported per case when simultaneous registration was employed, and two results were reported per case (one each for Anterior-Posterior (AP) and Lateral images) when sequential registrations were employed.

2.2 Clinical Studies

A comparison of simultaneous and sequential two-view registration was also performed on three clinical cases using AP and lateral angiographic images obtained during TIPS procedures. Preoperative images of the 3D liver vasculature were acquired by CT (a Siemens Somatom Plus system was used with collimation 0.56x0.56x2.5 mm) or MR (on a Siemens MagicVision 1.5T system with collimation 0.86x0.86x3 mm). Voxel size was variable, but around 1.5x1.5x3 mm.

Extraction of the portal venous tree from 3D image data involved 3 steps: definition of a seed point, automatic extraction of an image intensity ridge representing the vessel's central skeleton, and automatic determination of vessel radius at each skeleton point [7]. Vessels are represented as sets of 4-dimensional points with an (x,y,z) spatial position and an associated radius.

A Siemens Neurostar biplane digital angiographic unit was used to obtain x-ray angiograms as biplane views, separated by approximately 90°. The fields of view ranged from 8.7° to 16.5°. Images were captured and stored as 8-bit 884x884 pixel images. Fig. 4 shows sample clinical images.

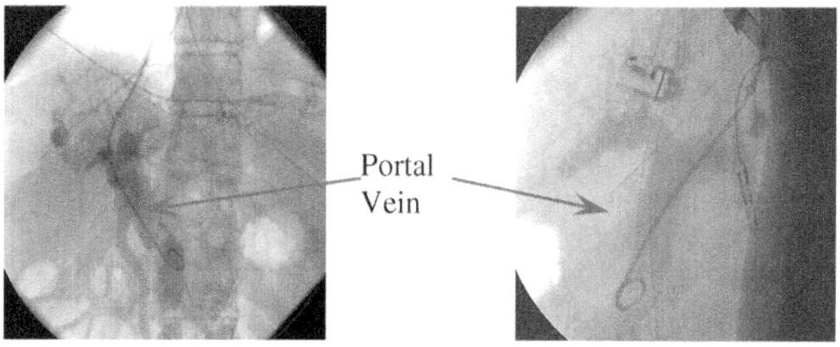

Fig. 4. AP (left) and lateral (right) abdominal angiograms obtained intra-operatively. Note the noisiness of the data and the significant projection overlap induced by wide-diameter vessels.

For patient studies, the relationship between the two fluoroscopic views was calibrated using a Plexiglas phantom containing a known arrangement of 5 mm diameter metallic spheres. The projection matrix for each view was calculated by taking an x-ray image of the phantom and minimizing the distance between observed pixel coordinates and ideal projection of each control point [8]. Intrinsic camera parameters were calculated using the same phantom.

Validation of Registration Results

The evaluation of clinical results is difficult since ground truth is unknown. Registration accuracy was estimated in these cases by reconstructing into 3D, a point that could be identified in both AP and lateral views, and comparing the location of this reconstructed 3D point to that of its corresponding point in the 3D model following registration. One subject ('Patient 1' in Table 2) had a metal clip in the liver as a result of previous surgery, and this clip was visible in the preoperative CT and on both projection views. The same subject also had 2 vessel branch-points that, with the help of an expert radiologist, could be associated on the AP and lateral projection views. Patients 2 and 3 had 3 and 2 vessel branch-points, respectively, that could similarly be associated on the AP and lateral views.

3 Results

3.1 Phantom Studies

For each test case, registration errors are presented for ideal pseudoangiograms, noisy pseudoangiograms and noisy pseudoangiograms without one-to-one vessel correspondences. For each of these pseudoangiogram pairs, accuracy is reported for simultaneous, sequential AP, and sequential lateral registrations.

Addition of noise to the image obscures small vessels and distorts vessel shape, making an accurate registration harder. The lack of one-to-one vessel correspondence is another source of error. For example, the image on the left in Fig. 5 shows a trimmed 3D model registered with the pseudoangiogram. On the right, the model has all branches present. The dark curves identify the position of previously deleted branches, thus highlighting the error.

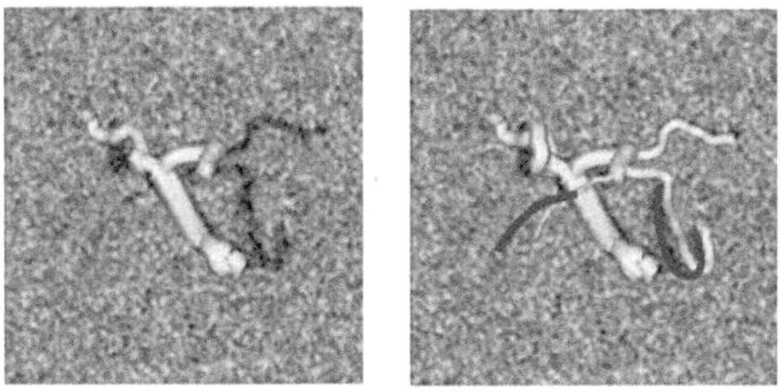

Fig. 5. Registration difficulties in presence of noise and without one-to-one correspondence

Vessel registration errors for the phantom studies, presented in Tables 1 and 2 and Fig. 6, 7 and 8, are calculated as described in section 2.1.

3.2 Clinical Studies

Table 3 contains the registration accuracy data for the clinical trials, calculated as detailed in section 2.4. For patient 1, the registration error given is the mean of the error over three points - a surgical clip and two vessel branch-points. For patients 2 and 3, the mean registration error for 3 and 2 branch-points, respectively, is presented.

Table 1. Registration errors for phantom studies for the ideal and noisy pseudoangiograms. Errors are in mm and are presented in the 'mean (maximum)' format.

Case	Ideal pseudoangiograms			Noisy pseudoangiograms		
	Sequential Registration		Simult-aneous Regn.	Sequential Registration		Simult-aneous Regn.
	AP	Lateral		AP	Lateral	
1	1.1 (2.1)	1.1 (2.1)	0.3 (0.6)	4.3 (4.8)	0.7 (1.7)	0.5 (1.9)
2	3.1 (3.9)	1.1 (2.0)	0.3 (0.6)	2.1 (3.6)	1.1 (2.0)	0.7 (1.1)
3	1.0 (2.2)	0.3 (0.5)	0.3 (0.5)	1.4 (2.0)	5.0 (5.5)	0.9 (1.2)
4	2.8 (2.9)	3.7 (4.1)	0.7 (0.9)	6.3 (6.9)	1.3 (1.4)	1.0 (1.2)
5	3.1 (5.3)	1.1 (1.5)	0.2 (0.2)	1.7 (2.2)	1.7 (2.2)	1.1 (1.6)
6	4.1 (4.2)	3.8 (5.3)	0.2 (0.2)	2.0 (4.4)	1.9 (3.8)	1.0 (2.6)
7	0.6 (1.0)	0.6 (1.0)	0.2 (0.2)	8.2 (9.2)	3.4 (4.5)	1.1 (1.4)
8	0.5 (1.0)	1.0 (1.7)	0.4 (0.6)	2.3 (3.8)	4.9 (6.1)	0.6 (0.7)

Table 2. Phantom registration errors in mm for noisy pseudoangiograms without one-to-one correspondence

Case	Noisy pseudoangiograms without 1-to-1 correspondence		
	Sequential Registration		Simultaneous Registration
	AP	Lateral	
1	1.1 (2.9)	1.9 (2.2)	0.5 (1.1)
2	3.4 (5.5)	1.1 (2.0)	1.1 (2.3)
3	1.4 (4.5)	6.8 (7.0)	1.0 (1.4)
4	5.3 (7.4)	5.0 (6.9)	1.0 (1.5)
5	7.3 (8.2)	6.0 (6.9)	1.2 (2.0)
6	3.8 (5.4)	7.7 (8.7)	1.1 (2.9)
7	8.7 (9.3)	8.0 (8.8)	0.8 (1.4)
8	1.2 (1.9)	4.2 (6.8)	0.6 (0.9)

Table 3. Registration errors in mm for clinical trials. Errors are in 'mean (maximum)' format.

Patient	Sequential Registration	Simultaneous Registrations
1	6.1 (7.2)	1.9 (2.12)
2	5.5 (9.6)	2.6 (3.7)
3	4.0 (4.8)	2.4 (2.5)

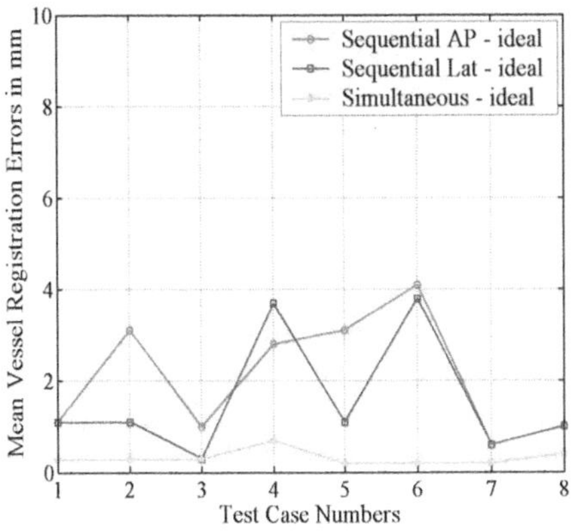

Fig. 6. Mean registration errors for the phantom studies with ideal angiograms

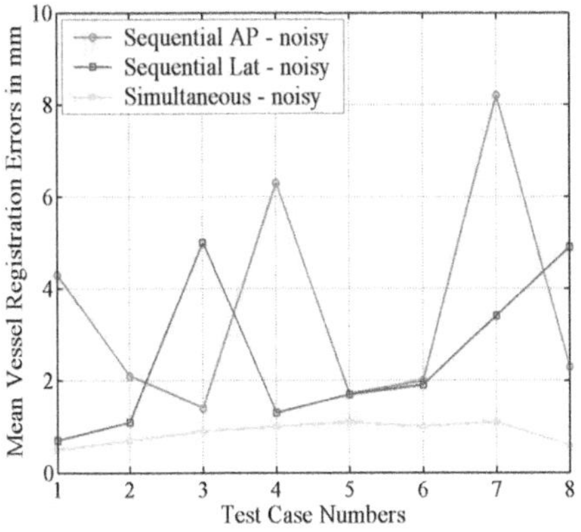

Fig. 7. Mean registration errors for the phantom studies with noisy angiograms

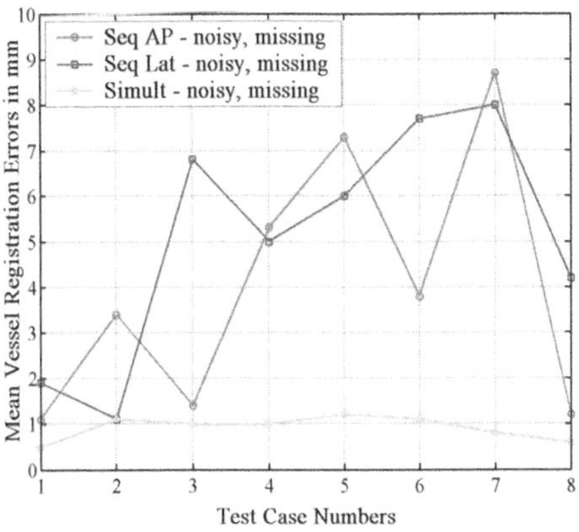

Fig. 8. Mean errors for phantom studies with noise and without one-to-one correspondence

4 Discussion and Conclusion

This paper compares the accuracy of simultaneous and sequential two-view registration in both phantom and clinical images of abnormal hepatic vasculature. The magnitude of the error we report for sequential-view registration is larger than the 1-2 mm error generally described in the literature [3,4,5]. Almost all prior studies evaluating 2D-3D vessel registration accuracy have used noiseless images, thin vessels, and one-to-one vessel correspondence, however. As shown by Figure 1, the images generated during TIPS are often of low quality and many vessels are thick - the main branch of the portal vein may be over 1 cm wide. Thick vessels increase projection overlap and complicate both centerline and branch-point definition. The difficulty of accurate 2D-3D registration is thus high in this actual clinical situation.

The current study details the behavior of the two registration methods with changes in image quality. Even under ideal conditions, one might expect simultaneous two-view registration to perform superiorly since with single-view registration, translation of an object along the depth axis produces relatively little change on projection. Simultaneous use of two orthogonal views allows each registration to correct the depth estimate of the other. Our phantom studies confirm this hypothesis, with improvement of accuracy by simultaneous registration even under ideal conditions.

The difference between the two approaches becomes more pronounced under conditions of noise and lack of one-to-one vessel correspondence – factors incorporated both in our phantom studies and in clinical data. Indeed, in two of the three clinical cases, the error in simultaneous registration was more than twice the magnitude of the error for sequential registration. This finding may result from the ability of one view to compensate for regional ambiguities in the other.

We conclude that simultaneous, two-view registration produces significantly more accurate results than sequential view registration. These findings should be applicable to a variety of 2D-3D registration metrics, and are of interest to those involved in the guidance of endovascular surgery.

Acknowledgements

This work was supported by R01 HL69808 NIH-HLB.

References

1. J.M. LaBerge, E.J. Ring, R.L. Gordon, J.R. Lake, M.M. Doherty, K.A. Somber, J.P. Roberts, N.L. Ascher, "Creation of Transjugular Intrahepatic Portosystemic Shunts with the Wallstent Endoprosthesis: Results in 100 Patients", *Radiology, 187(2):413-20, May 1993*
2. J. Feldmar, G. Malandain, N. Ayache, S. Fernández-Vidal, E. Maurincomme and Y. Trousset, "Matching 3D MR Angiography Data and 2D X-ray Angiograms", *CVRMed-MRCAS 1997, Grenoble, France, pp.129-138*
3. H.M. Chan, A.C.S. Chung, S.C.H. Yu, W.M. Wells, "2D-3D Vascular Registration between Digital Subtraction Angiographic (DSA) and Magnetic Resonance Angiographic (MRA) Images", *IEEE International Symposium on Biomedical Imaging: From Nano to Macro, April 2004*
4. Y. Kita, D. Wilson, J.A. Noble "Real-time Registration of 3D Cerebral Vessels to X-ray Angiograms" *MICCAI 1997, pp. 1125-1133*
5. A. Liu, E. Bullitt, S. Pizer "3D/2D Registration via Skeletal Near Projective Invariance in Tubular Objects", *Medical Image Computing and Computer-Assisted Intervention, LNCS 1496: 952-963, MICCAI 1998*
6. Y. Kita, D. Wilson, J.A. Noble, N. Kita "A quick 3D-2D Registration Method for a Wide-Range of Applications", *Proceedings of the International Conference on Pattern Recognition,* pp. 981-986, *ICPR 2000*
7. S. Aylward, E. Bullitt "Initialization, noise, singularities and scale in height ridge traversal for tubular object centerline extraction", *IEEE-TMI* 21:61-75, 2002
8. O. Faugeras "Three-Dimensional Computer Vision: A Geometric Viewpoint", *MIT Press 1996*

Interpolation Artefacts in Non-rigid Registration

P. Aljabar[1], J.V. Hajnal[2], R.G. Boyes[3], and D. Rueckert[1,*]

[1] Department of Computing, Imperial College London, U.K
[2] Robert Steiner MRI Unit, Imaging Sciences Department, Clinical Sciences Centre, Hammersmith Hospital Campus, Imperial College London, U.K
[3] Dementia Research Group, Institute of Neurology, University College London, U.K

Abstract. Voxel based non-rigid registration of images involves finding a similarity maximising transformation that deforms a source image to the coordinate system of a target image. In order to do this, interpolation is required to estimate the source intensity values corresponding to transformed target voxels. These interpolated source intensities are used when calculating the similarity measure being optimised. In this work, we compare the extent and nature of artefactual displacements produced by voxel based non-rigid registration techniques for different interpolators and investigate their relationship to image noise and global transformation error. A per-voxel similarity gradient is calculated and the resulting vector field is used to characterise registration artefacts for each interpolator. Finally, we show that the resulting registration artefacts can generate spurious volume changes for image pairs with no expected volume change.

1 Introduction

A common step in medical image processing is the application of voxel based registration techniques to 3D image volumes. Non-rigid registration is increasingly used to produce displacement fields that, with the emergence of deformation based morphometry [1] [6], have been used to provide data for further analysis. For example, the transformations estimated by registration can be used to generate Jacobian determinant maps in order to estimate volume changes [2] [6] [9]. Clearly, errors during non-rigid registration can lead to artefacts in the resulting transformations or in subsequent data. This implies a need to characterise the extent and nature of such artefactual displacement.

When registering images, interpolation of intensities at non-grid locations plays a part in the generation of artefacts and this has been the subject of a variety of previous studies [11] [21] [10] [7] [13] [23] [15]. It is possible, for example, to study interpolators in spectral terms in order to determine how close they are to the ideal low pass filter [11]. Generalised interpolation is described in [21]

* The authors would like to thank Dr Nick Fox and the Dementia Research Centre for their aid in this study.

J. Duncan and G. Gerig (Eds.): MICCAI 2005, LNCS 3750, pp. 247–254, 2005.

where interpolators are assessed using approximation theory and according to performance. A review of the literature on interpolator performance in various image processing tasks is given in [10] where the kernels and spectral properties are described. In the context of registration, interpolators have been been studied in a variety of ways. It is possible to assesses interpolators for artefacts by identifying local optima in the similarity metric under known misregistrations [23]. The effect of grid alignment under misregistration on joint histogram dispersion is investigated in [15] to demonstrate how optima in the similarity metric can be created (linear and partial volume interpolation). Mutual information in particular has been shown [12] to be less susceptible to false local optima using partial volume interpolation in comparison with linear and nearest neighbour interpolation during rigid registration.

Previous work on registration artefacts has, as far as we are aware, focused on rigid and affine transformations where local optima in the similarity metric are identified as a single affine parameter varies. Non-rigid registration, however, can generate small localised displacements suggesting an increased chance of artefact. An example could be a sharp contrast boundary, blurred by a linear interpolator, being sharpened by local (artefactual) contraction. In this paper we characterise interpolation artefacts in non-rigid registration. We show that the gradient of the similarity metric can be used to indicate the degree of artefacts. We have also assessed the effects of noise and global registration error in non-rigid registration. Finally, using repeat MR scans for 11 subjects, we demonstrate that non-rigid registration can generate spurious volume change where they are not expected.

2 Methods

Theoretically, registering an image pair created by sampling the same underlying continuous signal at different locations should produce no displacement. This can only occur if the constraints of the sampling theorem are met and the interpolator used has ideal spectral properties (uniformly one in pass-band and zero elsewhere). Thus, the departure of the registration from the ideal behaviour (zero displacement) can be used to measure the extent of interpolation artefacts. In most non-rigid registration algorithms the course of the registration is determined by the gradient of the similarity metric. Thus, the gradient of the similarity metric provides an alternative measure to characterise interpolation artefacts. In particular, this measure is independent of the particularities of any non-rigid registration algorithm such as the representation of the displacement field. In this paper the similarity metric investigated is the sum of squared differences (SSD).

Similarity Gradient. Many non-rigid registration algorithms rely on the minimization of a similarity measure like sums of squared differences using gradient descent techniques [4] [22] [14]. Let S and T be the images to be registered such that S is the interpolated source image and T is the target image. For a current transformation estimate f, from T to S, the SSD is calculated using a set of grid locations x_i in image T and their transformed locations $f(x_i)$ in image S.

$$SSD = \frac{1}{n}\sum_{i=1}^{n}(S(f(x_i)) - T(x_i))^2$$

where the $S(f(x_i))$ and $T(x_i)$ represent the intensities at the corresponding locations in S and T. Generally, $S(f(x_i))$ represents an interpolated intensity. The chain rule can be used to derive the SSD gradient with respect to displacements of individual voxels

$$\nabla SSD = \frac{\partial(SSD)}{\partial S}\nabla S|_{f(x_k)} = \frac{2}{n}(S(f(x_k)) - T(x_k))\nabla S|_{f(x_k)} \quad (1)$$

The estimate for the source image gradient $\nabla S|_{f(x_k)}$ is obtained using central differences from the transformed source image $S(f(x_i))$.

Interpolators. In this paper we investigated four different interpolators: Linear, piece-wise continuous cubic (PCC) spline [8,16], cardinal spline (based on a cubic B-Spline kernel) [24] and a sinc-based interpolator that was apodised using a width 12 Hanning window and was renormalised [20].

3 Results

We have used simulated and real data to assess non-rigid registration artefacts. In addition we have used data from a routine clinical study to assess non-rigid registration artefacts by estimation of global volume changes.

Simulated Data. For our simulations we used a 2D slice from the Montréal Neurological Institute (MNI) simulated MR image [5] to create a second image with sample locations offset by half a pixel in the x direction. This was done by applying a linear phase shift to the Fourier spectrum of the original image so that, as far as possible, both images have the same spectral content. Using the global transformation of a half voxel shift along the x axis and each of the interpolators, the SSD gradient field was calculated for the simulated image pair. The magnitudes of the field are shown in figure 1 as a cumulative frequency curves for each interpolator. If the cumulative frequencies for an interpolator reach high percentiles quickly, the SSD gradient magnitudes tend to be low indicating a low artefact potential. Figure 1 shows a clear order for the interpolators from best to worst as : sinc, cardinal, PCC then linear.

For comparison, the images were registered using a non-rigid registration algorithm [17]. The magnitudes of the resulting displacements are shown as cumulative frequencies in the left of figure 1. The clear separation of the interpolators is preserved and their order matches that shown by the SSD gradient. However, the cumulative frequency curves for the displacements appear smoothed relative to those for the SSD gradient, something that can be explained by the intrinsic smoothness of displacement fields represented by B-splines [17].

Separate experiments were conducted to determine the robustness of the relative ordering of the interpolators with respect to noise. The order of the interpolators remained stable until high SNR values are reached (≈ 12). Beyond

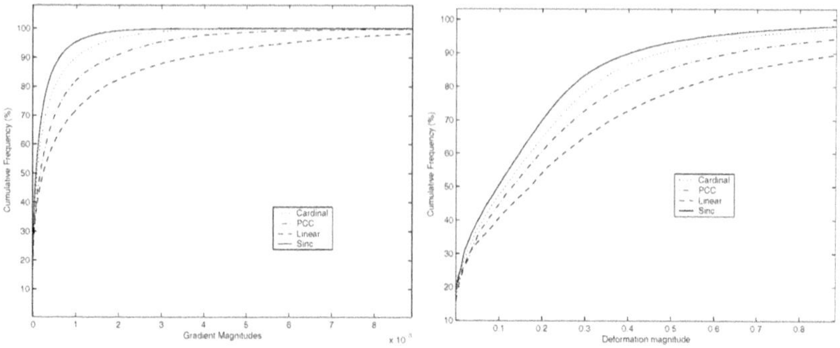

Fig. 1. Left: Cumulative frequency curves showing the distribution of magnitudes for the SSD gradient fields evaluated from the simulated MR image pair using each of the interpolators. Right: Cumulative frequency curves for the displacement fields obtained by registering the same images.

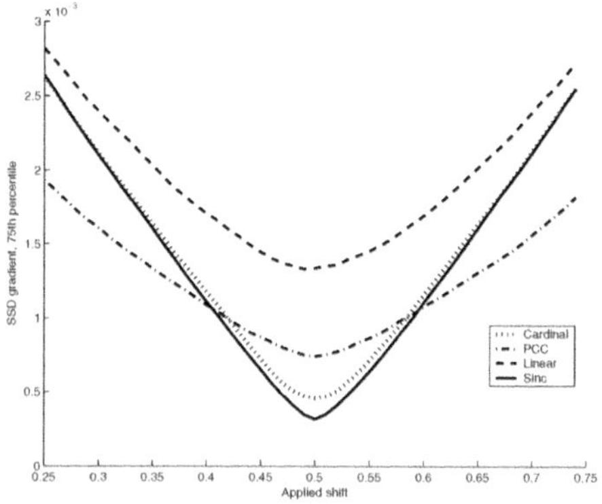

Fig. 2. A graph to show the effect of global registration error on the 75th percentile of the SSD gradient field. The horizontal axis shows the shift used as the global transformation estimate when calculating the SSD gradient. A shift of 0.5 voxels represents the 'true' transformation.

this point the linear interpolator performs best, something that can be explained by the relatively high degree of blurring it performs.

The effect of global misregistration was tested by varying the transformation estimate in equation (1). The size of the SSD gradient field, represented by its 75th percentile, is plotted against the applied shift in figure 2 where, for example, it can be seen that at an applied shift of 0.6, an error in the global transformation of a tenth of a voxel, there is little to distinguish the sinc, PCC and cardinal interpolators.

Real Data. To assess non-rigid registration artefacts in real data, two T1 weighted volumes were used that were acquired from a single subject on the same day. They were acquired on a 3T Intera system (Philips Medical Systems,

Best, The Netherlands) using an MP-RAGE sequence with an acquired resolution of $0.937 \times 1.15 \times 1.2mm^3$ reconstructed to $0.9375 \times 0.9375 \times 1.2mm^3$ voxels. A single rigid registration was carried out using a linear interpolator to obtain an estimate for the global transformation prior to calculating the SSD gradient field.

Each of the grids for the real images, after global transformation, varies in its alignment relative to the other. This contrasts with the simulated images for which the relative grid alignment is uniform at all locations. Because the differences between interpolators are clearer where the image grids are misaligned, an 'interpolation map' was created showing the distance from each globally transformed target voxel to the nearest source voxel. High values in the interpolation map indicate regions where the interpolation plays a more significant role.

The statistics of the SSD gradient were calculated where the brain region intersected the interpolation map thresholded at 75%. Figure 3 shows part of the resulting cumulative frequencies. Again, this correlates very well with the displacements generated from a non-rigid registration of the volumes (figure 3, right). The order of performance of the interpolators is well preserved. In both cases, the sinc and cardinal interpolators are however hard to distinguish, although both of these perform better than the PCC interpolator which in turn out-performs the linear interpolator.

Clinical Data. A common clinical application of non-rigid registration that could be affected by artefacts is the identification of volume differences between two sets of images. Recently, the use of transformations and their Jacobian determinants has been a useful tool in such volumetric approaches [2] [6] [9]. To test the effect of artefacts on volume change estimation a separate experiment was carried out using images from 11 subjects. All subjects were scanned twice on the same day using a 1.5T Signa Unit (GE Medical Systems, Milwaukee) with an IR-prepared spoiled GRASS sequence (TE, 6.4ms; TI, 650ms; TR 3000ms; Bandwidth 16KHz; 256x256x124 matrix; 240x240x186-mm FOV). Non-uniformity was corrected using N3 [19].

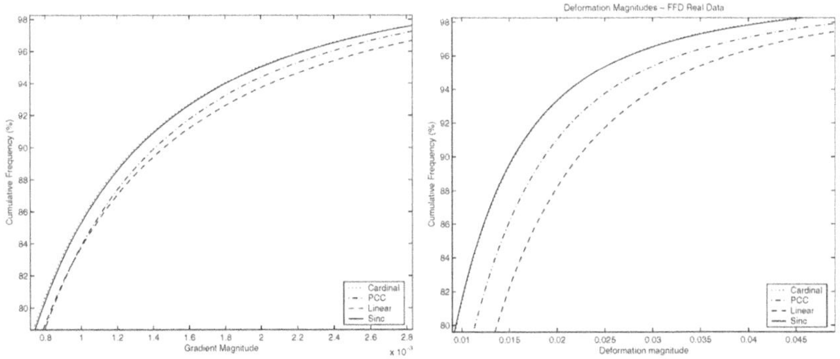

Fig. 3. Left: Cumulative frequency curves for the SSD gradient magnitudes derived using 2 acquired volumetric images. Each curve corresponding to a particular choice of interpolator. Right: The same curves for the displacement fields generated by registering the MR volumes.

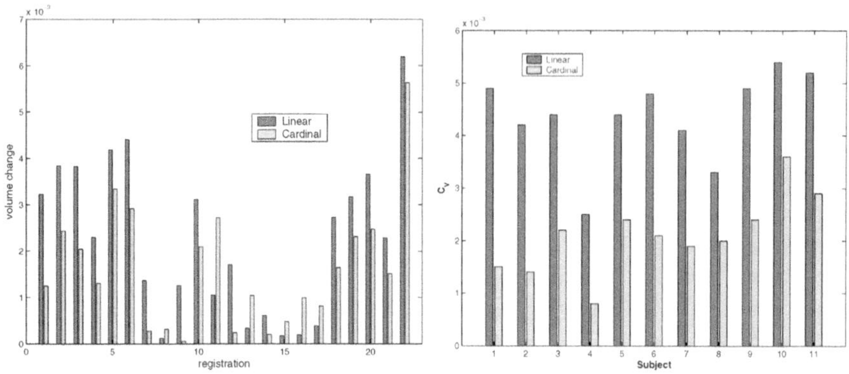

Fig. 4. Left: Volume changes generated by cardinal and linear based registrations for all 22 registrations (forward and reverse). Right: Volume consistency: Values of C_V calculated per subject for each of the linear (red) and cardinal (green) interpolators.

The departure of each registration from an expected zero volume change can be used to assess artefacts. The pairs were registered using the free-form deformation algorithm [17] in each direction producing 'forward' and 'reverse' transformations for both the linear and cardinal interpolators. The global volume change in the brain region was estimated for each transformation by integrating its Jacobian determinant (Figure 4 left). The mean volume changes were -0.22% and -0.11% for linear and cardinal interpolators respectively. A t-test showed this difference to be significant ($t = 12.5$, $p = 0.01$ gives critical value of $t = 2.5/2.8$ for 1/2 tailed tests). The volume changes were also highly correlated ($r^2 = 0.97$).

Given previous interest in registration consistency [18] [3], an estimate of volume change consistency was also calculated as a separate artefact measure. If D_{FR} represents the product of the forward and reverse volume changes then a measure of volume consistency C_V (symmetric for expansions and contractions) was defined as $C_V = |\log(D_{FR})|$. C_V should be zero for registrations that are truly volume consistent and higher values indicate increasing volume inconsistency. The values for all subjects are shown on the right of figure 4 which shows clearly better volume consistency for registrations using cardinal interpolation. Near identical results were obtained by evaluating the volume change directly from the composition of the forward and reverse transformations.

4 Discussion

In this paper we have shown how artefacts in non-rigid registration can be assessed using spectrally similar images the gradient of the similarity metric. Using SSD, the relative performance of different interpolators was assessed under 'ideal' conditions ('true' global transformation, zero noise) and under the effect of global misregistration and noise. This work has focused on interpolation artefacts in non-rigid registration while previous studies have concentrated on rigid and/or affine registration. The relative performance of the interpolators as indicated by the SSD gradient compares favourably with that indicated by the results of registration. The metric investigated here was SSD although we recognise that other metrics can be more appropriate depending on the circumstances. If intensity based measures (e.g. canonical cross correlation) are used, for example with single modality images of the same subject acquired months apart, then the method presented can be readily extended. Information theoretic measures (e.g. Mutual Information) are often used for inter-modality registrations, in this case the definition of the similarity gradient (for example whether it has an analytic or numeric representation) will depend on how the measure is implemented. Registrations using an optimisation method other than first order gradient descent would require a modified version of an artefact estimator. For example, the Hessian should be a better estimator if second order descent is used.

In general, the results suggest that, for images with a reasonable noise level and a sufficiently accurate global registration step, there appears to be benefit in using more sophisticated interpolators (e.g. cardinal) over simpler ones (e.g. linear). The noise level also needs to be quite high before before interpolators become comparable in terms of artefact whereas a reasonably small global registration error can nullify the benefit of using a sophisticated interpolator. The results based on clinical data showed a significant difference between the volume changes generated by linear and cardinal interpolators. The high correlation of their volume changes indicates the degree to which image content determines artefactual effects. If the inter or intra-subject volume differences in a study are sufficiently small then the results can be affected by the choice of interpolator with the ability to discriminate groups better served by the use of a more sophisticated interpolator. Our results suggest that the use of the cardinal over the linear interpolator could mean a potentially shorter interval between scans in a longitudinal study or the use of fewer subjects in a cross-sectional study. Our results also show that registrations are more volume consistent using a cardinal interpolator compared to a linear interpolator.

References

1. J Ashburner, C Hutton, R Frackowiak, I Johnsrude, C Price, and K Friston. Identifying global anatomical differences: Deformation-based morphometry. *Human Brain Mapping*, 6(5):348–357, December 1998.
2. JP Boardman, K Bhatia, S Counsell, J Allsop, O Kapellou, Rutherford MA, AD Edwards, JV Hajnal, and D Rueckert. An evaluation of deformation-based morphometry in the developing human brain and detection of volumetric changes associated with pre-term birth. *MICCAI*, 2878:697–704, November 2003.
3. GE Christensen and HJ Johnson. Consistent image registration. *IEEE Trans. Med. Imaging*, 20(7):568–582, 2001.
4. GE Christensen, RD Rabbit, and MI Miller. A deformable neuroanatomy textbook based on viscous fluid mechanics. *Information Sciences and Systems*, pages 211–216, March 1993.
5. C.A. Cocosco, V. Kollokian, R.K.-S. Kwan, and A.C. Evans. Brainweb: Online interface to a 3d MRI simulated brain database. *NeuroImage*, 5(4):425, May 1997.

6. C Gaser, I Nenadic, BR Buchsbaum, EA Hazlett, and MS Buchsbaum. Deformation-based morphometry and its relation to conventional volumetry of brain lateral ventricles in MRI. *Neuroimage*, 13(6):1140–5, June 2001.
7. JV Hajnal, N Saeed, EJ Soar, and et al. A registration and interpolation procedure for sub-voxel matching of serially acquired MR-images. *JCAT*, 19(2):289–296, Mar-Apr 1995.
8. RG Keys. Cubic convolution interpolation for digital image processing. *IEEE Trans. Acoustics, Speech, And Signal Processing*, 29(6):1153, December 1981.
9. M Kubicki, ME Shenton, DF Salisbury, Y Hirayasu, K Kasai, R Kikinis, FA Jolesz, and RW McCarley. Voxel-based morphometric analysis of gray matter in first episode schizophrenia. *Neuroimage*, 17(4):1711–9, December 2002.
10. TM Lehmann, C Gonner, and K Spitzer. Survey: interpolation methods in medical image processing. *IEEE Trans. Med. Imaging*, 18(11):1049–1075, November 1999.
11. E Maeland. On the comparison of interpolation methods. *IEEE Trans. Med. Imaging*, 7(3):213–217, September 1988.
12. F Maes, A Collignon, D Vandermeulen, G Marchal, and P Suetens. Multimodality image registration by maximization of mutual information. *IEEE Trans. Med. Imaging*, 16(2):187–198, April 1997.
13. JL Ostuni, AKS Santha, VS Mattay, and et al. Analysis of interpolation effects in the re-slicing of functional MR images. *JCAT*, 21(5):803–810, September 1997.
14. X Pennec, P Cachier, and N Ayache. Fast non-rigid matching by gradient descent: Study and improvements of the demons algorithm. Technical Report 3706, INRIA, June 1999.
15. JPW Pluim, JBA Maintz, and MA Viergever. Interpolation artefacts in mutual information-based image registration. *Computer Vision and Image Understanding*, 77(2):211–232, February 2000.
16. SE Reichenbach and F Geng. Two-dimensional cubic convolution. *IEEE Trans. Image Processing*, 12(8):857, August 2003.
17. D Rueckert, LI Sonoda, C Hayes, DLG Hill, MO Leach, and DJ Hawkes. Non-rigid registration using free-form deformations: Application to breast MR images. *IEEE Trans. Med. Imaging*, 18(8):712–721, August 1999.
18. Oskar M. Skrinjar and Hemant Tagare. Symmetric, transitive, geometric deformation and intensity variation invariant nonrigid image registration. *ISBI*, pages 920–923, 2004.
19. JG Sled, AP Zijdenbos, and AC Evans AC. A non-parametric method for automatic correction of intensity nonuniformity in MRI data. *IEEE Trans. Med. Imaging*, 17(1):87–97, February 1998.
20. NA Thacker, A Jackson, D Moriarty, and et al. Improved quality of re-sliced MR images using re-normalized sinc interpolation. *Journal of Magnetic Resonance Imaging*, 10(4):582–588, October 1999.
21. P Thévenaz, T Blu, and M Unser. Interpolation revisited. *IEEE Trans. Med. Imaging*, 19(7):739–758, July 2000.
22. JP Thirion. Image matching as a diffusion process: An analogy with maxwell's demons. *Medical Image Analysis*, 2(3):243–260, 1998.
23. J Tsao. Interpolation artifacts in multi-modality image registration based on maximization of mutual information. *IEEE Trans. Med. Imaging*, 22(7):854–864, July 2003.
24. M Unser. Splines : A perfect fit for signal and image processing. *IEEE Signal Processing Magazine*, pages 22–38, November 1999.

Learning Based Non-rigid Multi-modal Image Registration Using Kullback-Leibler Divergence

Christoph Guetter[1,2], Chenyang Xu[1], Frank Sauer[1], and Joachim Hornegger[2]

[1] Imaging & Visualization Department, Siemens Corporate Research, Princeton, USA
{christoph.guetter, chenyang.xu, frank.sauer}@siemens.com
[2] Institute of Computer Science, Universität Erlangen-Nürnberg, Erlangen, Germany
joachim.hornegger@informatik.uni-erlangen.de

Abstract. The need for non-rigid multi-modal registration is becoming increasingly common for many clinical applications. To date, however, existing proposed techniques remain as largely academic research effort with very few methods being validated for clinical product use. It has been suggested by Crum et al. [1] that the context-free nature of these methods is one of the main limitations and that moving towards context-specific methods by incorporating prior knowledge of the underlying registration problem is necessary to achieve registration results that are accurate and robust enough for clinical applications. In this paper, we propose a novel non-rigid multi-modal registration method using a variational formulation that incorporates a prior learned joint intensity distribution. The registration is achieved by simultaneously minimizing the Kullback-Leibler divergence between an observed and a learned joint intensity distribution and maximizing the mutual information between reference and alignment images. We have applied our proposed method on both synthetic and real images with encouraging results.

1 Introduction

Non-rigid multi-modal image registration in medical applications has become increasingly important to physicians in recent years. The fusion of complimentary image information has been shown to be particularly beneficial to physician's diagnosis. Furthermore, new imaging techniques such as molecular imaging pose a huge demand for multi-modal image registration in order to show functional, anatomical, and/or molecular image information in a single fused image.

Multi-modal image registration is a challenging problem. It has been strongly influenced by the introduction of an information theoretic similarity measure, the well-known mutual information (MI), into the medical registration domain in 1995 [2, 3]. Amongst others, MI has been applied successfully to rigid as well as non-rigid multi-modal registration of medical images. Surveys regarding this topic have also been published recently [4, 5]. Nevertheless, drawbacks of MI became apparent especially when the underlying transformation is not originated from a low dimensional parameter space, i.e. for non-parametric or non-rigid transformation models. Both the non-convexity of MI and an unconstrained transformation model make non-rigid multi-modal image registration a

J. Duncan and G. Gerig (Eds.): MICCAI 2005, LNCS 3750, pp. 255–262, 2005.

very challenging problem. Extensive research along this direction has been performed in recent years including variational formulations using advanced regularizers [6, 7], and local similarity maximization [6, 8]. Most non-rigid multi-modal registration work proposed so far focuses on methods that do not consider the underlying context of the registration such as the intensity mapping relationship of the class of images to be registered, statistics of modalities to be registered, and other prior information about the registration problem. It has been suggested by Crum et al. [1] that the context-free nature of these non-rigid registration methods is one of the main limitations for them to be clinically useful and that moving towards context-specific methods by incorporating prior knowledge of the underlying registration problem is necessary to achieve accurate and robust registration results.

In the case of rigid multi-modal image registration several approaches have been proposed to use prior information during optimization [9, 10, 11]. Leventon and Grimson were the first to use a prior learned joint intensity distribution [9], where the registration is obtained by maximizing the log likelihood of the images to be registered. Zöllei et al. showed that this method makes some implicit assumptions about the desired solution which do not always hold [12]. Chung et al. found empirically that the minimization of the Kullback-Leibler (KL) divergence between an observed and a learned joint intensity distribution is superior to maximizing the log likelihood [10, 11]. For non-rigid multi-modal image registration, however, very few work has been published so far. In [6], Hermosillo et al. proposed a supervised non-rigid registration algorithm using ML. Although KL divergence has been used in context-free non-rigid registration work [13], context-specific non-rigid multi-modal registration using KL divergence, to the best of our knowlege, has not been reported to date.

In this paper, we propose a variational formulation that incorporates prior knowledge by minimizing the KL divergence between an observed and a learned joint intensity distribution. In addition to the KL divergence term, our formulation also incorporates a regularization term that regularizes the displacement field and a term that maximizes the MI between reference and alignment images. Our work can be seen as an extension to the variational formulation work by Hermosillo et al. [6].

The outline of the paper is as follows. Section 2 describes the proposed method, the derivatives used for the optimization process, and its implementation. In Section 3, experiments on both synthetic and real images are presented to validate the proposed method. We conclude in Section 4 with a discussion and future developments.

2 Description of Method

2.1 Registration by Driving Mutual Information with Prior Knowledge

In order to non-rigidly match images from two different modalities, several strategies have been proposed in the past. Generally speaking, there are two categories of solutions available. The first approach, studied extensively in recent years, considers maximizing one or multiple similarity measures defined on both reference and alignment images such as intensity, gradient, edges, landmarks, shapes, and so on. The second approach uses prior knowledge obtained from pre-registered trained data to get a solution that is more meaningful in the clinical context. Our proposed method combines both perspectives into a unified formulation by simultaneously encouraging the observed joint intensity distribution to resemble the expected joint intensity distribution learned a priori and maximizing a similarity measure. This can be intuitively understood as guiding a context-free similarity measure by prior knowledge.

We define our combined registration framework as the minimization of the following cost functional

$$\mathcal{J}(\mathbf{u}) = \alpha\,\mathcal{I}_{\mathbf{MI}}(\mathbf{u}) + (1-\alpha)\,\mathcal{I}_{\mathbf{KL}}(\mathbf{u}) + \lambda\mathcal{R}(\mathbf{u}), \qquad \alpha \in [0,1], \lambda \in \mathbb{R}_+ \qquad (1)$$
$$\hat{\mathbf{u}} = \operatorname{argmin} \mathcal{J}(\mathbf{u}),$$

where $\mathbf{u}$ is a displacement field, $\mathcal{R}$ defines regularization or smoothing on $\mathbf{u}$, and λ is a positive constant that decides the amount of regularization. $\mathcal{I}_{\mathbf{KL}}$ measures the KL divergence between observed and learned data, and $\mathcal{I}_{\mathbf{MI}}$ denotes an expression for MI of the observed data. Here, we realize the role that prior knowledge plays. A displacement field that maximizes MI is being steered by prior information to achieve accurate alignment. The factor α controls the amount of guidance through prior knowledge. For $\alpha = 0$ the registration problem is solely based on the prior information. For $\alpha = 1$ the registration is defined as the classical optimization of MI without any prior information. For $\alpha \in (0,1)$, the maximization of MI is driven by clinical context in the form of prior knowledge captured by the minimization of the KL divergence.

This prior knowledge can be acquired in several ways and has become more accessible recently. One can use the expert knowledge of a physician who manually aligns the images or one can leverage the fused imaging data acquired using the dual-modality (PET/CT, SPECT/CT), also known as hybrid, scanners. The latter provide extensive amounts of pre-registered data, which is very important for avoiding patient specific training data. In order to increase robustness, one may learn a joint density distribution that represents a mean prior information of n pre-aligned images. But it has to be examined carefully as most scanners cannot correct the misalignment due to organ movement.

2.2 Derivative of Kullback-Leibler Divergence and Mutual Information

In the following we will refer to the two images that are to be registered by the functions $f_1 : \Omega \subset \mathbb{R}^n \mapsto \mathbb{R}$ and $f_2 : \Omega \subset \mathbb{R}^n \mapsto \mathbb{R}$. The images are registered by retrieving the underlying displacement field. Given the images, a displacement field can be modeled by a mapping $\mathbf{u} : \Omega \mapsto \Omega$. Without loss of generality, we can denote f_1 as the reference image and f_2 as the alignment image during the registration process.

We indicate by $p_1^o(f_1)$, $p_2^o(f_2)$ and $p_{\mathbf{u}}^o(f_1, f_2)$ the marginal and joint intensity distributions estimated from $f_1(\mathbf{x})$ and $f_2(\mathbf{x} + \mathbf{u}(\mathbf{x}))$ respectively. $p^\ell(f_1, f_2)$ is an estimate for the joint intensity distribution of the training data. In practice, the distributions are estimated by using a non-parametric Parzen window estimator with a Gaussian as the windowing function.

We incorporate prior knowledge by minimizing the KL divergence between observed and trained data. The KL divergence for a given displacement field $\mathbf{u}$ can be expressed as:

$$\mathcal{I}_{\mathbf{KL}}(\mathbf{u}) = \int_\Omega p_{\mathbf{u}}^o(i_1, i_2) \ln \frac{p_{\mathbf{u}}^o(i_1, i_2)}{p^\ell(i_1, i_2)} d\mathbf{x} \tag{2}$$

where $i_1 = f_1(\mathbf{x})$ and $i_2 = f_2(\mathbf{x} + \mathbf{u}(\mathbf{x}))$. The MI-based objective function is defined as the negate MI between the reference image and the alignment image transformed by $\mathbf{u}$ and can be expressed as:

$$\mathcal{I}_{\mathbf{MI}}(\mathbf{u}) = -\int_\Omega p_{\mathbf{u}}^o(i_1, i_2) \ln \frac{p_{\mathbf{u}}^o(i_1, i_2)}{p_1^o(i_1) p_2^o(i_2)} d\mathbf{x}, \tag{3}$$

We notice that MI can be viewed as the KL divergence between the observed joint density and the product of the observed marginals, whereas in $\mathcal{I}_{\mathbf{KL}}$ the product of the marginal densities is replaced by the prior knowledge learned from training data. Note that we use the negate of the MI here to define a cost.

The minimum of (1) can be found by means of variational calculus. We may descend the gradient of the combined functional with respect to the displacement field. The gradient of (1) is defined as,

$$\nabla_{\mathbf{u}} \mathcal{J} = \alpha \nabla_{\mathbf{u}} \mathcal{I}_{\mathbf{MI}} + (1 - \alpha) \nabla_{\mathbf{u}} \mathcal{I}_{\mathbf{KL}} + \lambda \nabla_{\mathbf{u}} \mathcal{R} \tag{4}$$

The gradient of MI has been derived by Hermosillo et al. in [6]. To derive the gradient of the KL divergence, we use the definition for a non-parametric Parzen density model. After some manipulation, $\nabla_{\mathbf{u}} \mathcal{I}_{\mathbf{KL}}$ can be written as follows,

$$\begin{aligned} \nabla_{\mathbf{u}} \mathcal{I}_{\mathbf{KL}} = & -\frac{1}{\mathrm{N}} \left[\left(\frac{\partial_2 p_{\mathbf{u}}^o(i_1, i_2)}{p_{\mathbf{u}}^o(i_1, i_2)} - \frac{\partial_2 p^\ell(i_1, i_2)}{p^\ell(i_1, i_2)} \right) * \mathrm{G}_\sigma \right] (f_1(\mathbf{x}), f_2(\mathbf{x} + \mathbf{u}(\mathbf{x})) \\ & \cdot \nabla f_2(\mathbf{x} + \mathbf{u}(\mathbf{x})). \end{aligned} \tag{5}$$

Here, G_σ is a two-dimensional Gaussian with standard deviation σ, ∂_2 is the partial derivative of a function with respect to its second variable, and N is a normalizing constant. We immediately notice the term $\frac{\partial_2 p_{\mathbf{u}}^o(i_1,i_2)}{p_{\mathbf{u}}^o(i_1,i_2)} - \frac{\partial_2 p^\ell(i_1,i_2)}{p^\ell(i_1,i_2)}$ as the comparison function of our registration method. This comparison function is evaluated repeatedly during the registration. In fact, alignment is achieved by continous adjustments of the joint intensity model until it resembles the learned joint intensity distribution. Furthermore, this assessment shows the central difference of our KL-based approach from the ML approach in [6], where the observed joint intensity distribution remains static.

2.3 Implementation

Variational calculus allows us to compute the minimizing displacement field by descending along the gradient $\nabla_{\mathbf{u}}\mathcal{J}$. We get the classical gradient flow:

$$\begin{aligned} \mathbf{u}_t &= -\nabla_{\mathbf{u}}\mathcal{J} \\ \mathbf{u}(\cdot,0) &= \mathbf{u}_0 \end{aligned} \tag{6}$$

with $\mathbf{u}_0$ being a suitable initial guess for the displacement field. In this paper, we use a *Tikhonov* model for regularization, i.e. $\mathcal{R}[\mathbf{u}] = \frac{1}{2}\int_\Omega |\nabla \mathbf{u}(\mathbf{x})|^2 \, d\mathbf{x}$. Its gradient expression is: $\nabla_{\mathbf{u}}\mathcal{R}[\mathbf{u}] = \mathrm{div}\left(\frac{\mathcal{R}'[\mathbf{u}]}{|\nabla \mathbf{u}|}\nabla \mathbf{u}\right) = \mathrm{div}(\nabla \mathbf{u}) = \Delta \mathbf{u}$, where Δ denotes the Laplace operator. Starting from an initial guess, we will follow a gradient descent strategy to find a solution for (1). In order to recover a larger class of deformations, to decrease computational cost, and to avoid irrelevant extrema of the non-convex functional, we pursue a coarse to fine scheme, i.e. consecutively smoothing and subsampling the images.

3 Experiments

Phantom Registration. The following phantom images were created to point out the importance of using context-specific information. Figure 1 visualizes an ambiguous setting for non-rigid registration. A circle is registered non-rigidly to another one that is of different intensity. However, its location is chosen such that there is an overlap with two other circles, a smaller and a larger circle, in a joint image. This setup suggests that there are at least two eqivalent optima for a context-free distance measure to align the circles. We compare two methods, i.e. minimizing (1) with $\alpha = 1$ and $\alpha = 0$ respectively. We train that the circle should align to the small circle. The MI method, $\alpha = 1$, finds an optimum in registering to the big circle, Figs. 1(d) and 1(e), whereas the KL approach, $\alpha = 0$, registers to the small circle, Figs. 1(f) and 1(g). Note that using the KL approach, we could also train the algorithm to align to the big circle.

T1 - T2 MRI Registration. We tested the KL method ($\alpha = 0$) on a simulated T1/T2 MRI brain data set acquired from the Brain Web Simulated Brain

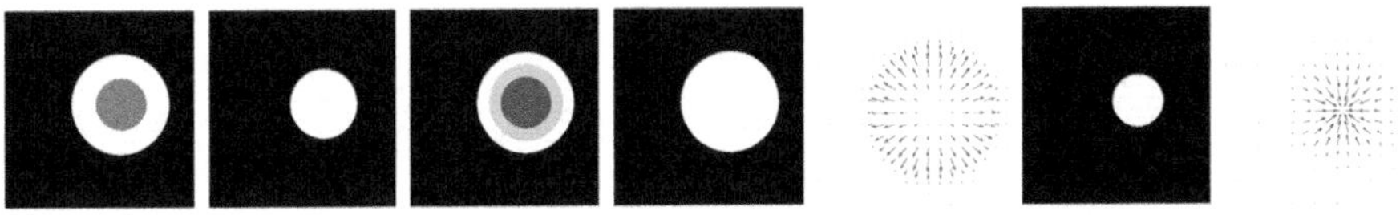

(a) (b) (c) (d) (e) (f) (g)

Fig. 1. (a) reference image (512x512), (b) alignment image, (c) difference image, (d) image (b) aligned using MI criterion only, (e) retrieved displacement field for (d), (f) image (b) aligned using prior information only, and (g) retrieved displacement field for(f)

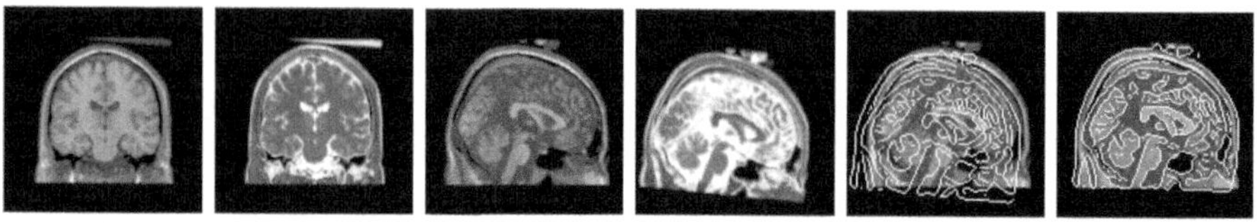

(a) (b) (c) (d) (e) (f)

Fig. 2. (a), (b) Training slices for T1-T2, (c) reference image, (d) alignment image, (e) edge map of unregistered T2 slice superimposed on T1 slice, and (f) registered result

Database [14]. The coronal slices, Fig. 2(a) and 2(b), were used for training whereas registration was performed on the sagittal slices, Fig. 2(c) and 2(d). The T2 image has been deformed by an artificially created displacement field. This experiment shows the strength of training joint intensity distributions that are used successfully for non-rigid registration.

SPECT - CT Registration. Our next experiment is performed on two corresponding slices of a SPECT/CT data set acquired by a Siemens Symbia T2 SPECT/CT hybrid scanner. We generate our prior knowledge from those two slices and deform the SPECT slice by an artificial displacement field. MI ($\alpha = 1$) and KL ($\alpha = 0$) are compared for performance and the final registration results are visualized in Fig. 3. Since we have the ground truth, we computed the difference between the warped SPECT images and the original image for visual evaluation. From the difference images we notice that although we are using a multi-resolution strategy, the MI-based approach gets trapped in an irrelavant local minimum possibly due to its insensitivity to local deformation. This experiment demonstrates the potential benefit of incorporating prior knowledge for registration in clinical applications.

PET - CT Registration. Our last experiment describes a PET/CT registration from clinical practice involving a visual evaluation by an expert. The imaging data acquired from a 70 year old male patient with multiple lesions in the lung and was acquired by a Siemens Sensation 10 (CT) and a Siemens Ecat 926 (PET). The PET was acquired 6 days after the CT. According to the

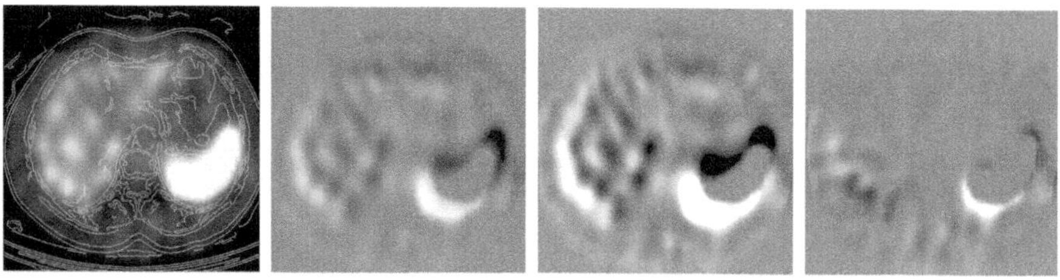

(a) (b) (c) (d)

Fig. 3. (a) Edge map of CT slice overlayed on SPECT slice as acquired from scanner, (b) deformed SPECT difference image, (c) SPECT difference image for MI based approach, (d) SPECT difference image for KL based approach

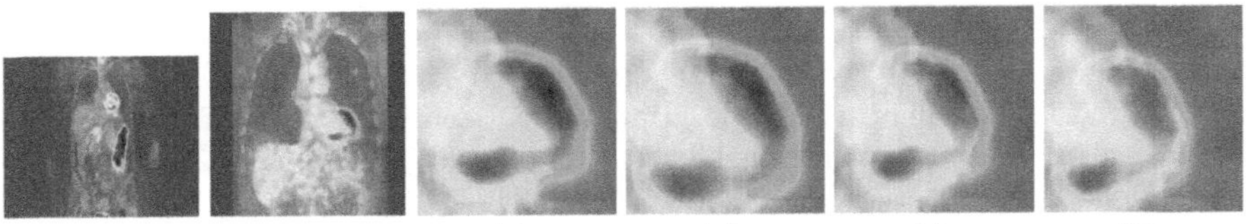

(a) (b) (c) (d) (e) (f)

Fig. 4. Blended PET/CT images showing (a) training data, (b) misaligned slices, (c) misaligned slices (zoomed), (d) pure MI registration (zoomed), (e) pure KL registration (zoomed) (e) combined result (zoomed), 40% MI and 60% KL

evaluation of an expert physician, only parts of the volume were registered accurately by a preceding manual fusion. For our experiment, we trained on two slices that have been classified as good registration and performed our approach on a misaligned slice. Figure 4 shows a collection of overlayed CT and corresponding PET images. In addition to a strong misalignment of the cardiac ventricle, an alignment deficit in the contours of the liver, the mediastinum and the thorax can be seen in Fig. 4(b). Figures 4(d) and 4(e) show the results for both the pure MI- ($\alpha = 1$) and the pure KL-based ($\alpha = 0$) registration, whereas Fig. 4(f) illustrates the registration result for our combined approach ($\alpha = 0.4$). The physician evaluated the combined approach as the most accurate one among all three registration results due to its accuracy not only in the alignment of the heart but also in the matching of the thoracic, mediastinal and hepatical (liver) outlines.

4 Discussion and Conclusion

We presented a novel approach to non-rigid multi-modal image registration by using prior information. The proposed framework allows flexible adjustment for the available quality of prior knowledge. Preliminary experiments on synthetically created phantoms and on real MRI, SPECT/CT, and PET/CT data show that prior knowledge can be crucial for retrieving the correct underlying displacement field. In addition, we have shown that our method has improved performance over a context-free registration. Future directions of research include the extension of our approach to 3D, an adaptive selection of the steering parameter α across different levels of resolution, and an investigation of a more comprehensive training data representation, which goes beyond using the mean joint intensity distribution. In order to confirm the robustness and the accuracy of this approach for multi-modal datasets, a more complete qualitative and quantitative experimental study must be carried out.

Acknowledgements. The authors would like to thank Christophe Chefd'Hotel, Lilla Zöllei, Daniel Cremers, and Klaus Kirchberg for helpful discussions. We are grateful to Gabi Wolz for her expert clinical knowledge in validating our results. The authors gratefully acknowledge the financial support by Dr. Jim Williams at Siemens Corporate Research Inc. and the Deutsche Forschungsgesellschaft (DFG) through grant SFB 603, TP C10.

References

[1] Crum, W., Griffin, L., Hill, D., Hawkes, D.: Zen and the art of medical image registration: correspondence, homology, and quality. NeuroImage **20** (2003) 1425–1437

[2] Wells, W., Viola, P., Atsumi, H., Nakajima, S., Kikinis, R.: Multi-modal volume registration by maximization of mutual information. MIA **1** (1996) 35–51

[3] Maes, F., Collignon, A., Vandermeulen, D., Marchal, G., Suetens, P.: Multimodality image registration by maximization of mutual information. IEEE TMI **16** (1997) 187–198

[4] Pluim, J.P.W., Maintz, J.B.A., Viergever, M.A.: Mutual-information-based registration of medical images: a survey. IEEE TMI **22** (2003) 986–1004

[5] Maes, F., Vandermeulen, D., Suetens, P.: Medical image registration using mutual information. In: Proceedings of the IEEE. Volume 91., IEEE (2003) 1699– 1722

[6] Hermosillo, G., Chefd'Hotel, C., Faugeras, O.: Variational methods for multimodal image matching. IJCV **50** (2002) 329–343

[7] D'Agostino, E., Modersitzki, J., Maes, F., Vandermeulen, D., Fischer, B., Suetens, P.: Free-form registration using mutual information and curvature regularization. In: WBIR. (2003) 11–20

[8] Gaens, T., Maes, F., Vandermeulen, D., Suetens, P.: Non-rigid multimodal image registration using mutual information. In: MICCAI. (1998) 1099–1106

[9] Leventon, M., Grimson, E.: Multi-modal volume registration using joint intensity distributions. In: MICCAI, Springer-Verlag (1998) 1057–1066

[10] Chung, A.C.S., Wells, W.M., Norbash, A., Grimson, W.E.L.: Multi-modal image registration by minimising Kullback-Leibler distance. In: MICCAI (2). (2002) 525–532

[11] Gan, R., Wu, J., Chung, A.C.S., Yu, S.C.H., III, W.M.W.: Multiresolution image registration based on Kullback-Leibler distance. In: MICCAI (1). (2004) 599–606

[12] Zöllei, L., Fisher, J.W., III, W.M.W.: A unified statistical and information theoretic framework for multi-modal image registration. In: IPMI. (2003) 366–377

[13] Lorenzen, P., Davis, B., Gerig, G., Bullitt, E., Joshi, S.C.: Multi-class posterior atlas formation via unbiased Kullback-Leibler template estimation. In: MICCAI (1). (2004) 95–102

[14] Collins, D., Zijdenbos, A., Kollokian, V., Sled, J., Kabani, N., Holmes, C., Evans, A.: Design and construction of a realistic digital brain phantom. IEEE TMI **17** (1998) 463–468

Deformable Registration of Brain Tumor Images Via a Statistical Model of Tumor-Induced Deformation

Ashraf Mohamed[1,2], Dinggang Shen[1,2], and Christos Davatzikos[1,2]

[1] CISST NSF Engineering Research Center,
Department of Computer Science, Johns Hopkins University
[2] Section for Biomedical Image Analysis, Department of Radiology,
University of Pennsylvania School of Medicine
{ashraf, dgshen, christos}@rad.upenn.edu

Abstract. An approach to deformable registration of three-dimensional brain tumor images to a normal brain atlas is presented. The approach involves the integration of three components: a biomechanical model of tumor mass-effect, a statistical approach to estimate the model's parameters, and a deformable image registration method. Statistical properties of the desired deformation map are first obtained through tumor mass-effect simulations on normal brain images. This map is decomposed into the sum of two components in orthogonal subspaces, one representing inter-individual differences, and the other involving tumor-induced deformation. For a new tumor case, a partial observation of the desired deformation map is obtained via deformable image registration and is decomposed into the aforementioned spaces in order to estimate the mass-effect model parameters. Using this estimate, a simulation of tumor mass-effect is performed on the atlas to generate an image that is more similar to brain tumor image, thereby facilitating the atlas registration process. Results for a real and a simulated tumor case indicate significant reduction in the registration error due to the presented approach as compared to the direct use of deformable image registration.

1 Introduction

Deformable registration of normal brain images into a common stereotactic space makes possible the construction of statistical atlases that are based on collective morphological, functional, and pathological information [1]. Similar atlases constructed from tumor patients' images can act as tools for optimal planning of therapeutic and neuro-surgical approaches that deal with tumors by statistically linking functional, and structural neuroanatomy to variables such as tumor size, location, and grade to the surgical or treatment approach and outcomes [2,3,4,5].

A major hurdle preventing the construction of such brain tumor atlases is the unsuitability of currently available deformable registration methods for adapting a tumor-bearing image to the stereotactic space of a normal neuro-anatomy atlas image. This is due to the substantial dissimilarity between the two images

J. Duncan and G. Gerig (Eds.): MICCAI 2005, LNCS 3750, pp. 263–270, 2005.

resulting from topological differences, tissue death and resorption, the confounding effects of edema and tissue infiltration, and severe deformation in the vicinity of the tumor beyond natural anatomical variability.

To account for topological differences between the atlas and the patient's images, Dawant et al. [4] proposed the introduction of a tumor "seed" in the atlas image and relied on image features to drive the registration. Bach Cuadra et al. [5] extended this idea with the use of a radially symmetric model of tumor growth. The lack of a physically realistic model of tumor-induced deformation, as well as the approximate determination of the seed location results in limited accuracy of these approaches for large tumor cases. Kyriacou et al. [2] used a biomechanical model of the deformation caused by tumors to register images of tumor patients to anatomical atlases. However, this approach was only implemented in 2D and relied on a computationally expensive regression procedure to solve the inverse problem of estimating the tumor location in the atlas.

In order to register brain tumor images to a normal anatomical brain atlas, here we present an approach that requires the integration of 3 components. The first, is a biomechanical 3D model for the soft-tissue deformation caused by the bulk tumor and peri-tumor edema. This model is implemented using the finite element (FE) method and is used to generate a number of examples of deformed brain anatomies due to tumors starting from normal brain images. The second component is a statistical model of the desired deformation map which approximates this map via the sum of two components in orthogonal subspaces with different statistical properties. For any particular tumor case that should be registered to the atlas, a partial observation of the desired deformation map is obtained via a deformable image registration method, which is the third component of the presented approach. Based on the constructed statistical model of the deformation, this partial observation is used to estimate the corresponding mass-effect model parameters that would have produced such a deformation. Finally, the desired deformation is obtained by applying the mass-effect model to the atlas image and the use of deformable image registration to match it to the subject's image. Details of the proposed approach are presented in Sect. 2.

In Sect. 3, we demonstrate our approach on real and simulated tumor cases, and we show that the registration error decreases significantly with our approach compared to the direct use of a readily available image registration method. The paper is concluded with a discussion of future work in Sect. 4.

2 Methods

The proposed approach is explained with the aid of Fig. 1. The subject's brain B_{SD} includes regions T_{SD} (bulk tumor), and possibly D_{SD} (peri-tumor edema). The main goal of the deformable registration problem is to find the homeomorphism $\chi_f : B_A \backslash T_A \rightarrow B_{SD} \backslash T_{SD}$ which maps points with coordinates $\boldsymbol{X}_A$ in the atlas image to points with coordinates $\boldsymbol{X}_{SD}$ in the subject image. Another goal is to identify T_A, which corresponds to brain tissue that is no longer present in the subject's image (died or invaded by tumor).

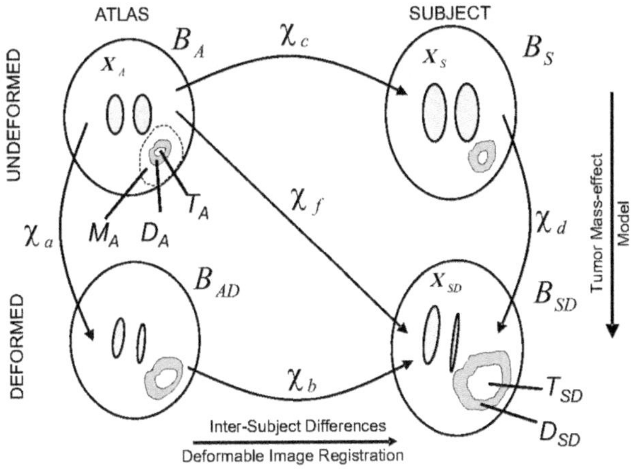

Fig. 1. Illustration of the deformation maps involved in the proposed approach. χ_f is the map from the atlas to a subject's tumor-bearing image. Regions T_{SD} and D_{SD} denote the bulk tumor and edema regions in the subject's images, and T_A, D_A are the corresponding regions in the atlas. χ_c is the mapping from the atlas to the subject's image before tumor mass-effect simulation (B_S is not known for non-simulated cases), and χ_d is that obtained through the simulation of tumor mass-effect. Simulating the tumor mass-effect on the atlas results in χ_a and a deformed atlas image which can then be registered to the deformed subject's image through χ_b.

If an accurate model of the deformation induced by the tumor is available, it can be used to simulate this deformation in the atlas and obtain χ_a, followed by the application of deformable image registration to get χ_b, and therefore $\chi_f = \chi_b \circ \chi_a$. A model of the mass-effect caused by tumor growth is described in Sect. 2.1. Estimates of region T_A as well as the other parameters affecting the model's behavior, such as the extent of peri-tumor edema and the mass-effect of the bulk tumor, are still needed in order to apply this approach. Here, we solve this inverse estimation problem by exploiting the statistical dependency between χ_f and the mass-effect model parameters. Although an approximation of χ_f obtained by the direct application of deformable image registration is incorrect in and around the tumor (region M_A in Fig. 1), the pattern of this deformation outside that region can guide the estimation of the tumor model parameters. In Sect. 2.2, we explain the collection of the statistics on $\chi_f = \chi_d \circ \chi_c$ through tumor mass-effect simulations on images of normal subjects. Estimation of the mass-effect model parameters is explained in Sect. 2.3.

2.1 Tumor Mass-Effect Model

This model is initialized with a 3D normal brain image (free of tumor) and it produces an estimate of the deformation due to the mass-effect of a simulated tumor. We explain the model by assuming that it is applied to the atlas image, although as explained later, the model may also be applied to other normal images for statistical training.

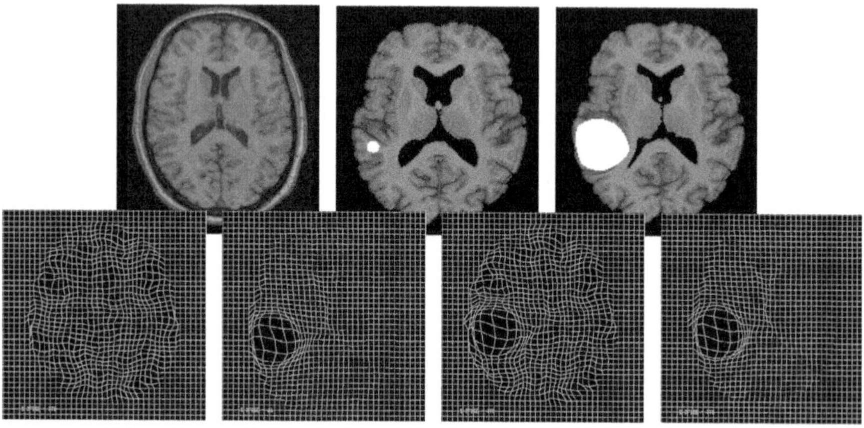

Fig. 2. Illustration of a tumor mass-effect simulation and the associated displacement maps. Upper row (left to right): atlas image, normal subject's MRI with an introduced small tumor, and resulting image after simulation of tumor mass-effect. Lower row (Left to right): displacement map $\boldsymbol{u}_c$, displacement map $\chi_d - \boldsymbol{X}_S$, displacement map $\boldsymbol{u}_f$, and displacement map $\boldsymbol{u}_d$.

With the assumption that the mass-effect is due to the bulk tumor and the peri-tumor edema only, regions T_A and D_A are defined in the undeformed (normal) atlas image. These correspond to the bulk tumor and peri-tumor edema regions in the deformed atlas at the end of the simulation. Although these regions are highly variable for different tumor cases and are not known in general, here for tractability, we assume that T_A and D_A are spherical and concentric with center $\boldsymbol{c}_t$ and radii r_t and r_d respectively. It is important to note that this does not restrict our approach to dealing with spherical tumors only since final simulated tumors need not be spherical (see Fig. 2) and also these regions are later refined through the deformable image registration component of our approach.

Brain tissue swelling due to edema is restricted to white matter in D_A and a volume expansion of 250% is used. Swelling is simulated by analogy to thermal expansion. We further assume that the expansive force of the bulk tumor may be approximated with a pressure P normal to the boundary of T_A [6]. With these assumptions, appending the necessary boundary conditions at the falx cerebri and the brain surface [7], and using the material constitutive model suggested in [8] for brain tissues, a mechanical problem is formulated and solved using the FE method. More details on this tumor mass-effect model can be found in [9]. The model parameters are collectively referred to by $\Theta \equiv (\boldsymbol{c}_t, r_t, r_d, P)$. The values of these parameters are not known for a real tumor case, but are estimated using the statistical model of the deformation explained next.

2.2 Statistical Model Training

The goal of this step is to create a statistical model for the deformation χ_f that will aid in the estimation of Θ for a particular tumor image. First, the deformation maps $\chi_{c_i}, i = 1,..,n_s$ between the atlas and MRI images of n_s normal subjects are obtained using a deformable image registration approach [10]. Simulations of the mass-effect of tumor growth are then conducted for each subject i for values $\Theta_j, j = 1,..,n_m$ covering a range of the model parameters to produce the deformations $\chi_{d_{i,j}}, i = 1,..,n_s, j = 1,..,n_m$.

A problem preventing the collection of statistics on $\chi_{d_{i,j}}$ directly is that the domains of these maps are different for different values of i and j. This precludes the point-to-point comparison of these deformation maps. To overcome this problem, for all tumor model simulations, regions T_{A_j} and D_{A_j} are defined in the atlas space based on Θ_j and mapped to each subject's space via $\chi_{c_i}, i = 1,..,n_s$. Next, for $\boldsymbol{X}_A \in B_A \backslash T_{A_j}, i = 1,..,n_s, j = 1,..,n_m$, we define

$$\boldsymbol{u}_{d_{i,j}}(\boldsymbol{X}_A) \equiv \chi_{f_{i,j}}(\boldsymbol{X}_A) - \chi_{c_i}(\boldsymbol{X}_A) = \chi_{d_{i,j}}(\chi_{c_i}(\boldsymbol{X}_A)) - \chi_{c_i}(\boldsymbol{X}_A) \quad (1)$$

$$\boldsymbol{u}_{c_i}(\boldsymbol{X}_A) \equiv \chi_{c_i}(\boldsymbol{X}_A) - \boldsymbol{X}_A \quad (2)$$

$$\boldsymbol{u}_{f_{i,j}}(\boldsymbol{X}_A) \equiv \chi_{f_{i,j}}(\boldsymbol{X}_A) - \boldsymbol{X}_A = \boldsymbol{u}_{c_i}(\boldsymbol{X}_A) + \boldsymbol{u}_{d_{i,j}}(\boldsymbol{X}_A). \quad (3)$$

For different $i = 1,..,n_s$, but the same $j = 1,..,n_m$, the domains of $\boldsymbol{u}_{d_{i,j}}$ are the same. An example of a tumor model simulation and the involved displacement maps is shown in Fig. 2.

We construct discrete versions of the displacement maps $\boldsymbol{u}_{c_i}$ and $\boldsymbol{u}_{d_{i,j}}$ by sampling their cartesian components for all voxels in the atlas in $B_A \backslash M_A$ to yield vectors $\boldsymbol{U}_{c_i}$ and $\boldsymbol{U}_{d_{i,j}}$ respectively. Assuming that $\boldsymbol{U}_{c_i}, i = 1,..,n_s$ are independent realizations of a Gaussian random vector, principal component analysis (PCA) is applied to these vectors to yield the mean $\boldsymbol{\mu}_c$ and the matrix $\mathbf{V_c}$ whose columns are eigenvectors corresponding to the first m_c principal components ($m_c \leq n_s - 1$). Next, we compute the component of $\boldsymbol{U}_{d_{i,j}}$ in the subspace orthogonal to the columns of $\mathbf{V_c}$ as

$$\boldsymbol{U}'_{d_{i,j}} = \boldsymbol{U}_{d_{i,j}} - \mathbf{V_c}\mathbf{V_c}^T \boldsymbol{U}_{d_{i,j}}. \quad (4)$$

We further assume that, for each j, $\boldsymbol{U}'_{d_{i,j}}, i = 1,..,n_s$ are independent realizations of a Gaussian random vector and we perform PCA on these vectors to yield the mean $\boldsymbol{\mu}_{d_j}$ and the matrices $\mathbf{V}_{d_j}$ whose columns are eigenvectors corresponding to the first m_{d_j} principal components ($m_{d_j} \leq n_s - 1$). Now, we can approximate the discrete displacement map $\boldsymbol{U}_f$ between the atlas and a subject with a simulated tumor with parameters $\Theta_j, j = 1,..,n_m$ as follows:

$$\boldsymbol{U}_f \approx \boldsymbol{\mu}_c + \mathbf{V}_c \boldsymbol{a} + \boldsymbol{\mu}_{d_j} + \mathbf{V}_{d_j} \boldsymbol{b}_j. \quad (5)$$

The vectors $\boldsymbol{a}$ and $\boldsymbol{b}_j$ each follows a a Gaussian distribution with decorrelated components, with that of $\boldsymbol{b}_j$ denoted by $f_j(\boldsymbol{b}_j)$.

2.3 Statistical Estimation

Given an approximate deformation map $\tilde{\chi}_f$ (between a real tumor patient's images and the atlas) obtained by the direct use of deformable image registration, the goal of the methods presented here is to obtain an estimate $\hat{\Theta}$ of the tumor model parameters. The displacement map $\tilde{\boldsymbol{u}}_f$ defined in a similar manner to eqn. 3 is also discretized over all the atlas voxels in $B_A \backslash M_A$ and represented by a vector $\tilde{\boldsymbol{U}}_f$. Owing to the orthogonality of $\mathbf{V}_{d_j}$ to $\mathbf{V}_c$ for all j, we can compute the component of this displacement that is caused by the tumor by projection as

$$\tilde{\boldsymbol{U}}_d = \tilde{\boldsymbol{U}}_f - \boldsymbol{\mu}_c - \mathbf{V}_c \tilde{\boldsymbol{a}}, \tag{6}$$

where $\tilde{\boldsymbol{a}} = \mathbf{V}_c^T(\tilde{\boldsymbol{U}}_f - \boldsymbol{\mu}_c)$. The likelihood of having $\tilde{\boldsymbol{U}}_d$ be generated with tumor model parameters Θ_j is defined as $L_j \equiv f_j(\tilde{\boldsymbol{b}}_j)$, where $\tilde{\boldsymbol{b}}_j = \mathbf{V}_{d,j}^T(\tilde{\boldsymbol{U}}_d - \boldsymbol{\mu}_{d,j})$, for $j = 1, .., n_m$. We estimate the tumor model parameters as

$$\hat{\Theta} = (\sum_{j=1}^{n_m} L_j \Theta_j)/(\sum_{j=1}^{n_m} L_j) \tag{7}$$

3 Experiments and Results

Results of applying the approach described above are reported here for two cases. The first is an MRI of patient with a glioma and a large region of peri-tumor edema. The second is a simulated tumor image obtained by applying the mass-effect model described in Sect. 2.1 to an MRI of a normal subject. All images used are T1-weighted MRI. The atlas image dimensions are 256x256x198 and a voxel size of 1x1x1mm. Other images used are of dimensions 256x256x124 and voxel size 0.9375x0.9375x1.5mm.

The FE tumor mass-effect model simulations are the most computationally intensive step of the presented approach. In order to make the statistical training step tractable, we performed tumor simulations on $n_s = 20$ MRI brain images of normal subjects. For each subject $n_m = 64$ simulations were performed with 2 values of each of the six model parameters covering the range expected for the real tumor case. The parameter values were $r_t \in \{3, 5\}mm$, $r_d \in \{20, 27\}mm$, $P \in \{2, 5\}kPa$ and corners of a cube in the atlas for the simulated tumor center locations. For the results reported here, all principal components of the displacement $\boldsymbol{U}_c$ were retained and we used $m_{d_j} = 1, j = 1, .., n_m$.

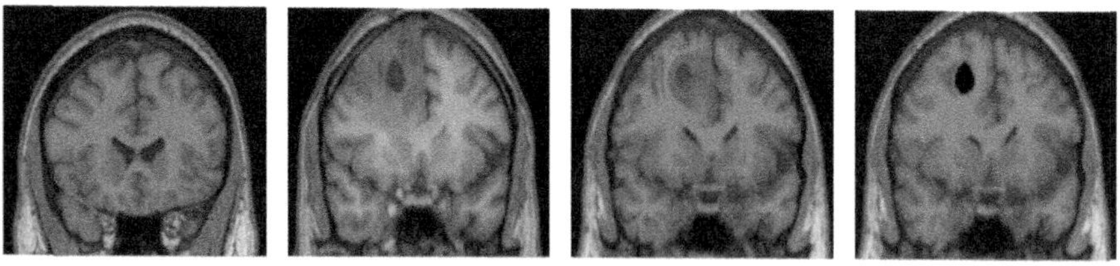

Fig. 3. Results of applying the proposed approach to register the real tumor case to the atlas. Left to right: Atlas image, subject's image, warped atlas image in the subject's space with the use of deformable registration directly between the two images, and the warped atlas image in the subject's space with the use of the proposed approach.

Table 1. Deformable registration error statistics for landmark points in the real tumor (RT) and simulated tumor (ST) cases. For each case, the errors are provided for the direct deformable image registration to the atlas (No Model), and the registration using the approach described in this paper (with Model). 21 landmark points were used for RT and 25 were used for ST.

	Minimum	Mean	Maximum	Standard Deviation
RT no Model, mm	1.06	8.70	24.87	6.19
RT with Model, mm	0.47	3.69	7.19	1.83
ST no Model, mm	2.54	6.39	10.91	2.62
ST with Model, mm	0.61	3.90	7.79	2.01

In Fig. 3, the result of applying our approach to the real tumor subject is demonstrated. With the use of deformable registration to directly register the (normal) atlas image to the subject's MRI, the warping result is innaccurate in the tumor area. Gray matter from the right cingulate region and adjacent cortical CSF in the atlas were stretched to match the intensity of the tumor and the surrounding edema in the patient's image. The estimated tumor model parameters were $\hat{\mathbf{c}}_t$=(109, 86, 126), $\hat{r}_t$=3.9mm, $\hat{r}_d$=24mm and $\hat{P}$=3.55kPa.

In order to quantitatively assess the improvement in the registration accuracy due to the proposed model, 21 landmark points were selected around the tumor area in the subject and corresponding points were identified by an expert in the atlas. The point coordinates were mapped through the resulting transformation with direct deformable registration and with our approach and the results are presented in Tab. 3. The maximum error was reduced by 71% by the use of our approach while the mean error was reduced by 57.6%.

Similar deformable registration experiments were performed for a simulated tumor case based on an MRI scan of a normal subject. The simulation parameters were $\mathbf{c}_t$=(106, 86, 128), r_t=4.5mm, r_d=21mm and P=4.5kPa. Using the approach described above, the estimated values of these parameters were $\hat{\mathbf{c}}_t$=(109, 85, 128), $\hat{r}_t$=4.1mm, $\hat{r}_d$=23mm and $\hat{P}$=3.6kPa. To evaluate the registration error in this case, 25 points were selected arbitrarily in the area around the simulated tumor, and their corresponding coordinates (found through $\chi_d \circ \chi_c$ which is available in this case) were computed in the atlas image and treated as ground truth. The errors for the direct deformable registration and that obtained by the proposed approach are also presented in Tab. 3. The maximum error was reduced by 29% using the proposed approach and the corresponding average error was reduced by 39%.

4 Discussion and Future Work

We introduced an approach for deformable registration of atlas to brain tumor images. The approach utilizes a 3D biomechanical FE model of tumor-induced deformation to introduce and simulate the tumor in the atlas followed by the use of a readily available deformable image registration approach. To solve the inverse problem of determining the model parameters, we proposed a statistical approach that relies on the decomposition of the desired deformation map into the sum of two maps defined on the same domain, but with different statistical properties that are learned via PCA from a number of training samples. These maps are modeled via two orthogonal subspaces which allows the estimation of the tumor model parameters via projection of a rough estimate of the required deformation map on the subspace representing tumor induced-deformation.

The results of applying the proposed approach on a real tumor case and a simulated one indicate significant reduction in the registration error. These experiments should be regarded as a proof-of-concept study. More validation experiments are need to asses the viability of the proposed approach for a variety of tumor cases of different grades, types and sizes. In addition, the sensitivity of the statistical estimator of the model parameters to the number of used principal components and the number of training samples also will be investigated.

Acknowledgments

The authors would like to thank Dr. Nick Fox at the University College London, UK for providing the tumor patient's images. This work was supported in part by the National Science Foundation under Engineering Research Center grant EEC9731478, and by the National Institutes of Health grant R01NS42645.

References

1. Davatzikos, C.: Spatial transformation and registration of brain images using elastically deformable models. CVIU, Spec. iss. on Medical Imaging **66** (1997) 207–222
2. Kyriacou, S.K., Davatzikos, C., Zinreich, S.J., Bryan, R.N.: Nonlinear elastic registration of brain images with tumor pathology using a biomechanical model. IEEE Trans. Med. Imag. **18** (1999) 580–592
3. Mohamed, A., Kyriacou, S.K., Davatzikos, C.: A statistical approach for estimating brain tumor induced deformation. Proc. of IEEE Workshop on MMBIA (2001) 52–59
4. Dawant, B.M., Hartmann, S.L., Pan, S., Gadamsetty, S.: Brain atlas deformation in the presence of small and large space-occupying tumors. Computer Aided Surgery **7** (2002) 1–10
5. Cuadra, M.B., Pollo, C., Bardera, A., Cuisenaire, O., Villemure, J.G., Thiran, J.P.: Atlas-based segmentation of pathological MR brains using a model of lesion growth. IEEE Trans. Med. Imag. **23** (2004) 1301–1314
6. Wasserman, R., Acharya, R.: A patient-specific in vivo tumor model. Mathematical Biosciences **136** (1996) 111–140
7. Miga, M., Paulsen, K., Kennedy, F.E., Hartov, A., Roberts, D.: Model-updated image-guided neurosurgery using the finite element method: Incorporation of the falx cerebri. In: MICCAI 1999. (1999)
8. Miller, K., Chinzei, K.: Mechanical properties of brain tissue in tension. Journal of Biomechanics **35** (2002) 483–490
9. Mohamed, A., Davatzikos, C.: Finite element modeling of brain tumor mass-effect from 3D medical images. In: Proceedings of MICCAI 2005. (2005)
10. Shen, D., Davatzikos, C.: HAMMER: Hierarchical attribute matching mechanism for elastic registration. IEEE Trans. Med. Imag. **21** (2002) 1421–1439

Myocardial Motion Estimation in Tagged MR Sequences by Using αMI-Based Non Rigid Registration

E. Oubel[1], C. Tobon-Gomez[1], A.O. Hero[2], and A.F. Frangi[1]

[1] Computational Imaging Laboratory, Pompeu Fabra University, Barcelona, Spain
{estanislao.oubel, catalina.tobon, alejandro.frangi}@upf.edu
[2] Dept. of EECS, The University of Michigan, Ann Arbor (MI), 48109-2122, USA
hero@umich.edu

Abstract. Tagged Magnetic Resonance Imaging (MRI) is currently the reference MR modality for myocardial motion and strain analysis. NMI-based non rigid registration has proven to be an accurate method to retrieve cardiac deformation fields. The use of αMI permits higher dimensional features to be implemented in myocardial deformation estimation through image registration. This paper demonstrates that this is feasible with a set of Haar wavelet features of high dimension. While we do not demonstrate performance improvement for this set of features, there is no significant degradation as compared to implementing the registration method with the traditional NMI metric. We use Entropic Spanning Graphs (ESGs) to estimate the αMI of the wavelet feature vectors WFVs since this is not possible with histograms. To the best of our knowledge, this is the first time that ESGs are used for non rigid registration.

1 Introduction

Tagged magnetic resonance imaging (MRI) is a well established technique used to obtain regional information about the deformation of the left ventricle (LV)[1,2], and thus potentially help to diagnose cardiovascular diseases. Basically, this technique consists in perturbating the magnetization of the myocardium in a specified spatial pattern at end-diastole. These perturbations appear as dark stripes or grids when imaged immediately after application of the tag pattern. Since the myocardium retains knowledge of this disturbance, the dark grids experience the same deformation the heart does as it contracts, allowing local strain parameters to be estimated.

Several methods have been proposed to retrieve LV deformation field: optical flow [3,4], Harmonic Phase (HARP) MRI [5,6], tag detection and tracking [7,8,9,10] and image registration [11,12]. The use of registration to estimate cardiac motion has proven to overcome many drawbacks existent on previous approaches.

The use of αMI permits higher dimensional features to be implemented in myocardial deformation estimation and registration problems. In this paper,

J. Duncan and G. Gerig (Eds.): MICCAI 2005, LNCS 3750, pp. 271–278, 2005.

we aim to evaluate the performance of αMI based registration methods with respect to gold standard measurements and with respect to NMI based image registration. Specifically, we use Haar wavelet coefficients at each pixel as feature vectors (FVs) and ESGs to estimate the αMI of these vectors.

This paper is organized in six sections. Section 2 explains how to estimate cardiac deformation fields by using image registration. In this section, the concept of αMI and its estimation by using ESGs is also presented. Section 3 describes the dataset used for the experiments. Results are presented in Section 4 and discussed in Section 5. Finally, the conclusions can be found in Section 6.

2 Method

The registration algorithm we used, is based on the method originally developed by Rueckert *et al.* [13] for detection of cancerous lesions in contrast enhanced MR breast images. We modified this algorithm by replacing NMI with αMI computed from Wavelet Feature Vectors (WFVs). The main problem derived from using vectors instead of intensity values, is that the curse of dimensionality forbids the use of histograms for probability density function (pdf) estimation. Therefore, in order to compute the αMI of these vectors, we used kNN graph estimators which completely bypass pdf estimation [14].

2.1 Motion Estimation

To track cardiac motion throughout multiple time frames we used Multilevel Free Form Deformations (MFFDs) as suggested by Schnabel *et al.* [15], where the transformation $\mathbf{T}(\mathbf{u}, t)$ is represented as the sum of a series of local FFDs:

$$\mathbf{T}(\mathbf{u}, t) = \sum_{p=1}^{t} \mathbf{T}_{local}^{p}(\mathbf{u}, t) \quad (1)$$

Thus, the motion estimation starts registering the first two frames of the sequence $I(\mathbf{x}, 0)$ and $I(\mathbf{x}, 1)$, and a single FFD is obtained. Then, for the next frame $I(\mathbf{x}, 2)$, a new FFD is added and the frame is registered to $I(\mathbf{x}, 0)$ taking as initial transformation the one obtained for $I(\mathbf{x}, 1)$. This process is repeated for the remaining frames $I(\mathbf{x}, t)$ in the cardiac cycle. Once all the frames are registered to the first one, the MFFD consists of N FFDs that model the myocardium deformation.

2.2 Similarity Measure

To recover the deformation field at time t, the image $I(\mathbf{x}, t)$ is registered to $I(\mathbf{x}, 0)$ by optimizing some cost function. Let I_s and I_t be random variables representing the source and target image, with pdfs $p_s(I_s)$ and $p_t(I_t)$ respectively. Let $p_{st}(I_s, I_t)$ represent the joint pdf of I_s and I_t. The α mutual information (αMI) of I_s and I_t is defined as:

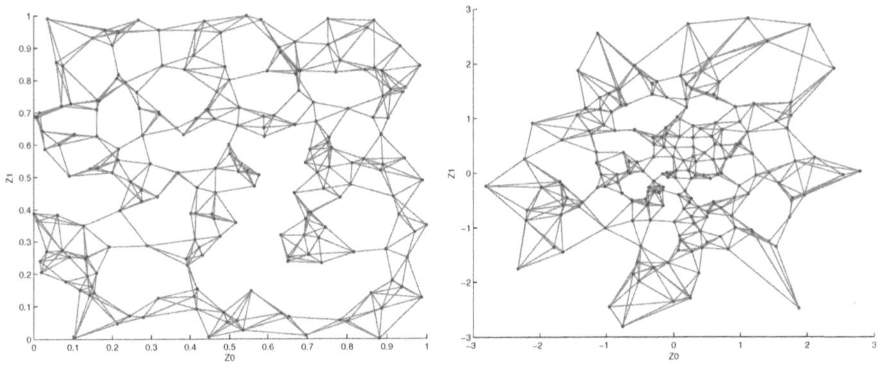

Fig. 1. kNN graphs for a set of 200 points in the plane and k=5. (a) Uniform distribution (SD=1). (b) Gaussian distribution (SD=1).

$$\alpha MI = D_\alpha(p_{st}(I_s, I_t) \parallel p_s(I_s)p_t(I_t)) \\ = \frac{1}{\alpha-1}\log\int p_{st}^{\alpha}(I_s,I_t)p_s^{1-\alpha}(I_s)p_t^{1-\alpha}(I_t)dI_s dI_t. \quad (2)$$

When $\alpha \to 1$, αMI converges to the standard (Shannon) MI

$$MI = \int p_{st}(I_s,I_t)\log\left(\frac{p_{st}(I_s,I_t)}{p_s(I_s)p_t(I_t)}\right)dI_s dI_t. \quad (3)$$

According to Equation (2), αMI can be interpreted as a measure of dependency between variables I_s and I_t, which is expected to be maximum at registration.

2.3 αMI Estimation

Given a set $\mathcal{Z} = \{z_1, \ldots, z_n\}$ of n vectors in $\mathbb{R}^d$, the k-Nearest Neighbor Graph (kNN Graph) is formed by the points z_i and the edges with their k nearest points $\mathcal{N}_{k,i}(\mathcal{Z})$. This graph belongs to a particular class of graphs known as Entropic Spanning Graphs (ESGs), whose relationship to alpha entropy is described in [14]. Figure 1 shows two examples of kNN graphs for different distributions.

Let I_s and I_t be two images from which the sets of feature vectors $\mathcal{Z}_s = \{z_{s1}, \ldots, z_{sn}\}$ and $\mathcal{Z}_t = \{z_{t1}, \ldots, z_{tn}\}$ have been extracted. kNN graphs allow for estimating αMI between these images as [16]

$$\widehat{\alpha MI} = \frac{1}{\alpha-1}\log\frac{1}{n^\alpha}\sum_{i=1}^{n}\sum_{p=1}^{k}\left(\frac{\|e_{ip}(z_{si},z_{ti})\|}{\sqrt{\|e_{ip}(z_{si})\|\;\|e_{ip}(z_{ti})\|}}\right)^{2\gamma}, \quad (4)$$

where $\|e_{ip}(z_{si},z_{ti})\|$ is the distance from the point $(z_{si},z_{ti}) \in \mathbb{R}^{2d}$ to its p-nearest neighbor in $\{z_{sj},z_{tj}\}_{j\neq i}$, and $\|e_{ip}(z_{si})\|$ ($\|e_{ip}(z_{ti})\|$) is the distance from the point $z_{si} \in \mathbb{R}^d$, ($z_{ti} \in \mathbb{R}^d$) to its p-nearest neighbor in $\{z_{sj}\}_{j\neq i}(\{z_{tj}\}_{j\neq i})$.

In this work we used $\alpha = 0.5$, $\gamma = 2$, $n \simeq 1000$ (it depends on the LV area), $k = 4$ and $\epsilon = 0.1$, the maximum allowed error between a point and its nearest neighbor.

2.4 Feature Vectors

There are many possible feature vectors (FV) to be used in αMI based techniques. In this work, in order to obtain the feature vector corresponding to the point $\mathbf{x}_0$, we applied the Discrete Wavelet Transform (DWT) to decompose the image $I(\mathbf{x})$ into four subimages $I_{LL}(\mathbf{x})$,$I_{LH}(\mathbf{x})$, $I_{HL}(\mathbf{x})$ and $I_{HH}(\mathbf{x})$. Then, we defined the FV of point $\mathbf{x}_0$ by taking the corresponding wavelet coefficients as:

$$\mathbf{z} = [I_{LL}(\mathbf{x})\ I_{LH}(\mathbf{x})\ I_{HL}(\mathbf{x})\ I_{HH}(\mathbf{x})] \tag{5}$$

This paper is not focused on finding the optimal feature for this particular application, but on evaluating the effect of introducing spatial information into the objective function. Therefore, for a first approach, we chose Haar wavelet coefficients owing to its well known ability for edge detection and simplicity. This basis was expected to perform well defining tags in MRI images and thus good for guiding the registration process.

3 Materials

3.1 Dataset

Two tagged 2D sequences were acquired with a GE Genesis Signa 1.5T MRI scanner. A cine breath-hold sequence with a SPAMM grid tag pattern was used, with imaging being done at end expiration. The in-plane image resolution was 1.56mm×1.56mm. Cardiac cycle was sampled by acquiring a total of 16 frames. However, only images from End of Diastole (ED) to End of Systole (ES) (systolic phase) were used in the experiments due to our interest on evaluating deformation during heart contraction. The length of this cardiac cycle segment is 5 frames.

3.2 Manual Measurements

In order to assess the method performance in tracking myocardial motion, tag-intersection points were marked manually in each frame by two observers in two independent sessions. For each sequence, 22 points were chosen to be tracked, and

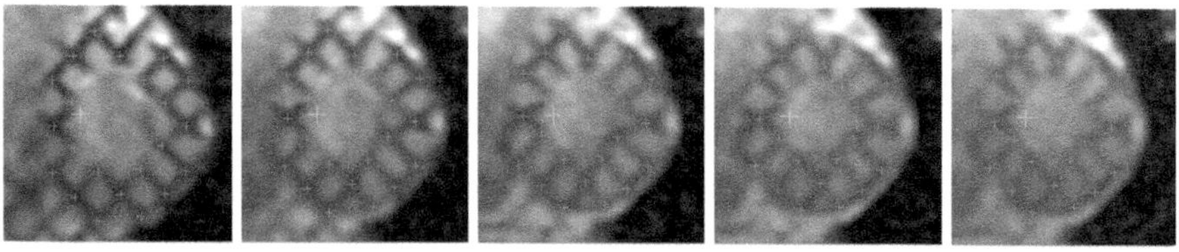

(1) (2) (3) (4) (5)

Fig. 2. Gold standard point positions in each frame from ED to ES for one of the sequences used in this work thus 110 (22×5) points were marked. Gold-standard measurements were derived for each tag-intersection point by taking the average of the measurements made by the observers. Figure 2 shows the gold-standard landmarks for each frame in sequence A.

4 Results

The mean error between the gold standard points and the corresponding positions assessed by the observers was calculated. Table 1 shows the intra and interobserver variabilities of manual landmarking.

The deformation field of the myocardium was calculated with the method explained in Section 2. The resulting transformations were then applied to the gold standard pointset at ED to map these points to each phase. The mean error between these mapped points and the actual positions according to the gold standard was calculated. Figure 3 shows this error from ED to ES. With both methods, subpixel accuracy was obtained for all the phases in patient A and for the two first phases in patient B. Figure 4 shows the initial frames of both sequences, along with an arrow plot showing the displacement field in the myocardium during systole.

Table 1. Accuracy of manual measurements. Bias and standard deviation of the differences, corrected for repeated measurements, between manual and gold standard measurements

	Observer A	*Observer B*	*Observer A and B*
Bias (mm)	0.01	0.06	0.03
SD (mm)	0.35	0.31	0.29

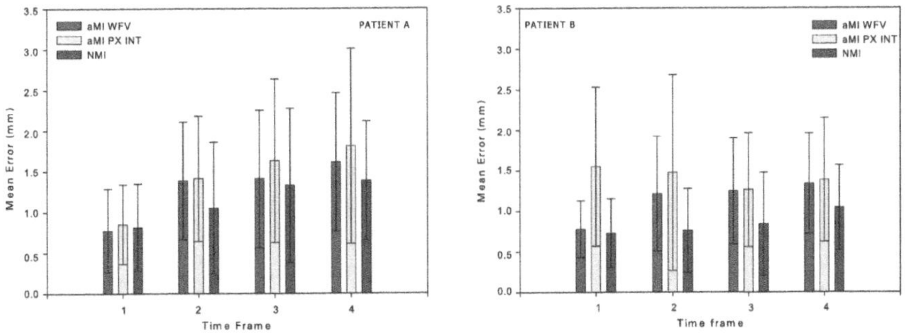

(*a*) (*b*)

Fig. 3. Mean error in landmark correspondence between the gold-standard position and the position of the landmarks in end-diastole after being transformed through the computed deformation field. Results for the different registration metrics is provided. (a) Patient A. (b) Patient B.

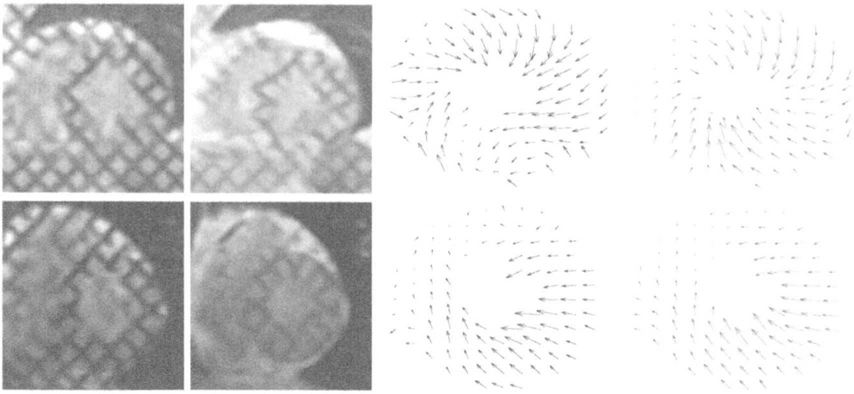

Fig. 4. Displacement of myocardium points during heart contraction by using non-rigid registration for sequence A (top row) and sequence B (bottom row). (a) ED frame. (b) ES frame. (c) Motion field close-up obtained by using αMI. (d) Motion field close-up obtained by using NMI.

5 Discussion

In this paper we have applied an ESG estimation of αMI for myocardial motion estimation. The results show low mean error values with respect to the gold standard measurements, which demonstrate that this method allows retrieving cardiac motion fields accurately.

For this particular application, and according to Figure 3, the use of NMI seems to give better results. However, the standard deviations of the errors are high, and therefore these differences are statistically not significant. A possible explanation for these differences may derive from the feature definition. In this work we have used Haar wavelet coefficients because of their well known ability for edge detection, which was expected to perform appropriately in detecting tag borders. However, Haar basis presents a lack of invariance to translation and rotation which can be corrected by using "cycle spanning" or complex wavelets. Haar basis also has an inherent lack of sensitivity to edge deformations which dominate the deformation feature space. Regarding this matter, a smoother basis like Daubechies or Curvelets might have better potential.

Another explanation for the differences with respect to NMI, is that estimating αMI in multidimensional spaces may introduce more local minima in the error surface than conventional NMI. Thus, the lower accuracy may arise as a consequence of using a local optimization like the downhill method used in this work. Finally, the image resolution of MRI may justify some of the disagreement between measurements. ESGs allow to estimate αMI accurately when the number of FVs used to calculate the graph is large. Given that the in-plane resolution is 1.56mm$\times$1.56mm and that only the LV was considered, less than 1000 points were available for αMI estimation.

Figure 4 shows a good agreement between estimated displacements fields of each metric for sequence B. For sequence A, there was clearly a different result in the lower-right portion of the image. The frame at ES for this patient shows completely vanished tags and poor image quality in the part of the myocardium where the motion field is altered. Therefore, it could be hypothesized that the incorporation of spatial features into the objective function makes the results more dependent on the presence of such features in the target and source images.

With respect to the extension of this work to the three dimensional case, the main drawback is that ESGs are computationally expensive. However, many algorithms have been developed to compute graphs in an approximated manner, allowing a significant speed up of the graph construction.

6 Conclusions

Entropic spanning graph estimation of αMI has been applied for non rigid registration for the first time and has proven to retrieve myocardial deformation fields accurately. Although the results were quite satisfactory, even lower errors have been obtained with NMI. However, the observed differences were statistically not significant and further research needs to be done to fully understand the reason of this behavior. ESGs offer an increased flexibility in the kinds of features one can use for these types of problems, and further research needs to be done regarding this matter.

Acknowledgements

This work was partially funded by Red IM3: Imagen Mdica Molecular y Multimodalidad (ISCIII G03/185), Redes Temticas Colaborativas, Ministerio de Sanidad y Consumo de Espaa (http://im3.rediris.es) and TIC2002-04495-C02 grant. The work of E. Oubel is supported by the Spanish Ministry of Education under a FPU Grant AP2003-1535. The work of A.F. Frangi is supported by the Spanish Ministry of Science and Technology under a Ramn y Cajal Research Fellowship. Special acknowledgements to Dra. Marina Huguet from Centro Cardiovascular Sant Jordi, Barcelona, Spain, for providing the images used in the experiments and to GridSystems S.A., Palma de Mallorca, Spain (http://www.gridsystems.com) for providing the InnerGrid Nitya Middleware for grid computing and technical support.

References

1. Axel, L., Dougherty, L.: MR imaging of motion with spatial modulation of magnetization. Radiology **171** (1989) 841–845
2. Zerhouni, E., Parish, D., Rogers, W.: Human heart: tagging with MR imaging - a method for non invasive assessment of myocardial motion. Radiology **169** (1988) 59–63

3. Prince, J., McVeigh, E.: Motion estimation from tagged MR image sequences. IEEE Trans. Med. Imag. **11** (1992) 238–249
4. Gupta, S., Prince, J.: On variable brightness optical flow for tagged MRI. In: Inform. Processing Med. Imag. (1995) 323–334
5. Osman, N., Kerwin, W., McVeigh, E., Prince, J.: Cardiac motion tracking using cine harmonic phase (HARP) magnetic resonance imaging. Magn. Reson. Med. **42** (1999) 1048–1060
6. Osman, N., McVeigh, E., Prince, J.: Imaging heart motion using harmonic phase MRI. IEEE Trans. Med. Imag. **19** (2000) 186–202
7. Kumar, S., Goldgof, D.: Automatic tracking of SPAMM grid and the estimation of deformation parameters from cardiac MR images. IEEE Trans. Med. Imag. **13** (1994) 122–132
8. Guttman, M., Prince, J., McVeigh, E.: Tag and contour detection in tagged MR images of the left ventricle. IEEE Trans. Med. Imag. **13** (1994) 74–88
9. Kraitchman, D., Young, A., Change, C., Axel, L.: Semi-automatic tracking of myocardial motion in MR tagged images. IEEE Trans. Med. Imag. **14** (1995) 422–433
10. Clarysse, P., Basset, C., Khouas, L., Croisille, P., Friboulet, D.: Two-dimensional spatial and temporal displacement and deformation field fitting from cardiac magnetic resonance imaging. Medical Image analysis **4** (2000) 253–268
11. Petitjean, C., Rougon, N., Prêteux, F., Cluzel, P., Grenier, P.: Measuring myocardial deformations from MR data using information-theoretic non rigid registration. In: Proceedings Second International Workshop on Functional Imaging and Modeling of the Heart (FIMH'2003), Lyon, France - Lecture Notes in Computer Science 2674, Heidelberg, Germany, Springer Verlag (2003) 162–172
12. Chandrasheckara, R., Mohiaddin, R.H., Rueckert, D.: Analysis of 3D myocardial motion in tagged MR images using non rigid image registration. IEEE Trans. Med. Imag. **23** (2004) 1245–1250
13. Rueckert, D., Sonoda, L.I., Hayes, C., Hill, D.L.G., Leach, M.O., Hawkes, D.J.: Nonrigid registration using free-form deformations: application to breast MR images. IEEE Trans. Med. Imag. **18** (1999) 712–721
14. Hero, A.O., Ma, B., Michael, O., Gorman, J.: Applications of entropic spanning graphs. IEEE Signal Processing Magazine (Special Issue on Mathematics in Imaging) **19** (2002) 85–95
15. Schnabel, J.A., Rueckert, D., Quist, M., Blackall, J.M., Castellano-Smith, A.D., Hartkens, T., Penney, G.P., Hall, W.A., Liu, H., Truwit, C.L., Gerritsen, F.A., Hill, D.L.G., Hawkes, D.J.: A generic framework for nonrigid registration based on non uniform multi-level free-form deformations. In Niessen, W.J., Viergever, M.A., eds.: Proc. 4th Int. Conf. Medical Image Computing and Computer Assisted Intervention, Utrecht, The Netherlands (2001) 573–581
16. Neemuchwala, H.F., Hero, A.O.: Entropic graphs for registration. In: Multi-sensor image fusion and its applications. Marcel-Dekker, Inc. (2004)

Iterative 3D Point-Set Registration Based on Hierarchical Vertex Signature (HVS)

Jun Feng[1] and Horace H.S. Ip[1,2]

[1] Image Computing Group, Department of Computer Science,
City University of Hong Kong, Tat Chee Avenue, Kowloon, Hong Kong
feng@cs.cityu.edu.hk
http://icg.cityu.edu.hk/ICGers/Judy/judy.htm
[2] Centre for Innovative Applications of Internet And Multimedia Technologies (AIMtech),
City University of Hong Kong, Tat Chee Avenue, Kowloon, Hong Kong
cship@cityu.edu.hk
http://icg.cityu.edu.hk/ICGers/hsip/hsip.htm

Abstract. Robust 3D point registration is difficult for biomedical surfaces, especially for roundish and approximate symmetric soft tissues such as liver, stomach, etc. We present an Iterative Optimization Registration scheme (IOR) based on Hierarchical Vertex Signatures (HVS) between point-sets of medical surfaces. HVSs are distributions of concatenated neighborhood angles relative to the PCA axes of the surfaces which concisely describe global structures and local contexts around vertices in a hierarchical paradigm. The correspondences between point-sets are then established by Chi-Square test statistics. Specifically, to alleviate the sensitivity to axes directions that often affects robustness for other global axes based algorithms, IOR aligns surfaces gradually, and incrementally calibrates the directions of major axes in a multi-resolution manner. The experimental results demonstrate IOR is efficient and robust for liver registration. This method is also promising to other applications such as morphological pathological analysis, 3D model retrieval and object recognition.

1 Introduction

Automatic and robust registration between 3D images is very important for medical image analysis. Three main purposes of this kind of registrations are: (1) Compare two organ shapes of the same patient in different periods for diagnosis. (2) Register tissue across individuals for physiological analysis. (3) Match 3D data of patients with anatomical atlas for shape representation [1]. The possible primitives of 3D shape registration include points, lines, curves, facets and surfaces [2]. Usually, point registration is also a key step to construct statistical deformable models [3].

The majority of the previous work dealing with 3D point-set registration came from the computer vision community. Most of them were based on shape matching. For example, a well-known method called "Iterative Closest Point" was proposed by Besl and Mckay [4]. It provides a general solution for registration by minimizing the distances between the nearest neighbors in an iterative procedure. However, the process is computationally expensive. Cyr and Kamal generated a number of typical sample 2D views from the 3D models and matched them against a given view [5].

J. Duncan and G. Gerig (Eds.): MICCAI 2005, LNCS 3750, pp. 279 – 286, 2005.

Sundar et al. encoded the topological information of 3D shapes in the form of a skeletal graph and matched them for registration [6]. Modal matching technique performs point registration between objects by their eigenmodes [7,8]. It provides a global to local description of shape deformation; however, the technique requires very expensive calculation for eigenmodes.

Another common approach for point-set registration is to match distinctive local features between surface points such as geometric invariants [9]; these often fail because of insufficient local information and different viewpoint that radically alter local feature appearance. Some authors resorted to stochastic approaches to let the registration process be immune to noise and small deformations. Belongie and Malik [10] introduced a 2D "*shape context*" which described the coarse distribution of shape with respect to a given point. This descriptor offers a globally discriminative characterization. Yamany et al. [11] presented a "*surface signature*" to capture the surface curvature information seen from certain points. Chin [12] proposed a "*point signature*" to describe the structural neighborhood of a point on the 3D surface. Statistics of the distance and relative angles are collected to characterize feature points.

However, these distributions cannot capture the location of the features and they are not always able to provide sufficiently distinctive information to achieve one-to-one point registration. This problem is more severe in medical/biomedical image analysis. Usually, shapes of biomedical tissues are very different from those of the man-made objects such as chairs, buildings, cars and aircrafts, etc., investigated in most computer vision applications. There exist large classes of nature objects in biomedical applications that are smooth, rounded, curved, and sometimes approximately symmetric such as livers, heart lenticels, stomachs and kidneys. Vertices on these kinds of organ surfaces frequently share similar geometric features, which often makes local geometric based matching fail.

In this paper, we propose an idea prompted by [11] and [12] to register point-sets defined in segmented biomedical sense data, especially for blobby and approximate symmetric soft tissues. The shapes of these tissues often differ from each other through some form of non-linear deformations. The challenge posed by such models is that it is frequently difficult to define landmarks or to obtain salient geometric features from the surfaces. We present an intuitively simple but very effective and robust feature descriptor called "**Hierarchical Vertex Signature**" (HVS) for describing the distribution of shape structures in the context of a surface point. Our proposed descriptor captures both global and local structures of the 3D surface from the point of view of any vertex by associating each vertex with a probability distribution of angles between vectors linking pairs of vertices and the major axes of the organs. Registration is then carried out based on the similarity between vertices on different surfaces. Our approach is different from [11] and [12] in: (1)We calculate angles relative to global axes (PCA axes) while they estimate angle values relative to local surface normals. Therefore, our method is more robust to noise and more insensitive to surface smoothness. More importantly, the extension of the relative angles (*RA*s) defined in a global canonical frame makes HSV has the ability to indicate orientation of a point relative to the whole surface. (2) We construct 1D signature for each point while both of them employ 2D signature feature images so our method is more efficient and the similarity comparison is more intuitive and accurate. (3) Our proposed signature is hierarchically defined in different neighborhood field of the vertex; therefore, it provides both local and global shape descriptions around a vertex. (4) Last but not least, we design an Iterative Optimization Registration scheme (IOR) to calibrate the global axes of surfaces continuously and in turn adjust the vertices' signatures. This procedure effectively alleviates the sensitivity of HVS to the major axes of the objects being matched that may be ambiguous across individuals.

The rest of the paper is organized as follows. We present the definition of the Hierarchical Vertex Signature (HVS) and describe the Iterative Optimization Registration (IOR) scheme in section 2. Experimental results in a liver database are shown in section 3, and we conclude the paper in section 4.

2 Method

2.1 Hierarchical Vertex Signature (HVS) in Canonical Coordinate Frame

We treat the coordinates of the points on a 3D shape as random variables. Three principal components (PCs) u_1 to u_3 are calculated from their covariance matrix C. They are used to build up a canonical PCA coordinate frame. Suppose there are N vertices on the surface, for each vertex v_i, $N-1$ spoke vectors $\overrightarrow{v_i v_j}$ are derived. A Relative Angle (*RA*) $\theta_j(v_i)$ is defined between the jth spoke vector of v_i and the first principal axis. Two base-planes Π_{12} ($e_2^T.v_i = 0$)and Π_{13} ($e_3^T.v_i = 0$) are formed, where e_2 and e_3 are the second and the third eigenvectors of C respectively. They are employed as reference planes to extend $\theta_j(v_i)$ from $[0,\pi]$ to $[-\pi,\pi]$. Furthermore, *RA*s are normalized to $0 \sim 2\pi$. For sake of paper space, please refer to our previous paper [14] to get the accurate formulation of $\theta_j(v_i)$.

Now what we want is investigating the distribution of these *RA*s in the different fields of the vertex's neighborhood. The neighborhood relationship can be constructed from the triangular meshes of surfaces. There are many standard algorithms to build triangular meshes for an unorganized point-set such as [13]. Actually, the strict definition and exact connectivity of the meshes are not necessary for our method. Please refer to [14] for the neighborhood construction. After obtain the neighborhood map of the point-set, the distributions of the relative angles in different fields of neighborhood are concatenated to form a Hierarchical Vertex Signature (HVS) for a given surface point (ordered from near neighborhood fields to distant neighborhood fields). Obviously, in this way, each HVS contains hierarchical shape description around a vexel in a concise form. Since the *RA*s are calculated with respect to the major axes of the organ, it captures the topological information of a point on a surface. We treat HVSs as sufficient and salient shape descriptors to register vertices between tissue surfaces. In practice, stochastic methods are employed to evaluate samples of HVSs, and histograms are constructed by counting how many samples fall into certain sized bins. Relative angles are rounded depended on the number of the histogram bins. Promisingly, HVS has the following properties:

(1) **Invariance:** One of the basic characteristics of angles is that they are invariant to scale and rigid motions. In addition, since the *RA*s are defined in the global canonical reference frame, they are translation and rotation invariant. Therefore, HVS can be directly employed for point registration without normalization.

(2) **Robustness:** As a bonus of stochastic methods, HVS is insensitive to noise, unsmoothness, small perturbations and points missing of organ surface, which are inevitably existed in 3D biomedical volumes recorded by different modalities.

(3) **Efficiency:** After obtaining the neighborhood map of a point-set, the complexity of HVS extraction is $O(N^2)$. The neighborhood map can be established and stored in advance prior to real-time registration.

(4) **Hierarchy:** HVS is a piecewise curve concatenated from the distributions in different neighborhood fields of a point. It expresses the local features of a surface when the layer of field is small, and represents the global shape when the layer becomes large. The last piece of HVS (See Fig.3) represents the distribution of the overall surface and provides a detailed and compact description of the global shape context. Therefore, we can claim that HVS captures both local and global spatial information around a given vertex in a hierarchical paradigm.

2.2 Iterative Optimization 3D Point-Set Registration (IOP) Based on HVSs

Our hypothesis is that HVSs of the correspondence pairs on tissue surfaces should be similar so the best matching distributions lead us to the most suitable point for registration. That is, we postulate that the HVSs associated with a pair of corresponding points possess the same theoretical form, even though they may be subjected to some forms of distortion and noise. As HVSs are represented as bins, it is natural to use Goodness-Of-Fit χ^2 test to measure the dissimilarity factor *df* between points:

$$df(v_i, v_j') = \sum_{k=0}^{2\pi} \frac{\left[(p_k(v_i) * S_l(v_i) - p_k'(v_j') * S_l'(v_j')\right]^2}{p_k(v_i) * S_l(v_l)} \qquad (1)$$

where v and v' are points in sample and target point-sets respectively. p_k is probability value of the k th bin, and S_l is the vertex number in the l th field. The range of *df* is [0,1], and the best registration result is achieved by searching for a point on the target surface which has the minimum *df* with a given point on the sample surface.

We observe that very close vertices in dense point-sets may have similar global *RA* distributions, but they have large differences between local structures (see the first piece of the distribution curve in Fig. 4). However, local distributions collected in the small neighborhood fields may contain much uncertainty and noise so they are not as robust as the global ones. Intuitively, HVSs of coarse point-set should be more distinctive since the vertices are sparse and distant so the spoke vectors of neighbors may not have similar orientations. Here, we propose an Iterative Optimization Registration scheme (IOR) for multi-resolution point-sets to perform accurate and robust registration in a hierarchical manner. The flowchart of IOS is elaborated in Fig. 1.

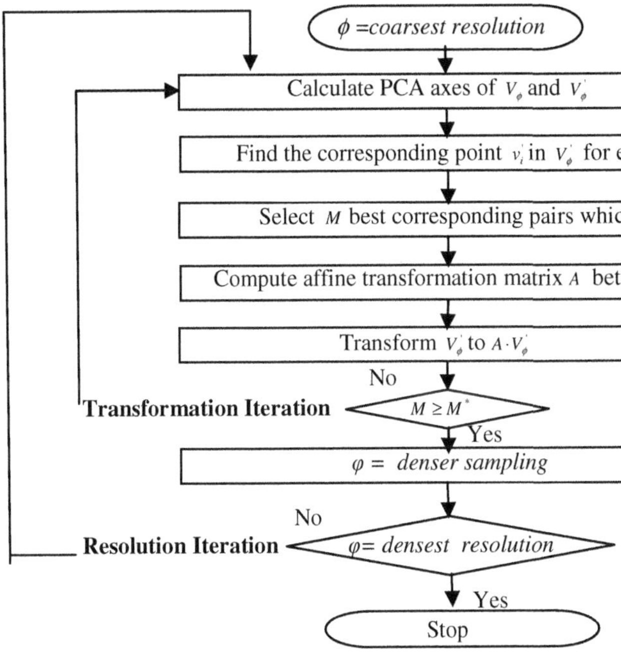

Fig. 1. The flowchart of the iterative optimization scheme for 3D point registration

Our approach consists of two main nested iterative schemes: resolution iteration and transformation iteration. During the **resolution iteration**, the registration begins with the coarsest point-sets [1] and the correspondence searching is conducted in the range of the whole surface. After finding M^* corresponding pairs and obtaining a rough alignment between surfaces by affine transformation, registration moves to denser sampling (higher resolution) data. At this stage, since the basic correspondence is established, the search range for a given vertex is limited to a small region. As we have mentioned, *RA*s are calculated relative to the global coordinate frame, slight deformation of shapes may change orientations of major axes and accordingly influence the distributions of surface points. To achieve robust registration, a **transformation iteration** is designed specifically to correct and adjust the PCA axes continuously for the target point-set based on its affine transformation (AI). The consistency of major axes improves significantly the matching of the corresponding HVSs match (See Fig. 2). In the transformation iteration, at least 10% of the best corresponding pairs are selected which are approximately evenly distributed over the surface. The affine transformation matrix is calculated in a minimum error sense by:

$$A = (V \cdot V'^T)(V' \cdot V'^T)^{-1} \tag{2}$$

[1] Please note that too much sub-sampling may make the blobby surface hard to find rotations.

3 Experiments and Results

We have implemented IOR using C++ on PCs (1.8 G CPU, 1G memory), and tested it in a liver image database. Each liver volume is defined by 20-30 CT slices. Livers are roundish and approximately symmetric soft tissues which frequently cause other registration techniques to fail. Imaging and analysis of the livers are also challenging due to potentially significant deformations among individuals and the lack of well-defined boundaries in the associated CT images. The shapes of the livers used in this work are semi-automatically segmented from the CT volumes. It has taken 5 minutes to generate the neighborhood map for the densest point-sets (1474 points). HVS extraction and point registration between two surfaces have taken less than 1 minute. The transform iteration usually converged after 3~5 iterations. Three different resolution point-sets (98, 370 and 1474) have been used for the evaluation by evenly sub-sampling the dense surfaces points. Fig. 2 shows an example of the alignment process between the PCA axes of the aligning livers during the lowest resolution point-set registration. The accuracy rates of the established point correspondence between the 12 livers used in the experiment and a sample are plotted in Fig. 2(d). The ground truth used here has been established in advanced by radiography specialists.

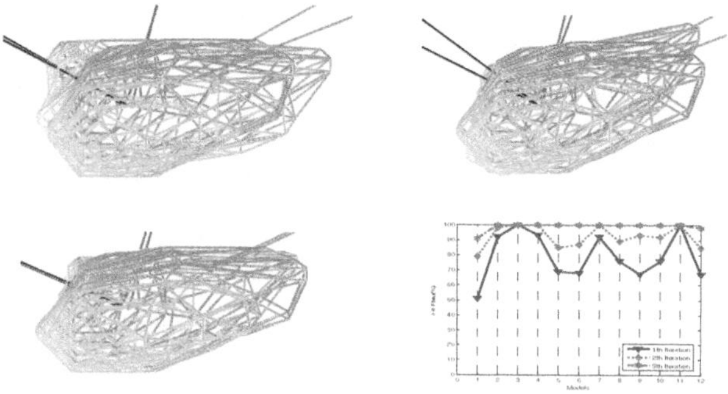

Fig. 2. (a-c) Alignment between PCA axes and affine transformation between the sample (yellow meshes) and the target surfaces (green meshes), red, blue and black axes are u_1 , u_2 and u_3 . (d) Accuracy rates comparison of point correspondence in different transformation iteration.

To demonstrate the highly discriminate ability of HVSs, in figure 3, we show the established point correspondences between a few selected vertices on the liver surfaces. For better visualization, the surfaces are rendered by standard method. The HVSs of point A and its registration partner A' are plotted in Fig. 3(b), 5 neighborhood fields and 72 bins are used. It is not difficult to discover that the resulting registration is visually correct, and their profiles of the HVSs match rather well. To verify that the distributions of corresponding points indeed follow the same theoretical function, we overlap the HVSs of the registration partners of point B on 14 liver surfaces, using 3 neighbor fields and 72 bins (Fig. 3c). The shapes of the curves are highly consistent.

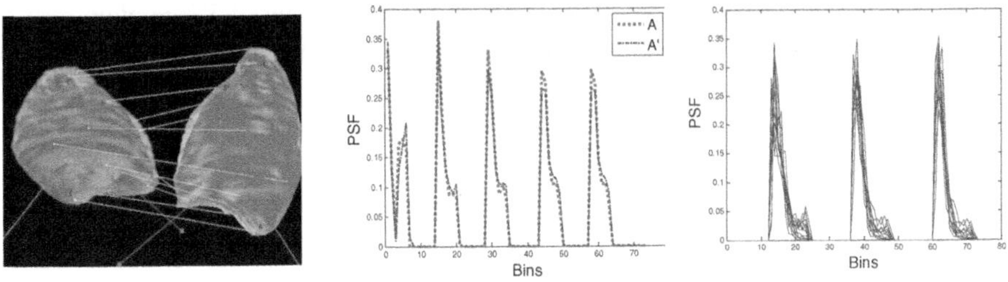

Fig. 3. (a) Point-set registration result (b) Overlapping HVSs of A and A'. (c) Overlapped HVSs of 14 corresponding points of B.

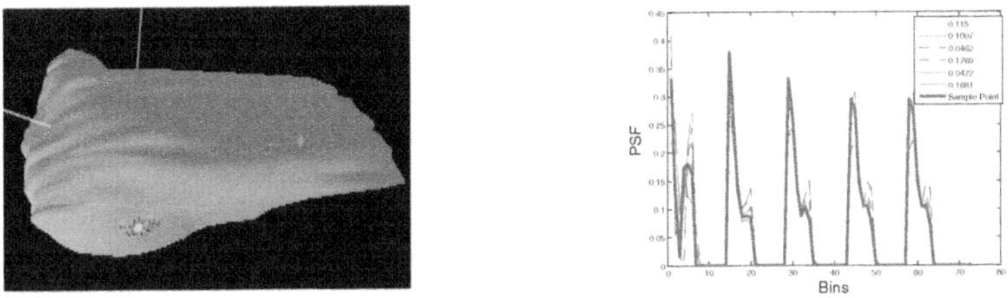

Fig. 4. (a) 12 vertices (pink dots) which have the lowest *df* with a sample vertex (yellow dot) (b) overlapping HVS curves of these vertices (Green curve is the distribution of sample vertex).

In Fig. 4a, we mark 12 vertices that have the lowest *df* value with a sample vertex. We can find that the vertices which have the most similar HVS distributions converge near the neighborhood of the sample vertex. The overlapping HVSs of these 12 vertices are plotted in Fig. 4b. The plots show high consistency in the global shapes (the last pieces of curves) but have large discrepancies in local structures, especially in the first neighbor field (the first piece of curves).

4 Conclusion

It is a fundamental yet still an open problem in computer vision to match two point-sets. In this paper, we propose a 3D point-set registration scheme for blobby biomedical objects. The angles (*RA*) of the spoke vectors derived from a vertex relative to PCA axes are defined and the concatenated distributions of the *RA*s in the different neighborhood fields around a vertex are used to describe a Hierarchical Vertex Signature (HVS). HVS has many good characteristics such as invariance, robustness and hierarchy. It is also computation efficient. We have also proposed an iterative optimization registration scheme (IOR) in which the directions of major axes if the surfaces are calibrated incrementally according to affine transformation alignment between multi-resolution point-sets. The experiments indicate that our algorithm produces robust registration results for deformable organs such as the liver.

The proposed techniques of registration and the establishment of 3D point correspondences are applicable to many other applications such as morphological or pathological analysis, 3D model retrieval and 3D object recognition.

References

1. Thirion, J.P., "Extremeal Points: Definition and Application to 3D image Registration", Proceedings CVPR '94, Pages: 587-592.
2. A. Liu, E. Bullitt, S. M. Pizer, "3D/2D Registration via Skeletal near Projective Invariance in Tubular Objects", Lecture Notes in Computer Science 1496: MICCAI 98, Springer, New York, 1998, Pages: 952-963.
3. T.F.Cootes, C.J.Taylor, D.H.Cooper and J.Graham et.al, "Active Shape Models-Their Training and Applications",CVIU Vol. 61 No. 1, 1995, Pages: 38-59.
4. P.J. Besl and N.D. McKay, "A Method for Registration of 3-D Shapes", PAMI Vol. 14(2), 1992, Pages: 239-256.
5. Cyr, C.M. Kamal, A.F. Sebastian, T.B. Kimia, B.B., "2D-3D registration based on shape matching", Proceedings of IEEE Workshop on Mathematical Methods in Biomedical Image Analysis, 2000, Pages: 198 – 203.
6. Sundar, H.; Silver, D.; Gagvani, N.; Dickinson, S, "Skeleton based shape matching and retrieval", Shape Modeling International, 2003, Pages:130 – 139.
7. Stan Scalroff et.al, "Modal Matching for Correspondence and Recognition", PAMI Vol. 17, No. 6, 1995, Pages: 545-561.
8. Marco Carcassoni et.al, "Correspondence Matching with Modal Clusters", PAMI Vol. 25, No. 12, 2003, Pages: 1609-1615.
9. Ehud Rivilin and Issac Weiss, "Local Invariants For Recognition", PAMI Vol. 17 No. 3, 1995, Pages: 226-238.
10. Belongie, S. Malik, J. Puzicha, J., "Shape matching and object recognition using shape contexts", PAMI, Vol. 24 No. 4, 2002, Pages: 509-522.
11. Yamany, S.M. Farag, A.A., "Surface signatures: an orientation independent free-form surface representation scheme for the purpose of objects registration and matching", PAMI Vol. 24 No. 8, 2002, Pages: 1105-1120.
12. Chin Seng Chua et.al, "Point Signatures: A New Representation for 3D Object Recognition", IJCV Vol. 25 No. 1, 1997, Pages: 63-85.
13. Hoppe, H. DeRose, T.,Duchamp, T. ScDonald, J and Stuetzle, W., "Surface Reconstruction from Unorganised Points", Computer Graphics, 26(2), 1992, Pages: 71-78.
14. Jun Feng, Horace H. S. Ip, "Chi-Square Goodness-of-Fit Test of 3D Point Correspondence for Model Similarity Measure and Analysis", Lecture Notes in Computer Science, CIVR 2005, LNCS 3568, Pages: 445-453.

Automatic Patient Registration for Port Placement in Minimally Invasive Endoscopic Surgery

Marco Feuerstein[1,2], Stephen M. Wildhirt[2], Robert Bauernschmitt[2], and Nassir Navab[1]

[1] Computer Aided Medical Procedures (CAMP) Group, TU Munich, Germany
[2] Department of Cardiothoracic Surgery, German Heart Center Munich, Germany

Abstract. Optimal port placement is a delicate issue in minimally invasive endoscopic surgery, particularly in robotically assisted surgery. A good choice of the instruments' and endoscope's ports can avoid time-consuming consecutive new port placement. We present a novel method to intuitively and precisely plan the port placement. The patient is registered to its pre-operative CT by just moving the endoscope around fiducials, which are attached to the patient's thorax and are visible in its CT. Their 3D positions are automatically reconstructed. Without prior time-consuming segmentation, the pre-operative CT volume is directly rendered with respect to the endoscope or instruments. This enables the simulation of a camera flight through the patient's interior along the instruments' axes to easily validate possible ports.

1 Introduction

Ideal port placement is one of the key issues in minimally invasive endoscopic surgery, particularly in robotically assisted surgery. The optimal choice of the instruments' ports provides full access to the whole operation region as well as adequate surgeon dexterity. This can avoid time-consuming new port placement, which is a strain on every patient.

In the current clinical work flow, the surgical staff selects all ports by palpation of external anatomic landmarks, primarily based on their previous experience. However, if these external landmarks do not correspond to the individual internal anatomy of each patient, a misplacement of ports can occur. Several methods have been proposed to improve and automate the optimal placement of ports [1,2,3,4]. They all have two major disadvantages: 1) They rely on the time-consuming manual or semi-automatic segmentation of pre-operative imaging data from CT or MRI, which is essential to reconstruct models of any involved anatomy, e.g. ribs, heart, and soft tissue. These 3D models are used to automatically compute the port locations. 2) They lack a practical and accurate way to transfer the planned port locations to the operating room, which is achieved by registering the patient to the pre-operative data.

In any case, the patient registration process is based on matching anatomical or artificial landmarks, which are visible on both the patient and its CT data.

J. Duncan and G. Gerig (Eds.): MICCAI 2005, LNCS 3750, pp. 287–294, 2005.

Adhami and Coste-Maniere use the end effectors of the da Vinci telemanipulator to point to fiducials, which are attached to the patient [1]. Due to their shape and intensity, the fiducials can be segmented automatically in the CT data. Intra-operatively, they move the robot arm's end effector to every single fiducial in order to get its position in the robot coordinate frame. This is a time-consuming and unnatural task. Similarly, Selha et al use the sensor of an additional electromagnetic tracking system [3] as a pointing device. However, they base their registration on anatomical landmarks. Both electromagnetic tracking and the use of anatomical landmarks introduce an inherent imprecision when determining corresponding landmarks.

We propose a fast, practical, and easy method to register the CT data to the patient. Spherical CT visible self-adhesive fiducials are stuck on the patient's skin. They are segmented automatically in its CT data. Intra-operatively, instead of pointing to the fiducials, we only move the tracked endoscope around the fiducials and acquire a set of images from differing, but arbitrary poses. To simplify the acquisition process, not all fiducials need to be seen by the camera in a single image. By automatically detecting the fiducials in these images, we reconstruct their 3D positions in the tracking (=world) coordinate frame. Point based registration methods enable us to match them with the CT data. For port placement, the surgical staff simply moves the tracked instruments or endoscope to the positions where it wishes to place their corresponding ports. A virtual camera is placed on top of the instruments' end effectors or the endoscope's camera center. It is able to simulate a flight through the patient's interior by rendering the CT volume as it would be seen by the endoscope. In this natural way, optimal port placements can easily be identified without prior segmentation of patient's anatomy or any tedious pointing device. Our method is applicable to any tracked endoscope, no matter whether it is tracked by an optical tracking system, a mechanical one such as da Vinci, or any other tracking system.

In order to reconstruct the 3D positions of the fiducials, the endoscope's pose and intrinsic parameters need to be determined. This is achieved by a one-time hand-eye calibration, as described in section 2. In section 3, we present our algorithms for 3D reconstruction and patient registration. Further details on the provision of volume rendering for port placement can be found in section 4. Our conducted experiments on a thorax phantom are described in section 5. We conclude in section 6 with an evaluation of our presented methods and a short outlook on future research.

2 Calibration of the Endoscope

For our application, the endoscope camera is rigidly attached to a sensor, e.g. to a marker target seen by an optical tracking system or an actuated robot arm as for da Vinci. The main purpose of calibrating the endoscope is to model the transformation of a 3D world point onto the camera's 2D image plane, so the projection of a fiducial onto the endoscope's image can be reproduced mathematically.

In detail, a point X_w in the world frame is first transformed into the sensor frame by ${}_wT_s$, from where it is transformed into the camera frame by ${}_sT_c$, and finally mapped onto the image plane by the camera's calibration matrix K. The transformation ${}_wT_s$ can be directly received from the tracking system. The rigid transformation ${}_sT_c$ from sensor to camera coordinate frame and the intrinsic camera parameters stored in K need to be computed once. Additionally, the rather large radial and tangential lens distortion of endoscopes needs to be corrected for.

To compute all unknowns, a classical hand-eye calibration approach is taken [5,6,7]. Therefore, a flat checkerboard pattern is placed arbitrarily. The tracked camera performs a series of n motions. At the pause of each motion, the camera acquires an image of the pattern and the pose of the attached sensor is recorded. Having at least two motions (rotations around distinguished axes) or three poses, respectively, the offset ${}_sT_c$ along with the camera's intrinsic parameters and distortion coefficients can be computed as follows:

First, the intrinsics, distortion coefficients, and camera poses in the pattern coordinate frame (${}_pT_c^1 \dots {}_pT_c^n$: the transformations from pattern to camera coordinate frame) are computed using the gold standard algorithms for camera calibration [8,9].

Second, the rigid offset between sensor and camera is computed. All transformations involved during a single motion from pose i to pose j can be seen on figure 1(a). The camera motions can be easily computed from previous results. Analogous, the sensor motions can be received from the recorded poses. To compute ${}_sT_c$, the following so-called hand-eye equation needs to be solved:

$$\forall i = 1 \dots n, j = 1 \dots n, i \neq j : {}_sT_c {}^iT_s^j = {}^iT_c^j {}_sT_c \quad (1)$$

This can be achieved by decomposing the involved matrices, as described by Tsai/Lenz and others [5,6,7].

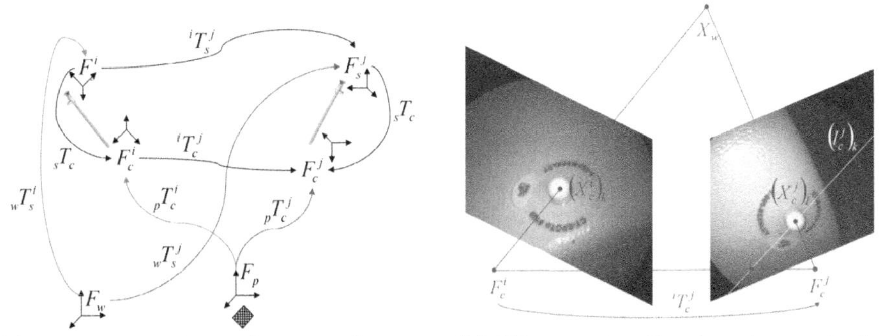

(a) Involved coordinate frames and transformations during hand-eye calibration

(b) 3D reconstruction based on epipolar geometry

Fig. 1. The principles of hand-eye calibration and epipolar geometry

3 Automatic 3D Reconstruction for Patient Registration

For patient registration, three essential steps are required: 1) All fiducials must be segmented in the CT volume to determine the positions of their centroids. 2) Their positions in the tracking coordinate frame need to be reconstructed using the images, which are acquired by the calibrated endoscope camera and show the fiducials. 3) The resulting point sets need to be matched in order to register the patient to its CT data set.

The automatic segmentation of the fiducials in the CT volume can be achieved by using standard image processing techniques based on thresholding, filling, morphology, and subtraction [10,11]. The centroids of all segmented fiducials can be computed very precisely by weighing their associated voxel intensities and incorporating partial volume effects.

For finding the 3D positions of the fiducials in the tracking coordinate frame, two iterations are performed for each image i containing an arbitrary number m of fiducials. First, the 2D positions $x_1^i \dots x_m^i$ of all visible fiducials are extracted automatically after undistortion of the image. Similar techniques as for the segmentation of the CT data are used, which also incorporate edge detection and color information of the fiducials and patient's skin [11]. Second, the properties of epipolar geometry are applied to reconstruct their 3D positions[9,12], as illustrated on figure 1(b).

Next, all 2D point pairs corresponding to the same 3D point are used to optimally reconstruct the 3D point. For all 2D points, their associated projection rays $r_1 \dots r_s$ are constructed, which intersect the camera center $C_r = {}_ct_w^i$ and the point's projection onto the image plane $P_r = {}_cR_w^i (X_c^i)_k + {}_ct_w^i$, where ${}_cR_w^i = ({}_wR_c^i)^T$ and ${}_ct_w^i = -({}_wR_c^i)^T {}_wt_c^i$. They can be represented using the camera center C_r as starting point and a directional unit vector d_r:

$$r_r = C_r + \lambda_r d_r = C_r + \lambda_r \frac{P_r - C_r}{\|P_r - C_r\|} \tag{2}$$

The associated midpoint X_w can be computed, which is closest in average to all s rays. Therefore, following overdetermined system of linear equations has to be minimized:

$$\sum_{r=1}^{s} \|C_r + \lambda_r d_r - X_w\|^2 \tag{3}$$

As stated by Sturm et al, this linear least squares problem may be solved using the Pseudo-inverse [13]. Finally, these results can be further improved by using the Levenberg-Marquardt iteration to minimize following equation:

$$\sum_{r=1}^{s} \left\| K \left[{}_sR_c | {}_st_c \right] \begin{bmatrix} ({}_wR_s)_r & ({}_wt_s)_r \\ 0 & 1 \end{bmatrix} \begin{bmatrix} X_w \\ 1 \end{bmatrix} - \begin{bmatrix} x_r \\ 1 \end{bmatrix} \right\|^2 \tag{4}$$

After the reconstruction of all 3D points from their associated 2D points, they need to be matched with the points segmented in the CT data set. Therefore, the correct point correspondences need to be identified and the transformation from the CT coordinate frame into the world coordinate frame, where the patient is registered in, needs to be computed. This can be done by a distance-weighted graph matching approach along with a point based registration algorithm [14,15]. Finally, the patient's CT volume is registered in the same coordinate frame as the patient.

4 Volume Rendered Port Placement

Once the CT volume is registered to the patient, it can be visualized with respect to any tracked instruments, overlaid onto the real images of the endoscope, displayed simultaneously with the real endoscopic images [16], or even be used to extend the endoscopic images to improve the surgeon's orientation. In our case, the CT volume is directly rendered as it would be seen by virtual cameras put in front of the tracked instruments or by the real endoscope camera. This can be used for placing the instruments and endoscope or their corresponding ports, respectively, in an optimal way. By virtually moving the camera in and out the volume along the instruments' or endoscope's main axes the surgeon can intuitively verify, whether the current poses of the instruments and the endoscope are ideal to reach the whole operating region.

For rendering the volume, pre-defined transfer functions are offered to assign specific colors and opacities to certain image intensities, which can be modified interactively to the surgeon's needs. This makes it easy to realistically visualize only the anatomy, which is essential for the success of the intervention, e.g. for cardiac surgery the bones, aorta, heart, and other main arteries such as the left and right arteria mammaria interna, which were contrasted for CT. To provide a fast and though detailed visualization during port placement in real time, our volume renderer is using the graphic card's GPU (graphical processing unit) to perform the computations for 3D texture mapping.

Utilizing this approach of direct volume rendering without prior segmentation and generation of polygonal 3D models of the patient's anatomy saves a noticeable amount of time for planning the ports and leaves the control to the surgical staff during port placement.

5 Experimental Results

For our experiments we used a 30 degrees laparoscope tracked by an optical tracking system, which has a root mean square error of 0.53 millimeters for the viewing axis and 0.32 millimeters for the other axes when tracking retroreflective markers. We implemented two classical hand-eye calibration methods by Tsai/Lenz and Daniilidis [5,6]. Tsai and Lenz combine two QR decompositions to determine the translation and rotation, whereas Daniilidis uses dual quaternions and a single singular value decomposition.

The intrinsic and extrinsic camera parameters were estimated from 32 frames. For hand-eye calibration, 3 to 32 endoscope poses and all possible motions between them were used to estimate the transformation from sensor to camera,

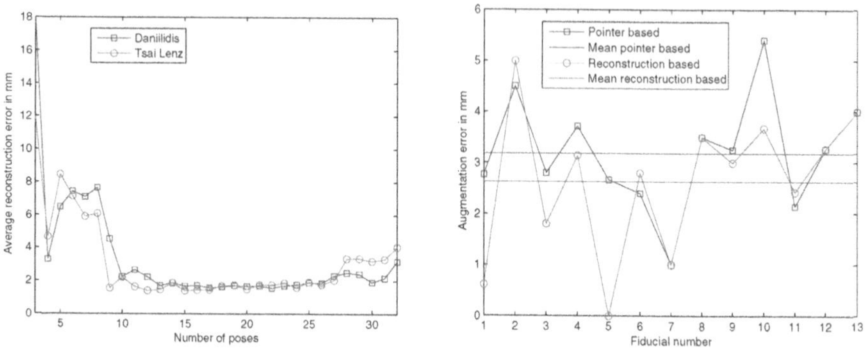

(a) Average reconstruction error for retroreflective markers depending on the hand-eye calibration method and number of poses

(b) The augmentation error for all 13 fiducials measured directly in the video

Fig. 2. Experimental reconstruction and augmentation error

resulting in 30 transformation matrices. To validate these matrices, the positions of 9 retroreflective spherical markers were reconstructed from 6 endoscopic images. These reconstructions were compared to the measurements of the optical tracking system. The average distance of the reconstructed points to the measurements of the tracking system was computed for each transformation matrix. As visualized in figure 2(a), a typical hand-eye calibration incorporating 10 to 25 poses gave errors between 1.4 and 2 millimeters. The described hand-eye calibration is done off-line, so above results remain valid for a long period of time and only need to be verified every now and then.

To determine the augmentation error during port placement, 13 CT visible spherical fiducials with a diameter of 4 mm were attached to a plastic thorax phantom containing a heart model. After a CT scan and segmentation of all fiducials, the phantom was placed arbitrarily. The 3D positions of 4 fiducials were reconstructed automatically by moving the tracked endoscope around them, using 3 to 4 images from differing poses for each fiducial. The other 9 fiducials were just used later for validating the augmentation from many different viewing directions, so in practice they are not needed. Next, the CT-to-tracking transformation of the 4 fiducials was computed.

Having the sensor-to-camera and CT-to-tracking transformations as well as intrinsic camera parameters and distortion coefficients, the endoscopic images can be undistorted and the CT volume can be augmented on them. To verify the augmentation, the distances of all 13 fiducials from the real images to a semi-transparent augmentation in an orthogonal view were measured. An average error of 2.6 mm could be determined. This is fully sufficient for a precise port placement. We also compared our automatic 3D reconstruction method to a pointer based approach. Therefore, a pointing device tracked by the optical tracking system was used to record the positions of the 4 fiducials. Again, the CT-to-tracking transformation was computed and used for the augmentation.

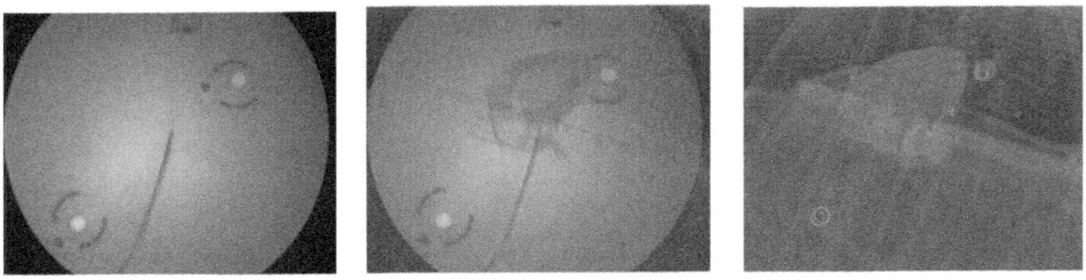

(a) Real (b) Augmented (c) Virtual

Fig. 3. 3 visualization modes for the same endoscope pose: 3(a): Real camera image, 3(b): Transparent augmented view outlining fiducials, ribs, and heart (the virtual green contours correctly match the white fiducials in the video image), 3(c): Purely virtual view, which can be used for port placement to move the camera in and out

With this method, we only achieved an average error of 3.2 mm, i.e. our method almost systematically performs better than the pointer based one. The comparison is visualized in figure 2(b).

A port placement application was implemented offering three visualization modes, as displayed on figure 3. In the first mode, the undistorted real endoscopic image is displayed. The second mode additionally augments the volume on the phantom in a half-transparent mode, so the accuracy of the overlay can be verified by the surgeon. In a third purely virtual mode the surgeon can switch the endoscope optics from 30 degrees to 0 degrees and move the camera in and out the volume along the endoscope's main axis to validate a possible port. The augmentation of a 512×512×444 CT volume and undistortion of the camera frames with a resolution of 800×600 pixels was achieved in real time (15 fps).

6 Conclusion

In this work we addressed and solved two substantial problems of current approaches dealing with the improvement and automation of port placement: Time-consuming segmentation of patient's anatomy and inadequate patient registration. Moreover, our technique not only supports the surgeon during port placement, it also enhances the endoscopic images by undistortion. Besides the tracking system used to determine the endoscope's pose no further tracking system is needed. We reckon that our technique can supplement the current clinical work flow easily, because we keep it simple and still leave the control to the surgeon during port placement. Apart from the pre-operative attachment of 4 fiducials to the patient and a short and intuitive intra-operative patient registration procedure we do not alter the conventional clinical work flow. Our method can be applied to any minimally invasive endoscopic procedure provided that pre-operative patient data is available.

This method is more precise than the usual method of pointing the robot or hand-held endoscope/instrument to each fiducial. It also fits more smoothly into the surgical work flow, as it only requires the surgical staff to move the endoscope camera over the patient's body. Our work does not address organ deformations and motions caused by the insufflation of carbon dioxide and respiratory as well as cardiovascular effects. In this sense, the system only provides an approximative result and relies on the surgeon's expertise for further considerations of possible deformations.

Acknowledgements. This work was supported in part by the German Research Foundation (DFG) within the Collaborative Research Centre SFB 453 on "High-Fidelity Telepresence and Teleaction". We like to thank A.R.T. GmbH for providing the tracking system.

References

1. Adhami, L., Coste-Manière, È.: A versatile system for computer integrated mini-invasive robotic surgery. In: MICCAI '02, Japan (2002) 272–281
2. Chiu, A.M., Dey, D., Drangova, M., Boyd, W.D., Peters, T.M.: 3-d image guidance for minimally invasive robotic coronary artery bypass. HSF **3** (2000) 224–231
3. Selha, S.D., Dupont, P.E., Howe, R.D., Torchiana, D.F.: Dexterity optimization by port placement in robot-assisted minimally invasive surgery. In: Proceedings of SPIE TTT VIII. Volume 4570. (2002) 97–104
4. Traub, J., Feuerstein, M., Bauer, M., Schirmbeck, E.U., Najafi, H., Bauernschmitt, R., Klinker, G.: Augmented reality for port placement and navigation in robotically assisted minimally invasive cardiovascular surgery. In: CARS 2004, Chicago, USA (2004) 735–740
5. Tsai, R., Lenz, R.: Real time versatile robotics hand/eye calibration using 3d machine vision. In: CRA88. (1988) 554–561
6. Daniilidis, K.: Hand-eye calibration using dual quaternions. The International Journal of Robotics Research **18** (1999) 286–298
7. Mourgues, F., Coste-Manière, È.: Flexible calibration of actuated stereoscopic endoscope for overlay in robot assisted surgery. In: MICCAI, Japan (2002) 25–34
8. Bouguet, J.Y.: Camera calibration toolbox for Matlab. `http://www.vision.caltech.edu/bouguetj/calib_doc/` (2004)
9. Hartley, R.I., Zisserman, A.: Multiple View Geometry in Computer Vision. Second edn. Cambridge University Press, ISBN: 0521540518 (2004)
10. Wang, M.Y., Maurer, C. R., J., Fitzpatrick, J.M., Maciunas, R.J.: An automatic technique for finding and localizing externally attached markers in ct and mr volume images of the head. IEEE Trans Bio Med Eng **43** (1996) 627–637
11. Nicolau, S., Garcia, A., Pennec, X., Soler, L., Ayache, N.: Augmented reality guided radio-frequency tumor ablation. CAVW **16** (2005)
12. Trucco, E., Verri, A.: Introductory Techniques for 3-D Computer Vision. Prentice Hall PTR (1998)
13. Sturm, P., Ramalingam, S., Lodha, S.K.: On calibration, structure-from-motion and multi-view geometry for panoramic camera models. In: Panoramic Photogrammetry Workshop, Berlin, Germany (2005)
14. Gold, S., Rangarajan, A.: A graduated assignment algorithm for graph matching. IEEE Trans. Pattern Anal. Mach. Intell. **18** (1996) 377–388
15. Walker, M.W., Shao, L., Volz, R.A.: Estimating 3-d location parameters using dual number quaternions. CVGIP: Image Underst. **54** (1991) 358–367
16. Shahidi, R., et al: Implementation, calibration and accuracy testing of an image-enhanced endoscopy system. IEEE Trans. Med. Imaging **21** (2002) 1524–1535

Hybrid Formulation of the Model-Based Non-rigid Registration Problem to Improve Accuracy and Robustness

Olivier Clatz[1,2], Hervé Delingette[1], Ion-Florin Talos[2], Alexandra J. Golby[2], Ron Kikinis[2], Ferenc A. Jolesz[2], Nicholas Ayache[1], and Simon K. Warfield[3]

[1] Epidaure Research Project, INRIA Sophia Antipolis, France
[2] Surgical Planning Laboratory, Harvard Medical School, Boston, USA
[3] Computational Radiology Laboratory, Brigham and Women's Hospital, Children's Hospital, Harvard Medical School, Boston, USA

Abstract. We present a new algorithm to register 3D pre-operative Magnetic Resonance (MR) images with intra-operative MR images of the brain. This algorithm relies on a robust estimation of the deformation from a sparse set of measured displacements. We propose a new framework to compute iteratively the displacement field starting from an approximation formulation (minimizing the sum of a regularization term and a data error term) and converging toward an interpolation formulation (least square minimization of the data error term). The robustness of the algorithm is achieved through the introduction of an outliers rejection step in this gradual registration process. We ensure the validity of the deformation by the use of a biomechanical model of the brain specific to the patient, discretized with the finite element method. The algorithm has been tested on six cases of brain tumor resection, presenting a brain shift up to 13 mm.

1 Introduction

1.1 Image-Guided Neurosurgery

The development of intra-operative imaging systems has contributed to improving the course of intracranial neurosurgical procedures. Among these systems, the intra-operative magnetic resonance scanner offers the possibility to acquire full brain MR images in less than 4 minutes.

Intra-operative measurements show that the deformation of the brain is an important source of error that needs to be considered. Indeed, imaging the brain during the procedure makes the tumor resection more effective, and provides additional guidance for the complete resections in critical brain areas. However, even if the intra-operative MR scanner provides significantly more information than any other intra-operative imaging system, it is not clinically possible to

J. Duncan and G. Gerig (Eds.): MICCAI 2005, LNCS 3750, pp. 295–302, 2005.

acquire image modalities like diffusion tensor MR, functional MR or high resolution MR images in a reasonable time during the procedure.

Non rigid registration algorithms provide a way to overcome the intra-operative acquisition problem: instead of a time consuming acquisition of images during the procedure (dt-MRI, f-MRI or high resolution MRI), the intra-operative deformation is estimated based on fast acquisition of intra-operative images. This transformation is then applied to match the pre-operative images on the intra-operative data.

1.2 Non-rigid Registration for Image-Guided Surgery

Simplified biomechanical linear models have been used to interpolate the full brain deformation based on the measure of surface displacements (brain, ventricles). Audette [1] measured the visible intra-operative cortex shift using a laser range scanner. Ferrant [2] extracted the full cortex and ventricles surfaces from intra-operative MR images. These interpolation-based registration methods however suffer from a decrease of accuracy when reaching internal structures far from the measured surface.

These models are introduced through the energy minimization formulation of the registration problem as a regularization component. In 1998, Yeung [3] showed impressive registration results on a phantom using an energy minimization formulation combining ultrasound speckle tracking with a mechanical finite element model. Rohr et al. [4] combined elastic regularization with an improved block matching (BM) algorithm relying on relevant anatomical landmarks and taking into account the anisotropic matching error. In 2001, Rexilius [5] combined feature point correspondences with a finite element biomechanical model in an approximation formulation to capture brain shift.

2 Method

We have developed a patient-specific registration algorithm to measure the brain deformation based on two images acquired before and during the brain surgery. This algorithm can be decomposed into three main parts. The first part consists in building a biomechanical model specific to the patient corresponding to his position in the open-magnet scanner. The second part is the block (or template) matching computation for selected blocks. The third part is the new iterative hybrid solver which alternates an energy minimization step with an outlier rejection step.

In addition, we address the problem of discriminant information distribution in the images (known as the aperture problem in computer vision) to make the registration process dependent on the spatial distribution of the information given by the structure tensor (see Section 2.1 for definition).

In the following section, we propose a description of the algorithm sequence, making a distinction between off line (before the first MR acquisition to be registered) and on-line computations.

2.1 Pre-operative MR Image Processing

Segmentation. We use the *Brainvisa* software[1] to automatically segment the brain in the pre-operative images (see Figure 1, B). The tumor segmentation is manually delineated by the physician for the pre-operative planning.

Rigid Registration. An initial intra-operative MR image is acquired at the very beginning of the procedure, before opening the dura-mater. This image is used to compute the rigid transformation between the two positions of the patient in the pre-operative image and the intra-operative image.

Biomechanical Model. The patient-specific brain tetrahedral mesh is build from the previous segmentation using the GHS3D mesher [6]. The mesh generated has an average number of 1700 vertices (the surface mesh is displayed on figure 1, B), which shows to be a reasonable trade-off between the number of degrees of freedom and the number of matches.

We rely on the finite element theory and consider a quasi-incompressible linear elastic constitutive equation to characterize the mechanical behavior of the brain parenchyma: $E = 694Pa$ and $\nu = 0.45$. Even if CSF is incompressible, the CSF is free to flow between the ventricles and the subarachnoid space. We thus assume very soft and compressible volumes for the ventricles: $E = 10Pa$ and $\nu = 0.05$.

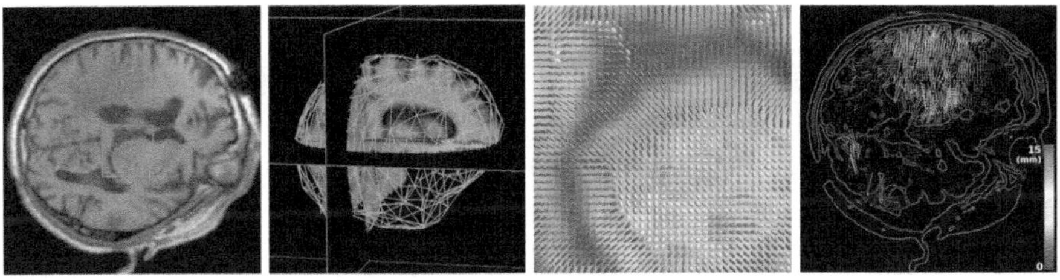

A B C D

Fig. 1. Illustration of the pre-operative processes. (A) pre-operative image. (B) segmentation of the brain and mesh generation (we only represent the surface mesh for visualization convenience). (C) Structure tensor visualization as ellipsoids (zoom on the square area), the color encodes the fractional anisotropy. (D) Example of a sparse displacement field computed with the block matching (BM) algorithm (5 % of the total voxels are selected as blocks centers). Color encodes displacement.

Block Selection. The relevance of a displacement estimated with a block matching (BM) algorithm depends on the presence of highly discriminant structures in this block. We use the variance of the block to measure its relevance, and only select a fraction of all potential block positions based on this criterion. In addition, we introduce the notion of prohibited connectivity between two block centers to prevent two selected blocks to be too close from each other. We obtained best results using the 26 connectivity, preventing two distinct blocks of $7 \times 7 \times 7$ voxels to share more than 42% overlapping voxels.

[1] `http://www.brainvisa.info/`

Computation of the Structure Tensor. We consider the normalized structure tensor T_k defined in the image I at position O_k by:

$$T_k = \frac{G * (\nabla I(O_k))(\nabla I(O_k))^T}{trace\left[G * (\nabla I(O_k))(\nabla I(O_k))^T\right]} \tag{1}$$

Where G defines a convolution kernel (chosen constant in a block). Considering the classical ellipsoid representation, the more the underlying image resembles to a sharp edge, the more the structure tensor elongates in the direction orthogonal to this edge (see Figure 1, C).

2.2 Block Matching Algorithm

The block matching (BM) algorithm makes the assumption that a global deformation results in translation for small parts of the image: considering a block $B(O_k)$ in the reference image centered in O_k, and a similarity metric between two blocks $M(B_a, B_b)$, it consists in finding the positions O'_k that maximize the similarity:

$$\arg\max_{O'_k} \left[M\left(B\left(O_k\right), B\left(O'_k\right)\right)\right] \tag{2}$$

In our algorithm, the BM is performed once and only in the sgmented brain, thus restricting the displacements to the intra-cranial area (see Figure 1, D). Considering the mono-modal (MR-T1 weighted) nature of our registration problem, the correlation coefficient appears as a natural choice for the similarity measure.

2.3 Iterative Hybrid Algorithm

The approximation problem can be formulated as an energy minimization, composed of a mechanical and a matching (or error) energy:

$$W_{approx} = \underbrace{U^T K U}_{Mechanical\ energy} + \underbrace{(HU - D)^T S (HU - D)}_{Matching\ energy} \tag{3}$$

with:

- U the displacement vector (of mesh vertices), of size $3n$, with n number of vertices.
- K the mesh stiffness matrix of size $3n \times 3n$.
- H is the linear interpolation matrix in tetrahedra of size $3p \times 3n$.
- D the block-matching computed displacement vector of size $3p$, with p number of matched points. Note that $HU - D$ defines the estimated displacement error vector.
- S is a block-diagonal matrix composed of 3×3 sub-matrices $S_k = \frac{\alpha}{p} c_k T_k$. The influence of a block thus depends on two factors:
  1. the value of the coefficient of correlation (c_k): the better the correlation is (coefficient of correlation closer to 1), then the higher the influence of the block on the registration will be.

2. The direction of matching with respect to the tensor of structure (T_k): we only consider the matching direction co-linear to the orientation of the intensity gradient in the block.

The $\frac{1}{p}$ factor is used to make the global matching energy independent of the number of selected blocks.

The approximation formulation however entails a systematic error: the final displacement of the brain mesh is a trade-off between the pre-operative rest position and the BM positions. An alternative approach is the interpolation formulation. The problem is turned into a mechanical energy minimization under the constraint of minimum data error, formalized with the Lagrange multipliers stored in the vector $\tilde{F}$ as:

$$\tilde{W}_{interp} = U^T K U + \tilde{F}^T H^T S \left(HU - D\right) \tag{4}$$

However, when some of the BM displacements are outliers, the minimization of Equation 4 may lead to unrealistic deformations.

Therefore, we propose a new iterative formulation of the registration problem:

$$\begin{cases} F_i \Leftarrow KU_i \\ U_{i+1} \Leftarrow \left[K + H^T SH\right]^{-1} \left[H^T SD + F_i\right] \end{cases} \tag{5}$$

which first solves the approximation problem (Equation 3) and gradually converges toward the interpolation solution (Equation 4). Equation 5 is iterated until the displacement modifications are smaller than a threshold. At each iteration, outliers are rejected, such that we get a more robust and unbiased estimate of the displacement. Note that H, S and D thus have to be recomputed at each iteration i.

Outlier Rejections. We introduced a robust block-rejection step based on a least-trimmed squares (LTS) estimator [7]. The LTS rejects a fraction of the total blocks based on an error function ξ_k measuring for block k the error between the current mesh displacement and the matching target:

$$\xi_k = \frac{\| S_k \left[(HU)_k - D_k\right] \|}{\lambda \, \|(HU)_k\| + 1} \tag{6}$$

D_k, $(HU)_k$ and $[(HU)_k - D_k]$ respectively define the BM displacement, the current mesh-induced displacement and the current displacement error for block k. λ is a parameter of the algorithm tailored to the error distribution on matches. With such a cost function, the rejection criterion is more flexible with points that account for larger displacements. In practice, this parameter was set to 0.5 for all our registrations. Although the least trimmed squares estimator is a robust estimator up to 50% of outliers [7], we experienced that a cumulated rejection representing 25% of the total initial selected blocks is sufficient to reject every significant outlier. The last parameter remaining in the algorithm is the matching stiffness α. We chose a matching stiffness $\alpha = \frac{trace(K)}{n}$, reflecting the average vertex stiffness (note that this value does not depend on the number of vertices used to mesh the volume), so that at least half of the displacement is already recovered after the first iteration step.

Algorithm 1 Registration scheme

Get the number of rejection steps n_R from user
Get the fraction of total blocks rejected f_R from user
for $i = 0$ to n_R **do**
  $F_i \Leftarrow KU_i$
  $U_{i+1} \Leftarrow \left[K + H^T SH\right]^{-1} \left[H^T SD + F_i\right]$
  for all Blocks k **do**
    Compute error function ξ_k
  end for
  Reject $\frac{f_R}{n_R}$ blocks with highest error function ξ
  Recompute $S,\ H,\ D$
end for
repeat
  $F_i \Leftarrow KU_i$
  $U_{i+1} \Leftarrow \left[K + H^T SH\right]^{-1} \left[H^T SD + F_i\right]$
until Convergence

Implementation Issues and Time Constraint. We developed a parallel version of the algorithm, reducing the computation time from 162 to 25 seconds on an heterogeneous group of 15 PCs.

3 Results

3.1 Experiments

We evaluated our algorithm using the same parameters on 6 pairs of pre and intra-operative[2]. Figure 2 presents the results for the slice showing the largest displacement, in depth results can be seen on: `http://splweb.bwh.harvard.edu:8000/pages/ppl/oclatz/registration/results.html`. The quantitative accuracy of the algorithm has been evaluated by a medical expert selecting 54 corresponding feature points in the registration result image and the intra-operative image. This landmark-based error estimation has been performed on every image for 9 different points. Figure 3 shows the distribution of the landmark-based registration error as a function of the displacement of the tissue (left) and of the distance to the tumor (right). The average error on the 54 landmarks (0.75 mm) indicates that this algorithm is valuable for image guided therapy. The error however tends to increase in the area close to the tumor (right graph, Figure 3). We can observe that the quality of the brain segmentation has a direct influence on the deformed image, for example patient 3 of Figure 2 had a brain mask eroded on the frontal lobe which induces a missing part in the registered image. The deformation field however does not suffer from the mask inaccuracy, since the brain segmentation is not directly used to guide the registration. The assumption of local translation assumed in the block-matching

[2] $256 \times 256 \times 58$ slice (0.86 mm, 0.86 mm, 2.5 mm) acquired with the 0.5 T open magnet system of the Brigham and Women's hospital.

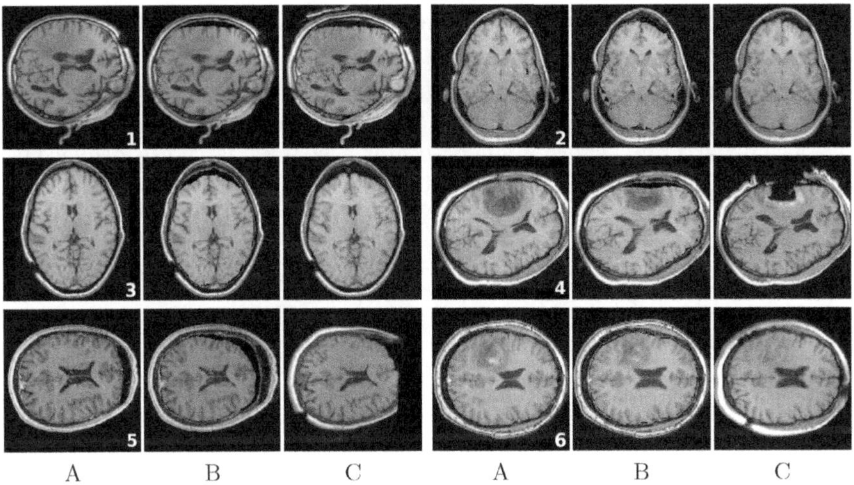

Fig. 2. Result of the non rigid registration of the pre-operative image on the intra-operative image for the 6 patient of our dataset. For each patient, column A shows the pre-operative image, column B shows the result of the registration and column C shows the intra-operative image (target image). The algorithm could recover large displacements (#5), and demonstrates robustness in presence of large resection (#4).

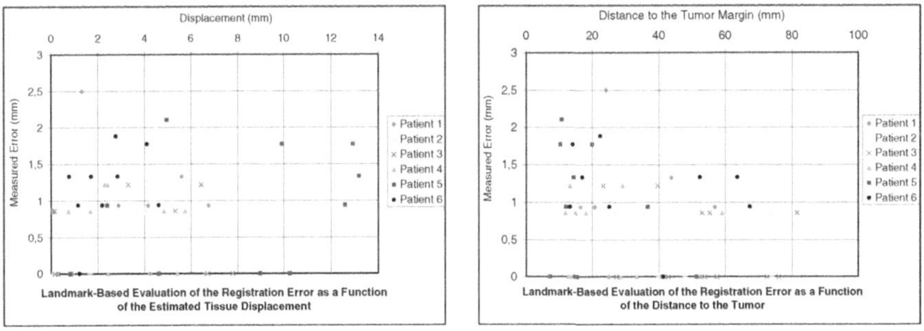

Fig. 3. Measure of the registration error for 54 landmarks. (Left) as a function of the initial arror. (Right) as a function of the distance to the tumor margin. Characteristic figures: average displacement = 3.77 mm, maximum displacement = 13.18 mm, average error = 0.75 mm, maximum error = 2.50 mm.

algorithm seems to be well adapted to the motion of the brain parenchyma. It somehow shows limitations for ventricles expansion (patient 4 and 6 of Figure 2) or collapse (patient 5 of Figure 2), where the error is approximately between two and three millimeters.

3.2 Conclusion

We presented in this article a new registration algorithm designed for robust non-rigid registration of intra-operative MR images. The algorithm has been motivated by the concept of using robust estimators to gradually move from an approximation to an interpolation formulation of the non rigid registration problem.

The results obtained with the six patients demonstrate the applicability of our algorithm to clinical cases. This method seems to be well suited to capture the mechanical brain deformation based on a sparse and noisy displacement field, limiting the error in critical regions of the brain (such as in the tumor segmentation). The remaining error may be due to the limitation of the linear elastic model.

In the future, we wish to adapt multi-scale methods to our problem, to compute near real-time deformations.

Acknowledgments. This investigation was supported by NIH grants R21 MH67054, R01 LM007861, P41 RR13218, P01 CA67165 and by a research grant from the Whitaker Foundation.

References

1. Audette, M.: Anatomical Surface Identifcation, Range-sensing and Registration for Characterizing Intrasurgical Brain Deformations. PhD thesis, McGill University (2003)
2. Ferrant, M., Nabavi, A., Macq, B., Black, P., Jolesz, F., Kikinis, R., Warfield, S.: Serial registration of intraoperative MR images of the brain. Medical Image Analysis **6** (2002) 337–360
3. Yeung, F., Levinson, S., Fu, D., Parker, K.: Feature-adaptive motion tracking of ultrasound image sequences using a deformable mesh. IEEE Transactions on Medical Imaging **17** (1998) 945–956
4. Rohr, K., Stiehl, H., Sprengel, R., Buzug, T., Weese, J., Kuhn, M.: Landmark-based elastic registration using approximating thin-plate splines. IEEE Transactions on Medical Imaging **20** (2001) 526–534
5. Rexilius, J., Warfield, S., Guttmann, C., Wei, X., Benson, R., Wolfson, L., Shenton, M., Handels, H., Kikinis1, R.: A novel nonrigid registration algorithm and applications. In: Medical Image Computing and Computer-Assisted Intervention (MICCAI'01). Volume 2208 of LNCS., Springer (2001) 923–931,
6. Frey, P.J., George, P.L.: Mesh Generation. Hermes Science Publications (2000)
7. Rousseeuw, P.: Least median-of-squares regression. Journal of the American Statistical Association **79** (1984) 871–880

Automatic Registration and Fusion of Ultrasound with CT for Radiotherapy

Wolfgang Wein[1], Barbara Röper[2], and Nassir Navab[1]

[1] Computer Aided Medical Procedures (CAMP) Group, TU Munich, Boltzmannstr. 3, 85748 Garching, Germany
{wein, navab}@cs.tum.edu

[2] Clinic and Policlinic of Radiation Oncology, Klinikum Rechts der Isar, TU Munich, Ismaninger Str. 22, 81675 Munich, Germany
barbara.roeper@lrz.tum.de

Abstract. We present a framework for rigid registration of a set of B-mode ultrasound images to a CT scan in the context of Radiotherapy planning. Our main focus is on deriving an appropriate similarity measure based on the physical properties and artifacts of ultrasound. A combination of a weighted Mutual Information term, edge correlation, clamping to the skin surface and occlusion detection is able to assess the alignment of structures in ultrasound images and simulated slices generated from the CT data. Hence a set of ultrasound images, whose relative transformations are given by a magnetic tracking device, can be registered automatically to the CT scan. We validated our methods on neck data of patients with head and neck tumors and cervical lymph node metastases.

1 Introduction

Overview. Registration of ultrasound images to three-dimensional tomographic modalities such as CT and MRI is receiving a lot of attention in the past few years. On one hand, many intra-operative procedures, especially in neurology and orthopedics, can be guided with ultrasound while integrating pre-operative information from CT/MRI. On the other hand, data fusion for diagnosis and treatment planning can improve the outcome as well.

In the particular application of radiation treatment planning for inoperable head and neck cancer the identification of metastatic neck lymph nodes is mandatory for the correct target volume delineation. This can be achieved with a reported accuracy of 80-95% using high-frequency ultrasound [1]. However, the target volume definition is done on individual slices of a planning CT scan. In direct comparison with ultrasonography, diagnostic CT was equally predictive in revealing lymph node size, but performed worse in depicting internal nodal architecture, leading to a lower sensitivity and specificity than ultrasonography [2]. As in planning CTs for radiotherapy contrast medium is usually omitted, their diagnostic properties are particularly poor. Therefore, transferring the diagnostic information from ultrasound onto the CT data could yield a more precise treatment.

J. Duncan and G. Gerig (Eds.): MICCAI 2005, LNCS 3750, pp. 303–311, 2005.

In general, registration of multimodal data is especially desirable if they provide complementary information. At the same time, this complementary nature hampers image-based registration algorithms, which try to align structures present in both modalities. In our work, we will try to overcome some of these problems for ultrasound-CT registration.

Related Work. Due to the very different characteristics of ultrasound imaging with respect to CT / MRT, a lot of research has been carried out on using features extracted from the ultrasound images, in order to align them with corresponding structures in other modalities. Possible anatomical features comprise vessels [3,4], bone surfaces [5], organ surfaces [6]. Pure intensity-based registration has been performed mainly for 3D ultrasonic data. Roche et al. [7] use an adapted correlation ratio similarity measure in order to register the ultrasonic data simultaneously to both the intensity and the gradient information of a MRI scan. A registration involving an automatic mapping of MR and Ultrasound data to Vessel probability values and successive registration of this information is proposed in [8]. Using a CT data of a kidney, where the intensity values are enhanced with strong edges from the gradient, a registration with freehand 3D ultrasound is performed in [9]. Voxel-based registration of MRA scans with Power Doppler ultrasound has been evaluated in [10].

2 Methods

2.1 Simulation from CT

Instead of a realistic simulation of ultrasound, we need an intelligent and efficient intermediate representation of the CT data at arbitrary cut-planes, such that an iterative registration can be performed in an acceptable time. These slices have multiple components containing intensity, gradient and edge information, which are used to derive various parts of a similarity metric, so that the correspondence of anatomy contained therein with structures in 2D B-mode ultrasound images can be determined.

In our approach, first the three-dimensional gradient vector values are computed from the CT data set by convolution with a sobel filter cube. They are stored in a 4-channel volume together with the original voxel intensity. The interpolated slices contain four channels as well. For each pixel, the 4-vector is computed from the volume using trilinear interpolation. In the first channel of the slice, the original CT intensity is stored. The 3D gradient vector is scalar multiplied with each of the vectors indicating the horizontal and vertical slice plane directions, respectively. The resulting values, corresponding to the 2D gradient of the CT intensity within the slice, are stored in the second and third channel.

The 2D slice gradient values are then used to perform Canny edge-detection on the slice data, storing the result in the fourth channel. The most time-consuming steps within the Canny algorithm for 2D images are the computation of the 2D gradients, as well as filtering them with a sufficiently large Gaussian kernel for smoothing. As we compute the 2D gradients directly from the pre-computed 3D gradient values, we do not need to run a 2D filtering for gradient computation. In addition, those gradients are very smooth, as they originate from a three-dimensional Sobel filter using a 27-neighborhood. This makes further Gaussian filtering unnecessary. The two remaining steps for the Canny algorithm, non-maxima suppression and hysteresis thresholding, can be performed each in one traversal of the 2D slice. The horizontal gradient is weighted with a user-defined factor between 0 and 1, as the ultrasound data tends to show mainly vertical edges.

Thus we are able to construct intermediate slices from the CT data at estimated transformations of the US scan plane in very little time[1]. The individual components of the slice pixels are then used to compute a similarity metric with the ultrasound data.

2.2 Occlusion Handling

If an ultrasonic pulse hits bony structures, all image intensities in the ultrasound image further along the specific ray are occluded, and mainly determined by noise. Therefore, all ultrasound intensity values on a ray below such an occlusion should be disregarded in the registration method. In our implementation, we scan the US image from bottom to top, updating the variances for all ultrasonic pulse rays. Where they exceed a threshold (which is easily determined in the user interface), the first pixel to be considered is defined. Thus, our Region of interest Ω is expressed by the following equations:

$$\Omega = \{(x,y) \mid (y < y_{top}) \wedge (y \geq b(x))\} \tag{1}$$

$$b(x) = \min y \left| \frac{1}{y}\sum_{i=0}^{y-1} U(x,y)^2 - \left(\frac{1}{y}\sum_{i=0}^{y-1} U(x,y)\right)^2 < \sigma_y^2 \right. \tag{2}$$

By applying a median filter on the bottom function $b(x)$, discontinuities are removed before defining the ROI. In addition, we discard all pixels which are located above $y_{top} = \frac{9}{10} size_y$, as we observed that the anatomy is highly compressed there due to the probe pressure on the patients skin. This compressed region is very distinct from the remaining anatomical structures, its size ($3.6mm$) being consistent on all data we obtained from patients (figure 1). This ROI definition is similar to the ones used in [8] and [9].

2.3 Similarity Measure

Based on both the physical properties of the imaging modalities, as well as the visible appearance of their images, we developed several components for a similarity measure, which can in turn be weighted to form a cost function value with respect to the transformation parameters.

[1] $1.1ms$ for a 128^2 pixel slice, interpolated from a $512^2 \cdot 100$ CT/gradient volume, on an AMD Opteron 2.4 Ghz machine.

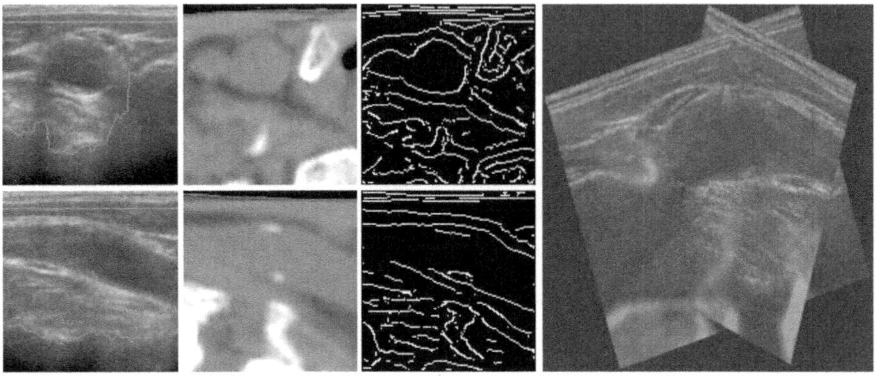

Fig. 1. Two ultrasound images with ROI (red lines) and target, corresponding CT slices, edges from CT, and overlay in 3D. The physical image size is $4 \times 4cm$.

Skin Surface Clamping. In the compressed fraction of the ultrasound image, the interpolation from CT is done with 6 times the vertical scaling (figure 1 on top). As result, the interface between skin and air always has to be within that region, producing a large vertical gradient in the interpolated slice. When all vertical gradient pixels are summed to t, high and low thresholds t_h, t_l can be defined in order to decide if the skin surface lies inside, outside or close to the compressed region:

$$f(t) = \left\{ \begin{array}{cc} 1 & if \quad t > t_h \\ 0 & if \quad t < t_l \\ (t - t_l)/(t_h - t_l) & otherwise \end{array} \right\}; \quad S_0 = 3f(t)^2 - 2f(t)^3 \tag{3}$$

A cubic polynomial is used instead of the linear rise in order to avoid discontinuities. Used as a cost function component, S_0 penalizes transformations which are physically impossible, as the patients skin is always on top of the ultrasound images.

Edge Alignment. As we have detected the edges in the simulated images, we would like to derive a similarity estimate based on the distance to edge structures in the ultrasound images. The straight-forward approach would be to 1) compute an edge-detection for the ultrasound images, 2) compute a 2D distance map for those edges and 3) sum over the distance map values at the locations indicated by the edges of the simulated data. Steps 1) and 2) need to be performed once for each ultrasound slice, while 3) establishes a similarity metric and thus has to be computed for each simulated slice during pose estimation.

However, due to the very different nature of CT and ultrasound data, detected edges do not correspond in general. We therefore propose to skip the edge detection from ultrasound data, instead using the original ultrasound intensity just as indicator for edges.

Given a binary edge image, the distance of an image point $\boldsymbol{x}$ to the edge structures $Y = \{\boldsymbol{y_i}\}$ is $d(\boldsymbol{x}) = \min_i |\boldsymbol{x} - \boldsymbol{y_i}|$. Instead of the euclidian distance, we can also express the proximity to edges by using a Gaussian expression, which allows us to adjust the sensitivity of the cost function value with respect to the distances, using σ^2:

$$d(\boldsymbol{x}) = \max_i \exp - \frac{(\boldsymbol{x} - \boldsymbol{y_i})^2}{\sigma^2} \tag{4}$$

Taking into account that we do not have precise edge information, a proximity value can be defined as

$$d(\boldsymbol{x}) = \sum_i p_i \exp - \frac{(\boldsymbol{x} - \boldsymbol{y_i})^2}{\sigma^2} \tag{5}$$

where $p_i \in [0 \dots 1]$ is the probability for the image pixel $\boldsymbol{y_i}$ being an edge. Assuming that the ultrasound image intensity directly scales with the edge probability, a two-dimensional proximity function $p(\boldsymbol{x})$ can be computed by just convoluting the ultrasound image with a large gaussian kernel. The similarity measure component arises from this as $S_1 = (\overline{p_e} - \overline{p})/\sigma_p$, where $\overline{p}$ is the mean of all values in the proximity image, $\overline{p_e}$ the mean of just the pixels at locations where an edge is present in the simulated image, and σ_p the standard deviation of the proximity image values.

Statistical Correspondence. Different tissues in the anatomy cause different scattering characteristics for ultrasonic waves. Higher scattering in turn causes a larger portion of the ultrasound pulse to be reflected back to the transducer, resulting in higher intensities in the ultrasound image. It is therefore applicable to assess the statistical dependance of the CT intensities, which classify the tissue according to the X-Ray attenuation property, with the intensity in the ultrasound image. We therefore use Mutual Information on the CT and ultrasound intensities. The Normalized Mutual Information term uses the entropies of the combined and individual images, which are computed with the Shannon entropy from probability distributions of the image intensities:

$$\begin{aligned} NMI(U,S) &= 2 - 2H(U,S)/(H(U) + H(S)) \\ H(U) &= -\sum_j p_u(j) \log p_u(j); \quad H(S) = -\sum_i p_s(i) \log p_s(i) \\ H(U,S) &= -\sum_i \sum_j p(i,j) \log p(i,j) \end{aligned}$$

Here U denotes an ultrasound image, and S the corresponding simulated image, i.e. the slice interpolation of CT attenuation values. The probability distributions can be estimated using histogram information from the images:

$$p_u(i) = \frac{1}{n_\Omega} |\{(x,y) \in \Omega | U(x,y) = i\}| \tag{6}$$

$$p_s(j) = \frac{1}{n_\Omega} |\{(x,y) \in \Omega | S(x,y) = j\}| \tag{7}$$

$$p(i,j) = \frac{1}{n_\Omega} |\{(x,y) \in \Omega | U(x,y) = i \wedge S(x,y) = j\}| \tag{8}$$

Here we assume that each intensity value is mapped into one histogram bin, and $n_\Omega = |\Omega|$ is the number of pixels in the region of interest. An equivalent formulation for constructing the probability distribution from a histogram can be written using a binary count function c_u

$$p_u(i) = \frac{1}{n_\Omega} \sum_{(x,y)\in\Omega} c_u(x,y,i); \quad c_u(x,y,i) = \left\{ \begin{matrix} 1\, if \quad U(x,y) = i \\ 0\, otherwise \end{matrix} \right\} \tag{9}$$

Due to the various physical effects in ultrasound imaging, both the chance that an image intensity reflects the anatomy, as well as the Signal to Noise Ratio (SNR), decrease with the distance from the ultrasound transducer. Thus we would like to give more emphasis on image pixels which are closer to the probe, i.e. with higher y values. In our approach, we introduce an integer weighting for assembling the distribution:

$$p'_u(i) = \frac{1}{n'_\Omega} \sum_{(x,y)\in\Omega} (y + c_0) c_u(x,y,i) \tag{10}$$

$$n'_\Omega = \sum_{x=0}^{n_x - 1} \sum_{y=b(x)}^{y_{top}-1} (y + c_0) \tag{11}$$

Every intensity value is inserted $y + c_0$ times into the histograms and the joint histogram. For $c_0 \to \infty$ the original Mutual Information notation is obtained. Our weighted Mutual Information component NMI' of the similarity measure is assembled by inserting all used ultrasound slice images and the corresponding simulations into one histogram, as it increases the statistical significance of the derived entropy terms.

Cost Function. The final similarity measure from a set of n ultrasound slices $\{U_i\}$ and their CT simulations $\{S_i\}$ is

$$cf = w_0 \frac{1}{n} \sum_{i=1}^{n} S_0(U_i, S_i) + w_1 \frac{1}{n} \sum_{i=1}^{n} S_1(U_i, S_i) + w_2 NMI'(\{U_i\}, \{S_i\}) \tag{12}$$

2.4 Registration

In order to manually navigate the stack of ultrasound images to the desired position within the CT data, the user picks a reference slice k, whose position and orientation is changed by left-multiplication with a rigid transformation matrix. At the same time, all other transformations are updated in order for the relative locations to stay fixed, as they originate from the tracker.

For automatic registration, a non-linear optimization method maximizes the cost function cf iteratively with respect to the parameters of a rigid transformation (6 DOF, translation and Euler angles), which is initialized with zero and affects the location of all slices. We used three optimization schemes: simple hill climbing, Powell-Brent and an exhaustive hill climbing. The latter one evaluates all combinations of [forward, keep, backward] for all parameters, using the best result of all $3^6 = 729$ evaluations as estimate for the next iteration.

3 Results

Three head and neck cancer patients with metastatic lymph node involvement were thoroughly examined with a 11 MHz linear array ultrasound probe. The images were recorded using a frame grabber card, while an Ascension microBIRD^{TM}magnetic tracking sensor provided the spatial encoding. A set of 3-10 slices from the right carotid artery of each patient was picked for registration. Figure 1 depicts two slices from the first patient alongside the registered CT data.

A ground truth registration pose was established with manual registration by the physician. This could be done with an estimated precision of $1mm$ in the first data set, as the calcifications in the carotid artery (figure 1) represented good anatomical landmarks.

In order to evaluate the robustness and accuracy of the automatic registration, 200 registrations were launched from initial transformations randomly displaced up to $5mm/5°$ in each parameter around the ground truth pose. The following table denotes both the root mean squared (RMS) error in the translational and rotational components, as well as the target registration error (TRE) for the lymph node (figure 1) picked as target. This evaluation was done for all three used optimization schemes on the data of patient 1.

	trans.	rot.	TRE	iterations	time
Hill Climbing	$1.2mm$	$3.7°$	$2.0mm$	242	$3s$
Powell-Brent	$1.0mm$	$2.8°$	$1.8mm$	4	$8s$
Exhaustive H.C.	$0.8mm$	$2.5°$	$1.2mm$	189	$144s$

All optimization methods are able to converge precisely to the ground truth registration, so that the registered data can be used reliably for therapy planning. To do so, the slices from the original CT data set, which are used to outline

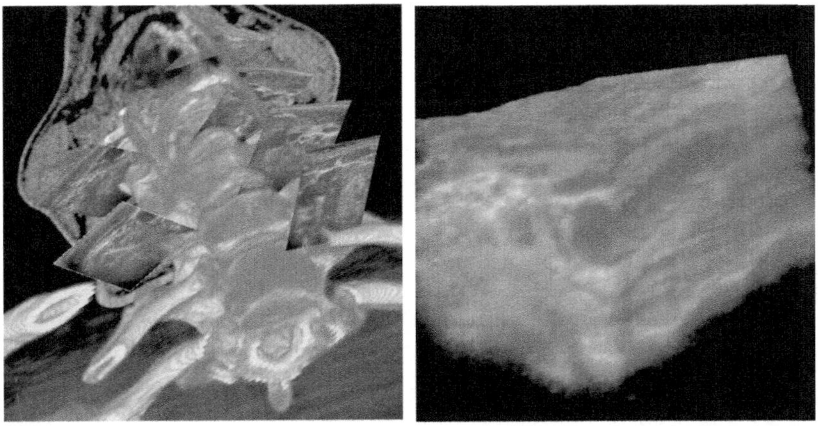

Fig. 2. Left: Overlay of registered ultrasound images, a slice from the CT data set, and CT volume rendering. Right: Volume rendering of compounded 3D ultrasound.

the target volume, are visualized together with the registered ultrasound slices and optionally volume rendering of both the CT and a 3D ultrasound volume spatially compounded from the tracking data (figure 2).

4 Conclusion

We developed methods which allow automatic registration of a set of ultrasound slices to a CT scan, despite the very difficult characteristics for registration of both modalities. The similarity metric is derived from the physical properties of ultrasound imaging, rather than from the particular anatomy used in our experiments. Therefore the algorithms are also applicable on any other part of the human body scanned with an external ultrasound probe. The registration is performed within a few seconds, and is therefore capable of supporting real-time applications, such as intra-operative navigation, as well. We evaluated our methods in the context of radiotherapy for head and neck cancer, where the use of registered data is beneficial for the treatment planning.

Acknowledgements. This research was funded by an academic grant from Siemens Corporate Research, Princeton, USA. The authors would like to thank in particular Frank Sauer and Ali Khamene for their continous support.

References

1. Yonetsu, K., Sumi, M., Izumi, M., Ohki, M., Eida, S., Nakamura, T.: Contribution of doppler sonography blood flow information to the diagnosis of metastatic cervical nodes in patients with head and neck cancer: assessment in relation to anatomic levels of the neck. AJNR Am J Neuroradiol **22** (2001) 163–169
2. Sumi, M., Ohki, M., Nakamura, T.: Comparison of sonography and CT for differentiating benign from malignant cervical lymph nodes in patients with squamous cell carcinoma of the head and neck. AJR Am J Roentgenol **176** (2001) 1019–1024
3. Penney, G.P., Blackall, J.M., Hayashi, D., Sabharwal, T., Adam, A., Hawkes, D.J.: Overview of an ultrasound to CT or MR registration system for use in thermal ablation of liver metastases. In: Proc. Medical Image Understanding and Analysis. (2001) 65–68
4. Porter, B., Rubens, D., Strang, J., Totterman, S., Parker, K.: Three-dimensional registration and fusion of ultrasound and MRI using major vessels as fiducial markers. IEEE Transactions on Medical Imaging **20** (2001) 354–359
5. Amin, D., Kanade, T., Gioia, A.M.D., Jaramaz, B.: Ultrasound registration of the bone surface for surgical navigation. Computer Aided Surgery **8** (2003) 1 – 16
6. Wu, R., Ling, K.V., Shao, W., Ng, W.S.: Registration of organ surface with intraoperative 3D ultrasound image using genetic algorithm. In: MICCAI 2003 Proceedings. (2003) 383–390
7. Roche, A., Pennec, X., Malandain, G., Ayache, N.: Rigid registration of 3D ultrasound with MR images: a new approach combining intensity and gradient information. IEEE Transactions on Medical Imaging **20** (2001) 1038 – 1049

8. Penney, G., Blackall, J., Hamady, M., Sabharwal, T., Adam, A., Hawkes, D.: Registration of freehand 3D ultrasound and magnetic resonance liver images. Medical Image Analysis (2004) 81 – 91
9. Leroy, A., Mozer, P., Payan, Y., Troccaz, J.: Rigid registration of freehand 3D ultrasound and CT-Scan kidney images. In: MICCAI Proceedings. (2004) 837ff
10. Slomka, P., Mandel, J., Downey, D., Fenster, A.: Evaluation of voxel-based registration of 3-D power doppler ultrasound and 3-D magnetic resonance angiographic images of carotid arteries. Ultrasound Med. Biol. **27** (2001) 945–955

Lung Deformation Estimation and Four-Dimensional CT Lung Reconstruction

Sheng Xu[1], Russell H. Taylor[1], Gabor Fichtinger[1], and Kevin Cleary[2]

[1] Engineering Research Center, Johns Hopkins University, Baltimore, MD 21218, MD USA
{sheng, rht, gabor}@cs.jhu.edu
[2] Imaging Science and Information Systems (ISIS) Center, Department of Radiology, Georgetown University Medical Center, Washington, DC 20007, USA
cleary@georgetown.edu

Abstract. Four-dimensional (4D) computed tomography (CT) image acquisition is a useful technique in radiation treatment planning and interventional radiology in that it can account for respiratory motion of lungs. Current 4D lung reconstruction techniques have limitations in either spatial or temporal resolution. In addition, most of these techniques rely on auxiliary surrogates to relate the time of CT scan to the patient's respiratory phase. In this paper, we propose a novel 4D CT lung reconstruction and deformation estimation algorithm. Our algorithm is purely image based. The algorithm can reconstruct high quality 4D images even if the original images are acquired under irregular respiratory motion. The algorithm is validated using synthetic 4D lung data. Experimental results from a swine study data are also presented.

1 Introduction

In radiation oncology, 4D CT is one technique that can account for respiratory motion during treatment planning. 4D CT may allow for the reduction of target volume margin to achieve increased tumor dose and decreased normal tissue dose [1]. While the radiation dose to the patient may be an issue, particularly if multiple 4D datasets are considered, in general the CT dose will be much less than the treatment dose delivered during radiation therapy. 4D CT may also be used to investigate the motion correlation between the internal tumor and external fiducials such as skin markers. The tumor position could then be estimated during the treatment by tracking the external fiducials. With sufficient 4D CT datasets, a respiratory model might also be constructed to parameterize the respiratory motion.

Most 4D lung reconstruction algorithms reported in the literature can be grouped into the following two approaches. The first approach requires controlling the patient's breath during image acquisition [2]. The respiratory cycle is divided into several phases (usually 7-11). The respiration is halted in each phase while a 3D CT volume is taken. A related technique is to use breathing tracking strategies such as active breathing control [3], [4], [5] to monitor the patient's breath at each phase. The 4D data acquired by this method has high spatial resolution, but very poor temporal resolution. This low temporal resolution limits its usefulness in analyzing the anatomical motion.

J. Duncan and G. Gerig (Eds.): MICCAI 2005, LNCS 3750, pp. 312 – 319, 2005.

The second approach does not try to monitor or control the patient's breath. The patient is allowed to breath freely on the CT table [2], [7]. The table is moved in small increments and a continuous free CT scan is taken at each table position to cover at least one complete respiratory cycle. Some external devices may be used during the scan to synchronize the CT scanning time with the respiratory phase [6], [7]. After image acquisition, all the free scan images are sorted into a sequence of 3D volumes according to their respiratory phase and table positions. This method has high temporal resolution at each table position. The major problem with this method is that respiratory motion is not completely repeatable, so the time stamp of the free scan image may not correlate well with the regular respiratory motion. In such a case, the image quality of the 3D data reconstructed at each respiratory phase will be very poor. It is usually very difficult to stitch these 3D volumes together into a 4D dataset.

Unlike prior methods, we propose a new 4D lung reconstruction method that has good temporal resolution and high reconstruction quality. In addition, our method does not rely on any external gating / tracking devices to synchronize the time of CT scan and the respiratory phase. Therefore problems caused by the discrepancy between the respiratory motion and the auxiliary surrogates are avoided.

2 Method

The outline of our 4D CT lung reconstruction method is as follows. First, a reference 3D CT volume is obtained under a long breath hold. Next, a continuous scan is taken at every table position to obtain a series of 2D images, while the patient is breathing freely. The 2D image series at every table position covers at least one complete respiratory cycle. Using deformable registration, each 2D image is registered to the reference volume to estimate the displacement field of the 2D image with respect to the reference volume. The respiration signal is extracted from the displacement field of each 2D image. This respiration signal is used to synchronize the 2D image series to the respiratory cycle at every table position. After the synchronization, the displacement field for the entire lung volume at every selected respiratory phase is reconstructed, interpolated and smoothed. The 4D lung images are reconstructed by a deformable transformation of the reference volume for the entire respiratory cycle.

2.1 Registration of 2D Image to Reference CT Volume

To calculate the deformation of the 2D image with respect to the reference volume, we divide the 2D image into small overlapping disk regions, and register each of the small regions piece by piece to the reference volume. The local registration algorithm is based on minimizing the Zero Mean Sum of Squared Differences (ZSSD) between a small region in the 2D image and a corresponding one in the reference volume. Quadratic transformation is used to model the deformation between the two regions. As a result, thirty parameters are estimated while the objective function is optimized. The details of the local registration are described in [8].

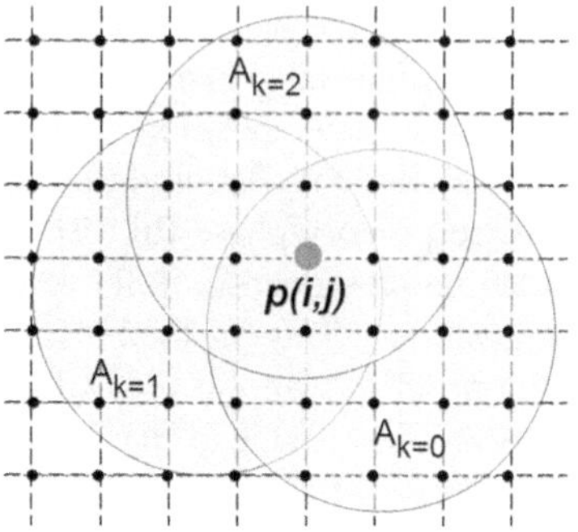

Fig. 1. Propagation of local registration

Since the registrations are performed at each local region, there is no guarantee that all the local registrations converge correctly. A global regularization of the registrations is necessary to remove outliers. In an example shown in Fig. 1, the regions are partially overlapped on each other. Since pixel p is included in all the disk regions A0, A1 and A2, the deformation of pixel p can be calculated from every one of these regions. As shown in equation (1), the final deformation of pixel p is the weighted average of all deformations obtained from the overlapped regions.

$$\hat{d}(i,j) = \sum_k r_k c_k w_k(i,j) d_k(i,j) \tag{1}$$

where d_k is the pixel displacement obtained from the kth region; $\hat{d}$ is the weighted average of the displacement; r_k is a function of the registration error of kth region. r_k will be assigned a large value for small registration error, and vice versa. r_k will be zero if the registration error of a region is above a threshold. c_k is a function of the registration consistency in the overlapping area between the current region k and the previously registered region. c_k will be large if the consistency is high, otherwise c_k will be small. c_k will be zero if the difference between current registration results and the previous registration results is too large. The assumption is that the results from previous registrations are more likely to be correct, because they are the weighted averages of many local registrations. w_k is a Gaussian window function that is centered on the center of region k, allowing the registration results of central pixels to have larger weight. As a result, Equation (1) filters out failed and bad registrations, and assigns large weight to good registrations. Unlike other registration techniques going from coarse to fine resolution, this registration goes from local to global. The algorithm iteratively propagates its local registrations, allowing the regions without enough local texture to be correctly estimated. This is an advantage over the spline-based registration [9] methods that rely on the local information of the control points. This procedure also makes the displacement field of the whole lung very smooth.

The region-based algorithm assumes the pixels of the region to have approximately the same type of motion. It is necessary that all the pixels in the region are lung pixels. If the region includes other pixels such as heart pixels (Fig.2 (b)), the registration is prone to fail, because the selected deformation models cannot explain the pixel motion of the analysis window. For the same reason, the region cannot have chest wall pixels (Fig.2 (a)), nor can the region have pixels from both the left and right lungs (Fig.2 (c)). Therefore, accurate lung segmentation is necessary before the registration, and the left and right lungs should be separated in the 2D images.

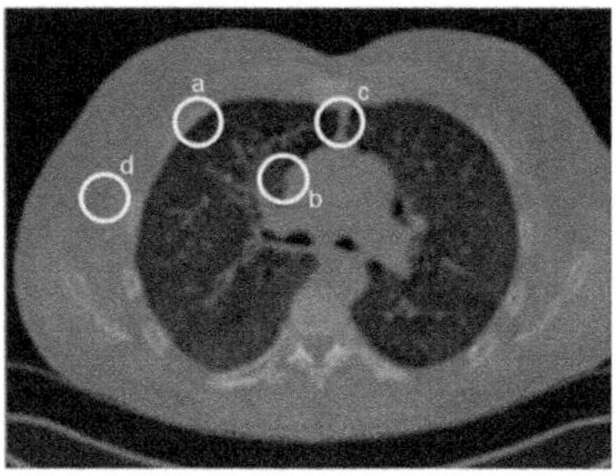

Fig. 2. Undesired regions: (a) both lung pixels and chest-wall pixels are included; (b) both lung pixels and heart pixels are included; (c) both left and right lungs are included (d) non-lung pixels are included

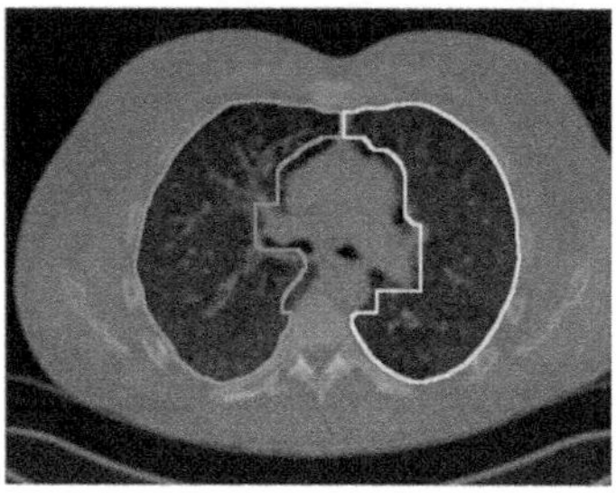

Fig. 3. The result of lung segmentation. Note that (a) the blood vessels are preserved; (b) the heart and chest-wall are removed; (c) the left and right lungs are separated; and (d) the marginal pixels are removed from the heart-lung boundary.

We adopted the techniques of Hu [10] to automatically segment the lungs in the 2D image. Base on their work, morphological closing is executed on the lung area to keep the small to middle blood vessels in the lungs. Extra margin is also introduced in the heart-lung boundary to exclude the artifact caused by the cardiac motion. The result of lung segmentation is shown in Figure 3.

2.2 Four-Dimensional Lung Reconstruction

After all the 2D images are registered to the preoperative lung volume, the average deformation of each image with respect to the reference volume is calculated, yielding a 3D motion vector. For the images taken at the same table position, a sequence of motion vectors is obtained. This vector sequence can be used as the respiration signal to synchronize the 2D image series at different table positions. It is assumed that there is no phase difference of respiratory motion in the craniocaudal direction. Since the tumor's respiratory motion is limited in a few centimeters, this assumption is valid. As a result, the two sequences of motion vectors at two adjacent table positions can be correlated to synchronize the scanning time at the two table positions with respect to the respiratory phase. The correlation is calculated using the following formula:

$$S = \arg\max_{j} \sum_{k=0}^{N-1} \left(\Delta x_k \Delta x'_{j+k} + \Delta y_k \Delta y'_{j+k} + \Delta z_k \Delta z'_{j+k} \right) \tag{2}$$

where N is the total number of frames to be correlated; $(\Delta x_k, \Delta y_k, \Delta z_k)$ is the average deformation of the kth 2D image at the a table position; $(\Delta x'_k, \Delta y'_k, \Delta z'_k)$ is the average deformation for the kth image at another table position; *S* is the number of frame shift between the two image sequences. By repeating this procedure at all table positions, all the 2D images can be synchronized.

Using principal component analysis, the principal axis of the motion trajectory can be obtained. By projecting the average motion on the principal axis, the one-dimensional respiration signal can be extracted. Fig. 4 shows the extracted respiration

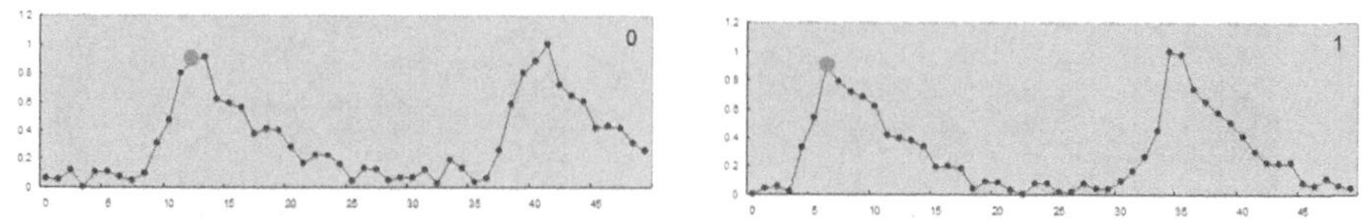

Fig. 4. Respiration signal at two adjacent table positions extracted from swine study. The vertical axis is normalized respiratory phase and the horizontal axis is time in frame number.

signals of two CT fluoroscopy image series obtained in a swine study at two adjacent table positions with an interval of 4mm. It can be observed that the CTF scan time of the two sequences was different with respect to the respiratory cycle. The two dots on the peaks of the respiration signals show the result of synchronization.

After all the 2D image series are synchronized, the 4D lung can be reconstructed by sorting the 2D images. As mentioned in Section 2, the 2D images come from different respiratory cycles. Since the respiratory motion is not completely reproducible, the direct 4D reconstruction by sorting the 2D images can result in very poor image quality. Especially in the coronal and sagittal views, fuzzy edges are usually observed. In response to this problem, we reconstruct the displacement field of the lung volume. In section 2.1, the displacement field of each 2D image has already been calculated from the deformable registration. Each 2D image has also been assigned to a respiratory phase. We generate a displacement field for the entire lung volume by combining the displacement fields of 2D images according to the table position and respiratory phase. The resulting displacement field of the reference volume may not be smooth because it is obtained from different respiratory cycles. However, the displacement field can be smoothed. We use the cubic B-spline [9] to smooth and interpolate the displacement in the cranial-caudal direction to obtain a very smooth displacement for the reference volume. As a result, the 3D volume at any respiratory phase can be computed from a deformable transformation of the reference volume.

3 Experimental Results

We used synthetic 4D data to validate the algorithm. The synthetic 4D data was generated from two lung volumes obtained at the end of inspiration and the end of expiration respectively. The two lung volumes were registered at Siemens Corporate Research using 3D/3D deformable registration. The displacement field between the two volumes was interpolated along the time axis such that the trajectory of each pixel is a 3D curve in space instead of a straight line [11]. The resulting 4D data was used as the ground truth to validate the reconstruction algorithm. The synthetic 2D free scan image series was obtained by sampling the 4D data at the selected table position. With the 2D image series and the lung volume at the end-of-expiration as the reference volume, we ran the algorithm to recover the lung deformation. The pixel size of both the preoperative CT volume and the 2D images was 0.7422mm. The slice thickness of the preoperative CT volume was 1.25mm, and 3.75mm for the synthetic 2D free scan images. The results were first compared to the ground truth to validate the deformable 2D/3D registration.

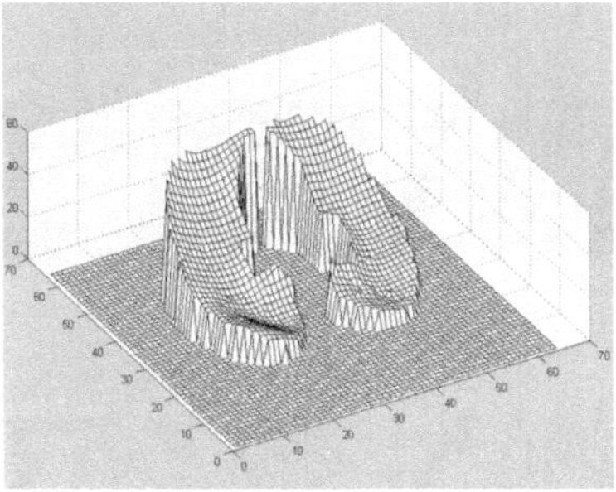

Fig. 5. Displacement magnitude of a CT fluoroscopy image with respect to the reference CT volume in mm

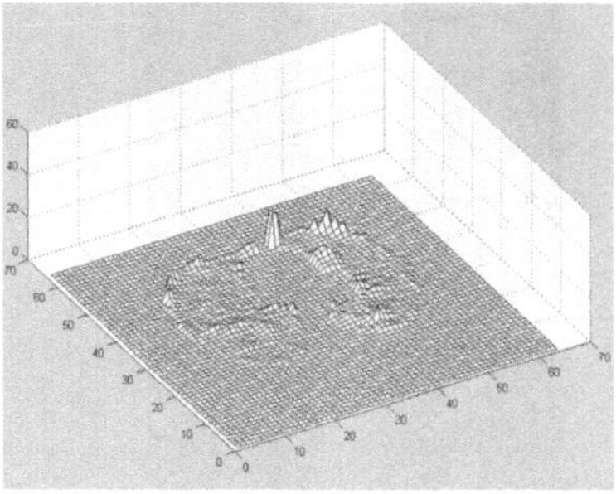

Fig. 6. Magnitude of reconstruction error in mm

Fig. 5 shows the deformation magnitude of a 2D image taken at the end-of-inspiration, when the 2D image has the largest deformation with respect to the reference CT volume. As shown in Fig. 6, most of the poor registrations happen on the boundary pixels of the lung. This problem has three causes. First, for the region-based algorithm, the registration accuracy is usually higher for the pixels near the center of the analysis window. The boundary pixels of lung are usually far from the center of the analysis window. Second, the boundary pixels (especially the boundary pixels near the top of image) have larger deformation than the average. Third, and perhaps most importantly, the areas near the lung boundary often have very little texture information, which may not be enough for the local image registration.

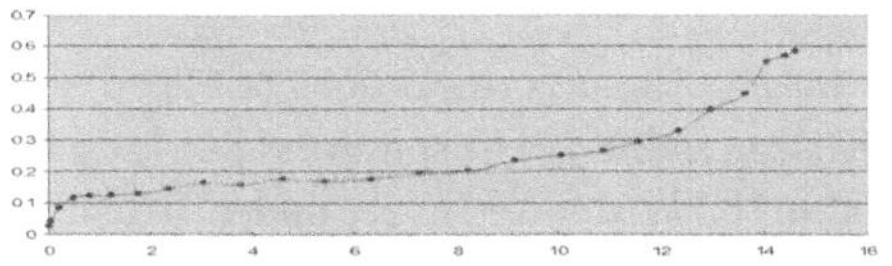

Fig. 7. Average reconstruction error vs. average displacement in mm

Fig. 7 shows the average reconstruction error of the lung pixels compared to the average lung deformation. The maximum average error is 0.6mm. For the respiratory phase with large respiratory motion, the average registration error is below 5% of the average lung deformation.

The algorithm was also tested on the data collected from a swine study as part of an approved animal protocol. This study was done at Georgetown University Medical Center on a Siemens Volume Zoom four-slice CT scanner. The reference volume was obtained at the end-of-expiration using a 1 mm slice thickness. While the animal was mechanically ventilated, for the image acquisition the ventilator was stopped and the animal was temporarily paralyzed to minimize any breathing artifacts. The 2D image series were acquired using CT fluoroscopy with a sample rate of 6Hz and a slice thickness of 4mm. Ten 2D image series were acquired. Fig. 8 and Fig. 9 show the reconstruction results at the end-of inspiration which is the respiratory phase of the maximum deformation with respect to the reference volume. As shown in the figures, the reconstruction result of our algorithm is much smoother compared to the standard image sorting method.

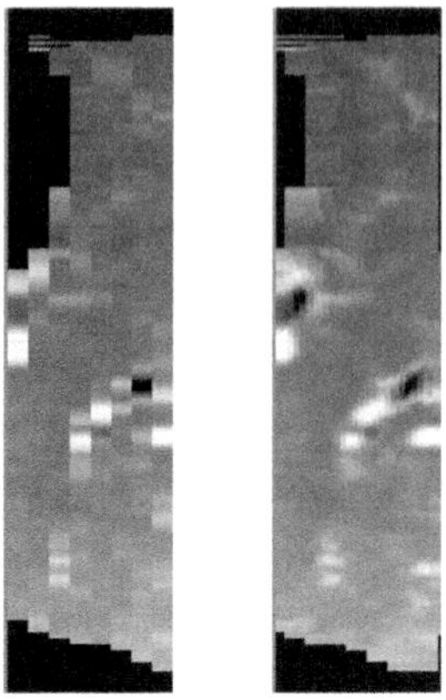

Fig. 8. Sagittal view of 4D reconstruction Left image: image sorting method Right image: our method

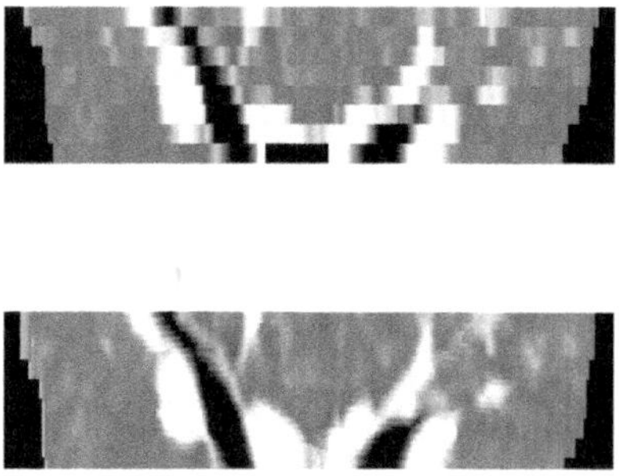

Fig. 9. Coronal view of 4D reconstruction Top image: image sorting method Bottom image: our method

4 Discussion and Conclusions

This paper presents a new methodology to reconstruct the 4D lung image. The temporal resolution of the method is high and the reconstruction provides good quality images. Based on a synthetic CT data set, the average reconstruction /registration error is under 5% of the average lung deformation, which is less than or equal to 0.6mm of respiratory motion. Results from a swine study also showed good correlation.

The algorithm is automated and software based. The algorithm does not need any auxiliary surrogates to synchronize the CT scan with the respiratory phase. The image reconstruction quality of the algorithm is very high even under irregular respiratory motion. The drawback of the algorithm is that it is time consuming. It takes about 5 minutes to register each 2D image to the reference volume. If improved processing speed is needed, the algorithm can be implemented on a parallel processing machine.

Although the algorithm was only tested on the synthetic data of the single slice CT and in one swine study, it can be easily extended for use with multi-slice CT. Since multi-slice CT allows the local region registration to have more texture information, it is expected to see higher accuracy and better robustness of the algorithm.

Acknowledgement. The authors gratefully thank Frank Sauer, Ph.D., Ali Khamene, Ph.D. and Christophe Chefd'hotel, Ph.D. at Siemens Corporate Research for providing the lung dataset. The dataset was originally obtained by the EMC in Rotterdam. The authors also thank David Lindisch, RT, for his assistance with the experiments at Georgetown University. The work was supported by U.S. Army grants DAMD17-99-1-9022 and W81XWH-04-1-0078, NSF Engineering Research Center 9731478.

References

1. Keall, P.: 4-dimensional computed tomography imaging and treatment planning. Semin Radiat Oncol. 14 (2004) 81-90
2. El Naqa, I. M., Low, D. A., Christensen, G. E., Parikh, P. J., Song, J. H., Nystrom, M. M., Lu, W., Deasy, J. O., Hubenschmidt, J. P., Wahab, S. H., Mutic, S., Singh, A. K., Bradley, J. D.: Automated 4D lung computed tomography reconstruction during free breathing for conformal radiation therapy. In: Amini, A. A., Manduca, A. (eds.): Medical Imaging 2004: Physiology, Function, and Structure from Medical Images, Vol. 5369. SPIE (2004) 100-106
3. Boldea, V., Sarrut, D., Clippe, S.: Lung Deformation Estimation with Non-rigid Registration for Radiotherapy Treatment. In: Ellis, R. E., Peters, T. M. (eds.): Medical Image Computing and Computer-Assisted Intervention. Lecture Notes in Computer Science, Vol. 2878. Springer-Verlag GmbH (2003) 770-777
4. Vedam, S. S., Keall, P. J., Kini, V. R., Mostafavi, H., Shukla, H. P., Mohan, R.: Acquiring a four-dimensional computed tomography dataset using an external respiratory signal. Phys Med Biol. 48 (2003) 45-62
5. Underberg, R. W., Lagerwaard, F. J., Cuijpers, J. P., Slotman, B. J., van Sornsen de Koste, J. R., Senan, S.: Four-dimensional CT scans for treatment planning in stereotactic radiotherapy for stage I lung cancer. Int J Radiat Oncol Biol Phys. 60 (2004) 1283-90
6. Pan, T., Lee, T. Y., Rietzel, E., Chen, G. T.: 4D-CT imaging of a volume influenced by respiratory motion on multi-slice CT. Med Phys. 31 (2004) 333-40
7. Ford, E. C., Mageras, G. S., Yorke, E., Ling, C. C.: Respiration-correlated spiral CT: a method of measuring respiratory-induced anatomic motion for radiation treatment planning. Med Phys. 30 (2003) 88-97
8. Xu, S., Fichtinger, G., Taylor, R. H., Cleary, K. R.: 3D motion tracking of pulmonary lesions using CT fluoroscopy images for robotically assisted lung biopsy. In: Galloway, R. L., Jr. (ed.): Medical Imaging 2004: Visualization, Image-Guided Procedures, and Display, Vol. 5367. SPIE (2004) 394-402
9. Unser, M.: Splines - A perfect fit for signal and image processing. Ieee Signal Processing Magazine. 16 (1999) 22-38
10. Hu, S., Hoffman, E. A., Reinhardt, J. M.: Automatic lung segmentation for accurate quantitation of volumetric X-ray CT images. IEEE Trans Med Imaging. 20 (2001) 490-8
11. Xu, S., Fichtinger, G., Taylor, R. H., Cleary, K. R.: Validation of 3D motion tracking of pulmonary lesions using CT fluoroscopy images for robotically assisted lung biopsy. In: Galloway, R. L., Jr., Cleary, K. R. (eds.): Medical Imaging 2005: Visualization, Image-Guided Procedures, and Display, Vol. 5744. SPIE (2005) 60-68

Automatic Parameter Optimization for De-noising MR Data

Joaquín Castellanos[1], Karl Rohr[2], Thomas Tolxdorff[3], and Gudrun Wagenknecht[1]

[1] Central Institute for Electronics, Research Center Jülich, Germany
j.castellanos@fz-juelich.de
[2] Dept. Intelligent Bioinformatics Systems IPMB, University of Heidelberg and DKFZ Heidelberg, Germany
[3] Institute of Medical Informatics, Biostatistics and Epidemiology, Charité - University Medicine Berlin, Germany

Abstract. This paper describes an automatic parameter optimization method for anisotropic diffusion filters used to de-noise 2D and 3D MR images. The filtering process is integrated into a closed-loop system where image improvement is monitored indirectly by comparing the characteristics of the suppressed noise with those of the assumed noise model at the optimal point. In order to verify the performance of this approach, experimental results obtained with this method are presented together with the results obtained by median and k-nearest neighbor filters.

1 Introduction

High-resolution MR images are often affected by noise, causing undesired intensity overlapping of represented tissues, making its posterior segmentation and classification difficult. Traditional linear filters, such as mean or Gaussian filters, commonly used to reduce the noise, do not consider the boundaries originated from regions with different intensities, producing smoothing of these edges and suppression of sharp details. As a result, the produced images are blurred and diffuse.

Anisotropic diffusion filters overcome these shortcomings by adjusting the smoothing (diffusion) strength to the boundaries, thus reducing the noise while preserving edges. The anisotropic diffusion approach arose from the use of the Gaussian filter in multi-scale image analysis [1]. Perona and Malik [2] modified the isotropic diffusion equation (Eq. 1) by making the diffusion coefficient term $c(\bar{x},t)$ a function of the magnitude of the gradient of the image intensity,

$$\frac{\partial}{\partial t} I(\bar{x},t) = div\left(c\left(\bar{x},t\right)\nabla I(\bar{x},t)\right) \qquad (1)$$

where $I(\bar{x},t)$ stands for the processed image at time t, $\bar{x} = (x,y,z)$ the space coordinates, t the iteration step (time) and ∇I the image gradient.

The diffusion coefficient was defined as a monotonically decreasing function $c(\bar{x},t)=f(|\nabla I(\bar{x},t)|)$ of the gradient, which becomes small when the magnitude of

J. Duncan and G. Gerig (Eds.): MICCAI 2005, LNCS 3750, pp. 320–327, 2005.

the gradient is large and approaches one when the gradient is close to zero. Perona and Malik [2] proposed two such diffusion functions, PMAD1 and PMAD2.

$$c_1(\bar{x},t) = \exp - \left(\frac{|\nabla I(\bar{x},t)|}{k} \right)^2 \qquad c_2(\bar{x},t) = \frac{1}{1 + \left(\frac{|\nabla I(\bar{x},t)|}{k} \right)^2} \tag{2}$$

Gerig et al. [3] introduced a discrete anisotropic (non-linear) diffusion algorithm for de-noising MR images. Other diffusion functions were reported by Black et al. [4] and Weickert [5]. Weeratunga et al. [6] assessed the de-noising performance of several diffusion functions using medical and non-medical images. Suri and Wu [7] give an overview of current trends and outlook on future development of the anisotropic diffusion field.

The main parameters which control the behavior of the smoothing process in anisotropic diffusion are the *number of iterations (it)* and the *diffusion factor* k (Eq. 2), which determines the level of gradient intensity where diffusion is at its maximum. For de-noising applications, the *diffusion factor* needs to be adjusted according to the noise level. The noise is usually estimated with some statistical methods that determine global characteristics (e.g. Black et al. [4] used the median absolute deviation), or by hand-picking some homogeneous areas and measuring the local variance. The *number of iterations* determines how many times the smoothing process is repeated. This parameter is often adjusted manually but it can also be done using an auto-stop criterion. In the latter case, the program can consider the number of pixel (voxel) modifications which occurred between the last two iterations to stop execution [4]. Either way, selecting an appropriate set of parameters is generally quite complicated and time-consuming.

In this work, an iterative method is presented that automatically adjusts these two main parameters. In contrast to previous approaches the estimation of the noise level is only used to determine the initial value of k. The optimization of the parameter k is driven by the feedback output from an evaluation method until a maximum response is reached. The novel evaluation method estimates indirectly the improvement of the image by analyzing the suppressed information and comparing its characteristics with those expected at the optimum. This is repeated several times for different values of *it*. The best combination of the two parameters, according to the evaluation method response, is then selected to finally process the image. Figure 1 shows a diagram of the method described here. The following sections will explain in detail our method and will present achieved experimental results.

2 Method

The three basic modules of the automatic iterative system proposed here are the *de-noising filters*, the *evaluation method* and the *adjustment rules* (Fig. 1). The *de-noising filters* module contains several anisotropic diffusion functions for data processing (e.g., PMAD2) as well as a set of anisotropic diffusion filters modeled

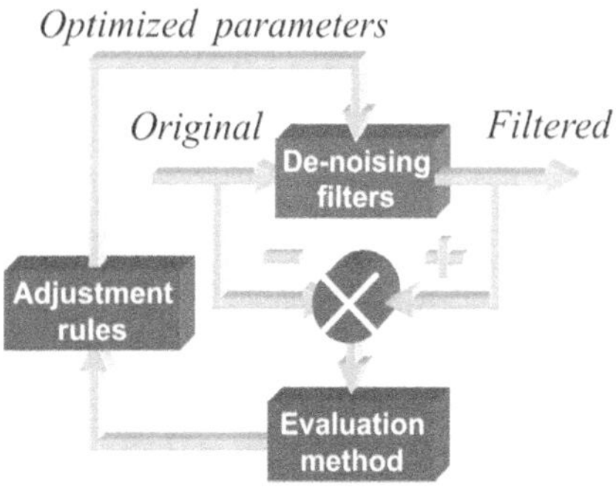

Fig. 1. Diagram of the automatic anisotropic filter system

after Nordström's [8] biased anisotropic formulation (e.g., PMAD2_bias). All the filters use a regularized (smoothed) version of the gradient to estimate the position of the edges [5] which should not be smoothed by the anisotropic filtering process.

The key component of the system, the *evaluation module*, gives feedback on image improvement or degradation during processing. Unlike other techniques, such as *image compression*, de-noising techniques do not have access to uncorrupted reference images to minimize the error between the reference and the processed image. Also, since this method is used for pre-processing, the only information available to it is that contained in the source image and that obtained during processing, so that no a priori anatomical knowledge is used to process the image. These conditions were set to keep the method as flexible and independent as possible.

MR images can be seen as the combination of the intensity information of the examined tissues and the noise generated during the measurement. After processing an MR image with an ideal filter configured using ideal parameters, the processed image would be perfectly clean of noise and only contain tissue information. Hence, the residual image, obtained by subtracting the source image from the processed one (Fig. 2), would consist only of the noise of the source image. The evaluation method takes advantage of this residual information to analyze the characteristics of the suppressed noise.

The characteristics of the noise for magnitude MR images are sufficiently known and therefore used as reference. In this case, the noise has a Rice distribution and its strength is homogeneous across the entire data set [9]. The closer the parametrization of k and it is to optimum, the more the residual image will approximate the characteristics of the initial noise. The images on the bottom row of Figure 2b were obtained by processing the image using successively increasing k values. The great variation in texture between the left and the right image suggest that either the source image needed more filtering or it was strongly smoothed and some anatomical structure have started to emerge in the residual image. The image in the middle was obtained using near-optimum parameters.

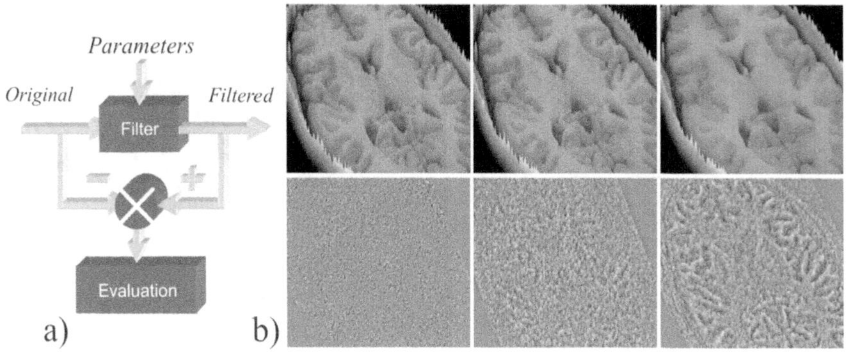

Fig. 2. Residual information used to monitor the noise reduction; a) diagram; b) processed (top) and residual images (bottom). The three pairs correspond to slightly smoothed (left), near optimally smoothed (middle) and heavily smoothed MR images (right).

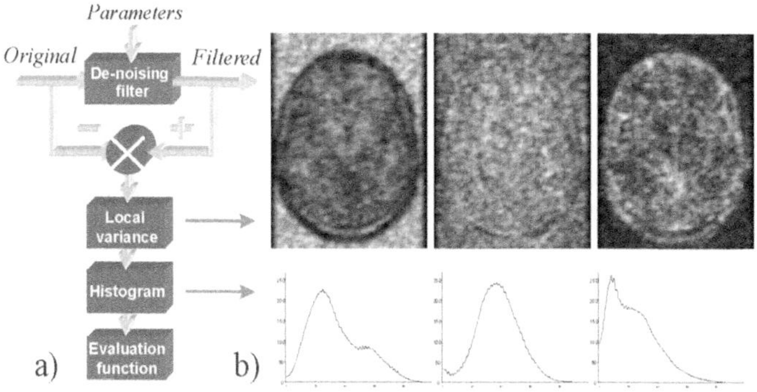

Fig. 3. a) Diagram of the evaluation method; b) results of the *local variance* (top) and from the *histogram* (bottom) modules. The three images correspond to slightly smoothed (left), near optimally smoothed (middle) and heavily smoothed MR images (right).

The *evaluation method* consists of three modules (Fig. 3a). The first one is a *local variance* operator which produces a picture of the noise, measuring the variance within a 3x3 (3x3x3) local region every third pixel (voxel). The local variance image is normalized to prevent bias during subsequent operations. The second module is a *histogram* which extracts the distribution information of the variance image. The results are smoothed with a low-pass filter to prevent discontinuities. The third module is an *evaluation function* of the histogram results which considers the maximum height, the width and the symmetry of the histogram to produce a noise reduction index. The *evaluation function* formula is shown in Equation 3.

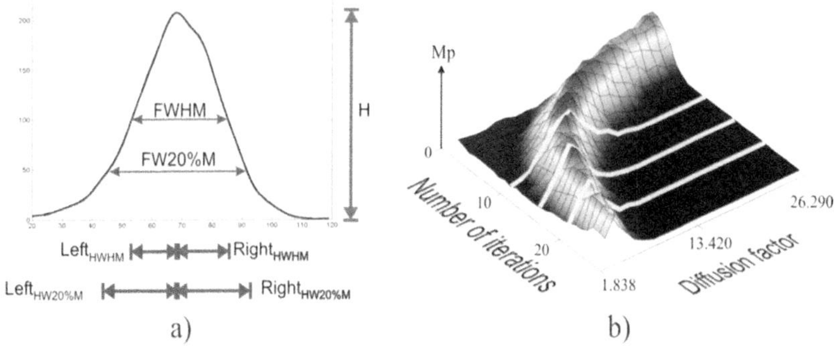

Fig. 4. a) Histogram characteristics considered by the *evaluation function* module; b) results of the *evaluation function*

Its first term H represents the maximum value of the histogram. The inverse of the Full-Width at Half-Maximum (FWHM) and the inverse of the Full-Width at 20%-Maximum (FW20%M) terms are indicators of the variance dispersion, and the two exponential terms are functions of the histogram symmetry based on the right and left Half-Widths at 50% (HWHM) and at 20% (HW20%M) of the maximum (Fig. 4a). This *evaluation function* yields large values when the histogram function is close to a large and narrow Gaussian-type curve, reflecting a homogeneous distribution of the local variance values. Figure 4b shows the results of the *evaluation function* after evaluating part of the parameters interval (it=1 to 25, k=1.838 to 26.290).

$$Mp = H * \left(\frac{1}{\mathrm{FWHM}}\right) * \left(\frac{1}{\mathrm{FW20\%M}}\right) * \left(1 - \exp\left(-\frac{(\mathrm{Symm_{FWHM}})^3}{0.2}\right)\right) * \left(1 - \exp\left(-\frac{(\mathrm{Symm_{FW20\%M}})^3}{0.2}\right)\right) \tag{3}$$

where:

$$\mathrm{Symm_{FWHM}} = \frac{\mathrm{Left_{HWHM}}}{\mathrm{Right_{HWHM}}} \quad if \;\; \mathrm{Left_{HWHM}} \leq \mathrm{Right_{HWHM}}$$

$$\mathrm{Symm_{FWHM}} = \frac{\mathrm{Right_{HWHM}}}{\mathrm{Left_{HWHM}}} \quad if \;\; \mathrm{Left_{HWHM}} > \mathrm{Right_{HWHM}}$$

$$\mathrm{Symm_{FW20\%M}} = \frac{\mathrm{Left_{HW20\%M}}}{\mathrm{Right_{HW20\%M}}} \quad if \;\; \mathrm{Left_{HW20\%M}} \leq \mathrm{Right_{HW20\%M}}$$

$$\mathrm{Symm_{FW20\%M}} = \frac{\mathrm{Right_{HW20\%M}}}{\mathrm{Left_{HW20\%M}}} \quad if \;\; \mathrm{Left_{HW20\%M}} > \mathrm{Right_{HW20\%M}}$$

The pairs *diffusion factor-number of iterations* corresponding to the ridge values are considered to be close to optimum parameter configurations because the response corresponds to a homogeneous distribution of the *local variance*.

The *adjustment rules* module was implemented to avoid evaluating each combination of parameters on the surface while searching for the optimum. This search is greatly simplified if each parameter is analyzed independently. It is more convenient if the continuous variable k is optimized first while the discrete variable it is kept constant (represented as white lines in Fig. 4b). The optimum k value of each sample it is obtained through a successive approximation scheme which determines the new k based on its current and previous values and on the corresponding results produced by the *evaluation function.* This optimization is repeated several times with different it values. From the optimum k values obtained, the median k value and its respective *number of iterations* are used for the final filtering of the image.

3 Results

In order to evaluate the method proposed here, several real and simulated data sets were processed (Fig. 5). For evaluation, three corrupted 3D data sets with increasing noise intensity were generated. These data sets represent different overlapping intensity levels between the tissue types cerebrospinal fluid, gray and white matter. The reference image, taken from the Montréal Neurological Institute (MNI) database [10], was an averaged T1-weighted image of 27 scans of the same individual. Rician noise was added following the equation:

$$I = \sqrt{((I_0 + n1(\sigma))^2 + (n2(\sigma))^2)} \tag{4}$$

where I_0 is the original image and $n1(\sigma)$ and $n2(\sigma)$ are two independent 3D images with zero-mean Gaussian-distributed noise. The standard deviations used to produce three noisy data sets were σ=9.16, 13.75 and 18.33.

These data sets were processed with the automatic method using the second Perona-Malik function PMAD2 (c_2 in Eq. 2) and its biased implementation PMAD2_bias [8]. The same data sets were also processed using a median filter (1 iteration) and a k-nearest neighbor (kNN) filter with k=14 (3 iterations). In all cases, the data were processed using a 26 neighborhood. The PMAD2 filter approximated the original image quite well, although it failed to reduce some speckle noise (Fig. 5e). The kNN filter also gave good results (Fig. 5f), although not as smooth as those of the anisotropic filter.

The experimental results were evaluated together with the corrupted data using the original MNI data set as reference. The evaluation was done using the mean-absolute error (MAE), the root-mean-square error (RMSE), the signal-to-noise ratio (SNR), the peak-signal-to-noise ratio (PSNR) and the structural similarity index (SSIM) [11]. Figure 6 summarizes the obtained results. As can be seen there, the automatic parameterization of the second Perona-Malik function (PMAD2) gave the lowest errors (MAE and RMSE) and the greatest ratios (SNR, PSNR and SSIM). The biased implementation of the same filter (PMAD2_bias) gave comparable results to the k-nearest neighbor filter. Results obtained using the median filter were consistently inferior. The computing time for the MNI data set (181x217x181) was 47 min using a 2.6 GHz Pentium-4

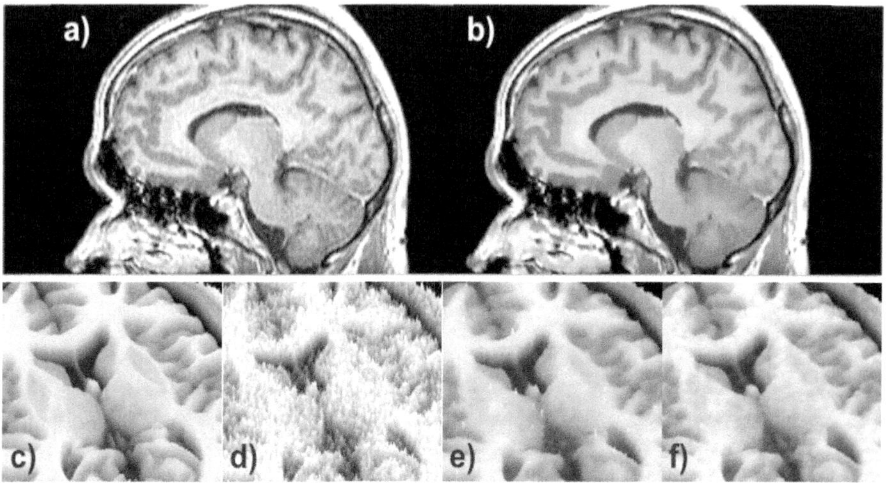

Fig. 5. a) Real MR image; b) after automatic filtering; c) reference MNI image; d) MNI image corrupted with Rician noise (σ=18.33); e) results from the anisotropic filter (PMAD2) using the parameters obtained with the automatic method (it=10, k=10.94); f) results from the k-nearest neighbor (kNN) filter

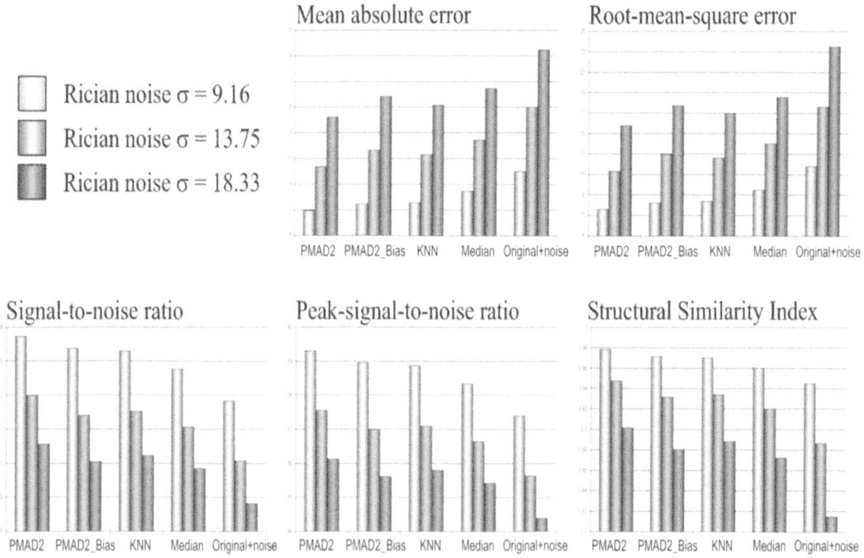

Fig. 6. Experimental results obtained comparing the original MNI data set with the corrupted and processed images

CPU. Each iteration took 1.8 seconds during the iterative optimization (using only 10 transaxial layers) and 33 seconds during the final filtering.

4 Discussion

The proposed evaluation function used to evaluate the filtering results is based on the characteristics of the expected noise model and therefore enables the implementation of a closed-loop system to automatically optimize the diffusion filter parameters. The obtained results, when compared to those obtained with median and k-nearest neighbor filters, indicate that our method is not only viable but also produces better results. In future work, we intend to incorporate adaptive versions of the diffusion filters into the *de-noising filters* module. These filters will locally adjust the global *diffusion factor* value according to the time (number of filter iterations) and to the local homogeneity of the image. In addition, we plan to optimize the behavior of the evaluation method according to the Rician noise model. We expect that these measures further increase the robustness and performance of the method.

Acknowledgment. The authors want to thank the German academic exchange service (DAAD) for financial support (reference no. A/02/11312). Thanks are also due to Alejandro Rodón for language editing.

References

1. Witkin, A.: Scale-space filtering. In: In Int. Join Conf. Artificial Intelligence. (1983) 1019–1022
2. Perona, P., Malik, J.: Scale-space and edge detection using anisotropic diffusion. IEEE Trans. In Pattern Analysis and Machine Intelligence **12** (1990) 629–639
3. Gerig, G., Kikinis, R., et al: Nonlinear anisotropic filtering of mri data. IEEE Transactions on Medical Imaging **11** (1992) 221–232
4. Black, M., Sapiro, G., et al: Robust anisotropic diffusion. IEEE Trans. Image Processing **7** (1998) 421–432
5. Weickert, J.: Anisotropic Diffusion in Image Processing. ECMI. Teubner (1998)
6. Weeratunga, S., Kamath, C.: A comparison of pde-based non-linear anisotropic diffusion technologies for image denoising. In: Image Processing: Algorithms and Systems. Algorithms and Systems II (2003)
7. Suri, J.S., Wu, D., et al: A comparison of state-of-the-art diffusion imaging technologies for smoothing medical/non-medical image data. In: Pattern Recognition. Algorithms and Systems II (2002)
8. Nordström, N.: Biased anisotropic diffusion - a unified regularization and diffusion approach to edge detection. In: 1st European Conf. on Comp. Vision. (1990) 18–27
9. Sijbers, J.: Signal and Noise Estimation from MR Images. Phd. thesis, University of Antwerp (1998)
10. Collins, D., Neelin, P., Evans, A., et al: Automatic 3d registration of mr volumetric data in standardized talairach space. J Comput Assist Tomogr **18** (1994) 192–205
11. Wang, Z., Bovik, A., Sheikh, H.: Structural similarity based image quality assessment. In: Digital Video Image Quality and Perceptual Coding. Marcel Dekker series in Signal Processing and Communications (2004)

Towards a Dynamic Model of Pulmonary Parenchymal Deformation: Evaluation of Methods for Temporal Reparameterization of Lung Data

Tessa A. Sundaram, Brian B. Avants, and James C. Gee

University of Pennsylvania, Philadelphia PA 19104, USA

Abstract. We approach the problem of temporal reparameterization of dynamic sequences of lung MR images. In earlier work, we employed capacity-based reparameterization to co-register temporal sequences of 2-D coronal images of the human lungs. Here, we extend that work to the evaluation of a ventilator-acquired 3-D dataset from a normal mouse. Reparameterization according to both deformation and lung volume is evaluated. Both measures provide results that closely approximate normal physiological behavior, as judged from the original data. Our ultimate goal is to be able to characterize normal parenchymal biomechanics over a population of healthy individuals, and to use this statistical model to evaluate lung deformation under various pathological states.

1 Introduction

The lung is a highly elastic organ composed of fibers connecting the large airways, intricate vasculature and pulmonary interstitium. Pathological processes that affect the lung typically alter the normal mechanical properties of lung tissue, and manifest as observable changes in lung morphology and function. Magnetic resonance (MR) imaging and other structural imaging modalities can be used to capture *in vivo* deformation of the lung between sequential images by harnessing the power of non-rigid registration algorithms, [1,2,3,4,5].

One of the challenges in evaluating the respiratory dynamics of multiple individuals lies in achieving temporal correspondence between physiologically similar points of the respiratory cycle. We refer to this process of establishing temporal correspondence as *reparameterization*. Solutions have been proposed that include extending the B-spline framework used to perform pairwise registrations to simultaneous spatio-temporal image matching, as well as applying translation and scaling in the temporal domain as a precursor to non-rigid registration in the spatial domain, [6,7].

We extend the technique of combining *capacity*-based reparameterization with shape and intensity averaging to establish a temporal correlation between sequences of lung images from different individuals, [8]. In earlier 2-D experiments, capacity was defined as the cross-sectional area of both lungs computed from coronal slices, and computed via interactive level-set segmentation, [9]. The

J. Duncan and G. Gerig (Eds.): MICCAI 2005, LNCS 3750, pp. 328–335, 2005.

data used in those experiments were acquired from human volunteers instructed to breathe slowly and deeply. Imaging was performed at a regular time interval; however, a consistent volume increment was not guaranteed between successive images in the sequence. One limitation of this study was computing lung capacity from 2-D lung MR images containing both a cross-section of parenchyma and portions of large blood vessels. In addition, there is inherent uncertainty associated with matching anatomy moving perpendicularly to the imaging plane.

In light of these confounding issues, we further investigate the reparameterization problem using 3-D whole-lung data. We evaluate the feasibility of two different interpolation techniques for the purposes of 1) reconstructing physiologically appropriate lung configurations between acquired images, and 2) using these reconstructions to establish temporal correspondences between sequences from different individuals. The latter aim lends itself to the construction of dynamic atlases of the normal lung, which is the ultimate goal of this research. We examine two approaches: direct shape averaging and interpolation of sequential images based on deformation computed within our non-rigid registration framework [10], and volume-based reparameterization via linear interpolation. We evaluate each method by comparing the expected *total* lung capacity (TLC) with the capacity in the reconstructed images. We also evaluate the methods by comparing the expected deformation between anatomies to the achieved deformation after reparameterization.

The goal of reparameterization is to establish a standard *physiologic time* axis between individuals who breathe at different rates and whose lungs undergo unique degrees of deformation. By developing this temporal correspondence between individuals, we can construct a dynamic atlas of normal parenchymal deformation and subsequently evaluate the lung motion of patients against this statistical norm.

2 Methods and Materials

2.1 Murine Data

The dataset used in these experiments was acquired using mechanical ventilation of a normal mouse weighing approximately twenty-six grams. First, tracheal cannulation of the anesthetized mouse was performed. The mouse was then connected to a small animal ventilator (FlexiVent, SCIREQ, Quebec, Canada) and mechanically ventilated at a rate of 120 breaths per minute. Four volumetric MR images were acquired using a 4.7T animal imaging system (Biospec 47/40, Bruker BioSpin, Karlsruhe, Germany) at the following physiologic time points: end-expiration, mid-inspiration, end-inspiration and mid-expiration. The first time point was duplicated to produce a dataset of five time points over a single murine breath (figure 1).

2.2 Method Summary

In these experiments we employ a variational registration algorithm with a linear elastic prior to quantify lung motion captured in serial image sequences, by

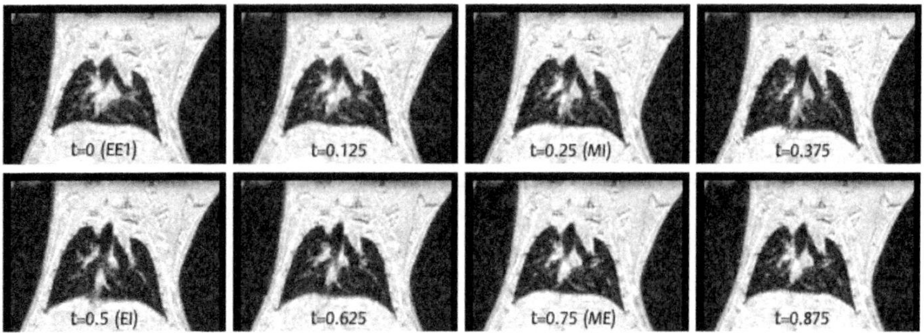

Fig. 1. Results of the reparameterization algorithm. Deformation of the murine lungs over one complete, reconstructed respiratory cycle (inspiration followed by expiration). Times are given in normalized units as described in the text. Odd images are original acquisitions, and are labeled with the appropriate physiologic phase of respiration; even images are intermediate images reconstructed from the anatomies at adjacent time points in the cycle.

registering sequential pairs of images I and J and examining the resulting displacement fields, [5]. We impose the linear elastic behavior of the image via a finite element mesh constructed over the domain of I. In related work, the original registration algorithm has been modified to yield the diffeomorphic fluid deformation framework which is assumed in this paper, [10]. The diffeomorphic component requires that the solution to the registration be continuous, differentiable and invertible. When combined with the fluid framework and approached from the Eulerian perspective, the total deformation between fixed image I and moving image J is considered to be a composition of incremental transformations, each of which is diffeomorphic.

First, we perform pairwise registration between consecutive images using our fluid registration algorithm. The resulting set of deformation fields, $\{\mathbf{u}_1, \cdots, \mathbf{u}_4\}$, reveals not only the motion of the lungs between successive images, but also the change in volume between each image pair through the *total Jacobian* of the field, $\mathcal{J} = \int |J(\mathbf{u}_i)|d\mathbf{x}$ (here, J is the Jacobian matrix and Ω is the domain of the lung segmentation). By construction, A_{i+1}, the capacity of the lungs at the next time, is equal to $\int_\Omega |J(\mathbf{u}_i)|d\mathbf{x}$.

Lung volumes are estimated via segmentation with the region competition mode of ITK-SNAP, [9], an open-source, level set implementation of 3-D geodesic active snake segmentation, [11]. The segmentations are not post-processed in any way; the trachea and large vessels traveling between the heart and lungs are omitted from the calculation of lung tissue volumes. The large pulmonary arteries and veins appear as regions of high intensity within the pulmonary parenchyma, and are consistently excluded from the segmentations.

Total lung capacity is estimated at each of the five time points during the respiratory cycle, and shown in figure 2a. The plot demonstrates that the volume of the murine lungs follows a parabolic path during respiration, which is in

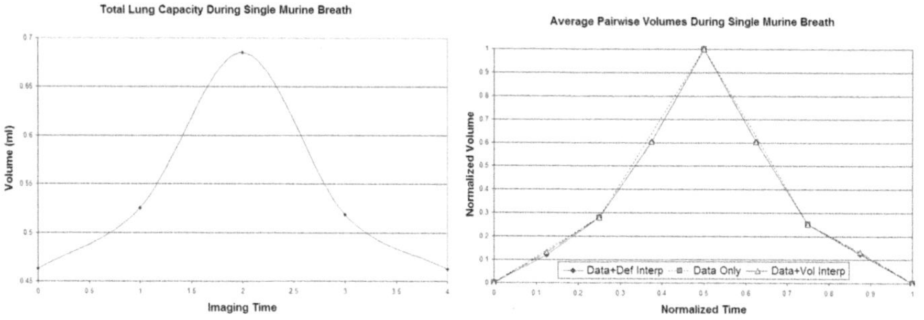

Fig. 2. (left) Trend of TLC during a single ventilator-dependent breath in a healthy mouse. (right) Comparison of normalized TLC in original image data to volume- and deformation-based interpolated images over the same breath. Note that the reconstructed anatomies bear TLC values that fall along the expected physiologic trend.

agreement with both the input to the ventilator as well as the expected pattern of respiration typically observed during tidal (passive) breathing via spirometry, [12]. The capacities computed from the original image data are subsequently used to evaluate the images reconstructed with our interpolation techniques.

2.3 Deformation-Based Reparameterization

We employ a shape and intensity averaging algorithm that computes an average anatomy by performing a simultaneous, symmetric registration of two images I and J, [13]. The registration simultaneously determines the diffeomorphism from I to J and J to I; the latter simulates a temporal path which can be sampled at specific intervals. The symmetric energy of the pairwise averaging problem is

$$\Pi_{sym}(I,J) = \inf_{\boldsymbol{v}_1} \inf_{\boldsymbol{v}_2} \int_0^1 \{\|\boldsymbol{v}_1\|_L^2 + \|\boldsymbol{v}_2\|_L^2 + (\|\boldsymbol{v}_1\|_L^2 - \|\boldsymbol{v}_2\|_L^2)^2 + \int_\Omega \Pi_\sim(I \circ \phi_1(\mathbf{X}), J \circ \phi_2(\mathbf{x}))\, d\Omega\}\, dt,$$

where $\boldsymbol{v}_i$ represents the speed and trajectory of the image voxels as they move through the Eulerian reference frame, $\Pi_\sim$ is the contribution of the similarity to the overall objective function, and $\mathbf{X}$ and $\mathbf{x}$ are the coordinate systems of I and J, respectively. Integration of $\boldsymbol{v}_i$ gives the flow ϕ_i in time, which can be used to map between the coordinate systems of I and J. Specifically, ϕ_1 pulls image I into the space of image J, while ϕ_2 provides the inverse mapping of image J into the space of image I. The symmetric solutions to the registration are given by $I \circ \phi_1$ and $J \circ \phi_2$, and the shape and intensity average of images I and J is represented by $\frac{1}{2}(I \circ \phi_1 + J \circ \phi_2)$. In our experiments, this anatomical mean at time t_j represents the average respiratory deformation between the lung configurations at times t_i and t_{i+1} (where $t_i < t_j < t_{i+1}$).

The effect of this approach is to reparameterize the image sequence by deformation, in order to reconstruct the lungs at intermediate configurations between the originally acquired images. The interpolated images are evaluated by calculating TLC at the intermediate times t_j and comparing them to the observed trend of lung capacity. In addition, the deformation between reconstructed lung configurations is also evaluated with respect to the deformation between the original anatomy.

2.4 Capacity-Based Reparameterization

Since the deformation between successive images at i and $i+1$ is small in this ventilator-assisted dataset, we define our capacity-based reparameterization to be a linear scaling of the deformation between successive images. For example, V_j, the reconstructed image between V_i and V_{i+1} (or images I and J, respectively), can be written as

$$V_j = V_{i+\alpha} = \frac{1}{2}(V_i \circ \alpha\phi_1 \ + \ V_{i+1} \circ (1-\alpha)\phi_2),$$

where α represents the desired capacity fraction between the image pair. Setting $\alpha = 0.5$ produces the anatomic configuration with an estimate of the average TLC between the known lung configurations.

2.5 Validation

TLC is computed at each of the five time points in our 3-D image sequence and shown in figure 2. We reconstruct deformation- and capacity-based ($\alpha = 0.5$) anatomic averages between sequential pairs of images (figure 1). The results are evaluated by comparing the capacities A_j of the successive average lung configurations V_j to the trend observed in the original data (figure 2).

In order to effectively validate the physiologic relevance of our two reparameterization schemes, we first generate a synthetic data sequence by densely sampling the inspiratory phase of our original dataset. This sequence of twelve images over the inspiratory phase of respiration is generated by shape interpolation between end-expiratory and end-inspiratory image volumes EE1 and EI, and serves as synthetic data from a second individual ("mouse" B) whose lung deformation we wish to correlate with that of our original individual (mouse A). Furthermore, we compute a third sequence of twelve images between EE1 and EI via volume reparameterization ("mouse" C). Lung capacities for sequences B and C are shown in figure 3a). Since the synthetic data was produced from the original respiratory endpoints, we have a ground-truth estimate against which to evaluate our method. However, since the trends of TLC in sequences B and C are not identical to that in mouse A, we are not artificially imposing a correct outcome by using this approach.

We normalize TLC to $[0, 1]$ such that capacity at end-inspiration becomes 1 and capacity at end-expiration becomes 0. We also normalize imaging time to $[0, 1]$ such that EE1=0, EI=0.5 and EE2=1. This enables us to make meaningful comparisons between individuals whose tidal volumes and breathing times will

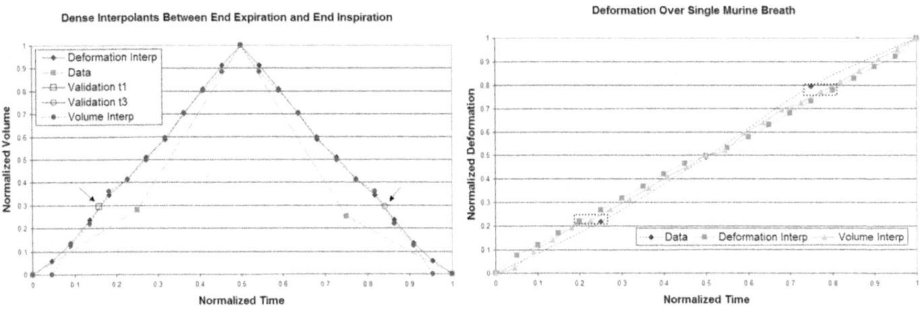

Fig. 3. (left) Comparison of normalized TLC from the original data (mouse A) with that from the deformation-based (B) and volume-based (C) interpolations. (right) Comparison of normalized deformation observed in the original data and the deformation- and capacity-based synthetic sequences. The dotted boxes highlight the anatomies with deformation coincident to that at MI and ME in mouse A.

naturally vary within some normal limits. Using the synthetic data, we attempt to reconstruct (via deformation- and volume-reparameterization in mice B and C, respectively) the anatomy that corresponds to the mid-inspiratory anatomic configuration of mouse A. First, we locate the image pair in sequence B whose normalized capacities are adjacent to the desired capacity in mouse A. Then, we compute the deformation-based average of this pair, and evaluate the capacity in this reconstructed image. It may be necessary to compute a set of shape interpolants between the adjacent images in order to find the best match to the target image. Additionally, we compare this deformation-based mean to the volume-based average estimated from the capacities of the two image neighbors in sequence C. This analysis is similarly performed for the mid-expiratory lung configuration in mouse A (figure 3a).

We also evaluate our reparameterization methods based on the expected deformation from a specific respiratory endpoint required to achieve a desired anatomic configuration. In this case, the total deformation over the entire breath is normalized such that 0 represents EE1, 0.5 the deformation required to arrive at EI and 1 the cumulative deformation to return to EE2 (figure 3b). Deformation is computed as the total magnitude of the gradient of the displacement field divided by the size of the image domain. First, we sum the incremental deformation pairwise between the original image volumes in mouse A. Next, we sum the incremental deformation computed pairwise between the synthetic image volumes in sequences B and C. The deformation required to deform the end-expiratory anatomy to the mid-inspiratory and mid-expiratory time points in mouse A is compared to the corresponding deformation in sequences B and C (figure 3b).

3 Results

Figure 2 compares the normalized capacity in the original data to those in the pairwise averages computed by our two interpolation techniques. Both methods produce virtually identical results, differing by 0.01 in the capacity estimates at normalized times $t = 0.125$ and $t = 0.875$ and by 0.001 in the estimates at $t = 0.375$ and $t = 0.625$. The error between the expected and achieved capacities was approximately 0.007 at $t = 0.125$ and $t = 0.875$ and 0.03 at $t = 0.375$ and $t = 0.625$.

The discrepancy in normalized TLC between the synthetic sequences computed via deformation- and capacity-based interpolation is approximately 0.002-0.03 per interpolant. However, the average configuration between the anatomies adjacent to the mid-inspiratory (open square) and mid-expiratory (open circle) configurations has a capacity within 0.0004 when computed by either method (figure 3a). The expected normalized lung capacity at MI was 0.281, while the reconstructed anatomy at MI had a capacity of 0.294. The computed normalized capacity at ME was 0.252.

Evaluation of both interpolation methods with respect to deformation is summarized in figure 3b. The corresponding mid-inspiratory and mid-expiratory anatomic configurations among sequences A-C are enclosed in the dotted boxes. The error in normalized deformation to arrive at MI is approximately 0.001, while the corresponding error to reach ME is approximately 0.025. The discrepancy between the deformation- and capacity-based approaches is approximately 0.003 at MI and 0.008 at ME. In addition, the closest image pair providing the matching deformation at MI and ME is the same image pair used to compute the deformation- and capacity-based average anatomies based on normalized TLC in figure 3a. This further validates the physiological basis of our approach.

4 Discussion and Future Work

We present an evaluation of two approaches toward the temporal reparameterization of dynamic lung data. Comparable results are achieved using both deformation-based shape and intensity averaging and volume-based linear scaling. The parenchymal deformation in this whole-lung mouse dataset is more uniform compared to that observed in 2-D data used in earlier experiments. In addition, the deformation between successive images is small, since the tidal volume in this animal is only around 0.2 ml. As a result, we plan to evaluate these methods on additional volumetric datasets acquired with non-zero and non-constant settings for positive end-expiratory pressure (PEEP).

Future analysis will also be extended to data acquired with breath-holding, since human imaging is typically not conducted with mechanical ventilation. Application of the techniques presented in this paper is not restricted to data acquired with ventilatory assistance; however, validation of the methods is augmented by the regular pattern of respiration imposed by the ventilator.

The ultimate goal of this research is to use temporal correspondences between individuals to provide comparisons of the biomechanical perturbation of the lung during respiration. Mechanics can be evaluated by computing finite strain over the respiratory cycle, and investigating regional variations in tissue character within as well as between individuals. By establishing temporally coincident anatomic points between individuals, it will be possible to assess the degree and distribution of strain required for these individuals to arrive at physiologically similar points in their respective respiratory cycles. Furthermore, various pulmonary pathologies are known to affect the mechanical properties of the lung tissue, and these changes can be quantified using the model described. Our work motivates the construction of dynamic atlases of normal lung motion, which will not only provide a statistical representation of normal parenchymal deformation but also a metric against which to evaluate changes introduced by the development and progression of pulmonary diseases.

References

1. Dougherty, L., Asmuth, J.C., Gefter, W.B.: Alignment of CT lung volumes with an optical flow method. Acad. Rad. **10** (2003) 249–254
2. Hatabu, H., Ohno, Y., Uematsu, H., Oshio, K., Gefter, W.B., Gee, J.C.: Lung biomechanics via non-rigid reg. of serial MR images. Rad. **221P** (2001) 630
3. Li, B., Christensen, G.E., Hoffman, E.A., McLennan, G., Reinhardt, J.M.: Establishing a normative atlas of the human lung: intersubject warping and registration of volumetric CT images. Acad. Rad. **10** (2003) 255–265
4. Sundaram, T., Gee, J., Nishino, M., Kiryu, S., Mori, Y., Kuroki, M., Takahashi, M., Hatabu, H.: 3-D Lung Motion Estimation Via Non-Rigid Registration Using Volumetric MR and CT. In: Proc. ISMRM 12th Mtg. (2004) 2609
5. Gee, J.C., Sundaram, T., Hasegawa, I., Uematsu, H., Hatabu, H.: Charac. of regional pulm. mechanics from serial MRI data. Acad. Rad. **10** (2003) 1147–1152
6. Ledesma-Carbayo, M.J., Kybic, J., Suhling, M., Hunziker, P., Desco, M., Santos, A., Unser, M.: Cardiac ultrasound motion detection by elastic registration exploiting temporal coherence. In: Proc. 1st IEEE ISBI. Volume 2. (2002) 585–588
7. Perperidis, D., Mohiaddin, R., Rueckert, D.: Spatio-temporal free-form registration of cardiac MR image sequences. In Barillot, C., Haynor, D.R., Hellier, P., eds.: Proc. 7th Intl. MICCAI. LNCS 3216 (2004) 911–919
8. Sundaram, T.A., Avants, B.B., Gee, J.C.: A dynamic model of average lung deformation using capacity-based reparameterization and shape averaging of lung MR images. In Barillot, C., Haynor, D.R., Hellier, P., eds.: Proc. 7th Int'l MICCAI 2004. Volume LNCS 3217., Springer (2004) 1000–1007
9. Yushkevich, P., Ho, S., Cody, H., Piven, J., Gerig, G.: Geodesic snakes for user-guided segmentation of 3-D anatomical objects: Significantly improved efficiency and reliability. In Submission (2005)
10. Avants, B., Ng, L., Sundaram, T., Duda, J.T., Gee, J.: Non-rigid image registration. In Yoo, T., ed.: Insight Into Images. AK Peters, Natick, MA (2004)
11. Zhu, S.C., Yuille, A.: Region competition: Unifying snakes, region growing, and bayes/mdl for multiband image segmentation. IEEE Trans. Pattern Anal. Mach. Intell. **18** (1996) 884–900
12. Townsend, M.C.: Spirometry in the occupational setting. J. Occupational & Environmental Med. **42** (2000) 228–245
13. Avants, B.B., Gee, J.C.: Geodesic estimation for large deformation anatomical shape averaging and interpolation. NeuroImage **Suppl. 1** (2004) S139–150

4D MR Imaging Using Internal Respiratory Gating

M. von Siebenthal[1], Ph. Cattin[1], U. Gamper[2], A. Lomax[3], and G. Székely[1]

[1] Computer Vision Laboratory, ETH, CH-8092 Zürich, Switzerland
{mvonsieb, cattin, szekely}@vision.ee.ethz.ch
[2] Institute of Biomedical Engineering, ETH, CH-8092 Zürich, Switzerland
[3] Paul Scherrer Institut, CH-5232 Villigen PSI, Switzerland

Abstract. Respiratory organ motion is a key problem in proton therapy and in many other treatments. This paper presents a novel retrospective gating method for 4D (dynamic 3D) MR imaging during free breathing to capture the full variability of respiratory organ deformation. In contrast to other imaging methods, a constant breathing depth or even strict periodicity are not assumed. 3D images of moving organs can be reconstructed for complete respiratory cycles by retrospective stacking of dynamic 2D images using internal image-based gating. Additional noise reduction by combining multiple images significantly increases the signal-to-noise ratio. The resulting image quality is comparable to breath-hold acquisitions. Although the method was developed for proton therapy planning, the new possibilities to study respiratory motion are valuable to improve other treatments and to assess gating techniques, which rely on stronger assumptions about the breathing pattern.

1 Introduction

Respiratory organ motion is a complicating factor in proton therapy and other treatments. Especially for dynamic dose delivery, exact knowledge of organ motion and its influence on the dose distribution is crucial. The aim of the proposed method was to provide realistic 4D data (dynamic 3D images) of organ motion for the evaluation of dose delivery methodologies in proton therapy and for the assessment of external gating techniques. Existing 4D imaging methods are limited to strongly simplified breathing patterns or achieve only modest spatial or temporal resolutions. In this paper we present a novel method that can capture the full variability of organ motion. The method, which is applicable to any organ affected by respiratory motion, will be shown for the liver as an example.

The main component of liver motion is a cranio-caudal shift, usually in the range of 0.5-2.5 cm for quiet breathing [1,2]. As quantified in [2], the liver additionally shows motion in anterior-posterior (1-12 mm) and left-right direction (1-3 mm) as well as non-rigid deformations (up to 2 cm). The breathing pattern

J. Duncan and G. Gerig (Eds.): MICCAI 2005, LNCS 3750, pp. 336–343, 2005.

may vary within short time scales in amplitude, frequency and shape. To capture this variability, we use MR Imaging. In contrast to CT, volunteers are not exposed to ionizing radiation and the orientation of the scanned slices can be chosen freely. Nevertheless, some gating methods are common for MR Imaging and CT, and therefore 4DCT is also considered in the following summary.

MR Imaging techniques are constantly evolving, but the required trade-off between resolution, acquisition speed and signal-to-noise ratio still prevents a detailed examination of organ motion in real-time. Dynamic 3D MR sequences like Fast Field Echo Planar Imaging (FFE-EPI) applied in [3] achieve high acquisition frequencies, but suffer from a reduced image quality and resolution if large regions like the lung or the liver are scanned. To overcome this trade-off, there are two main approaches, here denoted as *breath-hold imaging* and *slice stacking*. *Breath-hold imaging* uses static 3D volumes at different breathing depths determined for example with a stretch transducer [2] or a standard MR navigator [4]. One problem is that subjects may not be able to hold their breath for long periods like 40 s [4]. Additionally, breath-hold images do not capture how the organ is deformed during motion. Even if the breath-hold positions lie in the range of free breathing, the hysteretic organ deformation between inhalation and exhalation cannot be captured [3].

For *slice stacking*, one or a few 2D slices are scanned during a number of breathing cycles. Frames from these 2D sequences are retrospectively stacked to 3D images. The slice stacking methods found in the literature apply various gating methods, which use for example the tidal lung volume [5], infrared markers placed on the abdomen [6,7] or the abdominal skin detected in CT images [8]. In [7], an alternative internal gating method was proposed, which assumes a constant breathing amplitude.

To the author's knowledge, all gating methods that are currently used make strong assumptions on the regularity of the respiratory motion and parameterize this motion with a one-dimensional phase. Although respiration clearly shows a repetitive character, which is also exploited in this work, a reduction of the respiratory organ deformation to one parameter neglects all residual variability and may be a too coarse approximation in some cases. The purpose of the proposed imaging method is to overcome this issue and to reconstruct accurate 4D images from free-breathing sequences in an improved quality.

2 Methods

2.1 Data Acquisition

We propose an imaging method, which follows the slice stacking approach and captures the respiratory motion using free-breathing 2D MR images. In contrast to all techniques presented above, we use sagittal slices. This allows to track vascular structures during complete breathing cycles with minimal out-of-plane motion. Another advantage of this slice orientation is the reduction of blood flow artifacts in the liver region due to the beating of the heart.

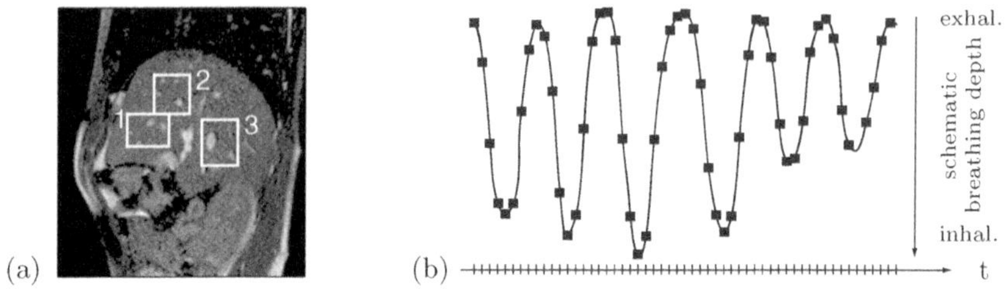

Fig. 1. (a) Navigator slice N_0. Regions 1-3 are considered for gating in Sect. 2.2. (b) Schematic acquisition sequence.

To illustrate the 4D reconstruction, we start with a 2D image sequence of a dedicated slice called the *navigator slice* N_0 (Fig. 1). Patient instruction ensures that this sequence captures a variety of different breathing depths. The aim is to reconstruct complete 3D images for all navigator frames in a complete breathing cycle. Therefore we need to acquire and identify fitting 2D images all across the liver. However, distant slices acquired during different breathing cycles are not directly comparable to the navigator slice. Different motion in distant slices can either reflect the relative motion in these regions or a change in the breathing pattern. To establish a relation between distant slices, we acquire pairs of slices, each pair containing the navigator slice, which is used for gating, and a *data slice* (Fig. 2a). The navigator slice stays at the same position for every pair p, whereas the position of the data slice is shifted across the liver. Each pair of slices is scanned for a certain time (Fig. 2b). The data and navigator frames of pair p acquired at times t_1 and t_2 are denoted D_{p,t_1} and N_{p,t_2}. $N_{0,t}$ is the pure navigator sequence, which is acquired twice as fast as the pairs of slices.

The 2D images were acquired on a 1.5 T Philips Intera whole body MR system (Philips Medical Systems, Best, NL) with a Steady State Free Precession sequence, SENSE factor 1.7 and halfscan, 192x192 pixel and 1.8x1.8 mm^2 in-plane resolution, flip angle 70°, TR=3.1 ms, 175 ms acquisition time per frame, with a coil array consisting of four rectangular elements. For pairs of slices, navigator and data frames were acquired alternately. At each of 30 slice positions we acquired 150 data frames and 150 navigator frames with 6 mm slice thickness and 3 mm overlap, yielding 3 mm through-plane resolution.

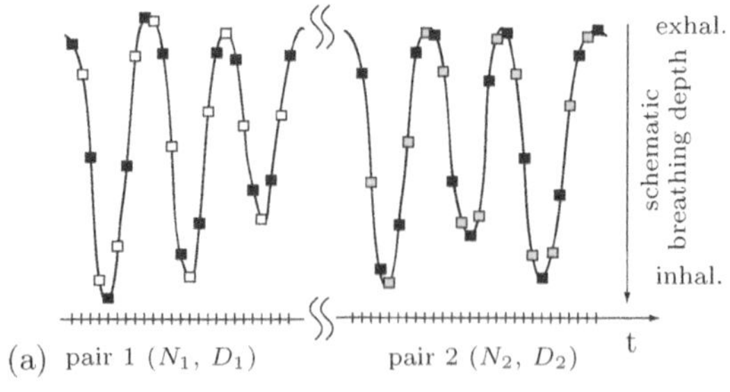

Fig. 2. Acquisition scheme. (a) Pairs of slices consisting of data slices D_p and a common navigator slice N_p. (b) Schematic acquisition sequences for two pairs of slices.

2.2 Internal Gating

To find matching 2D images, which can be stacked together to a 3D image, we propose an internal gating method based on the navigator images. This internal gating is less error-prone than external gating, which may fail to derive the accurate state of the organ from an external signal. To describe the proposed method, we consider a navigator frame $N_{0,i}$ acquired at time i, for which a matching data frame D_1 is searched. $N_{0,i-1}$ and $N_{0,i+1}$ are the neighboring navigator frames of $N_{0,i}$, whereas a candidate frame $D_{1,j}$ is embraced by the navigator frames $N_{1,j-1}$ and $N_{1,j+1}$ (Fig. 3). The proposed comparison is based on the assumption that the frames $N_{0,i}$ and $D_{1,j}$ show the same respiratory state, if the preceding navigator frames as well as the subsequent navigator frames are sufficiently similar. Thus, only navigator frames, which show the same slice of the liver, are compared to find fitting data frames. Therefore, different amplitudes or phase shifts at distant slices have no negative influence.

There are various possible similarity measures to compare the navigator frames. The evaluated options range from a simple sum of squared intensity differences to more sophisticated measures like the Mahalanobis distance in the eigenspace of the navigator frames. Since the goal is accurate slice fitting, a natural approach is to compare the position of prominent vascular structures and thus to directly quantify shift errors. This approach was chosen in the following and confirmed by the results. Figure 1a shows the three regions in the navigator frames that were considered in the presented example. The position of these regions was determined by template matching based on normalized cross correlation. Note that the apparent 2D translation detected by template matching may differ from the actual liver deformation, which in general has also an out-of-plane component. However, a similar apparent motion of all considered regions in both the preceding and the following navigator frames strongly indicates that the actual 3D deformation is similar as well.

To compare frames, we define a cost function $c(i,j)$, which should be small if the navigator frame $N_{0,i}$ and the data frame $D_{1,j}$ show the same respiratory state. Therefore, we require that each region r is at a similar position in the two preceding navigator frames $N_{0,i-1}, N_{1,j-1}$ and in the subsequent navigator

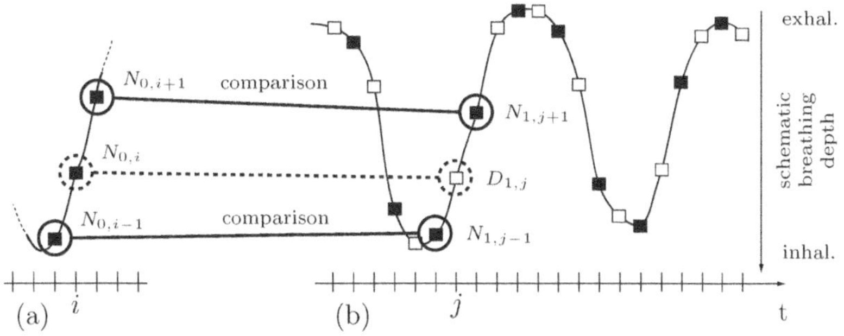

Fig. 3. (a) Navigator frame $N_{0,i}$, for which a matching data slice $D_{1,j}$ is searched in sequence (b) by comparing the neighboring navigator frames

frames $N_{0,i+1}, N_{1,j+1}$. The following cost function sums up the vectorially added deviations of the considered regions in the preceding navigator frames $\Delta\boldsymbol{X}^r_{-1}$ and the deviations in the subsequent navigator frames $\Delta\boldsymbol{X}^r_{+1}$. With coordinate axes in anterior-posterior and cranio-caudal direction, x^r_i and y^r_i are the coordinates of region r at time i. With P the number of tracked regions we define

$$c(i,j) = \sum_{r=1}^{P} \left\|\Delta\boldsymbol{X}^r_{-1} + \Delta\boldsymbol{X}^r_{+1}\right\| = \sum_{r=1}^{P} \left\| \begin{pmatrix} x^r_{j-1} - x^r_{i-1} \\ y^r_{j-1} - y^r_{i-1} \end{pmatrix} + \begin{pmatrix} x^r_{j+1} - x^r_{i+1} \\ y^r_{j+1} - y^r_{i+1} \end{pmatrix} \right\| . \quad (1)$$

Compared to the simple Euclidean distance, the vectorial displacements capture the actual motion more consistently and proved to be more robust. The best matching data frame D_{1,j^*} for a given navigator frame $N_{0,i}$ is found at time

$$j^* = \arg\min_j c(i,j) . \quad (2)$$

For the navigator frame $N_{0,i}$, the best matching data frames from each pair of slices D_{p,j^*}, $p = 1, 2, 3, \ldots$, are combined to a 3D stack. Such a stack is reconstructed for every navigator frame $N_{0,i}, N_{0,i+1}, N_{0,i+2}, \ldots$ in an entire breathing cycle to obtain a complete 4D data set with the temporal resolution of the pure navigator sequence N_0 (5.7 Hz).

2.3 Noise Reduction

The acquired images show a considerable amount of noise due to their short acquisition time and high spatial resolution. To improve the 4D reconstruction, a straight-forward noise reduction was applied. The developed gating method was used to find not only one but several frames showing possibly similar respiratory states. These frames were averaged, which artificially prolonged the acquisition time of the resulting image. Assuming additive noise, an averaging over M frames reduces the variance of the noise by a factor of M. The number of frames that can be averaged is limited by the duration of the acquisition session. In the presented example, the acquisition time was 30 min and five frames were averaged.

3 Results and Evaluation

The proposed imaging method was performed for six healthy volunteers. A 4D data set of a male volunteer is used to illustrate the method in the following. For comparison, Fig. 4a shows three cuts through a breath-hold image close to relaxed exhalation. A 3D image reconstructed from 30 free-breathing images using the proposed method is shown in Fig. 4b. The blood vessels and liver boundaries exhibit no major discontinuities. Note that Fig. 4b shows the reconstructed 3D image that is most similar to the breath-hold image. However, the free-breathing image looks different from the breath-hold image, because the latter cannot capture the shape of the moving organ, which undergoes a hysteretic deformation between inhalation and exhalation. Figure 4c shows the same free-breathing

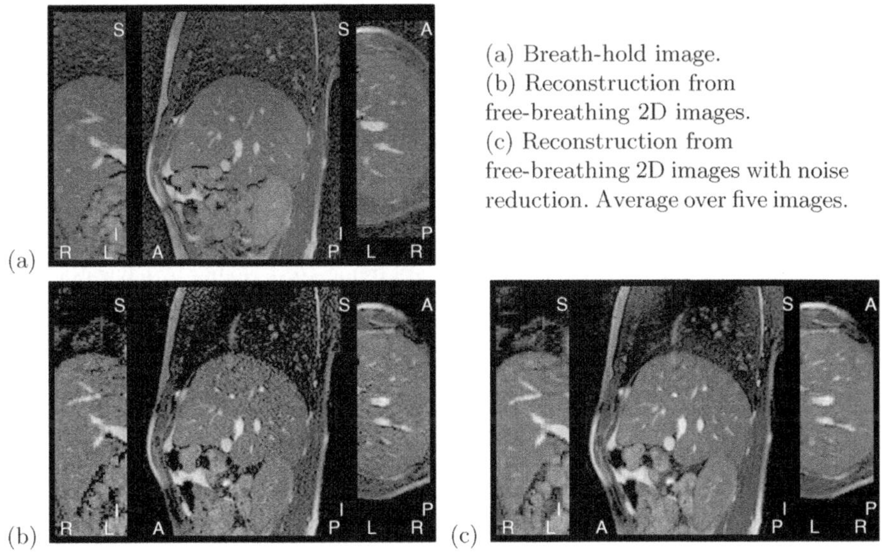

(a) Breath-hold image.
(b) Reconstruction from free-breathing 2D images.
(c) Reconstruction from free-breathing 2D images with noise reduction. Average over five images.

Fig. 4. Orthogonal cuts through 3D images of the right liver lobe

image with additional noise reduction as discussed in Sect. 2.3. The signal-to-noise ratio is remarkably improved and the resulting images achieve the quality of breath-hold acquisitions. The averaging of several images did not introduce significant blurring, which indicates that the number of acquisitions at each position was sufficient and enough similar frames were found. The darkband artifact through the dome of the liver can be shifted by proper shim adjustment.

In addition to the visual assessment of the reconstructed data sets, which showed well fitting 3D images, a rigorous validation is desirable but not straightforward. However, the proposed frame matching algorithm can be tested experimentally to evaluate the plausibility of the 4D data. To test if matching data frames are found, a leave-one-out experiment was performed. A sequence of navigator frames N_1 and data frames D_1 (288 frames in total) at 3 cm distance was considered. For each data frame $D_{1,i}$ in this sequence, the best matching data frame $D_{1,j}$ was searched among the remaining frames ($i \neq j$) according to the cost function $c(i, j)$ defined in Eq. (1). The similarity of the selected data frame D_{1,j^*} to the "ideal" left-out frame $D_{1,i}$ was quantified as the deviation of four selected regions within D_1 (Fig. 5) determined by template matching based on normalized cross correlation. While the respiratory motion ranged up to 11 mm in this example, the resulting mean deviations of the considered regions were in the range of 0.3-0.4 mm, which is less than half a voxel (0.9 mm).

4 Discussion and Outlook

The developed technique allows for the reconstruction of 4D data sets showing the detailed deformation of an organ during free breathing including the

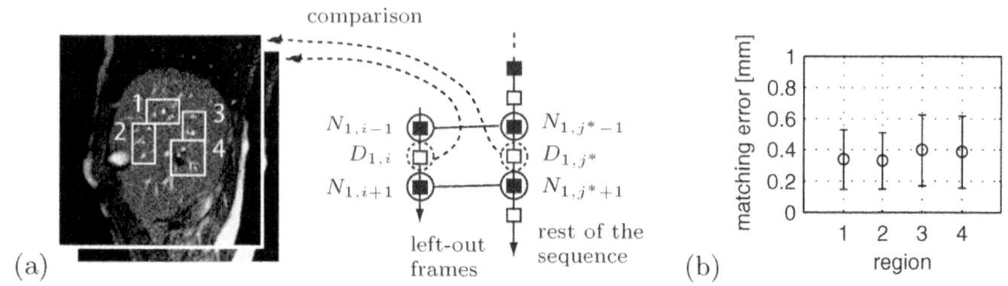

Fig. 5. Leave-one-out experiment. (a) The data frame D_{1,j^*} (found by navigator comparison) is compared to the "ideal" left-out frame $D_{1,i}$. (b) Mean error and its standard deviation for four regions.

hysteretic deformation between inhalation and exhalation. As opposed to other 4D imaging techniques, no strict assumptions on the regularity of the respiratory motion such as constant breathing depth or even periodicity are made. This allows to better study the intra-subject as well as the inter-subject variability of respiratory motion and to analyze these variations statistically. Provided that a sufficient amount of raw data was acquired, 4D data sets can be reconstructed for arbitrary amplitudes, frequencies and shapes of the breathing pattern.

Evaluation experiments have shown that the proposed gating method accurately finds fitting 2D images with minimal deviations based on the dedicated navigator slice, even if the considered slices are several centimeters apart. A gating scheme with overlapping pairs of neighboring slices as an alternative but would likely lead to error propagation from one overlapping pair to the next one.

For a rigorous validation of the proposed method, either experiments with a realistically deformable phantom or an in silico simulation of the entire data acquisition chain are possible. The second option will be investigated in the future work, for example to determine the maximum viable distance between a data slice and the navigator slice.

A common limitation for all slice stacking methods is that only breathing cycles can be reconstructed, for which all necessary frames were captured across the liver. If particularly deep breathing is only acquired at some of the slice positions, the method fails to reconstruct a complete 4D data set. This issue was addressed by instructing the volunteers to intentionally breath deeply during parts of each acquisition, which ensured that a variety of breathing depths was captured at each slice position.

Another observed issue was the drift of the exhalation position during the acquisition of most data sets. This drift ranged up to 7 mm in one case. On the one hand, this issue is aggravated by the long total acquisition time of half an hour in our studies. But on the other hand, the problem of variation beyond a regular breathing cycle is simply ignored by other 4D imaging approaches and can now be addressed specifically with the proposed method. Drift and other irregularities are recognized and handled by the internal gating technique. One possibility to alleviate the impact of organ drift is to change the acquisition sequence. The applied procedure selects a slice and completely captures its dynamic behavior before moving to the next spatial position. An interleaved sequence, which goes back and forth through all slices, would increase the probability that we acquire sufficient data for a complete 4D reconstruction before a major drift occurs.

Despite the discussed limitations, the obtained results demonstrate the potential of the proposed method for 4D imaging in surpassing quality. The technique is applicable to any organ that undergoes respiratory motion like the lung or the kidneys and can be implemented using a standard MR scanner without additional equipment. Although the proposed method was developed for proton therapy planning, the new possibilities to study realistic respiratory motion are valuable to improve many other techniques, first of all conventional radiation therapy planning. Other particularly interesting applications are the evaluation and the comparison of gating techniques that inherently rely on stronger assumptions about the respiratory motion. Furthermore, generic motion data, which is not patient specific, is useful for the evaluation of dose delivery methodologies and anatomical simulations or for advanced applications like model-based segmentation or tracking. Numerous research projects in these fields may profit from a more accurate and more reliable 4D imaging using the proposed method.

Acknowledgments. This work has been supported by the CO-ME/NCCR research network of the Swiss National Science Foundation (`http://co-me.ch`).

References

1. Davies, S., Hill, A., Holmes, R., et al.: Ultrasound quantitation of respiratory organ motion in the upper abdomen. Br. J. Radiol. **67** (1994) 1096–1102
2. Rohlfing, T., Maurer, C., Jr., O'Dell, W., Zhong, J.: Modeling liver motion and deformation during the respiratory cycle using intensity-based free-form registration of gated MR images. Proc. SPIE Med. Imaging 2001 **4319** (2001) 337–348
3. Blackall, J., Ahmad, S., Miquel, M., et al.: Modelling respiratory motion for optimisation of lung cancer radiotherapy using fast MR imaging and intensity-based image registration. In: Proc. Intl. Soc. Mag. Reson. Med. (2004) 12:2610
4. Blackall, J.: Respiratory Motion in Image-Guided Interventions of the Liver. PhD thesis, University of London (2002)
5. Low, D., Nystrom, M., Kalinin, E., Parikh, P., et al.: A method for the reconstruction of four-dimensional synchronized CT scans acquired during free breathing. Med. Phys. **30** (2003) 1254–1263
6. Ford, E., Mageras, G., Yorke, E., Ling, C.: Respiration-correlated spiral CT: A method of measuring respiratory-induced anatomic motion for radiation treatment planning. Med. Phys. **30** (2003) 88–97
7. Pan, T., Lee, T., Rietzel, E., Chen, G.: 4D-CT imaging of a volume influenced by respiratory motion on multi-slice CT. Med. Phys. **31** (2004) 333–340
8. McClelland, J., Chandler, A., Blackall, J., et al.: Feasibility study of a novel technique for constructing respiratory motion models, for use in 4D lung cancer radiotherapy planning. In: Proc. MIUA. (2004) 220–3

Anatomically Constrained Surface Parameterization for Cortical Localization

C. Clouchoux[1], O. Coulon[1], D. Rivière[2], A. Cachia[2], J.-F. Mangin[2], and J. Régis[3]

[1] Laboratoire LSIS, UMR 6168, CNRS, Marseille, France
[2] Equipe UNAF, SHFJ, CEA/DSV, Orsay, France
[3] Service de Neurochirurgie Fonctionnelle et Stéréotaxique, Marseille, France

Abstract. We present here a method that aims at defining a surface-based coordinate system on the cortical surface. Such a system is needed for both cortical localization and intersubject matching in the framework of neuroimaging. We propose an automatic parameterization based on the spherical topology of the grey/white matter interface of each hemisphere and on the use of naturally organized and reproducible anatomical features. From those markers used as initial constraints, the coordinate system is propagated via a PDE solved on the cortical surface.

1 Introduction

In the context of inter-subject brain data matching and localization, most methods deal with 3-dimensional images and consider the problem as a registration one, known as *spatial normalization* (e.g. [7]). Nevertheless there is great interest in analyzing data projected on the cortical surface [6]. The three-dimensional space does not provide any information about cortical organization. In this context, matching cortical surfaces implies facing several problems, the main one being the lack of an implicit coordinate system, such as the voxel grid in 3 dimensions. Instead of defining spatial normalization as a registration process, we can approach it in terms of localization. Few methods aim at building a surface referential by parameterizing the cortical surface in a reproducible way [6,16,5]. The method presented in [6] relies on the mapping of the cortical surface to a sphere. Resulting surfaces are aligned using a convexity measure, without any information on the cortical organization. In [16], the method presented allows a parameterization of the cortical surface from a geometric atlas, using a few anatomical constraints, but implying a deformation of the cortex, and a manual registration of the markers. Both methods require a warping of the surface to a sphere, which implies distortion on the shape and the distances on the surface.

In this framework, we propose here a method to automatically provide an anatomically meaningful parameterization, based on the definition of invariant and organized anatomical features, and which does not require any warping of the surface [4]. The paper is organized as follow : in section 2 we present the cortical anatomy theories we based our method on. Section 3 presents the method itself. Result and discussion are then detailed in section 4.

J. Duncan and G. Gerig (Eds.): MICCAI 2005, LNCS 3750, pp. 344–351, 2005.

2 Anatomical Background

The major problem in studying human brains is the great inter-subject variability. The pattern of a sulcus, even a major one, can have a different shape or different topology from one brain to another. One of the reasons of this variability is thought to be the result of the cortex folding process [11,2,16,14]. To provide invariant features, we have to understand the sulci organization over the cortical surface [8,16,14]. In [16], a geometric model of the cortical surface is proposed, which suggests an orthogonal organization scheme of main sulci. The idea of defining a geometric model of the cortical surface was introduced by [15]. In [13], a new approach is proposed to explain the sulci organization: the *sulcal roots* model. A key idea of this model is that the spatial stability of the deep sulcal cortex is greater than that of a superficial image of the sulci. This point led us to consider not only sulci, but deeply buried subparts of sulci as well, in order to generate the most generic set of anatomical features possible. The previous model provides this information: indivisible units, the so-called *sulcal roots*, corresponding to the first folding locations during antenatal life. This model raised the hypothesis of the presence of two major orthogonal directions of anatomical organization in the cerebral cortex. Figure 1 shows the some folding process results. Considering that and the spherical topology of each hemisphere led us to define a longitude/latitude coordinate system. Each sulcal root is surrounded by two meridians and two parallels of this gyral organization.

Although each sulcal root defines a cross point between longitude and latitude coordinates, several sulcal roots may be aligned on one sulcus, as shown in figure 1. The resulting fold defines then one coordinate, either meridian or parallel. Cortical folds corresponding to this criteria are thus considered as stable and reproducible markers. A consequence is that from the sulci point of view, sulcal roots are "specialized" in one coordinate. Hence, if a fold is considered to be a longitude constraint, it cannot and will not be used as a latitude constraint.

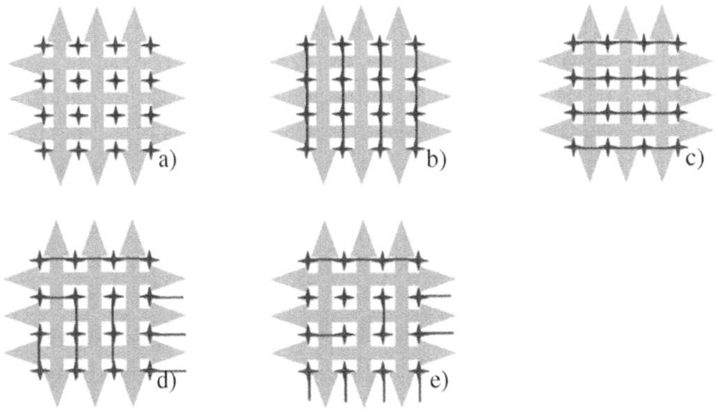

Fig. 1. Meridian/parallel organization around the sulcal roots. a) fœtal stage, b-e) different results of the folding process [13].

The correlation between sulcal-based representation and gyral-based representation has been established by [2]. In this context, sulci are considered as indicators of the meeting lines buried in the fold's depth between the two neighboring gyri. To define each gyrus borders, a set of sulci has been chosen, thought to be reliable and reproducible through individuals. In our work, a comparable process has been done. To obtain a reliable coordinate system over the cortical surface, we need to define some anatomical markers, present in every brain. The goal is to provide a generic set of those markers, which can be used as landmarks on every nonpathological mature brain. The next section details the choice of such constraints, and the algorithm used to obtain a parameterization of the whole cortical surface.

3 Method

The outline of our method is to *automatically* build a complete parameterization, in a longitude/latitude manner, starting from a few anatomical markers and propagating a coordinate system from those original constraints over the whole cortical surface of each hemisphere. All processings presented below are performed on the original cortical surface. Brains shown in figures are inflated for visualization purpose only.

3.1 Anatomical Markers

The first step of our method is the selection of anatomical markers. As explained above, a set of sulci, considered to be reproducible, can be defined. The set we built up is approximatively the same than the one used for the gyral-based representation in [2]. From MR anatomical images, a preprocessing stage provides a triangulation of the cortex hemisphere endowed with a spherical topology [9,10], corresponding to the interface between the gray and the white matter. From those images, an automatic recognition process provides the identification of the main sulci [14] (see figure 2).

At this stage of the process, the set of markers is chosen. To have a complete longitude/latitude coordinate system, two poles and an origin meridian are required. Latitude will be propagated from one pole to another, and longitude from one side of the origin meridian to another [1]. The poles are chosen as defined in [12]. One is the Insula. This area is the first folding zone appearing during the human brain growth. The other is an extension of the projection of the Corpus Callosum. The origin meridian is the one corresponding to the Central Sulcus. Indeed, this fold is one of the most stable sulci across individuals, and almost links the two poles together.

The sulci 3D representation is then used to get the projection of the bottom sulcal line on the cortical surface [2] of the set of sulci selected before, as shown in figure 2.

The diffusion process needs a complete origin meridian, i.e. linking one pole to another. The Central Sulcus projection is extended, using the shortest geodesic distance between the poles and the extremities of the sulcus projection.

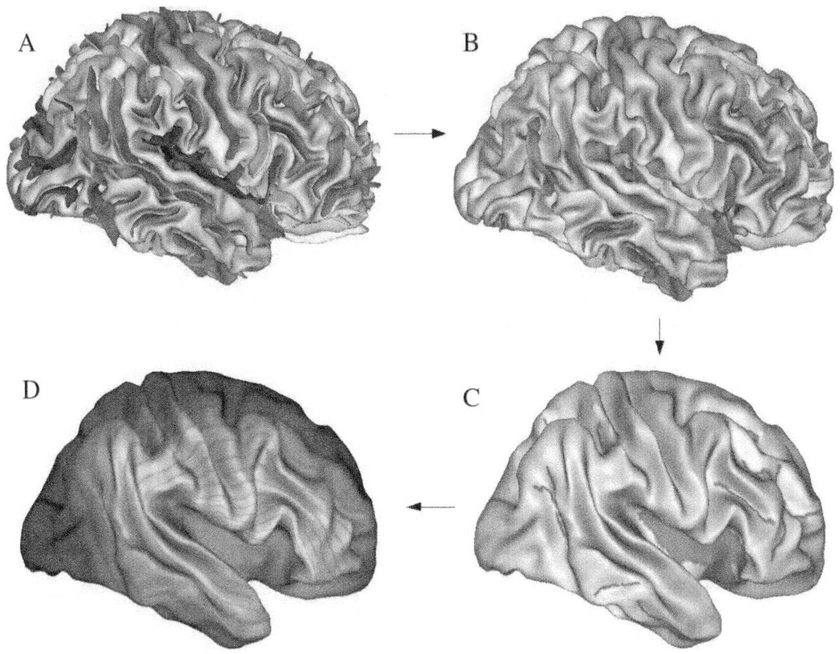

Fig. 2. Illustration of the main steps of the coordinates propagation: (A) Right hemisphere with all its sulci (each color represents a label). (B) Set of chosen constraints for latitude. (C) Constraints projection on smoothly inflated cortical mesh. (D) Resulting latitude coordinates *(All visualizations made with free package* **Brainvisa/Anatomist** - *http://brainvisa.info).*

Once we have defined the whole constraints set, including poles and origin meridian, each projection is attributed a constant longitude (meridians) or latitude (parallels). As we want an homogeneous spreading of the coordinates over the cortical surface, attention must be given to the coordinates values attributed to the constraints. A last step consists in removing some small branches of the projected sulci, in order to guaranty that each connected component is a simply connected object for the mesh topology.

3.2 Coordinates Propagation

The aim of the parameterization is to obtain a global coordinate system that complies with the initial anatomical constraints. To get such a result, we *propagate* the coordinates from the constraints. Markers are used as sources of a surfacic heat-equation diffusion process [1] that drives the propagation of both longitude and latitude over the whole hemisphere surface. Equation 1 shows a continuous heat diffusion process, where $\frac{\partial I(\overrightarrow{r},t)}{\partial t}$ represents the heat diffusion on the surface, t the time, ∇^2 the laplacian operator and K a constant conduction parameter.

$$\frac{\partial I(\boldsymbol{r},t)}{\partial t} = K\nabla^2 I(\boldsymbol{r},t) \tag{1}$$

As we are on a discrete domain, we use a finite element method to estimate $\nabla^2 I$ [3] and get the iterative numerical scheme shown in equation 2 :

$$I(\boldsymbol{r},t+\Delta t) = I(\boldsymbol{r},t) + \Delta t K\hat{\nabla}^2 I(\boldsymbol{r},t), \tag{2}$$

where $\hat{\nabla}^2 I(\boldsymbol{r},t)$ is a local estimate of the laplacian at time t. Stability is reached when $\hat{\nabla}^2 I(\boldsymbol{r},t) \to 0$. As presented in [3], $\hat{\nabla}^2 I$ is defined on each node of the surface mesh as a weighted sum of the nodes neighbours, taking into account the local geometry of the surface. Longitude and latitude are propagated separately, in an iterative process. First, the surface is initialized with the contraints and their mean value on the rest of the surface. The process then starts, iteratively updating the value at every node of the surface, except on the constraints, defined

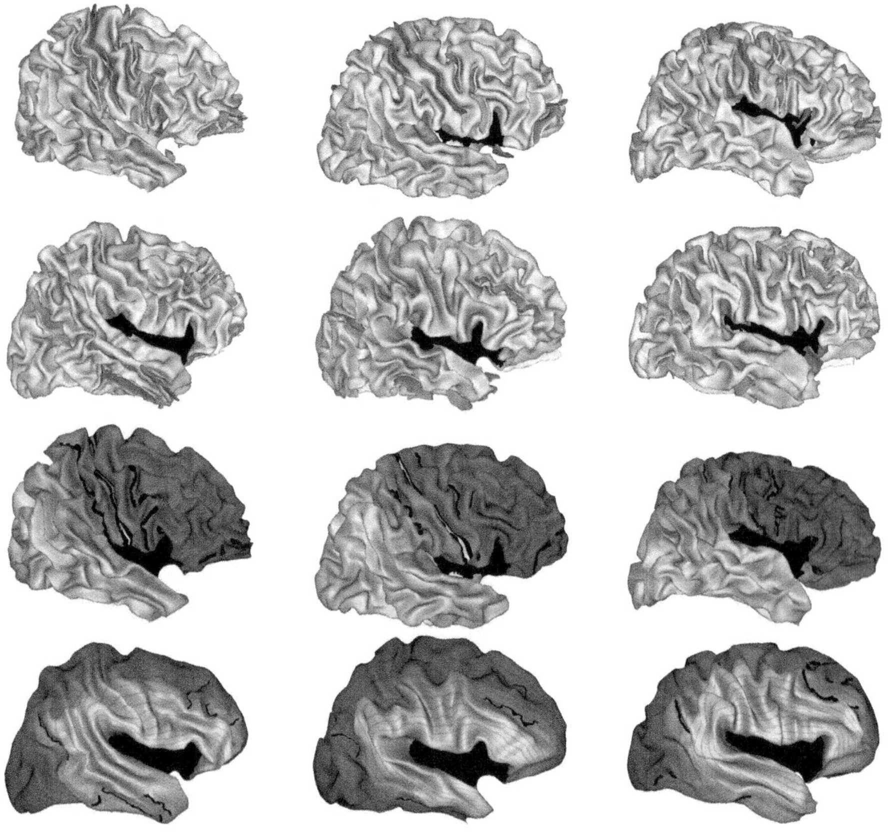

Fig. 3. Results of the coordinates propagation on six different brains. (Top row) Constraints for longitude and (second row) latitude. Resulting diffusion (constraints and isoparameter lines) for longitude (third row) and latitude (bottom row).

as constant heat sources. The result is obtained once the stability is reached, i.e. when $\hat{\nabla}^2 I \to 0$, leading to an homogeneous distribution of the coordinates values between the constraints.

4 Results and Discussion

We tested our algorithm on six nonpathological mature brains, taken from the ICBM database. Figure 3 shows the initial constraints we used and the resulting coordinate system, on the six brains. An exemple of detailed result is shown on figure 4.

The experiment led on 6 different brains shows a good behavior of the coordinate propagation. As we see on figure 4, iso-density lines of the coordinates system follows the global geometry of the surface, and locally complies with the anatomical constraints, included as axes over the surface. Coordinates are homogeneously spred all over the surface, between the constraints. Figure 5 shows in detail how the parameterization complies with the markers.

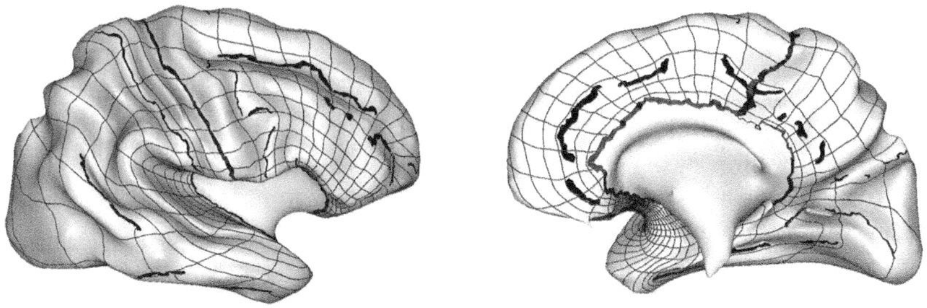

Fig. 4. Global obtained coordinate system on a right hemisphere, with resulting iso-density lines and latitude and longitude constraints

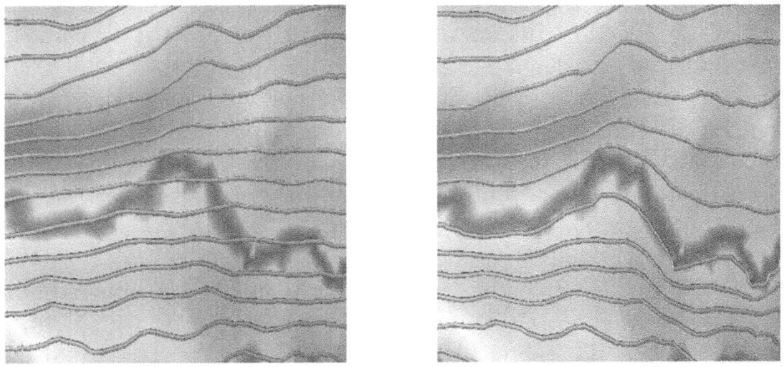

Fig. 5. Iso-density line complying with a sulcus projection. (left) Zoom on propagation result done *without any constraint.* (right) Propagation done *with constraint*, complying with the constraint (superimposed in red in both cases).

One of the problems we encounter is that parallels and meridians are propagated separately from each other. Because of this, we cannot guarantee theoretically the unicity of coordinate couples, although this problem can only be local.

We also must be aware of the influence of the inacurracy of some steps of our process, e.g. the automatic sulci recognition.

Currently, anatomical markers are subparts of reproducible sulci. A great improvement of our method would be the refinement of the definition of the markers, to match the sulcal roots model the best we could. That means we must be able to have a projection of sulcal roots. Such a process needs an important work on cortical anatomy, and is being studied at the moment.

5 Conclusion and Further Work

In this paper, we defined a process that aims at implementing an orthogonal coordinate system on every cortical surface. This parameterization relies on the theoretical orthogonal organization of the sulci. The algorithm used gives a global parameterization of the surface, that complies with anatomical markers.

From this work, several lines of research arise: refinement of the anatomical features used, the guarantee of the unicity of the parameterization which we are currently trying to solve by coupling the diffusion of longitude and latitude, and validation in a neuroimaging experimental context.

Our work could be also extended to a functional description of the surface, based on cortical folds. Other future applications are surface morphometry, or localization for the integration of modalities such as EEG and MEG.

References

1. Brechbuhler, C., Gerig, G., Kobler, O.: Parameterization of closed surfaces for 3d shape description. Computer Vision and Image Understanding **61** (1995) 154–170
2. Cachia, A., Mangin, J.F., Rivière, D., Papadopoulos-Orfanos, D., Kherif, F., Bloch, I., Régis, J.: A generic framework for parcellation of the cortical surface into gyri using geodesic voronoi diagrams. Medical Image Analysis **7** (2003) 403–416
3. Chung, M., Taylor, J.: Diffusion smoothing on brain surface via finite element method. In: IEEE International Symposium on Biomedical Imaging (ISBI). (2004)
4. Clouchoux, C., Coulon, O., Cachia, A., Rivière, D., Mangin, J.F., Régis, J.: Towards an anatomically meaningful parameterization of the cortical surface. In Barillot, C., Haynor, D., Hellier, P., eds.: Proc. of MICCAI'04. LNCS, Saint-Malo, France, Springer Verlag (2004)
5. Essen, D.V., Drury, H.: Structural and functional analyses of human cerebral cortex using a surface-based atlas. The Journal of Neuroscience **17** (1997) 7079–7102
6. Fischl, B., Sereno, M., Tootell, R., Dale, A.: Cortical surface-based analysis, ii: Inflation, flattening, and a surface-based coordinate system. NeuroImage **9** (1999) 195–207
7. Friston, K., Ashburner, J., Poline, J., Frith, C., Heather, J., Frackowiak, R.: Spatial registration and normalisation of images. In: Human Brain Mapping. Volume 2. (1995) 165–189

8. Lohmann, G., von Cramon, Y.: Automatic labeling of the human cortical surface using sulcal basins. Medical Image Analysis **4** (1999) 179–188
9. Mangin, J.F., Frouin, V., Bloch, I., Régis, J., López-Krahe, J.: From 3D magnetic resonance images to structural representations of the cortex topography using topology preserving deformations. Journal of Mathematical Imaging and Vision **5** (1995) 297–318
10. Mangin, J.F., Régis, J., Frouin, V.: Shape bottlenecks and conservative flow systems. In Press, I.C.S., ed.: IEEE Work. MMBIA, San Francisco, CA (1996) 319–328
11. Ono, M., Kubik, S., Abernathey, C.: Atlas of the cerebral sulci. Thieme Medical Publishers, Inc., New York (1990)
12. Régis, J., Mangin, J.F., Frouin, V., Sastre, F., Peragut, J.C., Samson, Y.: Generic model for the localization of the cerebral cortex and preoperative multimodal integration in epilepsy surgery. Stereotactic and Functional Neurosurgery **65** (1995) 72–80
13. Régis, J., Mangin, J., Ochiai, T., Frouin, V., Rivière, D., Cachia, A., Tamura, M., Samson, Y.: Sulcal roots generic model: a hypothesis to overcome the variability of the human cortex folding patterns. Neurol Med Chir **45** (2005) 1–17
14. Rivière, D., Mangin, J., Papadopoulos-Orfanos, D., Martinez, J., Frouin, V., Régis, J.: Automatic recognition of cortical sulci of the human brain using a congregation of neural networks. Medical Image Analysis **6** (2002) 77–92
15. Todd, P.: A geometric model for the cortical folding pattern of simple folded brains. J Theor Biol **97** (1982) 529 538
16. Toro, R., Burnod, Y.: Geometric atlas: modeling the cortex as an organized surface. NeuroImage **20** (2003) 1468–1484

Multiresolution Parametric Estimation of Transparent Motions and Denoising of Fluoroscopic Images

Vincent Auvray[1,2], Jean Liénard[2], and Patrick Bouthemy[1]

[1] IRISA/INRIA, Campus de Beaulieu, 35042 Rennes Cedex, France
[2] General Electric Healthcare, 283 rue de la Minière, 78530 Buc, France

Abstract. We describe a novel multiresolution parametric framework to estimate transparent motions typically present in X-Ray exams. Assuming the presence if two transparent layers, it computes two affine velocity fields by minimizing an appropriate objective function with an incremental Gauss-Newton technique. We have designed a realistic simulation scheme of fluoroscopic image sequences to validate our method on data with ground truth and different levels of noise. An experiment on real clinical images is also reported. We then exploit this transparent-motion estimation method to denoise two layers image sequences using a motion-compensated estimation method. In accordance with theory, we show that we reach a denoising factor of 2/3 in a few iterations without bringing any local artifacts in the image sequence.

1 Introduction

X-Ray fluoroscopic image sequences are widely used by cardialogists during interventional exams. Since radiation is kept as low as possible to protect the patient's health, the images are corrupted with a large amount of noise and must be processed. We are concerned with motion-compensated temporal filtering, which requires reliable motion estimation [1]. It is however difficult to directly apply motion estimation methods defined for video sequences to X-Ray images, since the image formation process is ruled by the phenomenon of transparency.

Unlike in usual video images, there is no occlusion in the image when an organ covers another but a grayvalue addition. The principle of brightness consistancy of points along their trajectories is in particular no longer valid. Motion estimation methods for X-Ray images have to explicitly tackle the transparency issue.

If some work have tried to directly extend usual motion estimation strategies to the transparency case [2], most of them model transparency in the spatial domain using the fundamental equation introduced by Shizawa and Mase [3], or its discrete version developed in [4]. The latter states that, if one considers the image sequence I as the superposition of two layers I_1 and I_2 ($I = I_1 + I_2$), respectively moving with velocities $v_1 = (v_{1x}, v_{1y})$ and $v_2 = (v_{2x}, v_{2y})$, we have:

$$\begin{aligned} r(x, y, v_1, v_2) = {} & I(x + v_{1x} + v_{2x}, y + v_{1y} + v_{2y}, t - 1) + I(x, y, t + 1) \\ & - I(x + v_{1x}, y + v_{1y}, t) - I(x + v_{2x}, y + v_{2y}, t) = 0 \end{aligned} \quad (1)$$

J. Duncan and G. Gerig (Eds.): MICCAI 2005, LNCS 3750, pp. 352–360, 2005.

It implicitly assumes that v_1 and v_2 are constant over time interval $[t-1, t+1]$. Even if the hypothesis of constant velocity remains problematic at a few specific instants of the heart cycle, Eq.(1) allows reliable estimations most of the time since the temporal velocity variations are usually reasonably smooth. This approach can be extended to n layers by considering $n+1$ images while extending the motion invariance assumption. We will focus on the two-layer case, but it is straightforward to extend our work to n-transparent layers.

This paper is organized as follows. In Section 2, we describe a parametric estimation method based on an efficient multiresolution minimization. Experimental results are given in Section 3 on realistic synthetic and real X-Ray images. We develop in Section 4 a motion-compensated denoising method for image sequences involving transparency. Finally, Section 5 contains concluding remarks.

2 Global Parametric Estimation

2.1 Transparent Motion Constraint with Parametric Models

A first category of methods estimate motions in transparency in the frequency domain [5], but these techniques have then to assume that the motion is constant over a large time interval (dozen of frames) and are therefore unapplicable to clinical image sequences involving time-variant movements.

To compute the velocity fields by solving equation (1) in the space domain, we have to minimize

$$J(v_1(.), v_2(.)) = \sum_{(x,y)\in\Im} r(x, y, v_1(x, y), v_2(x, y))^2 \tag{2}$$

where $r(x, y, v_1(x, y), v_2(x, y))$ is given by Eq.(1) and $\Im$ denotes the image grid.

Several methods have been proposed to solve this problem, making different assumptions on the velocity fields. The more flexible the hypothesis on the motions, the more accurate the estimations, but also the more complex the algorithm. Thus, a compromise has to be reached between measurement accuracy on the one hand and robustness to noise, computational load and sensitivity to the program tuning on the other hand.

In [6], dense velocity fields are computed by adding a regularization term to (2), allowing local motion variations to be correctly estimated at the price of a high sensitivity to noise and complex computations. On the contrary, strong assumptions on the velocities are made in [7] by considering v_1 and v_2 constant on blocks of the image (and therefore accounting for a limited range of motions), to allow fast and robust motion estimation. In [4], the velocities are decomposed on a B-spline basis, so that this method can account for complex motion, while staying relatively tractable. However, the structure of the basis has to be carefully adapted to every particular situation and the computational load becomes high if fine measurement accuracy is needed.

We propose instead to represent the velocity fields with 2D polynomial models, which can account for the considered motions (heart beating, lungs dilation, diaphragm translation), while requiring a few parameters for each layer. We believe that affine models describe the anatomic movements accurately enough, at least within a given area, while keeping the model simple to handle both the transparency issue and the high level of noise in the images. Our framework would also work with higher-order polynomial models, such as quadratic ones, if needed.

Hence, the velocity vector at point (x, y) for the layer i is given by:

$$v_{ix}(x, y) = c_{i,1} + a_{i,1}.x + a_{i,2}.y \quad \text{and} \quad v_{iy}(x, y) = c_{i,2} + a_{i,3}.x + a_{i,4}.y \tag{3}$$

Criterion (2) becomes a function of 12 parameters for the whole image:

$$J(\theta_1, \theta_2) = \sum_{(x,y)\in\Im} r(x, y; \theta_1, \theta_2) \text{ with } \theta_i = (c_{i,1}, c_{i,2}, a_{i,1}, a_{i,2}, a_{i,3}, a_{i,4}) \tag{4}$$

2.2 Multiresolution Transparent Motion Estimation

If the velocity magnitudes were small, we could consider a linearized version of (4), and then minimize it using an efficient iterative minimization scheme.

Since large motions can occur in practice, we introduce a multiresolution incremental framework exploiting Gaussian pyramids of the three consecutive images. At its coarsest level L, motions are small enough to allow for a minimisation using the conjugate gradient algorithm applied to the objective function (4) once linearized, which supplies first estimates of the two motions, denoted $(\hat{\theta}_1^L, \hat{\theta}_2^L)$.

At the level $L-1$, we initialize $(\theta_1^{L-1}, \theta_2^{L-1})$ with $(\tilde{\theta}_1^{L-1}, \tilde{\theta}_2^{L-1})$ where $\tilde{c}_{i,k}^{L-1} = 2\hat{c}_{i,k}^L$ $(k = 1, 2)$ and $\tilde{a}_{i,l}^{L-1} = \hat{a}_{i,l}^L$ $(l = 1, 4)$. We then write $\theta_i^{L-1} = \tilde{\theta}_1^{L-1} + \Delta\theta_i^{L-1}$, and we minimize the objective function $J(\theta_1, \theta_2)$ with respect to $\Delta\theta_i^{L-1}$, once J is linearized around $(\tilde{\theta}_1^{L-1}, \tilde{\theta}_2^{L-1})$. This incremental Gauss-Newton method is then iterated through the successive resolution levels until the finest one.

2.3 Initialisation with a Simplex Algorithm

Such a minimization scheme is efficient and fast, however it is also sensitive to the initialization, especially since we are dealing with medical X-ray images involving low contrast and high noise.

We resort to the downhill simplex method to provide an appropriate initialization at the level L. This minimization technique can be applied to nonlinear functions. For a function defined on a space of dimension n, it selects $n + 1$ samples. In our case, to minimize J in the 12-dimensional space of the affine motion parameters, it will involve 13 samples of parameters. At each iteration, it substitutes for the sample corresponding to the highest value of J a new sample found on a line perpendicular to the hyperplane containing the other n test points [8].

Computational load is limited since we use the simplex algorithm at the coarsest image resolution only.

3 Results of Transparent Motion Estimation

3.1 Image Simulation Process

Image Modeling. To synthetize images representative for X-Ray exams, we have modeled an imaging system as shown on Fig.1. The anatomy A attenuates the input dose R_{in} to give $R_{out} = R_{in}.A$. A part of the input radiation is also scattered, which is modeled by adding to R_{out} a part of a large low-pass version of R_{out}: $S = s.R_{out}^{LP}$ (s ranging from 10 to 50%). A Poisson quantic noise typical for radiation is added. Finally, the X-photons are converted into grayscale levels on the receiver screen, which has a given Modulation Transfer Function MTF.

Transparent Image Sequence Generation. To reproduce configurations typical of cardiac exams, we have formed one layer by taking a real image of an abdominal exam where the spine and ribs are visible, and the second layer with an X-Ray image of the heart (displayed on Fig.2).

To build the attenuation maps of these two images, we have inverted the chain described on Fig.1. We have thus transformed the grayscale image into the X-photonic image, compensated for the scatter, and inferred the attenuation maps from the dose used during the exams. Since we cannot invert the noise operator, we have chosen high radiation exams guaranteeing nearly noise-free images.

The two attenuation images were moved with the simulated velocity field and multiplied to generate the anatomy corresponding to the superposition of the two layers. A fluoroscopic acquisition was simulated following the image formation process given in Fig.1 to get realistic X-Ray images with two transparent layers undergoing known motions. Finally, to work with additive transparency instead of multiplicative one, we applied a log operator to the composite image.

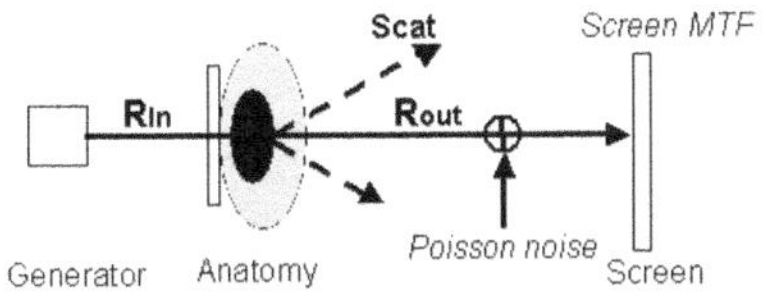

Fig. 1. Image formation model

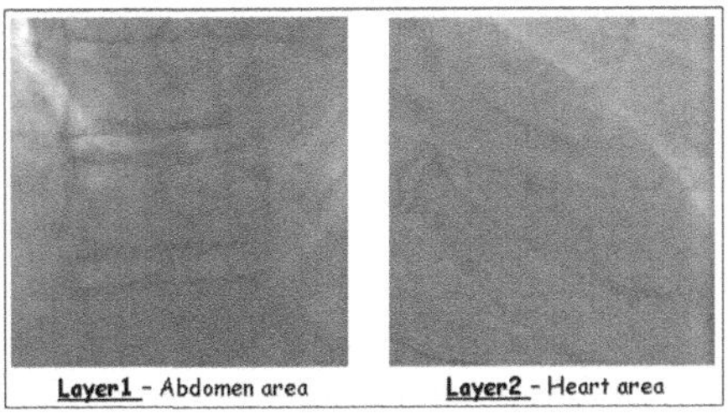

Fig. 2. Real X-Ray images used as layers for the image sequence generation

3.2 Results on Generated Examples

We have generated 250 image sequences of three frames as described above, the abdominal layer undergoing a translation and the heart layer an affine motion. The motion parameter values are randomly chosen while ensuring a displacement

Table 1. Mean estimation errors in pixels for the proposed framework, with different noise levels and scatter rate, with or without MTF addition (see main text)

	NoMTF		MTF	
Noise	10	20	10	20
No scatter	0.30	0.55	0.49	2.09
20% scatter	0.36	0.76	0.71	2.84
50% scatter	0.38	1.27	1.04	4.54

at each pixel in the range of -8 to 8 pixels. The images are coded on 12 bits, and their mean value is typically 500.

The estimation framework runs in 5 seconds for $288 * 288$ images on a Pentium IV (2.4 GHz and 1 Go). Tab.1 contains the mean estimation errors on the velocity vectors for different noise levels (standard deviation of $\sigma = 10$ or $\sigma = 20$ grayscale values), scatter rate and with or without MTF simulation.

The estimations are quite satisfactory if we do not take the MTF into account. Even with a large scatter rate, the mean velocities errors are below 1 pixel. However, the motion estimation method seems sensitive to the correlated noise introduced by the MTF. For images corresponding to a moderate radiation level (noise with $\sigma = 10$), the estimations remain reliable. Nevertheless, for a higher noise level which may be encountered in real images ($\sigma = 20$ and 20% scatter, 50% scatter being a quite extreme situation in practice), the velocities are affected by a mean error of about 2.5 pixels. This would imply some extention of the method to handle MTF effects in highly noisy situations.

3.3 Results on Clinical Image Sequences

We have also carried out experiments on real medical image sequences. X-Ray medical image sequences usually involves several layers as a whole, but only one or two layers at a time within delimited areas. The segmentation of the image into areas corresponding to two-layers-configurations is beyond the scope of this paper.

Therefore, we have selected a part of a cardiac fluoroscopic sequence corresponding to a two-layer transparency case. It represents an area of about 5cm x 5cm on the right of the heart, and was acquired at 30 Hz. Let us point out that these fluoroscopic exams are usually carried out without contrast media injection.

Two frames of this sequence are displayed on Fig.3 along with two computed transparent motion fields. The heart (appearing dark here) is beating on the right of the images over a static background corresponding to the spine and ribs. The bright tissues of the lungs are following the heart motion, so that an observer perceives only two "motions", one corresponding to the static background and the other to the group "heart+lungs". The magnitude of the motion over a cycle

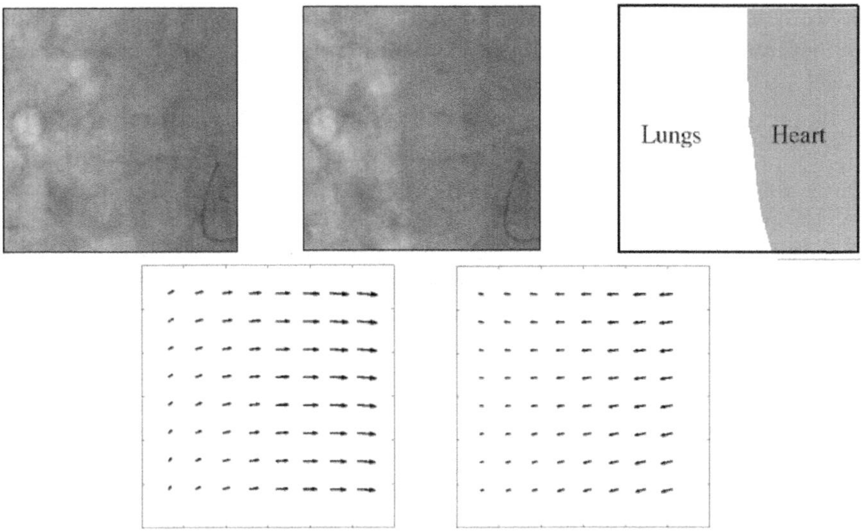

Fig. 3. Top: From left to right: Images at time instants 1 and 8 of the real fluoroscopic image sequence, anatomical moving regions. Bottom: computed velocities of the mobile layer with our parametric transparent motion estimation method during the diastole (at time 6), and during the systole (at time 13).

is 25 pixels. The images have a low contrast and are corrupted by an important noise ($\sigma \simeq 20$).

The estimated affine motion models are coherent with the movements observed on the sequence: the background is static (and therefore the corresponding velocity field is not plotted in Fig.3) and the (affine) motion of the heart matches the anatomic truth. Its magnitude is correctly decreasing in the lungs area with the distance to the heart.

The images are noisy, low contrasted and contain complex movements. Moreover, the motion is not perfectly constant over three consecutive images, which does not impair the estimation here. Even in this complicated situation, the proposed transparent motion estimation framework supplies convincing results.

4 Motion-Compensated Image Sequence Denoising with Transparency

4.1 Filtering Approach

Fluoroscopic images are acquired at a very low radiation level so that they need to be denoised to be tractable for the clinician. Their high aquisition rate (typically 30 Hz) is favourable to temporal filtering, whereas spatial filtering is difficult since noise correlation is very perceptible at such a high frame rate.

A direct application of motion-compensated temporal filter for video images (such as those reviewed in [9]) is impossible since it would require to have first separated the layers, which is a complex process. Instead, we propose a motion-compensated temporal filter adapted to transparent images. Rewriting (1) as:

$$I(x,y,t+1) = I(x+v_{1x}, y+v_{1y}, t) + I(x+v_{2x}, y+v_{2y}, t) - I(x+v_{1x}+v_{2x}, y+v_{1y}+v_{2y}, t-1) \quad (5)$$

we can note that, if the velocities v_1 and v_2 are available, the image at time $t+1$ can be predicted from the two previous images. If the estimated velocities are accurate enough, the predicted image $\hat{I}(x,y,t+1)$ is supposed to match the observed image $I(x,y,t+1)$ except for the noise realizations, thus providing the means to smooth out the noise.

4.2 Recursive Filtering Method

We adopt a temporally recursive linear filter technique specified as follows:

$$\tilde{I}_{t+1}(x,y) = \alpha(t).\hat{I}_{t+1}(x,y) + (1-\alpha(t)).I_{t+1}(x,y) \quad (6)$$

Let us note $(\sigma^2_{\tilde{I},t})_{t\in\mathbb{N}}$ the noise variance of the successive denoised images. From Eq.(5), we can infer that the noise variance of the predicted image equals $\sigma^2_{\tilde{I},t-1} + 2\sigma^2_{\tilde{I},t}$, so that (6) implies:

$$\sigma^2_{\tilde{I},t+1} = \alpha(t)^2\sigma^2_{\tilde{I},t-1} + 2.\alpha(t)^2\sigma^2_{\tilde{I},t} + (1-\alpha(t))^2\sigma^2_I \quad (7)$$

with σ^2_I the variance of the original noise. $\hat{\alpha}(t) = \sigma^2_I/(\sigma^2_{\tilde{I},t-1} + 2.\sigma^2_{\tilde{I},t} + \sigma^2_I)$ guarantees the smallest $\sigma^2_{\tilde{I},t+1}$. With this setting of $\alpha(t)$, the sequence $(\hat{\sigma}^2_{\tilde{I},t})_{t\in\mathbb{N}}$ has two positive fixed points: a repulsive one 0 and an attractive one 2/3.

4.3 Denoising Results

We have applied the proposed denoising scheme to 100 image sequences generated as explained in subsection 3.1, with MTF simulation and a scatter rate of 20%. Since we can in practice estimate the noise in the original images from acquisition parameters, we can recursively compute $\hat{\alpha}(t)$ for an optimal denoising. Our temporal filter used these settings of $\hat{\alpha}(t)$ (reported in Tab.2 with the theoretical denoising factor $\hat{\sigma}^2_{\tilde{I},t}/\sigma^2_I$) and the velocities estimated by the transparent motion estimation method of Section 2.

The difference between denoised and original image sequences is quite noticeable if visualized in a live manner at 30 Hz, but cannot be efficiently highlighted from two printed frames. Therefore, we rather present our simulation results in Tab.2. No local artifacts are observed on the denoised images: constrasts are preserved because of the motion compensation and no noise coloration nor structural artifacts have appeared.

Table 2. Noise reduction for a transparent image sequence with two layers. Theoretical values compared with experiments for different radiation configurations (MTF simulation and 20% scatter).

Frame t	n	0	1	2	3	4	5	6	7	8
Theoretical	$\hat{\alpha}(t)$	0.250	0.286	0.315	0.324	0.329	0.331	0.332	0.333	0.333
values	$\hat{\sigma}^2_{\tilde{I},t}/\sigma^2_I$	0.750	0.714	0.685	0.676	0.670	0.669	0.668	0.667	0.667
Simulations ($\sigma_I = 10$)	$\sigma^2_{\tilde{I},t}/\sigma^2_I$	0.653	0.648	0.659	0.661	0.655	0.655	0.657	0.655	0.657
Simulations ($\sigma_I = 20$)	$\sigma^2_{\tilde{I},t}/\sigma^2_I$	0.670	0.667	0.670	0.668	0.670	0.668	0.669	0.672	0.671

5 Conclusion

We have designed a novel and efficient multiresolution parametric framework to estimate transparent motions for two layers by using affine motion models. We have generated realistic X-Ray image sequences to assess the performance of our method with an available ground truth. The results on medium-level radiation images are quite satisfactory, and the performance smoothly decreases with higher noise and scatter unless the MTF effect is incorporated. Experiments on real clinical image sequences were also reported with convincing results.

An application of this method for temporal denoising transparent image sequences with two moving layers was also presented. Preliminary experiments have shown that we can reach in a few iterations a denoising factor of 2/3 without adding any local artifacts in the denoised image sequences.

We now plan to extend our method to handle the MTF effect and to carry out more experiments on real X-ray image sequences. We also plan to tackle the "*distributed two-layer configuration*". The proposed method will then be applicable if we can segment the image in its different regions of two layer configuration.

References

1. Dekeyser, F., Bouthemy, P., Pérez, P.: Spatio-temporal Wiener filtering of image sequences using a parametric motion model. In: IEEE Int. Conf. on Image Processing, Vancouver (2000)
2. Irani, M., Rousso, B., Peleg, S.: Computing occluding and transparent motions. International Journal of Computer Vision **12** (1994) 5–16
3. Shizawa, M., Mase, K.: Principle of superposition: A common computational framework for analysis of multiple motions. In: IEEE Workshop on Visual Motion, Princetown, New-Jersey (1991) 164–172
4. Pingault, M., Bruno, E., Pellerin, D.: A robust multiscale B-spline function decomposition for estimating motion transparency. IEEE Trans. on Image Processing **12** (2003) 1416–1426
5. Pingault, M., Pellerin, D.: Motion estimation of transparent objects in the frequency domain. Signal Processing **84** (2004) 709–719

6. Stuke, I., Aach, T., Mota, C., Barth, E.: Estimation of multiple motions: regularization and performance evaluation. Image and Video Communications and Processing 2003, SPIE **5022** (2003) 75–86
7. Stuke, I., Aach, T., Mota, C., Barth, E.: Estimation of multiple motions by block matching. In: 4th ACIS International Conference on Software Engineering, Artificial Intelligence, Networking and Parallel/Distributed Computing (SNPD 2003), Luebeck (2003) 358–362
8. Press, W., al: Downhill Simplex Method in Multidimensions. In: Numerical recipies in C : The Art of Scientific Computing. Cambridge university press (1988-1992) 408–412
9. Brailean, J., Kleihorst, R., Efstratiadis, S., Katsaggelos, K., Lagendijk, R.: Noise reduction filters for dynamic image sequences: A review. Proceedings of the IEEE **83** (1995) 1272–1292

Plaque and Stent Artifact Reduction in Subtraction CT Angiography Using Nonrigid Registration and a Volume Penalty

Dirk Loeckx[1], Stylianos Drisis[2], Frederik Maes[1], Dirk Vandermeulen[1], Guy Marchal[2], and Paul Suetens[1]

[1] Medical Image Computing (ESAT/PSI), Faculty of Engineering
[2] Department of Radiology, Faculty of Medicine,
University Hospital Gasthuisberg, Herestraat 49, B-3000 Leuven, Belgium
Dirk.Loeckx@uz.kuleuven.ac.be

Abstract. Computed tomography angiography (CTA) is an established tool for vessel imaging. Yet, high-intense structures in the contrast image can seriously hamper luminal visualisation. This can be solved by subtraction CTA, where a native image is subtracted from the contrast image. However, patient and organ motion limit the application of this technique. Within this paper, a fully automated intensity-based nonrigid 3D registration algorithm for subtraction CT angiography is presented, using a penalty term to avoid volume change during registration. Visual and automated validation on four clinical datasets clearly show that the algorithm strongly reduces motion artifacts in subtraction CTA. With our method, 39% to 99% of the artifacts disappear, also those caused by minimal displacement of stents or calcified plaques. This results in a better visualisation of the vessel lumen, also of the smaller vessels, allowing a faster and more accurate inspection of the whole vascular structure, especially in case of stenosis.

1 Introduction

Computed tomography angiography (CTA) is an established minimally invasive tool for imaging most major and also smaller vessels in the body [1]. Since its introduction more than 10 years ago, ongoing development of CT modalities resulted in shorter image acquisition time, a better spatial resolution and improved volume coverage.

New scanning protocols create an increasing amount of data, requiring a change in the way CTA studies are visualised and interpreted. Four main visualisation techniques are currently in use: multi- or curved planar reformat, maximum intensity projection (MIP), shaded-surface display and volume rendering [1,2]. Multiplanar or, preferably, curved planar reformat provides the most comprehensive cross-sectional luminal assessment, but extensive user interaction is required to accurately select the vessel of interest. Also, curved planar reformat can display only a single vessel at a time. MIP, shaded-surface display and volume rendering are true 3D visualisation methods, where the user can assess

J. Duncan and G. Gerig (Eds.): MICCAI 2005, LNCS 3750, pp. 361–368, 2005.

the whole vessel tree simultaneously. Using modern computer graphics hardware, high-resolution real-time interaction is possible. 3D methods render an in-depth view of the CT data, not only of the contrast-enhanced vessel tree, but of other structures as well. The presence of high-intense entities, like bone, heavy calcification or endoluminal stents can seriously hamper the luminal visualisation and/or require time-consuming manual editing [3].

This problem can be solved by recording a native image immediately before contrast administration. The native image is subtracted from the contrast image, resulting in a difference image that only visualises the contrast agent, which is since long the standard procedure in 2D DSA. The quality of the difference image is often deteriorated by motion-related artifacts due to patient or organ motion, especially when stents or calcified plaques are present in the vessel of interest. As proposed by several authors, this problem can be overcome by registration of the native to the contrast image. Most authors apply a rigid [4,5] or piecewise rigid [3,6] approach, which is often limited to correcting for intra-slice deformations only. However, those approaches can not remove motion artifacts caused by inter-slice motion or require prior selection and/or segmentation of the individual objects of interest.

In this paper, we present a fully automated intensity-based nonrigid 3D registration algorithm for subtraction CT angiography. A B-spline deformation mesh is used to calculate the local deformation in every voxel, using maximisation of mutual information of corresponding voxel intensities as similarity criterion [7]. By gradually increasing the number of mesh control points during optimisation, the deformation evolves from coarse to fine and becomes more and more local. A volume conservation penalty term is introduced to prevent physically impossible or improbable deformations, such as plaque shrinkage or enlargement. A similar approach was presented by Rohlfing *et al.* [8], but without proper validation. Also, we apply the registration to more difficult datasets containing severe artifacts near the vessel tree. Registration quality is evaluated based on a quantitative measurement of motion artifacts in the subtraction image. Both the automated measure and visual inspection consistently confirm the ability of our nonrigid registration scheme to create quasi artifact-free subtraction CT angiography images, especially in the presence of high intense structures such as bone, plaques, and stents.

2 Methods

2.1 Deformation Model

The nonrigid deformation is modelled by a B-spline deformation mesh [9,10]. A grid of mesh control points is positioned over the image. To model a more global deformation, the grid spacing is large, yielding a coarse mesh with few control points. A fine mesh has a small grid spacing and many control points, allowing a more local deformation. This approach allows a gradual refinement of the deformation mesh by decreasing the grid spacing.

2.2 Cost Function

The proposed cost function $E_c = E_s + \omega_p E_p$ consists of a similarity measure E_s and a penalty term E_p, using ω_p to modulate the influence of the penalty term. The similarity measure is the driving force behind the registration process and aims to maximise the similarity between the two images. As the contrast agent introduces local intensity differences between the images to be registered, similarity measures assuming identical intensity levels for corresponding structures, are inappropriate. Therefore, mutual information, which models the statistical dependence between the native and contrast image, is chosen [7]. The penalty term E_p is based on the Jacobian determinant, which models local compression or expansion, and penalises volume change. The volume penalty is $E_p(\boldsymbol{\mu}) = \frac{1}{V}\int_V \left(J_{\mathbf{g}}(\mathbf{r};\boldsymbol{\mu}) - 1\right)^2 d\mathbf{r}$, with $J_{\mathbf{g}}(\mathbf{r};\boldsymbol{\mu})$ the Jacobian determinant at location $\mathbf{r}$ for transformation parameters $\boldsymbol{\mu}$ and V the image volume.

2.3 Algorithm

A multiresolution optimisation algorithm is adopted [10], using 5 multiresolution stages. The algorithm gradually evolves from a coarsely sampled deformation mesh acting on downsampled images to a dense mesh at full image resolution. In stages one and two, the image is downsampled to half the original size, while stages 3 to 5 are calculated at full resolution. Initially, a B-spline mesh spacing of 64 voxels is used, that gradually decreases to 32, 16 and finally 8 voxels in stages 2, 4 and 5 respectively. The multiresolution approach increases processing speed by performing the initial calculations on subsampled data. Moreover, gradually decreasing the grid spacing will first recover more global deformations and progressively advance to finer deformations, thus avoiding local optima and creating a more realistic deformation field.

2.4 Validation Measure

Ideally, validation of medical image processing software should be performed by medical doctors on clinical applications. During the development of the algorithm, however, this is not always feasible. For a quick and reproducible evaluation of the influence of several registration settings an automated validation measure was developed. An automated measure also avoids intra-observer variations and the influence of the visualisation settings, thereby concentrating on the registration quality. The measure models image artifacts in the difference

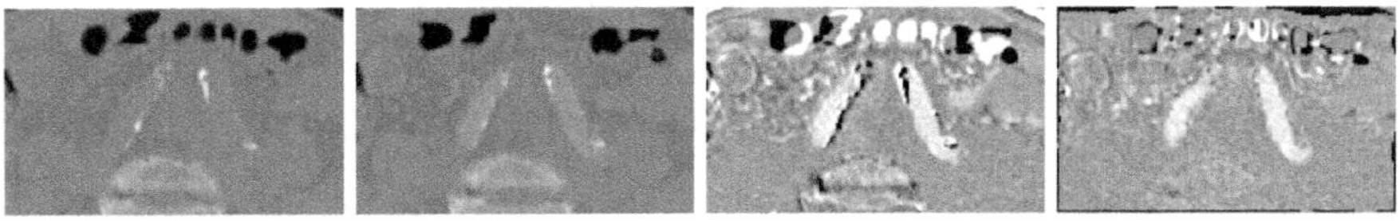

(a) (b) (c) (d)

Fig. 1. Example of a (a) native and (b) contrast image, and the resulting difference image with (c) rigid and (d) nonrigid registration. In (c), the dark and bright motion artifacts are clearly visible, whereas they have almost completely disappeared in (d).

Table 1. Overview of the intensity differences between the structures of interest in subtraction CT images (in HU)

	Contrast	*Soft Tissue*	*Vessel*	*Plaque*
Native		0	300	> 300
Soft Tissue	0	**0**	300	> 300
Vessel	0	0	**300**	> 300
Plaque	> 300	< -300	< 0	**0**

image. In the neighbourhood of the vessel, three important structures can be expected: soft tissue, vessel and high intense structures like calcified plaques or metal stents. An illustrative image is shown in Figure 1, and the expected intensities of these structures in the native, contrast and difference image are given in Table 1. For example, plaque voxels in the native image correctly registered to plaque voxels in the contrast image will yield an intensity difference of 0 Hounsfield units (HU) in the difference image. Plaque voxels incorrectly registered to soft-tissue in the contrast image will yield an intensity difference smaller then -300 HU, thus causing distinct dark artifacts.

For perfectly aligned datasets, only intensities on the diagonal of the table would appear in the difference image. The accepted intensities all lie in the range $0 \rightarrow 300$ HU. Due to tissue and contrast density fluctuations, noise and the partial volume effect, the actual intensity will differ from the expected one, especially along the upper limit. Therefore, we assume all voxels with intensity < -100 HU in the difference image to be misaligned. Misregistration also induces bright artifacts in the subtraction image, but these can not be distinguished from true enhanced vessel voxels. However, because of the volume preserving penalty, the number of voxels in the low and high intensity artifacts will be about the same. Hence, we define a region of interest (ROI) consisting of all voxels with intensity > 100 HU in the native image (i.e. calcified regions or stents) and intensity > -500 HU in the post-contrast image (to exclude air) and count the fraction of voxels in this ROI with a value < -100 HU in the difference image (i.e. dark appearing subtraction artifacts) to measure local misregistration in high-intense regions.

2.5 Visualisation

Besides the computed validation measure, we also performed visual inspection of the registered images. To obtain optimal results for the volume renderer, we simultaneously applied an intensity window to the transformed native image ($-50 \rightarrow 1000$ HU) and the contrast image ($100 \rightarrow 1000$ HU), showing only voxels that fall inside the specified window in both images. Finally, in the difference image, the intensities are clipped to ($-50 \rightarrow 400$ HU).

3 Experiments

The registration algorithm was applied to 4 datasets. P1 shows a healthy thoracic aorta, P2 and P3 show stented iliac arteries. P4 pictures a patient with an

Table 2. Dimension, voxelsize and registration time for the different image datasets

Data-set	*Dimensions (voxels)*	*Voxelsize (mm)*	*Time (h:m:s)*
P1	[91 136 411]	$0.74^2 \times 0.5$	3:05:20
P2	[158 187 261]	$0.70^2 \times 1.0$	2:14:08
P3	[114 177 144]	$0.68^2 \times 0.8$	0:24:24
P4	[221 129 151]	$0.74^2 \times 1.0$	2:49:48

Table 3. Influence of the volume preserving penalty on the artifact reduction (compared to rigid registration)

ω_p	*P1*	*P2*	*P3*	*P4*
0	98.93%	72.83%	29.89%	80.17%
0.01	98.92%	67.94%	27.17%	91.29%
0.1	98.67%	70.64%	32.02%	92.06%
1	**99.05%**	73.09%	38.53%	**95.23%**
10	98.98%	**75.21%**	**39.42%**	92.01%
100	97.51%	74.68%	38.56%	94.60%

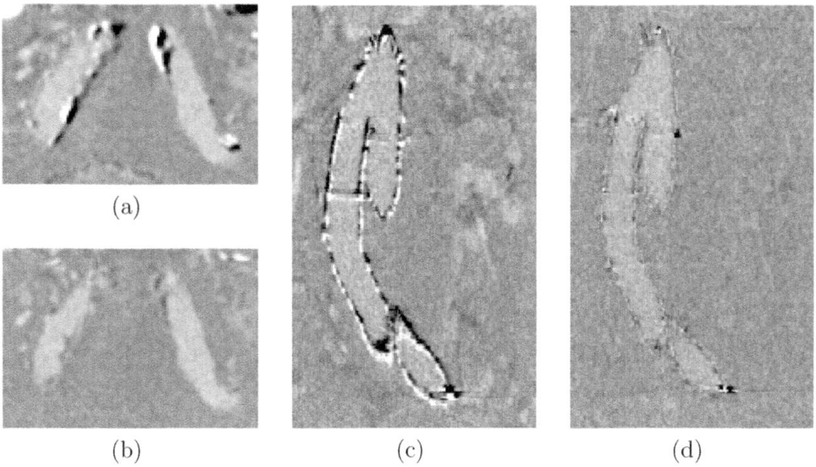

Fig. 2. (a,b) Axial slice of the highly calcified area at the aortic bifurcation of dataset P4; (c,d) sagittal slice of dataset P2 picturing a stent. These difference images show severe motion artifacts in case of rigid registration (a,c), appearing as dark and light areas near the vessel boundary. After nonrigid registration (b,d), the artifacts largely disappear.

aneurysma in the aorta abdominalis and heavy calcifications. An overview of the different datasets is given in Table 2.

The influence of the volume penalty on the artifact reduction is shown in Table 3. The artifact reduction is expressed as the artifact fraction after non-rigid registration compared to artifact fraction after rigid registration. The minimal remaining artifact fraction is 0.21%, 9.04%, 11.56% and 0.46% for P1, P2, P3 and P4 respectively. For visual inspection, we displayed the difference image slice by slice and in a volume renderer, allowing real-time interaction with the data. This inspection confirmed the results obtained by the validation measure. Figure 2 shows some representative slices of the difference image obtained with rigid and nonrigid registration. A volume rendering of all four datasets is shown in Figure 3.

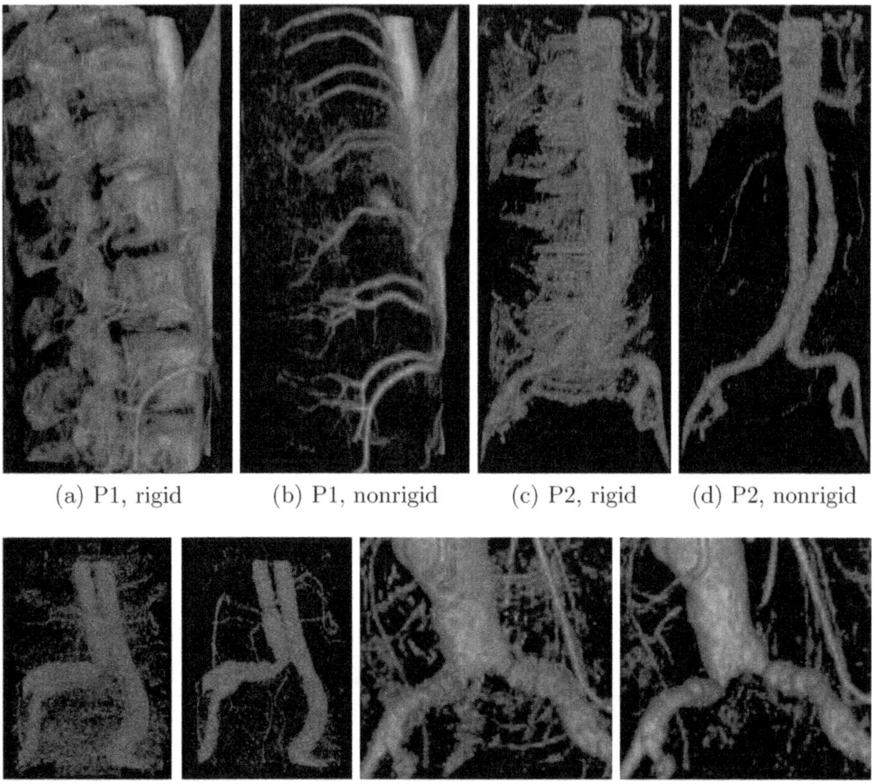

(a) P1, rigid (b) P1, nonrigid (c) P2, rigid (d) P2, nonrigid

(e) P3, rigid (f) P3, nonrigid (g) P4, rigid (detail) (h) P4, nonrigid (detail)

Fig. 3. Volume rendering of subtraction CT image for the different datasets using rigid and nonrigid registration. Nonrigid registration substantially reduces the motion artifacts. E.g., in (g), plaque artifacts obscure the stenosis at the bifurcation, whereas in (h) the narrowing is clearly visible.

4 Discussion

4.1 Artifacts

It is immediately clear from Figures 2-3 and Table 3 that nonrigid registration substantially reduces motion artifacts in the difference image. Artifacts caused by bone and calcified plaques almost disappear completely, enabling 3D visualisations, like volume rendering or MIP, to picture only the vessel lumen. This might strongly reduce reading time, as the radiologist can get a clear overview of the whole vessel. For example, in Figure 3(g), plaque artifacts obscure the stenosis at the bifurcation, requiring a slice-by-slice or planar reformat visualisation for proper diagnosis. In Figure 3(h), the narrowing is immediately clearly visible. The artifact reduction also allows the visualisation of smaller vessels, which otherwise would have not been discernable from the background noise, as can be seen in Figure 3(b).

Stent artifacts are also strongly reduced, although they are not removed completely. Due to the high attenuation difference between metallic stents and the surrounding tissue, stents will not only cause motion artifacts in the difference image, but also generate metal or streak artifacts in the native and contrast enhanced images. Especially in multi slice spiral CT, the appearance of these artifacts depends on small patient displacement and the x-ray tube starting angle [6]. Therefore, they can not be removed completely, as can be seen in Figures 3(d), 3(f) and 2(d).

4.2 Calculation Time

Depending on the size of the dataset, registration takes from 0.5 to 3 hours on a 2.8 Ghz Pentium 4 processor. For diagnostic clinical use, calculations can be performed off-line and therefore timing is not critical. If emergency or interventional applications are sought, several approaches are possible to reduce the calculation time. If timing is crucial, a trade-off of registration quality for registration time can be made using less multiresolution stages. Our experience shows that the larger artifacts mostly disappear after the first two stages, allowing a reduction of the required processing time down to 5 to 30 minutes. However, the final stages are necessary to cancel out smaller artifacts. A second possibility to speed up the registration is the manual selection of a smaller region of interest, thus reducing the size of the dataset to be registered. Also, some improvements might be made to the algorithm itself. For instance, the registration could be constrained to only account for the regions in and surrounding the vessel tree by prior crude segmentation of the original images.

4.3 Volume Preserving Penalty

The contrast agent introduces intensity differences between the native and the contrast enhanced images. Without a volume preserving penalty, the algorithm would be tempted to reduced these differences by increasing the plaque volume, especially when using a fine mesh. However, if the volume weigh ω_p is too high, the mesh will be too stiff to allow registration whatsoever. Using a sub-optimal volume penalty worsens the registration and fails to correct some smaller motion artifacts. This effect was most clear in datasets P1 and P4, while datasets P2 and P3 always showed some artifacts near the stents. Table 3 indicates that the optimal value of the volume weigh ω_p is rather independent of the acual datasets under study. Therefore, we propose a volume weight of $\omega_p = 1$.

5 Conclusion

In this paper, we showed that nonrigid registration can substantially reduce the artifacts in subtraction CT angiography, allowing for a clear 3D view of the vascular structure, also in the presence of calcified plaques and stents. We presented a quantitative validation of registration quality by evaluating the number of voxels that correspond to dark appearing artifacts in the difference image. Currently, the biggest concern of the algorithm is the calculation time, impeding real-time or emergency diagnostic use.

Acknowledgements

This work is part of K.U.Leuven/OF/GOA/2004/05 and FWO G.0258.02.

References

1. Napoli, A., Fleischmann, D., Chan, F., Catalano, C., Hellinger, J., Passariello, R., Rubi, G.: Computed tomography angiography: State-of-the-art imaging using multidetector-row technology. J Comput Assist Tomogr **28** (2004) S32–S45
2. Duddalwar, V.: Multislice CT angiography: a practical guide to CT angiography in vascular imaging and intervention. The Britisch Journal of Radiology **77** (2004) S27–S38
3. Beier, J., Oellinger, H., Richter, C., Fleck, E., Felix, R.: Registered image subtraction for CT-, MR- and coronary angiography. European Radiology **7** (1997) 82–89
4. Kwon, S.M., Kim, Y.S., Kim, T.S., Ra, J.B.: Digital subtraction CT angiography based on efficient 3D registration and refinement. Comput Med Imaging Graph **28** (2004) 391–400
5. Poletti, P.A., Rosset, A., Didier, D., Bachmann, P., Verdun, F.R., Rutschmann, O., Vallee, J.P., Terrier, F., Khatchatourov, G.: Subtraction CT angiography of the lower limbs: A new technique for the evaluation of acute arterial occlusion. American Journal of Radiology **183** (2004) 1445–1448
6. van Straten, M., Venema, H.W., Streekstra, G.J., Majoie, C.B.L.M., den Heeten, G.J., Grimbergen, C.A.: Removel of bone in CT angiography of the cervical arteries by piecewise mask bone elimination. Medical Physics **31** (2004) 2924–2933
7. Maes, F., Collignon, A., Vandermeulen, D., Marchal, G., Suetens, P.: Multimodality image registration by maximization of mutual information. IEEE Trans. Med. Imag. **16** (1997) 187–198
8. Rohlfing, T., Maurer, C.J., Beier, J.: Reduction of motion artifacts in three-dimensional CT-DSA using constrained adaptive multilevel free-form registration. In: Computer Assisted Radiology and Surgery (CARS 2001). (2001)
9. Rueckert, D., Frangi, A., Schnabel, J.: Automatic construction of 3D statistical deformation models using non-rigid registration. In: Proc. MICCAI. (2001) 77–84
10. Loeckx, D., Maes, F., Vandermeulen, D., Suetens, P.: Nonrigid image registration using free-form deformations with a local rigidity constraint. In: Lecture notes in computer science, vol. 3216, pp. 639-646, 2004 (Proceedings 7th international conference on medical image computing and computer-assisted intervention - MICCAI 2004, part I). (2004)

Respiratory Motion Correction in Emission Tomography Image Reconstruction

Mauricio Reyes[1], Grégoire Malandain[1], Pierre Malick Koulibaly[2], Miguel A. González Ballester[3], and Jacques Darcourt[2]

[1] Epidaure team, INRIA Sophia Antipolis, France
{Mauricio.Reyes_Aguirre,Gregoire.Malandain}@sophia.inria.fr
[2] Nuclear medicine department, Centre Antoine Lacassagne, Nice, France
[3] MEM center, University of Bern, Switzerland

Abstract. In Emission Tomography imaging, respiratory motion causes artifacts in lungs and cardiac reconstructed images, which lead to misinterpretations and imprecise diagnosis. Solutions like respiratory gating, correlated dynamic PET techniques, list-mode data based techniques and others have been tested with improvements over the spatial activity distribution in lungs lesions, but with the disadvantages of requiring additional instrumentation or discarding part of the projection data used for reconstruction. The objective of this study is to incorporate respiratory motion correction directly into the image reconstruction process, without any additional acquisition protocol consideration. To this end, we propose an extension to the Maximum Likelihood Expectation Maximization (MLEM) algorithm that includes a respiratory motion model, which takes into account the displacements and volume deformations produced by the respiratory motion during the data acquisition process. We present results from synthetic simulations incorporating real respiratory motion as well as from phantom and patient data.

1 Introduction

Respiratory motion during the data acquisition process leads to blurred images, making difficult an accurate diagnosis, planning and following. For instance, mislocalizations of lesions in the fusion of positron emission tomography (PET) and computerized tomography (CT) have been found [1]. Similarly, significant tumor motion has been reported in others studies (e.g. [2,3]) as well as significant volume increase of lung lesions in images reconstructed without respiratory motion compensation [4].

To our knowledge, motion correction in Emission Tomography (ET) has been seldom investigated in the literature. Current methods can be classified in four main categories: post-processing, Multiple Acquisition Frame (MAF), sinogram data selection based on detected motion, and sinogram correction.

- Post-processing methods are based on transformations performed either in projection-space (e.g [5]) or in image-space (e.g. [6]). However, the motion models used in projection-space are too simplistic (e.g. global scaling), and

J. Duncan and G. Gerig (Eds.): MICCAI 2005, LNCS 3750, pp. 369–376, 2005.

the transformations applied in image-space do not consider the true effects of motion on the acquired data.
- The MAF-based methods consist on regrouping the projections in smaller subsets according to the detected motion (either online or offline motion detection). Then, image reconstruction of each subset is performed independently followed by a realignment of the images. These approaches present the inconvenient that the signal-to-noise ratio increases for images reconstructed from smaller subsets of projections.
- Sinogram data selection based on motion detection, also known as gating, has been used to compensate for motion correction in ET [4]. Gating techniques have shown improvements, contributing to a better quantification of lesions. However, they require extra hardware or specific data acquisition modes and they discard part of the acquired projection data.
- Sinogram correction methodologies act directly on the projection data by repositioning the lines-of-response (LOR) when the motion is known [7,8]. However, these approaches are only applicable to rigid motions and require to deal with motion-corrected LOR's that may fall in non-valid positions, which decreases their practical interest.

The purpose of this paper is to describe a reconstruction algorithm that allows for a retrospective respiratory motion correction that operates directly over the complete projection data, without the need of additional acquisition protocols or discarding of data. To that end, we propose an extension to the MLEM reconstruction algorithm in which a motion model is plugged. We consider not only displacements but also local deformations.

The next sections present the methodology and results from phantom data and synthetic simulations incorporating real respiratory motion. For patient data, a preliminary approach of respiratory motion modelling and results of its use with the proposed motion correction methodology are also presented.

2 Method

2.1 Maximum Likelihood Expectation Maximization

First introduced in emission tomography by Shepp and Vardi [9], the MLEM algorithm is based on a *Poisson* model for the emission process. For a given emission element b the number of emissions f_b follows a Poisson law with mean λ_b. Besides, the projection matrix R (or called by some authors *system matrix* or *transition matrix*) gives the probability that a certain emission from voxel b is detected by the detector d (called *dexel* hereafter). Furthermore, the number of detections from dexel d (i.e., p_d) can be expressed in terms of the number of emissions f_b, $p_d = \sum_b f_b R_{db}$. This latter expression is important since it states the relationship between detections and emissions through the system matrix values. Later, this fact will be exploited in the motion correction step.

We are interested to find the mean value λ from the set of projections p. This can be done by searching the maximum likelihood of getting a set of measures p

given an image λ (i.e., $\hat{\lambda} = \arg\max_\lambda[P(p|\lambda)]$). It can be shown (see [9] for more details) that $\hat{\lambda}$ can be found by means of an iterative algorithm

$$\lambda_b^{<K+1>} = \frac{\lambda_b^{<K>}}{\sum_d R_{db}} \sum_d \frac{p_d R_{db}}{\sum_{b'} \lambda_{b'}^{<K>} R_{db'}} \tag{1}$$

where p_d stands for the number of detections of dexel d, λ_b is the mean number of emissions from voxel b, R_{db} is the probability that a particle emitted from voxel b is detected by the dexel d and K stands for the iteration number.

2.2 Incorporating Motion Correction into the MLEM Algorithm

We incorporate motion correction into the MLEM algorithm through the projection matrix R. We estimate the new contribution R^C_{db} of a voxel under motion b to every dexel d.

Let us consider a continuous motion modeled by the spatial transformations $\varphi_t : \mathbb{R}^3 \mapsto \mathbb{R}^3$, where $\varphi_t(m)$ denotes the position of point m at time t. This motion is observed from time $t = 0$ to $t = T$.

We first discretize this motion into a discrete set of spatial transformations φ_i, $i = 0 \ldots N$, the transformation φ_i being valid from $t = t_i$ to $t = t_{i+1}$. R^C_{db} expresses then the weighted sum of the contributions R^i_{db} of deformed voxels $\varphi_i(b)$ to d:

$$R^C_{db} = \sum_i w_i R^i_{db} \tag{2}$$

The weights $w_i = (t_{i+1} - t_i)/T$ allow to take into account the kinetic of the motion: $w_i T$ represents the duration where φ_t can be effectively approximated by φ_i.

2.3 Computation of System Matrix Terms

The voxels that contribute to a dexel d are assumed to intersect a 3-D line that stemed from d. Let us denote by l_{db} the length of the intersection of this line with the emission element b. We thus define the contribution of b to d by

$$\text{static: } R_{db} = \frac{l_{db}}{\sum_{d'} l_{d'b}} \quad \text{dynamic: } R^i_{db} = \frac{l^i_{db}}{\sum_{d'} l^i_{d'b}}. \tag{3}$$

In the static case, we model the emissions elements as spheres inscribed in the voxel space, which facilitates the calculation of Eq. (3): see Fig. 1a. The summation in each denominator of Eq. (3) acts as a normalization term.

If no deformations can be assumed for emission elements b during their motion, we could still have used the intersection of a line with a sphere for the computation of the contribution R^i_{db}. However, this will not be realistic. Indeed, it has been shown that the displacements in the thorax (due to the respiratory motion) present a non-linear and a non-homogeneous behavior [3]. Thus, we have to consider also the deformations of b. When under motion, the emission

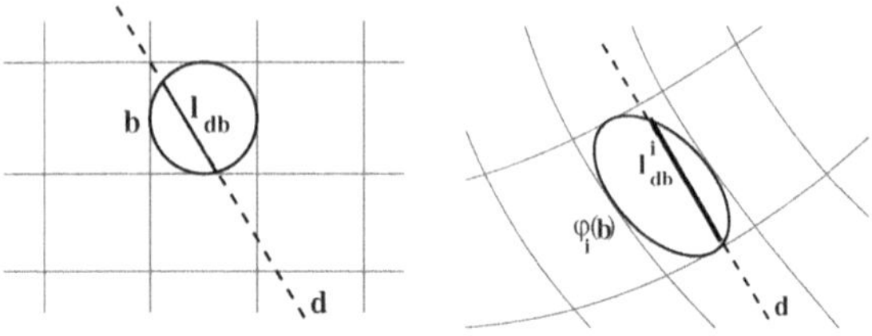

Fig. 1. The contribution of an emission element b to a dexel d represented by a dotted line is defined by the intersection (continuous line) of (a) a sphere with a line (static case) or (b) an ellipsoid (a deformed sphere) with a line (dynamic case)

element b will deform into $\varphi_i(b), i = 0 \ldots N$. As a first order approximation, a deformed sphere is an ellipsoid. The contribution of b at state i to d, *i.e.* $\varphi_i(b)$, is then similarly defined as the length intersection of the line d with this ellipsoid (see Fig. 1b).

The study of the matrix $\nabla\varphi_i$ allows to estimate the ellipsoid. Let us consider the singular value decomposition (SVD) of matrix $\nabla\varphi_i$, that is $\nabla\varphi_i = U\Sigma V^T$, where U and V are square and orthogonal matrices and $\Sigma = diag(\lambda_1, \lambda_2, \lambda_3)$, with $\lambda_j, (j = 1, 2, 3)$ the singular values of $\nabla\varphi_i$. It turns out that the columns of U are the eigenvectors of $\nabla\varphi_i\nabla\varphi_i{}^T$, and also give the preferred local deformation directions, while the λ_j are related to the magnitude of the deformations in the direction of the eigenvectors.

The modellization of the emissions elements as spheres that translate and deform locally into ellipsoids according to a known transformation, represents a novel contribution in this work. Furthermore, computations of the system matrix elements are faster than using classical methods of dexel-voxel intersection.

Since a dexel is defined by the path travelled by a single (e.g. SPECT) or by a pair of photons (e.g. PET), the method is independent of the type of ET modality, and thus can be used without further modifications.

2.4 Estimation of the Respiratory Motion

In practice, unless extra devices are used to measure the breathing pattern, the respiratory motion (transformation φ) is generally unknown.

A first approach to estimate this motion consisted in registering a known respiratory motion model on the data to be reconstructed. To build this model, two MRI images of a volunteer were acquired at breath holding in expiration and inspiration and then non-rigidly registered. This provides us with a volumic displacement vector field (DVF) $\mathbf{u}$. Transformations $\Phi_i(m)$ are then given by $\Phi_i(m) = m + i/N\mathbf{u}(m)$.

To adapt the transformation Φ_i to a patient, we first create an average image of the expiration and inspiration states (to simulate a non-corrected reconstruction) that is affinely registered against the non-corrected reconstructed patient's image. This provides us with an affine transformation T. We compose then the transformations to obtain $\varphi_i = T \circ \Phi_i \circ T^{-1}$.

Though this method is by no means a robust method, it provides a first insight of the results that can be achieved by using such an approximative model with the proposed motion correction technique. Further improvements are needed to assure a good estimation of the patient's respiratory motion model.

3 Results

3.1 Simulated Data

We simulated respiratory motion in a SPECT study of lungs. For this, we used the thorax phantom *NCAT* (*NURBS-based cardiac torso*) [10], to which a small lesion of 15 mm diameter was added. The model was then deformed with N φ_i transformations, estimated from a known real respiratory motion transformation Φ. Sinograms were then computed for each time state using the SimSET (*Simulation System for Emission Tomography*) library and combined into one single sinogram by a weighted sum.

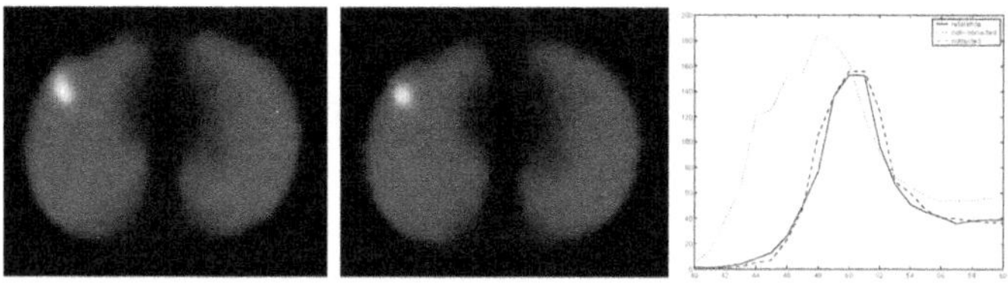

(a) Non-corrected (b) Corrected (c) Intensity profile

Fig. 2. Image reconstruction without motion correction (a) and with motion correction (b). The corrected profile (dashed line) show a close relationship with the reference profile (continuous line) in comparison with the non-corrected one (dotted line) (c).

Fig. 2 shows the reconstructed image with and without motion correction. As described in the literature, the lesion appears larger in the non-corrected reconstruction. A visual comparison of the intensity profiles (Fig. 2(c)) shows a good agreement between the motion-corrected reconstruction and the ground truth.

Two figures of merit were used to measure quantitatively the performance of the method, namely the coefficient of variability $CV = \sigma(lesion)/\mu(lesion)$ where $\mu(lesion)$ and $\sigma(lesion)$ denote the average and the standard deviation of the intensity values over the lesion, and the contrast recovery $CR = \mu(lesion)/\mu(background)$ [11]. For the reference volume CR and CV values are 5.80 and 0.14 respectively. The non-corrected volume presents CR and CV values of 3.20 and 0.13 respectively. After motion correction the CR value increased to 4.40 while the CV value remained in 0.13. From these results, it can be concluded that in the lesion area, noise properties are not affected by the motion correction. Higher CR values are found for the corrected cases in comparison with the non-corrected one (27±4% of increment), which demonstrates the deblurring effect of the motion correction.

3.2 Phantom Data

A phantom made of three spheres filled with 99mTc, having a concentration of $85\mu Ci/ml$ each and of 1.8, 3.2 and 1.3 cm diameters (Inserts numbers 1, 2 and 3 respectively) was acquired with a Millenium-VG SPECT camera. Five data acquisitions were performed, and for each acquisition, the phantom was translated 1 cm in the axial direction. By combining the sinograms, we simulate the acquisition of a moving phantom. Finally, one single acquisition of duration five times longer was performed in the reference position, to serve as ground truth.

Reconstructed volumes had dimensions 128^3 voxels with voxel size of 4.42 mm. Fig. 3 shows the corrected and non-corrected reconstructed volumes and the intensity profiles for insert number two.

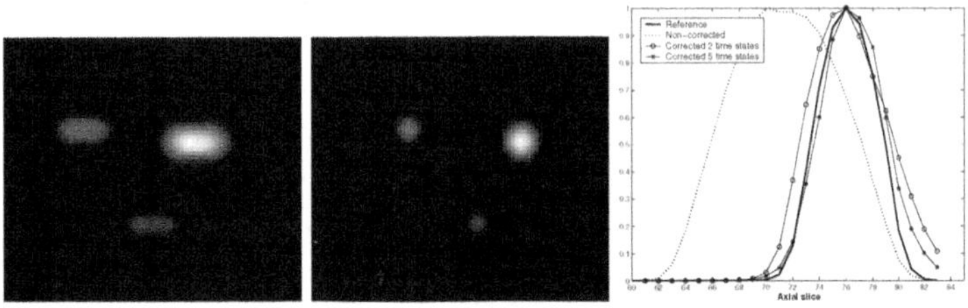

(a) Non-corrected (b) Corrected (c) Intensity profiles

Fig. 3. Axial translations of spherical sources during an ET study. Without motion correction (a), after motion correction (b) and the intensity profiles of reference, non-corrected and corrected volumes for insert number two (c).

For each insert, volume, CR, CV, Volume Error (VE), Volume Precision (VP), Centroid Error (CE) and Centroid Precision (CP) measurements were calculated to assess the quality of the motion correction in phantom data. VE and VP are defined as the relative error between the reference and non-corrected volumes and between the reference and corrected volumes, respectively. CE and CP are defined as the distance between reference and non-corrected centroids and between reference and corrected centroids, respectively. CR ratios are presented as CR_c (corrected contrast recovery) over CR_{nc} (non-corrected contrast recovery). Similarly for CV, we have CV_c/CV_{nc} (see Table 1). From Table 1 and Fig. 3 it can be seen that the motion correction method yields corrected volume size, spheres positions and improved contrast and noise properties.

Table 1. Results of motion correction for phantom data

Insert	VE	VP	CE (cm)	CP (cm)	CR_c/CR_{nc}	CV_c/CV_{nc}
1	350%	5,8%	2.0	0.16	2.2	0.58
2	125%	1%	1.96	0.21	1.62	0.89
3	166%	8%	1.85	0.21	2.57	0.48

3.3 Patient Data

Five patients, one lesion each, were used to test the methodology of motion correction in patient data. For each of them, image reconstruction with and without motion correction was performed. Gaussian regularization with filter full-width at half maximum (FWHM) of 8.5 mm every three iterations were set as main parameters. The reconstructed images had dimensions 128^3 with voxel size of 4x4x4 mm^3.

Table 2. Results of motion correction for patient dataset. The labels stand for: Non-corrected (NC), corrected (C), lateral (LR), anterior-posterior (AP) and cranial-caudal (CC).

Patient	Volume (C/NC)	Displacement (mm)			CR		CV	
		LR	AP	CC	NC	C	NC	C
1	0.95	2.00	3.20	3.20	4.78	5.42	0.22	0.23
2	0.64	2.60	3.60	5.10	5.04	6.06	0.24	0.20
3	0.98	0.30	2.62	4.23	7.47	7.49	0.26	0.22
4	0.86	0.45	1.20	1.74	3.66	3.90	0.18	0.16
5	0.77	2.50	0.60	2.33	4.92	5.70	0.09	0.09

From results presented in Table 2, it can be first noticed a volume reduction ranging from 2% to 36% after motion correction. Quantitative measures indicate improvements in contrast recovery after motion correction, which demonstrates the ability of the proposed method to compensate the blurring effects in the lesion area and its spatial activity distribution. Improvements in noise level are less significative. However, we did not find increases in noise level due to motion correction.

4 Conclusion

During an emission tomography study, induced motion due to patient breathing can lead to artifacts in the reconstructed image. This can produce less accurate diagnosis and more important, incorrect radiotherapy planning [3,4]. We have presented a methodology to correct for respiratory motion in the image reconstruction step. The method accounts for a respiratory motion model that takes place in the computation of each term of the system matrix, and takes into account displacements and deformations experienced by the voxels during respiratory motion.

The method was implemented in a parallel framework and tested with simulated, phantom and patient data. For simulated and phantom data, the results show the ability of the proposed method to compensate for motion, rendering images with improved spatial intensity distributions and corrected lesions's shapes. For patient data, we have addressed the problem when no information about the patient's breathing cycle is available. As a first approach, we have used a respiratory motion model created by adapting a known model to the patient's anatomy. Although this method lacks of robustness, we are convinced that this first approach yields images with lesser respiratory motion effects than those reconstructed without motion correction. Improvements of the figures of merit were found after motion correction, and volume reduction and lesions displacements are likely to occur according to findings of previous studies [3].

Some further improvements and work in progress consider the inclusion of breathing and anatomy subject variability into the respiratory motion model estimation (i.e. transition from an individual respiratory motion model to a statistical one) and validation of the proposed motion correction method against a ground truth (e.g. gating).

References

1. MM. Osman, C. Cohade, Y. Nakamoto, LT. Marshall, JP. Leal, and RL. Wahl. Clinically significant inaccurate localization of lesions with PET/CT: frequency in 300 patients. *J. Nucl. Med.*, 4(2):240–243, 2003.
2. S. Shimizu, H. Shirato, K. Kagei, T. Nishioka, X. Bo, H. Dosaka-Akita, S. Hashimoto, H. Aoyama, K. Tsuchiya, and K. Miyasaka. Impact of respiratory movement on the computed tomographic images of small lung tumors in three-dimensional (3D) radiotherapy. *Int J Radiat Oncol Biol Phys.*, 46(5):1127–33, Mar 2000.
3. Y. Seppenwoolde, H. Shirato, K. Kitamura, S. Shimizu, M. van Herk M, JV. Lebesque, and K. Miyasaka. Precise and real-time measurement of 3D tumor motion in lung due to breathing and heartbeat, measured during radiotherapy. *Int J Radiat Oncol Biol Phys.*, 53(4):822–34, July 2002.
4. SA. Nehmeh, YE. Erdi, KE. Rosenzweig, H. Schroder, SM. Larson, OD. Squire, and JL. Humm. Reduction of respiratory motion artifacts in PET imaging of lung cancer by respiratory correlated dynamic PET: Methodology and comparison with respiratory gated PET. *J. Nucl. Med.*, 44(10):1644–1648, 2003.
5. W. Lu and TR. Mackie. Tomographic motion detection and correction directly in sinogram space. *Phys. Med. Biol.*, 47(8):1267–84, April 2002.
6. O. Camara, G. Delso, and I. Bloch. Evaluation of a thoracic elastic registration method using anatomical constraints in oncology. In *2nd. Joint Conference of the IEEE Engineering in Medicine and Biology Society*, 2002.
7. A. Rhamim and P. Bloomfield. Motion correction in histogram-mode and listmode EM reconstructions. In *IEEE MIC*, 2003.
8. K. Thielemans, S. Mustafovic, and L. Schnorr. Image reconstruction of motion corrected sinograms. In *IEEE Medical Imaging Conf.*, 2003.
9. L. Shepp and Y. Vardi. Maximum likelihood reconstruction for emission tomography. *IEEE Trans. Med. Imag.*, 1(2):113–122, 1982.
10. W.P. Segars. *Development of a new dynamic NURBS-based cardiac-torso (NCAT) phantom.* PhD thesis, The University of North Carolina, 2001.
11. R. Levkovitz, D. Falikman, M. Zibulevsky, A. Ben-Tal, and A. Nemirovski. The design and implementation of COSEM, an iterative algorithm for fully 3-D listmode data. *IEEE Trans Med Imaging*, 20(7):633–42, July 2001.

Optimal Embedding for Shape Indexing in Medical Image Databases

Xiaoning Qian and Hemant D. Tagare

Yale University, New Haven CT 06520, USA

Abstract. Fast retrieval using organ shapes is crucial in medical image databases since shape is a clinically prominent feature. In this paper, we propose that 2-D shapes in medical image databases can be indexed by embedding them into a vector space and using efficient vector space indexing. An optimal shape space embedding is proposed for this purpose. Experimental results of indexing vertebral shapes in the NHANES II database are presented. The results show that vector space indexing following embedding gives superior performance than metric indexing.

1 Introduction

Content-based retrieval in medical image databases is critically dependent on efficient indexing techniques. There are two common indexing techniques: *vector space indexing*, and *metric space indexing*. If a feature has well defined coordinates, then *vector space indexing* techniques are used. If the feature does not have coordinates, then *metric space indexing* techniques are applicable.

In this paper, we propose techniques for efficient indexing of shape for 2-D medical image databases. We show that the 2-D *shape space* can be embedded in a vector space in such a way that the vector space metric best approximates the partial Procrustes distance in the shape space. With the optimal embedding, shapes can be indexed by classical vector space indexing techniques. We provide experimental results that compare the performance of the embedding strategy versus metric trees and show that the embedding strategy gives superior results.

All experiments reported in this paper use images from the NHANES II database. NHANES II has about 17,000 spine x-ray images. Spine disease is often manifest as *osteophyte*, which is bony prominence along the vertebral boundary. Because osteophyte changes the shape of the vertebra, retrieval by vertebral shape is important to NHANES II. Indexing vertebral shape in NHANES II is our main application.

The vertebrae are segmented using a dynamic programming template matching algorithm [11]. The output of this algorithm is a fixed set of m points placed on the vertebral boundary in a homologous manner. These points may be taken as landmarks along the boundary. By "shapes of vertebrae" we mean the shapes of these "landmark" points.

This paper draws on indexing theory and shape space theory – two theories that are quite different. In the limited space of this paper, we have opted to treat indexing rather briefly and present the shape embedding in more detail.

J. Duncan and G. Gerig (Eds.): MICCAI 2005, LNCS 3750, pp. 377–384, 2005.

2 Literature Review

The literature on shape analysis is vast. We briefly mention some of the related work. Shape descriptors may be boundary based or region based. For boundary based descriptors, Fourier and wavelet descriptors [9], scale space techniques [6], and shape matching techniques [2,7] are used. For region based description, different moment invariants [9] are used. When landmarks are available, the shape of the landmarks are described as elements of an appropriate shape space. We refer the reader to [3,4] for a complete discussion.

For indexing, we note that classical indexing structures for vector spaces are in [10], while classical indexing structures for metric spaces are in [1].

3 Indexing for Content-Based Retrieval

Content-based retrieval uses *range queries* and *nearest neighbor queries.* In a range query, the user has an example image with a feature u and asks the database to retrieve all images with features v, such that $d(u, v) \leq T$ for some threshold T. Here $d()$ is a metric in the feature space. A nearest neighbor query asks for k nearest neighbors to the example u according to the metric d. We concentrate on the nearest neighbor queries in this paper.

Queries can be answered by a linear search through the database. *Indexing trees* refer to techniques that can speed up the search by organizing the database into hierarchical trees. A brief, relevant summary of indexing is as follows:

1. Indexing hierarchically partitions the feature space and creates a cover for each partition. The covers are arranged in a tree; each node of the tree representing a cover.

   For vector space features, the covers are cubes with sides perpendicular to the coordinate axis [10]. For metric spaces, the covers are metric spheres. All leaf nodes point to the data that are contained in its cover.
2. Retrieval starts from the root node and proceeds by testing whether the cover at a node intersects the metric sphere defined by the query. If a node passes this *node test*, then the procedure is applied to the children of the node. If the node fails the node test, then the entire subtree rooted at the node is rejected since its children cannot contain any data that intersect the query sphere.
3. One performance measure for indexing trees is the average number of node tests per query. This measures the computation cost during retrieval. A theoretical expression for the performance was derived in [12].
4. The performance of an indexing tree becomes poor if its nodes increasingly survive the node test. In [12], we proposed a *greedy* algorithm that traverses and eliminates inefficient nodes.

   In [8], we reported an algorithm that *optimally* eliminates nodes. The algorithm is a dynamic program over all possible node eliminations. We call these procedures *tree adaptation procedures* since they adapt the tree to the data distribution.

4 Shape Spaces and Shape Queries

4.1 Configuration, Preshape, and Shape Space

As mentioned in section 1, vertebrae in NHANES II are segmented by an algorithm that gives a set of m points along the boundary. Representing each point as a complex number, every boundary can be considered as an element of $\mathbb{C}^m$, the complex vector space of dimension m. $\mathbb{C}^m$ is the *configuration space*. Two boundaries $z_i, z_j \in \mathbb{C}^m$ have the same shape if there exists a translation, rotation, and (non-zero) scaling that aligns them, i.e. if there exist complex numbers t, μ, with $\mu \neq 0$, such that $z_i = \mu z_j + 1_m t$, where $1_m = (1 \cdots 1)^T$. Here t is the translation and $\mu = re^{i\theta}$ is scaling by r and rotation by θ.

Following Kendall [4], we first consider only the action of scale and translation. For every $z \in \mathbb{C}^m$, define $\tilde{z} = \frac{z - \frac{1}{m} 1_m^T z}{|z - \frac{1}{m} 1_m^T z|}$ to be the *preshape* of z. Then, $\tilde{z}$ is simply z translated so its center of mass is at the origin and scaled so that the resulting scale is unity. All shapes that differ only by translation and scaling are mapped to the same preshape. The *preshape space* is the set of all preshapes, and is easily seen to be the unit sphere in the configuration space $\mathbb{C}^m$.

The map $z \to \tilde{z}$ from configurations to preshapes factors out translation and scaling. To get shape, it remains to factor out rotation. Suppose that a configuration z has preshape $\tilde{z}$. Rotating z by θ gives the configuration $ze^{i\theta}$ which has the preshape $\widetilde{ze^{i\theta}}$. It is easy to show that $\widetilde{ze^{i\theta}} = e^{i\theta}\tilde{z}$. Thus, all configurations that have the same shape as z fall on the one dimensional *orbit of $\tilde{z}$ in the preshape space* defined as $\breve{z} = \{e^{i\theta}\tilde{z}\}$. The orbit $\breve{z}$ is the *shape of z*.

Since each orbit is a shape, the set of all orbits is the *shape space*. Kendall showed that the shape space of m landmarks is a complex projective space of complex dimension $m - 2$. This is a non-Euclidean manifold.

The different spaces and relations between them are illustrated in figure 1.

Shape space has many natural metrics. The specific one we use is the *partial Procrustes metric* $d_P(z_i, z_j)$. It is defined as the minimum Euclidean distance between the preshape of z_i and the orbit of the preshape of z_j:

$$d_P(z_i, z_j) = \inf_\theta \parallel \tilde{z}_i - e^{i\theta}\tilde{z}_j \parallel .$$

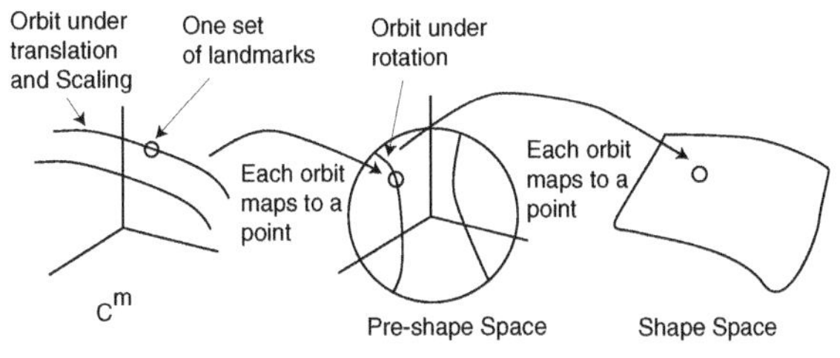

Fig. 1. Preshape and Shape Spaces

4.2 Metric Shape Indexing

Because shape spaces are curved manifolds and the partial Procrustes distance is non-Euclidean, one obvious choice for indexing shapes is to use metric indexing trees. Specifically, we use hierarchical clustering with the partial Procrustes metric to cluster shapes in a tree. Greedy node elimination and optimal tree adaptation are used to further increase the efficiency.

As mentioned in section 1, an alternative is to embed the shape space into a vector space and use vector space indexing. We discuss this next.

5 Shape Embedding

Let z_k be one of n configurations in the database, and let $\tilde{z}_k$ and $\breve{z}_k$ be its preshape and shape. Recall that the preshape space is a unit sphere in $\mathbb{C}^m$ and that the only variation left in the preshape space is rotation. Hence, it is reasonable to consider choosing one point on the preshape orbit of $\breve{z}_k$ to represent $\breve{z}_k$. That is, we choose the preshape with a particular orientation (yet to be determined) as the shape embedding. This is our key idea and is illustrated in figure 2.

Suppose we embed $\breve{z}_k$ as the point on the preshape orbit that is given by $[z_k] = e^{i\theta_k}\tilde{z}_k$ for some θ_k. This embedding gives a Euclidean shape distance:

$$d_s([z_i],[z_j]) = \|[z_i] - [z_j]\|, \tag{1}$$

where, $\|\ \|$ is the usual Euclidean norm in $\mathbb{C}^m$. In general, this shape distance will be different from the partial Procrustes distance, and we would like to choose an embedding such that the difference between them is as small as possible.

One measure of the difference between d_P and d_s is

$$J = \sum_i \sum_j \mid d_s^2([z_i],[z_j]) - d_P^2(z_i,z_j) \mid . \tag{2}$$

We would like to choose embeddings $[z_1] = e^{i\theta_1}\tilde{z}_1, [z_2] = e^{i\theta_2}\tilde{z}_2, \cdots$, or alternatively, choose the angles $\Theta = (\theta_1, \theta_2, \cdots, \theta_n)$ such that J is minimized as a function of Θ. From now on we will write J as $J(\Theta)$ explicitly showing dependence on Θ. We now derive an algorithm for minimizing $J(\Theta)$.

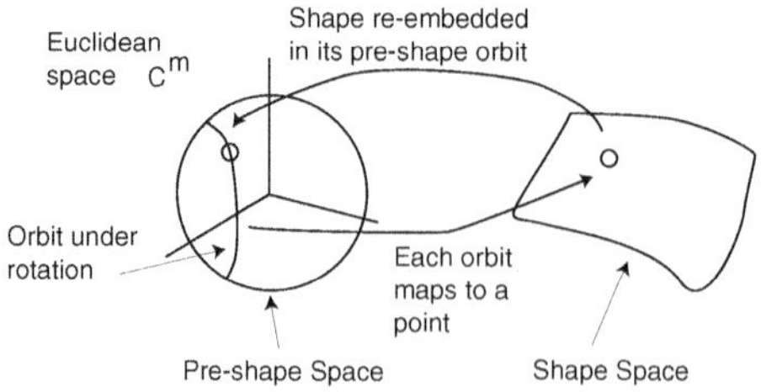

Fig. 2. Shape Embedding in Preshape Space

The first step is to show the following proposition:

Proposition 1: A Θ minimizes $J(\Theta)$ if and only if it minimizes

$$J_1(\Theta) = \sum_i \sum_j d_s^2([z_i], [z_j]). \tag{3}$$

Proof: First note that $d_s([z_i], [z_j])$ is the Euclidean distance between two fixed point $[z_i]$ and $[z_j]$ on the preshape orbits of $\widetilde{z}_i$ and $\widetilde{z}_j$. But $d_P(z_i, z_j)$ is the shortest distance between preshape orbits of $\widetilde{z}_i$ and $\widetilde{z}_j$. Thus, $d_s([z_i], [z_j]) \geq d_P(z_i, z_j)$, and therefore $\mid d_s^2([z_i], [z_j]) - d_P^2(z_i, z_j) \mid = d_s^2([z_i], [z_j]) - d_P^2(z_i, z_j)$. Note that the $d_P^2(z_i, z_j)$ term is independent of Θ and can be dropped from $J(\Theta)$, giving

$$J(\Theta) = \sum_i \sum_j d_s^2([z_i], [z_j]) = J_1(\Theta).$$

To proceed further, a simple algebraic manipulation of $J_1(\Theta)$ gives:

$$J_1(\Theta) = \sum_i \sum_j d_s([z_i], [z_j])^2 = 2n \sum_i \| [z_i] - \frac{1}{n} \sum_j [z_j] \|^2.$$

As a brief aside, consider a second objective function

$$H_1(\Theta, \mu) = 2n \sum_i \| [z_i] - \mu \|^2. \tag{4}$$

The minimizing μ of H_1 is known in the shape space literature as the *procrustean mean size-and-shape* of the preshapes $\widetilde{z}_i$. Conditions for a unique procrustean mean size-and-shape are given in [5]. Loosely speaking, a unique μ exists if the distribution of $\widetilde{z}_i$ is not too broad. In practice this condition almost always holds and a unique μ exists. We assume this to be the case and we have

Proposition 2: If $H_1(\Theta, \mu)$ has a minimizer (Θ^*, μ^*), Θ^* minimizes $J_1(\Theta)$.

Proof: For any fixed Θ, because $[z_i]$ are in the vector space $\mathbb{C}^m$, and $\| \ \|$ is the usual Euclidean norm, the function $H_1(\Theta, \mu)$ has a unique minimum with respect to μ, and the minimum is given by $\mu^* = \frac{1}{n} \sum_j [z_j]$. Thus,

$$\min_\mu H_1(\Theta, \mu) = 2n \sum_i \| [z_i] - \frac{1}{n} \sum_j [z_j] \|^2 = J_1(\Theta).$$

It follows that if $H_1(\Theta, \mu)$ has a minimizer (Θ^*, μ^*), Θ^* also minimizes $J_1(\Theta)$.

To obtain the optimal embedding, we minimize $H_1(\Theta, \mu)$ by alternately updating Θ and μ as follows:

1. Initialize $\Theta^{[0]} = (0, \cdots, 0)$, and $\mu^{[0]} = \frac{1}{n} \sum_k [z_k]$.
2. Update $\Theta^{[l]} = \arg_\Theta \min H_1(\Theta, \mu^{[l-1]})$, where $\Theta^{[l]} = (\theta_1^{[l]}, \cdots, \theta_n^{[l]})$ is given by

$$\theta_k^{[l]} = \arg \widetilde{z}_k^{\,*} \mu^{[l-1]}, \tag{5}$$

where, $\widetilde{z}_k^{\,*}$ is the complex conjugate transpose of $\widetilde{z}_k$.

Calculate $\mu^{[l]} = \arg_{\mu} \min H_1(\Theta^{[l]}, \mu)$. This is given by

$$\mu^{[l]} = \frac{1}{n}\sum_k [z_k] = \frac{1}{n}\sum_k e^{i\theta_k^{[l]}} \widetilde{z_k}. \tag{6}$$

3. Terminate if a fixed point is reached (i.e. if $(\Theta^{[l]}, \mu^{[l]}) = (\Theta^{[l-1]}, \mu^{[l-1]})$). Else, go to 2.

Let the terminating $(\Theta^{[l]}, \mu^{[l]})$ be denoted by $(\hat{\Theta}, \hat{\mu})$. Then, the optimal embedding is given by $[z_k] = e^{i\hat{\theta}_k} \widetilde{z_k} = \frac{\widetilde{z_k}^* \hat{\mu}}{\|\widetilde{z_k}^* \hat{\mu}\|} \widetilde{z_k}$ for all k.

5.1 Vector Space Indexing of Shape

Following optimal embedding, the embedded shapes can be indexed by any of the classical vector space indexing techniques. We choose to index by a kd-tree [10]. After embedding, shape similarity retrieval is carried out by using the d_s shape metric of equation (1).

6 Experiments

At the moment, a total of 2812 boundaries have been segmented. Each boundary is a consistent set of 34 landmarks.

We first evaluated the closeness of the embedding distance d_s to the partial Procrustes distance d_P. Recall that the optimal embedding was obtained by minimizing the absolute difference between d_s^2 and d_P^2 for all pairs of data in the database. To measure the similarity between the two we calculated fraction squared difference $FSD = |d_s^2([z_i],[z_j]) - d_P^2([z_i],[z_j])|/d_P^2([z_i],[z_j])$ as well as the fractional difference $FD = |d_s([z_i],[z_j]) - d_P([z_i],[z_j])|/d_P([z_i],[z_j])$. A set of 1000 vertebrae were randomly chosen from the database and the FSD and FD were calculated for all pairs of vertebrae from this set. The average and standard deviation of the FSD and FD are given in Table 1. From the table, it is clear that the Euclidean distance following embedding is very similar to the partial Procrustes distance.

We also compared the relative ranking of vertebrae according to the embedded Euclidean distance and the partial Procrustes distance. From the set of 1000 vertebrae used in the above experiment, 100 vertebrae were chosen as query vertebrae. For each query vertebra, the set of 20 nearest vertebrae was found according to the partial Procrustes distance d_P and the embedded Euclidean distance d_s. For 98 of 100 queries the sets of nearest neighbors were identical, and for 2 queries they differed by a single image.

Table 1. Mean and Variance of FSD and FD of pairs from a set of 1000 vertebrae

Quantity	Mean	Var.
FSD	9.19×10^{-4}	2.09×10^{-6}
FD	4.59×10^{-4}	5.21×10^{-7}

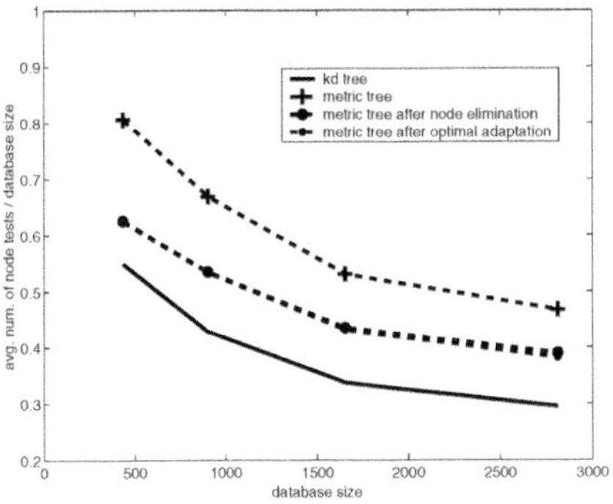

(a)

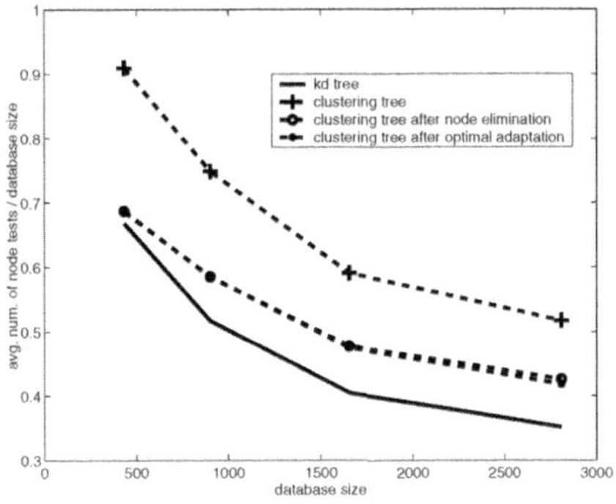

(b)

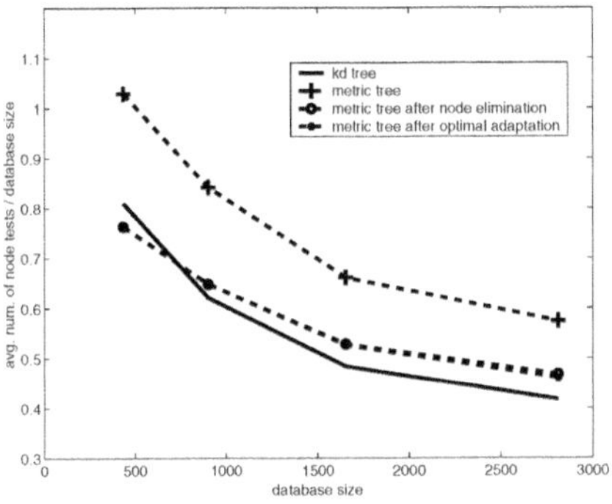

(c)

Fig. 3. Indexing performance comparison for (a) 5, (b) 10, and (c) 20-nearest neighbors

Finally, the 2812 shapes were randomly sampled into sets of size 434, 902, 1654 and 2812. Each set was indexed for shape with metric and vector indexing trees. The metric tree was used in its raw form, and to improve its performance also after greedy node elimination and optimal node elimination. Each vertebral shape in the database was used as query and 5, 10 and 20-nearest neighbor vertebral images were retrieved. The average number of node tests per query were recorded and expressed as a fraction of the total number of database points and plotted. Figure 3a-c show the results. From the figures, it is clear that

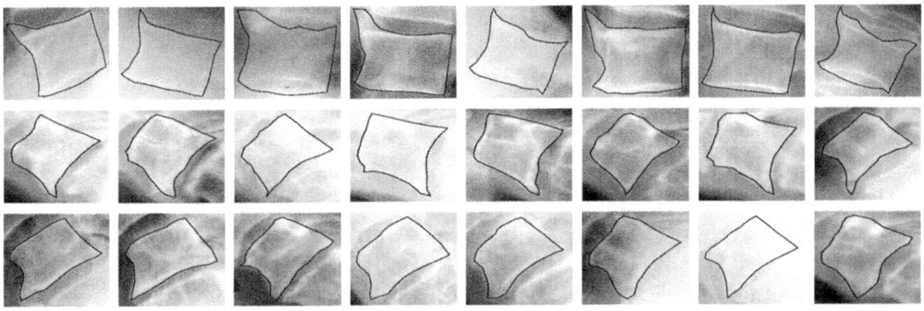

Fig. 4. Shape query samples

in all cases the kd-tree outperforms the raw metric tree. Further, except for the small database of 434 images and 20-nearest neighbors, the vector space indexing outperforms metric indexing with adaptation. Also, since the average number of node tests as a fraction of database size decreases with database size, kd-tree indexing has sub-linear complexity with respect to database size.

Three illustrative sample queries are given in figure 4. The left most image in each row is the query image and the successive images are the retrieved neighbors ranked in increasing shape distance from the query. The first query has an osteophyte near the top left corner. The other two have an osteophyte near the bottom left corner.

7 Conclusion

We proposed an embedding technique that optimally embeds shapes into a vector space. This allows the use of vector space indexing techniques for fast retrieval. Experiments show that the embedding does not significantly alter the metric or the nearest neighbor queries. Further, shape indexing efficiency using a kd-tree is significantly higher compared to the raw metric tree. It remains higher even when the metric tree is adapted.

Acknowledgment

This research was support by the grant R01-LM06911-05 from the National Library of Medicine.

References

1. E. Chávez, G. Navarro, R. Baeza-Yates, and J. L. Marroquin: Searching in Metric Spaces. *ACM Computing Surveys*, Vol. 33, No. 3, Sept., 2001, pp. 273–321.
2. T.F. Cootes and C.J. Taylor: Statistical models of appearance for medical image analysis and computer vision. *Proc. SPIE Medical Imaging*, 2001
3. I. L. Dryden and K. Mardia: Statistical Shape Analysis. *J. Wiley*, 1998.
4. D. G. Kendall, D. Barden, H. Le: Shape and Shape Theory. *Wiley Series*, 1999
5. H.-L. Le: Mean Size-and-Shapes and Mean Shapes: a Geometric Point of View. *Advances in Applied Probability*, 27, 1995, pp. 44–55
6. F. Mokhtarian, S. Abbasi, J. Kittler: Robust and Efficient Shape Indexing Through Curvature Scale Space. *Proceedings of BMVC*, 1996, pp. 53–62
7. S. M. Pizer, T. Fletcher, A. Thall, M. Styner, G. Gerig, S. Joshi: Object Models in Multiscale Intrinsic Coordinates via M-reps. *IVC*, 2000
8. X. Qian, H. D. Tagare: Optimal Indexing Trees for Medical Image Databases. *ISBI* 2002
9. Y. Rui, T. S. Huang, and S.-F. Chang: Image retrieval: current techniques, promising directions and open issues. *JVCIR*, Vol. 10, 1999, pp. 1–23
10. H. Samet: The Design and Analysis of Spatial Data Structures. *Addison-Wesley*
11. H. D. Tagare: Deformable 2-D Template Matching Using Orthogonal Curves. *IEEE Trans. on Med. Imaging*, Vol. 16(1), 1997, pp. 108–117
12. H. D. Tagare: Increasing Retrieval Efficiency by Index Tree Adaptation. *IEEE Workshop on Content-based Access of Image and Video Libraries*, 1997

Retrospective Cross-Evaluation of an Histological and Deformable 3D Atlas of the Basal Ganglia on Series of Parkinsonian Patients Treated by Deep Brain Stimulation

Eric Bardinet[1], Didier Dormont[1,2], Grégoire Malandain[3], Manik Bhattacharjee[5], Bernard Pidoux[6], Christian Saleh[2], Philippe Cornu[7], Nicholas Ayache[3], Yves Agid[4,5], and Jérôme Yelnik[5]

[1] CNRS UPR640-LENA, Hôpital Pitié-Salpêtrière, Paris, France
Eric.Bardinet@chups.jussieu.fr
[2] Department of Neuroradiology, Hôpital Pitié-Salpêtrière, Paris, France
[3] Epidaure group, INRIA, Sophia-Antipolis, France
[4] Centre d'Investigation Clinique, Hôpital Pitié-Salpêtrière, Paris, France
[5] INSERM U679, Hôpital Pitié-Salpêtrière, Paris, France
[6] Neurophysiology Dpt, Hôpital Pitié-Salpêtrière, Paris, France
[7] Department of Neurosurgery, Hôpital Pitié-Salpêtrière, Paris, France

Abstract. In functional neurosurgery, there is a growing need for accurate localization of the functional targets. Since deep brain stimulation (DBS) of the Vim thalamic nucleus has been proposed for the treatment of Parkinson's disease, the target has evolved toward the globus pallidus and subthalamic nucleus (STN) and the therapeutic indications have enlarged to include psychiatric disorders such as Tourette syndrome or obsessive compulsive disorders. In these pathologies, the target has been restrained to smaller functional subterritories of the basal ganglia, requiring more refined techniques to localize smaller and smaller brain regions, often invisible in routine clinical MRI. Different strategies have been developed to identify such deep brain targets. Direct methods can identify structures in the MRI itself, but only the larger ones. Indirect methods are based on the use of anatomical atlases. The present strategy comprised a 3D histological atlas and the MRI of the same brain specimen, and deformation methodology developpped to fit the atlas toward the brain of any given patient. In this paper, this method is evaluated in the aim of being applied to further studies of anatomo-clinical correlation. The accuracy of the method is first discussed, followed by the study of short series of Parkinsonian patients treated by DBS, allowing to compare the deformed atlas with various per- and post-operative data.

1 Introduction

Since Deep Brain Stimulation (DBS) has been proposed for the first time for the treatment of tremor [1], the precise localization of the target has proved to be a crucial condition for the success of this therapeutic approach. Nowadays, this

J. Duncan and G. Gerig (Eds.): MICCAI 2005, LNCS 3750, pp. 385–393, 2005.

technique is used for the treatment of Parkinsonian patients, the subthalamic nucleus (STN) being the optimal target [2], that provides significative clinical benefit to the patient. The STN is a very small biconvex lens-shaped central grey nucleus oriented obliquely with reference to the three anatomical planes. In addition to playing a role in the pathophysiology of Parkinson's disease, the STN is also considered as being involved in the development of non motor diseases such as obsessive compulsive disorders [3]. In such pathologies, it is believed that a non motor portion of the STN could receive associative and limbic information from the associative and limbic portions of the external globus pallidus. It is thus more and more important to being able to localize with a high degree of precision not even the STN and the other nuclei of the basal ganglia, but also the topography of their functional subdivision into sensorimotor, associative and limbic territories.

With the progressive development of magnetic resonance (MR) imaging techniques, MR based methods have been developed for targeting the STN in individual patients [4] but the resolution of the sequence used (T2-weighted) is not precise enough and electrophysiological and clinical per-operative testing still remain necessary. Also, contrast in an MR image is related to relaxation times, a property which does not reflect systematically the histological structure of the nervous tissue. Different strategies have been developed to identify deep brain targets. Direct methods can identify structures in the MRI itself, but only the larger ones. Indirect methods are based on the use of anatomical atlases. To obtain a detailed cartography of the basal ganglia of a given patient, the only possible strategy is to adapt an histological atlas to the patient MR image. Various histological atlases have been developed in the past. With printed atlases [5,6,7], atlas-MR adaptation is to be done mentally by the atlas user. In [8], the authors recently proposed a method in which a digitized version of the Schaltenbrand & Wahren (SW) atlas [7] is linearly coregistered interactively with the patient MR image. A similar technique [9] was previously applied to an atlas of the thalamus [6].

One motivation of the present work was to propose a tool allowing a better anatomical identification of the STN target. Our strategy was twofold. On the one hand, a three-dimensional (3D) anatomical atlas based on both histological and MR data of a postmortem brain specimen was constructed. Histological data were used to draw accurate contours of basal ganglia structures and functional territories. MR data were used to generate anatomically relevant 3D surfaces of these different structures by means of data fusion and contour optimization. On the other hand, image processing techniques were developed with which atlas surfaces could be deformed on an automatic basis onto any given patient's MR acquisition and could be sliced along any orientation. The most similar to the present study is [10] but it relied on the SW atlas, the contours of which are spatially inhomogeneous. In other methods there was no anatomical atlas but data acquisition through information learning [11,12,13,14].

In this article, basal ganglia histological mapping of Parkinsonian patients treated by DBS, achieved by automatic atlas deformation, is compared with various per- and post-operative data. Precisely, cross-evaluation is performed with per-operative electrophysiological recordings and with anatomical localization of therapeutic contacts obtained with an already published and clinically validated method [8].

2 Material and Methods

2.1 Atlas Construction

A human brain obtained at autopsy from body donation was submitted to T1- and T2-weighted MRI sequences 36 hours after death. After brain extraction, the left hemisphere was fixed in formalin solution for 24 hours, cut into 1.5-cm-thick frontal blocks that were fixed for 8 days and cut into 70-micron-thick frontal sections on a freezing microtome. Photographs of the frozen blocks were taken every ten sections. The 800 sections obtained were collected serially. One series of sections (every tenth section) was Nissl-stained. Another adjacent series was immunostained for calbindin. Contours of cerebral regions of the basal ganglia (striatum, globus pallidus, substantia nigra, subthalamic nucleus) and of their functional subterritories (sensorimotor, associative, limbic) and some related structures (thalamus, bed nucleus, pedunculopontine nucleus) were delimited on the basis of histological and immunohistochemical staining. Photographs of the frozen sections were aligned by using fiducial markers to obtain a geometrically consistent 3D cryo-block which was registered with the T1-MR and T2-MR sequences. Each histological section was registered onto the corresponding cryo-section, compensating for histological processing distortions, thus providing 3D histo-blocks. All registrations were performed by applying the same automatic intensity-based method to a region of interest centered on the basal ganglia. Tracing of the contours was optimized by confronting all co-registered atlas data. 3D consistency of atlas structures was also optimized at this stage. Such contours were considered as the best estimate of the actual 3D geometry of the atlas brain. Surfaces were generated from these serial contours, yielding a true 3D atlas of the basal ganglia which could be sliced in any orientation (e.g. an AC-PC based plane or an oblique surgical trajectory) [15].

2.2 Atlas Deformation

The histological 3D atlas was adapted onto the brain of a given patient by automatic registration of the patient's T1-weighted MR image with the atlas post-mortem T1-weighted MR image, following a hierarchical framework. First, a global registration was computed, consisting in a rigid transform completed by an isotropic scaling factor. On the atlas MR image, an Region of Interest wasq extracted once and for all, embbeding the basal ganglia of the left hemisphere (dorso-ventral limits: corpus callosum, pons; medio-lateral limits: mid-sagittal plane, Sylvian fissure; antero-posterior limits: corpus callosum). This ROI was automatically extracted on the globally registered patient MR image, both for the left and right hemispheres. Then non-rigid (affine) registration was performed between atlas ROI and patient ROIs, yielding two transformations which were used to map the atlas independantly on the two hemispheres of the patient's brain. All registrations were performed by an iconic robust multiscale block matching algorithm using correlation as similarity measure.

2.3 Evaluation

Qualitative evaluation of the deformation was first performed by constructing average normalized images. Then, evaluation was performed on two retrospective series of data related to Parkinsonian patients treated by DBS. The first series (six patients) consisted in pre-operative T1-weighted (3D IR-FSPGR) MR images, used for targeting in stereotactic conditions, and in per-operative microelectrode recordings interpreted by an electrophysiologist. The second series (ten patients) consisted in post-operative T1-weighted MR images and in clinical outcome obtained by stimulation of the definitive therapeutic contacts (each electrode comprises four contacts which can be tested and selected post-operatively on the basis of their therapeutic efficacy).

3 Results

3.1 Atlas Construction

Fig. 1 summarizes the different steps of the atlas construction.

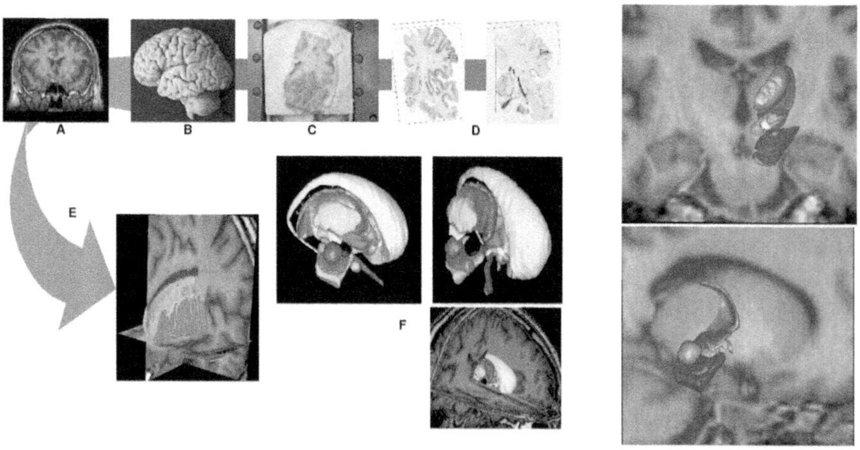

Fig. 1. Summary of atlas construction. Left block: A) MR (T1 and T2-weighted) acquisitions of the post-mortem specimen; B) brain extraction; C) frozen brain sectioning; D) histological colorations and contour tracing; E) coregistration of atlas data (cryo and histo 2D sections, MR images); F) resulting 3D meshes of the basal ganglia, after multimodal and 3D optimization. Right block: cerebral peduncle, substancia nigra, red nucleus, subthalamic nucleus, Forel field II, zona incerta and perithalamus with atlas T1-weighted MR image.

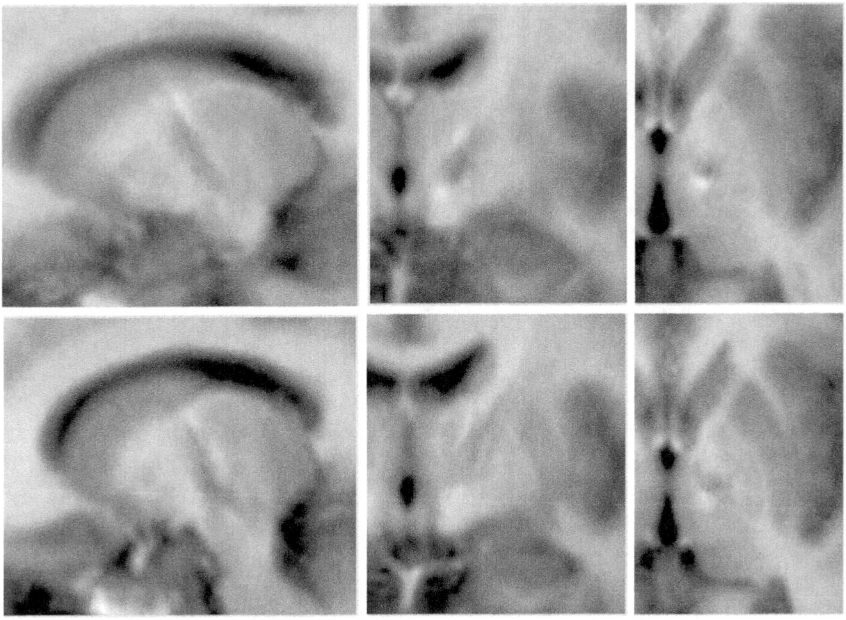

Fig. 2. Intensity normalized patient MR images averaged after ACPC (first row) and atlas spatial normalization (second row). Note that contours of the basal ganglia visible in MRI (caudate nucleus, putamen, thalamus) are sharper with the atlas normalization (only one hemisphere is presented, as the atlas is deformed indenpendantly on the 2 hemispheres).

3.2 Evaluation

Average Images. The 16 T1-weighted MR images of the patients included in this paper were normalized in intensity, spatially normalized and averaged. Spatial normalization was conducted following two distinct strategies (see Fig. 2). On the one hand, ACPC normalization was performed (the images were automatically aligned along their mid-sagittal planes, and scaling factors were applied along the antero-posterior direction to scale each image onto the AC-PC line of the first patient). On the other hand, atlas normalization was performed (using the transformation computed during atlas deformation - see section 2.2).

Comparison of Atlas-Based STN Contours Versus STN Revealed by Per-operative Electrophysiological Recordings. Before the operation, the target and trajectory angles were chosen using MRI imaging [4]. Electrophysiological activity was recorded during the operation using sets of two to four micro-electrodes, mounted on a microdrive attached to the stereotactic frame. Recordings were analyzed by the electrophysiologist every 0.5 mm, from 5.5 mm above the target to 3 mm deeper. For each point, the intensity of the signal and the structure identified by the electrophysiologist were noted. To

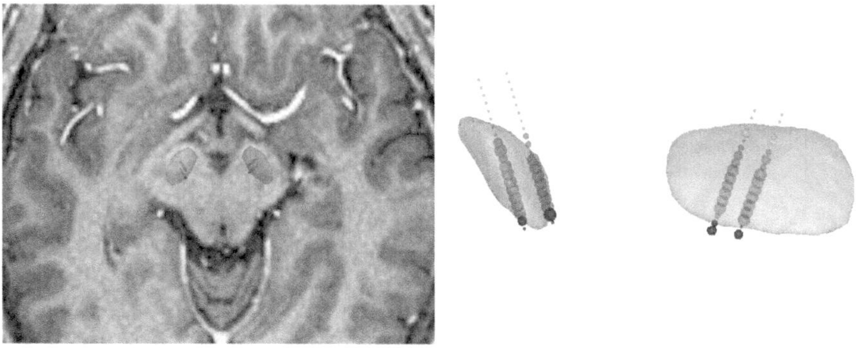

Fig. 3. Coregistration of the atlas structures and electrophysiological per-operative recordings in the patient's pre-operative MRI. The blue spheres represent the recordings of two microelectrodes by hemisphere identified as being within the STN by the electrophysiologist. Interval distance between two successive spheres is 0.5 mm.

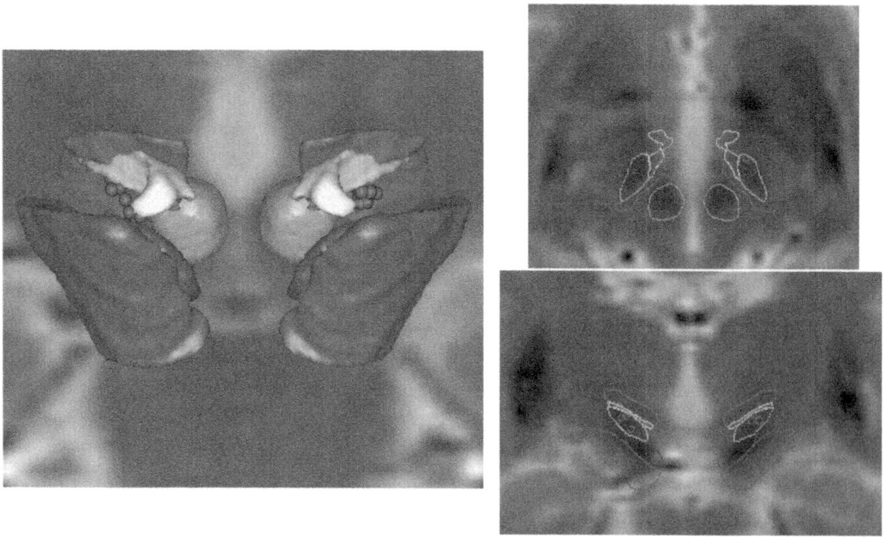

Fig. 4. Backprojection of the definitive therapeutic contacts in the atlas space. Left: STN surroundings - Cerebral Peduncle, Red Nucleus, Substancia Nigra, Zona Incerta, Forel Field II - the STN has been suppressed to allow visualization of the contacts (spheres); right: projection of the contacts onto the atlas T2 MR image (top: axial slice; bottom: coronal slice).Note that not all contacts are visible on these slices, as some contacts are located more dorsally or posteriorly.

be able to fuse this data with the atlas structures, the stereotactic frame was extracted from the T1 pre-operative MRI, then registered with a template of the frame to get the stereotactic referential. The stereotactic coordinates of the microelectrode recordings were converted to MRI coordinates, then each recording was encoded and displayed as a sphere, which size represents the intensity of the recorded signal, and which color represents the structure as identified by the electrophysiologist. For the six patients, 162 micro-electrode recordings were identified as STN by the electrophysiologist. Among them, 132 (81.5 %) were also inside the STN surface, obtained through automatic atlas deformation onto patient's T1-weighted pre-operative MR image. The remaining STN recordings were all located at less than 1 mm of the STN surface.

Anatomical position of therapeutic contacts in Parkinsonian patients treated by DBS Identification of the contacts on post-operative MR images was conducted following 2 steps: 1) MR images were reformatted along the electrodes trajectories; 2) the 3D atlas was deformed onto the post-operative MR images. This provided the anatomical position of the 4 contacts, including the therapeutic one. Fig. 4 presents all the therapeutic contacts backprojected into the 3D atlas space. For the 10 patients (meaning 20 therapeutic contacts), 14 contacts were located in the STN, 2 at the STH border, 2 in ZI (Zona Incerta) and 2 in H2 (Forel Field II).

4 Discussion

The average images illustrate that the atlas normalization is superior to the AC-PC normalization, as the resulting mean images are much less blurry. Moreover, particular features are only clearly visible in the atlas-based normalized images (such as the ventral part of the putamen).

Concerning the comparison between atlas-based STN and STN revealed by electrophysiological recordings, it should be pointed out that the microelectrode recordings coordinates were given by the electrophysiologist as the distance between the electrode and the target. This distance was given by the microdrive with a variable initial offset of at most 1mm. This offset could explain some of the mismatches between electrophysiological data and atlas STN surfaces.

Semi-automatic registration based on the SW atlas [8] led, for 10 patients (20 electrodes) to 15 contacts located in the STN, 2 at the STN border, 1 in ZI, 1 in H2 and 1 in the MRF. The results obtained with the new 3D atlas automatically deformed onto patients post-operative MR images were very similar (see section 3.2), suggesting that the automatic 3D atlas MRI registration technique is reliable. The observed difference is most likely to be due to differences in the drawing of the two atlases (in particular for ZI and H2). Moreover, the SW atlas is a printed histological atlas in which the number of sections is low (20 sections in the frontal series) and the spacing between adjacent sections very variable (1-4 mm). In the new 3D atlas there are 160 sections for a 0.35 mm spacing. This means that in [8] a section corresponding to the position of a contact had to be registered with the nearest section in the SW atlas, which implies approximations.

This study demonstrated a very good correlation between different methods for identifying the STN with an histological and deformable 3D atlas in different patients brains. In particular, comparison with STN revealed by microelectrode recordings led to good correspondance scores. Therefore it is concluded that this technique is reliable and that the current atlas/MRI coregistration could be used as a standard method of deep brain structures mapping. The method is currently validated through a large retrospective study of Parkinsonian patients treated by DBS.

References

1. Benabid, A.L., Pollak, P., Louveau, A., Henry, S., De Rougemont, J.: Combined (thalamotomy and stimulation) stereotactic surgery of the vim thalamic nucleus for bilateral parkinson disease. Appl. Neurophysiol. **50** (1987) 344–346
2. Limousin, P., Pollak, P., Benazzouz, A., Hoffmann, D., Broussolle, E., Perret, J.E., Benabid, A.L.: Bilateral subthalamic nucleus stimulation for severe parkinson's disease. Mov. Disord. **10** (1995) 672–674
3. Mallet, L., Mesnage, V., Houeto, J.L., Pelissolo, A., Yelnik, J., Behar, C., Gargiulo, M., Welter, M.L., Bonnet, A.M., Pillon, B., Cornu, P., Dormont, D., Pidoux, B., Allilaire, J.F., Agid, Y.: Compulsions, parkinson's disease, and stimulation. Lancet **360** (2002) 1302–1304
4. Bejjani, B.P., Dormont, D., Pidoux, B., Yelnik, J., Damier, P., Arnulf, I., Bonnet, A.M., Marsault, C., Agid, Y., Philippon, J., Cornu, P.: Bilateral subthalamic stimulation for parkinson's disease by using three-dimensional stereotactic magnetic resonance imaging and electrophysiological guidance. J. Neurosurg. **92** (2000) 615–625
5. Mai, J.K., Assheuer, J., Paxinos, G.: Atlas of the human brain. Academic Press, San Diego (1997)
6. Morel, A., Magnin, M., Jeanmonod, D.: Multiarchitectonic and stereotactic atlas of the human thalamus. J. Comp. Neurol. **387** (1997) 588–630
7. Schaltenbrand, G., Wahren, W.: Atlas for stereotaxy of the human brain. Georg Thieme Verlag, Stuttgart (1977)
8. Yelnik, J., Damier, P., Demeret, S., Gervais, D., Bardinet, E., Bejjani, B.P., Franois, C., Houeto, J.L., Arnulf, I., Dormont, D., Galanaud, D., Pidoux, B., Cornu, P., Agid, Y.: Localization of stimulating electrodes in parkinsonian patients by using a three-dimensional atlas-magnetic resonance imaging coregistration method. J. Neurosurg. **99** (2003) 83–93
9. Niemann, K., Mennicken, V.R., Jeanmonod, D., Morel, A.: The morel stereotactic atlas of the human thalamus: atlas-to-mr registration of internally consistent canonical model. Neuroimage **12** (2000) 601–616
10. St-Jean, P., Sadikot, A., Collins, D., Clonda, D., Kasrai, R., Evans, A., Peters, T.: Automated atlas integration and interactive 3-dimensional visualization tools for planning and guidance of functional neurosurgery. IEEE Trans. Med. Imaging **17** (1998) 672–680
11. Nowinski, W., Belov, D., Benabid, A.: An algorithm for rapid calculation of a probabilistic functional atlas of subcortical structures from electrophysiological data collected during functional neurosurgery procedures. Neuroimage **18** (2003) 143–155

12. D'Haese, P., Cetinkaya, E.and Kao, C., Fitzpatrick, J., Konrad, P., Dawant, B.: Toward the creation of an electrophysiological atlas for the pre-operative planning and intra-operative guidance of deep brain stimulators (dbs) implantation. In: MICCAI 2004, Proceedings. Volume 3216 of LNCS., Springer (2004) 729–736
13. Duerden, E., Finnis, K., Peters, T., AF, S.: A method for analysis of electrophysiological responses obtained from the motor fibers of the human internal capsule. In: MICCAI 2003, Proceedings. Volume 2878 of LNCS., Springer (2003) 50–57
14. Finnis, K., Starreveld, Y., Parrent, A., Sadikot, A., Peters, T.: Three-dimensional database of subcortical electrophysiology for image-guided stereotactic functional neurosurgery. IEEE Trans. Med. Imaging **22** (2003) 93–104
15. Bardinet, E., Ourselin, S., Dormont, D., Malandain, G., Tandé, D., Parain, K., Ayache, N., Yelnik, J.: Co-registration of histological, optical and MR data of the human brain. In: MICCAI 2002, Proceedings. Volume 2488 of LNCS., Springer (2002) 548–555

Anatomical and Electrophysiological Validation of an Atlas for Neurosurgical Planning

M. Mallar Chakravarty[1], Abbas F. Sadikot[1,2], Jurgen Germann[1], Gilles Bertrand[1,2], and D. Louis Collins[1]

[1] McConnell Brain Imaging Centre
[2] Division of Neurosurgery, Montreal Neurological Institute,
3801 University Street, Montreal, Quebec, Canada, H3A 2B4

Abstract. Digital brain atlases can be used in conjunction with magnetic resonance imaging (MRI) and computed tomography (CT) for planning and guidance during neurosurgery. Digital atlases are advantageous, since they can be warped nonlinearly to fit each patient's unique anatomy.

Two atlas-to-patient warping techniques are compared in this paper. The first technique uses an MRI template as an intermediary to estimate a nonlinear atlas-to-patient transformation. The second, is novel, and uses a pseudo-MRI volume, derived from the voxel-label-atlas, to estimate the atlas-to-patient transformation directly. Manual segmentations and functional data are used to validate the two methods.

1 Introduction

Print atlases were the first visualization tools used to identify surgical targets for functional neurosurgery [16,18]. In order to better visualize patient anatomy, digital atlases derived from print atlases are used in conjunction with imaging data to further enhance the visualization of targets in the subcortical nuclei [2,17,15,10,5]. Despite recent advances in medical imaging which allow improved visualization of the thalamus [7,14], most clinical MRI volumes lack the contrast and resolution required for proper visualization of all subcortical nuclei.

Groups who have developed atlas-to-patient warping techniques have used linear transformations in order to match the atlas to pre-operative patient MRI volumes [2,15]. Recently, nonlinear atlas warping has been used to account for local differences between the atlas and patient anatomy [17,5], and used for neurosurgical planning, to analyze intra-operative electrophysiological data in the thalamus and the internal capsule[8,9], and the analysis of thalamic lesions[1]. This paper analayzes the two different nonlinear atlas-to-subject warping techniques to determine which is most accurate for surgical planning.

In this paper, we use a new high resolution atlas that contains multiple registered represenions of the 105 atlas structures [4,5]. The atlas is derived from a single set of segmented serial histological data taken from a single subject. The segmentation contours are used to derive a voxel-label-atlas, whose intensities are modified to create a pseudo-MRI. Figure 1 shows the histological volume,

J. Duncan and G. Gerig (Eds.): MICCAI 2005, LNCS 3750, pp. 394–401, 2005.

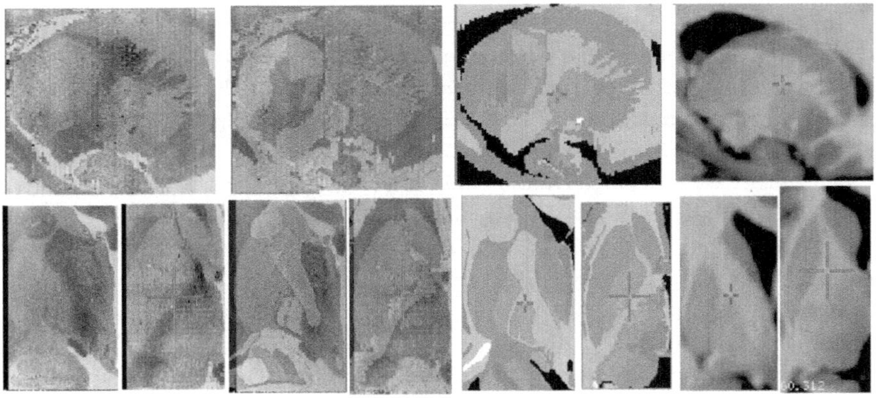

Fig. 1. From Left to Right: Reconstructed histological volume, histological volume with voxel-label-atlas overlaid, pseudo-MRI, and the Colin27 MRI average.

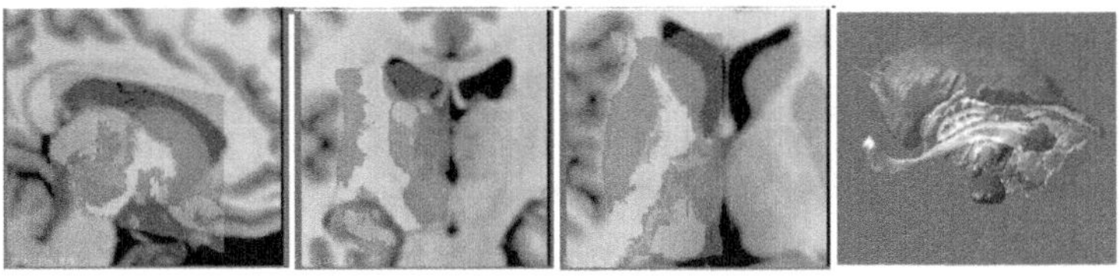

Fig. 2. First three panels: Voxel-label atlas warped to fit the Colin27 MRI average. **Right:** 3D geometric atlas.

the histological volume with the voxel-label-atlas overlaid, and the pseudo-MRI. Figure 2 shows the voxel-label-atlas warped onto the Colin27 MRI average template [13] and the 3D geometric atlas [5].

This paper evaluates the accuracy of two different atlas-to-patient nonlinear warping techniques presented in Section 2. Section 3 discusses the anatomical and electrophysiological validation criteria. The results of this evaluation are given in Section 4.

2 Atlas-to-Patient Warping Techniques

Two atlas-to-patient warping techniques have been developed to warp the atlas described in [5] to patient data. Both techniques begin by estimating a 9 parameter linear transformation (consisting of 3 translations, 3 rotations, and 3 scales) to transform the atlas into the native space of the MRI data. This transformation is used as the input for the nonlinear transformation estimation.

Nonlinear warping is used in order to account for any local differences between the anatomy of the atlas and patient data. Both techniques use the ANIMAL algorithm to estimate the nonlinear transformation used to warp the atlas to fit patient data (see section 2.1).

In the first technique, described in Section 2.2, the Colin27 MRI average is used as an intermediate template in order to estimate a nonlinear transformation. In the original work of St-Jean [17], a thin plate spline was used to align the digital atlas data to the Colin27 template [13]. To address limitations of the previous landmark-based technique, the ANIMAL intensity-based image registration technique was used to align the the new atlas with the Colin27 template. Since similar intensities between the atlas and template images were required, a pseudo-MRI was created from the voxel-label-atlas by mapping each label to an intensity from the analogous structure found in the Colin27 MRI average template volume (see Fig. 1). This procedure is validated in section 3.1.

The use of an atlas-based pseudo-MRI inspired the second atlas-to-patient customization technique, presented in Section 2.3. This technique estimates a nonlinear atlas-to-patient transformation directly, without using any intermediate steps.

2.1 The ANIMAL Registration Algorithm

ANIMAL is an iterative algorithm [6] which estimates a 3D deformation field which matches a source volume to a target volume. The algorithm is divided into two steps. The first step is the outer loop, where large deformations are estimated on data which has been blurred using a Gaussian kernel with of large full-width-at-half-maximum (FWHM). These larger deformations are then input to subsequent steps where the fit is refined by estimating smaller deformations on data blurred with a smaller FWHM.

Each step in the outer loop contains an inner-loop where the the nonlinear transformation which maximizes the similarity between a source and a target volume is estimated. The inner loop consists of two steps: calculating a deformation at each node which will maximize the local similarity measure, and the second is a smoothing step to ensure that a continuous deformation field has been estimated. For further details on ANIMAL's parameters, the reader is referred to [5,6]. For each step in the warping techniques presented in Sections 2.2 and 2.3 the same weight, stiffness, and similarity values are used (1, 1, and 0.3 respectively), and use the cross-correlation objective function.

2.2 MRI Template Based Warping

As mentioned in Section 1, the atlas has been nonlinearly warped to the Colin27 MRI average [13], which now serves as a template for atlas-to-patient registration. Here, ANIMAL is used to compute the nonlinear transformation required to align the Colin27 template MRI volume with the patient's MRI. The standard parameters used for the registration strategy are shown in Table 1. Once the transformation is estimated, it is applied to the atlas to customize it onto the patient's anatomy. This can be seen in the top path of the flowchart of Fig. 3.

Table 1. ANIMAL parameters used for template based atlas-to-subject nonlinear transformation estimation

FWHM (mm)	Step Size (mm)	Sub Lattice Diameter	Sub Lattice	Iterations
8	8	24	6	30
8	4	12	4	30
4	2	6	6	10

2.3 Pseudo-MRI Based Warping

In the novel customization procedure, the atlas pseudo-MRI is used as the source image in order to estimate the atlas-to-patient nonlinear transformation. Since the pseudo-MRI is derived directly from the anatomy of the atlas, any errors incurred by warping the atlas to an intermediate template are now eliminated. During the nonlinear transformation step, small deformations are estimated to warp the atlas to the target patient MRI volume. No blurring is required due to the homogeneous intensities for each structure represented in the pseudo-MRI. A hierarchical registration strategy is still used. The nonlinear transformation estimation procedure can be seen in the bottom path of the flowchart in Fig. 3. The registration parameters are shown in Table 2.

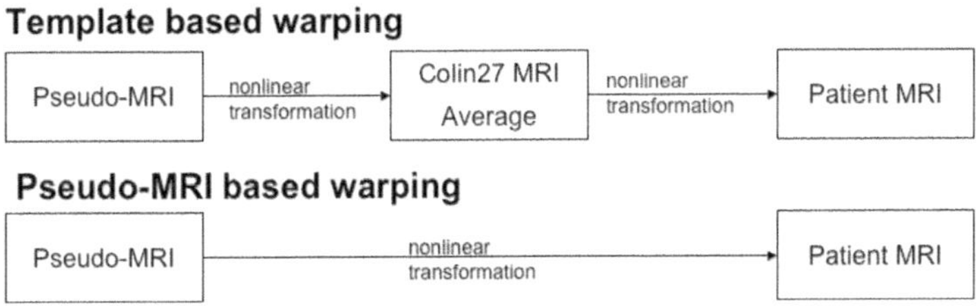

Fig. 3. Flow chart for atlas-to-patient nonlinear transformation estimation. The top path shows the template based atlas-to-patient warping technique. The atlas is registered to the Colin27 MRI template using the pseudo-MRI. The template-to-patient transformation is estimated and then applied to the atlas. The bottom path, demonstrates how the pseudo-MRI based technique bypasses the need to register the atlas to a patient MRI volume by directly estimating an atlas-to-patient transformation.

Table 2. ANIMAL parameters used for template based atlas-to-subject nonlinear transformation estimation

Step	Step Size (mm)	Sub Lattice Diameter	Sub Lattice	Iterations
1	4	8	6	10
2	2	6	6	10
3	1	6	3	10

3 Atlas-to-Patient Warping Evaluation

The atlas to patient warping techniques presented in Sections 2.2 and 2.3 were evaluated using clinical T1-weighted pre-operative image data from 10 surgical candidates: 5 subthalamic stimulation cases (5 males) and 5 thalamotomy (3 males and 2 females, 3 left and 2 right thalamotomy) cases with stereotactic headframe attached. All MRI volumes were acquired between 1997 and 2002. The following sections present anatomical and functional validation for each estimated atlas-to-patient transform.

3.1 Anatomical Validation

Since a gold standard for anatomical validation was not available, manual structure segmentations were used. To estimate inter-rater variability, three expert raters identified the striatum, the thalamus, and the globus pallidus in the MRI data. For each structure in each MRI volume, the consensus label (ie: all voxels labelled by at least two raters for each structure) was considered as "the ground truth". This consensus label was verified against the analogous atlas structure by determining the Kappa score (κ):

$$\kappa = \frac{2a}{(2a + b + c)}, \qquad (1)$$

where a is the number of voxels common to the rater and the warped atlas, and $b + c$ represents the sum of the voxels uniquely identified by either the rater or the atlas warping technique.

The Kappa score is extremely sensitive to changes in two different labels. Figure 4 shows the striatum from the atlas shown in Figs 1 and 2. If the striatum is translated by 0.5mm in all three dimensions, the Kappa score decreases from 1 (for the label on itself) to 0.87. If the striatum if translated by 1mm in all three dimension, then the Kappa score decreases further to 0.81. Typically, scores

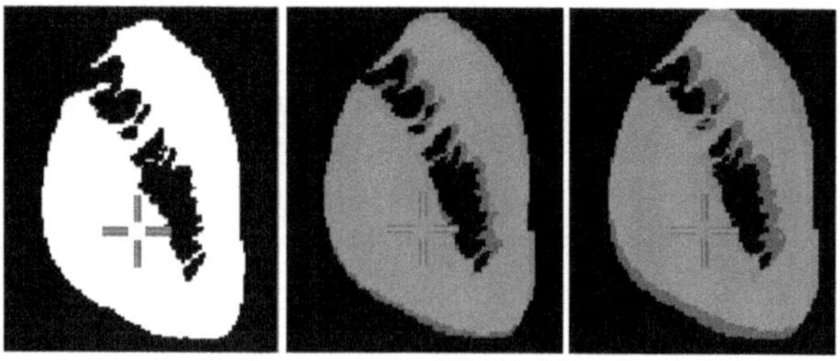

Fig. 4. Changing Kappa values for a displaced Striatum. From left to right Coronal slice through the original striatum defined by the atlas, the striatum translated by 0.5mm in all three dimension ($\kappa = 0.87$), and striatum displaced by 1mm in all three dimensions ($\kappa = 0.81$). In the middle and right most images, the label in red represents the original striatum, and the label in green represents the translated striatum, and yellow, the overlap between the two.

greater than 0.7 are deemed acceptable in the segmentation and classification literature.

Two validations were completed. The first quantifies the pseudo-MRI based customization of the atlas data on the Colin27 target, and thus establishes an upper bound for atlas-to-patient warping quality when using the Colin27 MRI template-based warping method. The second anatomical validation was done using the pre-operative data from the 5 subthalamic stimulation cases.

3.2 Functional Validation

The functional validation uses intra-operative recordings from the 5 patients who underwent thalamotomies to relieve symptoms of Parkinsons disease. In order to determine the lesion location, surgeons typically locate the sensory thalamus using electrical stimulation. By assessing the patients response to different levels of electrical stimulation (1V, 0.75V, 0.5V, 0.25V), the location of the sensory thalamus can be established within the coordinate system established by the stereotactic frame mounted on the patient's head. Using the surgical guidance software [17], the lesion target location, the extension of the electrical stimulator, angles of declination and azimuth, and the probe location frame-space coordinate, the framespace coordinates of the tip of stimulator can be found. For both atlas-to-subject warping techniques, the locations of stimulation point were warped onto the Colin27 MRI average or the pseudo-MRI using the inverse atlas-to-subject transformation. Points from patients who underwent right thalamotomies were reflected to the left side of brain. Only stimulations eliciting a sensory response were used for this validation, yielding a total of 36 functional data points. The warped functional data points were analyzed by determining how many fell inside the 3D boundary defined by the sensory thalamus, and by comparing the distance between the centroid of the warped data points and the center of gravity of the volume defined by the sensory thalamus.

4 Results

The first anatomical validation compares the atlas label to manual rater labels of the the Colin27 MRI template to validate the initial atlas-to-template warp. To establish a baseline, each of the raters labels is compared to the consensus label and shown in the first row of Table 3. Kappa scores show excellent agreement between raters for the striatum and thalamus, however the globus pallidus appears to be more difficult to manually segment as demonstrated by the lower kappa value, probably due to difficulty in identification of the posterior border that has lower contrast in the MRI image. Comparisons between the consensus label and the warped atlas, also show excellent agreement for the striatum and the thalamus, but as in the case for the manual raters, it is difficult to reach a consensus on the location of the globus pallidus. These scores indicate how well raters agree with the atlas structures defined on the Colin27 MRI template and serve as the upper limit in the kappa value when comparing the patient-customized atlas labels below.

Table 3. Top: Kappa scores to assess the overlap between initial warp to the Colin27 template and the rater-defined consensus label. The mean kappa is comparing the rater label overlap to the consensus label is also given. **Bottom:** The mean kappa comparing the rater label overlap to the mean label is also given.

Structures	Striatum	Thalamus	Globus Pallidus
Rater-to-Template ($\bar{\kappa}$)	0.95	0.95 (.93-.96)	0.82 (.76-.96)
Pseudo-to-Template (κ)	0.88	0.82	0.69

Structure	Striatum	Thalamus	Globus Pallidus
Rater-to-Consensus ($\bar{\kappa}$)	0.88	0.88	0.69
Pseudo-to-Consensus ($\bar{\kappa}$)	0.79	0.74	0.68
Template-to-Consensus ($\bar{\kappa}$)	0.80	0.71	0.63

The second validation compares the template-based and the pseudo-MRI based warping procedure against the manual rater labels on each of the 5 sub-thalamic stimulation cases. All comparison are done against the baseline established by consensus labels. Kappa values for these comparisons are shown in the top row of the second table in Table 3. Once again kappa values show excellent agreement between raters, except for in the globus pallidus. Comparisons between the results of the pseudo-MRI based warping technique and template-based warping technique are compared against the consensus label and show that the techniques are equivalent for the striatum, but the pseudo-MRI based technique yields better results for both the thalamus and the globus pallidus.

The functional validation for both warping techniques yields 31 of 34 (89%) data points falling inside the atlas definition of the sensory thalamus. The data points warped using inverse atlas-to-template transformation yielded a centroid which was 2.5mm away from the center of gravity of the sensory thalamus of the atlas. The points warped back to the atlas space using the inverse pseudo-MRI based transformations yielded a centroid which was 2mm away from the center of gravity the sensory thalamus. These results suggest the the pseudo-MRI based method yields a better atlas-to-patient customization.

5 Conclusions and Future Work

In this paper we have presented two different techniques to warp an atlas derived from serial histological data to fit clinical patient MRI volumes. The first relies on a template created from the Colin27 MRI average to estimate an atlas-to-patient warp. The second technique uses a pseudo-MRI derived from a voxel-label-atlas and has a contrast similar to the Colin27 MRI average. Both techniques were evaluated using anatomical and electrophysiological data from pre-operative clinical data from Parkinson's patients. The analysis comparing the atlas label to manual labels shows that the pseudo-MRI based warping technique may be better than the template based technique for the striatum, thalamus, and globus pallidus. An analysis of pre-operative electrophysiological data also suggests the pseudo-MRI based technique offers increased accuracy over the template based technique.

Additional data will be required to determine if the pseudo-MRI based non-linear atlas-to-patient warping technique is statistically better than the the Colin27 MRI template based technique, and is the subject of future work. We would like to continue the atlas validation using more intraoperative data, by classifying the electrophysiological data with respect to the strength of the stimulation and the strength of the sensory responses, and to create a probabilistic functional atlas of the basal ganglia and thalamus from this data.

References

1. J. Atkinson *et al.* *J. of Neurosurg.*, 96(5):672–680, October 2002.
2. G. Bertrand *et al.* *Trans Am Neurol Assoc*, 98:233–237, 1973.
3. F.L. Bookstein. *IEEE PAMI*, 11(6):567–585, 1989.
4. M.M. Chakravarty *et al.* In T. Peters and R. Ellis ed., *MICCAI* LNCS, 2003.
5. M.M. Chakravarty *et al.* *Neuroimage*, 2005. Submitted.
6. D.L. Collins and A.C. Evans. *IJPRAI*, pages 1271–1294, December 1997.
7. S.C.L Deoni *et al.* *MRM*, 53:237–241, 2005.
8. E.G. Duerden*et al.* In T. Peters and R. Ellis ed., *MICCAI* LNCS, 2003.
9. K.W. Finnis *et al.* *IEEE TMI*, 22(1), January 2003.
10. K.A. Ganser *et al.* *Med Image Anal*, 2004.
11. P. Gloor. *The Temporal lobe and the limbic system.* Oxford University Press, 1997.
12. T. Hirai and E.G. Jones. *Brain Res Brain Res Rev.*, 14(1), 1989.
13. C.J. Holmes *et al.* *J Comput Assist Tomogr*, 22(2), 1998.
14. H. Johansen-Berg *et al.* *Cereb Cortex*, 15, January 2005.
15. G.L. Nowinski *et al.* *IEEE TMI*, 19(1), January 2000.
16. G. Schaltenbrand and W. Wahren. *Atlas for Stereotaxy of the Human Brain.* Georg Thieme Verlag, 1977.
17. P. St-Jean *et al.* *IEEE TMI*, 17, May 1998.
18. J. Talairach and P. Tournoux. *Co-Planar Stereotaxic Atlas of the Human Brain.* Georg Thieme Verlag, 1988.

Construction of a 4D Statistical Atlas of the Cardiac Anatomy and Its Use in Classification

Dimitrios Perperidis[1], Raad Mohiaddin[2], and Daniel Rueckert[1]

[1] Visual Information Processing Group, Department of Computing, Imperial College, London, 180 Queen's Gate, London SW7 2BZ, United Kingdom
[2] Royal Brompton and Harefield NHS Trust, Sydney Street, London, United Kingdom

Abstract. In this paper we present a novel method for building a 4D statistical atlas describing the cardiac anatomy and how the cardiac anatomy changes during the cardiac cycle. The method divides the distribution space of cardiac shapes into two subspaces. One distribution subspace accounts for changes in cardiac shape caused by inter-subject variability. The second distribution subspace accounts for changes in cardiac shape caused by deformation during the cardiac cycle (i.e. intra-subject variability). Principal component analysis (PCA) have been performed in order to calculate the most significant modes of variation of each distribution subspace. During the construction of the statistical atlas we eliminate the need for manual landmarking of the cardiac images by using a non-rigid surface registration algorithm to propagate a set of pseudo-landmarks from an automatically landmarked atlas to each frame of all the image sequences. In order to build the atlas we have used 26 cardiac image sequences from healthy volunteers. We show how the resulting statistical atlas can be used to differentiate between cardiac image sequences from patients with hypertrophic cardiomyopathy and normal subjects.

1 Introduction

The early diagnosis and treatment of cardiovascular diseases is crucial in order to reduce mortality and to improve patients' quality of life. Recent advances in the development of magnetic imaging (MR) have enabled the acquisition of high resolution 4D cardiac image sequences which describe the cardiac anatomy as well as function. The acquisition of 4D cardiac image sequences drastically increases the amount of data to be interpreted by clinicians. Therefore, applications assisting the automatic interpretation of MR images are of high importance for increasing the clinical use of MR imaging.

A large number of approaches have been developed for the volumetric modeling of the heart. A comprehensive review of these approaches can be found in Frangi *et al.* [1]. Biomechanical models of the heart have been developed by combing surface information and motion information [2] and by using a deformation model inspired by continuum mechanics [3]. In contrast to these biomechanical models a number of researchers have developed statistical models (e.g. Active Shape Models) of the cardiac anatomy [4] [5] and statistical models of the appearance of the heart (e.g. Active Appearance Models) [6] [7]. For example, Frangi *et al.* have presented an approach for the construction of three-dimensional statistical shape models of the cardiac anatomy

J. Duncan and G. Gerig (Eds.): MICCAI 2005, LNCS 3750, pp. 402–410, 2005.

[8]. This approach eliminates the need for landmarking by using non-rigid registration to propagate landmarks from an automated landmarked atlas to the rest of the images. The resulting model includes the left and right ventricle. The approach developed by Lötjönen *et al.* goes one step further: In this work, statistical shape models of the atria, ventricles and epi-cardium from short-axis and long-axis MR images are constructed and used for the segmentation of cardiac images [9]. In addition a variety of methods which model shape variability have been explored including PCA, ICA and LPD. However, in both cases the statistical shape models describe only the 3D cardiac anatomy at a single time point and ignore the shape variation during the cardiac cycle. Although cardiac modeling of the anatomy is relatively well investigated, very few attempts have been made to build a computerized atlas which captures functional variability of the heart across a group of subjects. Rao *et al.* suggested a framework for building an atlas of the myocardial motion [10] by using tagged MR image sequences to calculate the cardiac motion. Then, the calculated motion fields of different subjects are mapped into the same coordinate system using a vector field transformation technique which accounts for differences in the size, orientation and shape of the heart.

In this paper we present a novel method for building a 4D statistical atlas describing the cardiac anatomy and how the cardiac anatomy changes during the cardiac cycle. In previous work we developed 4D probabilistic atlases of the left ventricle, the myocardium and the right ventricle describing the anatomy and function of a healthy heart [11]. While these probabilistic atlases contain information about the degree of variability at every voxel, statistical atlases provide additional information about the type of variability. The key contribution of our work is the construction of 4D statistical model of the heart that subdivides the distribution space of cardiac shapes into two subspaces: One distribution space accounts for changes in cardiac shape due to deformations throughout the cardiac cycle and the other distribution space accounts for the changes in cardiac shape due to variability across the population. Furthermore, we have used these statistical models to differentiate between cardiac image sequences from patients with hypertrophic cardiomyopathy and normal volunteers.

2 Building a 4D Statistical Atlas

Segmentation of Cardiac MR Image Sequences. The method developed by Lorenzo-Valdés *et al.* [12] has been used to segment the image sequences. In this method the first frame of each image sequence is segmented manually and then the segmentation is propagated to the subsequent frames using a non-rigid registration algorithm. The images sequences are segmented into three anatomical structures: the left ventricle, the myocardium and the right ventricle. After segmenting the image sequences, shape based interpolation is used to resample the images to isotropic voxels of size $1\text{mm} \times 1\text{mm} \times 1\text{mm}$.

Mapping the Image Sequences to the Same Spatio-Temporal Coordinate System. The second stage in the construction procedure of the atlas is to use a spatio-temporal registration method to align the image sequences into the same spatio-temporal coordinate system. The registration method is similar to one which we have previously introduced [13] and has also been used for the construction of a probabilistic atlas of the cardiac anatomy and function [11]. It uses a 4D mapping which has been resolved into decoupled spatial and temporal components $\mathbf{T}_{spatial}$ and $\mathbf{T}_{temporal}$ respectively.

The spatial transformation used is an affine transformation with 9 degrees of freedom which accounts for spatial differences caused by orientation, translation and scaling. The temporal transformation consists of a global part which scales the image sequences to match the end-systolic and end-diastolic time points and a local part which deforms the temporal characteristics of each image sequence to follow the same motion pattern with the reference image sequence. The local temporal transformation is modeled by a free-form deformation using a 1D B-spline:

$$\mathbf{T}_{temporal}^{local}(t) = \sum_{l=0}^{3} B_l(u)\phi_{t_{i+l}} \tag{1}$$

where Φ denotes a set of n_t control points ϕ_t with a temporal spacing δ_t and B_l represents the l-th basis function of the B-spline. The optimal spatial and temporal transformation is found by maximising a voxel based similarity measure, the normalized mutual information (NMI). The NMI of two image sequences can be calculated directly from the joint intensity histogram of the two sequences over their spatio-temporal domain of overlap.

Building the Statistical Atlas of the Heart. After obtaining the spatio-temporal mappings, the segmented image sequences are transformed to the common spatio-temporal coordinate system. Then, the transformed images are blurred with a Gaussian kernel to compensate for low out-of-plane resolution of the images which results in significant partial volume effects in the segmentation. In our approach we eliminate the need for manual landmarking by using a method similar to the one introduced by Frangi *et al.*[8]. In this method, a set of pseudo-landmarks are propagated from an automatically landmarked atlas to all the frames of each image sequence.

Landmark Extraction and Propagation. After blurring the image sequences with a Gaussian kernel, the *marching cubes* [14] algorithm is used to generate a dense triangulation (pseudo-landmarks) of the boundary surfaces of each anatomical structure (the left ventricle, the myocardium and the right ventricle) of all the frames of each image sequence. In order to perform any statistical analysis correspondence between the pseudo-landmarks of each image needs to be established. This is achieved by using a surfaced based registration method based on B-Splines. The end-diastolic frame of the image sequence used as reference during the construction of the atlases is also used as the reference surface in these registrations. After registering all surfaces, we use the obtained transformations to propagate the pseudo-landmarks of the reference surface to each frame.

Modeling Shape Variability. Let $\{\mathbf{q_{ik}}; i = 0...n_p; k = 0...n_f\}$ denote n shapes (n_p subjects with n_f frames each). Each shape consists of m 3D landmarks, $\mathbf{p_j} = (p_{1j}, p_{2j}, p_{3j}; j = 1....m)$. Each vector $\mathbf{q_{ik}}$ will consist of the landmarks $(p_{11}, p_{21}, p_{31}, p_{12}, p_{22}, p_{32}, ..., p_{1m}, p_{2m}, p_{3m})$. The aim of the statistical analysis is to approximate the distribution of the landmarks with a linear model of the form:

$$\mathbf{q} = \bar{\mathbf{q}} + \Phi \mathbf{b} \tag{2}$$

where $\bar{\mathbf{q}}$ is the average landmark vector, $\mathbf{b}$ is the shape parameter vector of the model, and Φ is a matrix of eigen-vectors. The matrix Φ is obtained by performing a principal component analysis (PCA) to the covariance matrix $\mathbf{C}$. During the principal component analysis, the principal components of $\mathbf{C}$ are calculated as its eigenvectors ϕ_i and the corresponding eigenvalues λ_i are also calculated (such that $\lambda_i < \lambda_{i+1}$).

The aim of our statistical analysis is to identify what changes in the cardiac anatomy occur due to the cardiac cycle and what changes occur due to shape variation across the population. Therefore, we want to use principal components analysis (PCA) to find the estimate of two subspaces of the overall distribution. In order to achieve this we perform two separate principal component analysis. The covariance matrices for the total shape distribution is given by:

$$\mathbf{C}_{total} = \frac{1}{n_f n_p} \sum_{i=1}^{n_p} \sum_{k=1}^{n_f} (\mathbf{q_{ik}} - \bar{\mathbf{q}})(\mathbf{q_{ik}} - \bar{\mathbf{q}})^T \tag{3}$$

where n_f is the number of frames of each image sequence, n_p the number of images sequences and $\bar{\mathbf{q}}$ is the mean shape.

The covariance matrix of the shape differences occurring due to the cardiac cycle is given by:

$$\mathbf{C}_{within} = \frac{1}{n_f n_p} \sum_{i=1}^{n_p} \sum_{k=1}^{n_f} (\mathbf{q_{ik}} - \bar{\mathbf{q}}_\mathbf{i})(\mathbf{q_{ik}} - \bar{\mathbf{q}}_\mathbf{i})^T \tag{4}$$

where $\bar{\mathbf{q}}_\mathbf{i}$ is the mean for the subject i (the image sequences contain the same number of frames since they are registered in the temporal domain) and $\mathbf{q_{ik}}$ is the shape of frame k of subject i.

The covariance matrix which described the shape differences occurring across the population is given by:

$$\mathbf{C}_{between} = \frac{1}{n_p} \sum_{i=1}^{n_p} (\bar{\mathbf{q}}_\mathbf{i} - \bar{\mathbf{q}})(\bar{\mathbf{q}}_\mathbf{i} - \bar{\mathbf{q}})^T \tag{5}$$

where, as in eq. 4, n_p is the number of image sequences and $\bar{\mathbf{q}}$ is the total mean.

In order to find the principal components of each subspace the eigen values and vectors of each covariance matrix (eq. 4 and 5) are calculated. A similar decomposition of the total distribution to subspaces has been used by Costen *et al.* for the automatic extraction of the face identity-subspace [15]. New shape examples can be generated by varying the parameters b of equation 2. Assuming that the distribution of the data follows a multidimensional Gaussian distribution (this assumption has some limitations), the variance of the ith parameter of $\mathbf{b}$ across the training set is given by λ_i. If we apply limits in the variation of b_i such that $b_i \leq \pm 3\sqrt{\lambda_i}$ we ensure the generated shape is similar to those contained in the training class.

3 Results

Materials. In order to produce the atlas we have acquired 26 untagged MR image sequences from healthy volunteers. The images have been acquired using a Siemens

Sonata 1.5T scanner using TrueFisp pulse sequence in a form of a series short-axis images. Seven of the images were acquired using retrospective gating acquisition while the rest were acquired using prospective gating acquisition. One of the image sequences was selected to be the reference subject of the spatio-temporal registration. Care was taken to ensure that the reference subject was a normal representative of the population. The reference subject had in-plane resolution of 192×256 with pixel size of $1.48 \times 1.48mm$ and a slice thickness of 10mm (which is the typical pixel size used in these acquisitions). After the shape based interpolation the slice thickness was reduced to 1mm. The images covered the entire left-ventricle form base to apex.

Statistical Model of the Variability Across Subjects. These models describe the significant changes in the shape of the left ventricle, the myocardium due to subjects' different heart shape. Figure 1 shows the three most significant modes of variation for the left ventricle (a) and the myocardium (b). For the left ventricle, the three most significant modes of shape variation describe the differences in the size of the left ventricle (mode 1), the variation of the position of the apex of the heart (mode 2) and the elongation of the apex of the heart (mode 3). For the myocardium, the three most significant modes of variation describe the size of the myocardium (mode 1), the thickness of the myocardium (mode 2) and the direction of the myocardium long-axis (mode 3). In order to describe 90% of the shape variability of the inter-subject distribution subspace 13 (of 26) modes of shape variation are required.

Statistical Model of the Variability Across the Cardiac Cycle. These models describe the most significant changes in the shape of the left ventricle and the myocardium which occur due to the cardiac cycle. Figure 2 shows the three most significant modes of variation of the left ventricle (a) and the myocardium (b). For the left ventricle, the

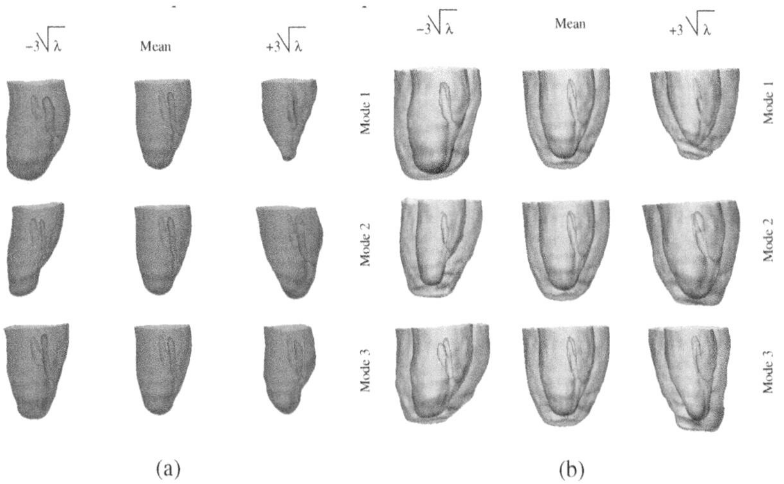

Fig. 1. The significant modes of variation across subjects of (a) left ventricle and (b) myocardium. Animations of all the atlases and also of atlases of the right ventricle can be found at: http:/www.doc.ic.ac.uk/~dp1/Research/StatisticalAtlases/

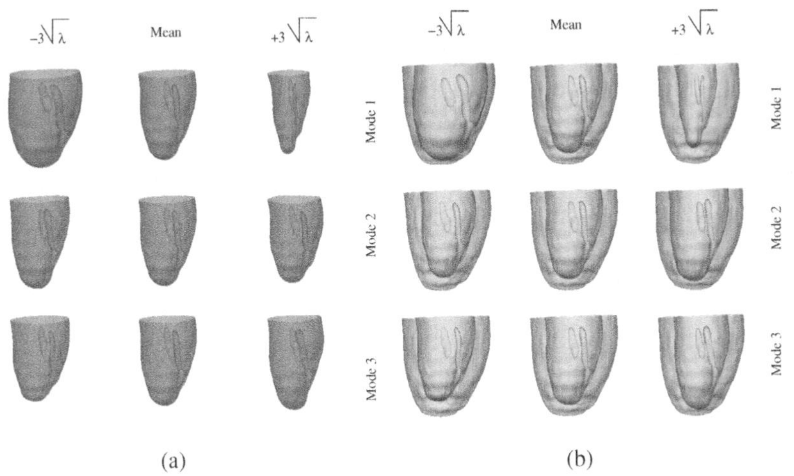

Fig. 2. The significant modes of variation across the cardiac cycle of (a) left ventricle and (b) myocardium

three most significant modes of variation (fig. 2(a)) describe the differences in the volume of the left ventricle during the cardiac cycle (mode 1), the twisting of the heart during the contraction phase (mode 2) and the changes in the position of the apex of the left ventricle and also the position of the papillary muscles (mode 3). For the myocardium, the three most significant modes of variation (fig. 2(b)) describe the changes in the size of the left ventricle and the thickening of the myocardium, the twisting of the myocardium during the contraction phase (mode 3) and the movement of the cardiac wall (mode 3). In order to describe 90% of the shape variability of the intra-subject distribution subspace 16 (of 468) modes shape variation are required.

4 Classification Using the 4D Statistical Atlas

In this section we demonstrate a possible use of the statistical atlases for the classification of cardiac data. We used the above statistical models to classify cardiac data from normal volunteers and patients with hypertrophic cardiomyopathy (a condition in which the myocardium has an excessive thickening). In order to perform this classification we have excluded six subjects from the model (i.e. the model has been constructed from only 20 healthy subjects) and we have acquired MR image sequences from 8 patients with hypertrophic cardiomyopathy. The same processing steps for the registration and pseudo-landmark extraction and propagation were used for these image sequences as for ones used for the construction of the statistical models (see section 2). Then, for each image sequence the mean surface (over the cardiac cycle) was calculated. These mean surfaces were projected into the shape space of the statistical models. Figure 3 shows the projections of the subjects' myocardium to the space of the across population atlas (a) and across cardiac cycle atlas (b) . We clearly see from the distribution of the data that a simple classifier will enable the correct differentiation between normal and hypertrophic subjects.

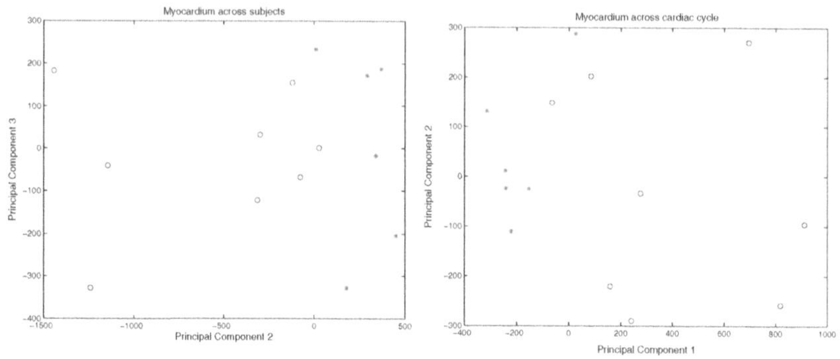

(a) (b)

Fig. 3. Projection of the myocardium to the space of the (a) across the subjects atlas and (b) across the cardiac cycle atlas (the circles on the figures are the subjects with hypertrophic cardiomyopathy while the stars the normal ones)

Table 1. Accuracy of the classification using the statistical model of the myocardium describing changes in the anatomy due to the cardiac cycle (model A), due to inter-subject variation (model B) and a combination of both

	Model A	**Model B**	**Model A and B**
Normal	83%	100%	100%
Hypertrophic cardiomyopathy	100%	87.5%	87.5%

In order to classify the data we used a *k-weighted NN-classifier.* A leave one out experiment was performed. The first 4 principal components were employed when using the statistical atlas describing the cardiac shape variability due to cardiac cycle, while the second and the third principal components were employed when using the statistical atlas describing the inter-subject shape variability. In this case, the first principal component was not used in the classification since it describes the size of the myocardium in the base to apex direction. Furthermore, the combination of these principal components (from both models) were also used for data classification. The classification results are reported in table 1.

5 Conclusions

In this paper we presented a novel method for building a 4D statistical atlas describing the cardiac anatomy and how the cardiac anatomy changes during the cardiac cycle. Contrary to probabilistic atlases, the statistical atlases provide not only information regarding how much variability exists in the data but also what the variability is. In order to build the atlas we have used 26 cardiac image sequences from normal volunteers. The method separates the distribution space of the cardiac shape into two subspaces. One distribution subspace accounts for the changes in cardiac shape caused by inter-subject variability. The second distribution subspace accounts for the changes in cardiac shape caused by deformation in the cardiac cycle (i.e. intra-subject variability). Principal component analysis (PCA) has been performed in order to calculate the most significant modes of variation of each distribution subspace. Moreover, our method eliminates the need for manual landmarking of the cardiac images by using a non-rigid registration algorithm to propagate landmarks from an from an automatically landmarked to each image. We have also demonstrated a possible use of the statistical atlases by using them to differentiate between cardiac image sequences from patients with hypertrophic cardiomyopathy and normal subjects.

References

1. A. F. Frangi, W. J. Niessen, and M. A. Viergever. Three-dimensional modeling for functional analysis of cardiac images: A review. *IEEE Transactions on Medical Imaging*, 20(1):2–25, 2001.
2. P. C. Shi, A. J. Sinusas, T. Constable, and J. S. Duncan. Volumetric deformation analysis using mechanics-based data fusion: Applications in cardiac motion recovery. *International Journal of Computer Vision*, 35(1):87–107, 1999.
3. X. Papademetris. *Estimation of 3D Left Ventricular Deformation from Medical Images Using Biomechanical Models*. PhD thesis, Yale University, 2000.
4. J. Lötjönen, J. Koikkalainen, D. Smutek, S. Kivistö, and K. Lauerma. Four-chamber 3D statistical shape model from cardiac short-axis MR images. In *Sixth Int. Conf. on Medical Image Computing and Computer-Assisted Intervention (MICCAI '03)*, number 2878 in Lecture Notes in Computer Science, pages 491–498. Springer, 2003.
5. P. Horkaew and G. Z. Yang. Optimal deformable surface models for 3D medical image analysis. In *Information Processing in Medical Imaging: Proc. 18th International Conference (IPMI'03)*, number 2732 in Lecture Notes in Computer Science, pages 13–24. Springer, 2003.
6. S. C. Mitchell, B. P. F. Lilieveldt, R. J. van der Geest, H. G. Bosch, J. H. C. Reiber, and M. Sonka. Multistage hybrid active appearance model matching: Segmentation of left and right ventricles in cardiac MR images. *IEEE Transactions on Medical Imaging*, 20(5):415–523, 2001.
7. S. C. Mitchell, J. G. Bosch, B. P. F. Lelieveldt, R.J . van der Geest, J. H. C. Reiber, and M. Sonka. 3D active appearance models:segmentation of cardiac MR and ultrasound images. *IEEE Transactions on Medical Imaging*, 21(9):1167–1178, 2002.
8. A. F. Frangi, D. Rueckert, J. A. Schnabel, and W. J. Niessen. Automatic construction of multiple-object three-dimensional statistical shape models: Application to cardiac modeling. *IEEE Transaction on Medical Imaging*, 21(9):1151–1165, 2002.
9. J. Lötjönen, S. Kivistö, J. Koikkalainen, D. Smutek, and K. Lauerma. Statistical shape model of atria, ventricles and epicardium from short- and long-axis MR images. *Medical Image Analysis*, 8(3):371–386, 2004.
10. A. Rao, G. I. Sanchez-Ortiz, R. Chandrashekara, M. Lorenzo-Valdés, R. Mohiaddin, and D. Rueckert. Comparison of cardiac motion across subjects using non-rigid registration. In *Fifth Int. Conf. on Medical Image Computing and Computer-Assisted Intervention (MICCAI '02)*, number 2488 in Lecture Notes in Computer Science, pages 722–729. Springer, 2002.
11. D. Perperidis, M. Lorenzo-Valdés, R. Chandrashekara, A. Rao, R. Mohiaddin, G. I. Sanchez-Ortiz, and D. Rueckert. Building a 4D atlas of the cardiac anatomy and motion using MR imaging. In *2004 IEEE International Symposium on Biomedical Imaging: From Nano to Macro*, 2004.

12. M. Lorenzo-Valdés, G. I. Sanchez-Ortiz, A. Elkington, R. Mohiaddin, and D. Rueckert. Segmentation of 4D cardiac MR images using a probabilistic atlas and the EM algorithm. *Medical Image Analysis*, 8(3):255–265, 2004.
13. D. Perperidis, R. Mohiaddin, and D. Rueckert. Spatio-temporal free-form registration of cardiac MR image sequences. In *Seventh Int. Conf. on Medical Image Computing and Computer-Assisted Intervention (MICCAI '04)*, number 3216 in Lecture Notes in Computer Science, pages 911–919. Springer, 2004.
14. W. E. Lorensen and H. E. Cline. Marching cubes: a high resolution 3D surface reconstruction algorithm. In *Computer Graphics: SIGGRAPH'87 Conference Proceedings*, volume 21, pages 163–169, 1987.
15. N. P. Costen, T .F. Cootes, G. J. Edwards, and C. J. Taylor. Automatic extraction of the face identity-subspace. *Image and Vision Computing*, 20(5-6):319–329, 2002.

Unbiased Atlas Formation Via Large Deformations Metric Mapping

Peter Lorenzen[1], Brad Davis[1], and Sarang Joshi[1,2]

[1] Department of Computer Science
[2] Department of Radiation Oncology, University of North Carolina,
Chapel Hill, NC 27599, USA
{lorenzen, davisb, joshi}@cs.unc.edu

Abstract. The construction of population atlases is a key issue in medical image analysis, and particularly in brain mapping. Large sets of images are mapped into a common coordinate system to study intra-population variability and inter-population differences, to provide voxel-wise mapping of functional sites, and to facilitate tissue and object segmentation via registration of anatomical labels. We formulate the unbiased atlas construction problem as a Fréchet mean estimation in the space of diffeomorphisms via large deformations metric mapping. A novel method for computing constant speed velocity fields and an analysis of atlas stability and robustness using entropy are presented. We address the question: how many images are required to build a stable brain atlas?

Keywords: Computational anatomy; Brain Atlases; Image Metric Space.

1 Introduction

Computational anatomy is the study of anatomical variation [1]. For a set of images representing a population, a natural problem in computational anatomy is the construction of an atlas — an image that serves as a representative for the population. Such an atlas must represent the anatomical variation present in the image population [2]. A major focus of computational anatomy has been the development of image mapping algorithms [3,4,5,6] that map and transform a single brain atlas onto a population.

In the recent and related work of [7], the authors developed a large deformation template estimation algorithm by averaging velocity fields. Most other previous work [8,9] in atlas formation has focused on the small deformation setting in which arithmetic averaging of displacement fields in well defined. We do not make this small deformation assumption.

To generate the deformations for producing atlases, we apply the theory of large deformation diffeomorphisms [10,4]. We simultaneously estimate the unbiased atlas and the transformations which map the atlas to each population image. Linear averaging cannot be applied directly to the large deformation setting as, under the large deformation model, the space of transformations is not a vector space, but rather the infinite dimensional group $\mathcal{H}$ of diffeomorphisms

J. Duncan and G. Gerig (Eds.): MICCAI 2005, LNCS 3750, pp. 411–418, 2005.

of an underlying coordinate system Ω. In our previous work [11], we address this problem by posing anatomical atlas creation as a statistical estimation problem where the notion of simple intensity averaging is extended to general metric spaces first proposed by Fréchet [12]. In [11], we developed a method for unbiased construction of atlases based on an iterative greedy method for generating large deformation diffeomorphisms.

In this paper, we present a complete large deformations metric mapping (LDMM) methodology introduced by [13]. Both the greedy and LDMM implementations provide large deformation coordinate system transformations. In [11], the solution to the atlas formation problem generates paths through the space of diffeomorphisms, the length of which cannot be used to define a metric as the method provides a locally optimal rather than full space-time solution. In contrast, the variational optimization of the atlas formation cost function in the LDMM algorithm, gives geodesic paths on the manifold of diffeomorphic transformations, $\mathcal{G}$, the lengths of which places the orbit of transformed images into a metric space. In this way, we build a geodesic atlas.

We use the entropy of voxel intensities to measure the robustness and stability of unbiased atlases. In the context of in MR images, entropy is often used to assess the degree to which an image differs from an ideal where an ideal image intensity histogram consists of a small number of modes representing tissue classes [14,15]. We study the stability of atlases produced by our method by building atlases, of increasing population size, using multiple permutations of images from a database of images.

The remainder of this paper is organized as follows: in Section 2, the unbiased atlas formation problem is developed; in Section 3, the Euler-Lagrange equations used to characterize the LDMM and implementation details and a novel method for constant velocity computation are presented; and in Section 4, an analysis of the atlas stability and robustness using entropy are reported.

2 Method

In our previous work [11], we exemplify the atlas estimation problem by first considering a population of N images $\{I_i\}_{i=1\ldots N}$ acquired by the same imaging modality which have been rigidly aligned. We seek the representative image, $\hat{I}$, that requires the minimum amount of energy to deform into each population image I_i. In the spirit of [13], we define dense transformations, from the infinite dimensional group of diffeomorphisms $\mathcal{H}$, and fluid flow vector fields in the following manner: the group elements of the change of coordinates φ_i such that $\hat{I} = \varphi_i^{-1} I_i = I_i \circ \varphi_i$ are generated as the end-points $\varphi_i = \phi_i(1)$ of the flows of time-dependent vector fields $v_i(\cdot, t)$, $t \in [0,1]$ from the space of smooth vector fields V via

$$\dot{\phi}_i^v(t) = \frac{d}{dt}\phi_i^v(t) = v_i(\phi_i^v, t)$$

where the superscript v in ϕ_i^v is used to explicitly denote the dependence of ϕ_i on the associated velocity field v. The terminal point of the curve ϕ_i^v at $t = 0$ is

$\phi_i^v(0) = e \in \mathcal{G}$ where e is the identity transformation $e(x) = x$, $\forall x \in \Omega$. The end point of the curve ϕ_i^v at $t = 1$ is the particular diffeomorphism $\phi_i^v(1) = \varphi_i \in \mathcal{G}$ that links the images $\hat{I}$ and I_i such that $\hat{I} = \varphi_i^{-1} I_i = I_i \circ \varphi_i$. The transformations φ_i are generated by integrating velocity fields, v_i, forward in time.

Given $\mathcal{H}$, with associated metric $D : \mathcal{H} \times \mathcal{H} \to \mathbb{R}$, along with an image dissimilarity measure $E(I_1, I_2)$, we wish to find the image $\hat{I}$ such that

$$\{\hat{\varphi}_i, \hat{I}\} = \underset{\varphi_i \in \mathcal{H}, I}{\operatorname{argmin}} \sum_{i=1}^{N} \left(E^2(I, I_i \circ \varphi_i) + D^2(e, \varphi_i) \right). \tag{1}$$

We induce a metric on $\mathcal{H}$ by a Sobolev norm via a partial differential operator L on the velocity fields. Let φ be a diffeomorphism isotopic to the identity transformation e, that is, there exists a continuous family of diffeomorphisms from e to ϕ. We define the squared distance $D^2(e, \varphi)$ on the space V of smooth velocity vector fields on the domain Ω, as

$$D^2(e, \varphi) = \min_{v:\dot{\phi}(t) = v(\phi^v, t)} \int_0^1 ||Lv(t)||_V^2 dt.$$

The distance between any two diffeomorphisms is defined by

$$D(\varphi_1, \varphi_2) = D(e, \varphi_1^{-1} \circ \varphi_2).$$

This distance satisfies all the properties of a metric [16].

Having defined a metric on $\mathcal{H}$, the minimum energy template estimation problem described by Equation 1 is formulated as

$$\{\hat{\varphi}_i, \hat{I}\}_{i=1\ldots N} = \underset{v_i:\dot{\phi}(t) = v(\phi^v, t), I}{\operatorname{argmin}} \sum_{i=1}^{N} \left(E^2(I, I_i \circ \varphi_i) + \int_0^1 ||Lv_i(t)||_V^2 dt \right).$$

Throughout this paper we use the square error dissimilarity metric. Under this metric, the template estimation problem becomes

$$\{\hat{\varphi}_i, \hat{I}\}_{i=1\ldots N} = \underset{v_i:\dot{\phi}(t) = v(\phi^v, t), I}{\operatorname{argmin}} \sum_{i=1}^{N} \left(\frac{1}{\sigma^2} ||I - I_i \circ \varphi_i||_{L^2}^2 + \int_0^1 ||Lv_i(t)||_V^2 dt \right) \tag{2}$$

where σ models the noise in the image match term. Smaller values of this parameter increase the penalty of image mismatch leading to exact matching when $\sigma \to 0$; this comes at the expense of smoothness in the estimated maps φ_i.

This minimization problem can be simplified by noticing that for fixed transformations φ_i, the image $\hat{I}$ that minimizes Equation 2 is given by the voxel-wise arithmetic mean of the deformed images

$$\hat{I} = \frac{1}{N} \sum_{i=1}^{N} I_i \circ \varphi_i. \tag{3}$$

Combining Equations 2 and 3 results in following optimization, in terms of velocity fields,

$$\{\hat{v}_i\}_{i=1\ldots N} = \operatorname*{argmin}_{v_i:\dot{\phi}(t)=v(\phi^v,t)} E(v_i) \doteq \sum_{i=1}^{N}\left(\frac{1}{\sigma^2}\left|\left|\left(\frac{1}{N}\sum_{j=1}^{N} I_j \circ \varphi_j\right) - I_i \circ \varphi_i\right|\right|_{L^2}^2 + \int_0^1 ||Lv_i(t)||_V^2 dt\right) \quad (4)$$

For each individual velocity field, the minimizer of Equation 4 is constant speed, that is, $||v_i(t)||_V = c_i$, since it is a geodesic. Note that the solution to this minimization problem is independent of the ordering of the N images.

3 Implementation

We use the full space time strategy presented in [13]. Since the minimization problem is independent of the ordering of the N images we use an algorithm that estimates, on a per iteration basis, each φ_i in turn. The optimization described by Equation 4 is implemented by an iterative steepest descent algorithm given by

$$v_i^{k+1}(t) = v_i^k(t) - \epsilon \nabla_{v_i^k(t)} E \quad (5)$$

where ∇E is the Gâteaux differential of the energy of the objective function giving the Euler-Lagrange condition. The Euler-Lagrange equation for the solution of the variational problem in 4, in space of smooth velocity fields V, becomes

$$v_i(t) = \frac{1}{\sigma^2} K\left(|D\phi_i^v(t,1)|(I \circ \phi_i^v(t,0) - I_i \circ \phi_i^v(t,1))\nabla(I \circ \phi_i^v(t,0))\right) \quad (6)$$

where $\phi_i(s,t) = \phi_i(t) \circ (\phi_i(s))^{-1}$ and $I = \frac{1}{N}\sum_{j=1}^{N} I_j \circ \varphi_j$. The operator K is the Green's function of the differential operator $L^\dagger L$ used to define the norm $||\cdot||_V$. In our implementation, L is a modified Navier-Stokes operator [10]. Note that the stable point of Equation 6 satisfies the Euler-Lagrange equation $\nabla E = 0$.

3.1 Constant Speed Velocity

The optimal velocity fields $\hat{v}_i$, given by Equation 4, each define a geodesic path on the space of diffeomorphisms. As geodesics have constant speed, the velocity fields have constant norm over time. Given ∇E, we enforce this geodesic constraint by calculating adaptive per-iteration time steps $\epsilon_i^k(t)$ such that for all time steps t, the norms $\int_\Omega ||Lv_i^k(t)||_2^2 dx$ are equal. We formulate the inductive hypothesis: $\int_\Omega ||Lv_i^k(t)||_2^2 dx = \rho_i^k$, a constant and solve for $\epsilon_i^{k+1}(t)$ such that

$$\int_\Omega ||Lv_i^{k+1}||_2^2 dx = \int_\Omega ||L[v_i^k - \epsilon_i^{k+1}(t)\nabla_{v_t^{k+1}} E]||_2^2 dx = \rho_i^{k+1}$$
$$\Rightarrow \rho_i^{k+1} = \rho_i^k(t) - 4\lambda_i^{k+1}(t)\epsilon_i^{k+1}(t) + 4\nu_i^{k+1}(t)\left(\epsilon_i^{k+1}(t)\right)^2 \quad (7)$$

where

$$\nu_i^{k+1}(t) = \rho_i^k - \frac{2}{\sigma^2}\int_\Omega \langle v_i^k(t), b_i^{k+1}(t)\rangle dx + \frac{1}{\sigma^4}\int_\Omega \langle b_i^{k+1}(t), K(b_i^{k+1}(t))\rangle dx$$

$$\lambda_i^{k+1}(t) = \rho_i^k - \frac{1}{\sigma^2}\int_\Omega \langle v_i^k(t), b_i^{k+1}(t)\rangle dx$$

$$b_i^{k+1}(t) = |D\phi_i^v(t,1)|(I \circ \phi_i^v(t,0) - I_i \circ \phi_i^v(t,1))\nabla(I \circ \phi_i^v(t,0)).$$

After choosing an appropriate value for the difference $\rho_i^{k+1} - \rho_i^k$, we solve Equation 7 for $\epsilon_i^{k+1}(t)$ using the quadratic formula for the positive solution which yields,

$$\epsilon_i^{k+1}(t) = \frac{1}{2\nu_i^{k+1}}\left(\lambda_i^{k+1}(t) + \sqrt{\left(\lambda_i^{k+1}(t)\right)^2 - \nu_i^{k+1}(t)\left(\rho_i^k - \rho_i^{k+1}\right)}\right).$$

We begin by specifying an initial value for one of the $\epsilon_i^{k+1}(t)$ and solve for $\rho_i^{k+1} - \rho_i^k$. Note that the integrated velocity norm $\int_\Omega ||Lv_i^{k+1}(t)||_2^2 dx$ does not have to be computed since it starts at zero and increases at iteration by $\rho_i^{k+1} - \rho_i^k$, which is known at each iteration.

4 Results

To evaluate the performance of this method, we consider the question: how many images are required to represent a population? To address this question, we build atlases of increasing population size and analyze their stability with respect to image intensity entropy. Entropy has often been proposed as a good measure of image quality [14,15] where sharp images have relatively low entropy. Let X be a random variable associated with the intensities for a given image and let p_X be the probability mass function associated with X. Discrete entropy is defined as the expected uncertainty in X,

$$H(X) = \mathcal{E}_{p_X}[-\log p_X(x)] = -\sum_{x\in X} p_X(x)\log p_X(x)$$

where the logarithm, in our case, is take with base two yielding entropy measured in bits. The uniform distribution maximizes entropy for random variables defined without moment constraints, such as image intensities [17]. That is, a blurry image, with a relatively flat histogram, will have greater entropy than a sharp image. We are interested in the entropy introduced by the atlas creation method rather than the intrinsic entropy associated with images of individual brain anatomy.

4.1 Atlas Formation

Our image database contains fourteen brain images that have been provided by the UNC autism image analysis group. These images have been intensity normalized and rigidly aligned. Due to the high memory demands of our implementation, we apply our algorithm to 2D mid-axial slices, although the methodology is generalizable to 3D. These images are show in Figure 1. There is noticeable large deformation variation between these anatomies, especially in lateral ventricles.

To quantify the stability of the estimated atlases, we generate eleven atlas cohorts, $\{C_l\}_{l=2...12}$, each with twenty atlases derived from l images randomly

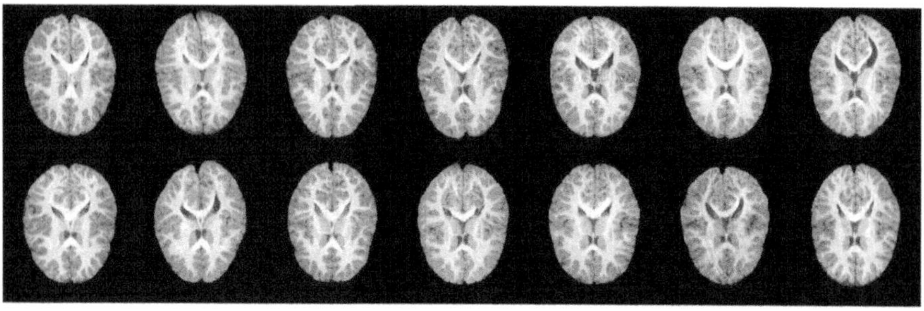

Fig. 1. Image Database: 2D mid-axial slices from MR images of fourteen subjects

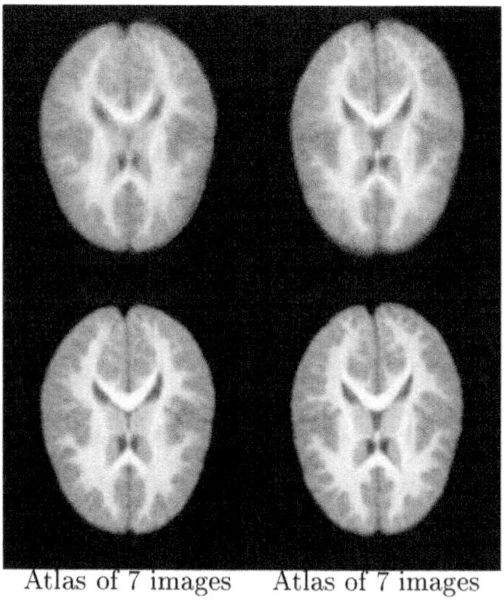

Fig. 2. Mutually Exclusive Atlases: each column represents an individual atlas constructed by both arithmetically averaging rigidly aligned images (top row) and estimating a Fréchet mean atlas after 100 iterations (bottom row). These two atlases were formed from completely separate sets of images.

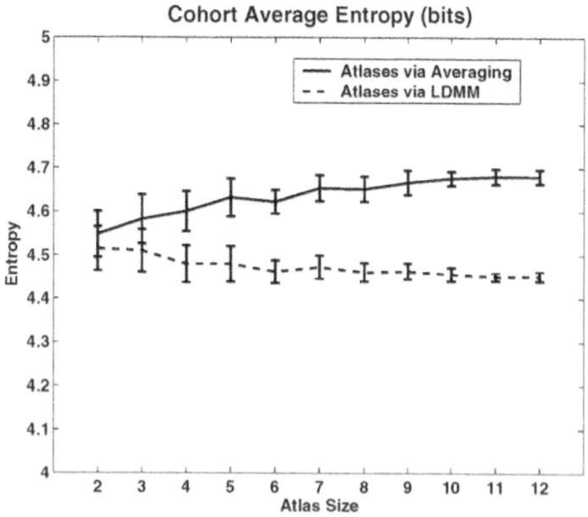

Fig. 3. Average Entropy: for comparison, the average entropy of the original fourteen images is 3.91 bits with standard deviation 0.08 bits. The error bars represent one standard deviation from the mean. Prior to computing entropy, we shift all atlases by half a pixel to compensate for the entropy introduced by the linear interpolation used to reconstruct images during registration.

selected from the original database of fourteen images. Two mutually exclusive atlases from C_7 are shown in Figure 2 for both simple averaging and the LDMM method. The rigidly aligned atlases are blurry since they are arithmetic averages of varying individual neuroanatomies. Ghosting is evident around the lateral ventricles and near the boundary of the brain. In the final Fréchet atlases, these regions appear much sharper.

4.2 Atlas Convergence

To evaluate the robustness and stability of our atlases we first compute the mean and standard deviation of the entropies of the original fourteen images. To this we compare the mean and standard deviation of the atlas cohort entropies that have been created both by simple arithmetic averaging of the rigidly aligned images and those produced by the LDMM method. These results are summarized in Figure 3. From this plot we notice that as atlas size increases, the average atlas entropy increases for atlases formed by simple intensity averaging, where as the average entropy decreases for atlases created via LDMM. The atlases also become more stable with respect to entropy as the standard deviation decreases with atlas size. After cohort C_{10}, the atlas entropy means appear to converge. To answer our original question, given these fourteen subjects, we need about ten images to create a stable atlas representing neuroanatomy.

5 Conclusion

A novel method for unbiased atlas formation involving large deformations metric mapping has been presented. The LDMM implementation has also been improved by new constant speed velocity reparameterization constraint. The preliminary results show that this method produces stable atlases with respect to the entropy image quality measure. A possible direction for future work is to explore the stability and robustness in the presence of much larger initial population databases.

Acknowledgments

This work was supported by NIBIB-NIH grant R01 EB000219, NIH-HLB grant R01 HL69808, DOD Prostate Cancer Research Program DAMD17-03-1-0134, NIMH grant MH064580 Longitudinal MRI Study of Brain Development in Fragile X, and the NDRC.

References

1. Grenander, U., Miller, M.: Computational anatomy: an emerging discipline. Quarterly of Applied Mathematics **56** (1998) 617–694
2. Toga, A.W.: An Introduction to Brain Warping. Academic Press, San Diego (1999)

3. Gee, J.C., Reivich, M., Bajcsy, R.: Elastically deforming an atlas to match anatomical brain images. Journal of Computer Assisted Tomography **17** (1993) 225–236
4. Miller, M.I., Younes, L.: Group actions, homeomorphisms, and matching: A general framework. Internation Journal of Computer Vision (IJCV) **41** (2001) 61–84
5. Rohlfing, T., Russakoff, D.B., Calvin R. Mauerer, J.: Extraction and application of expert priors to combine multiple segmentations of human brain tissue. In: Proceedings of Medical Image Computing and Computer-Assisted Intervention (MICCAI). Volume 2732., Springer-Verlag (2003) 578–585
6. Thompson, P.M., Toga, A.W.: A framework for computational anatomy. Computing and Visualization in Science **5** (2002) 13–34
7. Avants, B., Gee, J.C.: Geodesic estimation for large deformation anatomical shape averaging and interpolation. NeuroImage **Supplement 1** (2004) S139–S150
8. Bhatia, K.K., Hajnal, J.V., Puri, B.K., Edwards, A.D., Ruekert, D.: Consistent groupwise non-rigid registration for atlas construction. In: Proceedings of IEEE International Symposium on Biomedical Imaging (ISBI). (2004) 908–911
9. Guimond, A., Meunier, J., Thirion, J.P.: Average brain models: a convergence study. Computer Vision and Image Understanding **77** (2000) 192–210
10. Joshi, S., Miller, M.I.: Landmark matching via large deformation diffeomorphisms. IEEE Transactions on Image Processing (TIP) **9** (2000) 1357–1370
11. Joshi, S., Davis, B., Jomier, M., Gerig, G.: Unbiased diffeomorphic atlas construction for computational anatomy. NeuroImage: Supplement issue on Mathematics in Brain Imaging **23** (2004) S151–S160
12. Fréchet, M.: Les elements aleatoires de nature quelconque dans un espace distancie. Annales De L'Institut Henri Poincare **10** (1948) 215–310
13. Beg, M.F.: Variational and Computational Methods for Flows of Diffeomorphisms in Image Matching and Growth in Computational Anatomy. PhD thesis, The Johns Hopkins University (2003)
14. Guillemaud, R., Brady, M.: Estimating the bias field of MR images. IEEE Transactions on Medical Imaging (TMI) **16** (1997) 878–886
15. Atkinson, D., Hill, D.L.G., Stoyle, P.N.R., Summers, P.E., Keevil, S.F.: Automatic correction of motion artifacts in magnetic resonance images using an entropy focus criterion. IEEE Transactions on Medical Imaging (TMI) **16** (1997) 903–910
16. Twining, C., Marsland, S., Taylor, C.: Measuring geodesic distances on the space of bounded diffeomorphisms. In: Proceedings of the British Machine Vision Conference (BMVC), BVMA Press (2002) 847–856
17. Cover, T., Thomas, J.: Elements of Information Theory. John Wiley and Sons, Inc., New York (1991)

Least Biased Target Selection in Probabilistic Atlas Construction

Hyunjin Park[1], Peyton H. Bland[1], Alfred O. Hero III[2], and Charles R. Meyer[1]

[1]Department of Radiology, University of Michigan, Ann Arbor, MI, USA
{hyunjinp, bland, hero, cmeyer}@umich.edu
[2]Department of Electric Engineering and Computer Science,
University of Michigan, Ann Arbor, MI, USA

Abstract. Probabilistic atlas has broad applications in medical image segmentation and registration. The most common problem building a probabilistic atlas is picking a target image upon which to map the rest of the training images. Here we present a method to choose a target image that is the closest to the mean geometry of the population under consideration as determined by bending energy. Our approach is based on forming a distance matrix based on bending energies of all pair-wise registrations and performing multidimensional scaling (MDS) on the distance matrix.

1 Introduction

The probabilistic atlas has been widely used to bring useful prior information to segmentation and registration tasks of human organs, especially for brain. In the segmentation task, atlas information may be used as prior information in the Bayesian formulation [1]. Atlas information guides segmentation algorithms where there is little grayscale value information available.

A common approach to building an atlas is to first pick a target image and map other images onto that target so that statistical processing can be done in the same spatial frame. Methods for registration (i.e., mapping) in terms of degrees of freedom (DOF) and geometric interpolant have to be the same for all registration tasks to ensure consistent construction and use of the atlas. The resulting atlas is inherently biased towards the chosen target image. If the target image happens to be an extreme case of the population, then the atlas created does not reflect the population correctly. In that case, bringing an arbitrary image to the atlas space, i.e., registering a test image onto the atlas, maybe difficult since the geometric distance the test image has to travel to reach the atlas has been increased compared to the case of reaching an atlas which resides at the mean geometry of the population. The whole process of mapping other images onto the target may be repeated with the target replaced with an average image from the previous registrations until the average image converges [2]. In this case, the bias towards the initially picked target image may be reduced.

Studholme et al. proposed a method to jointly register all images simultaneously to a target space that is very close to the mean geometry to reduce the bias of the target space [3]. It employs a cost function encouraging mean displacement field from the target onto other images to be zero while minimizing the joint entropy of all images.

J. Duncan and G. Gerig (Eds.): MICCAI 2005, LNCS 3750, pp. 419–426, 2005.

All displacement fields to other images have to be known to compute the mean displacement field, thus the method requires registration of all images simultaneously increasing the optimization space tremendously. There are nontrivial issues in how to compute the high dimensional probability density function needed to evaluate the joint entropy. Joshi et al. used an atlas construction independent of choosing a specific target image [4]. They first construct an atlas by mapping other images onto a target image and performing statistical processing. After the atlas is constructed on the target image space, the atlas is warped onto a space where there is less bias towards the rest of the images. As a result they can choose any target image and arrive at the same atlas space since the atlas calculated on a specific target image space is always going to be warped onto another space where there is less bias. The above approach needs to satisfy certain constraints that will be discussed in section 4. Marsland et al. proposed to construct the atlas on a target image that is the closest to the mean geometry [10]. They choose the target image such that sum of distances from the target image to the rest of the images is minimized. Our work shares a similar approach to Marsland's paper. Improvements resulting from using our approach will be discussed.

Here we present a method to choose a target image that is the closest to the mean geometry. We acknowledge the existing work on unbiased atlas construction and provide an alternative method based on novel statistical machinery. Our approach is based on forming a distance matrix based on bending energies of all pair-wise registrations and using multidimensional scaling (MDS) on the distance matrix to find the closest target.

2 Methods

In this paper we choose the most common atlas construction method, mapping other images onto a chosen target image and performing statistical processing on the target image space. Our contribution is how to choose a target image that is the least biased considering all the other images.

2.1 Pair-Wise Registration

The task of mapping one image onto the other image is carried out by registration. Registration has been well discussed [5]. In short, two main components need to be determined for any registration method: the similarity measure which measures degree of alignment between images, and the geometric interpolant which defines the geometric transform. We choose mutual information (MI) as the similarity measure and thin-plate splines (TPS) as the geometric interpolant [6]. A simple histogram with fixed bin width is used to calculate the probability mass function of grayscale value distributions to compute MI. The process of registration can be formulated as maximizing the chosen similarity measure (i.e., MI) under a hypothetical geometric transform.

2.2 Distance Measure

Registration between two images yields a geometric transform optimized to maximize a certain cost function (e.g., MI). The geometric distance, hereafter called distance, between two images is often measured by the roughness of the geometric transform. In addition, having zero distance for a simple affine transform is desirable. We define distance between two images as the sum of squared second partial derivatives of the geometric transform,

$$d^2 = \iint (\frac{\partial^2 f_x}{\partial x^2})^2 + 2(\frac{\partial^2 f_x}{\partial x \partial y})^2 + (\frac{\partial^2 f_x}{\partial y^2})^2 + (\frac{\partial^2 f_y}{\partial x^2})^2 + 2(\frac{\partial^2 f_y}{\partial x \partial y})^2 + (\frac{\partial^2 f_y}{\partial y^2})^2 dxdy \tag{1}$$

f_x; displacement in x f_y;displacement in y.

Above formulation is for 2D and can be easily extended for 3D. This distance is often called the bending energy. Analytic formula for calculating bending energy is available for TPS [7]. For other geometric transforms, the bending energy may need to be calculated numerically. The defined distance is not strictly a metric since the distance between two different images can be zero if the two images can be registered by an affine transform.

2.3 Multidimensional Scaling (MDS)

Multidimensional scaling (MDS) is a technique to produce relative positional locations from a collection of pair-wise distances [8]. For example, given pair-wise Euclidean distances between North American cities, MDS will yield a map of relative locations (i.e., up to an arbitrary rotate-translate transform) of those cities. For N cities, N(N-1)/2 (i.e., N choose 2) pair-wise distances are needed. The distances used in MDS need not be metric; non-metric distances (e.g., ranking) can be used. Thus, our distance defined in section 2.2 is valid in MDS settings. Given a set of distances in the distance matrix D, whose element d_{ij} refers to the distance between objects i and j, MDS outputs a set of coordinates in a user specified dimension that reproduces the distance matrix best in the least square fashion. The dimension of MDS output should be based on the eigen structure of the distance matrix. The output coordinates are in the standard Euclidean space of the user supplied dimension.

2.4 Target Selection Based on MDS

An ideal target image is the one that resides at the mean geometry of the population. For the ideal target image, the sum of distances to other images from the atlas space (i.e., target space) is minimized. For a target image space that is far away from the mean geometry, the sum of distances to other images will be greater. Often there may not be an image at the mean geometry thus the best approach in picking a target image, which yields the minimum distance to other images, is to choose the image that is the closest to the mean geometry. The described approach works only if we know all the relative locations of images of the population. MDS identifies all the relative locations of the images from the distance matrix. Here the elements of the distance matrix are determined by the distances of pair-wise registrations. In summary, we select the target image which is the closest to the mean geometry with the aid of information of relative locations provided by MDS. MDS in turn requires a distance matrix whose elements are calculated from pair-wise registrations. The following is the procedure for N images,

```
1. Perform N(N-1)/2 pair-wise registrations
2. Calculate bending energies from the registrations
3. Form distance matrix D
4. Apply MDS and find relative locations of images
5. Calculate mean location of the images
6. Choose target image that is the closest to the mean.
```

Once the best (i.e., least biased) target is selected, all other images can be mapped on to the chosen target, this is trivial since all pair-wise registrations have been computed previously to fill the distance matrix.

2.5 Distance Matrix

The distance matrix is either symmetric or asymmetric. For a symmetric distance matrix, distance between object i and j is order independent. In atlas construction, it implies that the distance between image i as the reference image and image j as the floating image is the same as the distance between images i and j switching the role of the reference image and the floating image. In practice with TPS based registrations, switching the order of images in the registration task may yield a different geometric transform thus it may yield a different distance value, but the discrepancy in distance value is quite small provided that the degrees of freedom (DOF) of TPS is high enough. Christensen et al. proposed a registration method where both forward and inverse transform are estimated such that switching the order of reference and floating images has little effect [11]. In this case, symmetric distance matrix is ensured. Even for an asymmetric distance matrix, distance matrix can be made symmetric by using the average value of d_{ij} and d_{ji}. Here we assume a symmetric distance matrix thus we only calculate upper half of the distance matrix and replicate the lower half. The diagonal elements of the distance matrix are zero by definition.

3 Experiments

Synthetic experiments are carried out in 2D to show the feasibility of our approach. A synthetic MRI slice, 256x256 dimension and 1x1 mm^2 resolution, is obtained from BRAINWEB simulation [9]. It is deformed in a known way using a 6x6 grid of B-splines resulting in 50 deformed images. Deformations are applied by randomly choosing a knot and displacing the knot by the amount determined by zero mean Gaussian of variance 100 pixels in both x and y direction. After the image's geometry is deformed, a zero mean Gaussian noise of variance 16 is added to the image's grayscale values. Six images of the known 50 deformed images are shown in Figure 1. The atlas is constructed with these 50 deformed images. Geometric distances from the original undeformed image (i.e., BRAINWEB slice) to all 50 images are calculated given all the known synthetic deformations and are shown in Table 1. With these distances, ground truth on what is the best target image can be established. The best target image is the image that is the closest to the original image (i.e., the least distance from the original image). In addition, the quality of all potential target images can be rank ordered according to the distance from the original image.

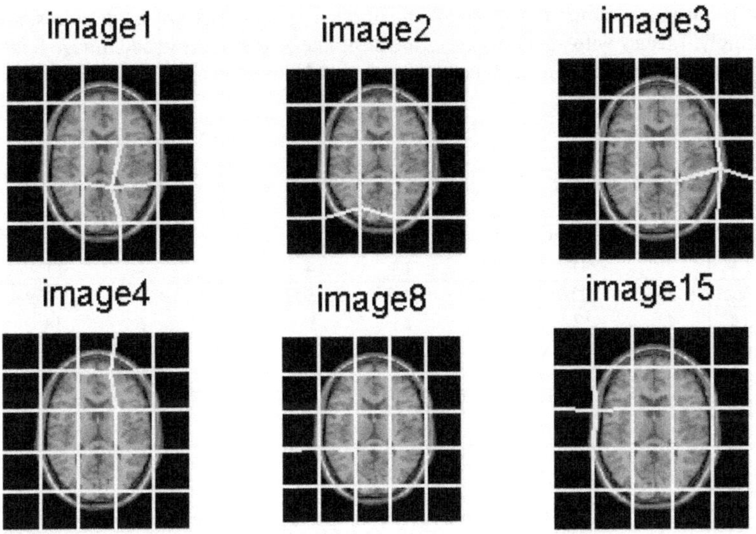

Fig. 1. Six images of the known 50 deformed images. Grid lines show the applied B-spline deformations. Image 8 and 15 have very small deformations compared to other images shown.

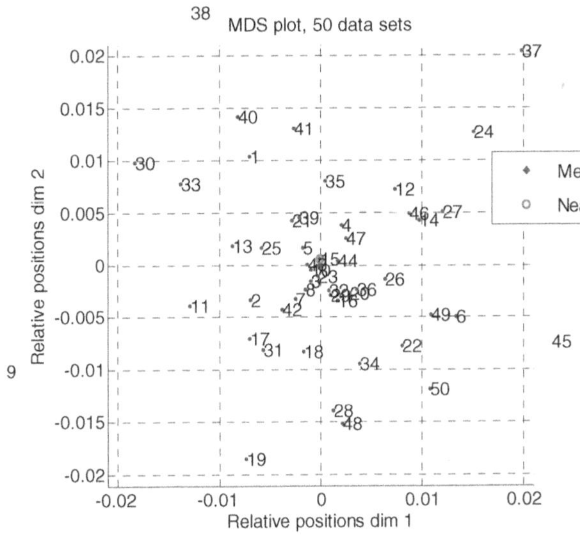

Fig. 2. Relative locations of 50 images by MDS. Mean location is at (0,0,0,0) and the closest image to mean is determined to be image 15. Only a 2 dimensional plot (out of 4) is given here for space constraints. Mean is marked with '+' and the nearest image to the mean is marked with 'o'.

Pair-wise registrations of the 50 images are performed using 25 uniformly spread control points. There are 1225 (i.e., 50 choose 2) pair-wise registrations required to fill up the symmetric 50x50 distance matrix. MDS is performed with 4 dimensions.

Table 1. Distances from the original undeformed image. Geometric distances are sorted ascendingly. Images with small distances are desirable as the target image. Image 8 is the most desirable target image and image 9 is the least desirable target image.

Distance	0.0046	0.0055	0.0121	0.0152	0.0203	0.0209	0.0251	0.0321	0.0325
Image #	8	10	29	15	32	44	5	36	47
Distance	0.0363	0.0598	0.0601	0.0777	0.0900	0.1170	0.1276	0.1350	0.1381
Image #	16	20	43	4	21	46	42	35	17
Distance	0.1409	0.1483	0.1499	0.2146	0.2182	0.2279	0.2288	0.2322	0.2416
Image #	26	18	31	13	14	1	34	11	49
Distance	0.2532	0.2581	0.2592	0.2785	0.2802	0.2881	0.2909	0.3289	0.3454
Image #	41	2	7	23	3	25	6	48	27
Distance	0.3611	0.3660	0.3734	0.3860	0.4176	0.4704	0.4805	0.5009	0.5158
Image #	40	19	50	12	39	24	22	28	33
Distance	0.5802	0.7047	0.8666	1.0827	1.3786				
Image #	45	30	37	38	9				

Table 2. MDS results. Image number is sorted by the distance from the location of mean geometry. Distances are sorted ascendingly. The order of image number is very similar to the order of image number in Table 1. RMS (root mean squared) error between the order of images by MDS and order of images of the ground truth is computed on the bottom row.

Order	1	2	3	4	5	6	7	8	9
Image #	15	8	5	32	44	29	10	43	47
Order	10	11	12	13	14	15	16	17	18
Image #	36	16	4	20	21	26	42	35	46
Order	19	20	21	22	23	24	25	26	27
Image #	18	17	34	1	31	14	7	3	2
Order	28	29	30	31	32	33	34	35	36
Image #	13	25	11	49	23	41	27	6	12
Order	37	38	39	40	41	42	43	44	45
Image #	40	50	19	48	33	39	28	24	22
Order	46	47	48	49	50	Error			
Image #	45	30	38	37	9	0.3970			

The dimension is determined by observing the eigenvalue trend (i.e., abrupt drop in eigenvalues) of the distance matrix. Output of the MDS is 50 coordinates in 4 dimensions representing the 50 images in the Euclidean space. Two dimensional projections of these coordinates are shown in Figure 2. The location of mean geometry is calculated by taking the arithmetic mean of 50 coordinates, which is set to be the origin (i.e., (0,0,0,0)). The image whose coordinate is the closest to the mean geometry is chosen to be the best target image. Distances from the mean geometry (i.e., origin) to the images (i.e., MDS coordinates) are sorted in Table 2 starting from the closest image to the furthest image. The best target image (i.e., the first image in Table 2) is image 15 while the ground truth (i.e., Table 1) indicates image 8 to be the best target. Image 8 and 15 have bending energies 0.0046 and 0.0152 respectively according to Table 1. The difference of bending energies between image 8 and 15,

0.0106, is relatively small compared to the possible variation of bending energies from 0.0046 to 1.3786 (i.e., bending energies of image 8 and 9). Thus our selected target is reasonably close to the mean geometry if not the closest target. Moreover comparison of order of images in Table 1 and 2 indicates that MDS results, order of images in Table 2, are very similar to the ground truth's order of images in Table 1. We are able to replicate the order of images reasonably well from MDS results, not just the closest image to the mean geometry. In fact, the root mean squared error between the rank orders of images of Tables 1 and 2 is computed to be 0.3970. MDS coordinates are tested for multi-variate normal distribution and satisfy 4 dimensional normality test with p = 1 and alpha = 0.05. It implies that the origin (i.e., (0,0,0,0)) represents the undeformed image and that the distribution is not skewed.

4 Discussions and Summary

Our target selection method based on MDS enables us to choose a target that is very close to the mean geometry. One potential reason for not arriving at the closest target may come from inaccuracies in the pair-wise registration processes. If the registration process is not accurate, then the distance matrix contains inaccurate elements. Thus, MDS results may be affected. Our approach is independent of the choice of the pair-wise registration methods. User can choose any reasonable combination of similarity measure and geometric interpolant, not just MI and Thin-plate splines. Relative locations of the images can be found as well as the closest image from the mean geometry.

Our method is potentially faster than the iterative atlas construction method if the iterative method needs many iterations (i.e., at least N/2 iterations) to converge [2]. Our approach requires N(N-1)/2 pair-wise registrations and the iterative construction method requires (N-1)x(# of iterations) pair-wise registrations for N images. Joshi's approach requires only N-1 pair-wise registrations and is independent of choosing a target image [4]. It assumes that the geometric transform has certain "small deformation" properties and is sensitive to pair-wise registration results requiring displacement fields to be accurate (i.e., almost no registration error). Our approach and Marsland's approach share a common theme, i.e., finding a target image that is the closest to the mean geometry [10]. Their method tries to minimize not only the sum of distances to all other image but also the sum of similarity measure between the target and other images. They start with an initial guess of the target image and try to update the target image if the sum of distances decreases and the sum of MI increases. We believe target should be chosen solely on distances. For example, if the ideal target image at the mean geometry happens to be noisy, under Marsland's approach it will never be selected as the target since choosing the ideal target will surely decrease the sum of MI. Their method is tied to a specific geometric interpolant, clamped-plate spline, while our approach can be applied to any geometric interpolant.

We have shown a method to choose the target image that is very close to the mean geometry. It is based on information of relative locations provided by MDS. MDS requires a distance matrix whose elements are calculated from pair-wise registrations.

Acknowledgements. This work is supported by the NIH grant 1P01CA87634.

References

1. H. Park, P. H. Bland, and C. R. Meyer, "Construction of an abdominal probabilistic atlas and its application in segmentation," *IEEE Trans. Med. Imaging.*, vol. 22, pp. 483-492, 2003.
2. W. Toga and P. M. Thompson, "The role of image registration in brain mapping," *Image and Vision Computing*, vol. 19, pp. 3-24, 2001.
3. C. Studholme and V. Cardenas, "A template free approach to volumetric spatial normalization of brain anatomy," *Pattern Recognition Letters*, vol. 25, pp. 1191-1202, 2004.
4. S. Joshi, B. Davis, M. Jomier, and G. Gerig, "Unbiased diffeomorphic atlas construction for computational anatomy," *NueroImage*, vol. 23, pp. s151-s160, 2004.
5. D. L. G. Hill, P. G. Batchelor, M. Holden, and D. J. Hawkes, "Medical image registration," *Physics in Medicine and Biology*, vol. 46, pp. r1-r45, 2001.
6. C. Meyer, J. Boes, P. Bland, K. Zasandy, P. Kison, K. Koral, K. Frey, and R. Wahl, "Demonstration of accuracy and clinical versatility of mutual information for automatic multimodality image fusion using affine and thin plate spline warped geometric deformations," *Medical Image Analysis*, vol. 3, pp. 195-206, 1997.
7. F. L. Bookstein, "Principal warps: thin-plate splines and the decomposition of deformations," *IEEE Trans. Pattern Anal. Mach. Intell.*, vol. 11, pp. 567-585, 1989.
8. F. W. Young and R. M. Hamer, *Theory and application of Multidimensional sclaing*: Eribaum Associates, 1994.
9. D. L. Collins, A. P. Zijdenbos, A. P. Kollokian, J. G. Sled, N. J. Kabani, C. J. Holmes, and A. C. Evans, "Design and Construction of a Realistic Digital Brain Phantom," *IEEE Trans. Med. Imaging*, vol. 17, pp. 463-468, 1998.
10. S. Marsland, C. J. Twining, and C. J. Taylor, "Groupwise non-rigid registration using polyharmonic clamped-plate splines," in MICCAI 2003, *LNCS*, vol. 2879, p.771-779, 2003.
11. G. E. Christensen and H. J. Johnson, "Consistent image registration," *IEEE Trans. Med. Imaging.*, vol. 20, pp. 568-582, 2001.

Automatic Selection of DBS Target Points Using Multiple Electrophysiological Atlases

Pierre-Francois D'Haese [1,2], Srivatsan Pallavaram[1], Ken Niermann[4], John Spooner[3], Chris Kao[3,5], Peter E. Konrad[3], and Benoit M. Dawant[1]

[1] Department of Electrical Engineering and Computer Science, Vanderbilt University, Nashville, TN, USA
[2] Université Catholique de Louvain, Louvain-la-Neuve, Belgique
[3] Departments of Neurosurgery, Vanderbilt Medical Center, Nashville, TN, USA
[4] Departments of Radiology, Vanderbilt Medical Center, Nashville, TN, USA
[5] Sentient Medical Systems, Cockeysville, MD 21030

Abstract. In this paper we study and evaluate the influence of the choice of a particular reference volume as the electrophysiological atlas on the accuracy of the automatic predictions of optimal points for deep brain stimulator (DBS) implants. We refer to an electrophysiological atlas as a spatial map of electrophysiological information such as micro electrode recordings (MER), stimulation parameters, final implants positions, etc., which are acquired for each patient and then mapped onto a single reference volume using registration algorithms. An atlas-based prediction of the optimal point for a DBS surgery is made by registering a patient's image volume to that reference volume, that is, by computing a correct coordinate mapping between the two; and then by projecting the optimal point from the atlas to the patient using the transformation from the registration algorithm. Different atlases, as well as different parameterizations of the registration algorithm, lead to different and somewhat independent atlas-based predictions. We show how the use of multiple reference volumes can improve the accuracy of prediction by combining the predictions from the multiple reference volumes weighted by the accuracy of the non-rigid registration between each of the corresponding atlases and the patient volume.

1 Introduction

Deep brain stimulation is a way to stimulate parts of the brain that cause movement disorders like Parkinson's disease, in order to minimize or eliminate disease symptoms without damaging the brain. This is done by placing electrodes in specific nuclei of the brain and stimulating them with electrical impulses. Such functional neurosurgical procedures of targeting small areas deep in the brain require precise targeting. Traditionally, this is done in two steps. An approximate target location is first selected pre-operatively. The target position is then adjusted intra-operatively. Manual localization of the target is achieved pre-operatively by registering an anatomic atlas such as the Schatelbrand-Wahren atlas to a pre-operative MR scan of the patient. This step is required because the precise boundaries of structures of interest in DBS surgeries are either not or poorly visible in the pre-operative MR scans. The anatomic information afforded by the atlas is thus used as a guide. Intra-operative adjustment is based

J. Duncan and G. Gerig (Eds.): MICCAI 2005, LNCS 3750, pp. 427 – 434, 2005.

on microelectrode recordings (MER) obtained by passing a recording electrode in the brain towards the pre-operatively planned target and on patient's response to stimulation as a stimulating electrode moves towards the planned target. Stimulation is provided by applying electrical impulses and the responses to such stimulation include improvement in disease symptoms, occurrences of side effects, etc. Intra-operative adjustment is necessary because of known limitations of available anatomical atlases (e.g. hemispheres that pertain to different subjects, discontinuities between slices, etc.), limited accuracy achievable when registering an MR volume to these atlases, and because available atlases provide only anatomic information while the position of the final target point is chosen based on the electrophysiology. To address these issues and to simplify the procedure, we created a three dimensional electrophysiological atlas that can be used for pre-operative planning and intra-operative guidance [2, 3].

Over the last several years we have also developed fully automatic 3D non-rigid registration algorithms that allow us to register accurately 3D MR brain volumes to each other and we use these algorithms to develop our atlas. In the operating room, we acquire MER signals, information about stimuli (in volts), response(s) to these stimuli, and the positions at which these data are recorded. We acquire these positions in CT coordinates via the stereotactic system used for the procedure (StarFix micro-Targeting Platform®, FHC Inc., Bowdoinham, ME). Using our registration algorithms, we then map the positions at which intra-operative information is gathered from each patient onto the corresponding positions in one MR volume chosen as a reference. This reference volume is referred to as the atlas. In this way all the intra-operative information gathered from the patients can be mapped onto the atlas for future use. The atlas thus becomes a repository that allows us to store information acquired from any number of patients in a normalized space.

Rohlfing et al. have shown that the choice of the atlas has a substantial influence on the quality of registration-based segmentation [4, 5]. Moreover, they demonstrated that by using multiple atlases, the segmentation accuracy could be improved over that obtained using a single atlas. Here, we investigate the effect of the atlas on the accuracy of our approach to predict the position of DBS targets. We also investigate a method by which using a combination of the atlases leads to improvement in accuracy of automatic prediction.

2 Data Set

With IRB approval (Vanderbilt University IRB # 010809) a set of CT and MRI pre-operative scans and a CT post-operative scan is acquired for each patient. CT and MR volumes are acquired with the patient anesthetized and head taped to the table to minimize motion. Typical CT images are acquired at kvp = 120 V, exposure = 350 mas, 512x512 pixels. In-plane resolution ranges from 0.49 to 0.62 mm, and slice thickness from 1 mm to 2 mm. MR images are 3D SPGR volumes, TR: 12.2 ms, TE: 2.4 ms, dimension 256x256x124 voxels; voxels dimensions are typically 0.85x0.85x1.3 mm^3. Fourteen patients who underwent STN (subthalamic nucleus) stimulation were used in the study presented herein. The patients were treated over a period ranging from December of 2003 to April of 2005. Patients included in this study are different from the ones used in our earlier work [2, 3]. Therefore, although results are qualitatively similar, quantitative comparison between results presented in this work and those presented earlier is not meaningful.

3 Method and Results

Four volumes were manually selected as reference volumes (atlases) based on their morphological characteristics. These volumes were not from the test set of 14 patients used in this study. They were of earlier DBS patients. They were selected to have a variety in the sizes and symmetry/asymmetry of the ventricles. Because the nuclei of interest in this study are either not or poorly visible in current image acquisition sequences, registration is driven by the surrounding structures such as the ventricles, the thalamus, or the putamen, which are visible. The size and shape of the ventricles and more particularly the size of the third ventricles were chosen as the criteria for the selection of the atlases.

3.1 Registration Algorithms

Two types of registrations algorithms are needed to process our data: rigid and non-rigid. The rigid registration algorithm is required to register MR and CT volumes of the same patient. The algorithm we have used for this is an independent implementation of a standard MI-based algorithm [10]. Non-rigid registration is required to register patient data to an atlas and vice-versa. In this study, non-rigid registration is always performed on MR image volumes using an algorithm we proposed recently [1].

3.2 Influence of the Choice of the Atlas on the Prediction Accuracy

In this work, we used the method that we described in [2, 3] to create an electrophysiological atlas based on the final positions of the implants. Because we now use four atlases, the process is repeated four times. Briefly, for each case we registered the MR patient volume to each the four atlases using the registration algorithms described in section 3.1. The registration parameters used for registration onto each of the four atlases were kept the same. We then projected final implant positions from each of the patients onto the four atlases, thus creating two clouds of points (one for the left and the other for the right STN) on each of the atlases. Figure 1 shows the results we have obtained for the left STN. Similar clusters were obtained for the right STN. To provide the reader with a better sense for the locations and spreads of the clusters we have superimposed contours obtained from the Schaltenbrand-Wharen (SBW) [9] atlas onto the MR images (the four atlases). Registration between each of the four atlases and the SBW atlas was performed based on a piecewise affine transformation using the Voxim software (IVS Solutions, AG, Chemnitz, Germany). This is known to be a difficult and inaccurate process. Thus, contour lines shown on the images in figure 1 may not exactly correspond to the true boundaries of the structures. The structure surrounding the core of each cluster is the STN. The structure above the STN is the thalamus with all its sub-nuclei; the structure below the STN is the substantia nigra (SNr).

To quantify the spread of the cluster in each atlas, we have computed the Euclidian distance from the points in each cluster to their corresponding centroid. Table 1 reports this average distance (Dc) for each of the atlases for the left and the right sides. It can be seen from table 1 that atlas0 is the best in terms of the tightness of the clusters.

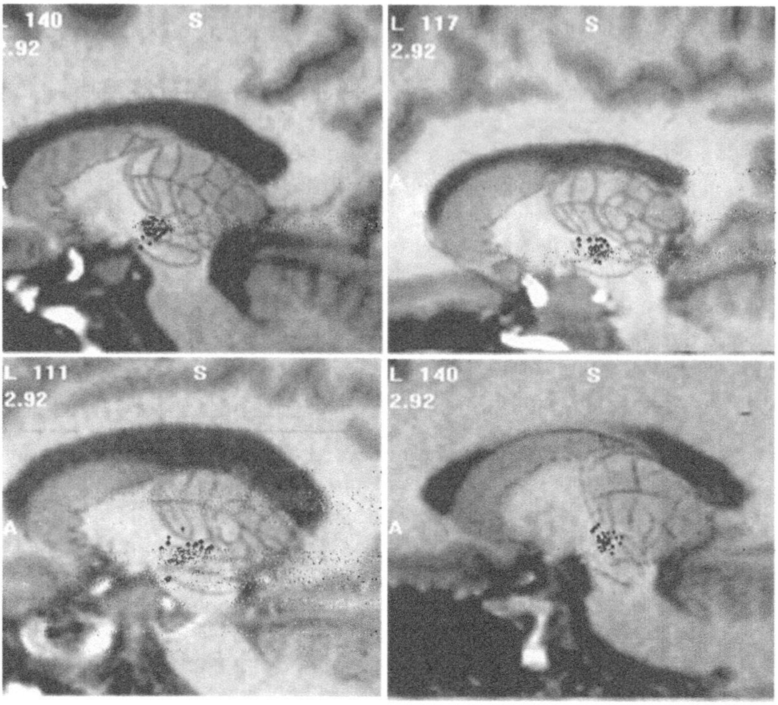

Fig. 1. Sagittal views of the right clusters on the 4 atlases (atlas 0 top left, atlas 1 bottom left, atlas 2 top right, atlas 3 bottom right). Contours extracted from the Shaltenbrand-Wahren atlas have been superimposed on the images to show the location and extent of the projected clusters with respect to anatomic structures seen in the SBW atlas.

Table 1. Euclidian distance (mm) of cluster points with respect to the corresponding cluster centroid on each of the atlases (Dc)

Atlas	RMS spread left side (mm)	RMS spread right side (mm)	Tightness ranking of atlases
0	2.01	2.05	1
1	3.19	4.35	4
2	3.06	3.11	3
3	2.42	2.71	2

The tightness of the cluster depends on the quality of the non-rigid registration between each of the atlases and the patient volume, which depends in large parts on the morphological similarity between the volumes being registered. A single patient volume will be registered with a higher accuracy on the most similar atlas. To study the effect of the choice of the atlas on the prediction of the optimal position for the placement of the implant we selected the centroids of the clusters in each of these atlases as the optimal implant positions in the corresponding atlases. These points were then projected using the transformations computed with the registration algorithms back onto each of the patients. On each of the patients this projection resulted in four possible optimal positions for the implant, each related to one of the atlases. To quantify the effect of the atlas on target prediction accuracy, we computed what we call the pre-operative placement error. This error is defined as the Euclidean distance between the final intra-operative position selected by the surgical team and the position chosen pre-operatively. It is thus the distance by which the surgical team would need to adjust the position of the electrode during the procedure. Table 2 shows the mean and standard deviation of this error for both automatic (atlas based) and manual predictions, over the 14 volumes included in this study. Columns titled *Atlas0, Atlas1, Atlas2 and Atlas3* correspond to the distances between the automatically predicted points using the corresponding atlases and the final (intra-operative) implant position, averaged over all the patients. The column titled *Centroid* represents the deviation between the centroid of the four predictions and the final implant position, averaged over all the patients. The column titled *Manual* represents the deviation between the target predicted pre-operatively by the surgeon and the final implant position, averaged over all the patients. Table 2 shows that the choice of atlas has a direct impact on the accuracy of prediction of optimal position of implant. In earlier work, we have shown that pre-operative target points obtained automatically were closer to the corresponding final points than the pre-operative target points obtained manually. This remains true in the results shown in table 2. Moreover, what table 2 shows is that the pre-operative placement error could be reduced substantially if we could select automatically the best atlas for the case at hand, thus incurring minimum prediction error. We cannot, of course, use the pre-operative placement error as a criterion to select this atlas since the intra-operative position is not known at the time of planning. In the next section, we describe a method we propose to select the best atlas (or an optimal combination of the atlases) for a given patient.

Table 2. Prediction errors incurred for atlas based predictions using individual atlases, centroids of atlas based predictions, sensitivities of individual structures based predictions, sensitivities of combination of structures based predictions and manual selection of targets. SD: Standard Deviation, T: Thalamus, TV: Third Ventricle, P: Putamen.

Side	Statistic	Deviation from final implant (mm)									
		Using individual atlases				Using combination of multiple atlases					Manual
						Centroid	Sensitivities weighted				
		Atlas0	Atlas1	Atlas2	Atlas3		T	TV	P	T+TV	
Left	Mean	2.01	1.99	1.72	1.9	1.8	1.8	1.71	1.93	1.66	2.23
	SD	0.85	0.94	1.11	0.99	0.93	0.93	0.89	0.85	0.92	1.17
Right	Mean	1.92	2.21	2.13	2.09	1.97	1.87	1.98	2.34	1.74	2.5
	SD	0.69	1	0.97	0.99	0.83	0.8	0.87	0.85	0.74	1.41

3.3 Multiple Atlases Based Prediction

The easiest way to combine the predictions is to compute the centroid of the four predicted points and use it as the best automatic prediction. Prediction accuracy using the centroid of the cluster is substantially better than that based on manual predictions as can be seen in table 2. However, it is still not as good as that achievable using the best atlas for every patient. For instance, it was found that for the left side, using the best atlas for each of the 14 patients the pre-operative error was 1.46 mm averaged over the patients, while the same based on the centroid of the cluster was 1.8 mm and that based on manual predictions was 2.23 mm. To select one atlas (or perhaps a subset of atlases) for a particular case, we need to find a way to estimate the likelihood that the atlas is more accurately registered to the patient than any other atlas. We achieve this through atlas-based segmentation of structures surrounding the target of interest. As discussed above, the STN is poorly visible in MR images. But surrounding structures such as the ventricles, the thalamus and/or the putamen can bee seen and have relatively well defined boundaries. To take advantage of this, the major basal ganglia structures (the putamen, the thalamus, the ventricles, the third ventricle, the red nuclei and the globus pallidus) were manually segmented on each of the four reference volumes by an expert. These segmented structures were projected from the four atlases onto the patients, resulting in four different segmentations for each structure on every patient. These contours were then used to estimate the specificity and sensitivity of each of the four segmentations for every structure using the STAPLE algorithm proposed by Warfield et al. [7, 8]. The computed sensitivity parameters were used, in turn, to weigh the contributions of the atlases to the prediction. We used a simple weighted average of the predictions made by the four atlases to arrive at the final automatic prediction.

The weights are the sensitivities of the segmented structures for the four atlases. Sensitivities below 95% of the highest sensitivity were set to zero. Let *P0*, *P1*, *P2* and *P3* be the predictions based on atlases *0*, *1*, *2* and *3* respectively and sensitivity be denoted by *p*. Let the sensitivity for the left thalamus of the patient with respect to *atlas0* be *p_thal_left_0*, that for the right thalamus with respect to atlas0 be *p_thal_right_0* and that for the third ventricles with respect to atlas0 be *p_third_ventricles_0*. A similar nomenclature for sensitivities with respect to atlases 1, 2 and 3 is used. Now, the average sensitivity of the structures on the patient volume with respect to *atlas0* is given by

$$SEN_0 = \frac{p\_thal\_left\_0 + p\_thal\_right\_0 + p\_third\_ventricles\_0}{3}$$

Similarly, SEN_1, SEN_2 and SEN_3 are computed. Next we define the set of indices IND such as

$$\text{IND} = \left\{ \text{k} \,\middle|\, \text{SEN}_\text{k} \geq 0.95 * \max(\text{SEN}_0, \text{SEN}_1, \text{SEN}_2, \text{SEN}_3) \right\}.$$

Then, the final prediction is given by,

$$P = \frac{\sum_{k \in IND} SEN_k \,.\, P_k}{\sum_{i \in IND} SEN_i}$$

In doing this, we eliminate the contributions of atlases that produce low sensitivity values for the structures, i.e., atlases that lead to poor segmentation results for structures surrounding the structure of interest. Table 2 also shows the prediction error when the sensitivities of the thalamus, the third ventricle, and the putamen are individually used. These results show that, though predictions based on sensitivities of a surrounding structure are better than manual predictions, the use of sensitivities of the putamen has shown to increase the error compared to the use of the centroid. Similarly, it can be seen that the use of sensitivities of the thalamus improves the accuracy of prediction for the right side, while the use of third ventricles improves the accuracy of prediction for the left side, both compared to the use of centroid. This suggests that combining the sensitivities of the thalamus and of the third ventricles could further improve the results as corroborated in table 2.

4 Discussion and Conclusion

From table 2, it can be seen that, using the sensitivities of the thalamus and the third ventricles together, the pre-operative error for the left side decreased to 1.66 mm compared to 1.8 mm when the centroid of the cluster was used and 2.23 mm when manual prediction was done. Similarly, for the right side, the errors were 1.74 mm, 1.97 mm and 2.5 mm respectively. These results are clinically important because they could improve the quality of DBS surgeries both in terms of accuracy and time.

The quality of segmentations achieved on the patient volume based on each of the atlases is a direct indication of the accuracy with which each of the corresponding atlases has been non-rigidly registered to the patient volume. Since the segmentations used are from regions around the (poor contrast) STN, our method serves as an approach to assessing the quality of non-rigid registrations in regions of low contrast in a patient volume. In our multi-atlas approach to prediction of optimal points for implants in DBS surgeries, we use the above method of assessing the quality of registrations to determine the contributions of the four atlases to the prediction process. It is conclusive from our results that the use of multiple atlases helps improve the accuracy of automatically predicting optimal positions for DBS implants. This scheme can easily be extended to other targets by changing the visible structures used to evaluate the quality of the registration. For instance, in the prediction of the target points for Globus Pallidus Internus (GPi), the putamen can be expected to play a key role due to its close proximity to GPi.

Acknowledgments

Pierre-François D'Haese is working towards a Ph.D. degree with awards from FRIA and FNRS (Belgian Science Foundation) (also supported by the Walloon Region by the MERCATOR grant). Part of this work has been supported by a Discovery grant from Vanderbilt University.

References

1. Rohde G.K., Aldroubi A., Dawant B.M., "The adaptive bases algorithm for intensity based non-rigid image registration." *IEEE Trans Med Imaging, 2003* Nov; 22(11): 1470-9.
2. Dawant B.M., Li R., Cetinkaya E., Kao C., Fitzpatrick J.M., and Konrad P.E., "Computerized Atlas-Guided Positioning of Deep Brain Stimulators: A Feasibility Study", *J.C. Gee et al. (Eds.): WBIR 2003*, LNCS 2717, pp. 142 –150, 2003.
3. D'Haese P.F., Cetinkaya E., Kao C. , Konrad P.E. and Dawant B.M. "Computer-aided Placement of Deep Brain Stimulators: From Planning to Intra-operative Guidance" *IEEE Trans Med Imaging, Special Issue on Computer Aided Surgery,* 2005 (In Press).
4. T.Rohlfing, C. Maurer, Jr., "Multi-Classifier framework for atlas-based image segmentation", *Proceedings of IEEE Computer Society Conference on Computer Vision and Pattern Recognition, Washington D.C., USA,* June 27-July 2, 2004, pp. 255-260, IEEE Press, 2004.
5. T.Rohlfing, D. B. Russakoff, C. Maurer, Jr., "Performance-based classifier combination in atlas-based image segmentation using Expectation-Maximization parameter estimation", *IEEE Transactions on Medical Imaging*, vol. 23, pp. 983-994, 2004.
6. Ebru Cetinkaya, Pierre-Francois D'Haese, Peter E. Konrad, Chris Kao, and Benoit Dawant. "Method for identifying brain nuclei from micro-electrode signals". *ASSFN* 2004, Cleveland, USA, Oct', 2004.
7. S. K. Warfield, K. H. Zou, W. M. Wells, "Validation of image segmentation and expert quality with an Expectation-Maximization algorithm", Lecture Notes in Computer Science, *MICCAI 2002*, pp. 298-306, 2002.
8. S. K. Warfield, K. H. Zou, W. M. Wells, "Simultaneous Truth and Performance Level Estimation (STAPLE): An algorithm for the validation of image segmentation", *IEEE Transactions on Medical Imaging*, vol. 23, no. 7, pp. 903-921, 2004.
9. G. Schaltenbrand and W. Wahren, "Atlas for Stereotaxy of the Human Brain" Stuttgart, Germany; *Thieme*, 1977.
10. Li R., "Automatic placement of regions of interest in medical images using medical image registration", *Master's thesis*, Vanderbilt University, Dec' 2001.

Nonrigid Shape Correspondence Using Landmark Sliding, Insertion and Deletion

Theodor Richardson and Song Wang

Department of Computer Science and Engineering,
University of South Carolina,
Columbia, SC 29208, USA
{richa268, songwang}@cse.sc.edu

Abstract. The growing usage of statistical shape analysis in medical imaging calls for effective methods for highly accurate shape correspondence. This paper presents a novel landmark-based method to correspond a set of 2D shape instances in a nonrigid fashion. Different from prior methods, the proposed method combines three important factors in measuring the shape-correspondence error: landmark-correspondence error, shape-representation error, and shape-representation compactness. In this method, these three important factors are explicitly handled by the landmark sliding, insertion, and deletion operations, respectively. The proposed method is tested on several sets of structural shape instances extracted from medical images. We also conduct an empirical study to compare the developed method to the popular Minimum Description Length method.

1 Introduction

Most anatomical structures posses a unique shape, which plays a critical role in modern medical image analysis. Statistical shape analysis (SSA) [2,5,8] is a very powerful tool for identifying and representing the underlying shape information of a certain structure. Particulary, SSA can construct a statistical shape model, usually from a set of individual shape instances, to describe the deformation space of the underlying shape. In 2D cases, each shape instance is in the form of a continuous curve. For convenience, we refer to this ground-truth continuous form of a shape instance as a *shape contour*.

Many researchers [6,3] have pointed out that the accuracy of the shape correspondence greatly affects the accuracy of SSA. In addition, most current SSA methods operate on a set of sparsely sampled landmarks along the shape contours. Therefore, our goal of shape correspondence is to find a way to locate a small set of corresponded landmarks along each shape instance. As in most SSA methods, landmarks discussed in this paper refer to a set of sampled points along the shape instances and may not coincide with anatomically critical points.

For the landmark-based shape correspondence, the following three important factors are critical in order to correctly model the shape-correspondence

J. Duncan and G. Gerig (Eds.): MICCAI 2005, LNCS 3750, pp. 435–442, 2005.

error: *landmark-correspondence error*, *representation error*, and *representation compactness*. In general, a small shape-correspondence error implies a small landmark-correspondence error, a small representation error, and a high representation compactness. Landmark-correspondence error should be small because we use it as an approximation of the underlying shape-correspondence error. This is a factor that has been widely considered in most prior shape-correspondence methods [4,1,6]. Small representation error is also important because the above approximation is accurate only when the sampled landmarks well represent the underlying shape contour. High representation compactness means that the landmark sampling should be as sparse as possible, which is desired in most SSA methods. Clearly, small representation error and high representation compactness are contradictory and require a balance.

With a set of roughly-corresponded landmarks, Bookstein [3] presents an algorithm to move these landmarks along the tangent directions of the shape contour to achieve a minimum landmark correspondence error that is defined by the thin-plate bending energy. However, the resultant landmarks may not be located on the underlying shape contour and, therefore, the representation error may be large. Wang, Kubota, and Richardson [11] address this problem by adding a step of projecting the landmarks back to the shape contour. This, however, is still not sufficient to achieve small representation error. Representation compactness is not considered in either of these two methods. Minimum Description Length (MDL) [6] is arguably the state-of-the-art method for landmark-based shape correspondence. The shape-correspondence error in MDL is measured by the required bit-length to transmit these shape instances. Genetic algorithms are usually used to locate the optimal landmarks in MDL. Recent efforts have been made to incorporate the factor of representation error into MDL [10,9].

In this paper, we develop a new method to explicitly consider the three factors listed above. More specifically, the proposed method combines three operations: *landmark sliding*, *landmark insertion*, and *landmark deletion*, which explicitly address the above three factors, respectively.

2 Problem Formulation

In this paper, we consider 2D shape correspondence, i.e., each shape instance is in the form of a shape contour, which can be open or closed. For simplification, we describe the shape-correspondence algorithm based on closed-curve shape instances, which can be easily extended to deal with open-curve shapes. Denote the given set of closed-curve shape instances to be $S = \{S_1, S_2, \ldots, S_n\}$. Each shape instance S_i is in the form of an arc-length parameterized curve $\mathbf{s}_i(t_i) = (x_i(t_i), y_i(t_i))$, $0 \leq t_i \leq L_i$, where L_i is the perimeter of S_i and t_i is the traversed curve length from $\mathbf{s}_i(0)$ to $\mathbf{s}_i(t_i)$. The goal of the landmark-based shape correspondence is to identify the same number m landmarks $\mathbf{s}_i(t_{i1}), \mathbf{s}_i(t_{i2}), \ldots, \mathbf{s}_i(t_{im})$ along each shape instance S_i such that for any k, the n landmarks $\mathbf{s}_i(t_{ik})$, $i = 1, 2, \ldots, n$, are corresponded across these n shape instances. For brevity, we denote $\mathbf{v}_{ik} = \mathbf{s}_i(t_{ik})$ as a landmark and $V_i = \{\mathbf{v}_{i1}, \mathbf{v}_{i2}, \ldots, \mathbf{v}_{im}\}$ to be the sampled landmark set along S_i. For convenience, we further assume that the m landmarks in V_i are sampled sequentially along S_i, as shown in Fig. 1(a).

As mentioned above, we need to define the measures for landmark-correspondence error, representation error, and representation compactness to fully model the underlying shape-correspondence error. For representation compactness, the measure is simply the number of landmarks m, i.e., we desire the number m to be as small as possible. The representation error measures the error of using these m landmarks to represent the underlying shape contour. As shown in Fig. 1(a), let $R(V_i, S_i)$ be the total discrepancy area (shown as dark gray regions) between the underlying shape contour S_i and the polygon formed by sequentially connecting the m landmarks in V_i for shape instance i. We define representation error as

$$\alpha(V_i, S_i) = \frac{R(V_i, S_i)}{R(S_i)},$$

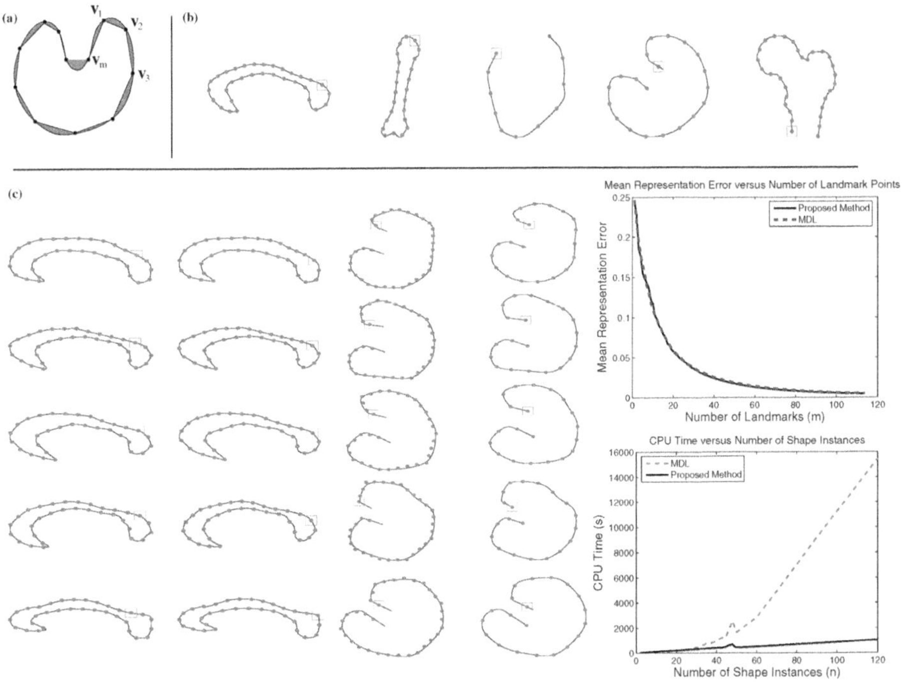

Fig. 1. (a) Illustration of shape representation error, (b) select shape instances from D1 to D5 respectively with landmarks resulting from the proposed method, and (c) selected correspondence results on D1 (corpus callosum) and D4 (kidney) with MDL results on the left and results from the proposed method on the right. See Tables 1 and 2 for statistical results on D1 and D4. Both graphs indicate further experiments in representation error and CPU time on D1.

where $R(S_i)$ indicates the area enclosed by the shape contour S_i. The normalization keeps this measure invariant to the shape size.

Thin-plate models [7] have been widely used for biological shape analysis for its capability of describing nonrigid shape deformations [2]. In this paper, we use the thin-plate bending energy to model the landmark-correspondence error. Specifically, we calculate the mean shape $V_T = \frac{1}{n}\sum_{i=1}^{n} V_i$ as the template and the landmark-correspondence error from V_q is defined as the thin-plate bending energy [7] from V_T to V_q, i.e.,

$$\beta(V_T \rightarrow V_q) = \frac{1}{8\pi}(\mathbf{x}_q^T \mathbf{M}_T \mathbf{x}_q + \mathbf{y}_q^T \mathbf{M}_T \mathbf{y}_q),$$

where $\mathbf{x}_q$ and $\mathbf{y}_q$ are columnized vectors of x- and y-coordinates of landmarks in V_q, and $\mathbf{M}_T$ is the bending matrix calculated from V_T [7]. One important property of the thin-plate bending energy is its invariance to affine transforms. The total landmark-based correspondence error can thus be defined as $\sum_{i=1}^{n} \beta(V_T \rightarrow V_i)$. Since the landmark sets $V_i, i = 1, 2, \ldots, n$ are continually updated in our algorithm, the template shape also needs to update accordingly.

Combining these three factors, we define the shape-correspondence problem as identifying a set of m landmarks V_i from the shape contours S_i, $i = 1, 2, \ldots, n$ such that: (a) $\sum_i \beta(V_T \rightarrow V_i)$ is minimized; (b) $\alpha(V_i, S_i) \leq \epsilon$ for $i = 1, 2, \ldots, n$, where ϵ is a preset allowed representation error; (c) m, the number of landmarks in V_i, is minimized given condition (b) is satisfied. In the next section, we develop an algorithm to achieve these goals.

3 Algorithm

To solve the problem formulated in Section 2, we propose an algorithm that combines three operations: landmark sliding, landmark insertion, and landmark deletion. To start the algorithm, we perform a landmark initialization that aims to find an initial estimate of V_i, $i = 1, 2, \ldots, n$. There are many ways to achieve an initial rough landmark-based correspondence, like those successfully used for shape recognition and retrieval [4,1]. In this paper, we use the initialization method in [11]: uniformly sampling each shape instance into the same number of landmarks and then finding the matching across them by minimizing the thin-plate bending energy.

3.1 Landmark Sliding

In the landmark sliding, we slide the landmarks in V_q along the shape contour S_q so that the landmark-correspondence error with the template landmark set V_T is minimized. The sliding operation consists of two steps: sliding and projection. In the sliding step, all the landmarks in V_q are moved along the tangent directions of S_q so that the resultant landmarks V_q' have the minimal landmark-correspondence error $\beta(V_T \rightarrow V_q')$. Let $\mathbf{r}_{qk}$ be the unit tangent direction at the landmark $\mathbf{v}_{qk}$, then we have

$$\mathbf{v}'_{qk} = \mathbf{v}_{qk} + \gamma_{qk} \cdot \mathbf{r}_{qk} \tag{1}$$

where $\mathbf{v}'_{qk}$ is the k-th landmark after sliding and γ_{qk} is the sliding distance which we want to find. Note that $\mathbf{v}'_{qk}$ is usually not located on the shape contour S_q.

In the projection step, the landmarks $\mathbf{v}'_{qk}$, $k = 1, 2, \ldots, m$ are projected back to S_q to construct a new version of V_q along S_q. This projection is achieved by updating the arc-length parameters for all landmarks:

$$t_{qk}^{(new)} \leftarrow t_{qk} + \gamma_{qk}. \tag{2}$$

One important problem here is to preserve the shape topology, i.e., no landmark is allowed to move across its neighbors along the underlying shape contour. Therefore, we have the constraint on the sliding distance γ_{qk}, $k = 1, 2, \ldots, m$,

$$(t_{q,k+1} - t_{q,k})|L_q - \gamma_{qk} + \gamma_{q,k+1} > 0, k = 1, 2, \ldots, m. \tag{3}$$

The $(m+1)$-th landmark is the same as the first landmark and $a|b$ is the modulus operation; $(t_{q,k+1} - t_{q,k})|L_q$ represents the traversed distance $\mathbf{v}_{q,k}$ to $\mathbf{v}_{q,k+1}$.

From these, we can see that the sliding distance γ_{qk}, $k = 1, 2, \ldots, m$, should minimize the landmark-correspondence error $\beta(V_T \rightarrow V'_q)$, subject to the linear constraints of Eqs. (1) and (3). This is a classical quadratic-programming problem that can be effectively solved.

3.2 Landmark Insertion and Deletion

Both the landmark-initialization and the landmark-sliding operations have no guarantee that the obtained landmark set V_q can represent the shape contour S_q within the allowed representation error ϵ. We address this problem by a landmark-insertion operation: If the shape-representation error $\alpha(V_q, S_q)$ is larger than the allowed threshold ϵ, we simply insert an additional landmark point at $\mathbf{s}_q(0.5 \cdot (t_{qk} + t_{q,k+1}))$, i.e., halfway between $\mathbf{v}_{qk}$ and $\mathbf{v}_{q,k+1}$, which contributes most to the total representation error. To keep the correspondence across shape instances, we insert an additional landmark along each of other shape instances, including the template, i.e., inserting landmark $\mathbf{s}_i(0.5 \cdot (t_{ik} + t_{i,k+1}))$ for each shape S_i. We repeat this landmark-insertion operation until all the shape instances are represented within the allowed error threshold ϵ.

Landmark deletion is the inverse process of landmark insertion that is used to improve the representation compactness and avoid the over-sampling of the shape instances. The basic idea is to delete k-th landmark from all the n shape instances (including the template), if the remaining landmarks can still represent all these n-shape instances within the allowed error threshold ϵ. In practice, we in fact set a larger allowed threshold ϵ_H for landmark insertion and a lower threshold ϵ_L for landmark deletion to reduce oscillation of the iterations and improve algorithm speed. Combining all the operations, the proposed shape-correspondence algorithm can be summarized as:

```
Choose one shape instance as the template V_T
Initialize the landmark sets V_q, q = 1,2,...,n
//Main loop
Repeat while ∀i,k,|γ_ik| > 0
     Repeat while α(·) > ε_H
          Landmark insertion
     Update the template V_T
     Loop over each shape instance
          Landmark sliding
     Repeat while α(·) < ε_L
          Landmark deletion
End
```

The stop condition of this algorithm is the convergence of all three operations, i.e., $|\gamma_{ik}| = 0$ and $\epsilon_L < \alpha(V_i, S_i) < \epsilon_H$, $\forall i, k$. In practice, we stop the algorithm when all $|\gamma_{ik}|$'s are sufficiently small.

4 Experiments

We implement the proposed method in Matlab and test it on five data sets extracted from medical images. These five data sets are: (D1) 120 corpus callosum shape instances; (D2) 24 metacarpal shape instances [10]; (D3) 50 cardiac shape instances; (D4) 50 kidney shape instances; and (D5) 32 femur shape instances [10], as shown in Fig. 1(b). Among them, D1 and D2 have closed-curve shapes, D3, D4, and D5 have open-curve shapes. For comparison, we choose the MDL implementation (also in Matlab) by Thodberg [9] and, in all experiments, MDL was run with 8 active nodes optimized over 40 passes. We test MDL on each data set with three settings where the number of landmarks along each shape instance is set to 16, 32, and 64, respectively. The proposed method is also run with three settings where the allowed representation error is set to match the average representation errors $E(\alpha)$ from the respective MDL runs ($\epsilon_L = E(\alpha) - std(\alpha)$, $\epsilon_H = E(\alpha) + std(\alpha)$). With similar representation error, we compare several other error/accuracy measures for MDL and the proposed method.

While it is very difficult to have an objective and comprehensive evaluation of the shape-correspondence performance, some quantitative measures have been developed in recent years. In this experiment, we compare the following measures: (a) $E(\beta)$ and $std(\beta)$: the mean and standard deviation of the thin-plate bending energy between the template and all the shape instances according to the identified landmarks; (b) λ_1, λ_2, and λ_3: the three principal eigenvalues of the covariance matrix of $V_i, i = 1, 2, \ldots, n$. In calculating the covariance matrix, the Procrustes analysis [2] is applied to normalize the size and orientation of all the shape instances. (c) m: the number of landmarks sampled in each shape instance, and (d) the total CPU time used for processing each data set, based on the specific implementations. In general, with a similar representation error, a good shape correspondence is expected to have small $E(\beta)$, λ_1, λ_2, λ_3, and m.

Table 1. Experimental results on D1(corpus callosum)

Measures	MDL $m = 16$	MDL $m = 32$	MDL $m = 64$	Proposed Method $\epsilon_L = 0.1880$ $\epsilon_H = 0.2669$	Proposed Method $\epsilon_L = 0.0199$ $\epsilon_H = 0.1442$	Proposed Method $\epsilon_L = 0.0090$ $\epsilon_H = 0.0885$
$E(\alpha)$	0.2275	0.0819	0.0487	0.2214	0.0637	0.0164
$std(\alpha)$	0.0394	0.0620	0.0397	0.0290	0.0090	0.0023
$E(\beta)$	1.0767	2.0420	2.4937	0.0661	0.2270	0.4063
$std(\beta)$	1.3434	1.8201	1.9548	0.0425	0.1509	0.1490
λ_1	0.0159	0.0155	0.0024	0.0150	0.0093	0.0016
λ_2	0.0016	0.0014	0.0017	0.0025	0.0016	0.0009
λ_3	0.0009	0.0010	0.0004	0.0014	0.0014	0.0004
m	16	32	64	16	32	64
CPU time(s)	1073.6	3853.0	15448.0	340.2	541.4	1027.8

Table 2. Experimental results on D4(kidney)

Measures	MDL $m = 17$	MDL $m = 33$	MDL $m = 65$	Proposed Method $\epsilon_L = 0.0501$ $\epsilon_H = 0.0977$	Proposed Method $\epsilon_L = 0.0331$ $\epsilon_H = 0.0764$	Proposed Method $\epsilon_L = 0.0194$ $\epsilon_H = 0.0663$
$E(\alpha)$	0.0739	0.0547	0.0428	0.0731	0.0366	0.0142
$std(\alpha)$	0.0238	0.0216	0.0234	0.0089	0.0045	0.0020
$E(\beta)$	0.4295	0.9501	1.4099	0.1099	0.1470	0.2217
$std(\beta)$	0.1450	0.2841	0.3627	0.0654	0.1441	0.0992
λ_1	0.0031	0.0029	0.0028	0.0025	0.0024	0.0022
λ_2	0.0014	0.0014	0.0012	0.0015	0.0016	0.0016
λ_3	0.0010	0.0009	0.0008	0.0012	0.0012	0.0009
m	17	33	65	14	20	34
CPU time(s)	298.6	764.3	1396.2	140.4	211.1	294.8

For conserving space, we only show the experimental results on D1 and D4 in Tables 1 and 2. Figure 1(c) shows the identified landmarks along several sample shape instances. We can see that, given similar representation error, the proposed method produces much smaller mean bending energy $E(\beta)$ than MDL. This is reasonable since minimizing the bending energy is one of our explicit goals. An interesting result is that, in all the experiments, the proposed method produces a correspondence with λ_1, λ_2, and λ_3 that are comparable to MDL (see Table 1), because minimizing the eigenvalues of the covariance matrix is a goal of MDL but not of the proposed method. In addition, we found that the proposed method usually runs faster than MDL, especially when the number of the shape instances increases, as in the bottom graph of Fig. 1(c). For the representation compactness, we found MDL and the proposed method sample each shape instance with similar numbers of landmarks given a similar representation error as in the top graph of Fig. 1(c). However, in the MDL implementation, m, the number of landmarks, is predetermined and kept unchanged in the algorithm, while in the proposed method, m is automatically determined by landmark insertion and deletion. We observed similar results on D2, D3, and D5.

5 Conclusion

In this paper, we developed a new landmark-based method for nonrigid shape correspondence, a prerequisite of accurate statistical shape analysis (SSA). This method considers three important factors in modelling the shape-correspondence error: landmark-correspondence error, representation error, and representation compactness. These three factors are explicitly handled by the landmark sliding, insertion, and deletion operations, respectively. The performance of the proposed method was evaluated on five shape-data sets that are extracted from medical images and the results were quantitatively compared with an implementation of the MDL method. We found that, within a similar allowed representation error, the proposed method has a performance that is comparable to or better than MDL in terms of (a) average bending energy, (b) principal variances in SSA, (c) representation compactness, and (d) algorithm speed.

References

1. S. Belongie, J. Malik, and J. Puzicha. Shape matching and object recognition using shape contexts. *IEEE Trans. PAMI*, 24(24):509–522, April 2002.
2. F. L. Bookstein. Principal warps: Thin-plate splines and the decomposition of deformations. *IEEE Trans. PAMI*, 11(6):567–585, June 1989.
3. F. L. Bookstein. Landmark methods for forms without landmarks: Morphometrics of group differences in outline shape. *Medical Image Analysis*, 1(3):225–243, 1997.
4. H. Chui and A. Rangarajan. A new algorithm for non-rigid point matching. In *Proc. Conf. Computer Vision and Pattern Recog.*, pages 44–51, 2000.
5. T. F. Cootes, C. J. Taylor, D. H. Cooper, and J. Graham. Active shape models - their training and application. *Comput. Vision Image Understanding*, 61(1):38–59, Jan. 1995.
6. R. Davies, C. Twining, T. Cootes, J. Waterton, and C. Taylor. A minimum description length approach to statistical shape modeling. *IEEE Trans. Med. Imag.*, 21(5):525–537, May 2002.
7. J. Duchon. Splines minimizing rotation-invariant semi-norms in sobolev space. In *Constructive Theory of Functions of Several Variables, Lecture Notes in Mathematics, 571*, pages 85–100, 1977.
8. C. G. Small. *The Statistical Theory of Shape*. Springer-Verlag, 1996.
9. H. H. Thodberg. Adding curvature to minimum description length shape models. In *British Machine Vision Conference*, volume 2, pages 251–260, 2003.
10. H. H. Thodberg. Minimum description length shape and appearance models. In *IPMI*, pages 51–62, 2003.
11. S. Wang, T. Kubota, and T. Richardson. Shape correspondence through landmark sliding. In *Proc. Conf. Computer Vision and Pattern Recog.*, pages 143–150, 2004.

Statistical Face Models for the Prediction of Soft-Tissue Deformations After Orthognathic Osteotomies

Sebastian Meller[1], Emeka Nkenke[2], and Willi A. Kalender[1]

[1] Institute of Medical Physics, University of Erlangen-Nürnberg, Germany
sebastian.meller@imp.uni-erlangen.de
[2] Department of Oral and Maxillofacial Surgery, University of Erlangen-Nürnberg, Germany

Abstract. This paper describes a technique to approximately predict the facial morphology after standardized orthognathic ostoetomies. The technique only relies on the outer facial morphology represented as a set of surface points and does not require computed tomography (CT) images as input. Surface points may either be taken from 3D surface scans or from 3D positions palpated on the face using a tracking system. The method is based on a statistical model generated from a set of pre- and postoperative 3D surface scans of patients that underwent the same standardized surgery. The model contains both the variability of preoperative facial morphologies and the corresponding postoperative deformations. After fitting the preoperative part to 3D data from a new patient the preoperative face is approximated by the model and the prediction of the postoperative morphology can be extracted at the same time. We built a model based on a set of 15 patient data sets and tested the predictive power in leave-one-out tests for a set of relevant cephalometric landmarks. The average prediction error was found to be between 0.3 and 1.2 mm at all important facial landmarks in the relevant areas of upper and lower jaw. Thus the technique provides an easy and powerful way of prediction which avoids time, cost and radiation required by other prediction techniques such as those based on CT scans.

1 Introduction

In oral and maxillofacial surgery one of the major issues is the correction of dentoskeletal deformities of the skull. The standard type of orthognathic surgery is to advance the upper jaw and to push back the lower jaw. Its aim is to establish a normal masticatory function along with an improvement in facial esthetics [1]. To obtain true informed consent of the patient in orthognathic surgery, the surgeon must effectively explain possible treatment outcomes to the patient. Unfortunately, up to now the few existing methods to predict the facial appearance changes that will result from orthognathic surgery are not reliable and require 3D imaging [2]. Computed tomography (CT) scans are often used as basic data for the prediction of the postoperative facial surface. Most

J. Duncan and G. Gerig (Eds.): MICCAI 2005, LNCS 3750, pp. 443–450, 2005.

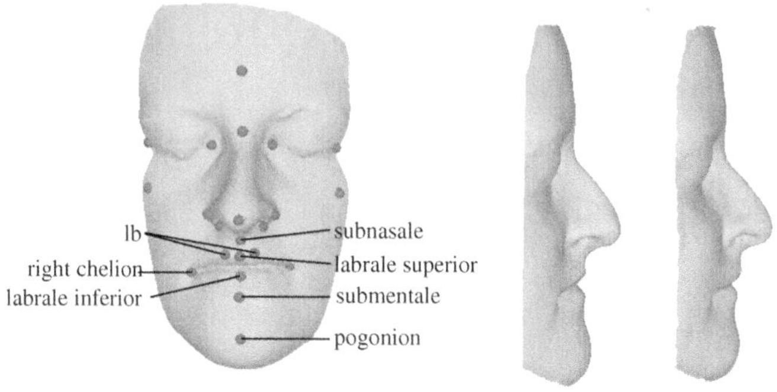

(a) (b) (c)

Fig. 1. Example for a typical input data set: a preoperative face acquired from an optical 3D sensor (a and b) with manually marked anatomical landmarks (a) and the postoperative face one year after surgery (c) in which the upper jaw has been moved forward and the lower jaw backwards.

of these methods try to model the soft tissue deformation with the aid of finite element or spring models based on the planned surgical change of the underlying bone structure. To date, there is little information available on the accuracy of these predictions [3,4,5]. Commercial applications exist that allow geometric deformations of photographs or scanned 3D models in order to plan the surgical outcome but there is no quantitative validation on how realistic these predictions are. It has been the aim of this study to introduce a new prediction approach avoiding time, cost and radiation introduced by the CT scan and to evaluate the accuracy of this approach. The presented method is based on a 3D statistical model built from a set of 3D surface scans of different patients before and 12 months after the same type of orthognathic surgery (see Fig. 1). The variety of preoperative facial morphologies as well as the corresponding postoperative deformations are both captured in the model. The model can be fitted to the face of a new patient whose facial morphology is partly known as a set of 3D positions on the face which can either be digitally acquired by 3D surface scans or from positions directly palpated using a tracking system. After this fitting process the prediction can simply be extracted from the model.

We will present our statistical models in section 2 and how the model was built from the given data in section 3. The model fitting algorithm is described in section 4, followed by an evaluation in section 5.

2 Extended Shape Models

Cootes and Taylor first presented the idea of deformable statistical models [6] for the purpose of image segmentation in 1992. The main assumption is that a class of shapes can be described by a relatively small number of linear variations of the average shape. Object shapes are described in a compact way as a vector of boundary point coordinates. A class of object shapes is modeled by an average shape and a linear combination of vectors that describe the possible variations of the shape compared to the average shape as deformation vectors. The model can be easily deformed by changing the weights of the deformation vectors within a limiting range keeping the shape always plausible, i.e. inside the given class of shapes.

Technically the shape of an object is described as a point set $\mathcal{F}_i$ of S points $\mathbf{p}_{ij}, j = 1 \ldots S$ on the object surface, given N objects ($i = 1 \ldots N$), in this case preoperative facial morphologies from different patients. Assuming at this point that a dense correspondence map between all shapes has already been defined and all shapes are already aligned in space, then we can describe each input shape as a vector $\mathbf{x}_i$ by concatenating the x-, y- and z-coordinates of the points, yielding a vector of dimension $M = 3S$. By applying an eigenvalue decomposition [7] to the covariance matrix of these vectors we get a number of eigenvalues λ_i with associated orthogonal eigenvectors $\mathbf{v}_i$. It can be shown that there are at most $N-1$ eigenvalues with $\lambda_k > 0$, if $N < M$ [6]. By defining a matrix $\mathbf{V}$ from the eigenvectors $\mathbf{v}_k$ associated to these eigenvalues, each of the input shape vectors $\mathbf{x}_i$ as well as arbitrary anatomically plausible shapes $\mathbf{x}$ can be described as a sum of the average shape vector $\bar{\mathbf{x}}$ plus a linear combination of these eigenvectors with a weight vector $\mathbf{b}$:

$$\begin{aligned} \mathbf{x} = \bar{\mathbf{x}} + \mathbf{V}\mathbf{b},\ \mathbf{V} = (\mathbf{v}_1, \mathbf{v}_2, \ldots, \mathbf{v}_{N-1}), \\ -3\sqrt{\lambda_k} < b_k < 3\sqrt{\lambda_k},\ k = 1 \ldots N-1 \end{aligned} \tag{1}$$

Since the eigenvalues are equal to the variance within the input data in direction of the associated eigenvector, we can assume plausible shapes generated by a linear combination of weights that are constrained to a variation of three standard deviations per eigenvector [6].

In order to include the transition between pre- and postoperative morphology into the model, we extended this original approach by adding the displacement vector field from pre- to postoperative facial morphology as a second part of the input vector: We assume at this point that preoperative and postoperative surfaces have already been registered and that a dense correspondence between them has been established. In other words, for each preoperative face point $\mathbf{p}_{ij}$ of a patient $\mathcal{F}_i$ there is a corresponding postoperative point $\mathbf{q}_{ij}$. The displacement vector field between pre- and postoperative face can thus be defined as $\mathbf{d}_{ij} = \mathbf{q}_{ij} - \mathbf{p}_{ij}$. The definition of the vector $\mathbf{x}_i$ is extended to contain the coordinates $\mathbf{p}_{ij}$ first and then the displacement vector field $\mathbf{d}_{ij}$, thus doubling the dimension M of the vector to $M = 6S$.

3 Model Generation

3.1 Data Acquisition

3D surface scans of 8 female and 7 male patients were acquired with an optical 3D sensor (SCAN3D, 3D-Shape GmbH, Erlangen, Germany), both preoperatively and one year after the surgery in which the upper jaw was moved forward and the lower jaw backwards, both between 3 and 7 mm (e.g. see Fig. 1). The postoperative scans were first rigidly registered to the preoperative scans as described by Maier et al. [8]. On all pre- and postoperative faces several important cephalometric landmarks were manually identified (see Fig. 1(a)).

3.2 Correspondence Mapping

A precondition for the statistical modeling is a dense correspondence between all input shapes. A manual correspondence mapping which involves marking mutually corresponding points on all input data sets is only feasible for a small subset of anatomical landmarks. Therefore several correspondence mapping algorithms have been proposed in the past [9,10,11]. We applied our own approach [12] that ensures smooth and dense correspondence mapping. It uses only moderate manual interaction and is based on the multiple deformation of a template surface to each of the input surfaces. The necessary non-rigid template-to-target registrations are performed in three steps: first, an affine registration based on the set of marked landmarks on both meshes [13] is performed, followed by second, a 3D thin plate spline deformation [14] which brings the template to exact alignment with the target mesh at the landmark positions. Thirdly, for refinement, a non-rigid iterative morphing approach is applied. It is based on four kinds of springs attached to the vertices of the template triangle mesh that determine the deformation of the template surface. Two of the springs minimize the surface distance to the target surface while the other two maintain the overall shape of the template surface by minimizing changes in inter-vertex edge lengths and inter-triangle edge angles compared to the original template surface. In each iteration for each of the template vertices a deformation vector is calculated composed of the four spring forces where each type of spring is weighted differently.

We applied the same technique for the inter-patient registration of a preoperative template face to each of the other faces and for the intra-patient registrations of each pair of pre- and postoperative facial morphologies. As a result all pre- and postoperative faces are described with the same mesh topology with mutually corresponding vertices.

3.3 Alignment and Model Calculation

In order to compensate for translation and rotation differences in the given data sets we applied an iterative Procrustes alignment [15], again based on the manually marked landmark sets for each patient. At this point the model is generated as described in section 2, including the displacement vector field to the postoperative facial morphology into the shape vector.

4 Model Fitting and Prediction

The preoperative part of the generated model can be fitted to given data from an arbitrary face. We assume that the data is given as a 3D set of points on the unknown preoperative face. These may either be single point positions at known anatomical landmarks or whole point clouds on the face. The fitting process thus involves the determination of a rigid transformation $\mathbf{T}_{\text{fit}}$ that transforms the model coordinates into the target coordinate system and the shape parameter vector $\mathbf{b}_{\text{fit}}$ that deforms the model surface such that it optimally fits the given point set. After the model-based deformation a further non-linear deformation can be applied (section 4.2).

4.1 Model Fitting

We partly applied the fitting algorithm described by Blanz et al. [16]. The method uses a linear matrix that maps the given vector $\mathbf{x}$ of model coordinates onto a subset of points and applies a linear transformation, in our case a rigid transformation that registers the model with the patient. Assuming the correspondences from given points to model vertices are known, the shape parameter vector $\mathbf{b}$ which generates the model face (according to (1)) that best fits the given points can be found in a closed solution by solving a linear equation system after applying a singular value decomposition [7].

In this study we only used the set of predefined landmarks for model fitting for which the corresponding vertices on the model surface are known. The approach can be extended to include the whole preoperative facial morphology by starting with an initial model fit defined by known landmarks. Correspondences for the remaining vertices can then be acquired by projection onto the already fitted model surface. Thus, the fitting can be iteratively refined.

4.2 Refinement Deformation

In order to perfectly fit the model surface to the given point set and consider shape variances not captured in the statistical model, a non-linear deformation can follow the fitting process described above. In this step a thin-plate spline warping is applied to the fitted model face based on the known pairs of corresponding landmarks between model and patient. In this way the preoperative model face perfectly fits the patient face at the landmark positions.

4.3 Face Prediction

The above fitting process defines a shape parameter vector $\mathbf{b}$ and therefore a vector $\mathbf{x}$ that represents in its first half an approximation of the given preoperative face. Since the displacement vector field to the postoperative face is stored in the second part of the same vector (see section 2) and is therefore determined by the same shape parameter vector according to (1), a prediction of the postoperative facial morphology can now be acquired by adding this adapted displacement vector field to the fitted preoperative face.

5 Evaluation Results

The evaluation was carried out in 15 leave-one-out tests. In each test one of the 15 data sets was defined as the test data set; the model was generated from the

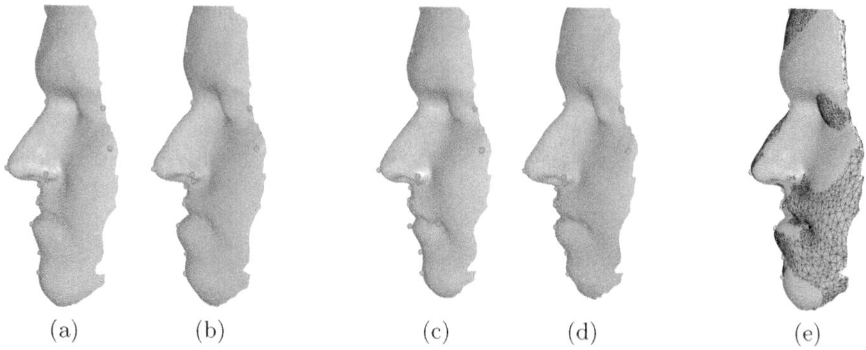

Fig. 2. Example for a prediction: A preoperative face of a patient (a) was landmarked and the statistical model generated without this patient was fitted to these landmarks as can be seen in (b). The actual postoperative outcome (c) one year after surgery can then be compared with the prediction (d) produced by the model, both combined in one image in (e).

14 remaining data sets and then tested against the test model (see example in Fig. 2).

We used the manually marked anatomical landmarks on the test data set in order to fit the model. The predicted postoperative face could then be compared to the known postoperative face. We measured the prediction error at a subset of the marked cephalometric landmarks:

- subnasale: point at the tip of the angle formed by colunella and upper lip
- labrale superior: most anterior point of the upper lip
- lb left and right: top of the cupid's bow of the upper lip
- chelion left and right: points located at the labial commissure
- labrale inferior: most anterior point of the lower lip

Table 1. Statistical evaluation of the average absolute prediction error in mm at certain anatomical landmarks from leave-one-out tests in 15 cases, compared to the maximum displacement caused by the surgeries at these landmarks.

Landmark	**Mean**	**SD**	**Max**	**Max. actual**
pogonion	1.2	1.2	3.8	8.5
submentale	1.0	1.1	3.4	7.5
labrale inferior	1.0	1.1	3.5	5.8
labrale superior	0.6	0.6	2.7	3.1
lb left	0.5	0.5	2.1	2.5
lb right	0.7	0.8	3.6	4.1
chelion left	0.8	0.5	1.9	2.6
chelion right	0.8	1.0	3.6	3.2
subnasale	0.3	0.4	1.6	2.3

- submentale: most posterior point between lower lip and chin
- pogonion: most anterior point of the chin

Results are shown in Table 1: The measured average prediction errors over all 15 cases at the landmarks with the greatest deviations (pogonion, submentale and labrale inferior) were about 1.2 mm $\pm$ 1.2 mm with rare outliers below 4 mm whereas the absolute displacements ranged from 2.3 mm to 8.5 mm. All other landmark positions showed average prediction errors below 1 mm.

6 Conclusions and Discussion

We showed how statistical face models that include the shape change between pre- and postoperative facial morphology can be successfully applied to predict the postoperative facial morphology after orthognathic surgery from sparse 3D data of a patient's preoperative face. Although sophisticated nonlinear finite element modeling may be an appropriate alternative, there is no proof from the current literature that these techniques generate valid predictions of the human face. The presented method avoids time, cost and radiation associated with other techniques that require a CT scan. It is fast and simple during application. The fit and prediction is calculated within a few seconds after minimal manual interaction. Even based on a relatively small data base of 15 male and female cases, the comparison between the real postoperative outcome of the facial surfaces and the predicted surfaces revealed that the average differences were below 1.5 mm for landmarks placed on the relevant areas of upper and lower jaw. This new type of prediction of the outcome of orthognathic surgery is favorable for several reasons: differences between facial surfaces below 1.5 mm cannot be easily distinguished by the normal observer and the thickness of the facial soft tissue already changes during the course of the day in this range. In addition, the facial surface is influenced by changes of body weight and aging. Therefore, it will be difficult to achieve a better prediction accuracy than the one shown in this study. Of course, the application of the method is restricted to the kind of surgery and the variability of facial morphologies covered in the data base. Thus, future work will include increasing the data base to more patient data sets from different types of surgeries, different ethnic groups and ages. The new method may also find its application in plastic facial surgery where well standardized procedures allow an accurate prediction by the proposed technique.

References

1. Xia, J., Ip, H., Samman, N., Wong, H., Gateno, J., Wang, D., Yeung, R., Kot, C., Tideman, H.: Three-dimensional virtual-reality surgical planning and soft-tissue prediction for orthognathic surgery. IEEE Trans Inf Technol Biomed **5** (2001) 97–107
2. Nkenke, E., Langer, A., Laboureux, X., Benz, M., Maier, T., Kramer, M., Häusler, G., Kessler, P., Wiltfang, J., Neukam, F.: Validation of in vivo assessment of facial soft-tissue volume changes and clinical application in midfacial distraction: a technical report. Plast Reconstr Surg **112** (2003) 367–80

3. Koch, R.M., Roth, S.H.M., Gross, M.H., Zimmermann, A.P., Sailer, H.F.: A framework for facial surgery simulation. In: SCCG '02: Proceedings of the 18th Spring Conference on Computer Graphics, ACM Press (2002) 33–42
4. Gladilin, E., Zachow, S., Deuflhard, P., Hege, H.C.: On constitutive modeling of soft tissue for the long-term prediction of cranio-maxillofacial surgery outcome. In Lemke, H.U., Vannier, M.W., Inamura, K., Farman, A.G., Doi, K., Reiber, J.H.C., eds.: Proc. CARS. Volume 1256 of ICS., London, Elsevier (2003) 3438
5. Westermark, A., Zachow, S., Eppley, B.: Three-dimensional osteotomy planning in maxillofacial surgery including soft tissue prediction. Journal of Craniofacial Surgery **16** (2005) 100–104
6. Cootes, T.F., Taylor, C.J., Cooper, D.H., Graham, J.: Training models of shape from sets of examples. In: Proc. BMVC, Berlin, Springer (1992) 266–275
7. Press, W., Flannery, B., Teukolsky, S., Vetterling, W.: Numerical Recipes: The Art of Scientific Computing. 2nd edn. Cambridge University Press, Cambridge (UK) and New York (1992)
8. Maier, T., Benz, M., Schön, N., Nkenke, E., Neukam, F., Vogt, F., Häusler, G.: Automatic coarse registration of 3D surface data in oral and maxillofacial surgery. In Buzug, T., Lueth, T., eds.: Perspective in image-guided surgery, Singapore, World Scientific (2004) 51–58
9. Hutton, T.J., Buxton, B.F., Hammond, P.: Dense surface point distribution models of the human face. In Staib, L., ed.: IEEE Workshop on Mathematical Methods in Biomedical Image Analysis. (2001) 153–160
10. Lamecker, H., Seebass, M., Hege, H.C., Deuflhard, P.: A 3D statistical shape model of the pelvic bone for segmentation. In Fitzpatrick, J., Sonka, M., eds.: Proceedings of SPIE Medical Imaging 2004: Image Processing. Volume 5370. (2004) 1341–1351
11. Fleute, M., Lavallée, S.: Building a complete surface model from sparse data using statistical shape models: Application to computer assisted knee surgery system. In: MICCAI. Volume 1496 of LNCS., Springer-Verlag (1998) 879–887
12. Meller, S., Kalender, W.: Building a statistical shape model of the pelvis. In Lemke, H.U., ed.: Computer Assisted Radiology and Surgery (CARS), Chicago, IL (2004)
13. Umeyama, S.: Least-squares estimation of transformation parameters between two point patterns. IEEE Trans. PAMI **13** (1991) 376–380
14. Bookstein, F.L.: Principal warps: Thin-plate splines and the decomposition of deformations. IEEE Trans. PAMI **11** (1989) 567–585
15. Goodall, C.: Procrustes methods in the statistical analysis of shape. Journal of the Royal Statistical Society **53** (1991) 285–339
16. Blanz, V., Mehl, A., Vetter, T., Seidel, H.P.: A statistical method for robust 3D surface reconstruction from sparse data. In: International Symposium on 3D Data Processing, Visualization and Transmission, Thessaloniki, Greece (2004)

Fully Automatic Shape Modelling Using Growing Cell Neural Networks

Luca Ferrarini, Hans Olofsen, Mark A. van Buchem,
Johan H.C. Reiber, and Faiza Admiraal-Behloul

LKEB - Leiden University Medical Center, The Netherlands
L.Ferrarini@lumc.nl
http://www.lkeb.nl

Abstract. In this paper, we present a new framework for shape modelling and analysis: we suggest to look at the problem from a pattern recognition point of view, and claim that under this prospective several advantages are achieved. The modelling of a surface with a point distribution model is seen as an unsupervised clustering problem, and tackled by using growing cell structures. The adaptation of a model to new shapes is studied as a classification task, and provides a straightforward solution to the point correspondence problem in active shape modelling. The method is illustrated and tested in 3D synthetic datasets and applied to the modelling of brain ventricles in an elderly population.

1 Introduction

Statistical shape modelling has been increasingly used during the last decade as a basis for image segmentation, interpretation and the studying of shape changes. Many successful 2D-applications have been described in literature [1]. The model building requires the establishing of correspondence between shape surfaces over a set of training examples. Defining correspondent points on different shapes is not trivial: in some 2D applications, manual landmark definition might be possible but it becomes unpractical when 3D/4D shapes are considered. Different techniques have been developed to address this problem: some solutions are rooted in computer graphics [2], others in signal/image processing [3], [4], [5], and some have used information theory [6], [7], [8]. An important distinction has to be made between *pairwise* and *groupwise* approaches (see [6] and [8]): *groupwise* analysis aims to optimize an objective function over the whole dataset while creating the statistical model, while *pairwise* solutions generally start with a good representative of the dataset and build up a model rooted on it. In the final discussion, we shortly present advantages and drawbacks of these approaches, justifying the research on the *pairwise* approach described in this work.

From a pattern recognition prospective, and considering a pairwise approach, the problem can be summarized in 3 questions: How many nodes are needed? Where should they be located? How can we define correspondence between them? The question "how many nodes are needed?" is tackled as an unsupervised learning (clustering) problem where the optimal number of clusters (nodes) has to be defined. To ensure an optimal location of the points, the clustering technique needs to be topology-preserving. We

J. Duncan and G. Gerig (Eds.): MICCAI 2005, LNCS 3750, pp. 451–458, 2005.

consider the point correspondence as a classification problem where the generalization aspect of a classifier is used to match unseen cases to similar previously seen points. We investigated the use of growing artificial neural networks to tackle all three questions. Most of the growing neural networks are variations of the growing cell structure (GCS) introduced by Fritzke in [9]. The GCS principle is based on Self Organizing Maps (SOM) (Kohonen [10]), which are known to be perfectly topology-preserving: the network preserves neighborhood relations in the data by mapping neighboring inputs onto neighboring nodes in the map. Recently, Marsland et al. presented a self-organizing network that grows when required (SONGWR) [11]: SONGWR proved to be (1) more data-driven while growing, and (2) faster in learning input representation, when compared with previous models.

In this paper we describe how the SONGWR is used to create a first point distribution model from a representative instance of the training set (a single case or an average). The adaptation phase of the SONGWR algorithm is then used to deform and match the obtained network to all the instances in the training set. We investigated the robustness and effectiveness of the method in synthetic data sets. Finally, we show a successful application of the algorithm in the modelling of brain ventricles in magnetic resonance images.

2 Method

Given a dataset of segmented objects $T = \{D_1, ..., D_n\}$, we detect the clouds of points $P_1, ..., P_n$ by selecting the boundary points of each instance. Afterwards, the method goes through two main phases: an unsupervised clustering is used to create a first model of a representative object P_i (chosen through visual inspection); subsequently, an adaptation phase adapts the model to the other clouds of points, keeping the point correspondence.

2.1 Unsupervised Clustering: How Many Nodes?

The unsupervised clustering algorithm (SONGWR) is fully described in [11]: we summarize it here, highlighting the main variations we introduced:

1. initialize a network M with 2 nodes at random positions
2. do
   (a) randomize the order of the points in P_i
   (b) for each point $p \in P_i$
      i. identify the two best matching nodes s, t in the network M:
         $s = arg\min_{n \in M} ||p - n||, \qquad t = arg\min_{n \in M-\{s\}} ||p - n||$
      ii. set $edge_{age_{s,t}} = 0$ (age of $edge_{s,t}$), or create the edge if not existing
      iii. evaluate the activity of s as: $\quad a = e^{-||p-s||}$
      iv. if $a < a_T$ and $s_{age} > age_T$
         – add a new node: $\quad r = (s + p)/2$
         – insert $edges_{r,s}$, $edge_{r,t}$, and remove $edge_{s,t}$
      v. else
         – adapt s position: $\quad s^{t+1} = w_{winner} * s^t_{age} * (p - s^t)$

- adapt nodes $i \in N_s$ in s'neighborhood: $i^{t+1} = w_d * i^t_{age} * (p - i^t)$, with $w_d = 0.1 * e^{-\frac{d^2}{2*0.42^2}}$, d = distance in steps between s and i

vi. update edges between s and $i \in N_s$: $edge_{age_{s,i}} = edge_{age_{s,i}} + 1$

vii. update s_{age} and $i_{age}, i \in N_s$

viii. delete edges with $edge_{age} > edge_T$

ix. delete nodes with no edges

(c) remove nodes which have never been selected as best-matching s in (b)

(d) evaluate new *accuracy* for M as the mean average distance between each node $p \in P_i$ and the correspondent best matching unit $s \in M$

while (*old_accuracy* - *new_accuracy* $\geq acc_T$)

3. evaluate the covariance matrix for each cluster (node of the network) by using the associated points from the cloud
4. repeat point 2. using the Mahalanobis distance instead of the Euclidian one in (b).i

The following thresholds and formulae have been used: $a_T = 0.1$, $edge_T = 50$, $acc_T = 0.001$, $age_T = 1 - \frac{1}{\alpha} * (1 - e^{\frac{-\alpha*5}{\beta}})$, $\alpha = 1.05$, $\beta_w = 3.33$, $\beta_n = 14.3$. As discussed in [11], the accuracy threshold a_T affects the final model, allowing for multi-scale analysis (although this aspect has not been investigated in this work). The growing steps (b).i-(b).ix follow the algorithm in [11], while points 3) and 4) are introduced to better represent the surface in points of high curvature, as also suggested in [2]. The model can be seen as a classifier, obtained by means of clustering techniques: the next paragraph shows how to adapt it to the other shapes of the training set T (only nodes of the final model are involved in the adaptation phase).

2.2 Point Correspondence: Adaptation Phase

In order to perform shape analysis, we need to adapt the model to the other clouds of points, keeping point correspondence. Adapting the network to a new pattern is equivalent to using the model as a classifier: for each given point in the new object, we find the best-matching cluster and adapt it. The process has similarity with SOMs, since there are no added/removed nodes. The segmented patterns D_i are considered already normalized for scaling, while we adjust for position and orientation during the process. The main parts of algorithm are summarized:

1. perform block 2 of the algorithm presented in paragraph 2.1, without adding/removing nodes (point correspondence granted, points 2.b(vii),2.b(ix),2.c skipped)
2. adapt the nodes which were never selected as best matching in the previous step (1)
   (a) move each node towards the closest node which was selected in (1)
   (b) average the node positions
3. repeat step (1), but using the points which were selected in (1) as new input (instead of the original cloud of points), and adapting only those nodes which were never selected as best matching (nodes involved in step (2))

Steps (2) and (3) are introduced in order to deal with non-closed objects. Performing the adaptation for all the clouds of the training set leads to n neural networks (models) $M_1, ..., M_n$. Summarizing the whole algorithm: while working on the first shape, the unsupervised clustering identifies the best location for nodes in order to optimize the representation of the cloud of points. During the adaptation phase, the nodes are moved towards those areas in the new shape where clusters are needed in order to better represent the new cloud of points. Since no nodes are added nor removed, by simply labeling the nodes on the first model and following them during the adaptation we obtain the desired correspondence.

3 Results

Results on synthetic datasets. The datasets created for the synthetic experiments are shown in figure 1.a. The algorithm introduced in 2.1 involves the randomization of the sequence of surface points (step 2.(a)); randomizing the sequence guarantees a more homogeneous growth for the network, but we have to assure stable results. For each shape, we run the algorithm 20 times using the same sequence of surface points, and evaluated the dissimilarity between models. Table 1 reports the results (*stability test*): the *accuracy* for a model, and the *dissimilarity* between two models M_i, M_j are defined as:

$$accuracy = \frac{1}{N_{points}} \sum_{j=1..N_{points}} ||p_j - w_j||, \tag{1}$$

$$d(i,j) = accuracy_{ij} + accuracy_{ji} + (1 - \frac{E_m}{E_M}), \tag{2}$$

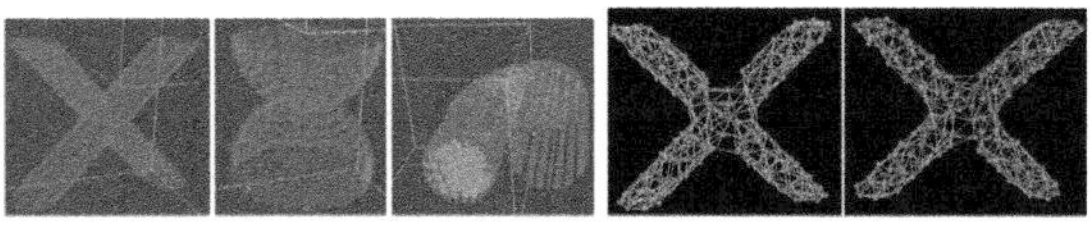

(a) (b)

Fig. 1. (a) Synthetic datasets (dimensions in voxel): from left to right: *XShape* (radius = 5, length = 30), *Chalice* (radius = 10), and *U-tube* (radius = 10, length = 105); (b) Overlapping for best (*Left*, diss. = 2.58) and worst (*Right*, diss. = 3.59) matching shapes: in both cases, one network has red nodes and white edges, the other has blue nodes and green edges. Even in the worst case the two networks nicely overlap.

Table 1. Results for *stability* and *noise* tests (*accuracy* and *dissimilarity* are given in voxel); results are averaged over 20 runs per shape and show the stability of the algorithm in relation to random effects and noise. Details on the applied randomization and noise are given in the text.

	Stability Test									Small Noise Test				
	Surf. Points	Avg. Diss.		Accur.		N nodes		N edges		Surf. Points	Avg. Diss.		Accur.	
		μ	σ	μ	σ	μ	σ	μ	σ		μ	σ	μ	σ
X shape	1464	2.84	0.68	2.18	0.005	146	0	372.95	7.72	1317	3.09	0.72	2.32	0.01
Chalice	1208	3.53	0.94	2.25	0.01	120	0	309.65	4.86	1087	3.04	0.71	2.39	0.03
U-Tube	2247	3.33	0.83	2.37	0.007	223.85	0.49	485.25	10.78	2022	3.12	0.74	2.53	0.03

where N_{points} is the number of surface points, and w_j is the best matching node in the model, given the p_j point of the surface sequence (the Euclidian distance is used). In $d(i,j)$, $accuracy_{ij}$ is the accuracy of the model M_i evaluated on the set of nodes of the model M_j (see eq. 1), $E_m = min(E_i, E_j)$, $E_M = max(E_i, E_j)$, and $E_k = \sum_{q=1..N^k_{edges}} ||edge_q||^2, k = i, j$. Figure 1.b shows a visual example for the dissimilarity between models. Tests on robustness to noise were performed: for each shape, starting with the original set of surface points, we built up 20 sequences by applying the following noise: 60% of the points were randomly moved in space (displacement in the range [-2,2] voxels for all the coordinates), and 10% of the nodes were removed. Table 1 (*small noise test*) shows the results. Finally, we tested the ability of the graph to adapt to different instances of a same class of shapes (capturing the main variations). We created a dataset of 40 tubes, where each tube varies in diameter and length following Gaussian distributions (radius r: $\mu_r = 10, \sigma_r = 2$ voxel, length l: $\mu_l = 125, \sigma_r = 40$ voxel). We generated an average tube and used it to train a growing neural network (first model); the model has then been adapted to the 40 tubes (average accuracy for the adaptation process: $\mu_{acc} = 2.37$, $\sigma_{acc} = 0.2$ voxel). We finally performed a PCA to analyze the performances of the PDM obtained with our algorithm. The properties we tested are the same presented in [6]. *Compactness* $C(M) = \sum_{m=1}^{M} p^m$ (percentage of variance covered by the first M modes); *reconstruction error* $E_r(M) = \frac{1}{N_s}\sum_{i=1}^{N_s} |S_i^{'}(M) - S_i|$ (average accuracy in approximating N_s shapes of the training set using M modes); *generalization ability* $G(M) = \frac{1}{N_s}\sum_{i=1}^{N_s} |S_i^{'}(M) - S_i|$: for a given i we build up a shape model without using S_i, and test the accuracy with which S_i is approximated by the model ($S_i^{'}(M)$); *specificity* $Sp(M) = \frac{1}{N}\sum_{i=1}^{N}[Diss(S_i(M), ObjCls)]$, with

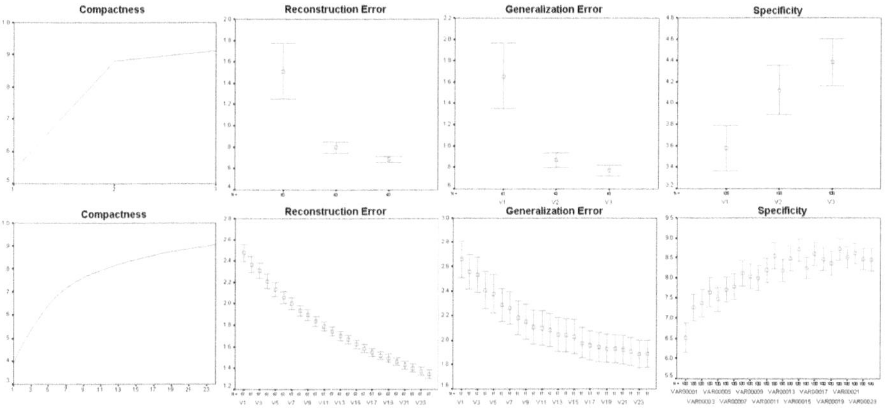

Fig. 2. First row: quantitative analysis for the *Tube-PCA*: compactness (in percentage), reconstruction error, generalization ability, and specificity (in voxel) are reported. The x axis shows the retained modes of variation. The error bar shows the confidential interval at 95% (see text for details). The model identifies the 2 main modes of variation. Second row: same analysis for brain ventricles (values are in mm): when the 24 modes of variation are used, the error values are particularly low, showing the good behaviour of the model: $E_r < 1.4$, $G_e < 2$, and $Sp < 9$.

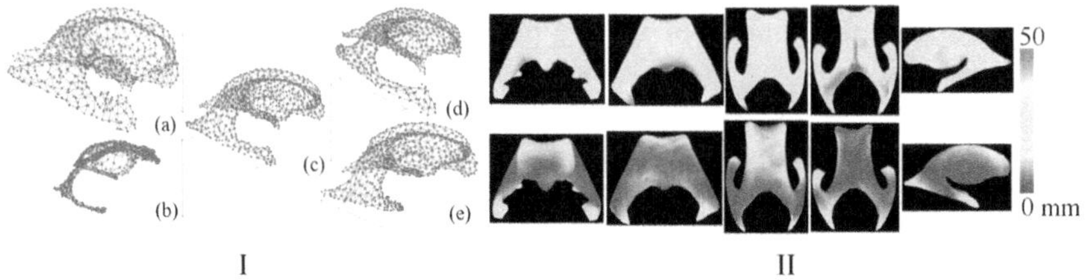

Fig. 3. Left image I: (a)-(b) 1st mode of variation, $\pm 3\sigma$; (c) mean shape; (d)-(e) 2nd mode of variation, $\pm 3\sigma$. The 1st mode presents a global shrinking/growing behaviour, while the 2nd mode shows elongation/compression of the temporal and occipital horns; Right image II: Color-coded maps for the amount of movement of each node. Top row: 1st mode $\pm 3\sigma$. Bottom row: 2nd mode $\pm 3\sigma$ (occipital and temporal horns mostly involved).

$Diss(S_i(M), ObjCls) = \frac{1}{N_s} \sum_{i=1}^{N_s} |S_i'(M) - S_i|$, where we create $N = 100$ instances of the object class and average the dissimilarity between them and the shapes in the training set. The results are shown in figure 2.

Results on a medical dataset. We applied the algorithm on a training set of 67, semi-automatically segmented, brain ventricles (T2-MRI, 91x109x91 voxels at 2x2x2 mm after normalization). After acquiring the clouds of points for each ventricle, we selected a representative one and build up a first model (see section 2.1): the optimal number of clusters (nodes) resulted in 755. The model was adapted to the other 66 clouds, and a PCA [1] was performed on the 67 models (average accuracy for the adaptation resulted in $\mu_{acc} = 2.06$, $\sigma_{acc} = 0.22$ mm). Results are reported in figure 2, while figure 3 shows the first 2 modes of variation. Although it was not the aim of the study, we tested the linear correlation between aging and first mode of variation. The dilation was significantly associated with aging ($p < 0.01$, $r^2 = 0.10$, older people showing a larger structure). The low value for r^2 is explained by the low variation in the population ($\mu = 75$, $\sigma = 5$ years).

4 Discussion

In Kaus et al. [2], the authors iteratively reduce the set of original surface points to a subset with high (sparse) dense point distribution in areas of high (low) curvature: a triangular mesh is then derived. In our method, all the surface points are used, and the unsupervised clustering detects the areas in which more clusters (nodes) are needed. Differently from [2], we adapt nodes as in SOM: once a node is moved, a parameter controls how many neighbors have to move, and a Gaussian function is used to determine the strength of movements. As in [2], we also make use of an elastically deformable model which avoids inverse transformations. In Gerig et al. [12], spherical harmonics are used to model a set of surface points. The main advantage is the multi-scale analysis which might highlight deformations not noticeable otherwise; drawback

[1] While applying the PCA, we adjusted for translation and rotation of shapes following the procedure suggested by Evangelos et al. in [13].

of the solution are pre-processing steps needed for *closing* the surface. We have not investigated the multi-scale feature, although we speculate it would be achievable by a reduction in the accuracy for the growing process (a_T). Our solution does not require a *closed* surface. Finally, the parameters used in our approach are the coordinates of the nodes: significant differences in shape are directly associated with positions, (in [12] a vision inspection is needed). In [8], Davies et al. highlight how critical some aspects are for the final model: the number of nodes, their locations, and the correspondence between them strongly influence the final performances. The authors suggest to use *descriptive functions* to identify correspondent points on different shapes, create a first model, and evaluate it through an objective function to be optimized: the search for the best descriptive functions is carried on through genetic algorithms. This approach leads to the distinction between *pairwise* and *groupwise* solutions. *Groupwise* approaches are known to provide better models, optimizing the results on the whole dataset; moreover, they do not require a first representative to start with. *Pairwise* approaches, like the one described in this work, need an initial shape to operate: thus, the final model can be influenced by such a choice. Nevertheless, *pairwise* approaches might overcome some drawbacks related with *groupwise* solutions. The optimization needed by *groupwise* solutions is often achieved by genetic algorithms (see [8]): although this improves the chances of getting a better model, an optimal result is not guaranteed. Genetic algorithms lead to heavy computation, surely a drawback if we aim to *learning* systems: how can we improve a given model when a new example becomes available? *Groupwise* solutions have to undertake the whole optimization process again, with a computation load which grows with the number of shapes. *Pairwise* and *groupwise* solutions should be seen as complementary for many aspects, and the results achieved in one field can improve the other. The results reported in sections 3 show the stability of our solution and its capability of generating good point distribution models (PDM) for statistical analysis (such as PCA). The stability has been tested on synthetic datasets both with and without noise, while the PDM has been tested both on synthetic dataset and on a medical training set of brain ventricles. The PCA could highlight the expected modes of variation for the synthetic data set and known variations in the aging brain ventricles due to brain atrophy.

5 Conclusions

In this paper, we presented a new solution, rooted in a pattern recognition framework, for a *pairwise* approach to the shape-modelling problem. An unsupervised clustering technique (SONGWR) automatically identifies the optimal number of nodes and their locations on the surface of a representative shape; the point distribution model (PDM), considered as a self-organized map (SOM), is then adaptated onto other datasets: the correspondence problem is solved by labeling the nodes in the first model and following them through the adaptation phase. The method has been thoroughly evaluated on synthetic datasets and its effectiveness has been proved in a challenging medical application. Due to its generality, the method can be applied to other anatomical structures (of any shape). Further investigation will be focused on the integration of the image intensities around the nodes in the model.

Acknowledgment

This work was supported by the Technology Foundation STW, applied science division of NWO and the technology programme of the Ministry of Economic Affairs, and by Medis medical imaging systems, Leiden, The Netherlands (www.medis.nl). The authors would like to thank W.M. Palm, M.D. for providing the medical dataset and for his help during the segmentation process.

References

1. T. F. Cootes, C. J. Taylor, D. H. Cooper, J. Graham, *Active Shape Models - their training and application*, Computer Vision and Image Understanding, Vol. 61, no. 1, January, pp. 38-39, 1995
2. M.R. Kaus, V. Pekar, C. Lorenz, R. Truyen, S. Lobregt, J. Richolt, J. Weese, *Automated 3D PDM Construction Using Deformable Models*, proceedings of the Eigth IEEE International Conference on Computer Vision (ICCV'01) pp. 566-572 vol.1
3. A. Pitiot, H. Delingette, A. W. Toga, P.M. Thompson, *Learning Object Correspondences with the Observed Transport Shape Measure*, IPMI 2003, pp. 25-37
4. S. Wrz, K. Rohr, *Localization of Anatomical Point Landmarks in 3D Medical Images by Fitting 3D Parametric Intensity Models*, IPMI 2003, pp. 76-88
5. D. Rueckert, A. F. Frangi, J. A. Schnabel, *Automatic Construction of 3-D Statistical Deformation Models of the Brain Using Nonrigid Resitration*, IEEE Transactions on Medical Imaging, vol. 22, no. 8, August 2003, pp. 1014-1025
6. R.H. Davies, C. J. Twining, P. D. Allen, T. F. Cootes, C. J. Taylor, *Shape Discrimination in the Hippocampus Using an MDL Model*, IPMI 2003, pp. 38-50
7. H. H. Thodberg, *Minimum Description Length Shape and Apperance Models*, IPMI 2003, pp. 51-62
8. R. H. Davies, C. J. Twining, T. F. Cootes, J. C. Waterton, C. J. Tayolr, *A minimum description length approach to statistical shape modelling*, IEEE Transactions on Medical Imaging Vol.21, pp.525-537, 2002
9. B. Fritzke, *Growing Cell Structures - A self-organizing Network for Unsupervised and Supervised Learning*, Neural Networks (1994), Vol. 7, No. 9, pp 1441-1460
10. B. Fritzke, *Kohonen Feature Maps and Growing Cell Structures - a Performance Comaprison*, NIPS 1992, Denver.
11. S. Marsland, J. Shapiro, U. Nehmzow, *A self-organizing network that grows when required*, Neural Networks 15 (2002), pp. 1041-1058
12. G. Gerig, M. Styner, D. Jones, D. Weinberger, J. Lieberman, *Shape analysis of brain ventricles using SPHARM*, Published MMBIA, IEEE Computer Society: 171-178, Dec. 2001
13. E. A. Coutsias, C. Seok, K. A. Dill, *Using Quaternions to Calculate RMSD*, Journal of Computational Chemistry, 2004, vol 25, pp. 1849-1857

Multiscale 3D Shape Analysis Using Spherical Wavelets

Delphine Nain[1], Steven Haker[2], Aaron Bobick[1], and Allen R. Tannenbaum[3]

[1] College of Computing, Georgia Institute of Technology, Atlanta, GA 30332-0280
delfin@cc.gatech.edu,
[2] Department of Radiology, Surgical Planning Laboratory,
Brigham and Women's Hospital, Boston, MA 02115
[3] Electrical Engineering, Georgia Institute of Technology, Atlanta, GA 30332-0250

Abstract. Shape priors attempt to represent biological variations within a population. When variations are global, Principal Component Analysis (PCA) can be used to learn major modes of variation, even from a limited training set. However, when significant local variations exist, PCA typically cannot represent such variations from a small training set. To address this issue, we present a novel algorithm that learns shape variations from data at *multiple scales and locations* using spherical wavelets and spectral graph partitioning. Our results show that when the training set is small, our algorithm significantly improves the approximation of shapes in a testing set over PCA, which tends to oversmooth data.

1 Introduction

Shape priors are commonly used to constrain shapes obtained during the segmentation and registration of biomedical images. Some of the first shape priors were based on local smoothness constraints [1] via elastic forces or combinations of global and local constraints [2] within the active contour framework. One limitation of these models is possible convergence to suboptimal shapes due to high flexibility in deformations. Statistical shape models were devised to overcome such drawbacks by learning a shape model from a training set. In [3] PCA was used in a framework called Active Shape Models (ASM) and has become a standard technique for segmentation tasks [4,3]. The advantage of using PCA as a shape prior is to restrict the segmentation task to a subspace of allowable shapes. However, it has two major limitations. First, it often restricts deformable shape too much, particularly if it has been trained on a relatively small number of samples. Second, finer, more local variations of shapes are often not encoded in eigenvectors representing the most global modes of variation in the shapes.

To address this issue, the authors in [5] have proposed a hierarchical active shape model framework for contours in 2D medical imagery using wavelets, with convincing results. We propose to extend this framework in two novel ways. First we describe a multiscale representation of surfaces in 3D medical imagery using conformal mapping and spherical wavelets. Further, we present a novel algorithm to discover optimal independent multiscale shape variations from the data. Spherical wavelets have been used primarily by the computer graphics community to generate multiresolution description of 3D shapes [6]. In [7], spherical

J. Duncan and G. Gerig (Eds.): MICCAI 2005, LNCS 3750, pp. 459–467, 2005.

wavelets are used to analyze a manifold not topologically equivalent to a sphere by doing a non-bijective mapping between the manifold and the sphere via the normals. This work does not conduct statistical analysis of a shape population and uses a basis defined on the sphere, not on the shape.

To the best of our knowledge, this is the first application of statistical analysis to a population of 3D surfaces using spherical wavelets. By using a spherical wavelet basis defined on the shapes and identifying independent multiscale shape variations, we build more accurate shape priors.

2 Shape Acquisition and Registration

In this paper, we used a dataset of 39 prostate gland shapes obtained from MR imaging. In these images [1] the prostate capsule is visible and was manually segmented by a radiologist. Each manual segmentation defined a 3D surface which was extracted as a triangulated surface using the Marching Cubes algorithm. We registered all prostate shapes in the dataset by re-triangulating the extracted surfaces in a consistent manner, providing a point-by-point registration of all surfaces in the dataset. This re-triangulation was done by first mapping each surface to the sphere using a conformal (angle-preserving) mapping technique as described in [8]. 6 Expert-specified landmark points were used to improve the consistency of the spherical mappings. Next, interpolation was used to find the coordinates of the original 3D surface at the vertices of a regular multiscale subdivision of the sphere, having an octahedral structure at its coarsest scale. Once corresponding points were identified, a Procrustes technique was used to align the shapes in the original coordinate system.

3 Shape Representation

Once registered, all shapes have N vertices and each shape can be described by its three coordinate functions, $x, y, z \in \mathbb{R}$ such that the kth shape S_k is a column vector of size $3N$: $S_k = [x_k(1), ..., x_k(N), y_k(1), ..., y_k(N), z_k(1), ..., z_k(N)]^T$.

Since all vertices in the shape population are registered, we interpret each entry of S_k as a random variable and each shape as a realization from a multivariate probability distribution. A population of K shapes can be described by a mean shape $\overline{S} = \frac{1}{K}(\sum_{k=1}^{K} S_k)$ and a set of transformations $T = [T_1, ..., T_M]$ that describe the variability observed in the population. Each transformation vector T_m is of size $3N$ where the ith entry is a transformation applied to the ith entry of the mean shape with a corresponding magnitude $\beta_m \in \mathbb{R}$.

Each transformation vector, or variation mode, can be characterized by *scale*, *spatial location* and *magnitude*. For scale, the variation can be *global*, meaning it applies to all vertices of the shape (all of its entries are non-zero) or *local*, meaning it is a sparse vector with a few non-zero entries. The non-zero entries determine the spatial location of the variation. Characterization of local variations could be important for shape analysis since a disease, such as cancer, could affect only

[1] Axial, T2-weighted, 120mm field of view, matrix size 256×256, 3.0mm thickness, 0.5mm gap, $1.5T$, using both endorectal and pelvic coil arrays.

a portion of an organ's surface. Therefore descriptive shape priors should discern shape variations at different scales and spatial location.

4 Limitation of PCA in Representing Finer Shape Details

Active shape models (ASM) [3] use principal component analysis (PCA) to discover *uncorrelated* shape variations from a training set. ASM assumes that training shapes have a multivariate normal distribution. The modes of variation are the eigenvectors of the data covariance matrix (major axes of the distribution).

If the training set is small, PCA favors discovery of significant *global* variations over *local* variations. Indeed, assuming a training set of K shapes with N vertices ($N \gg K$), the rank of the covariance matrix, and number of eigenvectors, will be at most $K - 1$. It can be shown that the eigenvectors associated with the largest eigenvalues of the covariance matrix describe the most significant modes of variation in the vertices [3]. This can be a feature of PCA, since it will enforce a global smoothness constraint on shapes, but also a limitation if shapes have important local variations, as will be shown in Section 6.

5 Multiscale Shape Prior Using Spherical Wavelets

In this Section, we describe our technique to model the full range of variation in a population. We first derive a *multiscale* analysis of the variation of shapes in section 5.1. Section 5.2 details our shape prior for multiscale statistical shape analysis. Section 6 shows our results and compares our technique with ASM.

5.1 Description of Spherical Wavelets

To address this limitation, we propose a shape prior that represents variations at different scales and spatial locations. This can be achieved with wavelet basis functions that are localized in space and characteristic scales and therefore match a wide range of signal characteristics, from high frequency edges to slowly varying harmonics [9]. Spherical wavelets are second-generation wavelets adapted to manifolds with non-regular grids. We briefly sketch their construction [10].

Subdivision: Spherical wavelets analyze signals on a mesh obtained from recursive partitioning of a mesh with spherical topology. With the technique described in Section 2, all shapes have the required mesh to conduct the analysis. We denote the set of all vertices obtained after j subdivisions with an index set $K(j)$. The $j + 1^{th}$ resolution mesh is obtained by introducing new nodes, identified by an index set $M(j)$ which subdivide existing edges (typically at their midpoint). The complete set of nodes in the $j + 1^{th}$ resolution mesh is given by $K(j+1) = K(j) \bigcup M(j)$ and shown in Figure 1(a) which represents a portion of a triangular surface mesh at resolution $j + 1$.

Representation of shape functions: Let S be a surface and let $\mathbf{x} \in \mathbb{R}^3$ be a point on S. To approximate a function f($\mathbf{x}$) we use a set of wavelet and scaling basis functions defined on the shape and modulated by coefficients. For each resolution level, $\varphi_{j,\cdot}(\mathbf{x})$ are hat-shaped scaling functions[2]defined at the nodes

[2] Varies linearly from value 1 at the vertex x_k to 0 at neighboring vertices.

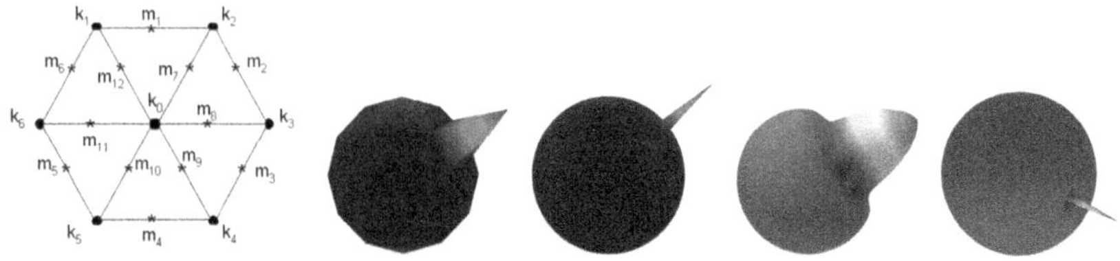

(a) grid (b) $j = 2$ (c) $j = 4$ (d) $j = 1$ (e) $j = 4$

Fig. 1. (a) Subdivision Grid. (b,c) Scaling (d,e) Wavelet Function for Different Nodes

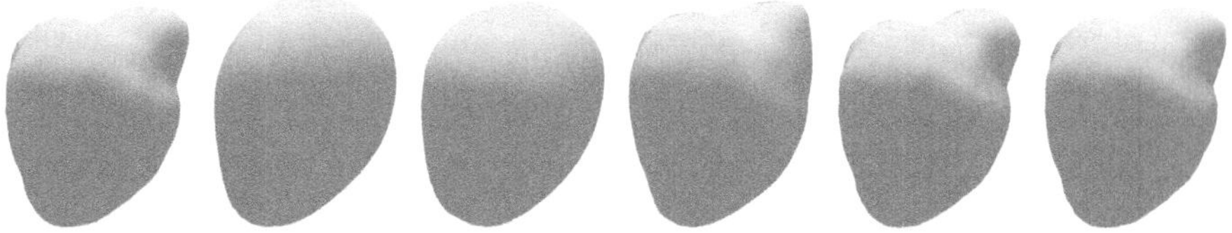

(a) shape (b) res. 0 (c) res. 1 (d) res. 2 (e) res. 3 (f) res. 4

Fig. 2. Shape at various resolution levels, see text for details

$k \in K(j)$ and $\psi_{j,\cdot}(\mathbf{x})$ are wavelet functions defined at nodes $m \in M(j)$. Wavelet functions capture finer features since they are composed of higher resolution $(j+1)$ scaling functions. Figures 1(b)- 1(e) show scaling and wavelet functions for different values of j,k and m. Note that the support of the functions becomes smaller as the resolution increases.

When a shape is transformed into the wavelet domain, its wavelet coefficients are calculated [3] *for all resolution levels*:

$$f(\mathbf{x}) = \sum_{k \in K(0)} \lambda_{0,k}\varphi_{0,k}(\mathbf{x}) + \sum_{0 \leq j} \sum_{m \in M(j)} \gamma_{j,m}\psi_{j,m}(\mathbf{x}). \qquad (1)$$

A shape is represented by its lowest resolution scaling coefficients and its wavelet coefficients at all higher resolution levels. The total number of coefficients calculated by the transform is equal to the number of points representing the shape. Each coefficient describes features at a particular scale and spatial location.

Wavelet transform of the Prostate Data: We have applied the wavelet transform to prostate data to analyze multiscale variations in the population. We first subtract the mean shape from all the shapes in the set. We then apply the transform independently to the residual x,y and z coordinates of the N vertices of the shape. The kth shape in a population of K shapes can be described by a vector of wavelet coefficients of size $3N$:

$$\Gamma_k = \{\lambda^x_{0,k}, \lambda^y_{0,k}, \lambda^z_{0,k}, \gamma^x_{j,m}, \gamma^y_{j,m}, \gamma^z_{j,m} | j = 0,..,4; m \in M(j); k \in K(0)\} \qquad (2)$$

Figure 2 shows a wavelet decomposition of a prostate. Figure 2(a) is the shape before decomposition. Each Figure 2(b)- 2(f) is the mean shape plus the cumulative signals up to that resolution. We observe more high frequency content as the resolution increases.

[3] By inner product with dual functions, see [10] for more details.

5.2 Spherical Wavelets and Construction of Shape Priors

The shape prior is the multivariate probability distribution of the coefficients, estimated from their covariance matrix $\Gamma\Gamma^T$. In our experiments, we have observed a very sparse covariance matrix with most of the dependency between coefficients at the same scale. Furthermore, for each scale we have observed clusters of correlated coefficients. This is consistent with the decorrelation property of the wavelet transform for real-world signals [9]. Given the sparseness of the covariance matrix, we approximate the joint distribution of coefficients with the product of distributions over smaller clusters of correlated coefficients.

Adaptive Band Selection by scale-space decomposition: For each scale, we cluster highly correlated coefficients into a *band*, with the constraint that coefficients across bands have minimum cross-correlation. Our technique is different from [5] where the authors perform a scale-space frequency decomposition of the coefficients by clustering coefficients of spatially adjacent bases into bands in each frequency plane. In this work, we cluster coefficients according to correlation to pick meaningful bands that indicate areas of variation. Such a decomposition can in itself be interesting for shape analysis.

To cluster correlated wavelet coefficients, we use a spectral graph partitioning technique [11]. We use a fully connected undirected graph $G = (V, E)$ where nodes V are wavelet coefficients for a particular scale. The weight on each edge $w(i, j)$ is the covariance between the wavelet coefficients at nodes i and j. A $cut(A, B) = \sum_{u \in A, v \in B} w(u, v)$ is the optimal partitioning of V into two disjoint sets A and B such that nodes within a partition have the highest covariance and nodes across partitions have the lowest covariance.

Using this technique, we do a recursive partitioning of the coefficients into bands. We use a stopping criteria based on the quality of the decomposition of each set, validating whether the subdivided band correspond to two independent distributions. Indeed, if we start with a graph G where we consider each coefficient to be a random variable and find a partition $A \cup B = G$, $A \cap B = \emptyset$, then

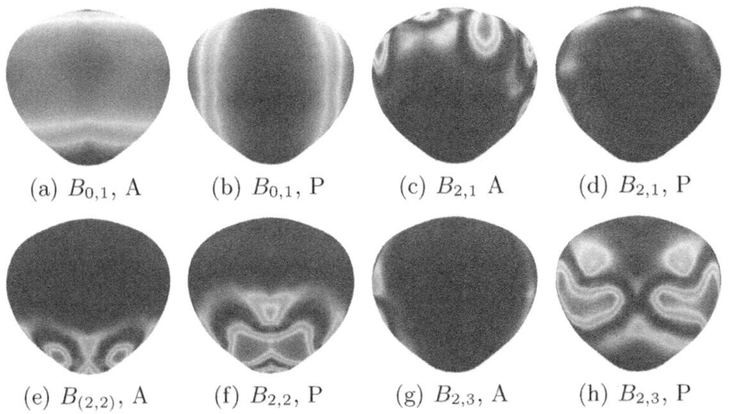

(a) $B_{0,1}$, A (b) $B_{0,1}$, P (c) $B_{2,1}$ A (d) $B_{2,1}$, P

(e) $B_{(2,2)}$, A (f) $B_{2,2}$, P (g) $B_{2,3}$, A (h) $B_{2,3}$, P

Fig. 3. Band Decomposition: various bands $B_{j,i}$, where j is the resolution and i is the band number, shown in Anterior view (A) and Posterior view (P), see text for color it is a good partition if $P(G) = P(A)P(B)$. We can test this with the Kullback-Leibler (KL) divergence between the joint and the product of the marginals.

In this work, we assume a multivariate Gaussian distribution for each partition and derived the KL divergence [12]:

$$D(P(G)||P(A)P(B)) = 1/2 \log(|\Sigma_A||\Sigma_B|) - 1/2 \log(|\Sigma_G|) \qquad (3)$$

where Σ_A is the covariance matrix of $P(A)$ and $|.|$ is the determinant [4]. If the distributions $P(A)$ and $P(B)$ are independent, then their KL divergence is 0. In practice, we do not accept a partition if $D(P(G)||P(A)P(B)) > 0.1$.

Band Visualization: To visualize the bands, we calculate the influence of all wavelet coefficient in band $B_{j,i}$ on each point $\mathbf{x}$ of the surface by setting those coefficients to 1 in (1) and others to 0. If $f(\mathbf{x}) = 0$, then the point is not affected and if $f(\mathbf{x}) > 0$ it is affected according to the magnitude of $f(\mathbf{x})$. Using this function as a colormap (blue= 0, red= 1), Figures 3(a)- 3(b) show the first band for the lowest scale. The second band is the complement of the first. As expected each band has a large spatial extent and indicate two uncorrelated shape processes on the prostate data: the variation of the anterior wall of the prostate (typically rounded) and the variation of the posterior wall of the prostate (typically flatter). Figures 3(c)- 3(h) show three bands for the scale 3. These bands are more localized. These are uncorrelated variations of the superior and inferior walls of the shape, as well as an uncorrelated variations of the anterior wall at that scale. Bands have compact support, though this is not a constraint of our technique. The symmetry in bands 2 and 3 is also interesting, showing that both the right and left side tend to co-vary similarly. This symmetry of variation is plausible for the prostate, and we plan to investigate this further. Notably a diseased organ could possibly be detected if there is a lack of symmetry.

Building the Prior: Each band of coefficients is modeled as a multivariate Gaussian that encodes a set of shape variations. To estimate their distribution from the data, we apply PCA analysis to the coefficients in each band. The eigenvectors and eigenvalues of lower scale bands represent relatively global aspects of shape variability, whereas bands at higher scales represent higher frequency and more localized aspects of shape variability. Hence, our technique discovers shape processes *at every scale*, where the processes are all the eigenvectors of all the bands, and does not favor the discovery of global processes over local processes. Additionally, our prior accurately encodes finer details even with small training sets, since there exists at least $B(K-1)$ eigenvectors for each scale with B bands.

6 Experiments

We compare our technique to PCA for the task of reconstruction. We partition our data randomly into T training samples and $39 - T$ testing samples, where $T = [5, 10, 20, 30]$ and learn a shape prior from the training set. The prior for

[4] In practice since Σ_A is often singular, we decompose it using SVD as $\Sigma_A = U\Sigma'_A U^T$ and estimate $log|\Sigma_A| = trace(log(\Sigma'_A))$, using only the positive entries of Σ'_A.

PCA consists of the mean shape, the eigenvectors and eigenvalues. The prior for our technique consists of the mean shape, the bands structure, the eigenvectors and eigenvalues for each band. We then reconstruct shapes in the testing set.

For PCA, we project the training shape coordinates onto the eigenvectors and translate the coordinates of the new shape to a point lying at a reasonable distance of the training data ($\pm$ 3 standard deviation) to obtain a reconstructed shape. For our technique, we transform the shape to its wavelet coefficients, project and correct the coefficients for each band separately, and transform the new coefficients back to a reconstructed shape. A mean squared error between the vertices of the ground truth and the reconstructed shape is calculated for all shapes in the testing set.

Figure 4 shows the reconstruction error with the multiscale prior (solid line). It is significantly smaller than for PCA (dashed line) across all training set sizes.

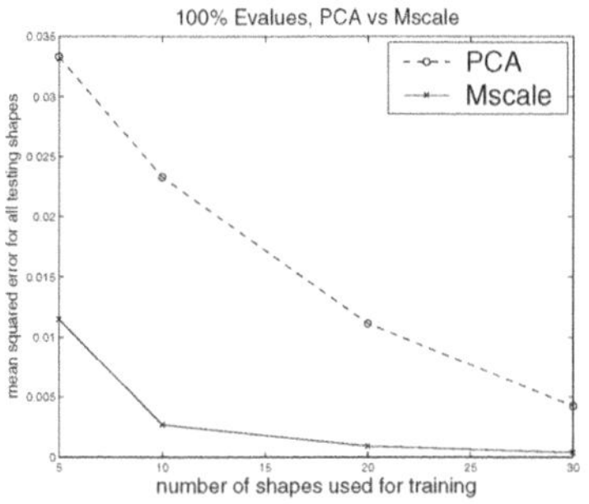

Fig. 4. Mean Squared Reconstruction Error for various training set sizes

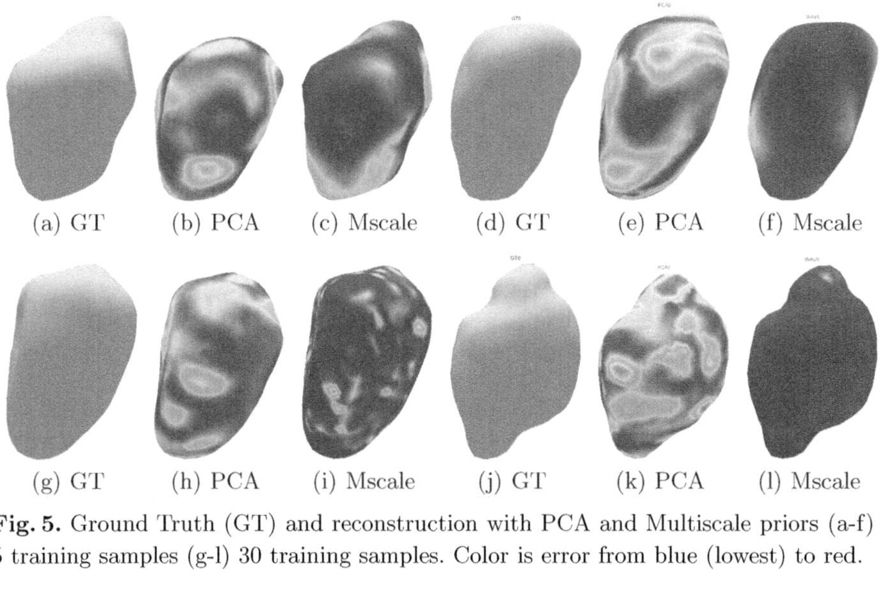

(a) GT (b) PCA (c) Mscale (d) GT (e) PCA (f) Mscale

(g) GT (h) PCA (i) Mscale (j) GT (k) PCA (l) Mscale

Fig. 5. Ground Truth (GT) and reconstruction with PCA and Multiscale priors (a-f) 5 training samples (g-l) 30 training samples. Color is error from blue (lowest) to red.

The error for PCA significantly increases when the training set size decreases, but only slightly increases for the multiscale technique.

Figures 5(a), 5(d), show a ground truth test shape and 5(b), 5(e), 5(c), 5(f), its reconstruction with the PCA and multiscale shape priors built from 5 training shapes. For PCA, the reconstruction is very smooth. Many of the finer details are lacking in the reconstruction. The multiscale technique incorporates both local and global details that PCA does not encode. Figures 5(g), 5(j) show a ground truth test shape and 5(h), 5(k), 5(i), 5(l) its reconstruction from 30 training shapes. For PCA, the reconstruction is more accurate, but still lacks some finer details, such as the sharper edges. Again, the multiscale technique incorporates both local and global details that PCA misses.

7 Conclusions and Future Work

We have demonstrated that our spherical wavelet based technique is a better shape prior than ordinary PCA when it is important to represent finer, more localized shape variation. Our novel method finds independent shape variation processes at multiple scales and multiple locations by adaptively clustering correlated wavelet coefficients. The visualization of the bands can, in itself, be an interesting tool for shape analysis. We plan in future work to compare this choice of L^2 basis to other natural bases such as spherical harmonics [13], as well as investigate the use of wavelet packets [14]. We also plan to use it for key imaging tasks such as segmentation. Further, we intend to build on this theory in order to derive a natural multiscale description for discriminative shape analysis. Localized processes cannot be overlooked when discriminating among populations, making this technique promising for localized lesions, such as tumors. Finally, we will be applying this methodology to other types of structures, in particular, to the caudate nucleus as part of our research in schizophrenia.

Acknowledgements. This work is part of the National Alliance for Medical Image Computing (NAMIC), funded through the NIH Roadmap for Medical Research, Grant U54 EB005149. A. Tannenbaum and D. Nain's work was also funded by NIH NAC grant P41 RR-13218 and S. Haker's work is supported by NIH grants R01CA109246, R01LM007861, R01CA1029246 and P41RR019703.

References

1. Kass, M., Witkin, A., Terzopoulos, D.: Snakes: Active contour models. Int. J. Comput. Vis **1** (1987) 321–331
2. Terzopoulos, D., Metaxas, D.: Dunamic 3d models with local and global deformations: Deformable superquadrics. IEEE Trans. Pat. Anal. Mach. Intell. **13** (1991)
3. Cootes, T., Taylor, C., Cooper, D., Graham, J.: Active shape models - their training and application. Computer Vision and Image Understanding **61** (1995) 38–59
4. Leventon, M., Grimson, E., Faugeras, O.: Statistical shape influence in geodesic active contours. Comp. Vision and Patt. Recon. (CVPR) (2000)
5. Davatzikos, C., Tao, X., Shen, D.: Hierarchical active shape models, using the wavelet transform. IEEE Trans. Medical Imaging **22** (2003) 414–423

6. Schröder, P., Sweldens, W.: Spherical wavelets: Efficiently representing functions on the sphere. Computer Graphics Proceedings (SIGGRAPH 95) (1995) 161–172
7. Greenshields, I.: 3d shape approximants via spherical wavelet decompositions. 14th Symposium on Computer-Based Medical Systems (2001) 31
8. Haker, S., Warfield, S., Tempany, C.: Landmark-guided surface matching and volumetric warping for improved prostate biopsy targeting. MICCAI (2004)
9. Mallat, S.: Wavelet Tour of Signal Processing. Academic Press (1999)
10. Schröder, P., Sweldens, W.: Spherical wavelets: Texture processing. In Hanrahan, P., Purgathofer, W., eds.: Rendering Techniques '95. Springer Verlag (1995)
11. Shi, J., Malik, J.: Normalized cuts and image segmentation. IEEE Transactions on Pattern Analysis and Machine Intelligence **22** (2000) 888–905
12. Papoulis, A.: Probability, Random Variables, and Stochastic Processes. McGraw-Hill (1991)
13. Styner, M., Lieberman, J.A., Pantazis, D., Gerig, G.: Boundary and medial shape analysis of the hippocampus in schizophrenia. Medical Image Analysis **8** (2004)
14. Mohamed, A., Davatzikos, C.: Shape representation via best orthogonal basis selection. MICCAI **1** (2004) 225–233

Discriminative Analysis of Brain Function at Resting-State for Attention-Deficit/Hyperactivity Disorder

C.Z. Zhu[1], Y.F. Zang[1], M. Liang[1], L.X. Tian[1], Y. He[1], X.B. Li[1], M.Q. Sui[2], Y.F. Wang[2], and T. Z. Jiang[1]

[1] National Laboratory of Pattern Recognition, Institute of Automation, Chinese Academy of Sciences, P.R. China
czzhu@nlpr.ia.ac.cn
[2] Institute of Mental Health, Peking University, P.R. China

Abstract. In this work, a discriminative model of attention deficit hyperactivity disorder (ADHD) is presented on the basis of multivariate pattern classification and functional magnetic resonance imaging (fMRI). This model consists of two parts, a classifier and an intuitive representation of discriminative pattern of brain function between patients and normal controls. Regional homogeneity (ReHo), a measure of brain function at resting-state, is used here as a feature of classification. Fisher discriminative analysis (FDA) is performed on the features of training samples and a linear classifier is generated. Our initial experimental results show a successful classification rate of 85%, using leave-one-out cross validation. The classifier is also compared with linear support vector machine (SVM) and Batch Perceptron. Our classifier outperforms the alternatives significantly. Fisher brain, the optimal projective-direction vector in FDA, is used to represent the discriminative pattern. Some abnormal brain regions identified by Fisher brain, like prefrontal cortex and anterior cingulate cortex, are well consistent with that reported in neuroimaging studies on ADHD. Moreover, some less reported but highly discriminative regions are also identified. We conclude that the discriminative model has potential ability to improve current diagnosis and treatment evaluation of ADHD.

1 Introduction

Attention-deficit/hyperactivity disorder (ADHD) is one of the most commonly diagnosed childhood behavioral disorders. According to related reports, 3~6% American and 5% Chinese school-age children are affected by ADHD. Developmentally inappropriate inattention, impulsivity, and hyperactivity are three core symptoms of ADHD. Children with ADHD have difficulty on controlling their behaviors or focusing their attentions which result in an adverse effect on academic performance and social function. Current available diagnosis and treatment evaluation of ADHD are mainly made from the levels of the core symptoms. Ranking of the symptoms is usually made by the parents or teachers of the children, which is unfortunately subjective. Therefore more objective approaches are highly desired.

J. Duncan and G. Gerig (Eds.): MICCAI 2005, LNCS 3750, pp. 468 – 475, 2005.

With the high spatial and temporal resolution as well as the non-invasive advantage, structural and functional magnetic resonance imaging (MRI) have been playing an increasingly important role in brain studies. Volumetric [1], morphological [2, 3] and functional [4, 5] brain properties have been studied on ADHD with MRI [6, 7]. Voxel-based structural and functional MRI studies on ADHD have suggested various brain abnormalities [7]. However such a group-level statistical difference is less helpful to diagnosis. Currently some promising studies on mental diseases [8, 9, 10, 11, 12] with multivariate statistical classifiers using neuroimaging information were reported. Unfortunately few were concerned on ADHD. Moreover, explanation of classification result in these studies is still unsatisfactory. In this work, an ADHD discriminative model which includes an ADHD classifier and an intuitive representation of discriminative pattern is proposed on the basis of Fisher discriminative analysis (FDA) of brain function obtained from resting-state fMRI.

The classification feature and classification algorithm will be detailed in Section 2 and 3 respectively. Materials are presented in Section 4. Experimental results and discussion are provided in Section 5. Section 6 is devoted to conclusion and some further directions.

2 Mapping of Brain Function at Resting-State

Low-frequency (0.01–0.08 Hz) fluctuation (LLF) synchrony among motor cortices was studied by Biswal at 1995, which indicated that LFF was physiologically meaningful [13]. Later some studies about diseases had been conducted using LFF synchrony [14, 15, 16]. As a mapping of brain function, regional homogeneity (ReHo) was first proposed to measure the regional synchrony of LFF voxel by voxel, and then employed to verify the default mode network (DMN) [17] successfully in [18]. ReHo has also been used to locate the ROIs automatically without a priori in a study of brain function connectivity [19]. Here, we used ReHo derived from fMRI series scanned at resting-state as a feature of classification. ReHo was defined at a given voxel as the temporal similarity of the LFF between the voxel and its neighbors, which was calculated with Kendall's coefficient as (1).

$$W = \frac{\sum (R_i)^2 - n(\bar{R})^2}{\frac{1}{12}K^2(n^3-n)} \tag{1}$$

where W is the Kendall's coefficient among given voxels, R_i the sum rank of the ith time point, $\bar{R}=((n+1)K)/2$ the mean of the R_i's, K the number of time series within a measured cluster and we used K=27 as in [18].

3 Pseudo-Fisher Discriminative Analysis

Fisher discriminative analysis (FDA) is a widely used technique in the domain of pattern recognition [20, 22]. Suppose there are two classes of samples with features of dimension D. Here, D is defined as the number of voxels in consideration. FDA is used to find a projective direction, $\omega^* \in \Re^D$, along which the two classes of projected samples are separated with maximal ratio of between-class distance and within-class variability. Mathematically, objective function (2) is to be maximized

$$J(\omega) = \frac{\omega^T S_b \omega}{\omega^T S_w \omega} \tag{2}$$

where $S_w = \sum_{i=1}^{N_1} (x_i^1 - m_1)(x_i^1 - m_1)^T + \sum_{i=1}^{N_2} (x_i^2 - m_2)(x_i^2 - m_2)^T$,

and $S_b = (m_1 - m_2)(m_1 - m_2)^T$

are between-class scatter matrix and within-class scatter matrix respectively; $x_i^1\big|_{i=1}^{N_1}$ and $x_i^2\big|_{i=1}^{N_2}$ are feature vectors, m_1 and m_2 mean feature vectors, N_1 and N_2 sample sizes. Theoretically, the optimal ω^* can be determined by:

$$\omega^* = S_w^{-1}(m_1 - m_2) \tag{3}$$

However, in case of small-sample ($N_1+N_2 << D$), which is common in brain image analysis, computing of inverse matrix of S_w is an ill-posed problem and therefore FDA would yield an unreliable result. While pseudo-Fisher discriminative analysis (pFDA), which is a variation of classical FDA, can solve the problem by using the pseudo-inverse of S_w to substitute the inverse of S_w [23, 24]. Briefly, principal component analysis (PCA) was firstly applied on sample features, $x_i \in \Re^D$, to find a linear subspace, $\Re^d$, spanned by all the eigenvectors, $\{\alpha_1, \alpha_2, \ldots, \alpha_d\}$, with non-zero eigenvalue. Representing an original sample feature, $x \in \Re^D$, with $\{\alpha_1, \alpha_2, \ldots, \alpha_d\}$ would result in a low-dimension feature, $y \in \Re^d$ ($d = N_1+N_2-1$), so that classical FDA and (3) can be directly used in the subspace to find $\omega^* \in \Re^d$. Projecting each sample, $y \in \Re^d$, onto $\omega^* \in \Re^d$ can result in a one-dimensional score of $z \in \Re^1$ by inner product operation, $z = \langle y, \omega^* \rangle$. Finally, the classification threshold, $z_0 \in \Re^1$, was determined by:

$$z_0 = (N_1 m_1^z - N_2 m_2^z)/(N_1 + N_2) \tag{4}$$

where m_1^z and m_2^z are centers of projective scores of the two classes.

4 Materials

To eliminate the impact of head motion on the calculation of ReHo maps, the subjects with head motion greater than 1.2 mm or rotation greater than 1.2° were excluded. The remained 9 ADHD and 11 controls (age range of 11-15 years and IQ > 80) were used for further analysis.

The imaging processes were undertaken on the SIEMENS TRIO 3-Tesla scanner in Institute of Biophysics, Chinese Academy of Sciences. For each subject we concerned the following two sets of imaging data: resting-state fMRI time cou rses and 3D structural MRI. Echo Planer Imaging (EPI) Blood Oxygenation Level Dependent (BOLD) images were acquired axially with the following parameters: 2000/30 ms (TR/TE), 30 slices, 4.5/0 mm (thickness/gap), 220 × 220 mm (FOV), 64 × 64 (resolution), 90° (flip angle), the whole session lasted for 480 seconds. 3D spoiled gradientrecalled whole-brain volume was acquired sagittally with the following parameters: 1700/3.92 ms (TR/TE), 192 slices, 1.0/0 mm (thickness/gap), 256 × 256 mm (FOV), 256 × 256 (resolution), 12° (flip angle).

Preprocessing procedures for fMRI signals included motion correction, within-subject registration, time aligning across slices, time series linear detrending, voxels resampling to 3×3×3 mm^3, spatially smoothing (FWHM = 4mm) and spatial normalization. All these processes were undertaken using SPM2 [25].

5 Experiments Results and Discussion

pFDA was performed on ReHo maps of the 9 ADHD and 11 controls, and an ADHD classifier and a representation of discriminative pattern were generated. First, the classifier was tested with the training samples to indicate the separability of the classifier on training set. Then leave-one-out (LOO) cross validation approach was employed to estimate the prediction ability of the model. Classification results are listed in the top row of Table 1, form which zero training error is achieved, and correct predictions performed on ADHD and controls are 78% and 91% respectively. The total correct prediction rate reaches 85%.

Table 1. Classification results

Discriminative model		Training set correct rate	LOO test correct rate		
			Controls	ADHD	Total
Functional information	ReHo Map	100%	91%	78%	85%
Structural information	Intensity	100%	38%	67%	53%
	Morphology	100%	50%	56%	53%

The distribution of projective scores of both the training and predicting samples in a 20-round LOO test are shown in Fig. 1, where white circles and squares represent normal controls and children with ADHD in the training set of LOO test respectively, and black circles and squares represent the control and patient for predicting respectively. The crosses indicate the corresponding classification thresholds determined by (4). As in Fig. 1, there are only one testing control and two testing patients located on the wrong sides of the classification boundary by the classifier. Moreover, within-class variations of projective scores of training samples are all close to zero, and between-class distances are quite large. This result convinces the objective of FDA.

With $\{\alpha_1, \alpha_2, \ldots, \alpha_d\}$, the optimal projective direction in subspace $\Re^d$ can be easily inversely mapped to the original space $\Re^D$. The projective direction in $\Re^D$ or Fisher brain, as a part of the discriminative model, was used to visualize the discriminative pattern of ReHo between the children with ADHD and normal controls. As illustrated in Fig.2, the larger the amplitude (positive or negative) of a voxel in the Fisher brain, the more the voxel contributes to the final discrimination. As shown in Fig.3, some highly discriminative regions are identified by the Fisher brain. Among these regions, prefrontal cortex and anterior cingulate cortex have been reported to be involved in

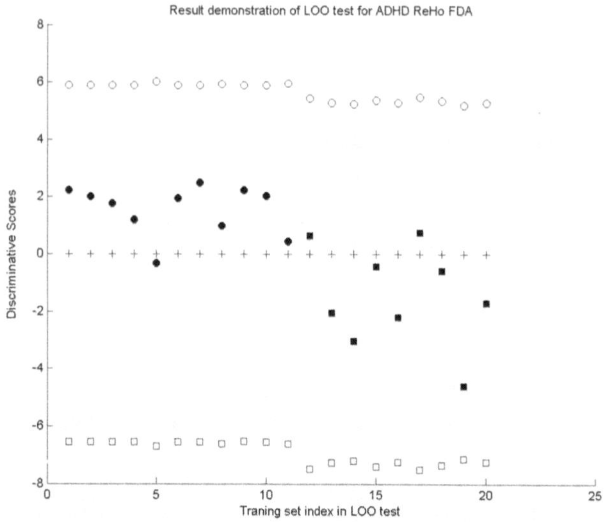

Fig. 1. Distribution of discriminative scores in LOO test

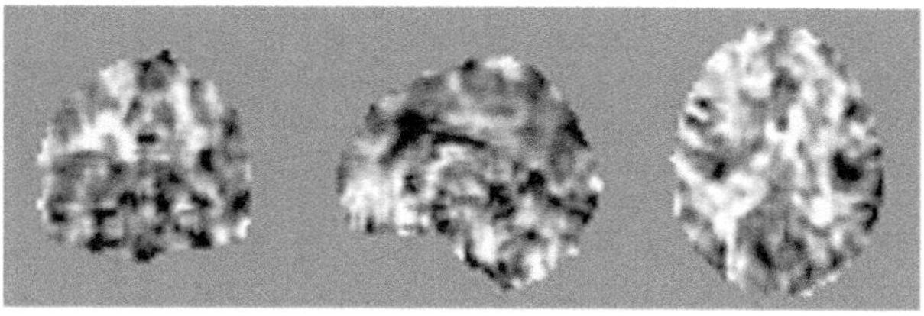

Fig. 2. Fisher brain to visualize the discriminative pattern

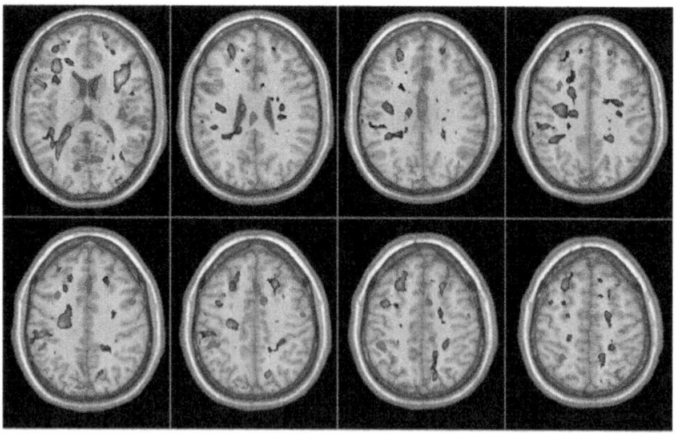

Fig. 3. Highly discriminative regions identified by Fisher brain. Red: ADHD>control; Blue: ADHD<control.

higher brain functions like attention and inhibition and abnormal for ADHD subjects [1, 2, 4, 7]. Moreover, some less reported but highly discriminative regions are also identified.

Our classifier was compared with other two typical linear classifiers, Batch Perceptron [20] and linear support vector machine (SVM) [21]. Table 2 lists the classification results of the three methods. Considering the stochastic property of Batch Perceptron algorithm, we repeated the 20-round LOO test for 10 times, each with a random initialization. Then the correct rates of 10 times of LOO tests were averaged as the final result of Batch Perceptron. From Table 2 we see that Batch Perceptron (54%) hardly yields a meaningful result. Though linear SVM has much better performance than Batch Perceptron, its classification rate (80%) is obviously lower than that of the proposed classifier (85%).

Table 2. Comparison of different linear classifer

Methods	LOO test correct rate		
	Controls	ADHD	Total
Batch Perceptron	62%	46%	54%
Linear SVM	100%	56%	80%
Proposed	91%	78%	85%

To compare the discriminative ability of functional brain information with that of structural brain information, FDA was also applied to 3D structural MR images. All 3D structural MR images were spatially normalized using SPM2 [25]. To comprehensively investigate the discriminative ability of structural brain information, both original 3D MR images and their tissue segmentation results were used as the classification features. Multi-context fuzzy clustering (MCFC) algorithm was used for tissue segmentation since it is insensitive to the intensity inhomogeneities [26]. The classification results of FDA using original MR images and segmented images are depicted in the second and third row of Table 1 respectively. Generally speaking, no significant difference in classification performance appears between intensity based approach and morphology based one, and none of them yield a meaningful classification result (53%). The results clearly demonstrate that ReHo map, as a mapping of brain function of resting state, is more effective for discrimination of ADHD than structural information of either the original MR intensity or the tissue segmentation result. More importantly, this implies that brain function may be more susceptible than brain structures for ADHD.

6 Conclusion

In this paper, a discriminative model of ADHD was proposed on the basis of Fisher discriminative analysis of ReHo map derived from fMRI scanned at resting state. The validation of the method was verified by experimental results. Compared with various classifiers and classification features, our method achieved much better classification performance. Furthermore, it yielded a significant representation for the discriminative pattern of brain function between the children with ADHD and the normal controls. Potential improvement of the diagnosis and treatment evaluation of ADHD can be realized based on the evidence given by the results of the discriminative model.

Evaluation of the proposed method with larger sample size and multi-center imaging data of children with ADHD is considered in future work. The statistic property of the Fisher brain is another issue to be addressed. Moreover, those less reported but highly discriminative regions found in this study will be further examined.

Acknowledgement. This work was partially supported by the Natural Science Foundation of China, Grant No. 30425004, the National Key Basic Research and Development Program (973) Grant No. 2003CB716103, and Natural Science Foundation of China, Grant No. 30470575.

References

1. S.H. Mostofsky, K.L. Cooper, and W.R. Kates, et al. Smaller prefrontal and premotor volumes in boys with attention-deficit/hyperactivity disorder. Biol Psychiatry 52(8):785-794, 2002.
2. E.R. Sowell and P.M. Thompson et al. Cortical abnormalities in children and adolescents with attention deficit hyperactivity disorder. THE LANCET, 362: 1699-1707, 2003.
3. P.C. Berquin, J.N. Giedd, L.K. Jacobsen, S.D. Hamburger, and A.L. Krain, et al. Cerebellum in attention-deficit hyperactivity disorder: a morphometric MRI study. Neurology 50:1087-1093, 1998.
4. G. Bush, J. A. Frazier, S. L. Rauch, and L. J. Seidman, et al, Anterior Cingulate Cortex Dysfunction in Attention Deficit/Hyperactivity Disorder Revealed by fMRI and the Counting Stroop. BIOL PSYCHIATRY 45:1542–1552, 1999.
5. C.J. Vaidya, G. Austin, G. Kirkorian, H.W. Ridlehuber, J.E. Desmond, G.H. Glover, and J.D. Gabrieli. Selective effects of methylphenidate in attention deficit hyperactivity disorder: A functional magnetic resonance study. Proc Natl Acad Sci U S A, 95:14494-14499, 1998.
6. M. Semrud-Clikeman, R.J. Steingard, P. Filipek, J. Biederman, K. Bekken, and P.F. Renshaw. Using MRI to examine brain-behavior relationships in males with attention deficit disorder with hyperactivity. J Am Acad Child Adolesc Psychiatry, 39:477-484, 2000.
7. L.J. Seidman, E.M. Valera, and G. Bush. Brain function and structure in adults with attention-deficit/hyperactivity disorder. Psychiatr Clin N Am, 27: 323-347, 2004.
8. P. Golland, W. E. L. Grimson, M. E. Shenton, and R. Kikinis, Deformation Analysis for Shape Based Classification.,In Proc. IPMI'2001, LNCS 2082, pp. 517-530
9. Z.Q. Lao, D.G. Shen, Z. Xue, B. Karacali S. M. Resnick, and C. Davatzikosa, Morphological classification of brains via high-dimensional shape transformations and machine learning methods, NeuroImage, 21 (2004) 46–57.
10. Y.X Liu. L. Teverovskiy, and O. Carmichael et al., Discriminative MR Image Feature Analysis for Automatic Schizophrenia and Alzheimer's Disease Classification, MICCAI 2004, LNCS 3216, pp. 393–401,2004.
11. J. Stoeckel, N. Ayache, and G. Malandain et al., Automatic Classification of SPECT Images of Alzheimer's Disease Patients and Control Subjects. MICCAI 2004, LNCS 3217, pp. 654–662, 2004.

12. D. Kontos, V. Megalooikonomou, and D. Pokrajac, et al., Extraction of Discriminative Functional MRI Activation Patterns and an Application to Alzheimer's Disease, MICCAI 2004, LNCS 3217, pp. 727–735, 2004.
13. B.B. Biswal, F.Z. Yetkin, V.M. Haungton, J.S. Hyde. Functional connectivity in the motor cortex of resting human brain using echo-planar MRI, Magn Reson Med., 34:537-541, 1995.
14. M.J. Lowe, B.J. Mock and J.A. Sorenson. Functional connectivity in single and multi,slice echoplanar imaging suing resting-state fluctuation, NeuroImage, 7:119-132. 1998.
15. D. Cordes, V.M. Haughton and K. Arfanakis et al. Mapping functionally related regions of brain with functional connectivity MR imaging. AJNR Am J Neuroradiol, 21:1636-1644. 2000.
16. S.J. Li, Z. Li, G.H. Wu, M.J. Zhang, M. Franczak and P.G. Antuono. Alzheimer Disease: Evaluation of a Functional MR Imaging Index as a Marker. Radiology, 225:253–259, 2002.
17. M. E. Raichle, A. M. MacLeod, A. Z. Snyder, W. J. Powers, D. A. Gusnard, and G. L.Shulman. A default mode of brain function. Proc. Natl. Acad. Sci. USA 98,676-682, 2001
18. Y.F. Zang, T.Z. Jiang et al,. Regional homogeneity approach to fMRI data analysis. NeuroImage, 22: 394-400 2004.
19. Y. He, Y.F. Zang, T.Z. Jiang and M. Liang, Detecting Functional Connectivity of the Cerebellum Using Low Frequency Fluctuations (LFFs). MICCAI 2004, LNCS 3217, pp. 907–915, 2004.
20. R. Duda, P. Hart, and D. Stork. Pattern Classification. John Wiley & Sons, New York, 2001.
21. V.N. Vapnik. Statistical Learning Theory. J. Wiley, New York. 1998.
22. P. N. Belhumeur, J. P. Hespanha and D. J. Kriegman. Eigenfaces vs. Fisherfaces: Recognition Using Class Specific Linear Projection. IEEE Trans. PAMI 19: 711-720, 1997.
23. S. Raudys and R.P.W. Duin. Expected classification error of the Fisher linear classifier with pseudo-inverse covariance matrix.Pattern Recognition Letters, 19:385–392, 1998.
24. J. Yang and J.Y. Yang. Why can LDA bc performed in PCA transformed space? Pattern Recognition 36,563 – 566, 2003.
25. K. J. Friston, A. P. Holmes and K. J. Worsley et al., Statistical parametric maps infunctional imaging: A general approach. Hum. Brain Mapp., 2:189–210, 1995.
26. C.Z. Zhu and T. Z. Jiang. Multicontext fuzzy clustering for separation of brain tissues in magnetic resonance images. NeuroImage, 18(3): 685-696, 2003.

Finding Landmarks in the Functional Brain: Detection and Use for Group Characterization

Bertrand Thirion[1], Philippe Pinel[2], and Jean-Baptiste Poline[1]

[1] Service Hospitalier Frédéric Joliot,
Département de Recherche Médicale - CEA - DSV
4, Place du Général Leclerc 91401 Orsay Cedex, France
{thirion, poline, pinel}@shfj.cea.fr
[2] Unité INSERM 562 "Neuroimagerie Cognitive",
Service Hospitalier Frédéric Joliot, CEA/DRM/DSV,
4, Place du Général Leclerc, 91401 Orsay cedex, France

Abstract. FMRI group studies are usually based on stereotactic spatial normalization and present voxel by voxel average activity across subjects. This technique does not in general adequately model the inter subject spatial variability. In this work, we propose to identify functional landmarks that are reliable across subjects with subject specific Talairach coordinates that are similar -but not exactly identical- between subjects. We call these Brain Functional Landmarks (BFLs), and define them based on cross-validation techniques using 38 subjects. We explore a dataset acquired while subjects were involved in several cognitive and sensori-motor processes, and show that this representation allows to classify subjects into sub-groups on the basis of their BFL activity.

1 Introduction

Across subjects variability of both the anatomical and functional organization of the brain is often observed in brain imaging [13] but rarely studied in depth. The causes of the observed fMRI variability are numerous and often difficult to discriminate. Some of it may be due to anatomical variability [7], and some to variation in the organization of the functional topography of our cognitive processes; part of it depends on the (current) physiological state of the subject at the time of scanning, and part is due to acquisition noise. The first two causes may well reflect both genetic or epigenetic factors. This leads to strong variability both in the *i) position* and in the *ii) activity level* (contrast to noise ratio: CNR) of the hemodynamic signal measured in fMRI.

This inter-subject variability strongly impacts the sensitivity of group studies [6,8], and currently the solution most widely adopted resorts to i) stereotactic normalization followed by spatial smoothing (often 12-14 mm Gaussian FWHM), and ii) assuming that voxel intensity follows a Gaussian distribution [1]. Both the current spatial and intensity models are probably suboptimal.

Global measures of the overall variability between subjects have been proposed and allow to address group homogeneity [11,4], but more local analyzes are needed to decompose the sources of variability. This combines with the need for

J. Duncan and G. Gerig (Eds.): MICCAI 2005, LNCS 3750, pp. 476–483, 2005.

sparser representation of brain activity that would open the way to techniques that are too computationally demanding in a dense (voxel based) representation of the functional activity. To some extent, thresholding activation maps turns a dense representation into a sparse one, but this operation is not robust to inter-session variations [8,10] and does not model the spatial variability.

The reduction of the volume-based information to a representation that retains the essential organization of the functional activity across subjects is crucial for many applications in the field of brain mapping, and the present paper is a step towards this goal. This reduction enforces the following constraints:

- Some cognitive processes (possibly not all) give rise to stable topographic organization across subjects [9].
- A common topographic organization may, however, result in different spatial positions when functional images are normalized to a standard template. Mild spatial variability across subjects should thus be modelled.
- Quantitatively, one can expect a relatively high inter-subject variability in the contrast magnitude or CNR. The relative activation magnitude (e.g. local maxima of the contrast maps) may thus better characterize the activation topography than across subject random effect tests.

The aim of the present work is to detect adapted landmarks, which we henceforth call Brain Functional Landmarks (BFLs). We propose to base our detection on the *reproducibility* of the occurrence of activations across subjects for some given contrasts. This analysis yields a topographic representation of the functional brain, and quantitative measurements of the spatial and contrast/CNR variability across subjects. We further use those results to classify subjects into subgroups with similar BFL activities.

The sequel of this paper is organized as follows. In section 2, we describe the dataset and the procedure that are used for the detection of BFLs. In section 3, we describe our results on the BFL detection and the use of BFLs to study the functional population variability. We discuss the technical aspects and implications of this work in section 4.

2 Materials and Methods

Datasets and pre-processing. We used an event-related experimental *Localizer* paradigm that comprises ten conditions. Subjects underwent a series of stimuli or were engaged in tasks such as passive viewing of horizontal or vertical checkerboards, left click after audio or video instruction, right click after audio or video instruction, computation (subtraction) after video or audio instruction, sentence listening and reading. Events were occurring randomly in time (mean inter stimulus interval: 3s), with ten occurrences per event type (except motor button clicks for which there were only five trials).

Thirty-eight right-handed subjects participated in the study. The subjects gave informed consent and the protocol was approved by the local ethics committee. Functional images were acquired on a 3T Bruker scanner using an EPI sequence (TR $= 2400ms$, TE $= 60ms$, matrix size$=64\times64$, FOV $= 24cm\times24cm$).

Each volume consisted of 34 $4mm$-thick axial slices without gap. A session comprised 130 scans. Anatomical T1 images were acquired on the same scanner, with a spatial resolution of $1 \times 1 \times 1.2\ mm^3$.

fMRI data pre-processing consisted in 1) temporal Fourier interpolation to correct for between-slice timing, 2) motion estimation. For all subjects, motion estimates were smaller than 1mm and 1 degree, so that no correction was performed on the datasets; 3) anatomo-functional image coregistration and spatial normalization of the functional images. This pre-processing was performed using the SPM2 software (see www.fil.ucl.ac.uk, [1]). Statistical analysis of the dataset was also carried out with the SPM2 software, using standard high-pass filtering and AR(1) whitening. For further analysis, we used the effect magnitude (GLM parameters) and significance (P-values) for each subject and contrast of interest.

Detection of BFLs. We define a Brain Functional Landmark (BFL) as a locus *around which* an activation can reliably be found across subjects.

An overall description of the BFL detection procedure is given in Fig. 1. We proceed as follows: Given N datasets (subjects), we smooth the parameter map of $(N-1)$ subjects and derive the corresponding random effect (RFX) map. We retain the maxima $M^i, i = 1..I$ of the maps that are above a rather liberal statistical threshold ($p_1 < 10^{-3}$, uncorrected). Then we find the nearest local maximum of the corresponding unsmoothed, thus bias free, statistical map in each subject. The positions $\tau_n^i, n = 1..N-1, i = 1..I$ of these local maxima define an area R^i. The region R^i is defined as a ball of center $c_i = \frac{1}{N-1}\sum_n \tau_n^i$ and radius $r_i = \sqrt{\frac{5}{3(N-1)}\sum_n \|c_i - \tau_n^i\|^2}$. This is equivalent to assuming a compactly supported, locally uniform spatial distribution of (τ^i) across the population. Then we perform the following test on the remaining dataset: if there is an activated voxel in the region R^i with corrected probability $p_2 < 0.05$, the locus c_i is retained as a potential BFL . We used the Bonferroni correction for multiple comparisons for the number of voxels in R^i.

This procedure is performed N times, one of the subjects being left out, and provides a collection of BFL candidates $c^i(n)$ (region i, subject n left out). This collection of BFL candidates is naturally redundant: if a candidate $c^i(l)$ is detected when subject l is left out, it -or a very close point $c^j(k)$- may also be detected when subject k is left out. Thus we perform an average link agglomerative clustering of the candidates, with a stopping criterion $\delta = 5mm$. The clusters of candidates are finally validated when they contain at least $\nu = N/2$ candidates. This procedure reduces the risk of false positives to $\alpha < V(\delta)p_1 p_2^\nu$, where $V(\delta)$ is the volume (in voxels) of a ball of radius δ, making it negligible in practice. Milder thresholds on ν, e.g. $\nu = N/4$, may be used when one is interested in finding landmarks on specific sub-groups of subjects. Therefore, ν, the number of candidates within a cluster, is a measure of the reproducibility of the BFL candidate. The BFLs are chosen on the basis of reproducibility and not contrast to noise ratio. Note that the algorithm adapts to the number of subjects N.

Despite smoothing, the initial RFX test in the detection procedure may contain several local maxima close to one another (possibly because of

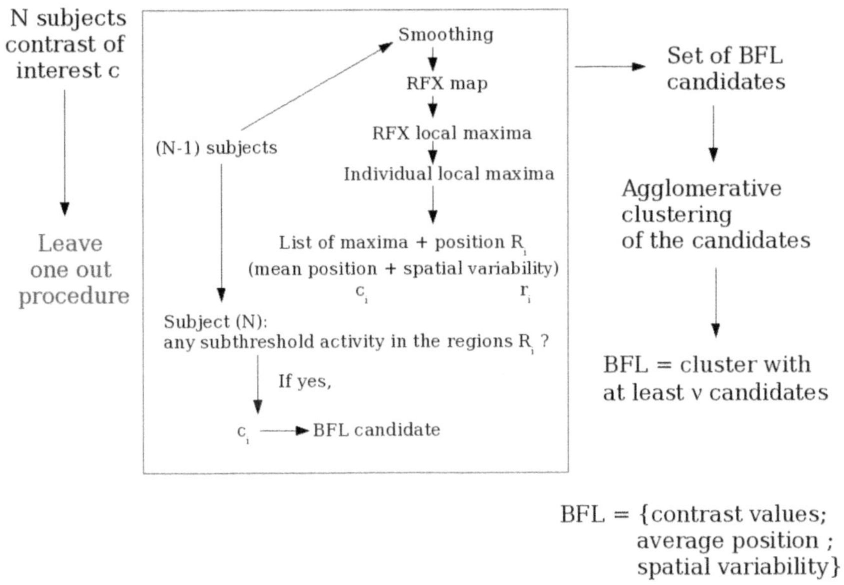

Fig. 1. Flowchart of our method for the extraction of Brain Functional Landmarks (BFLs). Of note, default choices for all the parameters can be easily set. This algorithm adapts to the number of subjects N; for each BFL and each subject, it yields a signal value and a position that can be further processed.

mis-registrations) which may yield confounding patterns. We avoid this by restricting our definition of local maxima to maxima within a rather large neighbourhood, $(5 \times 5 \times 5)$ voxels or greater, of the RFX map.

The information conveyed by BFLs. The definition of landmarks across a population provides a subject-specific representation of both the activation position foci and the magnitude of the effect. This allows an exploration of the activation pattern, and of the relative importance of the different regions across groups of subjects. While the contrast magnitude and statistical significance essentially classify subjects into groups activating weakly or strongly (data not shown), classification of the relative ranking (order statistics) of the different foci yields a more useful information. We use an agglomerative algorithm to check whether several subgroups can be defined in the population, and represent the average relative activation magnitude for each group.

3 Results

The BFLs found in the Localizer experiment. We applied BFL detection on the 38 subjects and the following contrasts: right click-left click; left-right click; audio

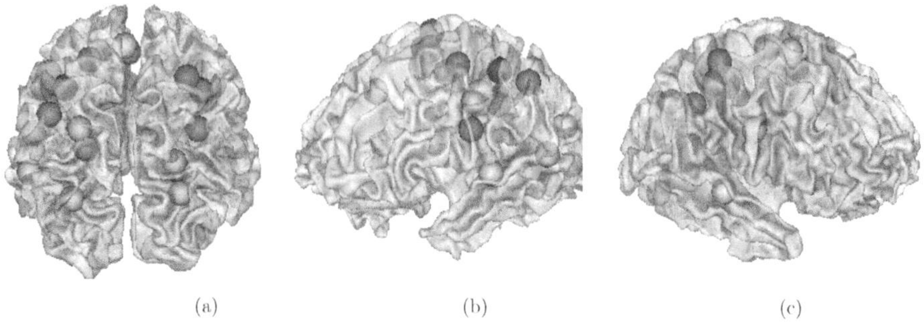

Fig. 2. Representation of the functional BFLs found on the group of subjects, on the left and right grey-white matter interface of an individual brain. (a) View from the occipital side, (b) left hemisphere, (c) right hemisphere. The color codes for the contrast associated with each BFL: Yellow BFLs for the *audio-video* contrast, green for the opposite contrast, dark blue for the *right-left click* contrast, red for the opposite, pink for the *computation-sentence understanding* contrast and light blue for the *reading-passive viewing* contrast. Note that subject specific loci could be reported on their own anatomy.

instructions-video instructions; video instructions-audio instructions; computation-sentence reading/listening; sentences reading-low level visual stimulation. The threshold ν is set to $\nu = N/2$. The BFL detection lasts about one minute per contrast with a C/Matlab code. The result is displayed in Fig. 2 on one subject grey-white matter interface, with respectively 2, 1, 9, 2, 6 and 3 BFLs for the above contrasts. This readily yields a topography of the functional brain.

Study of the relative activation magnitude in the population of subjects. Using the same experimental data, we chose to explore the *computation-sentence reading* contrast of interest. Lowering ν to $N/4$, we obtained 11 BFLs in the population for this contrast, located in the parietal and frontal cortices. For each subject, the BFLs are ranked according to their CNR, and a maximum link agglomerative clustering is applied to this rank data ; 3 clusters were found to be representative (data not shown). Fig 3(a) represents a 3D multidimensional scaling (MDS) plot of the rank data, and the three clusters formed by the algorithm. The size of the three subgroups are 14, 18 and 6 subjects respectively. The average network of activations in each subgroup is presented in Fig. 3(b-d).

Although these results are still preliminary and require more validations, recent work on computation [5] indicate that different activation strengths in the parietal cortex imply a stronger (Fig. 3d) or weaker (Fig. 3b) involvement of visual-spatial attention in the subtraction task; the strong dissymmetry of the parietal activation (group Fig. 3c) may indicate a stronger involvement of language areas in the task. Altogether, these three groups might thus represent different subjects strategies when computing (or reading).

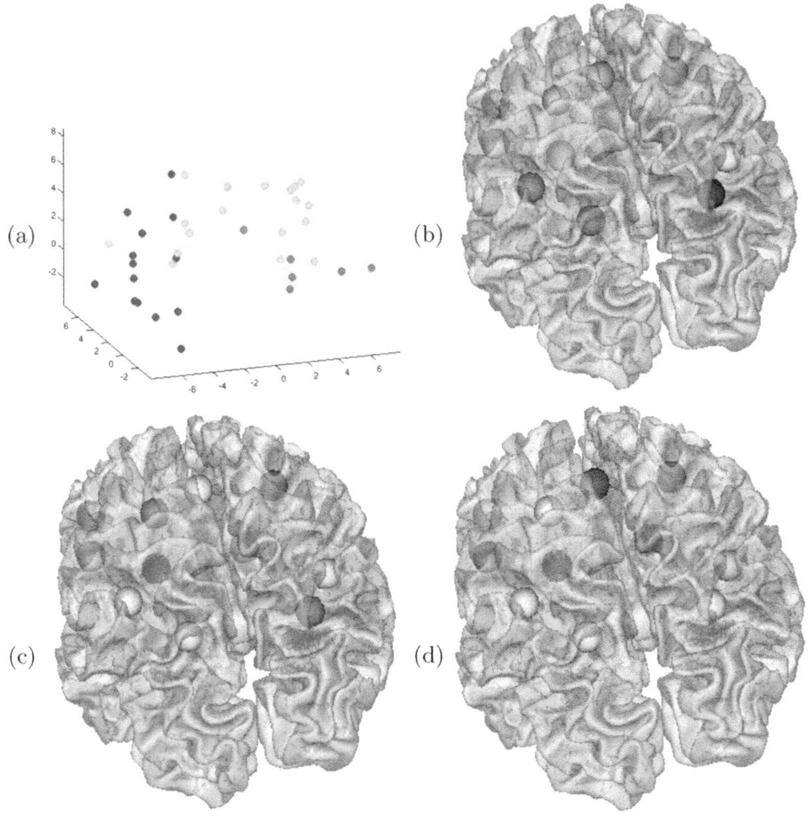

Fig. 3. Classification of the subjects according to the magnitude of their activity in different foci for the *computation- sentence reading* contrast. (a) 3-D MDS plot of the population. The maximum link clustering algorithm indicates a 3 classes structure. (b)(c)(d): Representation of the activation networks on the 11 foci defined by the BFLs. The color codes for the relative magnitude of activation, from weak (brown) to strong (yellow-white). These foci are superimposed on a standard grey-white matter interface.

4 Discussion and Conclusion

Dense versus sparse approaches in neuroimaging. So far, functional MR images have mainly been considered as unstructured fields of data from which information is extracted through statistical thresholding. Such a point of view is limited in the case of multi-subject studies, in which voxel-based inference treats different sources of variability as confounds and tries to reduce their impact by smoothing (see [1]). We propose here an alternative solution to extract and quantify what is common and what is variable across subjects. Obviously, this cannot be performed on dense data fields, and one has to turn to sparse representations. This is fortunate, since neuroimaging inference is generally concerned with extracting specific networks of regions, and not with each and every voxel in the whole brain volume.

Consequently, so long as brain anatomy should be better described by sulco-gyral or cytoarchitectonic structures, our results show that the brain can be endowed with some landmarks which can be used for a better and adaptable definition of regions of interests. To our knowledge, this is the first landmark-based approach in functional neuroimaging.

Detection of the BFLs. We have designed a BFL detection procedure that is robust to slight displacements of a focus of activation across subjects. Our method consists in a leave-one-out procedure, where learning is performed on second-level (inter-subject) statistics and test on first-level (intra-subject) statistics. This double thresholding has two advantages: it enables a relatively mild threshold at each step, and adapts to small populations. Since it is specifically based on the maxima of the map, unlike dense approaches, this procedure is not too sensitive to a particular choice of a P-value.

Although different approaches are possible, e.g. inter-subject clustering of the activated areas [12,9], the present method has the advantage of being computationally efficient, robust to displacement and easily interpretable. Moreover, it is controlled by reproducibility criteria that are more reliable than cluster selection techniques. While the method still requires further validations, it showed promising results on our data.

Use of BFL activity to characterize population subgroups. A tremendous advantage of sparse representations is that they allow an easy comparison of subjects activity: while distance between functional images provide very useful insight on the homogeneity of populations [11,4], the use of BFLs simplifies the picture by concentrating on informative regions that are not arbitrarily selected. In particular, our example in Fig. 3, shows interpretable subgroup structures for a contrast of interest. This study would greatly benefit from a more systematic comparison of the activation magnitude and significance across subjects and experimental conditions, that would clarify region-based inference [3]. We emphasize that such comparisons are precisely allowed by BFLs, whereas direct image comparisons may be confounded by the spatial variability of activated regions.

Conclusion and future work. The information carried out by fMRI activation images is seen in this work to have a topographic representation at least partially reproducible across subjects. This, together with functional localization studies [2,9] has led us to the concept of Brain Functional Landmark (BFL). We have shown that the detection of these landmarks, based on a reproducibility criterion, is relatively easy, and allows for sparse and thus manipulable representation of the brain functional information. Moreover, we have shown that such a sparse representation can be used to study, across individuals, the spatial topography of a cognitive network defined by computation minus sentence reading.

It can be noticed that robust detection of BFLs is a step forward in the representation of the population in a common referential (normalization).

Straightforward extensions of this work are *i)* the study of the warp implied by the spatial variability of BFLs across subjects *ii)* the comparison and the merge of BFLs with anatomical landmarks [7] and *iii)* the use of this information for spatial normalization and signal calibration.

Acknowledgments. We thank our colleagues S. Dehaene, A. Jobert, for their participation in this project for helpful discussions and ideas. This work was partly funded by the French ministry of research through concerted actions 'masse de données', 'neurosciences intégratives et computationnelles' and 'connectivité'.

References

1. J. Ashburner, K.J. Friston, and W. Penny, editors. *Human brain functions, 2nd Edition.* Academic press, 2004.
2. K. Grill-Spector, N. Knouf, and N. Kanwisher. The fusiform face area subserves face perception, not generic within-category identification. *Nat Neurosci*, 7(5):555–62, May 2004.
3. T. L Jernigan, A. C Gamst, C. Fennema-Notestine, and A. L Ostergaard. More "mapping" in brain mapping: statistical comparison of effects. *Hum Brain Mapp*, 19(2):90–5, Jun 2003.
4. F. Kherif, J.-B. Poline, S. Mériaux, H. Benali, G. Flandin, and M. Brett. Group analysis in functional neuroimaging: selecting subjects using similarity measures. *Neuroimage*, 20(4):2197–2208, January 2004.
5. C. Lemer, S. Dehaene, E. Spelke, and L. Cohen. Approximate quantities and exact number words: dissociable systems. *Neuropsychologia*, 41(14):1942–58, 2003.
6. M. Liou, H.-R. Su et al. Bridging functional MR images and scientific inference: Reproducibility maps. *Journal of Cognitive Neuroscience*, 15(7):935–945, 2003.
7. J.-F. Mangin, D. Rivière, A. Cachia, E. Duchesnay, Y. Cointepas, D. Papadopoulos-Orfanos, P. Scifo, T. Ochiai, F. Brunelle, and J. Régis. A framework to study the cortical folding patterns. *Neuroimage*, 23:S129–S138, 2004.
8. K. Murphy and H. Garavan. An empirical investigation into the number of subjects required for an event-related fMRI study. *Neuroimage*, 22(2):879–85, 2004.
9. O. Simon, F. Kherif et al. Automatized clustering and functional geometry of human parietofrontal networks for language, space, and number. *Neuroimage*, 23(3):1192–1202, 11 2004.
10. S. M Smith, C. F Beckmann et al. Variability in fMRI: a re-examination of intersession differences. *Hum Brain Mapp*, 24(3):248–57, Mar 2005.
11. S. C Strother, J. Anderson et al. The quantitative evaluation of functional neuroimaging experiments: the NPAIRS data analysis framework. *Neuroimage*, 15(4):747–71, Apr 2002.
12. B. Thirion and O. Faugeras. Feature detection in fMRI data: The information bottleneck approach. In *Proc. 6th MICCAI*, pages 83–91, Montreal, Nov 2003.
13. X. Wei, S.-S. Yoo, C. C. Dickey, K. H Zou, C. R G Guttmann, and L. P. Panych. Functional MRI of auditory verbal working memory: long-term reproducibility analysis. *Neuroimage*, 21(3):1000–8, 2004.

Topology Correction Using Fast Marching Methods and Its Application to Brain Segmentation

Pierre-Louis Bazin and Dzung L. Pham

Johns Hopkins University, Baltimore, USA

Abstract. We present here a new method for correcting the topology of objects segmented from medical images. Whereas previous techniques alter a surface obtained from the hard segmentation of the object, our technique works directly in the image domain, propagating the topology for all isosurfaces of the object. From an analysis of topological changes and critical points in implicit surfaces, we introduce a topology progagation algorithm that enforces any desired topology using a fast marching technique. Compared to previous topology correction techniques, the method successfully corrects topology while effecting fewer changes to the original volume.

1 Introduction

The topological properties of two-dimensional (2D) and three-dimensional (3D) objects are often very simple, regardless of the complexity of the geometric object. The cortex of the human brain is a striking example; despite its intricate folds, it is considered to have the topology of a sphere, without any holes or handle-like junctions. Most organs and sub-structures found in the human body also share this spherical topology.

Ideally, algorithms that extract objects from 2D or 3D images should respect the object topology. A major problem is that topology is a *global* property of the object, whereas most extraction techniques operate locally on the pixels or voxels of an image. One solution is to start from an object with the desired topology and deform it on the image to follow the shape of the object to extract [10,7,3]. However, surface segmentation algorithms that constrain the topology also require an initialization close to the object of interest. Correcting the topology of objects is therefore often necessary, either before or after the surface extraction from an initial segmentation. This initial segmentation is typically the result of a fuzzy or statistical classification algorithm [9,11]) that computes a normalized membership value for each class and each pixel that varies continuously between zero and one.

Current algorithms for topology correction, however, operate on a binary volume extracted from the classification of the image data [16,13,6,15], generally obtained by performing a threshold at the 0.5 level set of the membership function for the class. Two types of techniques can be found in the literature: graph-based analysis and correction [6,15], and distance function processing, inspired by level set methods [16,13]. In places where changes are needed to enforce the spherical topology, these methods must decide whether to cut a handle or fill a hole, and where to proceed, based solely on the geometry of the original surface. In brain segmentation applications, the binary volumes also require pre-procesing to remove isolated parts and close holes [16,6,15].

J. Duncan and G. Gerig (Eds.): MICCAI 2005, LNCS 3750, pp. 484–491, 2005.

Graph-based techniques convert the objects into graphs using either the 2D slices or a morphological opening to isolate sub-structures. The graph is then processed to identify cycles and remove them from the volume. The complexity of the analysis increases rapidly with the object size, and problems can occur at unusual configurations. Level set methods compute a distance function to encode the object shape, which changes when the volume is edited. In [13], candidate regions for addition or removal are identified and ranked through their distance function, so they must be recomputed whenever the object is modified and there is no guaranteed convergence. In all these methods, the intensity information available in the original image or in the membership function is largely ignored. If the object is highly convoluted, it may happen that the smallest change with regard to the geometry of the binary volume corresponds to including points with very low membership, or discarding points with very high membership.

In this work, we propose a new topology correction algorithm that can act directly on the membership function instead of the binary segmentation. The method propagates rigorous topological constraints on scalar 2D and 3D functions, even in the presence of noise. With a single computation of a modified fast marching method, the topology of the entire image is corrected. All isosurfaces extracted from the membership function or volumetric data will have the same topology, and we can even enforce non-spherical topologies, given an appropriate initialization. By working on the continuously-valued classification data rather than the binary segmentation, the amount of change effected by the topology correction is substantially reduced. The proposed method also provides greater flexibility in defining a desired surface. In some applications, isosurfaces at values other than 0.5 can be desirable [17]. Previous methods would require a separate topology correction for every desired isosurface value.

The paper is organized as follows. In Section 2, we study the topological properties of scalar fields and present a topology-preserving approximation algorithm for distance functions and membership functions. Section 3 details the topology correction algorithm, and Section 4 demonstrates its application to magnetic resonance brain images.

2 Topological Properties of Scalar Fields

Consider the general problem of extracting an object with a given topology from an image I in $\mathbb{R}^3$. The object is represented as a volume V bounded by a surface S, defined as the zero level set of a signed distance function d: $S = \{x \in \mathbb{R}^3 | d(x) = 0\}$. The image itself is a function of the object, and can be a distance function, membership function, or some other function. The image and the distance function are digital, so the values of x are defined on a regular grid of voxels. The topology of the surface is characterized globally by its Euler Number. This measure, however, does not account for the type, location or extent of local topology changes.

In scalar fields, topology changes occur only at critical points [8,18]. These points are the singular points of the implicit isosurfaces, an extension of the non-simple points of binary images[2,4,7]. They have been classified in [18] as *regular, flat, minimal, maximal* and *saddle* points, either *local* or *extended*. At any non-regular point or region made of extended non-regular points, topology changes may occur when the isovalue used to construct the surface is equal to the value at that point.

If the surface is moved away from its zero level set, it will keep the same topology until it reaches the value of a critical point. The changes are difficult to predict without a fine analysis of the critical point type (e.g. saddle points can have different effects). The only simple way to keep the topology invariant is to remove all critical points.

To identify critical points, consider the distance function $d(x)$ at a point x. We define positive, negative and equal regions to be connected regions of neighboring points y with $d(y) > d(x)$, $d(y) < d(x)$, $d(y) = d(x)$, respectively). The neighborhood of a point is defined as the set of 6,18 or 26-connected neighbors on the digital grid of x values. The numbers N_p, N_n and N_e of positive, negative and equal regions within a neighborhood determines the type of the point (see [1] for more details). The choice of connectivity will affect the shape of the object, as we will detail later. It is enough for the subsequent analysis to know if a point is regular or critical:

$$x \text{ is regular} \equiv N_p(x) = N_n(x) = 1, N_e(x) = 0$$

Regions of equal value are a practical problem, as globally regular or critical regions could have the same N_p, N_n and N_e in a small neighborhood (e.g. subsample the grid by a factor 2: all points have equal neighbors and become critical). We can remove that problem by grouping equal points within either positive or negative regions.

2.1 Topology-Preserving Distance Functions

To compute the distance function $d(x)$ efficiently, we rely on a fast marching method, implemented through a binary tree sorting technique [14]: all points outside of the initial surface S_0 are ranked into a binary tree depending on their distance $d(X)$ to the surface (initially, the distances are all equal to 1, but will increase as the algorithm evolves), then the surface is brought in front of the first of those points. Its neighbors (now in front of the surface) are added to the binary tree with an increased distance value, and the surface is moved again until the tree is empty. This method produces a distance function $d(x)$ accurate up to the grid scale, and the binary tree implementation provides $n \log n$ speed in the image size. To obtain a complete distance function, distances are propagated inside as well as outside S_0, with an inverse sign. With this distance function, arbitrary changes in the isosurface topology will occur when the isovalue is changed: parts will split or merge, holes will appear or disappear, etc (see Fig 1-b).

Using the previous analysis, we construct a modified distance function that will guarantee that the topology of the isosurface stays unchanged for all isovalues. The central idea is to detect critical points and change their distance while propagating the fast marching algorithm:

Algorithm: Topology-preserving distance function

1. *starting from volume V_k bounded by the surface S_k,*
2. *insert the points x on the outside boundary S_k of the volume V_k in the tree, ranked by their distance $d(x)$ (at first, $d(x) = 1$),*
3. *extract the first point x from the tree,*
4. *if the point has been previously labeled as critical, its distance function becomes $d(x) = \max\{d(y)\}$, for y inside the object and neighbors of x, otherwise $d(x)$*
5. *compute the number of positive and negative neighbors for x,*

6. *if x is regular, insert x into the volume and insert its neighbors outside the volume, regular or critical, into the tree with their distance $d(y) = d(x) + 1$*
7. *else, label x as critical and set it aside,*
8. *go back to step 3, until the tree is empty.*

This algorithm produces the regular distance function when the topology is invariant. Critical points are kept outside the volume until the neighboring distances make them regular: the algorithm not only isolates critical points but computes the exact amount of change needed to keep the volume regular while including them. This is illustrated in Figure 1-c: when the isovalue is low, the fingers stay connected from the bottom to the tip, until the distance is high enough in the middle to remove the finger completely. In the original geometric distance function, they split into several pieces before they disappear.

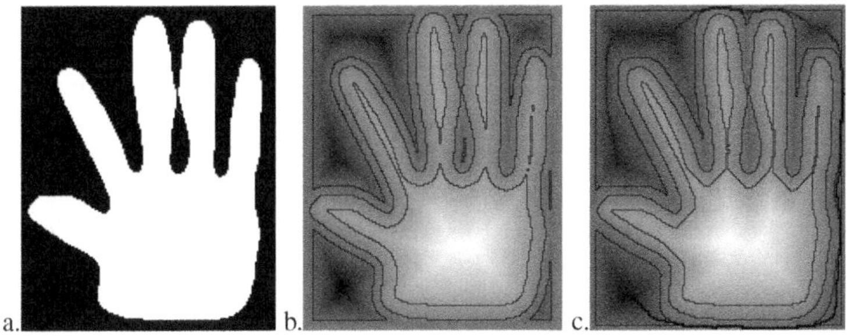

Fig. 1. Distance functions: a) the outline of a hand, b) the regular distance function started from the hand contour with three isocontours outlined, c) the topological distance function, with the same outlined isocontours. Note how the topology is different for the three regular isocontours. The topological distance function includes stronger skeleton-like features in the areas changed to maintain the correct topology, and all its isocontours have the same topology.

In the propagation, the object and background connectivity is controlled in step 5, when computing the number of positive and negative neighbors. If N_p, N_n are computed with 6/26 (resp. 6/18, 18/6, 26/6) connectivity, then the volume and background are 6/26, 6/18, 18/6 or 26/6 connected.

2.2 Topology-Preserving Membership Functions

We can extend the topology propagation from distance functions to general scalar fields. We replace the distance function $d(x)$ with a scalar field $f(x)$ to be approximated by a function $g(x)$. The same propagation algorithm applies to g:

Algorithm: Topology propagation on scalar fields

1. *start from $g(x) = f(x)$ everywhere,*
2. *consider the volume V_k bounded by S_k: $\{x|g(x) <= g_k\}$,*
3. *insert the points x on the boundary (and outside) of the volume V_k in the tree, ranked by their value $g(x)$,*
4. *extract the first point x from the tree,*

5. *if the point has not been labeled as critical, set the value as* $f(x)$*,*
6. *else, the field value becomes* $g(x) = \max\{g(y)\}$ *for* y *inside* V_k *and neighbor of* x*,*
7. *compute the number of positive and negative neighbors for* x*,*
8. *if* x *is regular, insert* x *into the volume (set* $g_k = g(x)$*) and insert its neighbors outside the volume or critical into the tree,*
9. *else, label* x *as critical and set it aside,*
10. *go back to step 2, until the tree is empty.*

This algorithm produces a scalar field as close as possible to $f(x)$, with the same topology as the starting volume V_0. As the changes are propagated along successive isovalues of the image, the technique is guaranteed to succeed in enforcing the original topology of V_0 in every isosurface of $g(x)$.

3 Topology Correction Algorithm

Topology correction aims at enforcing a chosen topology on the objects we want to extract. The correct or desired topology is known a priori, and depends on the application. Unlike previous techniques, our topology propagation technique will not just enforce spherical topology, but propagate through the distance or membership function any prior topology template. For spherical topology, a single point is enough to impose the sphericality constraint. For other topologies, different starting shapes can be used: a closed circle for doughnut or cylinder-like structures, a carved sphere for a hollow object, etc. Once we have chosen the appropriate template, we need to place it inside the object of interest. In the case of non-spherical topology, this step can be difficult as the holes and handles of the template should match those of the image. For spherical topology however, we just need to find a point inside the main object of interest. Starting from this point, we propagate the topology down from the highest membership values to the lowest:

Algorithm: Spherical topology correction
1. *threshold the membership function at the 0.5 isovalue, and select the largest connected region,*
2. *in this region, select one of the points of highest membership value,*
3. *from this original point in the membership function, use the topology propagation algorithm toward lower membership values, with proper connectivity.*

The initialization step ensures that we select a point inside the main structure of interest, except when dealing with several structures of similar size (in such case, it is necessary to select a point for each structure). The topology correction could as easily have started from a bounding box outside the image and converged toward the structure. From our experiments, we found that there is often more noise and outliers in the background area than holes in the high membership regions, and propagating the topology from the background would result in slightly more noise. This choice is consistent with the previous binary techniques that would only include the largest connected component. The corrected image with our algorithm is "included" in the original image: all corrected values can only be inferior or equal to the original ones. Methods to combine both directions of change are non-trivial, and would require to re-evaluate the topology at every change.

4 Experiments

We have gathered a set of 10 brains processed for the Baltimore Longitudinal Study on Aging [12] to test and validate the topology correction algorithm. These brains were first stripped, then segmented into gray matter, white matter and CSF, and the white matter memberships were further edited to fill the sub-cortical area [5]. The images all have a 1mm cubic resolution. We then perform the topology correction on the edited white matter memberships. The chosen connectivity is 18/6, so that we could compare with previous topology correction techniques evaluated on similar data [15,6].

In all cases, the topology correction succeeds. Even though the topology of every isovalue is guaranteed to be spherical, we verified it by automated graph-based analysis [15]. The corrected membership functions are very close to the original ones (cf. Table 1): the number of changed voxels over the entire image is around 10%, and the mean amount of change for these voxels (counting only changed voxels) is below 0.05 (the membership intensities are in $[0, 1]$). The changes counted on the 0.5 isosurfaces are similar to those of previous methods, as shown in Table 2. We obtained results from the GTCA method [6] for the same data, and compared them to our 0.5 isovalues. Even though the proposed method enforces the topology on all isovalues, it causes

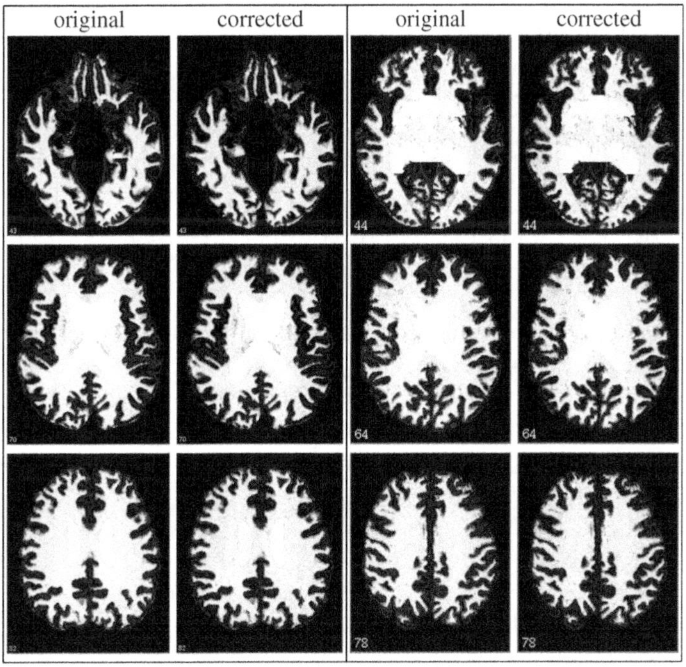

Fig. 2. Two examples of topology correction (brains number 4 and 7 of the experiments): three slices of the white matter membership function after filling of the internal parts, before and after the topology correction. Note the few visible changes: parts with high membership but disconnected from the white matter are removed, loops are cut (see top slices) and some patterns appear in the filled region due to remaining noise.

Table 1. Topology correction on a set of brains

Brain number	Computation time	Total voxels (x10^3)	Changed voxels (x10^3)	% of changed voxels	mean value of change
1	52s	2,997	334	0.111	0.0294
2	63s	3,370	412	0.122	0.0456
3	53s	3,153	352	0.112	0.0471
4	63s	3,654	409	0.112	0.0400
5	59s	3,371	387	0.115	0.0446
6	58s	3,407	383	0.113	0.0498
7	65s	3,449	406	0.118	0.0432
8	63s	3,425	416	0.121	0.0465
9	69s	3,969	467	0.118	0.0448
10	48s	2,862	316	0.110	0.0365

Table 2. Topology correction on a set of brains: extracted 0.5 isovalue

Brain	Initial Topology				Final Topology				Initial	Changed	% of brain	% of change
number	FP	FL	BP	BL	FP	FL	BP	BL	brain size	voxels	changed	with GTCA
1	243	125	20	86	1	0	1	0	607,236	1,422	0.234	0.190
2	368	177	136	112	1	0	1	0	662,357	1,964	0.297	0.253
3	464	380	207	220	1	0	1	0	636,077	2,650	0.417	0.308
4	281	114	150	81	1	0	1	0	708,954	1,279	0.180	0.171
5	373	171	177	149	1	0	1	0	632,431	1,761	0.278	0.237
6	441	218	46	174	1	0	1	0	594,337	2,166	0.364	0.314
7	380	207	36	153	1	0	1	0	700,270	2,174	0.310	0.230
8	483	273	53	231	1	0	1	0	710,775	2,320	0.326	0.245
9	425	245	35	141	1	0	1	0	775,059	2,592	0.334	0.262
10	196	118	17	68	1	0	1	0	522,015	1,182	0.226	0.190

fewer changes on a single isosurface than the graph-based technique. The only places of significant change are the regions close to 0 or 1 ("flat" areas, subject to higher topological noise). The processing times are usually below 1 minute on a Pentium 4 3Ghz PC. GTCA requires approximately 2 minutes on a similar machine. All the brains we have tested so far take about the same time to process, and the amount of change is very similar from one brain to any other.

5 Conclusions

We have introduced in this paper an algorithm for propagating topology over scalar fields. It offers an efficient way to correct the topology of objects with a complex geometry, using all the available information of their membership function. It improves over previous methods by acting on all isovalues rather than a binary volume, and allowing non-spherical topologies. The technique was successfully tested on the problem of cortical segmentation to enforce a proper spherical topology on the white matter/gray matter interface. The propagation algorithm provides fast and reliable results, always very close to the original data. All isovalues have the correct topology, and the changes made on the membership function take into account the geometry of the entire image. The method can be applied to any kind of scalar image data, is fairly robust to noise, and guarantees exact results, in a single fast marching propagation step. Beyond correcting topology for membership functions, it also has potential applications to topology-preserving level set evolution and volumetric segmentation.

References

1. P.-L. Bazin and D. L. Pham. Topology smoothing for segmentation and surface reconstruction. In *Proc. MICCAI'04*, St Malo, Sept. 2004.
2. G. Bertrand. Simple points, topological numbers and geodesic neighborhood in cubic grids. *Pattern Recognition Letters*, 15(10):1003–1011, Oct. 1994.
3. S. Bischoff and L. Kobbelt. Sub-voxel topology control for level-set surfaces. *Computer Graphics Forum*, 22(3):273–280, 2003.
4. M. Couprie, F. Bezerra, and G. Bertrand. Topological operators for grayscale image processing. *Journal of Electronic Imaging*, 10(4):1003–1015, 2001.
5. X. Han, D. Pham, D. Tosun, M. Rettmann, C. Xu, and J. Prince. Cruise: Cortical reconstructiong using implicit surface evolution. *NeuroImage*, 23(3):997–1012, 2004.
6. X. Han, C. Xu, U. Braga-Neto, and J. L. Prince. Topology correction in brain cortex segmentation using a multiscale, graph-based algorithm. *IEEE Trans. Med. Imaging*:109–121, 21(2), 2002.
7. X. Han, C. Xu, and J. L. Prince. A topology preserving level set method for geometric deformable models. *IEEE Trans. PAMI*, 25(6):755–768, June 2003.
8. J. C. Hart. Morse theory for implicit surface modeling. In H.-C. Hege and K. Polthier, editors, *Mathematical Visualization*, pp 257–268. Springer-Verlag, Oct. 1998.
9. K. V. Leemput, F. Maes, D. Vandermeulen, and P. Suetens. Automated model-based tissue classification of mr images of the brain. *IEEE Trans. on Med. Imaging*, 18(10), 1999.
10. J.-F. Mangin, V. Frouin, I. Bloch, J. Regis, and J. Lopez-Krahe. From 3d magnetic resonance images to structural representations of the cortex topography using topology preserving deformations. *J. Math. Imaging and Vision*, 5:297–318, 1995.
11. D. L. Pham. Spatial models for fuzzy clustering. *Computer Vision and Image Understanding*, 84:285–297, 2001.
12. S. M. Resnick, A. F. Goldszal, C. Davatzikos, S. Golski, M. A. Kraut, E. J. Metter, R. N. Bryan, and A. B. Zonderman. One-year age changes in MRI brain volumes in older adults. *Cerebral Cortex*, 10(5):464–472, 2000.
13. F. Segonne, E. Grimson, and B. Fischl. Topological correction of subcortical segmentation. In *Proc. MICCAI'03*, Montreal, Nov. 2003.
14. J. Sethian. *Level Set Methods and Fast Marching Methods*. Cambridge University Press, 1999.
15. D. W. Shattuck and R. M. Leahy. Automated graph-based analysis and correction of cortical volume topology. *IEEE Trans. on Med. Imaging*, 20(11), Nov. 2001.
16. A. Szymczak and J. Vanderhyde. Extraction of topologically simple isosurfaces from volume datasets. In *Proc. IEEE Visualization*, pp 67–74, Seattle, Oct. 2003.
17. D. Tosun, M. Rettmann, D. Naiman, S. Resnick, M. Kraut, and J. Prince. Cortical reconstruction using implicit surface evolution: Accuracy and precision analysis. *submitted to Neuroimage.*
18. G. H. Weber, G. Scheuermann, and B. Hamann. Detecting critical regions in scalar fields. In *Proc. EUROGRAPHICS - IEEE TCVG Symposium on Visualization*, Grenoble, May 2003.

New Ratios for the Detection and Classification of CJD in Multisequence MRI of the Brain

Marius George Linguraru[1,2], Nicholas Ayache[1], Miguel Ángel González Ballester[1,3], Eric Bardinet[4], Damien Galanaud[5,6], Stéphane Haïk[7,8,9], Baptiste Faucheux[7,8], Patrick Cozzone[6], Didier Dormont[4,5], and Jean-Philippe Brandel[7,9]

[1] EPIDAURE Research Group – INRIA Sophia Antipolis, France
[2] Division of Engineering and Applied Sciences, Harvard University, Cambridge MA, USA
[3] MEM-ISTB, University of Bern, Bern, Switzerland
[4] CNRS UPR640-LENA, Paris, France
[5] Department of Neuroradiology, La Pitié-Salpêtrière Hospital, Paris, France
[6] CRMBM UMR CNRS 6612, Faculty of Medicine, Marseille, France
[7] INSERM U360, La Pitié-Salpêtrière Hospital, Paris, France
[8] R. Escourolle Neuropathological Laboratory, La Pitié-Salpêtrière Hospital, Paris, France
[9] The National Reference Cell of CJD, La Pitié-Salpêtrière Hospital, Paris, France
mglin@deas.harvard.edu

Abstract. We present a method for the analysis of deep grey brain nuclei for accurate detection of human spongiform encephalopathy in multisequence MRI of the brain. We employ T1, T2 and FLAIR-T2 MR sequences for the detection of intensity deviations in the internal nuclei. The MR data are registered to a probabilistic atlas and normalised in intensity prior to the segmentation of hyperintensities using a foveal model. Anatomical data from a segmented atlas are employed to refine the registration and remove false positives. The results are robust over the patient data and in accordance to the clinical ground truth. Our method further allows the quantification of intensity distributions in basal ganglia. sCJD patient FLAIR images are classified with a more significant hypersignal in caudate nuclei (10/10) and putamen (6/10) than in thalami. Defining normalised MRI measures of the intensity relations between the internal grey nuclei of patients, we robustly differentiate sCJD and variant CJD (vCJD) patients, as an attempt towards the automatic detection and classification of human spongiform encephalopathies.

1 Introduction

The identification of diagnosis markers is a major challenge in the clinical care of patients with Creutzfeldt-Jakob Disease (CJD). This disease raises a number of questions to neuroradiological centres, due to the limited available knowledge that connects it to medical imaging. Some recent studies [1,5,13] found strong correspondences between the diagnosis of CJD and the detection of signal abnormality in the deep grey matter internal nuclei in Magnetic Resonance Imaging (MRI) of the brain. However, the observations describing the MRI ability to help in the diagnosis of CJD are in an early stage. Most of the studies are concerned with sCJD cases, which represent 80% of all forms of CJD. The first study cases describe

J. Duncan and G. Gerig (Eds.): MICCAI 2005, LNCS 3750, pp. 492–499, 2005.

hypersignals in T2-weighted images (and FLAIR-T2) with higher incidence in the basal ganglia in a bilateral symmetric form [1,6].

A great concern has been the occurrence in the United Kingdom of vCJD in the 1990s, a form of human environmentally acquired CJD. In FLAIR and T2 sequences, abnormal high signals are observed in the thalamus, mainly in the posterior pulvinar nucleus. Unlike in sCJD cases, in vCJD cases abnormal intensities are higher in the pulvinar when compared to striatum [13].

MR related image processing is an important tool in non-invasive CJD diagnosis [5,6]. At present time, MRI is not included as a diagnosis criterion for sCJD, which would be certainly useful to include, as for vCJD [13].

Leemput [12] proposes a method for automated quantification of MR intensity changes in images of CJD patients. A mixture model of normal distributions combined with the expectation-maximisation algorithm (EM) is proposed. However, the method does not detect signal abnormalities in all the CJD cases, while showing significant amounts of false positives (FP) along the interface between grey matter (GM) and cerebrospinal fluid (CSF).

Colchester, Hojjat *et al.* [3,7] analyse the putamen intensity gradient to separate CJD from normals and propose several ratios, (posterior thalamus to caudate and most notably to frontal white matter) to seclude vCJD from the rest. They use T2-weighted and Proton Density MRI for average intensities (no hyperintesnity analysis) and their segmentation is performed manually.

The image blurring due to motion artefacts in the set of images of patients suffering of dementia makes the use of statistical detection algorithms very difficult. They need good contrast between GM and white matter (WM) for stochastic analysis according to a general atlas context. The approach we propose is based on image normalisation and the use of a priori anatomical knowledge in the form of an accurately segmented and labelled image (e.g. the Zubal Phantom [12]) for precise segmentation and of a probabilistic atlas for intra- and inter-patient analysis. A feature detection technique based on a model of the Human Visual System (HVS) is employed for the depiction of hypersignals. We differentiate different types of human prion diseases (sCJD from vCJD) based on the lesions topographical distribution.

2 Pre-processing and Segmentation

The sequences used by our algorithm are: a T1-weighted acquisition for its higher contrast between GM and WM and higher image resolution; T2-weighted images for the good contrast between CSF and brain parenchyma; and a T2-weighted FLAIR sequence for the detection of CJD signs in the brain. We use a model of data normalisation and regularisation, which is required to put the images in the same general framework to reduce the number of parameters. A review of the different stages of our segmentation algorithm is shown in Figure 1.

Data registration to an atlas has become a common technique with the introduction of popular statistical algorithms for image processing. A well-known probabilistic atlas in the scientific community is the MNI Atlas from the Montreal Neurological Institute at McGill University [4] built using over 300 MRI scans of healthy individuals. We used a block matching-based affine transformation described in [10] to register the patient T1, T2 and FLAIR images to the MNI atlas.

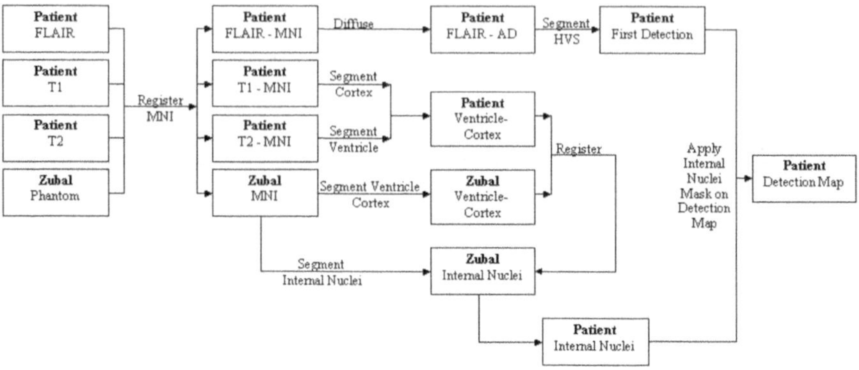

Fig. 1. Flowchart of the algorithm proposed for the detection of CJD-related abnormal hyperintensities in multisequence MRI of the brain

In addition to geometric variability, MR images may also exhibit intensity variations. Our method performs an affine equalisation using the joint histogram of two images [11]: a standard image (from our database) onto which we align the intensity distribution of the second image.

Our analysis is based on the abnormal MR intensities that can appear in the basal ganglia (including the thalamus) of CJD patients, which often show movement artefacts and therefore low contrast in images. The MNI atlas can provide a probabilistic segmentation of GM, which is not precise enough for our application. While avoiding direct non-rigid registration, the affine registration is approximate. We use instead a segmented anatomical atlas of the brain, the Zubal Phantom [12].

The Zubal atlas offers a precisely labelled segmentation of brain structures from the T1-weighted MR image of a single subject. First, the atlas must be aligned to our set of images; thus, we register the Zubal Phantom to the MNI template, again using the block-matching algorithm [10]

Some important anatomical landmarks in the brain that are easier to identify are the ventricles and cortex external boundary. We segment them by morphological opening on patient T1 and T2 images. Ventricles will give a good approximation of the deformation field around the internal nuclei, whereas the cortex boundary will impose the global spatial constraints and stabilise the deformation field inside the brain. We are now in the possession of two binary maps of ventricles and brain boundaries for each patient: one from the Zubal Phantom and the other from the patient. Non-rigid registration is used to align the two images and compute deformation fields, employing the iconic feature-based algorithm described in [2].

We create a mask with the pulvinar, "anterior thalamus" (the part of thalamus with small probability to show abnormal signals in CJD patients), putamen and head of the caudate - which will be referred as internal nuclei for the rest of this paper - from the Zubal Phantom registered on MNI. Then we apply the above computed patient-specific deformation fields to the mask of internal nuclei of the Zubal Phantom. The deformed mask is used to segment the internal nuclei on the patient image.

A foveal segmentation algorithm (HVS) [9] completes the detection of areas of CJD MR hypersignals in the brain. This is in essence an algorithm of adaptive thresholding, which uses a mathematical model of human vision. A simplified model for the computation of the adaptive threshold C_{min} is shown in equation (1), where c_{mpc} is the minimal perceivable contrast, b is constant, μ_N the mean value of the intensity of neighbourhood and μ_A a mean weighted value of neighbourhood and background (entire image).

$$C_{\min} = \frac{c_{mpc}}{\mu_N}\left(b + \sqrt{\frac{\mu_N^{\ 2}}{\mu_A}}\right)^2 \tag{1}$$

c_{mpc} must be computed as a function of the image gradient. In MR images of the brain, the intensity values of GM, WM and CSF can be regularised by intensity normalisation and c_{mpc} can be kept constant. Using an adaptive contrast measure both locally and globally, through the HVS foveal segmentation, our algorithm is less sensitive to artefacts, image quality and GM/WM contrast.

3 Intensity Quantitative Analysis

With the tools developed in this study, we can perform what seems to be the first computer-aided quantitative analysis between intensities in caudate nuclei or putamen, on one hand, and thalami (pulvinar nuclei and anterior thalami), on the other hand, for CJD patients. We will refer to it as Intensity Quantification Study (IQS).

We use the segmented putamen, caudate nuclei, pulvinar and anterior thalami on the patient images to compute the mean MR intensities in nuclei. We calculate the absolute values Δ_1 and Δ_2 as in equation (2) to represent the mean intensity differences for each patient and control, where $\overline{Pul}$, $\overline{Put}$, $\overline{CN}$ and $\overline{AT}$ represent the mean intensities respectively in the pulvinar, putamen, caudate nuclei and "anterior thalamus". M represents the maximum value of all Δ_1 and Δ_2 over all controls.

$$\Delta_1 = \left|\overline{Put} - \overline{Pul}\right|,\ \Delta_2 = \left|\overline{CN} - \overline{Pul}\right|,\ M = \max_{controls}(\Delta_1, \Delta_2) \tag{2}$$

We define a first CJD prompting ratio (*CP*) for the separation of CJD patients from healthy cases as in equation (3). *CP* reflects the value in each control that is closer to the patient data and therefore less discriminating, while in patients it highlights the most suspicious grey nuclei (as not all nuclei are affected in a patient and different types of CJD affect stronger different nuclei).

We further define a first CJD characterisation ratio (*CC*) to differentiate between sCJD and vCJD based on the lesions topographical distribution, as in equation (3). $\overline{HPul}$ and $\overline{HCN}$ represent the mean hyperintense (abnormal) values (lesion specific) in the pulvinar and caudate nuclei.

$$CP = \max_{case}(\overline{Pul} / \overline{AT}, \overline{Put} / \overline{AT}, \overline{CN} / \overline{AT}),\ CC = \overline{HCN} / \overline{HPul} \tag{3}$$

4 Results

The database comprises a total number of 23 MR image sets acquired in two major neuroradiological centres of France: 10 sCJD cases (5 definite and 5 probable cases);

5 vCJD cases (2 definite and 3 probable cases with detection of PrPres in tonsil biopsy); and 8 healthy controls of similar ages to the patients. The images collected in Paris were acquired using a 1.5 Tesla GE Signa scanner: T1 (TE=20, TR=500), T2 (TE=92, TR=3000) and FLAIR-T2 (TE=148.5, TR=10002, TI=2200). The CJD data collected in Marseille were acquired using a 1.5 Tesla Siemens Magnetom Vision scanner: T1 (TE=15, TR=644), T2 (TE=22, TR=4000) and FLAIR (TE=110, TR=8000, TI=2200). Through intensity normalisation and the use of normalised ratios we can treat all data together for hypersignal segmentation.

Two radiological experts annotated all patient images. Figure 2 shows detection results on two patients with post-mortem neuropathologically confirmed CJD. The main radiological characteristic of the ten sCJD patients is the presence of higher intensities in the caudate nuclei and putamen. Strong thalamic abnormal intensity distributions are present in all vCJD cases, especially in the pulvinar. No false positive (FP) in are detected the control images.

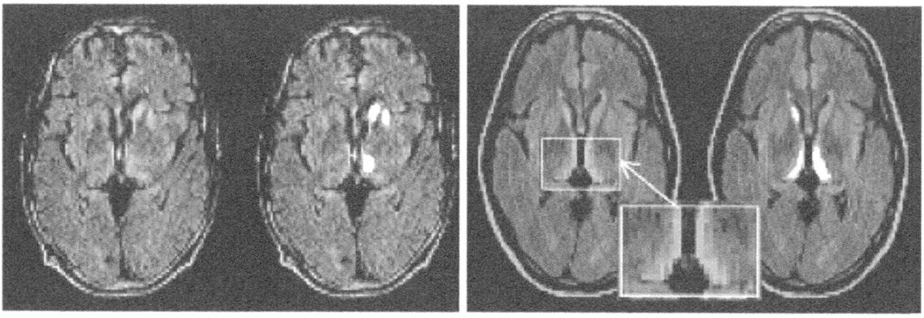

Fig. 2. Results on patient data – on the left an sCJD case with asymmetric lesions; on the right a vCJD case. We present a cross-section of each contrast-enhanced FLAIR MR data with abnormal hyperintensities in the internal nuclei; next to it we have the CJD detection map.

4.1 CJD Prompting

For the intensity quantification (IQS), we prefer using FLAIR images before intensity normalisation (which was used for the hypersignal segmentation) for the most accurate estimation of mean values in the segmented internal nuclei. This naturally leads to different intensity values for the Paris (M=9.48) and Marseille (M=25.63) databases, as a result of using different MR scanners and acquisition protocols. The results are consistent over the sCJD patients and conform to the clinical observations, where cases can be differentiated from controls judging by the Δ_1 and Δ_2 values higher than M. There is no significant difference between mean intensities in putamen or caudate nuclei versus pulvinar for our control data.

We further compute the *CP* normalised measure for the entire database. We select the values in patient data that are greater than the highest value of all ratios over the control data (which is 1.155). All patient data provide at least one suspicious value higher than 1.155. All 10 sCJD cases show significant values in the caudate ratio, while 8/10 in the putamen ratio too. Four out of five vCJD cases present significant values in the pulvinar ratio, while 3/5 in the putamen and caudate nuclei, when mean intensities (not hyperintensities) over the entire nucleus are computed.

We box plot the value of *CP* into two groups: 1 - CJD cases (sporadic and variant together) and 2 – controls, as shown in Figure 3. For each group of data (CJD patients or controls), the plot shows the group median value (the bold central line), the minimum and maximum values (at the end of the dotted lines), the lower and upper quartiles (which enclose the box around the median), and the outliers (in circles). Performing a Welch Two Sample t-test between the two groups we get a value of $p = 6.729e^{-6}$, which gives an excellent separation between patients and controls with ratio mean values of 1.266 for CJD patients and 1.092 for controls.

4.2 CJD Characterisation

It is important to compute mean intensities over the entire nucleus (i.e. pulvinar, putamen or caudate) to be able to distinguish patients from controls (who have no hyperintensities in the deep grey nuclei). The addressed internal nuclei do not show hyperintensities for all patients; the caudate appears to be the only nucleus constantly affected. Furthermore, only parts of a nucleus may show hyperintensities and therefore the mean value computed over the entire nucleus does not always reflect the degree of abnormality in the respective patient nucleus. Therefore the need to concentrate on the hyperintense areas, rather than the entire nucleus. The abnormal intensities we will refer to are the hyperintensities found by our detection algorithm based on a foveal model (HVS).

We compute the *CC* ratio for each patient. All 10 sCJD cases have CC ratios greater than 1, while all 5 vCJD cases have CC ratios lower than 1. These results prove in a quantitative form that vCJD patients present higher abnormal intensities in the pulvinar than putamen or caudate nuclei, whereas sCJD patients show stronger hyperintensities in the caudate nuclei or putamen than pulvinar.

The box plot of the two patient subgroups is presented Figure 3. The two distributions are clearly different, as shown by the result of the Welch Two Sample t-test with a p value of $5.865e^{-6}$. The ratio mean values of the two classes are 1.190 for the sCJD and 0.967 for the vCJD.

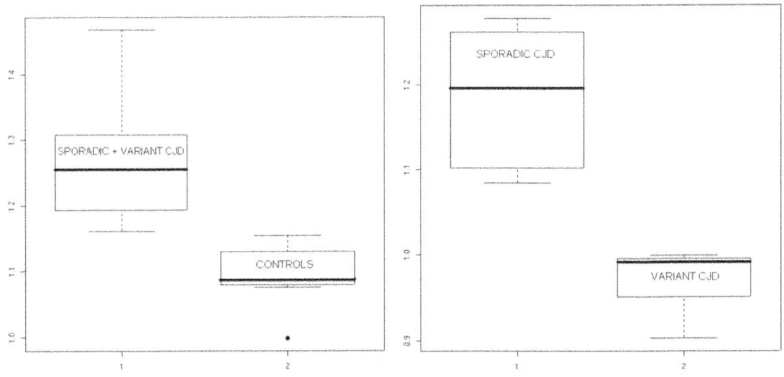

Fig. 3. Prompting and differentiating CJD: on the left the boxplot separating CJD patients (sCJD and vCJD together) from controls using the *CP* ratio shown on the vertical axis; on the right the boxplot separating sCJD patients from vCJD cases using the *CC* ratio shown on the vertical axis

The IQS separates on a first instance the CJD patients from healthy controls using the newly-defined *CP* ratio. Once the CJD cases isolated, we use the *CC* ratio to discriminate vCJD cases from sCJD. The IQS allows differentiating without ambiguity three distinctive classes: healthy controls, sCJD patients and vCJD patients. With a combination of HVS and IQS, we are able to prompt 15/15 prion disease cases with no FP amongst the controls and distinguish between sCJD and vCJD cases.

5 Discussion and Conclusion

We present a first attempt for quantitative numerical analysis of MR intensities of pulvinar versus putamen and caudate nuclei in FLAIR-T2 images of CJD patients. They accurately quantify the clinical remarks related to the possible classification of different types of human spongiform encephalopathies.

We define two new MRI-based ratios to prompt and differentiate CJD forms. All patients show abnormal intensities in the deep grey nuclei, which are correctly detected by our algorithm. All ten sCJD patients have higher mean intensities in the caudate nuclei and generally putamen. vCJD cases show more significant hyperintensities in the pulvinar than in the other deep grey nuclei, which makes them separable from the sCJD cases. All our experimental results are in complete accordance with the neurological findings in clinical practice and with the brain lesions profile described in each form of the disease.

In order to decrease the number of FP prompted by our detection algorithm, we refined the registration of the segmented data (the Zubal Phantom) on the patient specific data. We use intensity normalisation for the automated segmentation of hyperintensities, but the quantitative analysis is performed on the original values.

Quantifying the intensities in thalami, caudate nuclei and putamen, we show that there are always higher mean intensities in the caudate nuclei (10/10) and sometimes putamen (6/10) than the pulvinar of sCJD patients. The caudate nucleus is also of high intensity in the vCJD cases. This conclusion highlights the caudate nuclei as area of interest for the diagnosis of CJD, in complete agreement with the neuropathological findings. The relevance of caudate nuclei is also underlined by the decreased quantified mean ADC values in sCJD patients versus normal data (Diffusion Tensor and Diffusion Weighted images were available for some patients and controls in our database, but the results are preliminary).

The algorithm allows the study of asymmetries in CJD MR hypersignals, which has been long questioned by neuropathologists. Using basal ganglia masks, we also note that hypersignals are inhomogeneous over the nuclei.

We differentiate without ambiguity all CJD cases (sporadic and variant) from healthy controls and further characterise the CJD patients into two subgroups of human spongiform encephalopathies, sporadic and variant. More validation will be performed in future work, when more patient data are available.

The reader can refer to a detailed version of the methodology in this paper in [8].

We presented a method for the detection of hypersignals in grey matter internal nuclei from multisequence MR images. The particular context of our application is that of human spongiform encephalopathies, prion protein diseases referred as Creutzfeldt-Jakob Diseases (CJD). The technique employs intensity and spatial normalisation, foveal segmentation for the detection of hyperintensities and a priori anatomical information for refined registration and removal of false positives. We are able to prompt 15/15 prion disease cases with no FP amongst the controls. Our method further allows the quantification of intensity distributions in basal ganglia, as we introduce two MRI-based ratios that discriminate between patients and normals and differentiate between CJD forms. The caudate nuclei are highlighted as main areas of diagnosis of sCJD, in agreement with the histological data. In vCJD patients, we find more significant hyperintensities in the pulvinar than in the other internal nuclei, which confirms the visually-based radiological observations related to CJD.

Our method proves as reliable as the visual interpretation of radiologists for the detection of basal ganglia hypersignals. Moreover, it allows to automatically obtain quantitative data from MR patients with CJD, which could be used for the follow-up of patients and evaluation of the efficiency of therapeutic procedures. Our study demonstrates the value of MRI for a prospective non-invasive diagnosis of sCJD and the characterisation of prion diseases, as we clearly differentiate sporadic from variant CJD cases. This work was partially funded by the GIS-Prions project.

References

[1] J.P. Brandel: Clinical aspects of human spongiform encephalopathies, with the exception of iatrogenic forms. Biomed Pharmacother, 53:14-18, 1999.

[2] P. Cachier, E. Bardinet, D. Dormont, X. Pennec, and N. Ayache: Iconic feature-based nonrigid registration: The PASHA algorithm. CVIU 89(2-3):272-298, 2003.

[3] A.C.F. Colchester, S.A. Hojjat, R.G. Will and D. Collie: Quantitative Validation of MR Intensity Abnormalities in Variant CJD. In: J.Neurol.Neurosurg.Psychiatry 73(2): 213, 2002

[4] D.L. Collins *et al.*: Design and construction of a realistic digital brain phantom. IEEE Transactions on Medical Imaging, 17(3):463-468, 1998.

[5] M. Finkenstaedt, A Szudra, I. Zerr, S. Poser, J. Hise, J. Stoebner, and T. Wener: MR imaging of Creutzfeldt-Jakob disease. Radiology, 3:793-798, 1991.

[6] H.J Gertz, H. Henkes, and J. Cervos-Navarro: Creutzfeldt-Jakob disease: Correlation of MRI and neuropathologic findings. Neurology, 38(9):1481-1482, 1988.

[7] A. Hojjat, D. Collie, and A.C.F. Colchester: The putamen intensity gradient in CJD diagnosis. In MICCAI 2002, Vol. 2488 of LNCS, Springer, (2002) 524-531.

[8] M.G. Linguraru *et al.*: Automated Analysis of Basal Ganglia Intensity Distribution in Multisequence MRI of the Brain – Application to CJD. Res.Report RR-5276, INRIA, 2004.

[9] M.G. Linguraru, M. Brady, and R. English: Detection of Microcalcifications using SMF. In Peitgen, H.O. (ed.): Digital Mammography, Springer (2002) 342-346

[10] S. Ourselin, A. Roche, S. Prima, and N. Ayache: Block matching: A general framework to improve robustness of rigid registration of medical images. In A.M. DiGioia and S. Delp, editors, MICCAI 2000, volume 1935 of LNCS, Springer (2000) 557-566,.

[11] D. Rey, G. Subsol, H. Delingette, and N. Ayache: Automatic detection and segmentation of evolving processes in 3D medical images: Application to multiple sclerosis. Medical Image Analysis, 6:163-179, 2002.

[12] K. Van Leemput: Quantitative Analysis of Signal Abnormalities in MR Imaging for Multiple Sclerosis and Creutzfeldt-Jakob Disease. PhD thesis, Kath. Univ. Leuven, 2001.

[13] M. Zeidler *et al.*: The pulvinar sign on magnetic resonance imaging in variant Creutzfeldt-Jakob disease. The Lancet, 355:1412-1418, 2000.

[14] I.G. Zubal, C.R. Harrell, E.O. Smith, Z. Rattner, G. Gindi, and P.B. Hoffer: Computerized dimensional segmented human anatomy. Medical Physics, 21:299-302, 1994.

Statistical Representation and Simulation of High-Dimensional Deformations: Application to Synthesizing Brain Deformations

Zhong Xue, Dinggang Shen, Bilge Karacali, and Christos Davatzikos

Section of Biomedical Image Analysis, Department of Radiology,
University of Pennsylvania, Philadelphia, PA 19104
http://www.rad.upenn.edu/sbia

Abstract. This paper proposes an approach to effectively representing the statistics of high-dimensional deformations, when relatively few training samples are available, and conventional methods, like PCA, fail due to insufficient training. Based on previous work on scale-space decomposition of deformation fields, herein we represent the space of "valid deformations" as the intersection of three subspaces: one that satisfies constraints on deformations themselves, one that satisfies constraints on Jacobian determinants of deformations, and one that represents smooth deformations via a Markov Random Field (MRF). The first two are extensions of PCA-based statistical shape models. They are based on a wavelet packet basis decomposition that allows for more accurate estimation of the covariance structure of deformation or Jacobian fields, and they are used jointly due to their complementary strengths and limitations. The third is a nested MRF regularization aiming at eliminating potential discontinuities introduced by assumptions in the statistical models. A randomly sampled deformation field is projected onto the space of valid deformations via iterative projections on each of these subspaces until convergence, *i.e.* all three constraints are met. A deformation field simulator uses this process to generate random samples of deformation fields that are not only realistic but also representative of the full range of anatomical variability. These simulated deformations can be used for validation of deformable registration methods. Other potential uses of this approach include representation of shape priors in statistical shape models as well as various estimation and hypothesis testing paradigms in the general fields of computational anatomy and pattern recognition.

1 Introduction

Representing prior statistical knowledge of high-dimensional scalar or vector fields is of fundamental importance in a variety of scientific areas including computational anatomy, shape analysis, pattern recognition, and hypothesis testing applied to images or their deformations [1,2,3,4]. For instance, statistical study of deformations can be used to provide voxel-based morphological characterization of different groups; to incorporate prior knowledge of deformations from training samples into image segmentation and registration algorithms; to provide an efficient way of synthesizing new deformation fields for validation of registration

J. Duncan and G. Gerig (Eds.): MICCAI 2005, LNCS 3750, pp. 500–508, 2005.

and segmentation methods; to regularize deformations according to prior knowledge of sample deformations; and to estimate the missing parts of a deformation from parts that are observed.

The goal of this paper is to construct a statistical model of deformations from a limited number of training samples and to simulate deformations of MR brain images by sampling this model. By simulating deformations, we can synthesize respective images, which can then be used for validation of various segmentation and registration algorithms since the deformations are known [5]. Although many statistical shape modeling methods have been proposed in literature, they are often designed for 2-D or 3-D shapes that can be represented by a relatively small number of landmarks or outline points [2]. However, the high dimensionality of a variety of image warping methods of 3-D structural images renders simple PCA-based methods unable to properly estimate the statistics of deformation fields, from the typically limited number of training samples [6]. This is especially true for the finer local detail of a deformation.

This paper builds upon previous methods for estimating the covariance structures of high-dimensional distributions via scale-space decompositions [7,8,9]. In particular, the approach described herein utilizes an expansion to a wavelet packet basis [6] to rotate the high-dimensional coordinate system in which the discretized deformation field is defined, so that its covariance structure is close to a block-diagonal one; each block of this covariance matrix is approximated by its principal components via a scale-wise PCA, which captures spatial correlations among wavelet coefficients within a specific scale and band. The probability density function (pdf) of deformations can therefore be approximated by a product of the pdfs derived from the different wavelet-based PCA subspaces. This approach, referred to as the Wavelet-PCA (W-PCA) model, effectively implies the assumption of independence across different scales/bands. Although this assumption is not strictly true, it is found to lead to far more accurate estimation of the pdf of the deformation field, compared to global PCA. It is also motivated by the structural and functional correlations found among adjacent anatomical regions, at various scales. For example, in the brain adjacent neurons typically display dense connections among each other, and the same holds for adjacent anatomical regions at the substructure as well as at the between-structures level.

In this paper, the W-PCA model is applied not only to deformation fields but also to Jacobian determinants. The rationale is that the Jacobian determinant field is much smoother than the deformation field itself. Cortical gyri of the brain can have quite variable curvature patterns, but their volumes do not differ greatly, thereby leading to tighter pdfs of volumetric measurements and making them easier to estimate. Moreover, since the W-PCA model of deformations can introduce some unrealistic discontinuities emanating from the assumption of independence across wavelet bands, a valid deformation should also be a smooth field represented by a MRF. Therefore, a deformation field simulator is designed to synthesize a valid deformation via iteratively constraining a randomly sampled deformation so that it lies in the subspaces defined by the statistics of deformations and Jacobian determinants, and the MRF regularization.

The experiments synthesize deformations and respective images by randomly sampling the pdfs determined as above. Quantitative measures of generalization of the approach are evaluated and compared with those of the global PCA method. The results show that the proposed statistical model of deformations captures the prior knowledge of sample deformations well and generates realistic deformations and simulated warped images.

2 Methods

2.1 General Description

Wavelet-PCA (W-PCA) Statistical Priors. Let $\mathbf{f}(\mathbf{x})$ be a scalar or vector field defined over the template image domain Ω_t, $\mathbf{x} \in \Omega_t$. Trying to estimate the pdf of $\mathbf{f}$ from a relatively small number of training samples is a very difficult task. The commonly used PCA method (e.g. [1,2,4]) fails miserably when $\mathbf{f}$ is of very high dimensionality [6]. If $\mathbf{f}$ represents a 3-D warping transformation and it is to be estimated from 100 training samples, a global PCA model will capture mainly global size and shape characteristics that are of limited interest and value, especially for the purposes of simulating complex deformations to be used for validation purposes. In order to capture finer and more localized variations of $\mathbf{f}$, we follow and extend the framework proposed in [9], which decomposes $\mathbf{f}$ using the Wavelet Packet Transform (WPT), and subsequently captures within-scale statistics via hierarchically-organized PCA models. These PCA models are estimated from statistical distributions that are both of lower dimensionality, and more compact due to correlations among variables (*e.g.* the PCA model derived from a high-scale representation of $\mathbf{f}$ represents a very compact distribution due to the smoothing and down-sampling applied at each level of the wavelet packet decomposition; the distribution of high frequency detail within a local window is also easier to estimate due to its low dimensionality emanating from the small window size). PCA within each band at a given scale is important, due to correlations among wavelet coefficients corresponding to adjacent locations, something which is particularly prominent in smooth elastic-type of deformations, in contrast to, for example, acoustic signals. The fundamental assumption here is that the wavelet-based rotation renders the covariance matrix of $\mathbf{f}$ close to block-diagonal, thereby leading to a more accurate estimation compared to the usual sample covariance estimation. Generating a random sample from the pdf of $\mathbf{f}$ is then achieved by randomly sampling each PCA model in this hierarchy, and then using the inverse WPT.

"Valid Deformations" as the Intersection of Different Subspaces. In theory, if the W-PCA model described above captures the statistics of deformation $\mathbf{f}$ accurately, we can just generate sample deformations as described above. In practice, however, the assumption that the covariance matrix of $\mathbf{f}$ is block-diagonal in the wavelet packet basis does not hold exactly. Although it is well-known that for broad classes of signals, correlations across scales diminish rapidly, they are nonetheless non-negligible for adjacent scales. Therefore, the

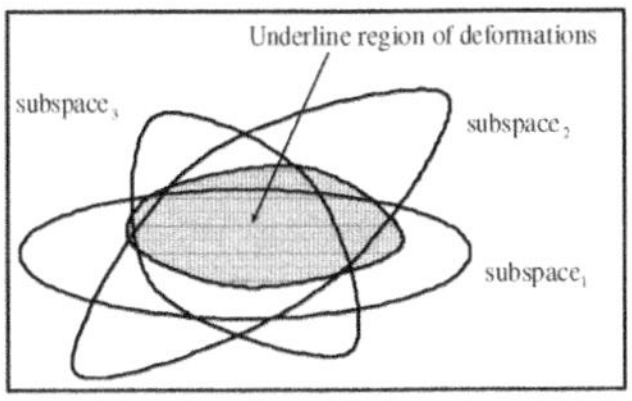

Fig. 1. The space of valid deformations are represented as the intersection of different subspaces reflecting different aspects of deformations

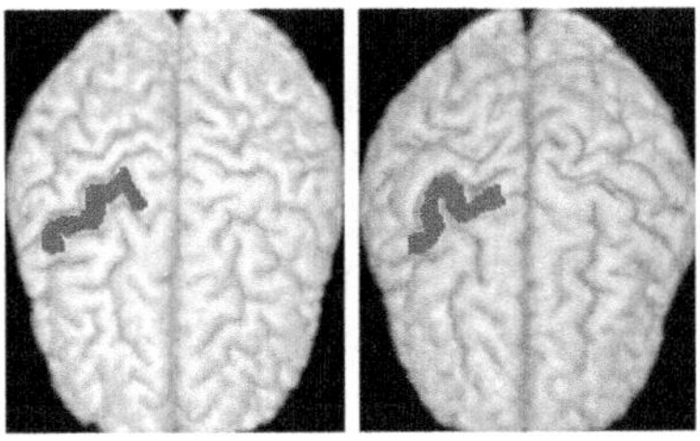

Fig. 2. Jacobians are less variable than displacement fields. *E.g.* the displacement fields of the precentral gyri are very different for these two brains, whereas the volumes of these gyri are very similar, leading to much less variable Jacobian determinants.

resulting deformation fields might have unrealistic discontinuities. In order to alleviate this problem, we observe that additional constraints imposed on the estimated deformation fields can be used to define subspaces in which the deformation must belong to. Therefore, we require that a valid deformation field simultaneously satisfies all available constraints, *i.e.* it belongs to the intersection of a number of subspaces, each of which satisfies some constraints on the deformation. The W-PCA model applied to the deformation field specifies one such subspace. In order to describe the second subspace, we first observe that if **f** represents a linear or nonlinear function of the deformation field that can be estimated more accurately, we can use it to further constrain the form of the deformation field. Herein we also use the determinant of the Jacobian of the deformation field in place of **f** in the W-PCA formulation above. The Jacobian determinant is not only of lower dimensionality, since it is a scalar field, but it is also much less variable across individuals, for the reason that is pictorially shown in Fig. 2. Accordingly, it can be estimated much more accurately from the typically limited training samples, using the W-PCA framework. In order to find the deformation field that satisfies a given Jacobian determinant, we use [10].

Hierarchical Regularization. The W-PCA model of deformations can introduce some unrealistic discontinuities emanating from the assumption of independence across different scales and bands. Such potential discontinuities can be eliminated by using a nested regularization scheme, which is applied sequentially to each level of the wavelet decomposition via a respective MRF that imposes spatial smoothness at different scales.

Summary of the Algorithm. An algorithm that samples the resulting pdfs is described next and detailed in the following sections.

- Step 1. Randomly sample the W-PCA model of deformation fields, thereby generating a tentative deformation.
- Step 2. Project the Jacobian of the deformation field onto the W-PCA model of valid Jacobian determinants.

- Step 3. Find the deformation field whose Jacobian matches the one generated in Step 2, using [10].
- Step 4. Apply the nested MRF regularization to impose spatial smoothness on the deformation at all scales.
- Step 5. Iterate above steps until convergence, *i.e.* until the smoothed deformation field belongs to the subspaces of valid Jacobians and deformations.

2.2 The Wavelet-PCA (W-PCA) Model

The W-PCA model is used to estimate the pdf of $\mathbf{f}$, which can be a deformation field or a Jacobian determinant field, using N samples. It first applies an L-level WPT to $\mathbf{f}$, and then constructs a PCA model of the wavelet coefficients of each wavelet band at level L, and finally it combines these pdfs together. Fig.3 illustrates the structure of 1-D WPT. For 3-D WPT, the wavelet coefficients at level l are represented by $\mathbf{w}^{(l,b)}, b = 0, 1, ..., B_l - 1$, where $B_l = 8^l$ and $l = 1, 2, ..., L$. At each level, $\mathbf{w}^{(l,0)}$ represents the low-pass wavelet coefficients. For

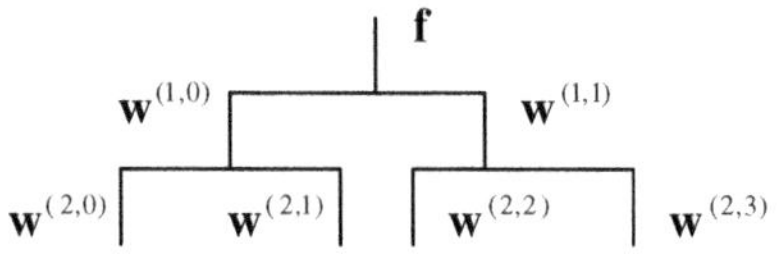

Fig. 3. Illustration of Wavelet Packet Transform (WPT)

simplicity, $\mathbf{f}$ is also referred to as $\mathbf{w}^{(0,0)}$. After L-level WPT, $\mathbf{f}$ can be represented by all the wavelet coefficients at level L, *i.e.* $\mathbf{w}^{(L,b)}$. Assuming that different bands in the wavelet subspaces are independent, the pdf of deformation $\mathbf{f}$ is,

$$p(\mathbf{f}) = \prod_{b=0}^{B_L-1} p(\mathbf{w}^{(L,b)}). \tag{1}$$

The pdf of each band (L, b), $p(\mathbf{w}^{(L,b)})$, can be estimated by applying PCA to the wavelet coefficients of N sample deformations $\mathbf{f}_s$ at that band, denoted as $\mathbf{w}_s^{(L,b)}$, $s = 1, 2, ..., N$. After performing PCA, we obtain the mean of the wavelet coefficients $\bar{\mathbf{w}}^{(L,b)}$ and the matrix $\Phi^{(L,b)}$ formed by the eigenvectors of the covariance matrix of these coefficients, which correspond to the largest $K_{(L,b)}$ eigenvalues $\lambda_j^{(L,b)}$, $j = 1, ..., K_{(L,b)}$, of that matrix. Therefore $\mathbf{w}^{(L,b)}$ can be represented by its projected vector $\mathbf{v}^{(L,b)}$ in the space spanned by the $K_{(L,b)}$ eigenvectors,

$$\mathbf{v}^{(L,b)} = \Phi^{(L,b)^T}(\mathbf{w}^{(L,b)} - \bar{\mathbf{w}}^{(L,b)}). \tag{2}$$

Then, the pdf of $\mathbf{f}$ in Eq.(1) is calculated by,

$$p(\mathbf{f}) = \prod_{b=0}^{B_L-1} c_{(L,b)} \exp\left\{ - \sum_{j=1}^{K_{(L,b)}} \frac{\mathbf{v}_j^{(L,b)2}}{2\lambda_j^{(L,b)}} \right\}, \tag{3}$$

where $c_{(L,b)}$ is the normalization coefficient. After obtaining $p(\mathbf{f})$, we can generate randomly new vectors $\hat{\mathbf{v}}^{(L,b)}$ according to the pdf in Eq.(3) and synthesize the wavelet coefficients of different wavelet bands using,

$$\hat{\mathbf{w}}^{(L,b)} = \Phi^{(L,b)}\hat{\mathbf{v}}^{(L,b)} + \bar{\mathbf{w}}^{(L,b)}. \quad (4)$$

A simulated deformation can therefore be generated by performing L-level Inverse WPT. This W-PCA model can not only be used to model statistics of deformations, but also be used to model other fields like the Jacobian determinants of deformations.

We stress the importance of using PCA within each band, which is in contrast to the commonly used independence assumption for wavelet coefficients. In particular, PCA is known to be the optimal linear expansion, provided that a good estimate of the covariance matrix is available. Although sample covariance is a very inaccurate estimate of the covariance of $\mathbf{f}$, the sample covariance at various scales provides a much better estimate of the covariance at that scale, for reasons that were detailed in Section 2.1. As a result, the W-PCA model can capture correlations between adjacent spatial locations at a given scale.

2.3 Hierarchical MRF Regularization

As mentioned in Section 2.1, if deformations are synthesized directly using the W-PCA model, some unrealistic discontinuities emanating from the assumption of independence across wavelet bands may occur. In order to eliminate such potential discontinuities, a nested MRF regularization scheme that imposes spatial smoothness at different scales is applied in conjunction with the inverse WPT. That is, $\mathbf{f}$ is regularized at different scales: at level $l, l = L-1, ..., 1, 0$, its wavelet coefficient $\hat{\mathbf{w}}^{(l,0)}$ is regularized.

Denoting the input low-pass coefficients as $\hat{\mathbf{w}}$ (which can be any of $\hat{\mathbf{w}}^{(l,0)}, l = L-1, ..., 0$), the MRF regularization estimates a "true" $\mathbf{w}_r$, by assuming that low-pass wavelet coefficients obey MRF conditions and $\hat{\mathbf{w}}$ is a degraded observation of $\mathbf{w}_r$ ($\hat{\mathbf{w}} = \mathbf{w}_r + \mathbf{n}$, $\mathbf{n}$ is the disturbance assumed to be zero-mean Gaussian noise with standard deviation (std) σ_N), and by using the Maximum *a posteriori* (MAP) framework [11,12], *i.e.*

$$\begin{aligned} \mathbf{w}_r &= \text{argmax}_{\mathbf{w}}\{p(\mathbf{w}|\hat{\mathbf{w}})\} \\ &= \text{argmax}_{\mathbf{w}}\{p(\hat{\mathbf{w}}|\mathbf{w})p(\mathbf{w})/p(\hat{\mathbf{w}})\}. \end{aligned} \quad (5)$$

Assuming the priors $p(\hat{\mathbf{w}}|\mathbf{w})$ and $p(\mathbf{w})$ are Gaussian distributions, we have $p(\hat{\mathbf{w}}|\mathbf{w}) \propto \exp\{-\frac{1}{2\sigma_N^2}\|\mathbf{w}-\hat{\mathbf{w}}\|^2\}$ and $p(\mathbf{w}) \propto \exp\{-\Psi(\mathbf{w})\}$, where $\Psi(\mathbf{w}) = \frac{1}{2}(\mathbf{w}-\bar{\mathbf{w}})^T\chi^{-1}(\mathbf{w}-\bar{\mathbf{w}})$. $\bar{\mathbf{w}}$ and χ refer to the mean and the covariance matrix of $\mathbf{w}$ respectively, and the structure of χ meets the MRF property. Thus $\mathbf{w}_r$ is solved by minimizing an energy function $E_r(\mathbf{w})$,

$$E_r(\mathbf{w}) = \frac{1}{2\sigma_N^2}\|\mathbf{w}-\hat{\mathbf{w}}\|^2 + \Psi(\mathbf{w}). \quad (6)$$

We use a simplified approach similar to [11,13] to minimize $E_r(\mathbf{w})$. First, we estimate $p(\mathbf{w})$ as a product of all the local (marginal) pdfs across the locations $\mathbf{x}$, *i.e.* $p(\mathbf{w}) \simeq \prod_{\mathbf{x}} G(\mathbf{w}_{\mathbf{x}}, \boldsymbol{\mu}_{\mathbf{x}}, \sigma_{\mathbf{x}})$, where $G(,,)$ represents a single Gaussian distribution with mean $\boldsymbol{\mu}_{\mathbf{x}}$ and std $\sigma_{\mathbf{x}}$. Then $\Psi(\mathbf{w})$ in Eq.(6) is estimated by $\hat{\Psi}(\mathbf{w}) = \sum_{\mathbf{x}}\{\frac{\|\mathbf{w}_{\mathbf{x}}-\boldsymbol{\mu}_{\mathbf{x}}\|^2}{2\sigma_{\mathbf{x}}^2}\}$, where $\boldsymbol{\mu}_{\mathbf{x}} = \frac{1}{|\delta(\mathbf{x})|}\sum_{\mathbf{y}\in\delta(\mathbf{x})}\mathbf{w}_{\mathbf{y}}$ and $\sigma_{\mathbf{x}}^2 = \frac{1}{|\delta(\mathbf{x})|}\sum_{\mathbf{y}\in\delta(\mathbf{x})}\|\mathbf{w}_{\mathbf{y}}-$

$\mu_{\mathbf{x}}\|^2$. $\delta(\mathbf{x})$ refers to a neighborhood centered on $\mathbf{x}$ but not including $\mathbf{x}$, and $|\delta(\mathbf{x})|$ is the cardinality of $\delta(\mathbf{x})$. Therefore, the regularized wavelet coefficients $\mathbf{w}_r$ can be obtained by minimizing Eq.(6) iteratively using Newton's method.

3 Results

In the experiments, the W-PCA models of deformations and the W-PCA models of their Jacobian determinants are first constructed, and then new deformations and their respective images are synthesized using the proposed deformation simulator. The dataset used in this experiment includes $N = 158$ MR brain images of different subjects. All the subject images were first rigidly transferred onto the space of the template image, and then the registration [14] was used to obtain the deformations from the template image to all the 158 rigidly-aligned subject images. After constructing the W-PCA models, we simulated randomly a large number (more than 50) of deformations and respective images using the deformation simulator described in Section 2.1. These deformations and images were visually evaluated and the simulated deformations were found realistic, smooth and also with quite significant variations. An example of the synthesized deformation fields and the respective image is given in Fig.4.

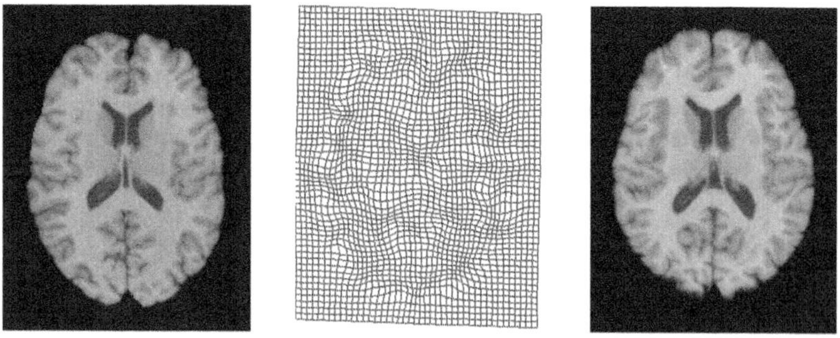

(a) the template image (b) a simulated deformation (c) the simulated image

Fig. 4. An example of the simulated deformation

We also used the generalization measure in [9,15] to evaluate the performance of our approach. The average and std of the generalization errors are calculated using the leave-one out method. The generalization error is defined as the mean of the absolute voxel-wise differences between a testing deformation field and its counterpart after projection to the intersection of the three subspaces (see Fig.1). We also compared the results using our approach with those using the global PCA. It turned out that the average and std of the generalization errors of the proposed approach are 2.3mm and 0.6mm respectively, which is a significant (P-value close to zero) improvement comparing to the results of the global PCA (mean 7.6mm and std 1.5mm).

4 Conclusion

We presented a method for estimating the statistics of deformations, which is then utilized by a deformation simulator to generate realistic deformations and images. The W-PCA models capture the statistics of deformations and their Jacobian determinants, and the nested MRF regularization eliminates possible discontinuities of deformations. A valid deformation is simulated by iteratively constraining a randomly generated deformation, so that it belongs to the intersection of these three subspaces. Better performance is observed by comparing to the global PCA approach using subjective and quantitative evaluations.

Acknowledgement

This work was partially supported by the Human Brain Project. The authors would like to thank Drs. David Rottenberg and Josh Stern from the University of Minnesota for discussions of application of this work to validation of warping algorithms and for financial support.

References

1. Cootes, T., Hill, A., Taylor, C., Haslam, J.: Use of active shape models for locating structures in medical images. Image and Vision Computing **6** (1994) 355–365
2. Cootes, T., Taylor, C., Cooper, D., Graham, J.: Active shape models - their training and application. Computer Vision and Image Understanding **61** (1995) 38–59
3. Staib, L., Duncan, J.: Boundary finding with parametrically deformable models. IEEE Trans. on Pattern Analysis and Machine Intelligence **14** (1992) 1061 –1075
4. Miller, M., Banerjee, A., Christensen, G., Joshi, S., Khaneja, N., Grenander, U., Matejic, L.: Statistical methods in computational anatomy. Statistical Methods in Medical Research **6** (1997) 267–299
5. Schnabel, J., Tanner, C., Castellano-Smith, A., Degenhard, A., Leach, M., Hose, D.: Validation of non-rigid registration using finite element methods: application to breast MR images. IEEE Trans. on Medical Imaging **22** (2003) 238–247
6. Mallat, S.: A wavelet tour of signal processing. Academic Press (1998)
7. Coifman, R., Wickerhauser, M.: Entropy-based algorithms for best basis selection. IEEE Trans. on Information Theory **38** (1992) 713–718
8. Davatzikos, C., Tao, X., Shen, D.: Hierarchical active shape models using the wavelet transformation. IEEE Trans. on Medical Imaging **22** (2003) 414–423
9. Mohamed, A., Davatzikos, C.: Shape representation via best orthogonal basis selection. In: MICCAI 2004, St. Malo, France (2004) 225–233
10. Karacali, B., Davatzikos, C.: Simulation of tissue atrophy using a topology preserving transformation model. Submitted to IEEE Trans. on Medical Imaging (2004)
11. Belge, M., Kilmer, M., Miller, E.: Wavelet domain image restoration with adaptive edge-preserving regularization. IEEE Trans. on Image Processing **9** (2000) 597–608
12. Geman, S., Geman, D.: Stochastic relaxation, Gibbs distributions, and the Bayesian restoration of images. IEEE Trans. on Pattern Analysis and Machine Intelligence **6** (1984) 721–741

13. Shen, D., Ip, H.: Markov random field regularization models for adaptive binarization of nonuniform images. IEE Proc. Vis. Image Signal Process. **145** (1998) 322–332
14. Shen, D., Davatzikos, C.: HAMMER: Hierarchical attribute matching mechanism for elastic registration. IEEE Trans. on Medical Imaging **21** (2002) 1421–1439
15. Styner, M.A., Rajamani, K.T., Nolte, L.P., Zsemlye, G., Szkely, G., Taylor, C.J., Davies, R.H.: Evaluation of 3D correspondence methods for model building. In: Information Processing in Medical Imaging. (2003)

Model-Based Parameter Recovery from Uncalibrated Optical Images

S.J. Preece[1], I.B. Styles[2], S.D. Cotton[1], E. Claridge[2], and A. Calcagni[2,3]

[1] Astron Clinica, The Mount, Toft, Cambridge CB3 7RL, UK
[2] School of Computer Science, University of Birmingham, Birmingham B15 2TT, UK
[3] Birmingham and Midland Eye Centre, City Hospital NHS Trust, Dudley Road, Birmingham B17 7QU, UK

Abstract. We propose a novel method for quantitative interpretation of uncalibrated optical images which is derived explicitly from an analysis of the image formation model. Parameters characterising the tissue are recovered from images acquired using filters optimised to minimise the error. Preliminary results are shown for the skin, where the technique was successfully applied to aid the diagnosis and interpretation of non-melanocytic skin cancers and acne; and for the more challenging ocular fundus, for mapping of the pigment xanthophyll.

1 Introduction

Optical imaging methods have recently assumed a much more important role in medicine: light is non-ionising and relatively safe; and increasingly powerful computers make it possible to implement detailed models of image formation. These can provide principled means of relating image values to physical properties of the tissues being imaged. A common problem is the interpretation of images taken under conditions of varying illumination. The magnitude of light reaching the detector depends on many factors not related to tissue properties, including the magnitude, direction and spectral composition of the incident light; the object geometry; the presence of other objects in the scene, etc. In some cases these factors can be controlled and compensated for by calibrating against objects with known reflectance, but this is impossible in many cases. We show how a physical model of image formation can be used to derive quantitative properties of tissue from uncalibrated optical images.

Earlier work [1,2] has laid down the foundations for a physics-based image interpretation method capable of deriving quantitative parameters characterising tissue histology from in vivo multi-spectral images. The method was first applied to skin imaging, and shown to be successful in the early detection of melanoma [1,3]. Although the principles of that work are generic, many human tissues present major additional challenges in comparison to the skin.

The existing approach assumes that the absolute reflectance of the tissue can be deduced from a simple measurement. This is usually accomplished by placing an object of known reflectance (a "standard") alongside the tissue, but this

J. Duncan and G. Gerig (Eds.): MICCAI 2005, LNCS 3750, pp. 509–516, 2005.

is inappropriate where the image is of a non-planar object; the illumination is spatially non-uniform; or when the tissue under investigation cannot be accessed in order to place the standard. We have developed a method for compensating for spatial variations in illumination and geometry in an image. The method does not require any form of reflectance standard to be used and is quite general. We provide objective criteria which ensure that parameter recovery from such uncalibrated images is both unique and of sufficient accuracy.

2 Compensating for Geometric Variations in Illumination

The proposed technique is based upon an analysis of the imaging process. When capturing an image on a CCD-based device, using a filter with transmittance $F_n(\lambda)$ at wavelength λ, the signal recorded at position $\mathbf{x}$ is

$$i_n(\mathbf{x}) = C \int_{\Lambda} I_0(\lambda, \mathbf{x}) R(\lambda, \mathbf{x}) F_n(\lambda) Q(\lambda) \mathrm{d}\lambda, \tag{1}$$

where $Q(\lambda)$ is the quantum efficiency of the CCD, $I_0(\lambda, \mathbf{x})$ defines the illuminant, and $R(\lambda, \mathbf{x})$ is the reflectance of the tissue. The constant C scales the signal onto the range of the detector and is determined by factory calibration. We have assumed that $F_n(\lambda)$ and $Q(\lambda)$ are spatially uniform. Clearly the reflectance of the tissue varies with position as its composition changes, and the intensity of illumination can also vary spatially due to surface irregularities, beam edge effects or surface curvature. We can generally assume all variations in system geometry can be included in $I_0(\lambda, \mathbf{x})$, and that these variations are independent of wavelength in diffuse imaging. We can therefore write $I_0(\lambda, \mathbf{x}) = A(\mathbf{x}) S(\lambda)$, a product of spatial $A(\mathbf{x})$ and spectral $S(\lambda)$ terms. The geometric properties of the system are then contained solely in $A(\mathbf{x})$. Substituting for I_0 in Eqn. (1), and noting that $A(\mathbf{x})$ does not depend on λ we obtain

$$i_n(\mathbf{x}) = C A(\mathbf{x}) \int_{\Lambda} S(\lambda) R(\lambda, \mathbf{x}) F_n(\lambda) Q(\lambda) \mathrm{d}\lambda. \tag{2}$$

All geometric information is contained in the pre-factor to the integral. We may therefore eliminate system geometry by considering quantities $q_{mn}(\mathbf{x}) = i_m(\mathbf{x})/i_n(\mathbf{x})$, the so-called *image quotients.* In the next section we will define objective criteria for the selection of image quotients, and show how they can be used to recover tissue parameters from appropriate images.

3 Modelling of Uncalibrated Imaging

In Ref. [2], Preece and Claridge described the process of image formation as a sequence of mappings. They assumed that the optical properties of tissue can be described by a vector of K parameters $\mathbf{p} = \{p_k\}_{k=1...K}$, $\mathbf{p} \in \mathcal{P}$, where P is the space of all possible parameter vectors for a given tissue type. The first stage in the imaging process is the formation of the reflectance spectrum of the tissue: $r = r(\lambda)$, $r \in \mathcal{R}$, where $\mathcal{R}$ is the space of all possible reflectance spectra. We define a mapping $a : \mathcal{P} \mapsto \mathcal{R}$ describing the relationship between tissue parameters and spectral reflectance. This mapping can be realised using Monte Carlo simulation [4].

Optical imaging devices typically acquire images by filtering the remitted spectra to generate a single image value per filter. For N filters $\{F_n(\lambda)\}_{n=1\ldots N}$, an image vector $\mathbf{i} = \{i_n\}_{n=1\ldots N}$, $\mathbf{i} \in \mathcal{I}$ is recorded, where $\mathcal{I}$ is the space of all possible image vectors for a given tissue. This is represented by a mapping $b : \mathcal{R} \mapsto \mathcal{I}$, defined by Eqn. (2).

We now introduce an additional step. Given an N-component image vector, we can form an $(N-1)$-component vector of independent image quotients, $\mathbf{q} = \{q_m\}_{m=1\ldots N-1} = \{i_m/i_N\}_{m=1\ldots N-1}$, $\mathbf{q} \in \mathcal{Q}$. The image quotients are independent of surface and illumination geometry, and remove the need for calibration. We represent this final stage as a mapping $c : \mathcal{I} \mapsto \mathcal{Q}$. The process of forming image quotients is then the composite function $f = a \circ b \circ c : \mathcal{P} \mapsto \mathcal{Q}$, relating the composition of the object described by a parameter vector $\mathbf{p}$ to image quotients $\mathbf{q}$ formed from an image captured by a set of optical filters $\{F_n(\lambda)\}_{n=1\ldots N}$. We can now, in principle, construct an inverse mapping $f^{-1} : \mathcal{Q} \mapsto \mathcal{P}$ which allows us, given a vector of image quotients $\mathbf{q}$, to deduce the vector of parameters $\mathbf{p}$ that describes the tissue at the point of interest.

There are two important criteria which f and f^{-1} should meet: f should be a unique, one-to-one (bijective) mapping between points in $\mathcal{P}$ and points in $\mathcal{Q}$; and when applied to a vector $\mathbf{q}$, f^{-1} should compute the corresponding parameter vector $\mathbf{p}$ with sufficient accuracy. Preece and Claridge [2] established objective criteria to ensure that these conditions are met, and our analysis is similar. We assume that the spectrum of the illuminating source $S(\lambda)$ and the quantum efficiency of the detector $Q(\lambda)$ are known, and that we have control over the filters $\{F_n(\lambda)\}$ used to acquire the image. We first check whether f is bijective using the criteria defined in Sect. 3.1. Sets of filters which do not meet this requirement are discarded. We then use an evolutionary algorithm [5] to select $\{F_n(\lambda)\}$ such that they minimise the mean error with which parameters can be computed from image quotients. This is described in Sect. 3.2.

3.1 Uniqueness of the Mapping

To determine the uniqueness of the forward mapping f, we compute the Jacobi matrix $\mathbf{J}$ with components $J_{ij} = \partial q_i / \partial p_j$ at each point at which the model is defined. We then compute the Jacobian $J = \det(\mathbf{J})$, and test the sign of J at all points in P. The mapping f is bijective if J is found to be of constant sign (and non-zero) throughout $\mathcal{P}$. An important consequence of this is that the number of image quotients must equal the number of object parameters, $N - 1 = K$.

3.2 Minimisation of Error in f^{-1}

Minimisation of error is essential in medical image analysis. The accuracy of a clinician's diagnosis depends on the quality of information that analysis of an image provides. We have identified three main sources of error: errors in f; errors in the imaging process; and errors in the construction of f^{-1}.

Errors in f can arise from several sources. The data used to characterise the tissue may not be known accurately; the characteristics of the imaging equipment may not be known exactly; and the model of tissue reflectance may not be deterministic. The main source of error in the imaging process is thermal noise in the CCD. This leads to a small error in the image values recorded by the camera, and hence in the recorded image quotients. Finally, f^{-1} cannot generally be computed exactly and an approximation is necessary (see Sect. 3.3). Each of these errors reduces the accuracy of the recovered tissue parameters. It is a simple exercise in error propagation to compute the error which which parameters can be recovered, given these known sources of uncertainty. The resulting measure of error is a function of the set of filters chosen, and is used in the optimisation process to determine optimal filters for the problem.

3.3 Construction of the Inverse Function

When processing an image using these ideas, an explicit implementation of f^{-1} will be required, but in general, we cannot compute f^{-1} directly. The forward model f is defined only at a finite number of points in $\mathcal{P}$, and there are a finite number of points in $\mathcal{Q}$. A natural approach to the construction of f^{-1} is to fit a multi-dimensional surface to the data, but both f and f^{-1} are often highly nonlinear, and finding an appropriate functional form for the surface is very hard. For the two-dimensional model of skin discussed in Sect. 4, a standard surface fitting algorithm provided good results, but models with higher dimensionality have proven to be much more difficult. In these cases, acceptable theoretical results have been obtained using a neural network.

4 Application: Non-contact Skin Imaging

The original parameter recovery method developed for skin imaging by Cotton and Claridge [1] requires calibrated, illumination-invariant image data. This is fairly simple to achieve for small areas of the skin by contact photography, but larger, curved or uneven surfaces cannot be imaged in this way.

We have implemented a system for uncalibrated non-contact imaging of the skin and have carried out a preliminary evaluation for a number of medical conditions including non-melanocytic skin cancers and acne. For practical reasons we have based the system on an off-the-shelf digital camera which involved making small departures from the generic interpretation scheme described above.

An accurate optical model of the skin requires three parameters: concentration of epidermal melanin, concentration of dermal blood and thickness of the dermal layer [6]. Appropriate ranges for each of these parameters were taken from Ref. [6]. For each parameter vector, the mapping $a : \mathcal{P} \mapsto \mathcal{R}$ was implemented using a Monte Carlo simulation. The standard RGB camera used provides only three filters $\{F_n(\lambda)\} = \{R, G, B\}$, allowing only two of the three parameters to be recovered. Blood and melanin were chosen because of their clinical importance, but also because of their significantly greater local variability in comparison with collagen. A constant value of collagen of 0.2mm was assumed [6]. The thickness of collagen does change the absolute magnitude of the reflectance spectrum, but has only a small effect on the relative magnitudes of the image quotients. Since $\{F_n(\lambda)\}$ were predefined, the optimisation was reduced to selecting one of the R, G or B bands to play a role of the denominator in the image quotients, and testing whether the uniqueness of the mapping is preserved. The quotients B/R and G/R were found to give the best unique mapping. The correctness of this mapping was tested by comparison with the original method, which does require calibration.

The imaging system uses a Cannon G5 Powershot digital camera capable of taking images ranging in size from half-body to 5mm patches. Illumination is provided by a ring flash mounted in the camera lens plane with a system of polarising filters to prevent flash artifacts. Images are taken under ambient illumination. Parametric maps are computed in ~ 2 seconds on a standard PC. Two pilot studies described here investigate the pre-therapeutic characterisation of non-melanocytic skin lesions, and the objective assessment of severity of acne.

Non-melanocytic skin cancers. Basal Cell Carcinoma (BCC) and Squamous Cell Carcinoma (SCC) are the most common forms of skin cancer. These can be difficult to differentiate from non-cancerous and non-invasive lesions. A non-invasive alternative to biopsy would reduce the likelihood of unnecessary surgery and patient trauma. In a pilot study 150 images of non-melanocytic skin lesions were obtained and parametric maps of blood and melanin were examined by a

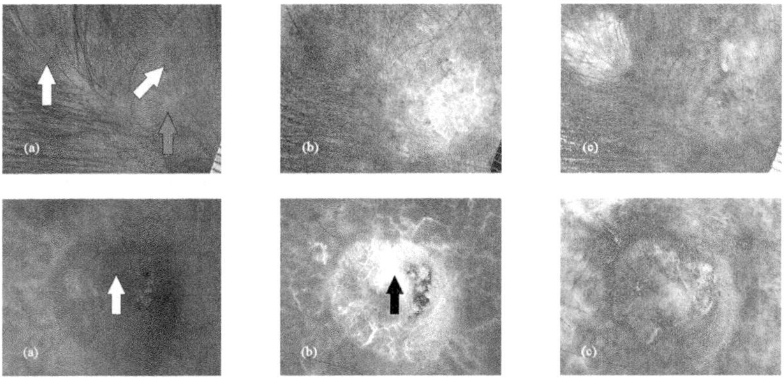

Fig. 1. First row: an infiltrative BCC, (a) colour image; (b) blood map; (c) melanin map. The lesion (dark arrow in (a)) shows increased vascularity and tortuous engorged vessels in (b). Two nearby lesions (seborrhoeic keratoses, marked by white arrows), show no increase in vasculature (b), and their pigment content contrasts with the non-pigmented BCC in (c). Second row: a moderately differentiated SCC: (a) colour image; (b) blood map; (c) melanin map. A nodular area (arrow in (a)) is highly vascular (arrow in (b)), possibly reflecting tumour activity. Low melanin values in (c) demonstrate the non-pigmented nature of this lesion.

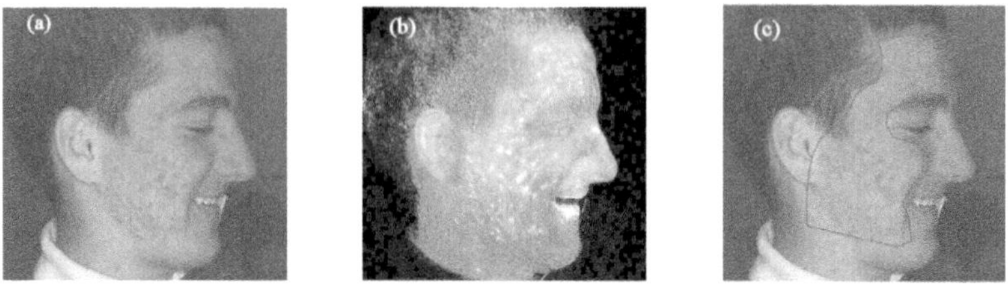

Fig. 2. Acne Lesions. (a) Colour photograph; (b) parametric map of blood; (c) extent of the lesions identified from (b) and overlaid on the original photograph.

dermatologist for diagnostically useful features. The tumour vascularity, clearly visible in the blood map shown in Fig. 1b (second row), was identified as a highly relevant sign of BCC. A combination of features in blood and melanin maps was useful in eliminating suspicious lesions as non-cancerous (Fig. 1, first row). An in-vivo examination of these histological, diagnostically relevant signs of cancer is at present not possible in any other way.

Acne. In acne, bacteria caught in the skin pores causes an inflammatory skin reaction. The treatment depends on the severity and extent of the condition, however the assessment of these factors is highly subjective. In a small study involving 20 patients, clinical scores were compared with scores derived from parametric maps of the blood distribution. The 'extent' score was computed as a percentage of skin with blood levels above the mean in the region of interest (outlined in Fig. 2c). The 'severity' score of the inflammation was computed as the mean of the blood level values in the affected area. The correlation between clinical and computer-derived scores was R2 = 0.82 for the severity and R2 = 0.8 for the extent, indicating good agreement.

It should be stressed that values recorded in the parametric maps correspond to real physical quantities. For example blood levels can be expressed in units of mmol/L. For this reason both, the 'extent' and 'severity' scores, are truly objective measures of inflammation which can be compared over time or over a population of patients. At present there are no other methods, neither clinical, nor photographic, capable of such objective assessment.

5 Application: Ocular Fundus Imaging

Age-related macular degeneration (ARMD) causes irreversible sight loss in elderly patients. Early identification may facilitate preventative treatments, but at present there are no objective screening methods. The pigment xanthophyll is thought to play a protective role in ARMD and decreasing levels may indicate the onset of the disease. Quantitative estimates of the pigment level may be of considerable clinical value. This section describes work in progress on quantitative interpretation of fundus images.

The model of fundus reflectance is described by five parameters: RPE melanin, choroidal blood, choroidal melanin, xanthophyll and retinal blood,

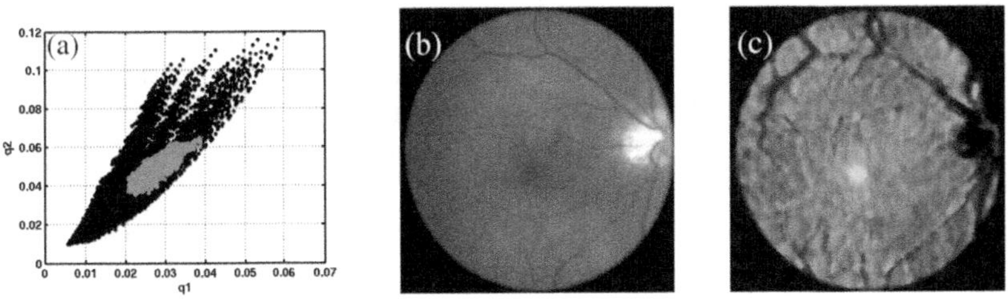

Fig. 3. (a) Projection of the model (black points) and image (gray points) onto the q_1-q_2 subspaces, where $q_1 = i(507\text{nm})/i(611\text{nm})$, $q_2 = i(525\text{nm})/i(611\text{nm})$. (b) A sample fundus image in the band centred at 507nm. (c) Distribution of xanthophyll in a healthy human subject recovered from fundus images.

based on the model proposed by Preece and Claridge [7]. Other properties of the tissue were assumed to be constant. The parameters were discretised within their respective ranges and tissue reflectance for each parameter vector was computed using a Monte Carlo simulation. The recovery of five parameters requires six images, and the optimisation procedure found that the best unique mapping was provided by filters with central wavelengths 507nm, 525nm, 552nm, 585nm, 596nm with the filter used in the denominator of the image quotients located at 611nm.

Xanthophyll absorbs light at $\lambda < 534$nm, and it is possible to recover its distribution using the quotients at 507nm, 525nm and 552nm. Fig. 3a shows an example of the relationship between the model vectors and image quotient vectors in a projected view. Images from twelve normal subjects were taken using a standard fundus camera coupled to a Retiga EXi monochrome camera and a VariSpec programmable LCD filter. The VariSpec filter was programmed to implement the selected filters.

When applied to a normal subject, the inverse mapping yields the distribution of xanthophyll shown in Fig. 3c. The pigment level shows a significant increase near the fovea, which is in agreement with the accepted distribution [8]. Areas showing no xanthophyll include the optic disk, which is not modelled in the current implementation, and large veins, which obscure the underlying tissue. Values of xanthophyll range from zero (in the black regions) to 0.6 mmol/L in the white regions. To our knowledge this is the first time that the distribution of a single ocular pigment has been deduced by digital imaging and computer modelling. These results are very encouraging and work is in progress to produce parametric maps showing the distribution of the remaining model parameters.

6 Discussion and Conclusions

We have developed a generic method for quantitative interpretation of optical images. The method uses image quotients to effectively normalise the intensity of illumination, allowing objects with complex geometries and/or large areas to be interpreted. This is similar to "discounting the illuminant", a process used to normalise pixel values prior to image segmentation and classification [9,10]. In this paper we have shown for the first time that it is possible to carry out *quantitative analysis* of tissue composition from *uncalibrated* images. This is a far more ambitious and difficult task than classification, and the merits of quantitative image interpretation methods in medical imaging are well recognised. A clinically important practical advantage of our method is that it does not require the use of calibration patches and can be used for non-contact imaging. This is vital when studying, for example, large burns, where the area of interest is likely to be highly sensitive to the touch and prone to infections.

The theoretical bases and computational methodology of our method are truly generic. We have demonstrated their successful application to aid the diagnosis and interpretation of several skin conditions and to compute the distribution of the pigment xanthophyll in the ocular fundus. The same method has also been applied to problems in x-ray astronomy [11], and fluorescein imaging of cancer cells [12] . We anticipate that in the future this work will yield much insight into the optical imaging of biological tissues in general, and that it will lead to the development of clinically useful systems.

References

1. Cotton, S.D., Claridge, E., Hall, P.N.: Noninvasive skin imaging. In: Information Processing in Medical Imaging (LNCS1230). (1997) 501–507
2. Preece, S.J., Claridge, E.: Spectral filter optimisation for the recovery of parameters which describe human skin. IEEE Trans. PAMI **26** (2004) 913–922
3. Moncrieff, M., Cotton, S., Claridge, E., Hall, P.: Spectrophotometric intracutaneous analysis - a new technique for imaging pigmented skin lesions. British Journal of Dermatology **146** (2002) 448–457
4. Prahl, S.A., Keijzer, M., Jacques, S.L., Welch, A.J.: A monte carlo model of light propagation in tissue. SPIE Insitute Series IS **5** (1989) 102–111
5. Yao, X., Liu, Y.: Fast evolution strategies. Control and Cyb. **26** (1997) 467–496
6. Anderson, R., Parrish, J.A.: The optics of human skin. J. Invest. Dermatol. **77** (1981) 13–19
7. Preece, S.J., Claridge, E.: Monte carlo modelling of the spectral reflectance of the human eye. Phys. Med. Biol. **47** (2002) 2863–2877
8. Hammer, M., Schweitzer, D.: Quantitative reflection spectroscopy at the human ocular fundus. Phys. Med. Biol. **47** (2002) 179–191
9. Healey, G.: Using colour for geometry-insensitive segmentation. J. Opt. Soc. Am. A **6** (1989) 920–937
10. Maloney, L., Wandell, B.: Color constancy: a method for recovering surface spectral reflectance. J. Opt. Soc. Am. A **3** (1986) 29–33
11. O'Dwyer, M., Claridge, E., Ponman, T., Raychaudhury, S.: Mapping the physical properties of cosmic hot gas with hyper-spectral imaging. In: Proceeding of the Seventh IEEE Workshop on the Applications of Computer Vision. (2005) 185–190
12. Claridge, E.: Optimal filter selection for quantitative interpretation of fluorescence microscopy images. Technical Report CSR-05-02, University of Birmingham, School of Computer Science (2005)

MRI Tissue Classification with Neighborhood Statistics: A Nonparametric, Entropy-Minimizing Approach

Tolga Tasdizen[1], Suyash P. Awate[1], Ross T. Whitaker[1], and Norman L. Foster[2]

[1] School of Computing, University of Utah
[2] Department of Neurology, University of Michigan

Abstract. We introduce a novel approach for magnetic resonance image (MRI) brain tissue classification by learning image neighborhood statistics from noisy input data using nonparametric density estimation. The method models images as random fields and relies on minimizing an entropy-based metric defined on high dimensional probability density functions. Combined with an atlas-based initialization, it is completely automatic. Experiments on real and simulated data demonstrate the advantages of the method in comparison to other approaches.

1 Introduction

Segmentation of magnetic resonance images (MRI) of the brain is an important problem in biomedicine; it has a number of applications including diagnosis, surgical planning and monitoring therapy. One of the fundamental tasks in brain MRI segmentation is the classification of volumetric data (3D images) into gray matter, white matter and cerebral-spinal fluid (CSF) tissue types. This classification is of great interest in the study of neurodegenerative disorders such as Alzheimer's Disease. It also has other applications such as the generation of patient-specific conductivity maps for EEG source localization. Manual segmentation of high-resolution 3D images is an extremely time consuming and subjective task; hence, automatic and semi-automatic brain tissue classification methods have been studied extensively in the field of biomedical image processing. Recent developments in automatic brain tissue classification have led to a class of systems that incorporate the following strategies:

1. Parametric statistical models of single-pixel image intensity for each tissue class,
2. Markov random field (MRF) type models of spatial smoothness,
3. Bias field correction, and
4. Digital brain atlas information.

In this paper, we propose a novel approach that combines the intensity and spatial smoothness models (items 1-2) using an unsupervised learning approach that incorporates nonparametric statistics of local neighborhoods. The proposed method is compatible with state-of-the-art segmentation methods that use probabilistic brain atlases [1,2] and bias field correction [3], but it uses an information-theoretic, data-driven approach to incorporate image neighborhood information. Validation studies on simulated data demonstrate that this approach offers significant advantages over the state-of-the-art.

J. Duncan and G. Gerig (Eds.): MICCAI 2005, LNCS 3750, pp. 517–525, 2005.

2 Related Work

This paper introduces a new approach for removing the effects of imaging noise in tissue classification using a statistical framework. Others have used non-linear diffusion for image denoising as a pre-processing step [4]. However, for probabilistic algorithms, it is intuitive to incorporate spatial smoothness constraints directly into the segmentation process via Markov random field (MRF) models [5,6,3,7,8]. These methods modify single-pixel tissue-probabilities with energies defined on local configurations of segmentation labels. Spatially smooth segmentations are assigned lower energies and therefore are more likely. However, such MRF models can over regularize the fine structured borders, e.g. the interface between gray and white matter; therefore, it is often necessary to impose additional, heuristic constraints [6,3]. Active contour models [9,10] have also been used to impose smoothness constraints for segmentation. These methods typically attempt to minimize the area of the segmentation boundary, an approach that also can over regularize interfaces. The method proposed in this paper formulates the segmentation problem in information-theoretic terms using probability density functions (PDFs) defined on the space of image neighborhoods. In contrast to MRF-type approaches to tissue classification regularization, which formulate neighborhood probabilities on discrete segmentation labels, the method relies on the discovery of regular patterns in the input data.

Lee *et al.*[11] analyze the intensity statistics of 3×3 pixel patches in optical images, in the corresponding high-dimensional spaces, and find the the data to be concentrated in clusters and low-dimensional manifolds exhibiting nontrivial topologies. Motivated by this observation, we use nonparametric density estimation. Consequently, we impose very few assumptions about the statistical structure of image neighborhoods. Popat *et al.*[12] were among the first to use nonparametric Markov sampling in images. They attempt to capture the higher-order nonlinear image statistics via cluster-based nonparametric density estimation and apply their technique for image restoration, image compression and texture classification. However, their method takes a *supervised* approach for learning neighborhood relationships. The proposed method builds on the work in [13], which lays down the foundations for unsupervised learning of higher-order image statistics. However, that work proposes reducing the entropy of image-neighborhood statistics as a method for removing image noise.

3 Method

A random field/process [14] is a family of random variables $X(\Omega;T)$, for an index set T, where, for each fixed $T = t$, the random variable $X(\Omega;t)$ is defined on the sample space Ω. If we let T be a set of points defined on a discrete Cartesian grid and fix $\Omega = \omega$, we have a specific realization of the random field as a deterministic function $x(t)$ – the image. In the case of 3D MRI data, t is a three-vector and T represents the set of pixels in the 3D image. Let $N_t \subset T$ be the set of pixels in the neighborhood of t. If we associate with T a family of neighborhoods $N = \{N_t\}_{t \in T}$ such that $u \in N_t$ if and only if $t \in N_u$, then N is called a neighborhood system for the set T. An example of such a neighborhood is a $3 \times 3 \times 3$ cube of pixels centered at t. We define a random vector $Z(t) = \{X(t)\}_{t \in N_t}$, denoting its realization by $z(t)$, corresponding to the set of intensities at the neighbors of pixel t. If the image is real-valued, then $z(t) \in \mathbb{R}^m$ where m is the number of pixels in the neighborhood.

3.1 Neighborhood Entropy

Let $p_k(Z = z)$ be the probability of observing the image neighborhood z given that the center pixel of the neighborhood belongs to the tissue class k. This PDF is called the *likelihood* function. The total entropy associated with a set of K tissue PDFs is

$$H = -\sum_{k=1}^{K} \int_{\mathbb{R}^m} p_k(Z = z) \log p_k(Z = z) dz, \tag{1}$$

where the integration is performed over $\mathbb{R}^m$, the domain of the random vector Z. Let the sets $\{T_k\}_{k=1}^{K}$ denote a mutually exclusive and exhaustive decomposition of T into K tissue classes. We assume that the random process X, limited to pixels belonging to a single class T_k, is stationary ergodic. Entropy is the expectation of negative log-probability, and for such processes it can be approximated with the sample mean [15]

$$H(T_1, \ldots, T_K) = -\sum_{k=1}^{K} \left(\frac{1}{|T_k|} \sum_{t \in T_k} \log p_k(z(t)) \right). \tag{2}$$

Piecewise stationarity is a better model for MRI, which is not truly stationary. In practice, the stationary ergodic assumption can be relaxed as shown in Section 3.2.

We consider the optimal decomposition (segmentation) to be the sets $\{\hat{T}_k\}_{k=1}^{K}$ for which H is minimum. If the PDFs $p_k(Z)$ are known, H can be minimized by assigning any pixel t to the class with the highest likelihood for that particular realization $z(t)$:

$$\hat{T}_k = \{t \in T \mid p_k(z(t)) \geq p_i(z(t)),\ \forall i \neq k\}. \tag{3}$$

In practice, the likelihood functions are not known a priori and have to be estimated as well. We propose to iteratively estimate the likelihood functions and update the segmentation sets $\{T_k\}_{k=1}^{K}$ until H converges. This approach is similar to the estimation of means and variances for Gaussian PDFs in the Expectation Maximization algorithm. However, Z is not well represented by a Gaussian PDF. For instance, consider the image neighborhood for a white matter pixel deep inside the white matter mass and for one close to the interface with gray matter. These two neighborhoods are drawn from a PDF with multiple modes. Hence, we use a nonparametric density estimation approach.

3.2 Nonparametric Multivariate Density Estimation

Entropy optimization on image neighborhoods entails the estimation of PDFs in sparsely populated, high dimensional spaces (the so-called *curse of dimensionality*). Despite theoretical arguments suggesting that density estimation beyond a few dimensions is impractical, empirical evidence is more optimistic [12,13]. We use Parzen-window density estimation [16] with an m-dimensional isotropic Gaussian interpolation kernel, G_m, with standard deviation σ for all dimensions. The density estimate for class k is

$$p_k(Z(t) = z(t)) \approx \frac{1}{|A_k(t)|} \sum_{t_j \in A_k(t)} G_m(z(t) - z(t_j), \sigma), \quad (4)$$

where $A_k(t)$ is a small subset of T_k, chosen randomly. For a truly stationary random process, it is sufficient to form a global sample $A_k(t)$ and use it to evaluate the PDF for all $z(t)$. For a piecewise stationary model, we estimate the PDF locally by choosing the locations in $A_k(t)$ from a spatial sampling Gaussian PDF centered at t.

Parzen-window density estimation involves the following parameters: the size of the set $A_k(t)$, the standard deviations of the spatial sampling Gaussian and the interpolation Gaussian kernel. The first two are not critical, and they can easily be fixed for a wide range of MRI. In all of our experiments, we fix the standard deviation of the spatial sampling Gaussian to 15 pixels. This also automatically determines the minimum number of required samples in $A_k(t)$ to be 1000 as explained in [13]. On the other hand, the standard deviation σ of the interpolation kernel in equation (4) is critical for successful density estimation in high dimensional spaces. The optimal choice for this parameter depends on the sparsity of the data which varies with various factors including the amount of noise present in an image. We choose σ to minimize the entropy of the associated PDF via a Newton-Raphson optimization scheme [13]. This choice for σ is consistent with our entropy minimization segmentation formulation.

3.3 MRI Brain Tissue Classification Algorithm

The algorithm segments four tissue classes: gray matter, white matter, CSF and non-brain tissue. Each class is represented with a non-parametric PDF. Since, the true PDFs are not known *a priori*, we use an iterative learning procedure. Another component in MRI brain tissue classification is the correction of intensity inhomogeneities. Various solutions to this problem have been proposed. The approaches in [20,21,3] are the most interesting because they propose a combined approach that iteratively updates the segmentation labels and the bias field correction. The focus of this paper is not on bias field correction; however, to show that our segmentation method is compatible with previous techniques, we have implemented a simplified version of the polynomial least-squares fit correction described in [3]. In summary, the segmentation algorithm carries out the following steps per iteration:

1. estimate likelihood functions from the current $\{T_k\}_{k=1}^{K}$ and bias field,
2. update $\{T_k\}_{k=1}^{K}$ according to the new likelihoods,
3. estimate the bias field from the new $\{T_k\}_{k=1}^{K}$.

The iterations are carried out until the reduction in entropy H computed from equation (2) drops below 0.1% of the current value of H.

The algorithm requires an initial partition of classes, which can be obtained by registering the MRI with a brain atlas. Digital brain atlases can be used to provide segmentation labels for a reference dataset [17,18] or prior tissue probabilities computed from a population of subjects [1,2,19]. In this paper, we use the ICBM probabilistic atlas [19], which provides probabilities of gray matter, white matter and CSF classes for each pixel. We register this atlas with the MRI by computing the affine transformation that maximizes a mutual information metric. The registered probability maps are then used to form an initial segmentation using equation (3). As in [1,2], we also treat these atlas probability maps as prior probabilities. However, we have found that while the priors help in the discrimination between brain tissues vs. non-brain tissues, they don't offer significant benefits for our method when choosing between the brain tissues. Hence, we sum the CSF, white matter and gray matter priors into a single brain-tissue prior map. The non-brain-tissue prior map is then obtained by subtracting this map from unity.

4 Results and Validation

We validate the proposed approach on simulated images with known ground truth. We use 1 mm isotropic T1-weighted images from the BrainWeb simulator [22] with varying amounts of noise and bias field. The neighborhood system is chosen to include the six adjacent pixels in the three Cartesian directions in addition to the center pixel. Hence, the PDFs exist in a seven dimensional space.

Van Leemput *et al.* [1] use the Dice metric [23] to evaluate the performance of their state-of-the-art Expectation Maximization and MRF based approach on images from the BrainWeb simulator. For comparison purposes, we use the same metric. Let $\tilde{T}_k$ denote the ground truth set of pixels in tissue class k, then the Dice metric for class k is defined as $2|\hat{T}_k \cap \tilde{T}_k|/(|\hat{T}_k| + |\tilde{T}_k|)$, where $|\cdot|$ denotes set size.

The first validation experiment is performed on simulated T1-weighted data without any bias field and with intensity noise levels in the range $0\% - 9\%$. The noise percentages are defined with respect to the mean intensity of each tissue class. Figure 1 plots the Dice metric for gray and white matter tissue classifications from the proposed algorithm and the corresponding values given in [1]. The Dice metric for combined brain tissues vs. non-brain tissues is consistently above 98% for both algorithms and is not shown in this paper due the lack of space. The proposed algorithm performs better at all noise levels for gray and white matter tissues. For 3% noise, which can be considered typical for real MRI, the performance gains are approximately 1.1% and 2.8% for gray and white matter, respectively. The proposed approach scales better with increasing noise amounts; the performance gain at 9% noise is 3.8% and 6.1% for gray and white matter, respectively. This property would be useful for segmenting clinical, fast acquisition MRI that can have high amount of noise. The use of image neighborhood

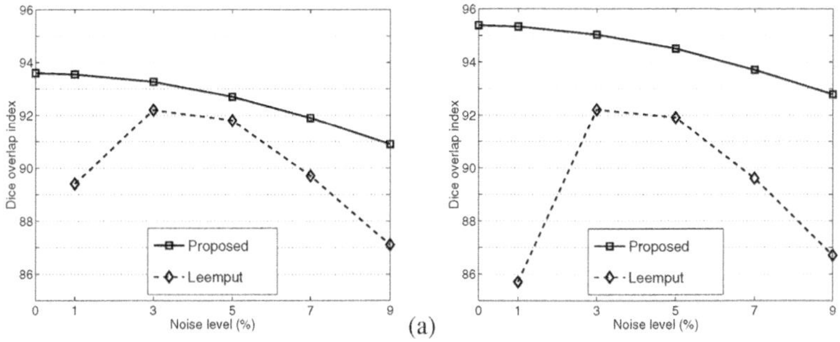

(a) (b)

Fig. 1. Dice metric as a function of noise level: (a) gray matter, and (b) white matter. Solid and dashed lines plot the performance of the proposed algorithm and [1], respectively.

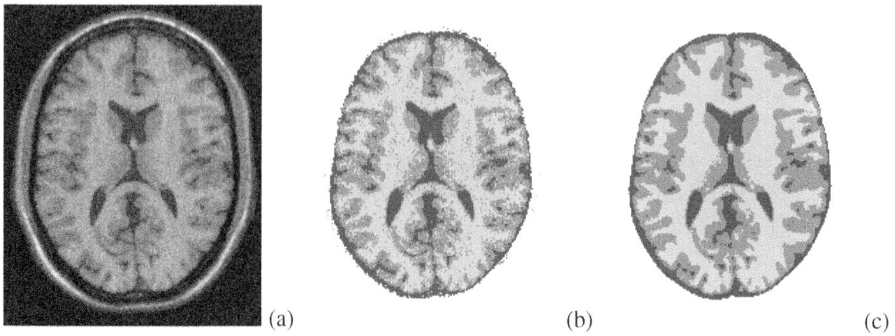

Fig. 2. (a) Simulated, noisy image. Tissue classification (b) without, and (c) with neighborhood information. Classification legend: CSF(black), gray matter(dark gray), white matter(light gray).

information is critical to the success of the proposed method. We repeated the segmentation experiments at the 9% noise level using only the center pixel of the neighborhood. In this case, the method learns single-pixel intensity PDFs in a nonparametric manner. The Dice metrics for gray and white matter were 82% and 85%, respectively, a drop of 8% from the neihborhood algorithm. Figure 2 visually demonstrates this same drop in performance using an axial slice from the 3D image with 9% noise.

For low noise levels, the performance of the parametric Expectation Maximization algorithm drops dramatically [1] because pixels close to the interface between gray and white matter are systematically assigned to the class which happens to have the larger amount of natural variability, i.e. gray matter. In contrast, nonparametric density estimation does not suffer from this drawback as can be observed in Figure 1.

The second validation experiment is performed on simulated T1-weighted data with 40% bias field, i.e. the multiplicative factor is in the range 0.8-1.2 over the brain area. Figure 3 plots the Dice metric with and without bias field correction for the proposed algorithm and the corresponding values given in [1]. These results point out the importance of performing bias field correction. Also, as in the previous experiment, the proposed method performs better at all noise levels for both tissue types. We use a 2nd degree polynomial least squares fit to the observed multiplicative factors between white matter pixel intensities and the white matter mean intensity. The Dice metric values obtained with this correction method are approximately 0.5% worse than the values

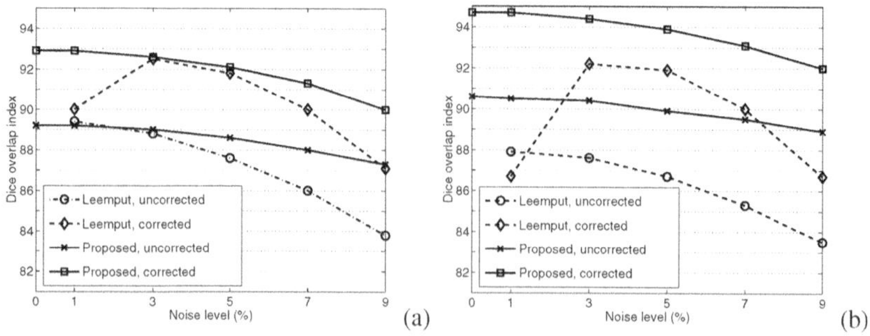

Fig. 3. Results on simulated data with 40% bias field. Dice metric as a function of noise level with and without bias field correction: (a) gray matter, and (b) white matter.

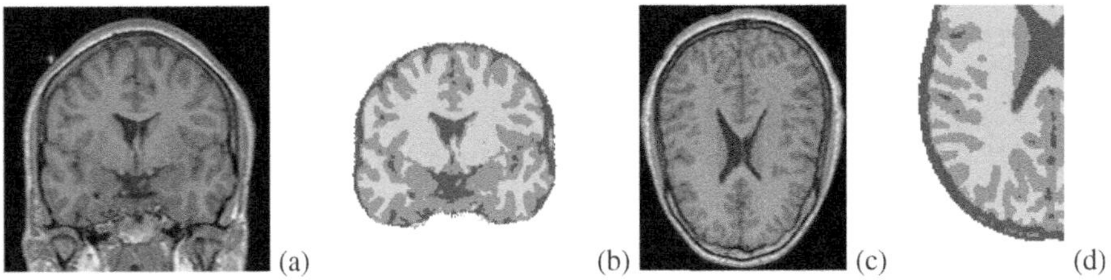

Fig. 4. Real data: (a) coronal slice, (b) classification, (c) close-up view of an axial slice, and (d) classification. Classification legend as in Figure 2.

shown in Figure 1 for data with no bias field. Van Leemput *et al.* use a 4th degree polynomial fit using all tissue types and obtain results that are effectively the same as their results for unbiased data. We expect that with better bias correction methods, such as the one used in [1], this difference can be made very small for our algorithm as well.

Figure 2 illustrates that our approach can remove the effects of noise from the classification results without over regularizing the interfaces between different tissue types. We have also tested the algorithm on a 1 mm isotropic real T1-weighted image. Figure 4 shows coronal and axial slices from this data with corresponding tissue classifications. In both of these cases, the fine structure of the interface between gray and white matter is preserved without the need of placing any additional constraints on the neighborhood PDFs learned by the algorithm.

The disadvantage of the proposed algorithm is the computational speed. For volumetric data with dimensions $181 \times 217 \times 181$, one complete iteration of the algorithm takes approximately 90 minutes to compute on an *Intel 2.7Ghz* processor. The algorithm requires 4-7 iterations to converge depending on the noise level in the data. The Parzen window density estimation is the bottleneck in computational speed; therefore, we plan to address computational issues by using fast density evaluation algorithms [24].

5 Conclusion

In this paper, we introduced a segmentation method that uses entropy minimization to learn nonparametric statistics of local neighborhoods from noisy data in an unsupervised manner . This segmentation framework is used in conjunction with the ICBM brain atlas and bias field correction methods from the literature in an automatic MRI brain tissue classification application. Validation studies on simulated 3D images compare favorably to a state-of-the-art parametric algorithm based on MRFs. Validation studies on real data is also necessary, and will be performed as a continuation of this work. Experiments on real and artificial data also demonstrate that noise is effectively removed without over regularizing interfaces between different tissue types.

The algorithm easily extends to larger neighborhood systems and multi-modal data. Preliminary experiments with 2D images demonstrate that the classification performance can be slightly improved in these cases. Also, we have not considered the partial voluming effect, which has been studied in several papers in the literature. In future work, we plan to generalize the entropy defined in equation (1) from tissue labels to mixture percentages; hence, treating the partial voluming effect in an explicit manner.

Acknowledgments

This work was supported in part by NIH NCRR P41 RR12553-04, NSF EIA 0313268, NIH U01-AG024904, the Louise Madsen Memorial Fund and the Rolan K. Schuholz Research Fund at the University of Michigan.

References

1. Leemput, K.V., Maes, F., Vandermeulen, D., Seutens, P.: Automated model-based tissue classification of mr images of the brain. IEEE Tr. Med. Imaging **18** (1999) 897–908
2. Pohl, K.M., Wells, W.M., Guimond, A., Kasai, K., Shenton, M.E., Kikinis, R., Grimson, W.E.L., Warfield, S.K.: Incorporating non-rigid registration into expectation maximization algorithm to segment mr images. In: Proc. MICCAI. (2002) 564–571
3. Leemput, K.V., Maes, F., Vandermeulen, D., Seutens, P.: Automated model-based bias field correction of mr images of the brain. IEEE Tr. Med. Imag. **18** (1999) 885–896
4. Gerig, G., Kubler, O., Kikinis, R., Jolesz, F.A.: Nonlinear anisotropic filtering of mri data. IEEE Tr. Med. Imaging **11** (1992) 221–232
5. Kapur, T., Grimson, W.E.L., Wells, W.M., Kikinis, R.: Segmentation of brain tissue from magentic resonance images. Med. Im. An. **1** (1996) 109–127
6. Held, K., Kops, E.R., Krause, B.J., Wells, W.M., Kikinis, R., Muller-Gartner, H.W.: Markov random field segmentation of brain mr images. IEEE Tr. Med. Imaging **16** (1997) 878–886
7. Pachai, C., Zhu, Y.M., Guttmann, C.R.G., Kikinis, R., Jolesz, F.A., Gimenez, G., Froment, J.C., Confavreux, C., Warfield, S.K.: Unsupervised and adaptive segmentation of multispectral 3d magnetic resonance images of human brain: a generic approach. In: Proc. MICCAI. (2001) 1067–1074
8. Zhang, Y., Brady, M., Smith, S.: Segmentation of brain mr images through a hidden markov random field model and the expectation maximization algorithm. IEEE Tr. Med. Imaging **20** (2001) 45–57
9. Kelemen, A., Szekely, G., Gerig, G.: Three-dimensional model-based segmentation of brain mri. In: Proc. IEEE Workshop Biomedical Image Analysis. (1998) 4–13
10. Atkins, M., Mackiewich, B.: Fully automatic segmentation of the brain in mri. IEEE Tr. Med. Imaging **17** (1998) 98–107
11. Lee, A., Pedersen, K., Mumford, D.: The nonlinear statistics of high-contrast patches in natural images. Int. J. Comput. Vision **54** (2003) 83–103
12. Popat, K., Picard, R.: Cluster based probability model and its application to image and texture processing. IEEE Tr. Image Processing **6** (1997) 268–284
13. Awate, S., Whitaker, R.: Higher-order image statistics for unsupervised, information-theoretic, adaptive, image filtering. SCI Institute Technical Report UUSCI-2005-004, University of Utah (2005) To appear in CVPR'05.
14. Dougherty, E.R.: Random Processes for Image and Signal Processing. Wiley (1998)
15. Viola, P., Wells, W.: Alignment by maximization of mutual information. In: Int. Conf. Comp. Vision. (1995) 16–23
16. Duda, R.O., Hart, P.E., Stork, D.G.: Pattern Classification. Wiley (2001)
17. Fischl, B., Salat, D.H., Busa, E., ALbert, M., Dieterich, M., Haselgrove, C., van der Kouwe, A., Killiany, R., Kennedy, D., Klaveness, S., Montillo, A., Makris, N., Rosen, B., Dale, A.M.: Whole brain segmentation: Automated labeling of neuroanatomical structures in the human brain. Neuron **33** (2002)
18. Collins, D.L., Zijdenbos, A.P., Barre, W.F.C., Evans, A.C.: Animal+insect: Improved cortical structure segmentation. In: Proc. An. Symp. Inf. Proc. in Med. Img. Volume 1613. (1999)

19. Rex, D.E., Ma, J.Q., Toga, A.W.: The loni pipeline processing environment. NeuroImage **19** (2003) 1033–1048
20. Wells, W.M., Grimson, W.E.L., Kikinis, R., Jolesz, F.A.: Adaptive segmentation of mri data. IEEE Tr. Med. Imaging **15** (1996) 429–443
21. Guillemaud, R., Brady, M.: Estimating the bias field of mr images. IEEE Tr. Med. Imaging **16** (1997) 238–251
22. Cocosco, C., Kollokian, V., Kwan, R.S., Evans, A.: Brainweb: Online interface to a 3d mri simulated brain database. NeuroImage **5** (1997)
23. Dice, L.R.: Measures of the amount of ecologic association between species. Ecology **26** (1945) 297–302
24. Yang, C., Duraiswami, R., Gumerov, N.A., Davis, L.: Improved fast gauss transform and efficient kernel density estimation. In: Int. Conf. Comp. Vision. (2003) 464–471

Robotic Assisted Radio-Frequency Ablation of Liver Tumors – Randomized Patient Study

A. Patriciu, M. Awad, S.B. Solomon, M. Choti, D. Mazilu, L. Kavoussi, and D. Stoianovici

The Johns Hopkins University, Baltimore MD 21224

Abstract. The minimally invasive treatment of liver tumors represents an alternative to the open surgery approach. Radio-frequency ablation destroys a tumor by delivering radio-frequency energy through a needle probe. Traditionally, the probe is placed manually using imaging feedback. New approaches use robotic devices to accurately place the instrument at the target. The authors developed an image-guided robotic system for percutaneous interventions using computed tomography. The paper presents a randomized patient study comparing the manual versus robotic needle placement for radio-frequency ablation procedures of liver tumors. The results of this study show that in our case robotic interventions were a very viable solution. Several treatment parameters such as radiation exposures and procedure-times were found to be significantly improved in the robotic case.

1 Introduction

Minimally invasive image guided procedures are increasingly popular due to their potential benefits such as reduced trauma and improved recovery time. In such procedures an instrument, usually a needle, is percutaneously placed to an anatomical target under image guidance. The imaging methods used for guidance include all types of imaging: ultrasound, X-Ray, computed tomography (CT), and magnetic resonance imaging (MRI). In the traditional approach the needle is manually placed by the physician. This requires a significant amount of training, hand-eye coordination, 2D to 3D extrapolation skills, and in the same time it can deliver a large amount of radiation to the patient and medical personnel if imaging uses X-Rays. To overcome these problems researchers proposed a number of needle guides, shields and even robotic manipulators. Robots have the advantage of operating in the digital space of the image, potentially have better manipulation performance, and are insensitive to radiation.

Robot manipulators for minimally invasive image guided interventions have been developed starting in the late 80's. Several robotic systems have been purposely developed for CT-guided interventions. A system named Minerva was designed for stereotactic neurosurgery at the Micro-engineering Laboratory of the Swiss Federal Institute of Technology Center [3]. Masamune et al. developed a minimally invasive surgical system for neurosurgery [6]. An MRI compatible needle driver was designed by the same group using ultrasonic motors and non-ferromagnetic materials [7].

J. Duncan and G. Gerig (Eds.): MICCAI 2005, LNCS 3750, pp. 526–533, 2005.

In recent years a growing effort was devoted to building robots that can work with magnetic resonance imaging (MRI). Chinzei et al. [1] developed an MR compatible robot that can work in an open magnet MR. Kaiser et al. developed a system for breast biopsy [4]. The system uses ultrasonic motors for actuation and a combination of laser range sensors and custom built optical rotation code transducers for position feedback.

Another device for MR guided interventions was developed by Krieger et al. [5] at the Johns Hopkins University. The manipulator was designed for transrectal prostate interventions. The position of the device in MR coordinates is computed using special design position coils. The system was used initially on animal studies and after the initial validation was redesigned and used on a patient pilot study.

The validation of a surgical system requires model studies, followed by cadaver or animal studies before the system can be clinically used. In order for a system to demonstrate an improvement over a traditional approach, it is commonly evaluated in a randomized patient study. The procedures outcome variables are compared for the robotic assisted and manual approaches. Despite the relatively large number of experimental surgical robotic systems, there are very few randomized patient studies that assess their functionality in real clinical environments. Cleary et al. [2] reported a randomized clinical study with twenty patients. The study compared the outcome of a joystick controlled robotic needle placement versus manual needle placement. The study showed that the robot can be at least as accurate as the human operator. Even though in the reported study the system did not include computer controlled image guidance, the study provided important validation methodologies for surgical systems in the interventional suite.

This paper reports the results of a randomized patient study comparing the robotic assisted versus manual needle placement. Both cases are performed under CT-guidance. The goal of the study is to evaluate wether or not the robotic system can improve the time, radiation exposure, and/or accuracy of the RF procedure.

2 Materials and Method

The interventional system comprises a surgical robot [10] attached to a CT-Scanner mobile table. The target is defined by the surgeon/radiologist in CT image space. In order to compute the position of the target in robot space it is necessary to compute first the transformation between the CT image space and the robot space - the registration transformation. This is computed using the laser system provided with the CT-scanner [8]. A short description of the surgical robot and of the registration technique is presented below.

2.1 Surgical Robot

The surgical robot (Figure 1) presents a bridge like structure comprising a XYZ cartesian stage and a PAKY-RCM robotic module connected through a 6DOF

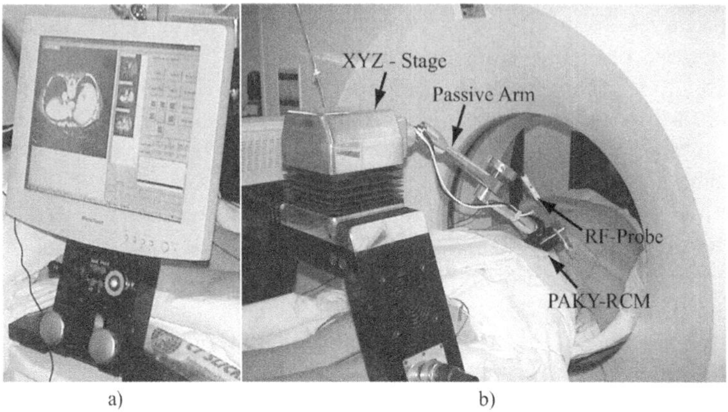

Fig. 1. AcuBot robot: a) User interface detail; b) Acubot in a robotic assisted CT guided RF Ablation

passive arm [10]. The RCM (Remote Center of Motion) module is capable of precisely orienting an instrument (needle) around a fixed point distal to the mechanism. PAKY (Percutaneous Access to the KidneY) is a needle driver allowing for the needle insertion to be performed after alignment with the target. The instrument is loaded initially with its point at the fulcrum. The PAKY-RCM ensemble is initially positioned using the passive arm such that the fulcrum is close to the desired entry point. The XYZ cartesian stage can be used for small adjustments in the initial robot positioning until the point of the needle is at the skin entry site.

The user interface includes an LCD mounted on the bridge adapter (Fig. 1) together with a joystick and an emergency stop button. The manipulator is controlled using an industrial PC fitted with a PCX-DSP Motion Engineering card. The manipulator can be attached to a CT table as well as an OR table, using special adapters.

2.2 CT-Registration and Targeting

The registration procedure involves two main steps, as follows:

Step 1. This step defines the current image plane (LP_1) in the robot coordinate system by using the laser alignment process (Fig. 2). The current image plane is defined in robot coordinates by placing the instrument/needle in two different positions contained in that plane. The robot is initially placed such that the needle point is in the image plane, then the instrument is rotated around its tip and placed in two different positions $\vec{v}_i$, $i = 1, 2$ contained in the image plane. In the current implementation, the containment condition is verified visually by the operator observing if the laser marker shines the end of the needle. In future implementations an optical sensor will be attached to the needle end for automatic plane detection. The cross product of $\vec{v}_1 \times \vec{v}_2$ defines the $\vec{z}$-axis of the CT-Scanner in robot space. At this stage, the

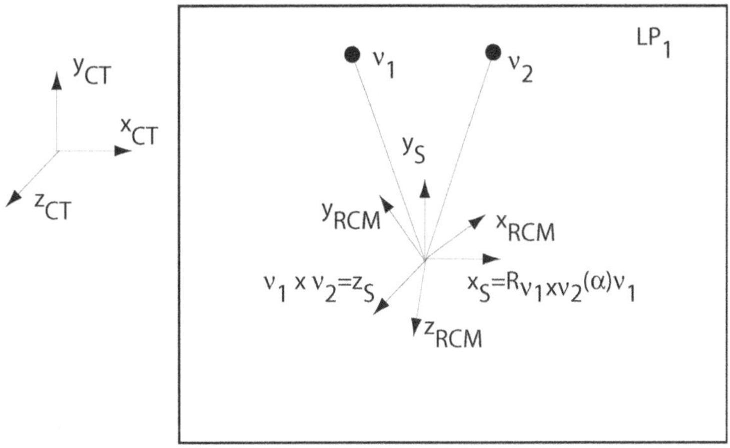

Fig. 2. Registration method and associated coordinates frames. xyz_{RCM} - RCM robot coordinate frame; xyz_{CT} - CT coordinate frame; xyz_s - auxiliary coordinate frame, parallel with xyz_{CT} and with the same origin as xyz_{RCM}

robot can be restricted to move in the LP_1 image plane. This could be used to remotely manipulate the needle in the image space in a similar way that radiologists presently perform CT fluoroscopy manual interventions.

Step 2. The remaining registration data is image-based and uses the image acquired for entry-point/target specification. An image is acquired at the $\vec{\nu}_1$ needle orientation. The angle between the image of the needle and the $\vec{x}$-axis of the CT is α. Then, the CT $\vec{x}$-axis in robot coordinates is $Rot_{\nu_1 \times \nu_2}(\alpha)\nu_1$, where $Rot_\delta(\theta)$ is a rotation matrix about the axis δ with the angle θ. This completes the necessary rotational registration data. The translational component is computed using the current position in the image of the tip of the needle which is also the origin of the robot space and the data stored in the DICOM image.

The physician selects the target in an intra-operative CT image displayed on the monitor of the robot. The image coordinates are transformed to robot coordinates using the registration transformation. The coordinates of the target are then used by the robot controller to accurately align and insert the needle at the specified location, if commanded by the physician.

2.3 Randomized Patient Study

The system accuracy and reliability were initially tested in a preclinical environment. The mean accuracy recorded over $n = 25$ trials was $1.7mm$ with a standard deviation of 0.8 [9]. While the preclinical study represents a good engineering validation of the system, a clinically usable system is more demanding; it is necessary to prove that the system improves the results of a real procedure. After the system obtained the authorization of the hospital, the performance of the system was objectively assessed using a randomized study involving fourteen patients undergoing radio-frequency ablation of the liver tumors. The patients were randomized to undergo the robot assisted RF probe placement or conventional CT guided manual probe placement.

For the manual needle placement the following steps were performed:

1. The patients were placed on the CT table. A volume scan was initially acquired to localize the lesion and plan the procedure. The entry site was cleaned with betadine; local lidocaine was administered over the planned entry site.
2. The needle was manually inserted at the desired location under CT fluoroscopy guidance. During the insertion the patient is instructed by the physician to hold his breath.
3. The radio-frequency ablation was performed.

In the robotic needle placement the following steps were performed:

1. The patients were placed on the CT table. A volume scan was initially acquired to localize the lesion and plan the procedure. The entry site was cleaned with betadine; local lidocaine was administered over the planned entry site.
2. The robot was placed such that the point of the needle entry point was at the planned entry point. The registration procedure was performed.
3. A CT image is acquired such that the target is contained in that image.
4. The robot automatically oriented the instrument.
5. The radiologist manually inserted the needle in with the amount specified by the targeting algorithm under patient breath-hold; the direction of the needle is maintained by the robot. The optimal approach would be to automatically insert the needle using the needle driver. In the current setting this is not possible due to a plastic insulation coating present on the RF needle barrel.

Table 1. Recorded treatment variables for CT guided RF ablation randomized patient study

#	Treatment Variable	Description
1	number of probe passes	How many times was the RF probe placement adjusted.
2	time to successful targeting	Time in minutes from the moment when the CT image used to define the target was acquired and the moment when the probe was at the desired location.
3	overall procedure time	The total duration of the procedure, including the RF teatment, measured in minutes.
4	patient radiation exposure	mrem
5	physician radiation exposure	mrem
6	complications	complications during or after the procedure
7	ablation completeness	did the treatment cover the entire tumor?

6. The radio-frequency ablation of the tumor is performed after a verification of the needle placement accuracy.

For all patients, the treatment variables presented in Table 1 were recorded. The accuracy of the procedure was characterized by the number of probe passes required to reach a satisfactory instrument placement. The radiation exposure of the patient was measured using a radiation badge placed in the proximity of the entry site. The radiation exposure of the physician was measured at the hand level using a radiation monitoring ring badge. The study was designed to evaluate the potential of the robot to reduce the procedure costs by reducing the overall procedure time, as well as, and the potential of the robot to reduce the radiation exposure of the patient and physician.

3 Results

The study shows that the number of passes to reach the target is lower in the robotic case ($p = 0.0006$). Also, the robotics approach delivers a smaller amount of radiation to the physician ($p = 0.0004$) and to the patient ($p = 0.0007$). The time to reach the target ($p = 0.0001$) and the overall procedure time ($p = 0.00005$) were lower in the case of robotic approach when compared to the manual case. All statistical tests were performed using Student's t-Test. Table 2 presents the mean values and standard deviations of the treatment variables measured. Furthermore, all ablative procedures were well tolerated in all patients with no difference in the ability to achieve complete ablation ($> 90\%$) in the two groups. RF ablation was considered successful if no local recurrence was detected by CT or MRI after 6 months of follow-up imaging (either CT or MRI). For all patients in both robotic and manual groups, no local recurrence was detected.

Table 2. Data statistics for the CT guided robotic versus manual RF ablations patient study

	Robotic				**Manual**			
	Mean	Std. Dev.	Max	Min	Mean	Std. Dev.	Max	Min
time to successful targeting (min)	3.57	1.13	4	2	8.57	1.99	12	6
overall procedure time(min)	44.57	6.68	53	36	67.57	8.28	57	78
number of probe passes	1		1	1	3.71	1.25	6	2
patient radiation exposure (mrem)	469.71	177.09	836	279	7075.71	3181.65	2923	12522
physician radiation exposure (mrem)	0				577.57	250.56	327	1097

4 Conclusion and Discussion

The paper presents a randomized study designed to assess the performances of robotic assisted CT guided RF-ablations procedures. The robotic assisted radio-frequency ablation was compared against the standard manual approach through several treatment variables. The study showed that the robotic assisted treatment of liver tumors is feasible, and it provides an improvement in terms of the procedure time, procedure accuracy, physician radiation exposure and patient radiation exposure.

Robotic assisted approaches present the potential to reduce costs by reducing the time of the procedure. The needle placement accuracy influences the outcome of the procedure; precise needle placement ensures that the tumor is destroyed with more reliable margins, while minimizing the healthy tissue damage. The reduction of radiation exposure is equally advantageous for patient and physician. Since there is a maximum amount of radiation that a human can tolerate the reduction in radiation exposure translates in the physician's ability to perform more procedures annually. The results of this study show that the robotic approach can be beneficial for CT-guided RF ablations procedures.

The proposed testing methodology can be used to validate the real performances of other robotic systems designed for minimally invasive procedures. Future developments will evaluate its potential application to other CT guided interventions.

Disclosure

"Under licensing agreements between ImageGuide and the Johns Hopkins University, the authors are entitled to a share of royalty received by the University on ImageGuide's sales of products embodying the robotic technology described in this article. Under a private license agreement, authors are entitled to royalties on ImageGuide's sales of products embodying the technology described in this article. The authors and the University own Image Guide stock, which is subject to certain restrictions under University policy. Dr. Stoianovici is a paid consultant to Image Guide and a paid member of the company's Scientific Advisory Board. Dr. Stoianovici's participation in the study was limited to technical maintenance of the robot. Dr. Stoianovici did not interact with patients and was not involved in clinical data analysis. The terms of this arrangement are being managed by the Johns Hopkins University in accordance with its conflict of interest policies."

Acknowledgements

This work was partially supported by grant No. CA88232 from the National Cancer Institute (NCI) and by the American Foundation of Urologic Disease (AFUD/AUER) Research Scholar Program and Dornier MedTech. Its contents are solely the responsibility of the authors and do not necessarily represent the official views of NCI and AFUD.

References

1. K. Chinzei, N. Hata, F. Jolesz, and R. Kikinis. Mr compatible surgical assist robot: System integration and preliminary feasibility study. In *Proceedings of Third International Conference On Medical Robotics, Imaging and Computer Assisted Surgery*, pages 921–930, Pittsburgh, 2000.
2. K. Cleary, V. Watson, D. Lindisch, A. Patriciu, D. Mazilu, and D. Stoianovici. Robotically assisted interventions: Clinical trial for spinal blocks. In *Medical Image Computing and Computer-Assisted Intervention - Miccai 2003, Pt 2*, volume 2879 of *Lecture Notes in Computer Science*, pages 963–964. 2003.
3. D. Glauser, H. Fankhauser, M. Epitaux, J.-L. Hefti, and A. Jaccottet. Neurosurgical robot minerva, first results and current developments. In *Proc. 2nd Int. Symp. on Medical Robotics and Computer Assisted Surgery*, pages 24–29, Baltimore, Maryland, 1995. MRCAS '95 Symposium, C/O Center for Orthop Res, Shadyside Hospital, Pittsburgh, Pa.
4. W. A. Kaiser, H. Fischer, J. Vagner, and M. Selig. Robotic system for biopsy and therapy of breast lesions in a high-field whole-body magnetic resonance tomography unit. *J. Investigative Radiology*, 35(8):513–519, 2000.
5. A. Krieger, R.C. Susil, C. Menard, J.A. Coleman, G. Fichtinger, E. Atalar, and L.L. Whitcomb. Design of a novel mri compatible manipulator for image guided prostate interventions. *Biomedical Engineering, IEEE Transactions on*, 52(2):306–313, 2005. TY - JOUR.
6. K. Masamune, L. H. Ji, M. Suzuki, T. Dohi, H. Iseki, and K. Takakura. A newly developed stereotactic robot with detachable drive for neurosurgery. In *Medical Image Computing and Computer-Assisted Intervention - Miccai'98*, volume 1496 of *Lecture Notes in Computer Science*, pages 215–222. 1998. Times Cited: 2 Article.
7. K. Masamune, E. Kobayashi, Y. Masutani, M. Suzuki, T. Dohi, H. Iseki, and K. Takakura. Development of an mri-compatible needle insertion manipulator for stereotactic neurosurgery. *Journal of Image Guided Surgery*, 1:242–248, 1995.
8. Alexandru Patriciu, Stephen Solomon, Louis R. Kavoussi, and Dan Stoianovici. Robotic kidney and spine percutaneous procedures using a new laser-based ct registration method. In WJ Niessen and M.A. Viergever, editors, *Medical Image Computing and Computer-Assisted Intervention*, volume 2208 of *Lecture Notes in Computer Science*, pages 249–258, Utrecht, Netherlands, 2001. Springer-Verlag.
9. S. B. Solomon, A. Patriciu, M. E. Bohlman, L. R. Kavoussi, and D. Stoianovici. Robotically driven interventions: A method of using ct fluoroscopy without radiation exposure to the physician. *Radiology*, 225(1):277–282, 2002.
10. D. Stoianovici, K. Cleary, A. Patriciu, D. Mazilu, A. Stanimir, N. Craciunoiu, V. Watson, and L. R. Kavoussi. Acubot: A robot for radiological interventions. *IEEE Transactions on Robotics and Automation*, 19(5):927–930, 2003. Times Cited: 0 Article.

New Approaches to Catheter Navigation for Interventional Radiology Simulation

S. Cotin[1,2], C. Duriez[1], J. Lenoir[1], P. Neumann[1,2], and S. Dawson[1,2]

[1] Sim Group, CIMIT, Cambridge, MA 02139
[2] Harvard Medical School, Boston MA 02114, USA
Cotin.Stephane@mgh.Harvard.edu

Abstract. For over 20 years, interventional methods have improved the outcomes of patients with cardiovascular disease. However, these procedures require an intricate combination of visual and tactile feedback and extensive training periods. In this paper, we describe a series of novel approaches that have lead to the development of a high-fidelity simulation system for interventional neuroradiology. In particular we focus on a new approach for real-time deformation of devices such as catheters and guidewires during navigation inside complex vascular networks. This approach combines a real-time incremental Finite Element Model, an optimization strategy based on substructure decomposition, and a new method for handling collision response in situations where the number of contacts points is very large. We also briefly describe other aspects of the simulation system, from patient-specific segmentation to the simulation of contrast agent propagation and fast volume rendering techniques for generating synthetic X-ray images in real-time.

1 Introduction

Stroke, the clinical manifestation of cerebrovascular disease, is the third leading cause of death in the United States. Each year, more than 700, 000 strokes result in over 200, 000 deaths [2]. Ischemic strokes can now be treated using interventional neuroradiologic therapies which rely on the insertion and navigation of catheters and guidewires through a complex network of arteries to restore blood flow. Because the treatment is delivered directly within the closed brain, using only image-based guidance, the dedicated skill of instrument navigation and the thorough understanding of vascular anatomy are critical to avoid devastating complications which could result from poor visualization or poor technique. This was the foundation for a recent decision by the FDA requiring all physicians who wish to treat carotid disease using catheter-based techniques to train to proficiency before performing high-risk procedures in the cerebral circulation. However, while most publications in the field of medical simulation have addressed issues related to laparoscopic training, few aspects of interventional radiology simulation have been explored. Aside of modeling the soft tissue deformation of arteries, other complex problems need to be solved to enable real-time, accurate simulation of such procedures. The one we address in this paper concerns

J. Duncan and G. Gerig (Eds.): MICCAI 2005, LNCS 3750, pp. 534–542, 2005.

the simulation of non-linear deformations of wire-like structures under a large number of non-holonomic constraints, and the definition of such constraints to confine the catheter inside the vascular network. We also briefly mention other results in the areas of real-time fluid flow computation, real-time synthetic X-ray rendering, and patient-specific segmentation. Although some of theses problems have been addressed in previous work [3,9,6,1], in particular in the areas of visualization and catheter modeling, many challenging problems remain, especially when trying to reach a higher level of fidelity and accuracy in the simulation.

2 Modeling of Wire-Like Structures

To control the motion of a catheter or guidewire within the vascular network, the physician can only push, pull or twist the proximal end of the device. Since such devices are constrained inside the patient's vasculature, it is the combination of input forces and contact forces that allow them to be moved toward a target. The main characteristics of wire-like structures that current models attempt to capture include geometric non-linearities, high tensile strength and low resistance to bending. We previously proposed a multibody dynamics model [5] where a set of rigid elements are connected using spherical joints [3], thus mimicking the basic behavior of such devices. Another interesting approach to modeling wire-like structures was introduced by [8]. In this model, a one-dimensional dynamic spline model is used, providing a continuous representation. Different constraints can be defined to control the model, such as sliding through fixed locations. Although real-time computation is possible, this model does not incorporate torsional energy terms. A virtual catheter model, based on a linear elasticity, was introduced by [9], using a set of finite beam elements. The choice of beams for the catheter model is natural since beam equations include cross-sectional area, cross-section moment of inertia, and polar moment of inertia, allowing solid and hollow devices of various cross-sectional geometries and mechanical properties to be modeled. The main issue is its inability at representing the large geometric non-linearities of the catheter or guidewire that occur during navigation inside the vascular network. Another approach also directly targeted at virtual catheter or guidewire modeling was proposed by [1]. In this model, only bending energies are computed, assuming no elongation and perfect torque control. The model has characteristics similar to a multi-body dynamics model but integrates more complex bending energies, as well as local springs for describing the intrinsic curvature of the catheter. Although based on a more ad-hoc representation, a good level of accuracy is obtained using this model. The main drawbacks are how collision response is handled during contact with the walls of the vessel, and computation times that are not compatible with real-time requirements.

To improve the accuracy of previously proposed models, and handle geometric non-linearities while maintaining real-time computation, we have developed a new mathematical representation based on three-dimensional beam theory, combined with an incremental approach that allows for highly non-linear behavior using a linear model, thus guarantees real-time performance. Further optimizations based on substructure decomposition are introduced. Finally, a new method for correctly handling contact response in complex situations where a large number of nodes are subject to non-holonomic constraints, is presented.

2.1 Incremental Finite Element Model

To model the deformation of a catheter, guidewire, we use a representation based on three-dimensional beam theory[10], where the elementary stiffness matrix K_e is a 12×12 symmetric matrix that relates angular and spacial positions of each end of a beam element to the forces and torques applied to them:

$$K_e = \frac{E}{l}\left[\begin{array}{cccccc|cccccc}
A & & & & & & [K_i]_{(1,1)} & & & & & [K_i]_{(1,2)} \\
0 & \frac{12I_z}{l^2(1+\Phi_y)} & & & & & & & & & & \\
0 & 0 & \frac{12I_y}{l^2(1+\Phi_z)} & & & & & & \mathit{Symmetric} & & & \\
0 & 0 & 0 & \frac{GJ}{E} & & & & & & & & \\
0 & 0 & \frac{-6I_y}{l(1+\Phi_z)} & 0 & \frac{(4+\Phi_z)I_y}{1+\Phi_z} & & [K_i]_{(2,1)} & & & & & [K_i]_{(2,2)} \\
0 & \frac{6I_z}{l(1+\Phi_y)} & 0 & 0 & 0 & \frac{(4+\Phi_y)I_z}{1+\Phi_y} & & & & & & \downarrow \\
\hline
-A & 0 & 0 & 0 & 0 & 0 & A & & & & & \\
0 & \frac{-12I_z}{l^2(1+\Phi_y)} & 0 & 0 & 0 & \frac{-6I_z}{l(1+\Phi_y)} & 0 & \frac{12I_z}{l^2(1+\Phi_y)} & & & & \\
0 & 0 & \frac{-12I_y}{l^2(1+\Phi_z)} & 0 & \frac{6I_y}{l(1+\Phi_z)} & 0 & 0 & 0 & \frac{12I_y}{l^2(1+\Phi_z)} & & & \\
0 & 0 & 0 & \frac{-GJ}{l} & 0 & 0 & 0 & 0 & 0 & \frac{GJ}{E} & & \\
0 & 0 & \frac{6I_y}{l(1+\Phi_z)} & 0 & \frac{(2-\Phi_z)I_y}{1+\Phi_z} & 0 & 0 & 0 & \frac{6I_y}{l(1+\Phi_z)} & 0 & \frac{(4+\Phi_z)I_y}{l(1+\Phi_z)} & \\
0 & \frac{6I_z}{l(1+\Phi_y)} & 0 & 0 & 0 & \frac{(2-\Phi_y)I_z}{1+\Phi_y} & 0 & \frac{-6I_z}{l(1+\Phi_y)} & 0 & 0 & 0 & \frac{(4+\Phi_y)I_z}{1+\Phi_y}
\end{array}\right]$$

with $G = \frac{E}{2*(1+\nu)}$ where E is the Young's modulus and ν is the Poisson's ratio; A is the cross-sectional area of the beam, and l its length; I_y and I_z are cross-section moments of inertia; Φ_y and Φ_z represent shear deformation parameters and are defined as $\Phi_y = \frac{12EI_z}{GA_{sy}l^2}$ and $\Phi_z = \frac{12EI_y}{GA_{sz}l^2}$ with A_{sy} and A_{sz} the shear area in the the y and z directions. For the entire structure describing a catheter or guidewire, the global stiffness matrix $[K]$ is computed by summing the contributions of each element, thus leading to the following equilibrium equation in the quasi-static case:

$$[K]U = F \tag{1}$$

where $[K]$ is a band matrix due to the serial structure of the model (one node is only shared by one or two elements). U represents a column matrix of displacements corresponding to external forces F. The matrix $[K]$ is singular unless some displacements are prescribed through boundary conditions. Such boundary conditions are naturally specified by setting the first node of the catheter (base node) to a particular translation or rotation imposed by the user.

There is, however, one main drawback in using directly such a model: it is linear and therefore cannot represent the geometric non-linearities that a typical wire-like object exhibits. Therefore we propose to update $[K_e]$ at every time step, by using the solution obtained at the previous time step. The new set of local stiffness matrices are then assembled in $[K_t]$. Here, we do not use the initial configuration as the reference state, but instead use the previously computed solution. By controlling when each new $[K_t]$ is going to be computed, we can ensure we remain in the linear domain for each incremental step, leading to a correct, global deformation. One potential drawback of this approach is that the model could exhibit a inelastic behavior, i.e. in the absence of forces or torques, the model would only return to the previous state, not the reference configuration. We overcome this problem by computing a force F_t defined as $F_t = -\alpha[K_t](X_t - X_0)$ with $0 < \alpha \leq 1$. This force is added to the external forces F before solving the linear system, and it can be shown that it acts as a damping force, where α relates to the damping coefficient of the model.

To simulate accurately a device such as a guidewire or catheter in the context of interventional neuroradiology, we need to have a large number (from 100 to 200) of beam elements in the model. Although solving linear systems with about 1,000 unknowns can be done in real-time using iterative methods, when integrating non-holonomic constraints, real-time computation on a single-processor workstation is no longer possible. To improve speed and handle accurately collision response, we propose the following optimizations.

2.2 Optimization Using Substructures Analysis

To optimize the computation of a wire-like object composed of multiple beams, we decompose the object in a set of substructures. Each substructure can be constituted of one or several beam elements, and is analyzed independently, assuming that all common boundaries (joints) with the adjacent substructures are fixed (see Figure 1*(a)*). By doing this, we isolate each substructure from the rest of the model. In a second phase, the boundary conditions are relaxed by propagating from the base to the tip of the catheter (see Figure 1*(b)*). The actual local compliance is determined from equilibrium equations at each boundary joint. The total deformation of the structure can be calculated from the superposition of two displacement such that:

$$U = U^l + U^c \tag{2}$$

By specifying the displacement of the first node of each beam to zero, one can compute the local displacement of the second node U^l, due to external force applied on it. Then, U^c represents the necessary corrections to allow boundary displacements. The FEM model of each beam i gives the stiffness between node i and node $i+1$:

$$\begin{bmatrix} (K_i)_{(1,1)} & (K_i)_{(1,2)} \\ (K_i)_{(2,1)} & (K_i)_{(2,2)} \end{bmatrix} \begin{bmatrix} U_i \\ U_{i+1} \end{bmatrix} = \begin{bmatrix} F_i \\ F_{i+1} \end{bmatrix} \tag{3}$$

Setting Boundary Conditions. When applying boundaries conditions to the first node of each beam, we obtain $U_i^l = 0$ in equation (3). Then, the local displacement of node $i+1$ subject to an external force F_{i+1} is:

$$U_{i+1}^l = [(K_i)_{(2,2)}]^{-1} F_{i+1} \tag{4}$$

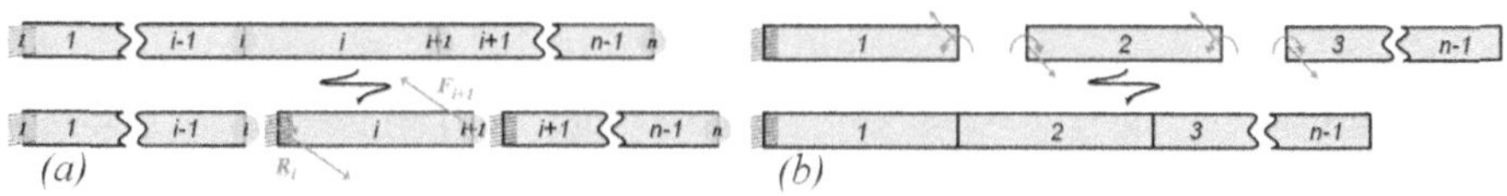

Fig. 1. *(a) Setting boundary conditions:* the object is split in a series of substructures, and local displacements and forces are computed after constraining the first node of each substructure; *(b) Relaxing boundary conditions:* correction displacements are applied recursively, starting from node 1, at each first node of each substructure.

And the reaction on point i, due to this displacement is:

$$R_i = [(K_i)_{(1,2)}]U_{i+1}^l = -\underbrace{(-[(K_i)_{(1,2)}][(K_i)_{(2,2)}]^{-1})}_{[H_i]^T}F_{i+1} \tag{5}$$

Relaxing Boundary Conditions. In this second phase, the external force applied at node $i+1$ has already been taken into account, therefore $F_{i+1}^c = 0$ and only R_i remains. The correction displacement at node $i+1$ is linked to the correction displacement at node i by equation (7):

$$F_{i+1}^c = [(K_i)_{(2,1)}]U_i^c + [(K_i)_{(2,2)}]U_{i+1}^c = 0 \tag{6}$$

$$U_{i+1}^c = \underbrace{-[(K_i)_{(2,2)}]^{-1}[(K_i)_{(2,1)}]}_{[H_i]}\ U_i^c\ ;\ U_i^c = -[K^{-1}]R_i \tag{7}$$

When relaxing boundary conditions, all joints are taken into account except the first node (base) of the model. Doing so eliminates rigid body motion and leads to a non-singular system.

Solving for the Entire Structre. Wire-like objects being composed of serially-linked elements, a bottom to top propagation strategy allows to solve the entire structure. The local compliance $[(K^{-1})_{(i,i)}]$ of each node i will be first computed (we recall that $U_i = [(K^{-1})_{(i,i)}]F_i$). Gathering equations (4), (5) and (7), we obtain:

$$[K^{-1}]_{(i+1,i+1)} = [(K_i)_{(2,2)}]^{-1} + [H_i]^T[(K^{-1})_{(i,i)}][H_i] \tag{8}$$

To initialize the computation, we note that since all 6 DOFs of the first node are fixed, $(K^{-1})_{(1,1)} = 0$. The beam model then leads to a global structural analysis: the force applied on one node induces the displacement of all other nodes. Then, a top to bottom function (Algorithm 1) computes the displacement contribution of each force F_i on the current and previous nodes, and a bottom to top function (Algorithm 2) computes the contribution on following nodes.

2.3 Contact Response

Another important problem in simulating catheter or guidewire navigation is solving the contacts between the virtual device and the vessels wall. Because

Algorithm 1: Force accumulation

Input: $[(K^{-1})_{(2,2)}]...[(K^{-1})_{(n,n)}]$, F, U
Output: U
$f_{acc} = 0$;
for $i = n \dots 2$ **do**
  $f_{acc} = f_{acc} + F_i$;
  $U_i = [(K^{-1})_{(i,i)}] f_{acc}$;
  $f_{acc} = [H_{i-1}]^T f_{acc}$;
end

Algorithm 2: Dpt accumulation

Input: $[(K^{-1})_{(2,2)}]...[(K^{-1})_{(n,n)}]$, F, U
Output: U
$u_{acc} = 0$;
for $i = 2 \dots n-1$ **do**
  $U_i = U_i + u_{acc}$;
  $u_{node} = [(K^{-1})_{(i,i)}] F_i$;
  $u_{acc} = [H_i](u_{acc} + u_{node})$;
end
$U_n = U_n + u_{acc}$;

sliding occurs at the point of contact, Lagrange multiplier techniques, simple penalty forces or quadratic programming approaches will not constrain the flexible body properly. To solve this problem, we compute the local compliance of the node in the contact space defined by $\boldsymbol{n}$, where $\boldsymbol{n}$ is the normal at each contact point. The local compliance of the contact α, at node i, is:

$$W_{\alpha\alpha} = [\boldsymbol{n}]^T (K^{-1})_{(i,i)} [\boldsymbol{n}] \tag{9}$$

The computation of $W_{\alpha\alpha}$ is very fast, as $(K^{-1})_{(i,i)}$ is already known from equation (8). The problem of multiple sliding contact, can be solved using a Gauss-Seidel like algorithm [4]. Considering a contact α, among m instantaneous contacts, one can write the linearized behavior of the catheter in the form:

$$\underbrace{\delta_\alpha - [W_{\alpha\alpha}] f_\alpha}_{\text{unknown}} = \underbrace{\sum_{\beta=1}^{\alpha-1} \underbrace{[W_{\alpha\beta}] f_\beta}_{\text{from algorithm 2}} + \sum_{\beta=\alpha+1}^{m} \underbrace{[W_{\alpha\beta}] f_\beta}_{\text{from algorithm 1}}}_{frozen} + \delta_\alpha^{\text{free}} \tag{10}$$

where $[W_{\alpha\beta}]$ is a compliance matrix that models the coupling between contact points α and β. For each contact α, this method solves the contact and friction equations by considering the others contact points ($\alpha \neq \beta$) "frozen". The solution of these equations (contact, friction) is non-linear and can be computed using an iterative method [7]. Contributions of frozen nodes are accumulated according to algorithms (1) and (2). By sorting nodes in decreasing order, the contribution of contact force f_α on the current and previous nodes is computed by algorithm 1. Its contribution on following nodes is computed at the end of Gauss-Seidel iteration, by using algorithm 2. This leads to a precise and very fast method for computing the entire structure.

3 Interventional Neuroradiology Simulation

In addition to the models and algorithms described previously, we have addressed several other aspects of the simulation of interventional radiology procedures. We briefly describe here these results, more details can be found in [11].

A first problem we addressed concerns arterial flow computation, which impacts both catheter navigation and contrast agent propagation. Blood flow in

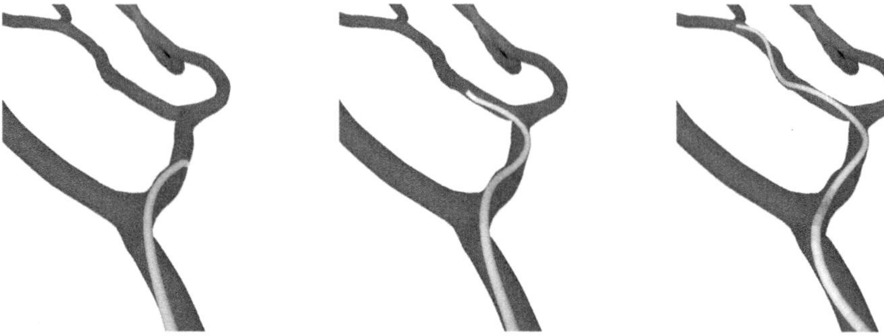

Fig. 2. Catheter navigation inside the cerebrovascular network. Complex, non-linear deformations are correctly represented by the incremental FEM model. Collision detection and collision response allow the catheter to stay within the lumen of the vessels.

each vessel is modeled as an incompressible viscous fluid flowing through a cylindrical pipe, and can be calculated from a simplified Navier-Stokes equation called Poiseuille's Law (11). It relates the flow Q in each vessel to the pressure gradient ΔP, viscosity of the fluid η, radius r, and length L of the vessel.

$$Q = \frac{\Delta P}{R} \quad with \quad R = \frac{8\eta L}{\pi r^4} \tag{11}$$

Solving this equation for the whole vascular system is equivalent to solving a linear FEM model, and, assuming there is no deformation of the vessels, the global resistance matrix $[R]$ can be pre-inverted, allowing for real-time simulation of vascular flow. An example of flow computation is illustrated in Figure 3.

Two other important aspects which relate to visual feedback are X-ray simulation and contrast agent propagation. Both are used during interventional procedures to visualize blood vessels, as well as the anatomy. Contrast agent propagation is simulated using an advection equation where the concentration of contrast agent $\mathbf{C}(x,t)$ is a function of the injection rate $r(t)$ and the averaged laminar flow velocity $u(x,t)$.

$$\frac{\partial C(x,t)}{\partial t} + u(x,t)\frac{\partial C(x,t)}{\partial x} = r(t) \tag{12}$$

We numerically solve (12) using a finite difference scheme. The resulting angiogram is visualized using 3D particles which intensity values are a function of $C(x,t)$. Similarly, we have developed a new volume rendering approach that can render CT datasets as fluoroscopic or X-ray images, in real-time. The X-ray attenuation process simulates X-ray beam attenuation as described by a discretized Beer's Law [11]. This method greatly reduces computation times by using OpenGL and specific texture map operations.

Finally, we propose a multi-modal representation of the vascular system, generated from skeletonization of patient specific CTA datasets, as a mean to ensure consistency in the simulation. The segmentation task is particularly challenging due to the small vessel diameter and the close proximity of vessels to the skull,

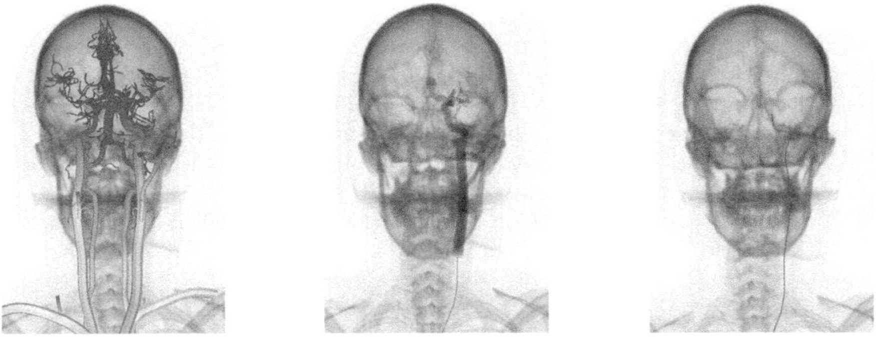

Fig. 3. *Left*: Color-coded vascular model obtained from patient data, warmer colors correspond to increased blood flow; *Center*: Contrast agent injection using particle-based rendering; *Right*: Real-time catheter navigation and fluoroscopic rendering

and thus remain semi-automatic. After applying a combination of anisotropic filtering and morphological operators, medial axis and local radius information is computed. This information is then used to automatically generate a graph of the vascular network for fluid flow computation, a set of 3D particles for contrast agent rendering, a discretization of the centerlines for contrast agent numerical computation, and a C1-continuous triangulation of the surface of the vasculature optimized for fast collision detection. An example of segmented vascular network is presented in Figure 3.

4 Conclusions and Future Work

In this paper we propose a series of new approaches for fast and accurate simulation of catheter or guidewire navigation within a vascular network. The model we introduce for simulating wire-like structures is able to represent the complex behavior of medical devices and handles collision responses in an effective manner. We also describe results related to the development of a full simulator for interventional neuroradiology. The system runs in real-time on a single processor machine and is capable of simulating realistically key aspects of a diagnostic procedure. Current results for a 100 node model show a computation time of 25 ms for one time step (including the computation of Ke, substructure analysis, collision detection, and contact response) on a Pentium 4 2.6 GHz processor. Going forward, we will address the issue of simulating devices such as stents and coils, and develop a set of metrics for measuring performance during training.

References

1. T. Alderliesten. *Simulation of Minimally-Invasive Vascular Interventions for Training Purposes*. PhD dissertation, Utrecht University, December 2004.
2. American Heart Association. Heart and stroke facts statistics: Statistical supplement. American Heart Association, Dallas, Texas, 1999.

3. S. Cotin, S. Dawson, D. Meglan, D. Shaffer, M. Ferrell, and P. Sherman. Icts, an interventional cardiology training system. In J.D. Westwood et al., editor, *Proceedings of Medicine Meets Virtual Reality*, pages 59–65. IOS Press, 2000.
4. C. Duriez, C. Andriot, and A. Kheddar. Signorini's contact model for deformable objects in haptic simulations. In *IEEE-IROS*, pages 3232–3237, 2004.
5. R. Featherstone. The calculation of robot dynamics using articulated-body inertias. *International Journal of Robotics Research*, 2(1):13–30, 1983.
6. U. Hoefer, T. Langen, J. Nziki, F. Zeitler, J. Hesser, U. Mueller, W. Voelker, and R. Maenner. Cathi - catheter instruction system. In *Computer Assisted Radiology and Surgery (CARS)*, pages 101 – 06, Paris, France, 2002.
7. F. Jourdan, P. Alart, and M. Jean. A gauss-seidel like algorithm to solve frictional contact problems. *Comp. Meth. in Appl. Mech. and Eng.*, pages 33–47, 1998.
8. J. Lenoir, P. Meseure, L. Grisoni, and C. Chaillou. Surgical thread simulation. In *MS4CMS (Proc. of ESAIM)*, volume 12, pages 102–107, 2002.
9. W.L. Nowinski and C.K. Chui. Simulation of interventional neuroradiology procedures. In *MIAR*, pages 87 – 94, 2001.
10. J.S. Przemieniecki. *Theory of Matrix Structural Analysis*. 1968.
11. X. Wu, V. Pegoraro, V. Lubos, P. Neumann, R. Bardsley, S. Dawson, and S. Cotin. New approaches to computer-based interventional neuroradiology training. In James D. Westwood et al., editor, *Proceedings of MMVR*, pages 602–607, 2005.

Hybrid Bronchoscope Tracking Using a Magnetic Tracking Sensor and Image Registration*

Kensaku Mori[1], Daisuke Deguchi[1], Kenta Akiyama[1], Takayuki Kitasaka[1], Calvin R. Maurer Jr.[2], Yasuhito Suenaga[1], Hirotsugu Takabatake[3], Masaki Mori[4], and Hiroshi Natori[5]

[1] Graduate School of Information Science, Nagoya University, Nagoya, Japan
{kensaku@is., ddeguchi@suenaga.m.is.}nagoya-u.ac.jp
[2] Department of Neurosurgery, Stanford University, Stanford, U.S.A
[3] Sapporo Minami-Sanjyo Hospital, Sapporo, Japan
[4] Sapporo Kosei Hospital, Sapporo, Japan
[5] School of Medicine, Sapporo Medical University, Sapporo, Japan

Abstract. In this paper, we propose a hybrid method for tracking a bronchoscope that uses a combination of magnetic sensor tracking and image registration. The position of a magnetic sensor placed in the working channel of the bronchoscope is provided by a magnetic tracking system. Because of respiratory motion, the magnetic sensor provides only the approximate position and orientation of the bronchoscope in the coordinate system of a CT image acquired before the examination. The sensor position and orientation is used as the starting point for an intensity-based registration between real bronchoscopic video images and virtual bronchoscopic images generated from the CT image. The output transformation of the image registration process is the position and orientation of the bronchoscope in the CT image. We tested the proposed method using a bronchial phantom model. Virtual breathing motion was generated to simulate respiratory motion. The proposed hybrid method successfully tracked the bronchoscope at a rate of approximately 1 Hz.

1 Introduction

A videobronchoscope consists of a flexible tube and a tiny camera installed at the tip. It is controlled by a physician who watches the camera image through a headpiece or on a video monitor. Bronchoscopy is currently the most commonly employed invasive procedure in the practice of pulmonary medicine and is used for a variety of diagnostic and therapeutic procedures. The physician guides the bronchoscope using only what he sees on the monitor and his knowledge of anatomy. The long-term goal of this research is to develop a bronchoscopic navigation system that provides information such as the planned path of the

* This research was supported in part by a Grant-In-Aid for Scientific Research from the Ministry of Education; the 21st-Century COE program; a Grant-In-Aid for Scientific Research from the Ministry of Education, Culture, Sports, Science, and Technology; the Japan Society for Promotion of Science; and a Grant-In-Aid for Cancer Research from the Ministry of Health and Welfare.

J. Duncan and G. Gerig (Eds.): MICCAI 2005, LNCS 3750, pp. 543–550, 2005.

bronchoscope, the current position of the bronchoscope, and augmented reality visualization of anatomical structures that lie beyond the surface of the bronchial airway. Tracking a bronchoscope is one of the fundamental functions required to build a bronchoscopic navigation system and is the short-term goal of this work.

One approach is image-based tracking in which the position of the bronchoscope is determined by registration of real bronchoscopic (RB) video images and virtual bronchoscopic (VB) images generated from a CT image acquired before the examination. Bricault *et al.* [1] reported the first such work. Their method, which uses the structure of the bronchial tree extracted from the CT image, has difficulty estimating the position of the bronchoscope in areas where no bifurcation appears and considers only the static registration of RB and VB images. Mori *et al.* [2] reported continuous image-based bronchoscope tracking. Good starting points for the image registration process are provided by epipolar geometry analysis of sequential video images. They later improved the tracking process using a sub-block matching algorithm [3].

Image-based tracking generally works very well, but one limitation is that when mistracking occurs in one frame, tracking of subsequent frames is difficult and the method often fails. The two most common causes of failure are quick motion of the bronchoscope and the appearance of bubbles. Another situation that can cause difficulty and failure is when the bronchoscope is both near the bronchial surface and pointing at the surface: the light from the source at the bronchoscope tip can saturate the image. To address this issue and make tracking more robust, we propose a hybrid method for tracking a bronchoscope that uses a combination of magnetic sensor tracking and image-based tracking (image registration). Rigid endoscopes have been tracked with magnetic and optical sensors, and one report uses sensor-based tracking to compare real and virtual endoscopy images [4]. Our proposed method is the first we are aware of to use magnetic sensor tracking for a flexible endoscope, in particular a bronchoscope, and to combine sensor-based tracking with image-based tracking. The position of a magnetic sensor placed in the working channel of the bronchoscope is provided by a magnetic tracking system. Because of respiratory motion, the magnetic sensor provides only the approximate position and orientation of the bronchoscope in the coordinate system of the CT image. The sensor position and orientation is used as the starting point for the registration of RB and VB images. We define coordinate systems and transformations, present the hybrid tracking method, and present preliminary experimental results using a bronchial phantom model with simulated respiratory motion.

2 Background

Bronchoscope tracking: The inputs of the proposed hybrid tracking method are: 1) CT image acquired before the examination, 2) RB video image, and 3) magnetic sensor tracking data. The output is the position and orientation of the bronchoscope, specifically the viewpoint and view direction of the bronchoscope camera model. Tracking consists in generating a sequence of outputs from a sequence of inputs. Synthetic VB images are generated from the CT image using the viewpoint and view direction of the camera. We use volume rendering of the CT image in this work rather than surface rendering of a bronchial surface model extracted from the CT image as in previous work [2]. We denote the k-th frame of a RB video sequence by $\mathbf{B}^{(k)}$ and the position (viewpoint) and orientation (view direction) of the camera by the homogeneous transformation matrix $\mathbf{Q}^{(k)}$ constructed from the rotation matrix $\mathbf{R}^{(k)}$ and the translation vector $\mathbf{t}^{(k)}$.

Magnetic tracking system and sensor: We use the Aurora magnetic tracking system (Northern Digital, Inc., ON, Canada) and a miniature magnetic sensor that is placed in the working channel of the bronchoscope. The measurement volume of the magnetic tracking system is $500 \times 500 \times 500$ mm. The sensor has a cylindrical shape with diameter 0.8 mm and length 8 mm. With this sensor, the tracking system provides only five of the six parameters required to fully describe position and orientation in 3D space. The missing parameter is the rotation angle about the longitudinal sensor axis, which means that the sensor does not provide the twist angle of the bronchoscope. Preliminary tests showed that the bronchoscope we use (BF-200, Olympus, Tokyo, Japan) has negligible effect on tracking accuracy when the sensor is placed in the working channel.

Coordinate systems and transformations: Figure 1 illustrates the various coordinate systems and transformations. We represent the position of a point in the bronchoscope camera coordinate system C as $\mathbf{p}^C$. The position of this point in the CT image coordinate system is represented as $\mathbf{p}^{CT}$. We consider the reference frame defined by a sensor attached to the patient (or phantom) as the world coordinate system W and the position of this point is denoted as $\mathbf{p}^W$. The transformation between $\mathbf{p}^C$ and $\mathbf{p}^{CT}$ is given by

$$\begin{aligned} \mathbf{p}^{CT} &= {}^{CT}_{W}\mathbf{M}\,\mathbf{p}^W = {}^{CT}_{W}\mathbf{M}\,{}^{W}_{F}\mathbf{M}^{(k)}\,{}^{F}_{S}\mathbf{M}^{(k)}\,{}^{S}_{E}\mathbf{M}\,{}^{E}_{C}\mathbf{M}\,\mathbf{p}^C \\ &= {}^{CT}_{W}\mathbf{M} \begin{pmatrix} {}^{W}_{S}\mathbf{R}^{(k)} & {}^{W}\mathbf{t}_S^{(k)} \\ \mathbf{0}^T & 1 \end{pmatrix} {}^{S}_{E}\mathbf{M}\,{}^{E}_{C}\mathbf{M}\,\mathbf{p}^C. \end{aligned} \tag{1}$$

The coordinate system at the tip of the sensor in the working channel of the bronchoscope is denoted as E and the transformation between C and E is ${}^{E}_{C}\mathbf{M}$. The coordinate system at the actual sensing point of the sensor is denoted as S and the transformation between E and S is ${}^{S}_{E}\mathbf{M}$. The coordinate system of the magnetic field generator is denoted as F and the transformations between S and F and between F and W for the k-th frame are ${}^{F}_{S}\mathbf{M}^{(k)}$ and ${}^{W}_{F}\mathbf{M}^{(k)}$. The transformation between S and W is ${}^{W}_{S}\mathbf{M}^{(k)} = {}^{W}_{F}\mathbf{M}^{(k)}\,{}^{F}_{S}\mathbf{M}^{(k)}$ and is obtained from the magnetic tracking system; Eq. (1) shows the rotation and translation components ${}^{W}_{S}\mathbf{R}^{(k)}$ and ${}^{W}\mathbf{t}_S^{(k)}$ of this transformation. The transformation ${}^{E}_{C}\mathbf{M}$ describes the relation between the bronchoscope camera and the tip of the sensor.

3 Hybrid Tracking Method

The tracking method consists of several steps: 1) magnetic sensor calibration, 2) image-to-physical registration, 3) estimation of camera pose for the first frame,

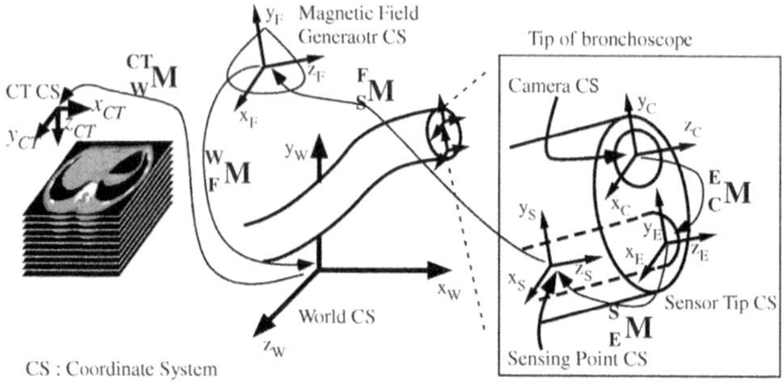

Fig. 1. Coordinate systems and transformations

and 4) updating of camera pose for additional frames. Steps 1 and 2 are performed once before a bronchoscopic examination. Step 3 is performed for the first frame. Continuous tracking is achieved by iterating step 4.

Magnetic sensor calibration: We need to determine the transformation ${}^{S}_{C}\mathbf{M} = {}^{S}_{E}\mathbf{M}\ {}^{E}_{C}\mathbf{M}$. If the sensor provided all six parameters necessary to describe pose in 3D space, the transformation ${}^{S}_{C}\mathbf{M}$ could easily be determined by recording sensor tracking data and RB images of a calibration grid while moving the bronchoscope to various positions and orientations. Since the sensor we use does not provide the rotation angle about the longitudinal sensor axis, we set ${}^{E}_{C}\mathbf{M} = \mathbf{I}$ and construct ${}^{S}_{E}\mathbf{M}$ by measuring the offset between the tip of the sensor and the actual sensing point of the sensor. The error of the identity transformation assumption is corrected during the image registration process.

Image-to-physical registration: We need to estimate the transformation ${}^{CT}_{W}\mathbf{M}$ between the coordinate systems W and CT. This is accomplished by point-based registration between corresponding points on the patient (or phantom) and the CT image. A set of N points $\mathbf{p}_i^{CT}$ $(i = 1, \ldots, N)$ are identified in the CT image. If we had a magnetically tracked probe, we could measure corresponding points on the patient by touching them with the probe and recording their positions. Since we do not have a tracked probe, we use the tip of our five-parameter sensor. The transformation ${}^{CT}_{W}\mathbf{M}$ is found by calculating the rigid transformation that minimizes

$$\sum_{i=1}^{N} \left| \mathbf{p}_i^{CT} - {}^{CT}_{W}\mathbf{M} \left({}^{W}_{F}\mathbf{M}_i\ {}^{F}_{S}\mathbf{M}_i\ {}^{S}_{E}\mathbf{M}\ \mathbf{p}_i^{E} \right) \right|^2, \quad (2)$$

where $\mathbf{p}_i^E = (0, 0, 0, 1)^t$ is the tip of the sensor.

Initial estimation of camera pose: Since the sensor does not provide the twist angle about the bronchoscope camera's viewing direction, we estimate the twist angle using a 1D image registration method for the first frame ($k = 0$). We modify Eq. (1) as

$$\mathbf{p}^{CT} = {}^{CT}_{W}\mathbf{M}\ {}^{W}_{F}\mathbf{M}^{(0)}\ {}^{F}_{S}\mathbf{M}^{(0)}\ {}^{S}_{E}\mathbf{M}\ {}^{E}_{C}\mathbf{M} \begin{pmatrix} \mathbf{r}(\theta) & \mathbf{0} \\ \mathbf{0} & 1 \end{pmatrix} \mathbf{p}^{C} = {}^{CT}_{C}\mathbf{M}(\mathbf{r}(\theta))\ \mathbf{p}^{C} \quad (3)$$

where $\mathbf{r}(\theta)$ is a rotation matrix that represents rotation about the z-axis by angle θ. The pose (viewpoint and view direction) of the bronchoscope camera is $\mathbf{Q}^{(0)} = {}^{CT}_{C}\mathbf{M}(\mathbf{r}(\theta))$. The twist angle $\theta_{\max}$ is found as the parameter generating the VB image $\mathbf{V}(\mathbf{Q}^{(0)})$ that is most similar to the RB image $\mathbf{B}^{(0)}$. This 1D image registration process is formulated as:

$$\theta_{\max} = \arg\max_{\theta} S\left(\mathbf{B}^{(0)}, \mathbf{V}\left({}^{CT}_{C}\mathbf{M}(\mathbf{r}(\theta))\right)\right), \tag{4}$$

where $S(\mathbf{B}, \mathbf{V})$ denotes the image similarity between $\mathbf{B}$ and $\mathbf{V}$ calculated by the method presented in Ref. [3]. The search is performed using Brent's algorithm [5]. Finally, the initial camera pose is $\mathbf{Q}^{(0)} = {}^{CT}_{C}\mathbf{M}(\mathbf{r}(\theta_{\max}))$.

Continuous tracking of camera pose: The sensor position and orientation is used as the starting point for the registration of RB and VB images. The output transformation of the image registration process is the pose of the bronchoscope camera in the CT image. For the k-th frame, we rewrite Eq. (1) as

$$\begin{aligned}\mathbf{p}^{CT} &= {}^{CT}_{W}\mathbf{M} \begin{pmatrix} {}^{W}_{S}\mathbf{R}^{(0)} & {}^{W}\mathbf{t}^{(k)}_{S} \\ \mathbf{0}^{T} & 1 \end{pmatrix} {}^{S}_{E}\mathbf{M}\, {}^{E}_{C}\mathbf{M} \begin{pmatrix} \mathbf{R}^{(k)} \ldots \mathbf{R}^{(0)} & \mathbf{t}^{(k)} \\ \mathbf{0}^{T} & 1 \end{pmatrix} \mathbf{p}^{C} \\ &= {}^{CT}_{C}\mathbf{M}(\mathbf{R}^{(k)}, \mathbf{t}^{(k)})\, \mathbf{p}^{C},\end{aligned} \tag{5}$$

where $\mathbf{R}^{(k)}$ represents rotation between frames $\mathbf{B}^{(k-1)}$ and $\mathbf{B}^{(k)}$, $\mathbf{R}^{(0)} = \mathbf{r}(\theta_{\max})$, and ${}^{W}_{S}\mathbf{R}^{(0)}$ is the rotation component of ${}^{W}_{S}\mathbf{M}^{(0)} = {}^{W}_{F}\mathbf{M}^{(0)}\, {}^{F}_{S}\mathbf{M}^{(0)}$. The updated camera pose is obtained by performing the following image registration process:

$$(\mathbf{R}^{(k)}_{\max}, \mathbf{t}^{(k)}_{\max}) = \arg\max_{\mathbf{R}^{(k)}, \mathbf{t}^{(k)}} S\left(\mathbf{B}^{(k)}, \mathbf{V}\left({}^{CT}_{C}\mathbf{M}(\mathbf{R}^{(k)}, \mathbf{t}^{(k)})\right)\right). \tag{6}$$

The search is performed using Powell's algorithm [5]. The camera pose is $\mathbf{Q}^{(k)} = {}^{CT}_{C}\mathbf{M}(\mathbf{R}^{(k)}_{\max}, \mathbf{t}^{(k)}_{\max})$. This process is iterated for frames $k \geq 1$.

4 Experiments and Results

Configurations: We tested the hybrid tracking method using a bronchial phantom model made of rubber. The phantom was fixed in a plastic box. We placed 24 acrylic tubes in the box and used them as fiducial markers. The tips of these tubes are used for estimating the image-to-physical transformation ${}^{CT}_{W}\mathbf{M}$. CT images were acquired using a multi-detector CT scanner. Image acquisition parameters of the CT image are: 512×512 pixels, 341 slices, 0.68 mm pixel size, and 1.25 mm slice thickness. The locations of the tips of the acrylic tubes were manually identified on the CT images. The distance between the magnetic field generator and the phantom was 200 mm. The computer used in these experiments was a PC workstation with dual 3.6 GHz Intel Xeon processors and 2 GB memory running Windows XP operating system. Intrinsic camera parameters of the bronchoscope camera were determined using a calibration grid and standard camera calibration software. Synthetic VB images are generated using a highly optimized software-based volume rendering method. The actual sensing point of the sensor was found to be 3.3 mm from the sensor tip.

Virtual breathing motion (VBM): The bronchoscope and the RB and VB images are in the coordinate system of the lung or the CT image of the lung. The lung of a living person moves during respiration and thus the lung and the bronchoscope move relative to the coordinate system of the magnetic field generator, which is fixed in the physical space of the treatment room. Even if the bronchoscope is stationary with respect to the lung (and the RB image does not change with time), the bronchoscope position will move relative to the magnetic field generator. Since the phantom we employed here does not simulate breathing motion, we added virtual breathing motion (VBM) to the sensor output. Here, we simplify breathing motion as motion in the axial direction of a human body. We assume that breathing motion in the axial direction is zero at the carina of the trachea and is sinusoidal at the diaphragm. We define the VBM as $\Delta\mathbf{p}(t) = (\Delta\mathbf{p}_x(t), \Delta\mathbf{p}_y(t), \Delta\mathbf{p}_z(t))^T$ and add this motion to Eq. (5) as

$$\mathbf{p}^{CT} = \begin{pmatrix} \mathbf{I} & \Delta\mathbf{p}(t) \\ \mathbf{0}^T & 1 \end{pmatrix} {}^{CT}_{W}\mathbf{M} \begin{pmatrix} {}^{W}_{S}\mathbf{R}^{(k)} & {}^{W}\mathbf{t}^{(k)}_{S} \\ \mathbf{0}^T & 1 \end{pmatrix} {}^{S}_{E}\mathbf{M}\, {}^{E}_{C}\mathbf{M}\, \mathbf{p}^{C}. \tag{7}$$

Since the z-axis of CT images is aligned with the cranial-caudal direction, we add VBM after the transformation between W and CT (${}^{CT}_{W}\mathbf{M}$). The VBM at positions between the carina and diaphragm is interpolated according to fractional axial position. Thus the VBM $\Delta\mathbf{p}(t)$ is defined as $\Delta\mathbf{p}_x(t) = \Delta\mathbf{p}_y(t) = 0$, $\Delta\mathbf{p}_z(t) = A_d \frac{z_c - z_{carina}}{z_d - z_{carina}} \times \sin(2\pi\frac{t}{T})$, where A_d is amplitude of breathing motion at the bottom of the diaphragm, z_c is the z-coordinate of the real camera position before adding VBM, z_{carina} is the z-coordinate of the carina of the trachea, and the z_d is the z-coordinate of the bottom of the diaphragm. These z-coordinates are represented in the CT coordinate system.

Effectiveness of image registration: We measured the changes of estimated RB camera motion caused by VBM. We fixed a bronchoscope at some position and recorded estimated camera positions. As a gold standard of the camera position, we used the estimated position obtained by only image registration. The breathing cycle was set to $T = 6$ s. The mean position errors and their standard deviations are measured. The results are shown in Table 1. Examples of VBM are shown in Fig. 2.

Continuous tracking: We performed bronchoscopic examination on the phantom model using the hybrid tracking method. Camera motion was continuously

Table 1. Position estimation error by adding virtual breathing motion

Amp. of VBM at diaphragm (mm)	Amp. of VBM at camera position (mm)	Avg. error of estimated position (mm)	Standard deviation(mm)
±5.0	±2.4	0.54	0.3
±10.0	±4.8	1.22	0.57
±15.0	±7.2	2.26	1.29

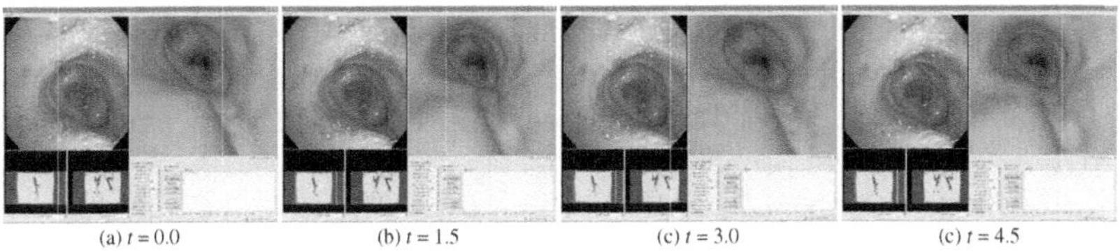

Fig. 2. Effect of virtual breathing motion (VBM). VB views are rendered by using only the sensor's outputs.

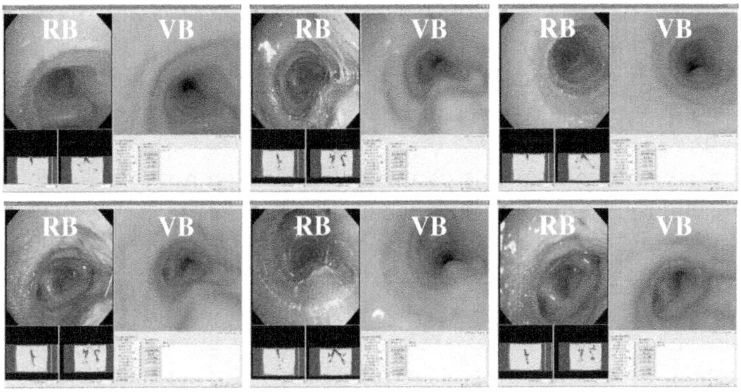

Fig. 3. Tracking results. VB views were rendered by using estimated RB camera position and orientation. VBM was generated during tracking.

tracked and estimated positions were displayed on CT images. VB images were generated using estimated results. In these experiments, VBM was added to the outputs of the magnetic sensor. Figure 3 shows examples of the tracking results. It was possible to update RB camera position and orientation every 1.2 s.

5 Discussion

In the experimental results shown in Table 1, the position estimation errors are much smaller than the VBM; the RB camera positions are satisfactorily estimated by image registration. Figure 3 illustrates that the proposed system successfully estimated RB camera motion in the presence of the VBM shown in Fig. 2. This is the main advantage of hybrid tracking. Although the sensor gives us only a rough estimation, precise estimation is done by image registration. Since the sensor's outputs are used for initial estimation of image registration, it is possible to make the tracking system robust and to reduce computation time. In previous work, e.g., the method in Ref. [2], camera motion is tracked only by image registration. The estimated position of the previous frame is used as the starting point of the iterative search for the current frame. When significant estimation failures occurred, tracking failed in subsequent frames. However, the proposed method in this paper continues to track after such failures. The proposed system tracked the RB camera at 0.8 frames per second. Because of the limited processing speed, the system failed in tracking when an operator inserted or pulled out a bronchoscope quickly. However, in such situations, when the operator kept the bronchoscope stationary at a bifurcation point, the system recovered to the correct estimated position.

We assumed that virtual breathing motion is motion in the axial direction. However, actual breathing motion is much more complicated. Further experiments are required to validate the proposed method. It would be useful to use a bronchial phantom that includes physical breathing motion. Because the Aurora sensor outputs only five pose parameters, we estimated only translation terms of ${}^{S}_{E}\mathbf{M}$ and assumed that the tip of the sensor is aligned with the optical center and direction of the bronchoscope camera (${}^{E}_{C}\mathbf{M} = \mathbf{I}$). The image registration process compensated for the error inherent in these assumptions and produced good results in actual tracking.

The work described in this paper is another step towards developing a fast, accurate, and robust method for tracking a bronchoscope. The results are preliminary but promising. Future work includes: 1) incorporating a magnetic tracking system and sensor that fits in the working channel of a bronchoscope and provides all six parameters necessary to describe pose in 3D space (e.g., Ascension microBird magnetic tracking system), 2) development of a better sensor calibration method, 3) development of better methods for estimating and correcting for breathing motion, 4) improvement of processing speed, and 5) testing with a bronchial phantom model that includes physical breathing motion and with data collected from patients.

References

1. I Bricault, G Ferretti, P Cinquin. Registration of real and CT-derived virtual bronchoscopic images to assist transbronchial biopsy. *IEEE Trans Med Imaging*, 17: 703–714, 1998.
2. K Mori, D Deguchi, J Sugiyama, et al. Tracking of a bronchoscope using epipolar geometry analysis and intensity-based image registration of real and virtual endoscopic images. *Med Image Anal*, 6: 321–336, 2002.
3. D Deguchi, K Mori, Y Suenaga, et al. New image similarity measure for bronchoscope tracking based on image registration. *Proc MICCAI 2003*, LNCS 2878: 309–406, 2003.
4. R Shahidi, MR Bax, CR Maurer Jr, et al. Implementation, calibration and accuracy testing of an image-enhanced endoscopy system. *IEEE Trans Med Imaging*, 21: 1524–1535, 2002.
5. WH Press, SA Teukolsky, WT Vetterling, BP Flannery. *Numerical Recipes in C: The Art of Scientific Computing*, 2nd ed. Cambridge University Press, 1992.

Toward Robotized Beating Heart TECABG: Assessment of the Heart Dynamics Using High-Speed Vision

Loïc Cuvillon[1], Jacques Gangloff[1], Michel de Mathelin[1], and Antonello Forgione[2]

[1] LSIIT / EAVR (UMR CNRS-ULP)*, Strasbourg I University, France
{loic, jacques, demath}@eavr.u-strasbg.fr
[2] IRCAD / EITS, University Hospital of Strasbourg, France

Abstract. Active robotic filtering is a promising solution for beating heart Totally Endoscopic Coronary Artery Bypass Grafting (TECABG). In this work, we assess the heart motion dynamics using simultaneously high speed imaging of optical markers attached to the heart, ECG signals and ventilator airflow acquisitions. Our goal is to make an assessment of the heart motion (shape, velocity, acceleration) in order to be able to make more accurate specifications for a dedicated robot that could follow this motion in real-time. Furthermore, using the 2 additional inputs (ECG, airflow), we propose a prediction algorithm of the motion that could be used with a predictive control algorithm to improve the tracking accuracy.

1 Introduction

Beating heart TECABG will probably bring a great improvement in coronary revascularization surgery. Current open surgery techniques on the beating heart make use of mechanical stabilizers to reduce the motion of the working area. But they still need a sternotomy which induces a long recovery period for the patient.

Totally endoscopic stabilizers begin to be commercially available (e.g. the Octopus TE from Medtronics) but due to their long size and the way they are attached, the residual motion is significant. So it seems that the best way to achieve good precision in TECABG on the beating heart is to have an active filtering system *e.g.* a robot that follows the heart motion in real time. Experiments with robotic prototypes and high speed cameras (500-1000Hz) demonstrate the feasibility of active compensation on pig's heart [1] [2]. However, the achieved tracking accuracy ($1mm$) remains greater than the minimum accuracy needed for grafting a medium sized coronary artery ($0.1mm$).

From these experiments, it comes out that a better knowledge of the dynamic behavior of the heart motion would greatly improve the design of the system for mainly 3 reasons : 1) the motion of the heart has some interesting properties that should be taken into account to predict its behavior in combination with a

* The authors wish to thank the Alsace Regional Council and Centre National de la Recherche Scientifique for the grant which support this research project.

J. Duncan and G. Gerig (Eds.): MICCAI 2005, LNCS 3750, pp. 551–558, 2005.

predictive control scheme. 2) a knowledge on how the heart moves (acceleration, amplitude, shape of the cycle) would certainly help defining more accurately the specifications of the dedicated mechanical structure. 3) the main concern in medical robotics is safety, so knowing the behavior of the heart with respect to redundant input signals should improve the robustness of the whole procedure.

Some previous studies have already dealt either with heart motion properties or its modeling. In 2004 [3], Cattin *et al.* assess the significance of the residual motion of a pig's beating heart after stabilization with an Octopus. The repeatability of the stabilized cardiac motions, providing that hemodynamics are constant, is underlined but no model is proposed. In [4], Ortmaier studies robust motion prediction of heart landmarks with ECG and respiration as additional robust landmark. In [5], Fourier coefficients of respiratory and cardiac components are estimated by a two-stage adaptive algorithm. A similar approach based on adaptive filtering to separate the two components and predict the future motion is presented in [1]. These frequential models assume that ventilation and heartbeat components are independent and invariant.

In this work, we assess the local motion properties of heart for the free and stabilized case. We take advantage of a high speed vision sensor to measure more precisely heart beating velocity, acceleration and their correlation with the ECG waves and ventilation airflow. The analysis of this data demonstrates that the heart global motion is not the result of two *independent* components : it shows that the shape of the cardiac cycle depends on the lung volume. Finally, we demonstrate that arrhythmic behavior of the heart can be predicted using ECG signals. In a second part, a model of the heart motion that takes into account this coupling is proposed in order to predict and anticipate future motion with a robotic device. This model, with biological signals as inputs, is then evaluated and compared with the frequential model found in the literature.

2 Materials and Methods

Experiments were carried out on a pig that underwent a sternotomy with general anesthesia. After positioning the chest retractor, a coronary artery was stabilized using an Octopus v4.3 tissue stabilizer from Medtronics. A rotating knob allows to modify the stiffness of the Octopus arm and so to free or constraint local motion of the heart.

To measure heart motion, a 500Hz high speed camera with a 256*256 pixel grayscale sensor (DALSA CAD6) is placed on a tripod, its lens focused on the stabilized area (figure 1). When its arm is free, the Octopus stabilizer can be used as a convenient way to simply attach visual markers to the heart. The pose of the myocardium area of interest is computed in the camera frame of reference using the modified version of the Dementhon algorithm for coplanar points.

ECG signals are acquired with a classical 3-leads cable and the CARDIOVIT AT-6 ECG from Schiller, which outputs analog amplified and filtered ECG signals. Due to built-in signal pre-processing, it exhibits an average group delay of $8ms$ between electrodes potentials and the ECG analog outputs. Two AWM700 airflow sensors from Honeywell are used for the real-time measurement of the

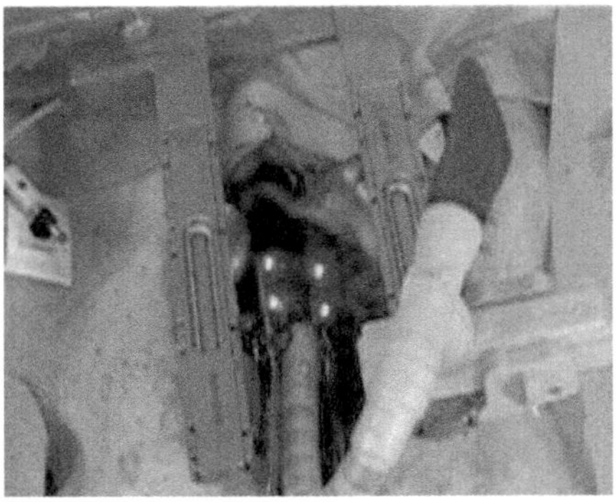

Fig. 1. The heart stabilizer OCTOPUS and its 4 visual markers

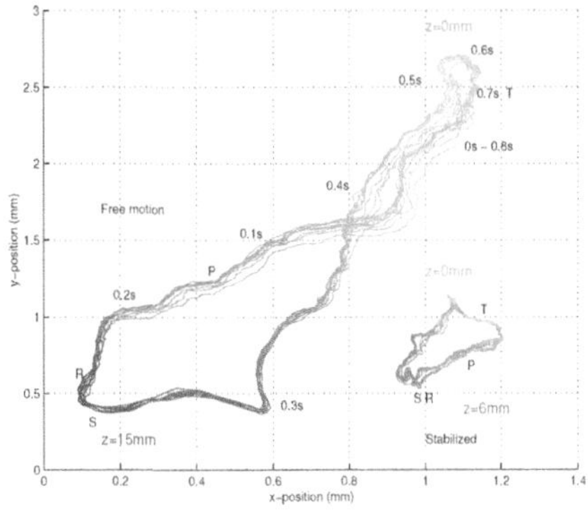

Fig. 2. Heart trajectories in absence of ventilation with timing and ECG waves

ventilator flow. This uni-directional sensor specially designed for biomedical use has a 6-millisecond response time.

Both ECG signals and airflow measurements are then acquired at 500Hz by a PCI acquisition board synchronized with the image acquisition. The whole acquisition software runs on RTAI, a real-time operating system, in order to ensure perfect synchronization and minimal jitter.

3 Motion of an Area of Interest (AOI) on the Heart

3.1 Heart Beating Motion in Absence of Ventilation

Stabilized residual motion. Trajectories of 10 consecutive heartbeats with and without stabilization are plotted in figure 2. It appears that the excursion range of the AOI is about $2.3mm$ in the frontal plane and $15mm$ in the sagital plane for the free motion case. With a constrained motion (maximum stiffness of the octopus arm), the amplitude of the heart motion is highly damped by the stabilizer: the excursion range is reduced to $500\mu m$ and $6mm$ respectively. These values of excursion ranges are similar to those reported in [3] for the residual motion of a stabilized AOI with constant hemodynamics.

Repeatability of the beating trajectory. The repeatability of heart beating trajectory in absence of ventilation and cardiac arrhythmia is a very interesting feature. In the plots of figure 2, for 10 heart beats, the maximum deviation and standard deviation around a mean trajectory on the free and stabilized case are reported in table 1. Thus, considering this perfect periodicity, a *repetitive* control scheme (an example is given in [1]) should give really good results if we assume that respiration can be stopped for a short amount of time. The standard and maximal deviation give then a clue on the accuracy such a system could achieve.

AOI velocity and ECG signal correlation. The heart local velocity is plotted in figure 3. Some markers are added to show the occurrences of T,P,R and S

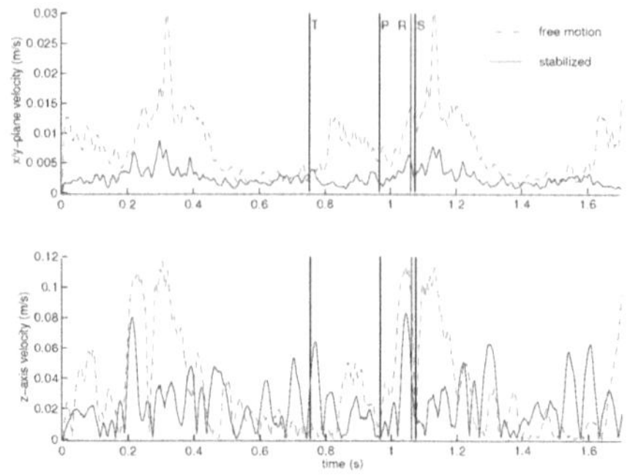

Fig. 3. Heartbeat velocity magnitude with ECG-waves timing in the frontal and sagital planes

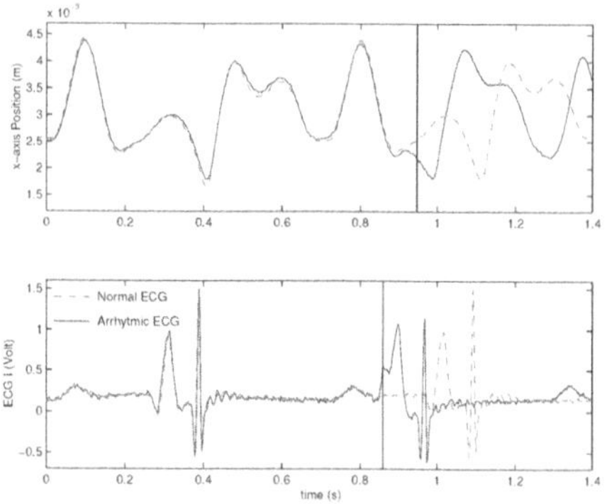

Fig. 4. Correlation between ECG and heart beating: arrhythmic case

Table 1. Deviations with respect to the mean trajectory of 15 consecutive heart beats

	frontal plane		sagital plane	
	max deviation	std deviation	max deviation	std deviation
free motion	146.6 μm	25.6 μm	1.6 mm	0.39 mm
stabilized	63.7 μm	14.7 μm	1.5 mm	0.4 mm

waves of the ECG. The cardiac period is $810ms$. Strong accelerations (therefore high velocities) occur $60ms$ after the T, P and QRS complex waves. On the other hand, heart rest (low velocities) covers a range from $200ms$ after the QRS complex to the next T waves. The maximum acceleration is $0.3m.s^{-2}$ measured in the frontal plane and $10m.s^{-2}$ measured in the sagital plane. These values should be taken into account when writing the specifications of an active robotic stabilizer. Moreover, after injection of a high dose of adrenaline, maximum velocities and maximum accelerations were doubled.

In figure 4, we assess the possibility of predicting arrhythmic behavior of the heart. The vertical cursors indicate in both plots the time when the error between arrhythmic ECG (resp. motion) in plain lines and normal ECG (resp. motion) in dashed lines becomes greater than 10% of the peak to peak amplitude. This figure shows that abnormal ECG can be detected $\approx 90ms$ before the abnormal motion (mean delay=$80ms$, std. deviation=$32ms$ on 12 arrhythmias) letting quite enough time to a robotic system to switch to a failsafe mode.

3.2 Heart AOI Motion Properties with Ventilation

Influence of ventilation on heart motion. During respiration, variation of the lung volume yields a motion of the heart within the chest. In figure 5, the motion of a heart AOI and the corresponding lung volume are recorded over a full respiration cycle with the following parameters : a tidal volume set to 600mL and a frequency of 21 breaths/min.

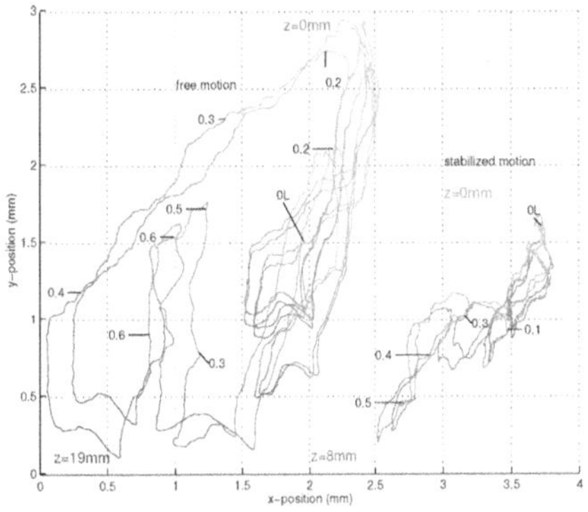

Fig. 5. Heart 3D trajectories with lungs volume information (depth z coded in color intensity)

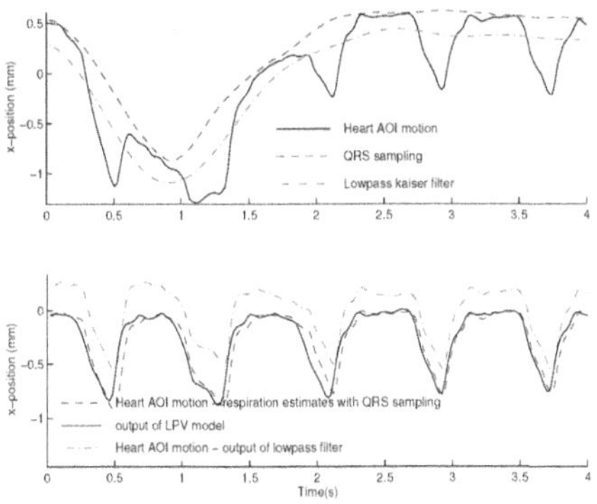

Fig. 6. Respiration and cardiac component over one ventilation period, extracted by proposed model and lowpass filtering

The slow motion component of the heart AOI appears to be directly correlated with the lung volume. Note the different paths followed by the AOI during forced inspiration and the free expiration. Moreover, for low lung volume, *i.e.* at the end of expiration, the 3D trajectory of the heart AIO during a heart beat is similar to the one observed in total absence of ventilation.

Extraction of the ventilation component. ECG signal acquisition can be used as a clock to sample the heart AOI position when *e.g.* the heart is 'at rest'. This way it is possible to suppress the heart beating motion and to access to the respiration component alone.

The detection of the QRS complex can be performed on-line by derivation and adaptive thresholding of the ECG signal. From the original ECG signal, a discrete clock signal $QRS[k]$ with impulses corresponding to QRS detection time is created. In order to increase precision, the previous clock can be delayed by half a cardiac period ($T_b/2$) to sample the respiration while the heart is at rest (when the velocity is slow, see fig 3). By interpolating between the respiratory samples, the respiration motion is reconstructed and subtracted from the global motion in order to isolate the heart beating motion.

The upper plot in figure 6 shows the reconstructed respiratory component and the lower plot shows the isolated heart beating component. The beating motion is very similar to the motion in absence of ventilation, however it is *modulated* by the lung volume. So we cannot assume that the beating is decoupled from respiration.

4 A Heart Motion Model Based on Biological Signals

4.1 Description of the Model

The proposed model is based on the extraction of the respiration component presented earlier. Both the integrated airflow, so the air volume, and QRS occurrences of the ECG signal are used. The proposed algorithm is a 2 stages component identification:

1) In a first step, the profile of the respiration component r is extracted with the approach described in the previous section. Let k be the current sample number and T_{ov} be the sample number corresponding to the beginning of a new respiration cycle. This beginning can be easily detected by a simple thresholding of the volume information. Then :

$$r[k] = Fr(k - T_{ov}) \tag{1}$$

where Fr is a spline function which interpolates one period of the respiration component.

2) In a second step, the heart beating component is extracted from the global motion by subtracting the respiration component. As it was shown before, the heart beating depends on lung volume. In order to take into account this coupling, a Linear Parameter Variant (LPV) Finite Impulse Response model is proposed. This model input is an impulse at each QRS occurrences and its parameters depend on lung volume. Let $v[k]$ be the lung volume and $QRS[k]$ the impulse signal corresponding to the QRS occurrence. The heart position due to cardiac beating $b[k]$ is then given by :

$$b[k] = Fb(v[k])\, QRS[k-1] \tag{2}$$

$$\triangleq \begin{pmatrix} a_{10} + a_{11}v[k] & a_{20} + a_{21}v[k] & \dots & a_{d0} + a_{d1}v[k] \end{pmatrix} \begin{pmatrix} QRS[k-1] \\ \vdots \\ QRS[k-d] \end{pmatrix} \tag{3}$$

where d, is the number of samples in one cardiac period. With this formulation, the coefficients a_{i0} represent the mean value of the beating position, i samples after the previous QRS complex and a_{i1} is the variation of this position related to lung volume. Identification of the coefficients $\{(a_{i0}, a_{i1}), i = 1 \dots d\}$ can be performed online via a recursive least mean square (RLS) algorithm for LPV systems, where the criterion of minimization is the error $e[k]$ between the model output and the reference signal [6].

This identification scheme is summarized in the upper part of the figure 7. The global motion $h[k]$ of the heart AOI at sample k is given by :

$$h[k] = r[k] + b[k] \tag{4}$$

$$= Fr(k - T_{ov}) + Fb(v[k])\, QRS[k-1] \tag{5}$$

4.2 Validation and Comparison with other Approaches

The output of the proposed model is used to predict the motion of the heart some steps ahead. We compare the accuracy of these predictions with respect to other methods found in the literature. We use a set of data down-sampled at 50Hz with a ventilation frequency of $f_r = 0.242Hz$ and a cardiac frequency $f_b = 1.23Hz$. We predict the motion $\Delta = T_b/2 = 20$ samples ahead, so 1/2 heart beat ahead.

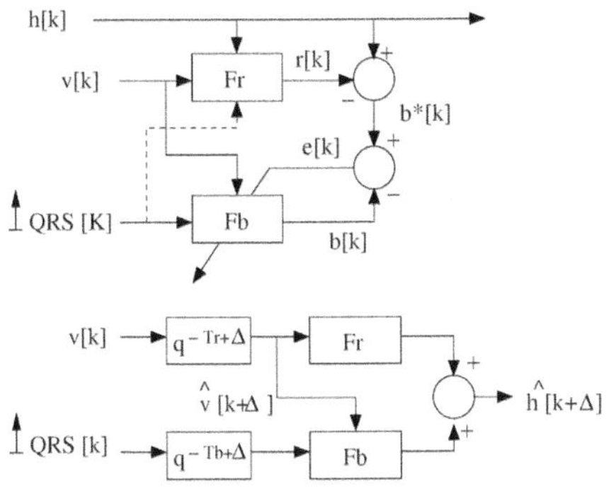

Fig. 7. Identification of the respiration component using QRS sampling method (top) and the corresponding prediction algorithm (bottom)

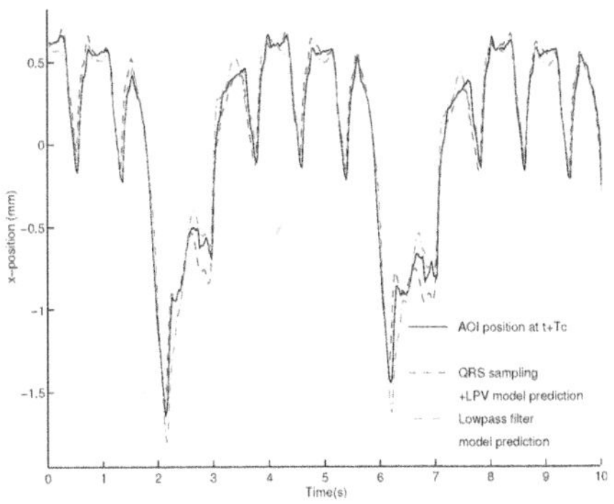

Fig. 8. Comparison of predictions with the lowpass filter approach and with the LPV approach

On one hand, the classical frequential approach filters the global motion to extract the respiration component. One can use a lowpass filter or adaptive filter [1], or also Fourier coefficient estimation [5] to suppress heart beating harmonics with equivalent results. In this study, a kaiser-FIR lowpass filter with a cut-off frequency located between the fundamental of the beating fb and the last significant harmonic of the respiration ($4fr$) is used to separate the 2 components. Predicting Δ steps in the future is then done with pure delays (q^{-1} operator) since the components are equal to themselves in the past with the assumption of perfect decoupling and quasi-periodicity.

On the other hand, in our approach, the prediction assumes only that biological signals (QRS complex and ventilation parameters) remain quasi-periodic over the next beating period (lower part of the figure 7). In figure 6, the respiration component extracted from the global motion with the two methods are plotted on the top whereas cardiac motion resulting from the LPV model output or from the lowpass filter output are presented on the bottom.

Finally, predictions of heart motion Δ steps ahead for both strategies are shown on the figure 8. The continuous line plots the real heart motion Δ steps in the future, whereas the other curves give the predictions with the 2 compared method. Standard deviation error of the prediction is $131\mu m$ (4.7% of the total amplitude) in the frontal plane and 530μ (2.8%) in the sagital plane for our proposed method. For comparative purpose, standard deviation of the error is respectively of $152\mu m$ (5.5%) in the frontal plane and $547um$ (2.9%) for the lowpass approach. If we compare the errors in the image plane (this is relevant when doing image-based visual servoing as in [1]), the standard deviation of the prediction error is 0.62 pixels along x and 0.78 pixels along y when using lowpass filtering whereas it falls to 0.37 and 0.41 pixels respectively with the LPV technique.

5 Discussion

This study shows that there is a *coupling* between the motion components of the heart : the shape of the beating is modulated by the state of the respiration. Furthermore, we measured that the cardiac beating component exhibits very sharp transients (up to $2g$ acceleration). We propose a new motion prediction algorithm using LPV techniques that takes into account this coupling. This approach improves prediction accuracy.

References

1. Ginhoux, R., Gangloff, J., de Mathelin, M., Soler, L., Sanchez, M.A., Marescaux, J.: Active filtering of physiological motion in robotized surgery using predictive control. IEEE Transactions on Robotics **21** (2004) 67–79
2. Nakamura, Y., Kishi, K., Kawakami, H.: Heartbeat synchronization for robotic cardiac surgery. In: Proc. of the IEEE International Conference on Robotics and Automation, Seoul, Korea (2001)
3. Cattin, P., Dave, H., Grünenfelder, J., Szekely, G., Turina, M., Zund, G.: Trajectory of coronary motion and its signicance in robotic motion cancellation. European Journal of Cardio-Thoracic Surgery **25** (2004) 786–790
4. Ortmaier, T.J.: Motion Compensation in Minimally Invasive Robotic Surgery. PhD thesis, Technische Universität München (2003) http://tumb1.biblio.tumuenchen.de/publ/diss/ei/2003/ortmaier.html.
5. Thakral, A., Wallace, J., Tomlin, D., Seth, N., Thakor, N.V.: Surgical motion adaptive robotic technology (s.m.a.r.t.): Taking the motion out of physiological motion. In: Proc. of the 4th Int. Conf. on Medical Image Computing and Computer-Assisted Intervention (MICCAI), Utrecht, The Netherlands (2001) 317–325
6. Bamieh, B., Giarr, L.: Identication of linear parameter varying models. In: Proc. 38'th IEEE Conference on Decision and Control. (1999)

Data-Fusion Display System with Volume Rendering of Intraoperatively Scanned CT Images

Mitsuhiro Hayashibe[1], Naoki Suzuki[1], Asaki Hattori[1], Yoshito Otake[1], Shigeyuki Suzuki[1], and Norio Nakata[2]

[1] Institute for High Dimensional Medical Imaging, Jikei Univ. School of Medicine, 4-11-1, Izumihoncho, Komae-shi, Tokyo 201-8601, Japan
haya@jikei.ac.jp
[2] Department of Radiology, Jikei Univ. School of Medicine, 4-11-1, Izumihoncho, Komae-shi, Tokyo 201-8601, Japan

Abstract. In this study we have designed and created a data-fusion display that has enabled volumetric MIP image navigation using intraoperative C-arm CT data in the operating room. The 3D volumetric data reflecting a patient's inner structure is directly displayed on the monitor through video images of the surgical field using a 3D optical tracking system, a ceiling-mounted articulating monitor, and a small size video camera mounted at the back of the monitor. The system performance was validated in an experiment carried out in the operating room.

1 Introduction

Recently, due to developments in clinical engineering, many types of equipment have become available in the operating room: vital signs monitors, anesthesia apparati, artificial respirators and electric cauteries to count a few. They are essential to collect intraoperative electrocardiograms, breath rates, body temperature and blood pressure, and by exerting their functions they proved to be integral to performing successful operations. Further, in laparoscopic surgery, additional equipment like high intensity light sources, carbon dioxide insufflators, monitors and video recorders have been used; though all have been crucial to carry out the laparoscopic procedures, they also required additional space in the operation theatre [1]. Regarding imaging devices, a plain X-ray imaging device and an ultrasonic imaging system are sometimes introduced and used during operations. Moreover, in recent years, surgery navigation systems that utilize magnetic sensors or precise optical position sensors such as OPTOTRAK (Northern Digital Inc., Canada) have been studied in a number of surgical settings. In such technologies, however, position sensors and additional monitors to provide guided information for surgeons have been necessary. Feasibility and effectiveness of such systems has been pointed out in the literature and they have successfully assisted surgeons and reduced their fatigue caused by long operation hours.

On the other hand, accuracy and speed of the intraoperative navigation systems are important factors to consider. However, before these factors are taken

J. Duncan and G. Gerig (Eds.): MICCAI 2005, LNCS 3750, pp. 559–566, 2005.

into account, usability of the whole system in the operating room environment, especially its ergonomic parameters and simplicity, require prioritazation, since in the cluttered OR and with growing complexity of operative procedures, simply increasing the number of devices would not facilitate operations. Ergonomics of the environment, especially providing navigation data, prevention of technical difficulties and comfort of the OR staff should be firstly considered.

In the present study, we designed a data fusion display system and when prototyping devices for clinical use, their ergonomics as well as an easy-to-understand intraoperative display of navigation images were taken into consideration. A novel interface for advanced operation planning that was based on the guided images with volume rendering of intraoperatively scanned CT images rather than preoperative ones was also proposed. In recent years, intraoperative navigation, in which the target position is provided to assist an intuitive understanding of the surgical field has been studied and applied in many clinical areas [2][3], mainly orthopedics and neurosurgery. Position measurements of a surgical field have been usually performed with magnetic and marker-type optical position sensors, and preoperatively scanned CT or MRI images have been commonly used to represent inner structures. We believe that the time gap between acquisition of inner structure data and the actual operative procedures should be as short as possible for the correct depiction of the operated site. In this study, a mobile C-arm type CT (Siemens-Asahi Medical Technologies, Ltd.) was applied to acquire the inner structure data in the operating room; this provided the source of information for surgery navigation. In the literature [4], registration-free navigation with scanned images obtained by C-arm CT has been reported. This paper attempts to design and implement a data-fusion LCD display system for surgical navigation, which involves combining Maximum Intensity Projection MIP-based volumetric rendering of CT data, which was acquired intraoperatively from mobile 3D-CT device, with real-time views. A preliminary experiment was performed to validate the system.

2 Method

The functions desirable for an image presentation device that would be used as an intraoperative surgery navigation system were thought to be as follows:

1. It would be preferable if the image presentation device itself never limited the space required by other surgical equipment.
2. The image presentation device and position sensors should not interfere with the operative space. The position of the display monitor should be easily changeable and the monitor should be easily removable from the operative field when not used.
3. The monitor should be located in the vicinity of the surgical field. And it also allows the assistant on the other side reference to the same navigation images.
4. In order for a surgeon to better understand the spatial relations and directions between the surgical field and navigation images, the line of sight

for observing the surgical field and that for the navigation image should be correspondingly adjusted.

5. It would be preferable if cabling for the surgery navigation devices was not installed on the operating room floor.

To fulfill the abovementioned requirements, we considered that monitors and the position measurement device should hang from the ceiling of the operating room. Fig.1 shows a 3D CAD image of the positional layout of an optical position sensor, its measurement area, 5 monitor arms, and 4 shadowless lamps. The data-fusion display and optical position sensor were originally built into the operating room. This design enabled the minimalization of the operating room clutter, even when devices for surgery navigation had been installed. The monitors were mounted on 5 degrees-of-freedom multi-joint arms so that they could be observed from various positions and angles. Further, the layouts of the

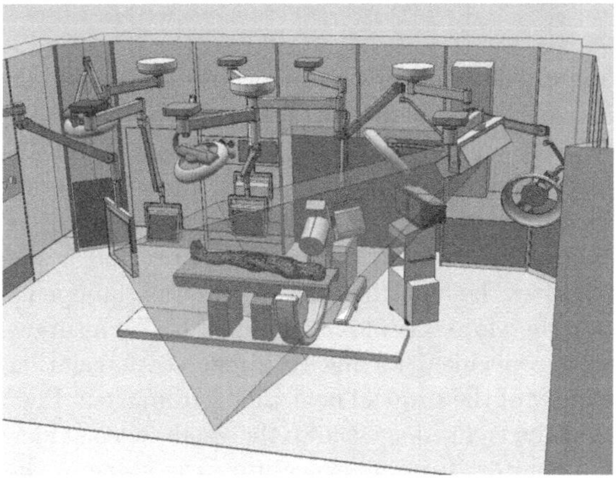

Fig. 1. 3D CAD layout of data-fusion display and measuring range of ceiling-mounted OPTOTRAK in the operating room

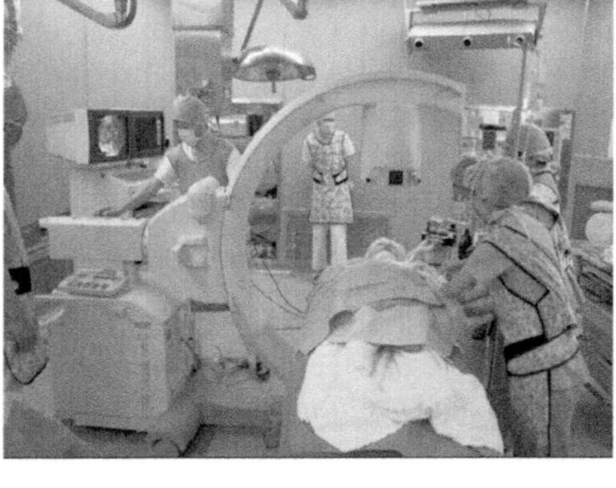

Fig. 2. The High-Tech Navigation Operating Room

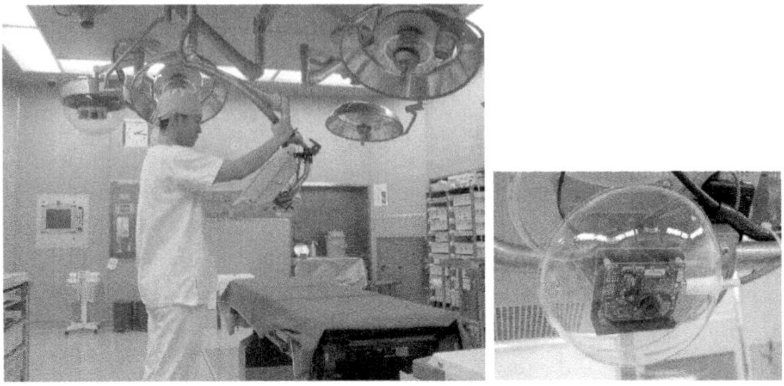

Fig. 3. The setup of a data-fusion display. The operator is grabbing and moving the monitor to the position from where he wants to observe the inner structure. A small video camera is inset in the backside of the monitor.

devices were carefully designed not to disturb the measurement area of the position sensor. The room was constructed as the High-Tech Navigation Operating Room in an operation building of the Dai-San Hospital, Jikei University, Tokyo, as shown in Fig.2. A report on the system was presented in MMVR13 [5].

The data-fusion display system was composed primarily of a 15-inch LCD monitor affixed to a ceiling-hung articulating arm and a small video camera installed at the back of the monitor. The system was equipped with a detachable sterilization lever; therefore it could be manipulated by a surgeon and positioned where it was most convenient for her to utilize the navigation data, i.e. in the immediate proximity of the surgical field. The left image in Fig.3 shows the data-fusion display and the right image shows the small video camera installed at the back side of the monitor. In order to capture the scene of the surgical field, a small color video camera, Dragonfly (Point Grey Research Inc., Canada) was used. Time-sequentially captured images were sent to a PC (Dual CPU: Xeon 2.8GHz, 2GB RAM, nVidia QuadroFX1000) through an IEEE1394 interface. This camera could collect stream VGA quality images at 30 frames per second without compression and was incorporated in the ceiling-hung LCD monitor thus providing "through"-the-monitor images for the operating surgeon. The position and direction of the monitor was constantly measured and tracked by the ceiling-hung optical 3D position sensor OPTOTRAK. Further, the system enabled surgeons to observe a patient's inner structure from the viewpoint of the monitor using VR augmentation with video see-through way during surgery.

In the present study, a mobile C-arm type CT was applied to acquire the inner structure data used as an information source for surgery navigation inside the operating room. To enable CT measurements during surgery, a non-metal operating table with dynamoelectric mobility characteristics (MAQUET GmbH & Co. KG) was incorporated. 3D volume data in 12 cm^3 was measured once with a scanning period of two minutes. The display of an acquired internal structure data was available immediately by volume rendering onto the video image of

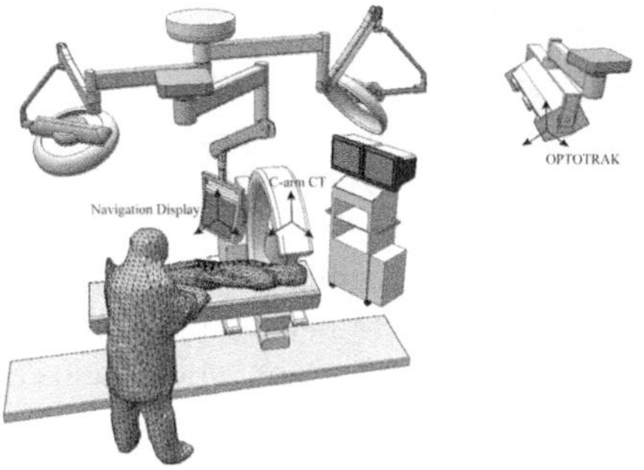

Fig. 4. Configuration of the navigation system and key coordinate systems

the surgical field. As shown in Fig.4, key coordinate systems are that of OPTOTRAK as a global basis, the navigation display, and the volume data obtained by the C-arm CT. An optical marker flag is attached to the C-shaped frame of the CT, and its position during the measurement of volume data is obtained. The positional relationship between the marker flag and the data position of the C-arm CT should be calibrated once in the operating room. A cube-shaped gypsum block was used for the calibration of the C-arm CT data position. The cube-shaped gypsum was created using a rapid prototyping system (Zprinter, Zcorporation) with powder lamination technology, its shape was designed with a 3D CAD system and the physical model directly created from the digital data. The gypsum block was measured by the C-arm CT as shown in Fig.5(a), and the calibration was conducted using the corner position in the measured data coordinate and the corner position in the physical space obtained by OPTOTRAK. Finally, the transformation matrix between the marker flag of the C-arm CT and the coordinate system of the C-arm data itself could be solved. Fig.5(b) shows the result of the cube registration and fusion representation of the segmented cube surface model on the video images of the data-fusion display. After this calibration, the measured data position of the C-arm CT becomes a known parameter until the marker flag attached to the C-arm is repositioned.

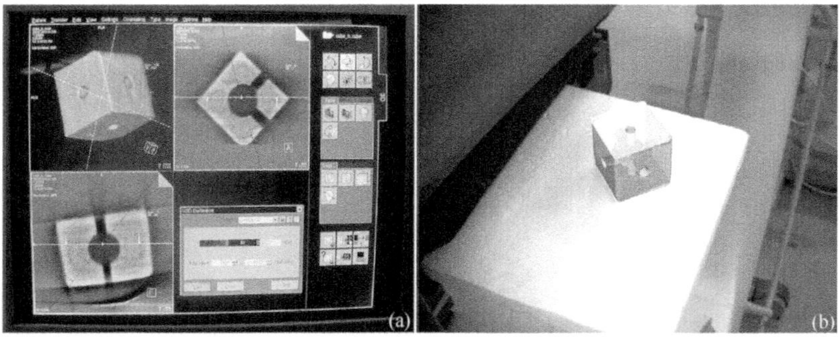

Fig. 5. (a) C-arm CT images of a gypsum block; (b) Results of the cube registration and fusion representation of the cube surface model on the video images

3 Results and Discussion

For camera calibration of the data-fusion display, a checkered board was used. Its position was changed in pre-set time intervals and the respective images captured. The internal camera parameters and positional relationship between the camera coordinate and the marker flag attached to the display could be instantly obtained by image processing and computer vision algorithm. This was a very useful in calibrating parameters that could be executed quickly and easily in the operating room. For details on calculations and algorithms applied, we referred to the reports of Tsai [6] and Zhang [7].

Fig.6 shows the differential error between the detected checkered board corners in the captured images and the re-projected corners of the computed projection matrix on the image plane. The calibration was performed at about 700-800 mm distance from the display, assuming that the object was placed as during an operation. The graph shows results of error calculations when the image resolution was set as 360 240 pixels. The RMS error was 0.126 pixel. 35 points of the grid per one frame and the calibration was done with 22 captured frames. We believe that such accuracy in calibration with perspective matrix is sufficient for video see-through navigation. When intraoperatively scanned CT data was loaded into the data-fusion system, the volume data at 256 256 256 resolution was transferred through a gigabit network into the computer located in the operating room. Parallel processing of the display position tracking and rendering of the volume data with a 3D texture technique was implemented, and this method allowed a 12 fps update rate of the surgical field video images and the superimposed volume data. The operator was able to intuitively confirm the intraoperative inner structure obtained by the C-arm CT just by observing through the display, as shown in Fig.7(a). Fig.7(b) represents the augmented navigation image for an elbow joint depicted on the data-fusion display.

Head-mounted displays have been very common as image presentation devices for augmented reality. However, their prolonged usage causes fatigue and they also obstruct the operator's view. For operating room applications and by using a mobile ceiling-hung arm, our system enabled a surgeon to intuitively ob-

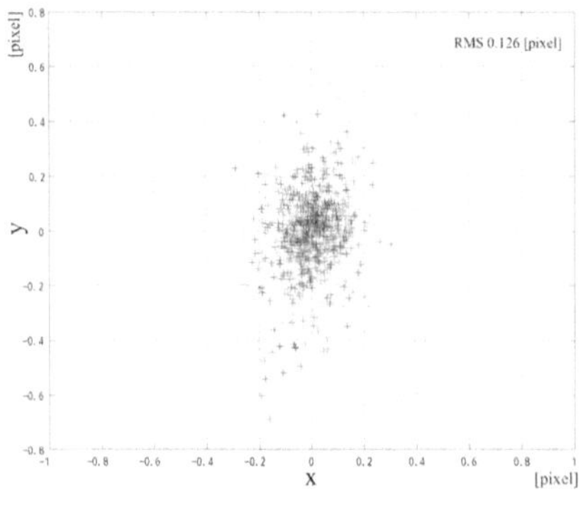

Fig. 6. Reprojection error of camera calibration

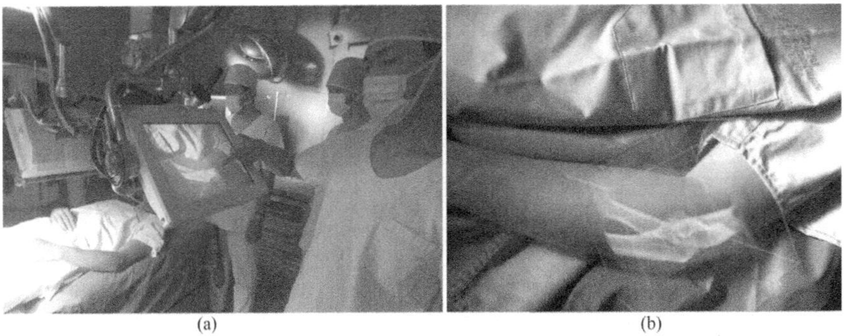

Fig. 7. Images of the volumetric navigation system for an elbow joint

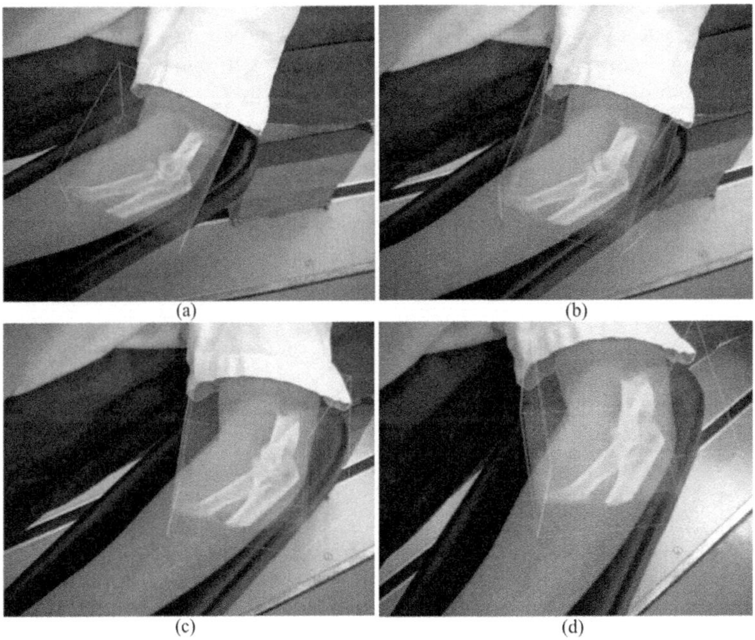

Fig. 8. Time-sequentially generated images in the data-fusion display. The volume data of the mobile 3D-CT was superimposed onto the live video image according to the varying direction of the display.

serve a patient's inner structure from his viewpoint. Further, the devices could be easily removed from the proximity of the surgical field when the navigation was not necessary. Fig.8 shows time-sequentially generated images on a data-fusion display while changing the viewing direction. The volume data of the mobile 3D-CT was smoothly superimposed onto the live video images accordingly with the varying directions of the display. We assumed that the subject was static and that updating the data was limited due to reduction of radiation exposure. Thus, the data acquisition was conducted fragmentarily and with the minimal possible amount of exposure. Furthermore, the time of one scanning time with the mobile 3D-CT was two minutes. In effect, the volume rendering image did not correspond to the deformation tracking. Even with such limitations, however, this kind of visual representation would be effective for intuitive confirmation of the static subject just after the performing the intraoperative measurements.

4 Conclusion

In the present study we designed and created a data-fusion display for clinical applications in the operating room. The system enabled volumetric MIP image navigation using intraoperative C-arm CT data. The 3D volumetric images reflecting a patient's inner structure were directly displayed on the monitor, which also simultaneously displayed the superimposed video images of the surgical field. In the system, a 3D optical tracking device, a ceiling-mounted articulating monitor and a small size video camera mounted at the back of the monitor were utilized. The system performance was validated in an experiment carried out in the operating room. In addition, it was very important and challenging for the system that the surgical navigation data was intraoperatively obtained and was not based on preoperative images. We think, however, that preoperative imaging will still be necessary because data resolution and measurement ranges were limited in the intraoperative imaging system. A combination of techniques that utilize several medical imaging modalities would be crucial for on-coming surgery navigation.

References

1. D. Hong and L.L. Swanstrom, Electronic and Computer-Integrated Operating Rooms, Primer of Robotic & Telerobotic Surgery, Lippincott Williams & Wilkins, pp.21-25, 2004.
2. T.J. Levison, J.E. Moody Jr., B. Jaramaz, C. Nikou, A.M. DiGioia, Surgical Navigation for THR: A Report on Clinical Trial Utilizing HipNav, Proceedings of MICCAI, pp.1185-1187, 2000.
3. A.Nabavi, N. Hata, et al., Image Guided Neurosurgery Visualization of Brain Shift, Navigated Brain Surgery, pp.17-26, 1999.
4. P.A. Grutzner, A. Hebecker, H. Waelti, B. Vock, L.-P. Nolte, A. Wentzensen, Clinical Study for Registration-Free 3D-Navigation with the SIREMOBIL Iso-C3D Mobile C-Arm, electromedica, Vol.71, No.1, pp.7-16, 2003.
5. N. Suzuki, A. Hattori, S. Suzuki, Y. Otake, M. Hayashibe, S. Kobayashi, T. Nezu, H. Sakai, Y. Umezawa, Construction of a High-Tech Operating Room for Image-Guided Surgery using VR, Proceedings of MMVR13, IOS Press, pp.538-542, 2005.
6. R.Y. Tsai, A versatile camera calibration technique for high accuracy 3D machine vision metrology using off-the-shelf TV cameras and lenses, IEEE J. Robotics Automat., Vol.RA-3, No.4, pp.323-344, 1987.
7. Z. Zhang, A flexible new technique for camera calibration, IEEE Transactions on Pattern Analysis and Machine Intelligence, Vol.22, No.11, pp.1330-1334, 2000.

A Hybrid Cutting Approach for Hysteroscopy Simulation

M. Harders[1], D. Steinemann[2], M. Gross[2], and G. Székely[1]

Swiss Federal Institute of Technology
[1]Computer Vision Lab
[2]Computer Graphics Lab
ETH Zentrum, CH-8092 Zürich, Switzerland
{mharders, szekely}@vision.ee.ethz.ch, {deniss, grossm}@inf.ethz.ch

Abstract. An integral element of every surgical simulator is the ability to interactively cut tissue. A number of approaches have been suggested in the past, the most important being mesh subdivision by introducing new elements and mesh adaptation by adjusting existing topology. In this paper we combine these two methods and optimize them for our training system of hysteroscopic interventions. The basic methodology is introduced in 2D, a first extension to 3D is presented and finally the integration into the simulator described.

1 Introduction

Therapeutic hysteroscopy has become a common technique in gynecological practice [4]. Nevertheless, a number of potentially dangerous complications exist - the most common being uterine wall perforation, intra-uterine bleeding, and mismanagement of distension fluid. In [19] the rate of complications for therapeutic interventions is reported as 17%. According to [14], 97% of hysteroscopic interventions are performed with resectoscopes, with up to 9% of them leading to perforations. The most critical situation is wall perforation with resectoscope electrodes during cutting procedures, since lesions of intra-abdominal organs are likely. In these cases hysteroscopy usually has to be stopped and an emergency abdominal intervention performed. Therefore, specialized training is necessary to reduce the rate of complications. Virtual Reality based surgical simulation [11] is one option to provide a corresponding learning environment. In contrast to existing systems and products [10,15,13], our work aims at achieving the highest possible realism. With this system, we intend to identify the necessary level of fidelity for achieving a specific training effect, by stepwise reduction of realism. As described above, a key element of training is the tissue ablation process. We currently focus on the resection of intra-uterine neoplasms. Myomectomy with loop electrodes has to be carried out by stepwise shaving. The process is depicted in Figure 3. Including these procedures in our simulator system necessitates updates of the underlying tissue model.

Different approaches for handling cutting have been proposed, which can be summarized into three major categories: straight-forward element deletion

J. Duncan and G. Gerig (Eds.): MICCAI 2005, LNCS 3750, pp. 567–574, 2005.

[2,7,5], mesh subdivision [12,16,8,3,1] and topology adaptation [20,17]. While the first method is not appropriate for a realistic simulator, the latter two have produced reasonable results. However, both of them still have significant limitations (e.g. increase of element count, reduced element sizes or degenerate elements), which will be discussed in more detail in the next section. In the following, we propose a hybrid approach, combining subdivision with mesh adaptation strategies. These are completed by a subsequent mesh optimization step. Our method is tailored for our hysteroscopic training system.

2 Previous Work

Cutting approaches are usually tailored to the applied deformation and visualization mesh representations. With only few exceptions, these are triangular or tetrahedral meshes, respectively. Straight-forward deletion of mesh entities has been applied in [2] and [5]. The idea is to remove elements, which are contacted by a cutting tool. Unfortunately, this leads to visual artifacts, since the cutting path can not be accurately approximated. Moreover, the principle of mass conservation is violated.

More appealing visual representations of incisions were made possible with mesh subdivision methods. These usually have in common the classification of a cut according to different rotational invariant intersection states. Predefined subdivisions of mesh elements will then be performed. In the context of medical applications, this was first introduced in [12] for cutting of tetrahedral meshes with predefined planes. This approach has been refined in [16], where partial incision of mesh elements as well as progressive cutting is taken into account. Finally, [1] discusses the use of a state machine to keep track of different incisions in tetrahedral meshes. All described approaches have in common the often considerable increase of element count, which is reported to range from five up to 17 new elements per incised tetrahedron. Moreover, introduction of new mesh elements often necessitates extensive model recalculations, for instance when using implicit FEM. Another negative factor is the reduction in element sizes. Deformation stability problems were reported [16], which required a significant reduction of the time step, thus rendering real-time simulation intractable.

Some of these problems could be ameliorated with topology adaptation approaches as suggested in [20] and [17]. The central idea is to approximate a cutting path with existing edges or surfaces. This enables mesh incisions without large increase of element count and occurrence of small elements. Unfortunately, problems arise due to degenerated elements, which can appear, if unconditional node displacement is carried out in the mesh. Also, the quality of incision approximation is limited by the initial mesh resolution.

3 Hybrid Cutting Approach in 2D

The key idea of our method is the combination of mesh adaptation by adjusting existing topology, and mesh subdivision by introducing new elements. This is complemented by subsequent local mesh optimization procedures to ensure a consistent overall mesh quality. Finally, similar deformation behavior is guaranteed by adjusting mechanical parameters. The basic concepts are first introduced in 2D, however, the strength of our approach becomes especially evident in the 3D case.

Generally, element count $\#E$, number of nodes $\#N$ and element size should be kept constant. Therefore, mesh adaptation should be applied whenever possible. To this end, edges are divided into regions, which define, whether displacement or subdivision is applied. Three general cases can occur as depicted in Figure 5. Depending on the intersection, one or two additional elements are created. In extreme circumstances, this still leads to an increase in element count. The situation, however, is rectified in the mesh optimization step described below. With the combined approach, small sized elements as well as degeneracies are avoided. Moreover, the process is easily applicable in progressive cutting, since only local edge intersection information is needed.

The method is further refined by extending the view beyond the current triangle. If two type 2 cases follow each other, element creation can be avoided with an edge flip. However, if the second displacement would involve a neighbor of the edge to be flipped, this can not be done. This case requires the addition of two new elements. Furthermore, a few other cases can appear, which need special treatment. Similar to the previous example, it can happen, that after a type 3 case, the displacement of a neighbor would require additional elements. This can be solved by displacing the node on the cut itself. The selected cases discussed are shown in Figure 4. Special treatment is also necessary for nodes on the object border. Displacement can only be performed within the border to preserve object shape. Moreover, this is only possible, if no prominent features, for instance sharp corners, are represented by the nodes. This is the case, if the angle between normals of neighboring border elements is small.

Succeeding several adaptation/subdivision steps, a mesh optimization process is performed. Although generally applicable, this step is optimized for a straight incision through several triangles. This is justified by the nature of the cutting process in myomectomy (see section 4). The optimization includes edge collapse and equal node distribution on the cut, as well as local mesh

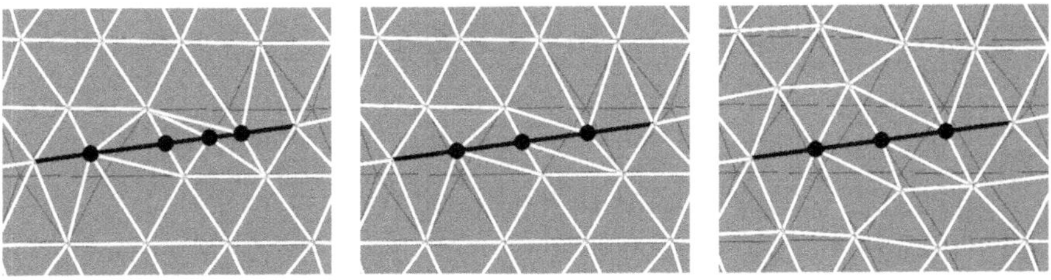

(a) Before optimization after initial cut. (b) Edge collapse and node distribution on cut. (c) Mesh after homogenization step.

Fig. 1. Mesh optimization process (cut line/nodes depicted in black) regularization. The latter is carried out by local computation of a combined mass-spring/particle system in the cut's vicinity. In this local system, nodes, which can be reached from cut nodes via one or two edge steps, are movable, while the remainder, including the cut nodes, is fixed. Mean local edge length is used to set mass-spring constants and particle system force profiles. Moreover, constant masses and high damping values are applied to avoid unnecessary oscillations. Positions $\boldsymbol{x}_{\tilde{i}}$ of the nodes proximal to the cut are adjusted by integrating the equation of motion.

$$m_{\tilde{i}}\ddot{\boldsymbol{x}}_{\tilde{i}} + c_{\tilde{i}}\dot{\boldsymbol{x}}_{\tilde{i}} + \left(\alpha \sum_j \boldsymbol{g}_{\tilde{i}j} + \beta \boldsymbol{f}_{\tilde{i}}^{int}\right) = 0, \qquad \tilde{i} \in \tilde{\mathcal{N}}$$

where $\tilde{\mathcal{N}}$ are indices of the proximal nodes. $\boldsymbol{g}_{\tilde{i}j}$ are spring forces, and $\boldsymbol{f}_{\tilde{i}}^{int}$ are forces resulting from the potential energy function of the particle system. The homogenization will be carried out, until node movement $x_{\tilde{i}}^{t} - x_{\tilde{i}}^{t-1}$ drops below 2% of mean edge length. Generally, about $4\tilde{n}$ steps have to be carried out, with $\tilde{n}$ being the number of elements intersected. All three optimization steps are displayed in Figure 1.

Table 1 shows results obtained with our proposed algorithm. The test meshes were created with the *DistMesh* tool described in [18]. The following statistical values were determined: number of nodes and elements, minimum, mean and standard deviation of element areas (A_{min}, A_μ, A_σ) and edge lengths (E_{min}, E_μ, E_σ), as well as mesh optimization time t. Moreover, a commonly used quality measure $q \in [0, \frac{1}{2}]$ (q_{min}, q_μ, q_σ) based on ratio between largest inscribed and smallest circumscribed circle, is also computed (triangles with $q > 0.25$ are considered to be well shaped). All values were determined for the initial mesh (*Initial*), as well as after remeshing with standard subdivision (*Stndrd*) and our hybrid approach (*Hybrid*). With our proposed method element and node count were kept almost constant. Also, the values of A_{min}, E_{min} and q_{min}, which have the strongest impact on deformation stability, remained favorable. Computation time increased in larger meshes, which is due to large incisions performed across

Table 1. Statistical values of test cases with two example meshes

Test		#N	#E	A_{min}	A_μ	A_σ	E_{min}	E_μ	E_σ	q_{min}	q_μ	q_σ	$t[ms]$
	Initial	88	59	88.93	113.64	11.06	12.63	16.26	1.81	0.393	0.473	0.028	
1a	**Stndrd**	107	70	0.23	93.46	38.27	0.66	14.64	4.07	0.012	0.433	0.108	
	Hybrid	88	59	72.45	113.64	18.31	10.30	16.31	2.25	0.361	0.465	0.032	10
1b	**Stndrd**	108	70	0.38	92.59	37.72	0.87	14.62	3.97	0.036	0.434	0.101	
	Hybrid	93	62	71.96	107.98	15.79	9.94	15.93	2.29	0.284	0.460	0.036	20
	Initial	519	298	4.10	5.09	0.28	2.75	3.45	0.27	0.398	0.487	0.015	
2a	**Stndrd**	587	335	0.03	4.50	1.40	0.05	3.23	0.68	0.011	0.461	0.086	
	Hybrid	521	299	2.19	5.07	0.43	2.19	3.45	0.32	0.332	0.483	0.021	190
2b	**Stndrd**	603	343	0.03	4.39	1.50	0.09	3.18	0.72	0.012	0.454	0.094	
	Hybrid	517	297	3.51	5.11	0.52	2.03	3.48	0.39	0.270	0.478	0.028	250

the complete mesh without any intermediate calculations. This can be alleviated by progressively carrying out regularization while the cut is being made.

Finally, we have to update the tissue model, since the underlying mesh has been changed. This is necessary to ensure a consistent deformation behavior. For the currently applied mass-spring system, node masses and spring constants need to be adjusted. The new mass distribution can be obtained via preservation of object mass moments p_{jk} up to second order as suggested in [6]. The moments are computed for the initial configuration.

$$p_{jk} = \sum_{i=1}^{n} x_i^j y_i^k m_i \qquad j + k \leq 2$$

where (x_i, y_i) and m_i are coordinates and masses of node i. This gives us the moment vector $\boldsymbol{p} = (p_{00}, p_{01}, ..., p_{20})^T$ for the initial mesh. After the remeshing process, the new mass coefficients $\boldsymbol{m}^*$ for the adjusted node coordinates can the be obtained via the precomputed moments. To this end, we have to solve the underdetermined system $\boldsymbol{A}\boldsymbol{m}^* = \boldsymbol{p}$, where $\boldsymbol{A}$ is the Vandermonde matrix of the new coordinates. This can be done, by introducing $\boldsymbol{B} = \boldsymbol{A}\boldsymbol{A}^T$. We first solve $\boldsymbol{B}\tilde{\boldsymbol{m}} = \boldsymbol{p}$, and in a second step, we obtain the new mass distribution according to $\boldsymbol{m}^* = \boldsymbol{A}^T\tilde{\boldsymbol{m}}$.

For setting of new spring constants k^*, a method was suggested in [9].

$$k_s^* = \frac{E \sum_E area(T_E)}{|s|^2}$$

where the sum is over elements T_E incident on edge s and E is Young's modulus. This was suggested for isotropic, homogeneous, linear elastic material.

4 Extension of Hybrid Cutting to 3D

The main elements of our hybrid approach have been implemented for incisions into tetrahedral meshes. In the current stage, subsequent mesh optimization has not been integrated. However, the mass-spring/particle regularization generalizes

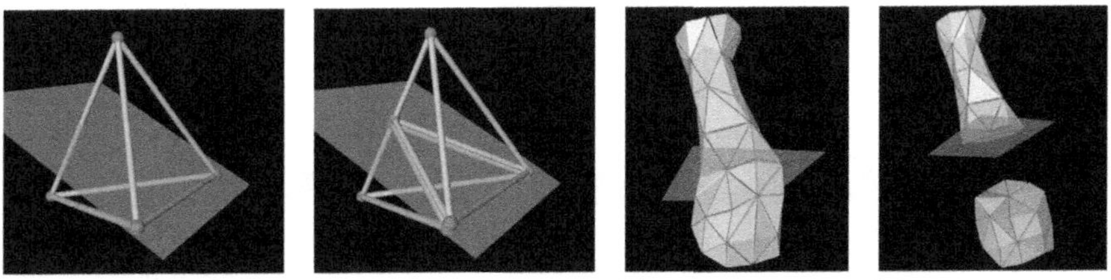

(a) Cut plane through one tetrahedron (b) After remeshing approach (c) Example mesh for a polyp (d) Excised tissue sample

Fig. 2. Examples of incisions into 3D meshes

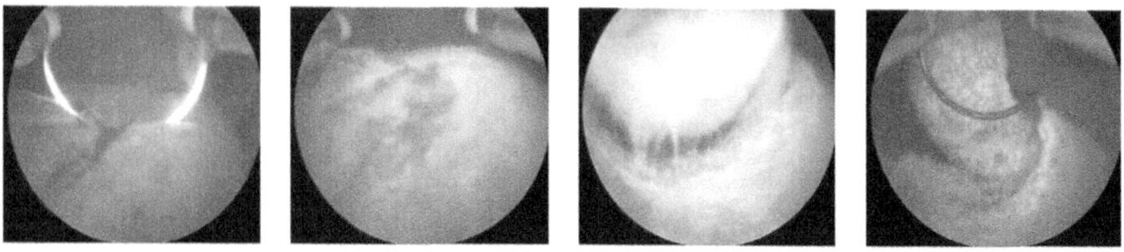

(a) Deformation with inactive electrode (b) Start of cut (c) Directly after end of cut (d) Excised tissue moved against fundus

Fig. 3. Steps of shaving process with loop electrode during myomectomy

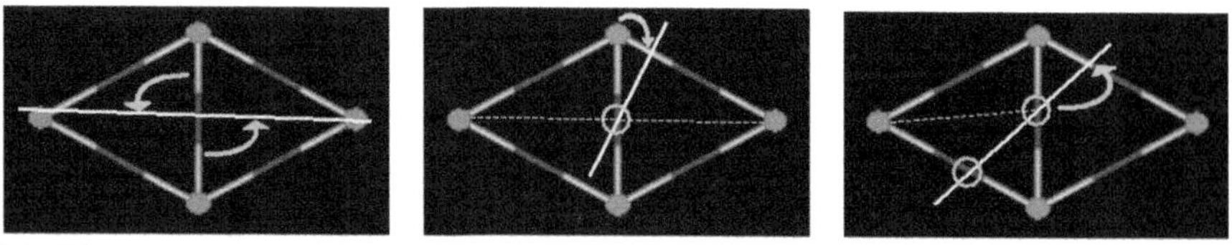

(a) Edge exchange possible in this configuration (b) Additional elements necessary (c) Cut node displaced

Fig. 4. Treatment of special cases

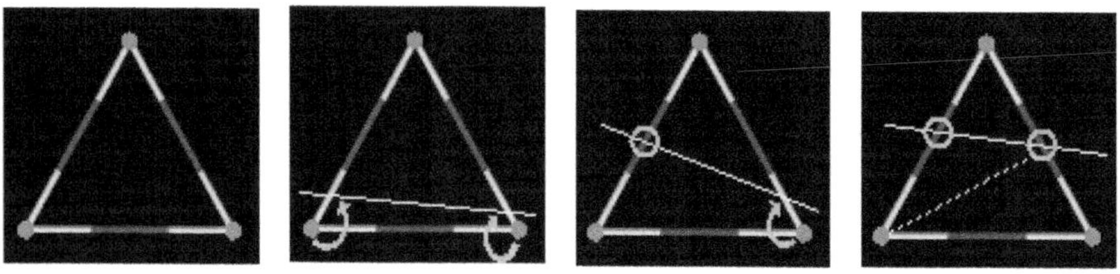

(a) Edge regions (b) Case 1: Two displacements (c) Case 2: Subdivision & displace (d) Case 3: Two subdivisions

Fig. 5. Cases for hybrid approach (cut line depicted in yellow)

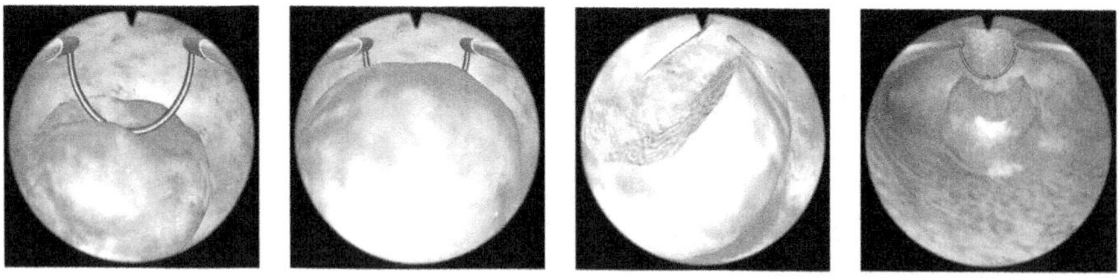

(a) Deformation with inactive electrode (b) Start of cut (c) Directly after end of cut (d) Excised tissue moved against fundus

Fig. 6. Steps of myoma shaving process in Virtual Reality

Table 2. Statistical values of test cases with a tetrahedral mesh

Test	#N	#E	V_{min}	V_μ	V_σ	E_{min}	E_μ	E_σ	q^*_{min}	q^*_μ	q^*_σ
Initial	69	136	3.54	37.07	15.80	3.14	7.19	1.99	0.017	0.21	0.06
Standard	319	620	$8.8x10^{-6}$	8.13	14.5	0.03	3.69	2.78	$3.2x10^{-3}$	0.09	0.09
Hybrid A	76	136	3.54	37.12	15.82	3.14	7.17	1.99	0.018	0.22	0.06
Hybrid B	88	145	2.96	34.77	16.29	2.82	7.06	1.96	0.017	0.21	0.06

well to 3D and its addition is straight-forward. Again, subdivision is carried out, if a cut plane is close to the middle of an edge. If the plane is close to a node, the incision is approximated by separating existing mesh nodes. This gives us four rotationally invariant cases, where zero to three nodes of a tetrahedra are separated. Examples of this process can be seen in Figure 2.

As in 2D, this approach allows for smooth cuts without considerably increasing node and element count, while mesh quality is kept in an acceptable range. Table 2 shows statistical values for example cuts in 3D. It contains the number of nodes and elements, minimum, mean and standard deviation of element volumes (V_{min}, V_μ, V_σ) and edge lengths. $q^* \in [0, \frac{1}{3}]$ is again a quality measure, this time denoting the ratio between radii of tetrahedra inspheres and circumspheres. All values were determined for the initial mesh, the mesh after remeshing with standard subdivision (*Standard*), as well as two different cuts using our hybrid approach ($HybridA/B$). Our approach prevents a considerable increase of element and node counts. The values of V_{min}, E_{min} and q_{min}, which have the strongest impact on deformation stability, remain again in acceptable ranges.

Since our application area is tissue ablation in hysteroscopy, we can make some assumptions about the cutting process. In the standard approach, the loop electrode is placed behind the pathology and then advanced towards the camera along a straight path (as depicted in Figure 3). This allows us to simplify the definition of the cutting surface by extruding the shape of the loop along the tool vector. Entry and exit position of the loop are registered in our collision detection routine. As soon as the tool leaves the tissue, our hybrid approach is carried out. Steps of this process, integrated into a simulator framework for hysteroscopy, are shown in Figure 6.

5 Conclusion and Future Work

We have presented a hybrid cutting approach combining mesh subdivision and topology adaptation. The approach was optimized for our specific application domain - simulation of tissue excision in hysteroscopic interventions. The method was introduced in 2D, followed by an extension to 3D. Future work will focus on integration of the mesh regularization process also in 3D. Moreover, the generalization of the cutting approach to arbitrary cut paths will be further investigated.

Acknowledgment

The authors would like to thank all developers of the hysteroscopy simulator project. This research has been supported by the NCCR Co-Me of the Swiss National Science Foundation.

References

1. D. Bielser et al. A state machine for real-time cutting of tetrahedral meshes. In *Proc. of Pacific Graphics*, pages 377–386, 2003.
2. M. Bro-Nielsen. Finite element modeling in medical VR. *Journal of the IEEE*, 86(3):490–503, 1998.
3. C. Bruyns and K. Montgomery. Generalized interactions using virtual tools within the spring framework: Cutting. In *Proc. MMVR02*, pages 23–26, 2002.
4. ACOG Tech. Bulletin. Hysteroscopy. Int J Gyn. Obstet., May 1994. 45(2): 175-180.
5. S. Cotin, H. Delingette, and N. Ayache. A hybrid elastic model allowing real-time cutting, deformations and force-feedback for surgery training and simulation. *The Visual Computer*, 16(8):437–452, 2000.
6. Oliver Deussen et al. Using simulated annealing to obtain good nodal approximations of deformable objects. In *Comp. Anim. and Simul.*, pages 30–43, 1995.
7. S. Frisken-Gibson. Using linked volumes to model object collisions, deformation, cutting, carving, and joining. *IEEE Trans on Vis. and Comp. Graphics*, 5(4), 1999.
8. F. Ganovelli et al. A multiresolution model for soft objects supporting interactive cuts and lacerations. *Computer Graphics Forum*, 19(3), 2000.
9. A. Van Gelder. Approximate simulation of elastic membranes by triangulated spring meshes. *Journal of Graphics Tools*, 3(2):21–42, 1998.
10. J.S. Levy. Virtual reality hysteroscopy. *J Am Assoc Gyn. Laparosc.*, 3 (4, Suppl.):25–26, 1996.
11. A. Liu et al. A survey of surgical simulation: Applications, technology, and education. *Presence: Teleoperators & Virtual Environments*, 12(6):599–614, 2003.
12. A. Mazura and S. Seifert. Virtual cutting in medical data. In *Proc. of Medicine Meets Virtual Reality*, pages 420–429., 1997.
13. Immersion Medical. AccuTouch system. Company webpage (visited Mar 2005).
14. L. Mencaglia and E. Hamou. Manual of gynecological hysteroscopy - diagnosis and surgery. Endo-Press, Germany, 2001.
15. K. Montgomery et al. Surgical simulator for hysteroscopy: A case study of visualization in surgical training. In *IEEE Visualization*, 2001.
16. A. Mor and T. Kanade. Modifying soft tissue models: Progressive cutting with minimal new element creation. In *MICCAI Proc.*, pages 598–607, 2000.
17. H.W. Nienhuys and A.F. van der Stappen. A surgery simulation supporting cuts and finite element deformation. In *MICCAI'01 Proc.*, pages 153–160, 2001.
18. P.O. Persson and G. Strang. A simple mesh generator in matlab. *SIAM Review*, 46(2):329–345, 2004.
19. S.B. Pinion et al. Randomised trial of hysterectomy, endometrial laser ablation, and transcervical endometrial resection for dysfunctional uterine bleeding. *British Medical Journal*, 309:979–983, October 1994.
20. D. Serby, M. Harders, and G. Szekely. A new approach to cutting into finite element models. In *MICCAI'01 Proc.*, pages 425–433, 2001.

Hydrometra Simulation for VR-Based Hysteroscopy Training

R. Sierra[1], J. Zátonyi[1], M. Bajka[2], G. Székely[1], and M. Harders[1]

[1] Computer Vision Laboratory, ETH Zürich, Switzerland
{rsierra, zatonyi, szekely, mharders}@vision.ee.ethz.ch
[2] Clinic of Gynecology, Dept. OB/GYN,
University Hospital of Zurich, Switzerland

Abstract. During hysteroscopy a hydrometra is maintained, i.e. the uterus is distended with liquid media to access and visualize the uterine cavity. The pressure and flow induced by the liquid are crucial tools for the gynecologists during surgery to obtain a clear view of the operation site. This paper presents two different aspects of hydrometra simulation, namely the distension of the uterine muscle and the liquid flow simulation in the cavity. The deformation of the organ's shape is computed offline based on finite element calculations whereas the flow is approximated on the fly by solving the simplified Navier-Stokes equations. The real-time capabilities of the presented algorithms as well as the level of fidelity achieved by the proposed methods are discussed.

1 Introduction

Hysteroscopy, the endoscopic inspection of the uterus, has become an established technique in gynecological practice [2]. A fundamental prerequisite of the method is the proper distension of the uterine cavity, also known as hydrometra. In general, a non-ionic solution will be used for therapeutic procedures. In- and outflow of the distension fluid is accomplished via the endoscopic tool and controlled with valves, while the pressure of the liquid is provided by a pump. It is essential to select correct pressure settings for the hydrometra according to muscle tone and uterine wall thickness [9]. Additional to the inflation of the uterus, the fluid flow also ensures a clear visibility in the cavity during interventions. Obscurations can be caused by endometrial bleeding, floating tissue fragments or air bubbles. It is the gynecologist's experience to correctly dose the in- and outflow through the valves that leads to a proper view of the scene. According to [7], a number of complications can be encountered related to the application of the distension fluid. Thus, the total amount of liquid loss should be strictly limited to 1500 ml, at which point the procedure has to be terminated.

Due to these reasons, the correct handling of the valves is a crucial skill that has to be an integral part of training for every gynecologist. Virtual Reality based surgical simulation offers a promising alternative to today's teaching approaches, which are largely based on interventions performed on real patients. In order to provide a suitable learning environment, the degree of realism necessary for

J. Duncan and G. Gerig (Eds.): MICCAI 2005, LNCS 3750, pp. 575–582, 2005.

effective training of complete surgical procedures with a simulator has to be identified. Our current research aims at the development of a simulator of highest possible realism for the procedural training of hysteroscopy. Key elements of this system are the proper cavity inflation, flow control of the distension fluid, pressure adjustment to handle small bleeding, and correct management of liquid pressure.

2 Related Work

In this paper an integrated approach for real-time simulation of various aspects of generating and maintaining of the hydrometra is presented. The authors are not aware of work with a similarly comprehensive approach. Nevertheless, related research exists, which focuses on individual aspects of our method.

A number of different approaches has been suggested for the description of the mechanical behavior of organic tissue. Usually, for these methods a trade-off has to be found between accuracy and computation time. Free-form deformation (FFD) techniques, stemming from Computer Graphics [11], have been applied in surgical simulation due to their efficiency. However, FFD procedures have only very limited physical meaning. More accurate deformations can be obtained with mass-spring models, initially introduced in [15]. Numerous projects have made use of this method, however, problems remain due to its limitations when approximating true physics. Nevertheless, an advantage of the method is its applicability in real-time simulations. Finally, rigorous representation of soft tissue physics can be achieved with continuum mechanics approaches, the most popular one being the Finite Element Method (FEM). Different levels of accuracy for deformation simulation have been realized with FEM, ranging from elastic linear [4] to nonlinear anisotropic systems [10]. Recently, a simulation of a hydrometra using FEM has been presented which, however, requires several hours of computation [17].

Physically-based real-time simulation of fluid flow in 3D has found increasing attention in recent years, mainly fueled by ever increasing computing power. In [3], discretized Navier-Stokes equations are solved using explicit finite differences and visualized with a so-called marker particle approach. The method requires relatively small time steps to ensure stable simulation, thus limiting its usage in real-time applications. A solver based on a semi-Lagrangian advection scheme has been presented in [14]. Its unconditional stability allows using larger time-steps, hence making fluid simulation in real-time possible. Recent work aims at efficient GPU-based implementations of fluid solvers to increase computational speed [6]. We previously reported on a method that combines the semi-Lagrangian solver with the marker particle approach to represent the blood flow in a simple geometry [18]. This combination allowed to achieve more realistic liquid-like behavior. However, the method was tailored to only visualize blood streams in a static environment. The results are extended in the following to consider the complex dynamic scene when regulating pressure and flow conditions during hydrometra.

3 Real-Time Deformation of the Uterine Cavity

The almost instantaneous response of the uterine cavity to pressure adjustments of the distension fluid exceeds by far the real-time capabilities of most known deformation models. Not only computationally intensive approaches, like FEM, are therefore completely infeasible, but even mass-spring methods proved intractable for the given problem. Firstly, the deformation accuracy of the latter is limited, and suitable model parameters can not easily be found. Secondly, in order to precisely approximate the shape of the uterus, still a large number of mesh elements is needed. As a result, the required mesh updates are currently beyond the capabilities of mass-spring methods. Therefore, free-form deformations seem to be better suited to solve the problem at hand. However, they do not provide the needed physical realism.

In order to achieve physically realistic real-time deformation of the uterine cavity, we suggest the combination of accurate FEM computations with FFD approaches. The underlying idea is to first carry out offline precomputations to obtain an accurate response of the tissue model to the fluid pressure. These data are then used during real-time interaction for model adjustments based on given pressure states. It is assumed that the boundary conditions of the deformation model do not change during the intervention. This is usually the case in hysteroscopic procedures, since the surrounding tissues are not directly accessible. Moreover, extreme modifications of the cavity wall should be avoided. This is also fulfilled, since cutting into the myometrium is limited to a relatively thin layer during surgery, otherwise risking the perforation of the wall leading to the immediate termination of the intervention. Hence we can assume, that the uterus' response to pressure differences stays relatively constant throughout the intervention.

Three major steps are needed for our approach: Data acquisition from real organs for model geometries and material laws, offline computations with a highly accurate FE approach, and real-time replay of these data during the intervention. The first step consists of a statistical model which encodes the natural variability of the healthy organ geometry which was segmented from MRI data obtained from a study with volunteers [13]. Based on a predefined set of parameters that are familiar to the gynecologists, new surface meshes of the uterus can be derived intuitively prior to training. Material parameters for the offline deformation computations are obtained in-vivo with a tissue aspiration device [8]. The obtained data are fed into the FE model in order to achieve a reasonable approximation of real deformation behavior. Both the FEM computation and the real-time simulation are based on homogeneous tetrahedral meshes. While in the former stage the mesh is required for calculating the deformations, the tetrahedral representation is needed for collision detection and haptic feedback in the latter step. The specific mesh generation approach employed is presented in [12]. In the second step, the offline computation enables the use of more advanced, and thus more accurate, tissue modeling techniques. We apply the FEM presented in [17], where homogeneous, isotropic and nonlinear hyper-elastic material laws are used. Based on the in-vivo aspiration experiment a polynomial strain-energy function of the form

$$\Psi(\bar{I}_1, J) = \sum_{p=1}^{N} \mu_p(\bar{I}_1 - 3)^p + \frac{1}{2}\kappa(J-1)^2$$

is used to describe the mechanical behavior of the particular soft tissue where $\bar{I}_1$ is the first reduced invariant of the right Cauchy-Green tensor, J the volume ratio, μ_p material parameters and κ the bulk modulus. $J \approx 1$, i.e. the material is assumed to be quasi-incompressible. The resulting equations are solved with the commercial package MarcMentat^{TM}. The organ model deformations are obtained for 100 different pressure settings. In the third step, the precomputed deformation states are loaded into the simulator and interpolated in real-time according to the applied fluid pressures. As the mesh topology does not change during deformation, only the vertex positions $\mathbf{x}$ of the tetrahedral mesh have to be updated based on the interpolation parameter t and a limited number n of precomputed instances $\mathbf{x}_i$: $\mathbf{x} = f(t, \mathbf{x}_0, ..., \mathbf{x}_n)$. Therefore, large meshes consisting of more than 30'000 tetrahedra and 50 interpolation samples can be updated in real-time. Already simple linear interpolation with as few as four precomputed samples proved to be sufficient for obtaining convincing visualizations.

4 Handling of Distension Fluid

The motion of liquid is described by the Navier-Stokes equations. For an incompressible fluid they take the form:

$$\nabla \cdot \mathbf{v}_f = 0 \qquad \text{and} \tag{1}$$

$$\frac{\partial \mathbf{v}_f}{\partial t} = -(\mathbf{v}_f \cdot \nabla)\mathbf{v}_f + \nu\nabla^2\mathbf{v}_f - \frac{1}{\rho}\nabla p + \mathbf{F} \tag{2}$$

where $\mathbf{v}_f$ is the velocity vector, p is the pressure, ρ is the density of the fluid, ν represents the kinematic viscosity coefficient and $\mathbf{F}$ corresponds to the vector of external body forces. The density and the temperature of the fluid are considered constant. Equation (1) represents the mass conservation in the fluid, while (2) is the momentum equation [1]. Equations (1) and (2) are solved numerically on a uniform Cartesian grid to evaluate the time dependent behavior of the fluid.

In order to solve the velocity field, proper boundary conditions have to be set. For hysteroscopy these are the endometrium as well as pathologies present in the scene, the in- and outflow according to the tool position, and their intensity according to the valve states. By labeling the voxels of the grid, these elements can be incorporated consistently into the numerical solver as discussed in [3]. As both the hydrometra and the pathologies may frequently change during simulation, the labeling of the voxels has to be updated accordingly. Therefore all voxels are re-labeled whenever the surfaces are modified in real-time [12]. For the inflow, constant velocity is set at the voxels corresponding to the tip of the tool. The outflow is represented by voxels that are set to velocities according to the outflow conditions at the respective positions.

Depending on the state of the valves, the properties of the liquid current vary in a wide range. The maximal flow speed of the distension liquid at fully opened valves reaches approximately $2\frac{m}{s}$ according to our measurements. Considering the small size of a normal cavity in the order of a few cm^3, the liquid flow is highly turbulent with a Reynolds number of about 30'000. However, the direct numerical simulation of turbulent flows is still a challenging task and physically based simulation approaches require extremely time-consuming calculations. In order to improve the simulation fidelity, the swirling motion within the fluid caused by the turbulence has still to be modeled. Therefore the velocity field $\mathbf{v}_f$ serves as a realistic approximation for moderate flow speed. For higher flow rates, artificial vortices can be added as needed. While this combination is not physically accurate, it provides a higher level of fidelity in real-time.

At the start of the simulation, we place the initial position of the vortices randomly within the fluid filled area. The orientation ω of the vortices is given by the curl of the velocity field $\mathbf{v}_f$ interpolated at the position of the vortex: $\omega = \nabla \times \mathbf{v}_f$. The Rankine vortex model is used, where a concentrated vorticity is simulated in the core region and combined with an exponential decay of the circumferential velocity as the distance from the core increases [5]. The velocity field represented by the Rankine vortex is divergent free, i.e. satisfies (1), and therefore provides a kinematically plausible velocity field. During simulation, the vortices are moved in each iteration according to their vorticity vector ω by a simple Euler step, i.e. ${\mathbf{p}_{vort}}^{t+1} = {\mathbf{p}_{vort}}^{t} + \Delta t_{vort}\omega$. The resulting flow velocity can finally be computed by superimposing the flow provided by the fluid solver and the velocity originating from the various vortices i: $\mathbf{v} = \mathbf{v}_f + \sum_{i=1}^{n} \mathbf{v}_{vorti}$.

5 Results and Discussion

The left image in Figure 1 illustrates a surface mesh of a uterus. The vertices are labeled according to their behavior during the subsequent deformations. The white vertices, highlighted with the ellipse, represent the portion of the surface protruding into the vagina which is fixed prior to surgery. The blue vertices (inner surface) represent the endometrium deforming according to the pressure induced by the fluid. The surrounding organs like the urinary bladder and the rectum can be considered as being quite soft compared to the uterus. Therefore, the remaining vertices colored in red (outer surface) are free to move. The uterus in the middle corresponds to the surface of the tetrahedral mesh consisting of

Table 1. Performance data

Δvoxel [cm]	#voxels total	#voxels fluid	CPU time [ms] no vortices	CPU time [ms] with vortices	Voxelization [ms]	Time to traverse [s]	Fidelity
0.06	191022	35179	100	112	77	5	+
0.09	62964	9528	26	30	42	2	++
0.12	27880	3813	10	12	28	1.5	++
0.15	15246	1818	5	6	19	1	−
0.18	9408	969	3	5	12	<1	−

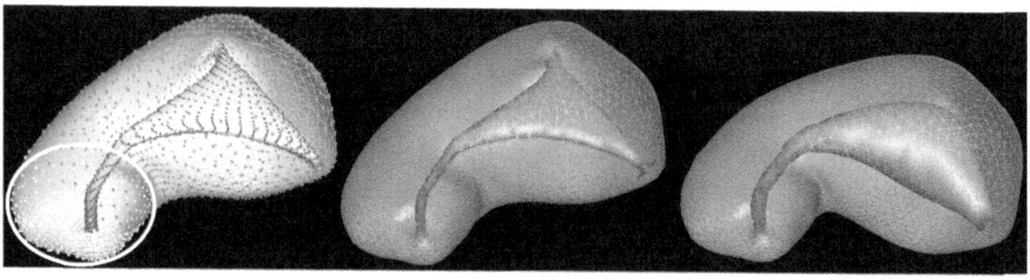

Fig. 1. Left: Uterus with labeled vertices. Middle: Corresponding surface of tetrahedra mesh. Right: uterus with hydrometra. In all cases the frontal surface has been rendered in wireframe mode to visualize the inner cavity.

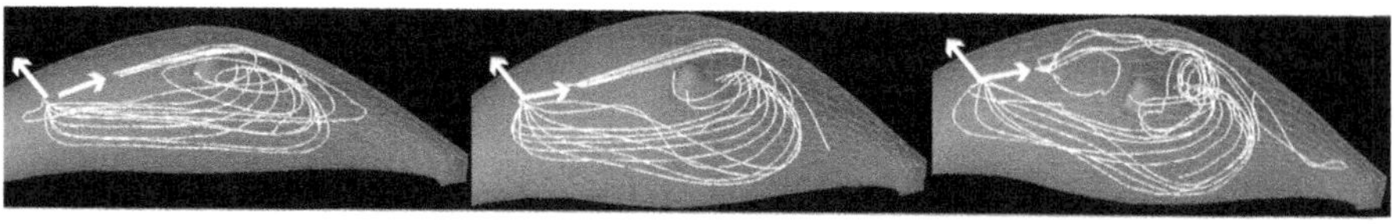

Fig. 2. Left: Visualization of the flow in the uterine cavity under limited pressure. Middle: Flow pathlines in a fully distended state. Right: Effect of additional vortices on the flow field.

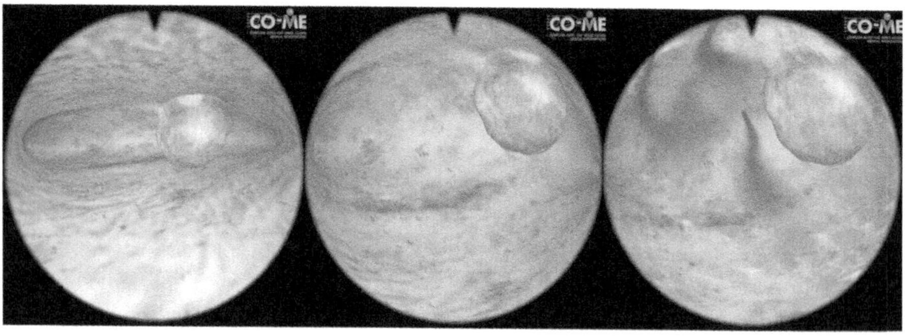

Fig. 3. Left: Low hydrometra in a cavity with a myoma. Middle: Same scene under maximal distension. Right: Scene with blood streams under the influence of both inflow and vortices.

approximately 35'000 tetrahedra. Finally, the uterus on the right illustrates the result of the FEM-based hydrometra simulation as presented.

During surgery the interaction is mainly restricted to the fundus of the uterus. Therefore, the simulation is confined to this region of interest. In Figure 2 the flow field is visualized by pathlines. Two different stages of hydrometra are shown in the first two images, while the third image illustrates the flow in the presence of 20 vortices. The arrows indicate the inflow and outflow directions. As can be seen, the pathlines clearly indicate the main flow streams from the inlet position to the outflow. The vortices clearly perturb the local behavior as desired, but do not disrupt the overall flow.

Table 1 compiles different performance measurements while using the presented algorithms on a standard 3.0 GHz PC. As the computational time for the deformation of the tetrahedral mesh can be neglected, the single parameter that determines the overall performance is the size of the voxels used for discretization. The table shows the values measured for increasing voxel dimensions. The total number of voxels in the bounding box of the organ are shown in the second column. The effective number of voxels used for flow simulation in the fully distended case are shown in the third column. Obviously, all calculations are faster for smaller hydrometra states. The next two columns indicate the CPU time for the flow field evaluation without and with up to 100 vortices. For every new state, the voxel representation has to be updated (6th column). While all these values prove that the update of the flow can be computed in real-time, the maximal flow speed that can be represented is limited by the time required to propagate a single particle across the cavity, indicated by the 'time to traverse'. The highest resolution is not optimal, as the numerical dissipation of the semi-Lagrangian method can be observed. Large voxel dimensions allow for the representation of faster flows, however, they are no longer able to accurately guide the particles from the in- to the outlet. In conclusion, an optimal voxel size of approximately 0.12 cm has been identified.

In order to validate the visual fidelity of the flow field we use blood streams as they are highly influenced by the distension liquid in real surgery. The blood streams are mostly computed on the GPU by using billboards and dynamic textures to represent the blood particles. Figure 3 shows three different snapshots of the simulator with a myoma attached to the upper wall. The dynamic behavior of the discussed images can be observed in the movie provided online (`www.vision.ee.ethz.ch/~rsierra/hydrometra.avi`).

As stated, the computation of fluid dynamics on the GPU is nowadays a field of intensive research. However, this approach is only of limited relevance in the current environment, as the information of the fluid field needs to be propagated to several other components of the simulator, such as the rendering of the blood streams, the displacement of floating tissue fragments or air bubbles. This requires copying of the results from the GPU to the CPU memory, an expensive operation in currently available hardware setups.

6 Conclusion and Future Work

In this paper we have presented the methods developed for the full simulation of hydrometra during hysteroscopy. Both the organ's deformation and the fluid flow in the cavity are modeled with highest possible realism while still meeting the real-time requirements of a simulator.

The fluid simulation will be further validated. We plan to perform an accurate flow simulation with exactly the same boundary conditions with an available commercial packages offline and quantitatively compare to our own results. The increased computational power of future hardware can be used to enhance the accuracy of the flow simulation. The Lattice Boltzmann Method [16] offers an appealing alternative to account for additional aspects of the underlying physics and will be implemented in the future.

The presented FEM computation is simplified in several respects. Many assumptions, e.g. quasi static behavior, may not hold for a realistic simulation. It might be necessary to resort to more complex models incorporating non-linear, anisotropic, and time dependent materials which approximate the real behavior of the myometrium more precisely. Therefore, a study is currently being performed where the hydrometra is generated in a surgically removed uterus in a CT scanner. This study will provide the necessary ground truth for the derivation of more advanced FEM models in the future.

Acknowledgment. This work has been supported by the NCCR CO-ME of the Swiss National Science Foundation. We are grateful to Stephan Weiss for his help with the FEM models and the use of MarcMentat™.

References

1. J. D. Anderson et al. *Computational Fluid Dynamics: The Basics with Applications.* McGraw-Hill, Inc., New York, 1995.
2. ACOG Tech. Bulletin. Hysteroscopy. Int J Gyn. Obstet., May 1994. 45(2): 175-180.
3. N. Foster and D. Metaxas. Realistic animation of liquids. *Graphical Models and Image Processing*, 58(5):471–483, 1996.
4. E. Gladilin et al. A biomechanical model for soft tissue simulation in craniofacial surgery. In *Medical Imaging and Augmented Reality*, pages 137–141, 2001.
5. M. Jiang, R. Machiraju, and D. Thompson. Geometric verification of swirling features in flow fields. In *Visualization '02*, pages 307–314, 2002.
6. Y. Liu, X. Liu, and E. Wu. Real-time 3D fluid simulation on GPU with complex obstacles. In *Pacific Graphics*, pages 247–256, 2004.
7. L. Mencaglia and E. Hamou. Manual of gynecological hysteroscopy - diagnosis and surgery. Endo-Press, Germany, 2001.
8. A. Nava et al. Evaluation of the mechanical properties of human liver and kidney through aspiration experiments. *Technology and Health Care*, 12(3):269–280, 2004.
9. J.C. Petrozza. Hysteroscopy. `http://www.emedicine.com/med/topic3314.html`, July 2004.
10. G. Picinbono et al. Non-linear and anisotropic elastic soft tissue models for medical simulation. In *Intl. Conf. on Robotics and Automation*, pages 1370–1375, 2001.
11. T. Sederberg and S. Parry. Free-form deformation of solid geometric models. *Computer Graphics*, 4:151–160, 1986.
12. R. Sierra et al. Coherent scene generation for surgical simulators. In *Proceedings of ISMS 2004*, pages 221 – 229. Springer Verlag, June 2004.
13. R. Sierra et al. Generation of variable anatomical models for surgical training simulators. *Medical Image Analysis*, to appear.
14. J. Stam. Stable fluids. In *Proceedings of the 26th annual conference on Computer graphics and interactive techniques*, pages 121–128, 1999.
15. D. Terzopoulus and K. Waters. Analysis and synthesis of facial image sequences using physical and anatomical models. *IEEE Trans. PAMI*, 15(6):569–579, 1993.
16. X. Wei et al. Blowing in the wind. In *Proceedings of the 2003 ACM SIGGRAPH/Eurographics Symposium*, pages 75–85, 2003.
17. S. Weiss et al. A finite element model for the simulation of hydrometra. *Technology and Health Care*, 12:259–267, 2004.
18. J. Zátonyi et al. Real-time synthesis of bleeding for virtual hysteroscopy. *Medical Image Analysis*, 9(3):255–266, June 2005.

Brain Shift Computation Using a Fully Nonlinear Biomechanical Model

Adam Wittek[1], Ron Kikinis[2], Simon K. Warfield[3], and Karol Miller[1]

[1] Intelligent Systems for Medicine Laboratory,
School of Mechanical Engineering, The University of Western Australia,
35 Stirling Highway, Crawley/Perth WA 6009 Australia
[2] Surgical Planning Laboratory,
[3] Computational Radiology Laboratory,
Brigham and Women's Hospital, Children's Hospital and Harvard Medical School,
75 Francis Street, Boston, MA02115, USA
Karol Miller: kmiller@mech.uwa.edu.au
http://www.mech.uwa.edu.au/ISML

Abstract. In the present study, fully nonlinear (i.e. accounting for both geometric and material nonlinearities) patient specific finite element brain model was applied to predict deformation field within the brain during the craniotomy-induced brain shift. Deformation of brain surface was used as displacement boundary conditions. Application of the computed deformation field to align (i.e. register) the preoperative images with the intraoperative ones indicated that the model very accurately predicts the displacements of gravity centers of the lateral ventricles and tumor even for very limited information about the brain surface deformation. These results are sufficient to suggest that nonlinear biomechanical models can be regarded as one possible way of complementing medical image processing techniques when conducting nonrigid registration. Important advantage of such models over the linear ones is that they do not require unrealistic assumptions that brain deformations are infinitesimally small and brain tissue stress–strain relationship is linear.

1 Introduction

Brain shift occurring during craniotomy distorts the preoperative anatomy and often leads to misalignment between the actual position of important brain structures and its position determined from the preoperative images. This is one of the key challenges faced by neurosurgery, and its importance is increasing with progress of therapeutic technologies. Important feature of the technologies that are entering medical practice now, such as e.g. gene therapy, nanotechnology devices, focused radiation, lesion generation and robotic surgery, is that they have extremely localized area of therapeutic effect [1]. Therefore, they have to be applied precisely in relation to the current (i.e. intraoperative) patient's anatomy, directly over specific location of anatomic/functional abnormality (e.g. tumor).

While the intraoperative imaging would be the most straightforward method when determining the current position of the tumor during surgery, its quality suffers from the constraints of the operating room. As a result of these constraints, spatial resolu-

J. Duncan and G. Gerig (Eds.): MICCAI 2005, LNCS 3750, pp. 583 – 590, 2005.

tion and contrast of intraoperative images are typically inferior to those of preoperative ones [2]. This problem is typically solved by aligning (i.e., registering) the preoperative data to scans of the brain acquired intraoperatively, which makes it possible to retain the preoperative image quality during the surgery. In order to achieve accurate alignment, the brain deformation must be taken into account, which implies nonrigid registration. In recent years, biomechanical models have been recognized and used as efficient tools for predicting the brain deformation. In most practical cases, such models utilize the finite element method [3] to solve sets of partial differential equations governing the deformation behavior of continua.

Selection of appropriate mathematical model governing the deformation is crucial to ensure realistic computer simulation of brain deformation. In nonrigid registration, linear elastic formulation is typically used [2], [4], [5]. In this formulation, the brain deformations are regarded as infinitesimal (i.e. geometric linearity) and brain tissue is treated as an elastic material in which the stress is a linear function of the strain (i.e. material linearity). Although nonrigid registration using linear biomechanical models has been an important achievement that significantly adds to the value of intraoperative imaging [2], it must be realized that neither the assumption about infinitesimally small brain deformation nor the one about brain stress–strain linear behavior is valid during brain shift. Craniotomy typically results in deformation of brain surface as large as 10 mm [6] (i.e. around 10% of distance between the left and right cortical landmarks) and rigid body movement of the brain, which implies that fully nonlinear finite element formulations and material models are needed when predicting deformation field within the brain during a typical brain shift.

Therefore, we propose that when conducting nonrigid registration, image analysis techniques should be complemented by biomechanical models based on fully nonlinear finite element formulations rather than linear ones. We demonstrate that such nonlinear models facilitate accurate prediction of deformation field within the brain even when simplified brain geometry and limited data about the brain surface deformation are used.

2 Methods

2.1 Construction of Finite Element Mesh for Patient Specific Brain Model

In the present study, a volumetric (i.e. three-dimensional) patient specific brain mesh was constructed from the segmented preoperative magnetic resonance images (MRIs) (Fig. 1). The segmentation was done using *3D Slicer* [7] — open-source software for visualization, registration, segmentation and quantification of medical data developed by Artificial Intelligence Laboratory of Massachusetts Institute of Technology and Surgical Planning Laboratory at Brigham and Women's Hospital and Harvard Medical School.

The mesh was built using 15036 hexahedron elements (i.e. 8-node "bricks") (Fig. 2). The hexahedron finite elements are known to be the most effective ones in nonlinear finite element procedures using explicit time integration. The construction of hexahedron grid for the present brain model has been described in our previous publication [8].

In order to simulate the pia matter, the brain surface was covered by a layer of 3522 membrane elements (thickness of 0.1 mm). The cerebral falx was also discretized using membrane elements: 436 such elements of thickness of 1 mm were used.

a) b)

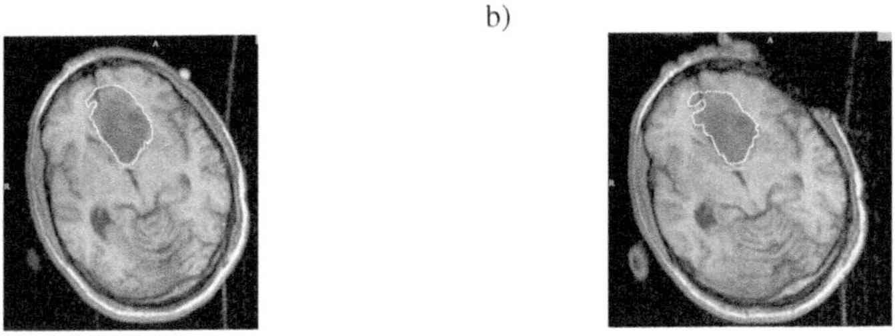

Fig. 1. Example of segmented MRIs of the head used when building patient specific brain mesh. The tumor segmentation is indicated by white lines in the anterior brain part. a) Preoperative; b) Intraoperative.

a) b)

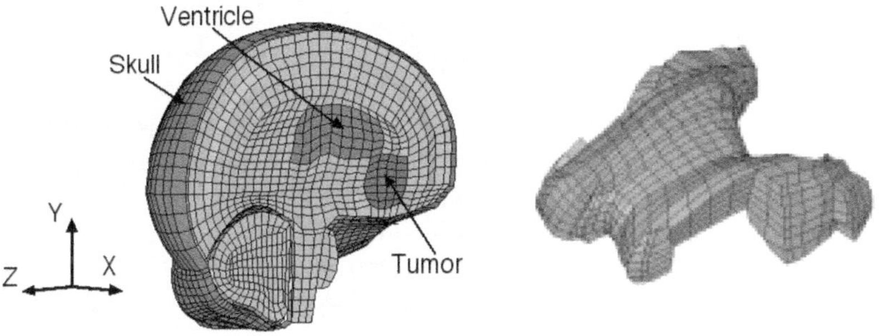

Fig. 2. Patient specific brain mesh constructed in the present study. a) Entire left brain hemisphere; b) Lateral ventricles.

2.2 Brain Shift Simulation

Equations of Mathematical Model. Detailed account of biomechanics of the brain including relevant equations was given by Miller [9]. In this section, the basic ideas are summarized.

From the perspective of surgical simulation, the brain can be considered a single-phase continuum undergoing large deformations. In the present analysis, the stresses and strains were measured with respect to the current configuration. Thus, energetically conjugate Almansi strain $\boldsymbol{e}$ and Cauchy stress $\boldsymbol{\tau}$ (i.e. forces per unit areas in the deformed geometry) were used:

$$\boldsymbol{e} = \frac{1}{2}[\boldsymbol{I} - (\boldsymbol{F}^{-1})^T(\boldsymbol{F}^{-1})], \tag{1}$$

where $\boldsymbol{F}$ is the deformation gradient and $\boldsymbol{I}$ is the identity matrix.

Using Almansi strain and Cauchy stress, the equation of equilibrium can be written in the following way:

$$\tau^{ij}_{,i} + \rho R_i = 0\,, \tag{2}$$

where ρ is a mass density, R_i is a body force per unit mass in direction i, and comma indicates covariant differentiation with respect to the deformed configuration. Repeated index summation convention was used.

Eqs. (1)-(2) must be supplemented by formulae describing mechanical properties of materials, i.e. appropriate constitutive models. Modeling of physical properties of the brain is still an uncovered area pioneered by a few only [10], [11], [12]. As shown by Miller and Chinzei [13], [14], the stress–strain behavior of the brain tissue is nonlinear. The stiffness in compression is significantly higher than in extension. One can also observe a strong stress–strain rate dependency. To account for these complexities, we used the model suggested by Miller and Chinzei [14]:

$$W = \frac{2}{\alpha^2}\int_0^t [\mu(t-\tau)\frac{\mathrm{d}}{\mathrm{d}\tau}(\lambda_1^\alpha + \lambda_2^\alpha + \lambda_3^\alpha - 3)]\mathrm{d}\tau\,, \tag{3}$$

$$\mu = \mu_0[1 - \sum_{k=1}^{n} g_k(1 - e^{-\frac{t}{\tau_k}})]\,, \tag{4}$$

where W is a potential function, λ_i's are principal stretches, μ_0 is the instantaneous shear modulus in undeformed state, τ_k are characteristic times, g_k are relaxation coefficients, and α is a material coefficient, which can assume any real value without restrictions. The model parameters are given in Table 1.

The cerebral falx was assigned Young's modulus of 3.4 MPa [15]. For pia, the Young's modulus of 1.1 MPa was used – a value derived from the studies on brain injury by Takhounts et al. [15] and Zhang et al. [16].

Table 1. List of material constants for constitutive model of brain tissue, Eqs. (3) and (4), n=2. The constants were taken from Miller and Chinzei [14]

Instantaneous response	μ_0=842 [Pa]; α=-4.7
k=1	Characteristic time τ_1=0.5 [s]; g_1=0.450
k=2	Characteristic time τ_2=50 [s]; g_2=0.365

Integration of Equations of Equilibrium. Integration of equations of equilibrium/dynamics (i.e. Eq. 2) can be done using either implicit or explicit methods [3]. The implicit integration methods are unconditionally stable but can be time consuming as iterations are conducted at each time step. Therefore, in the present study an explicit integration was used. In the explicit integration, no iteration is needed as the displacement at time $t+\Delta t$ is solely based on the equilibrium at time t.

The computations were conducted using the *LS-DYNA* code (Livermore Software Technology Corporation, Livermore, California, USA) [17], which is one of the explicit finite element codes routinely applied in car crash simulation. Fully nonlinear formulations are used in *LS-DYNA*, i.e. both geometrical and material nonlinearities are taken into account.

Boundary Conditions for Simulation of Brain Shift. The anterior parts of the preoperative and intraoperative cortical surfaces were discretized using consistent rectangular meshes of the same density. The distances between corresponding nodes of the preoperative and intraoperative cortical surfaces were calculated and used as displacement boundary conditions (i.e. prescribed nodal displacements) for the nodes located in the anterior part of the brain model surface. To define the boundary conditions for the remaining nodes on the brain model surface, contact interfaces were defined between the rigid skull model and parts of the brain surface where the nodal displacements were not prescribed.

The spine–spinal cord interactions and constraining effects of the spinal cord on the brain rigid body motion were simulated by rigidly constraining the spinal end of the model.

In biomechanical models for nonrigid registration, cerebral falx is typically not simulated. However, as suggested by Warfield [18], disregarding falx may lead to misregistration of the lateral ventricles on the side opposite to surgical intervention. Therefore, in the present study the falx was simulated as elastic membrane rigidly attached to the skull. The contact interfaces were defined between this membrane and inter-hemisphere surfaces.

3 Results

The craniotomy-induced displacements of the ventricles' and tumor's centers of gravity (COGs) predicted by the model agreed well with the actual ones determined from the radiographic images (Table 2). With the exception of the tumor COG displacement along the Y (i.e. inferior-superior) axis, the differences between the computed and observed displacements were below 0.65 mm. Important and not unexpected feature of the results summarized in Table 2 is that the displacements of the tumor's and ventricles' COGs appreciably differed. This feature can be explained only by the fact that the brain undergoes both local deformation and global rigid body motion, which implies that nonrigid registration had to be used.

Table 2. Comparison of craniotomy-induced displacements of ventricles' and tumor's centers of gravity (COGs) predicted by the present brain model with the actual ones determined from MRIs. Directions of X, Y and Z axes are given in Fig. 2a.

	Determined from MRIs	Predicted
Ventricles	$\Delta x = 3.40$ mm $\Delta y = 0.25$ mm $\Delta z = 1.73$ mm	$\Delta x = 3.06$ mm $\Delta y = 0.29$ mm $\Delta z = 1.65$ mm
Tumor	$\Delta x = 5.36$ mm $\Delta y = -3.52$ mm $\Delta z = 2.64$ mm	$\Delta x = 4.74$ mm $\Delta y = -0.40$ mm $\Delta z = 2.77$ mm

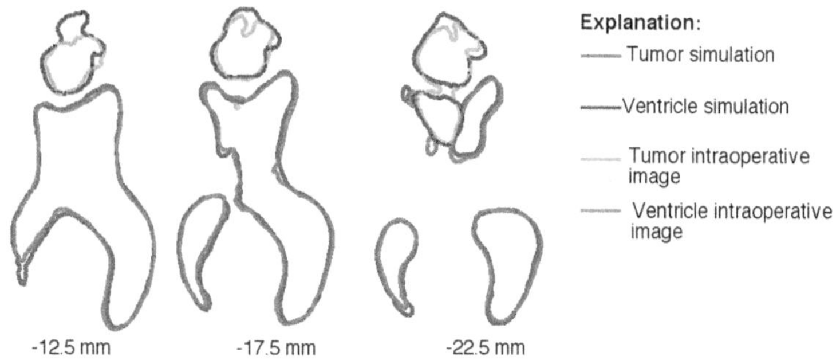

Fig. 4. Comparison of contours of axial sections of ventricles and tumor obtained from the intraoperative images with the ones predicted using the present brain model. Positions of section cuts are measured from the most superior point of parietal cortex (superior direction is positive).

Detailed comparison of cross sections of the actual tumor and ventricle surfaces acquired intraoperatively with the ones predicted by the present brain model indicates some local misregistration, particularly in the inferior tumor part (Fig. 4). However, the overall agreement is remarkably good.

4 Discussion and Conclusions

Instead of relying on unrealistic linearization (i.e. assumption about infinitesimally small brain deformation during craniotomy and linear stress – strain relationship of brain tissue) used in almost all biomechanical models for neurosurgical registration (with a notable exception of Xu and Nowinski [19]), we applied fully nonlinear (i.e. including both geometrical and material nonlinearities) finite element formulations to compute deformation field within the brain. These formulations made it possible to predict the displacement of the ventricles' and tumor's centers of gravity with around 0.5 mm accuracy (Table 2). This remarkable accuracy was achieved using displacement boundary conditions determined from very limited information about the brain surface deformation.

Detailed comparison of the calculated and image-determined cross sections of ventricles and tumor after craniotomy indicated local misregistration (Fig. 4), but the overall agreement was remarkably good. The local inaccuracies observed here could be related to simplifications of the brain geometry when building the finite element mesh and inability of our brain model to accurately account for various complex physiological phenomena, such as loss of fluid from ventricles, that could affect deformation field within the brain. A combined approach is needed in which nonlinear biomechanical models, such as the one developed in the present study, are applied together with traditional registration methods relying on image processing techniques, such as e.g. optical flow [20], mutual information-based similarity [21], entropy-based alignment [22] and block matching [23].

The presented results indicate that finite element analysis using fully nonlinear solid mechanics formulations is a powerful method for computing deformation field within the brain during craniotomy. As realistic prediction of deformation field within the brain is crucial for nonrigid registration, our results show that biomechanical models using fully nonlinear finite element formulations can be regarded as promising tool when complementing traditional image processing techniques used in image registration. Such models do not require unrealistic assumptions that the brain deformations are infinitesimally small and brain tissue stress–strain relationship is linear. Therefore, they can be seen as one possible way of improving reliability of image registration.

Acknowledgements

The financial support of the Australian Research Council (Grant No. DP0343112) is gratefully acknowledged.

The medical images used in the present study were obtained in the investigation supported by NSF ITR 0426558, a research grant from the Whitaker Foundation and by NIH grants R21 MH67054, R01 LM007861, P41 RR13218 and P01 CA67165.

The authors gratefully acknowledge collaboration of Toyota Central R&D Labs. (Nagakute, Aichi, Japan) in development of brain model.

References

1. Bucholz, R., MacNeil, W. and McDurmont, L.: The operating room of the future. Clinical Neurosurgery, Vol. 51 (2004) 228-237
2. Warfield, S. K., Talos, F., Tei, A., Bharatha, A., Nabavi, A., Ferrant, M., Black, P. McL., Jolesz, F. A. and Kikinis, R.: Real-time registration of volumetric brain MRI by biomechanical simulation of deformation during image guided surgery. Computing and Visualization in Science, Vol. 5 (2002) 3-11
3. Bathe, K.-J.: Finite Element Procedures. Prentice-Hall (1996)
4. Ferrant, M., Nabavi, A., Macq, B., Black, P. McL., Jolesz, F. A., Kikinis, R. and Warfield, S. K.: Serial registration of interoperative MR images of the brain. Medical Image Analysis, Vol. 6 (2002) 337-359
5. Hagemann, A., Rohr, K., Stiehl, H. S., Spetzger, U. and Gilsbach, J. M.: Biomechanical modeling of the human head for physically based, nonrigid image registration. IEEE Transactions on Medical Imaging, Vol. 18 (1999) 875-884
6. Miga, M. I., Sinha, T. K., Cash, D. M., Galloway, R. L. and Weil, R. J.: Cortical surface registration for image-guided neurosurgery using laser-range scanning. IEEE Transactions on Medical Imaging, Vol. 22 (2003) 973-985
7. 3D Slicer: Medical visualization and processing environment for research, http://www.slicer.org/
8. Wittek, A., Miller, K., Laporte, J., Kikinis, R. and Warfield, S. K.: Computing reaction forces on surgical tools for robotic neurosurgery and surgical simulation, in Proc. of Australasian Conference on Robotics and Automation ACRA, Canberra, Australia, (2004) 1-8
9. Miller, K.: Biomechanics of Brain for Computer Integrated Surgery. Warsaw: Publishing House of Warsaw University of Technology (2002)
10. Miller, K. and Chinzei, K.: Modeling of soft tissues deformation. Journal of Computer Aided Surgery, Vol. 1 (1995) 62-63
11. Bilston, L. E., Liu, Z. and Phan-Tien, N.: Linear viscoelastic properties of bovine brain tissue in shear. Biorheology, Vol. 34 (1997) 377-385

12. Prange, M. T. and Margulies, S. S.: Regional, directional, and age-dependent properties of the brain undergoing large deformation. ASME Journal of Biomechanical Engineering, Vol. 124 (2002) 244-252
13. Miller, K. and Chinzei, K.: Constitutive modelling of brain tissue; Experiment and Theory. Journal of Biomechanics, Vol. 30 (1997) 1115-1121
14. Miller, K. and Chinzei, K.: Mechanical properties of brain tissue in tension. Journal of Biomechanics, Vol. 35 (2002) 483-490
15. Takhounts, E. G., Eppinger, R. H., Campbell, J. Q., Tannous, R. E., Power, E. D. and Shook, S. S.: On the development of the SIMon finite element head model. Stapp Car Crash Journal, Vol. 47 (2003) 107-133
16. Zhang, L., Bae, J., Hardy, W. N., Monson, K. L., Manley, G. T., Goldsmith, W., Yang, K. H. and King, A. I.: Computational study of the contribution of the brain vasculature on the dynamic response of the brain. Stapp Car Crash Journal, Vol. 46 (2002) 145-163
17. Hallquist, J. O.: LS-DYNA Theoretical Manual, Livermore Software Technology Corporation (1998)
18. Warfield, S. K., Ferrant, M., Gallez, X., Nabavi, A., Jolesz, F. A. and Kikinis, R.: Real-time biomechanical simulation of volumetric brain deformation for image guided neurosurgery, in Proc. of SC 2000: High Performance Networking and Computing Conference, Dallas, USA, (2000) 1-16
19. Xu, M. and Nowinski, W. L.: Talairach-Tournoux brain atlas registration using a metal-forming principle-based finite element method. Medical Image Analysis, Vol. 5 (2001) 271-279
20. Beauchemin, S. S. and Barron, J. L.: The computation of optical flow. ACM Computing Surveys, Vol. 27 (1995) 433-467
21. Viola, P. A.: Alignment by maximization of mutual information. Artificial Intelligence Laboratory, Massachusetts Institute of Technology, Report AI-TR-1548 (1995)
22. Warfield, S. K., Rexilius, J., Huppi, P. S., Inder, T. E., Miller, E. G., Wells III, W. M., Zientara, G. P., Jolesz, F. A. and Kikinis, R.: A binary entropy measure to assess nonrigid registration algorithms, in Proc. of MICCAI 2001: Fourth International Conference on Medical Image Computing and Computer Assisted Intervention, Utrecht, The Netherlands, (2001) 266-274
23. Dengler, J. and Schmidt, M.: The dynamic pyramid - a model for motion analysis with controlled continuity. International Journal of Pattern Recognition and Artificial Intelligence, Vol. 2 (1988) 275-286

Finite Element Model of Cornea Deformation

Jessica R. Crouch[1], John C. Merriam[2], and Earl R. Crouch III[3]

[1] Computer Science Dept., Old Dominion University, VA, USA
jrcrouch@odu.edu
[2] Department of Ophthalmology, Columbia, New York, NY, USA
[3] Department of Ophthalmology, Eastern Virginia Medical School, Norfolk, VA, USA

Abstract. Cornea surgeons have observed that changes in cornea curvature can follow cataract surgery and cause astigmatism. The placement of surgical incisions has been shown to influence these curvature changes. Though empirical data has been collected about this phenomenon, a biomechanical model has not been employed in predicting post-surgical outcomes. This work implemented an incised finite element model of the eye to investigate factors influencing corneal shape after surgery. In particular, the effects of eye muscle forces and intra-ocular pressure were simulated. Cornea shape change was computed via finite element analysis, and the resulting change in cornea curvature was measured by fitting quadratic curves to the horizontal and vertical meridians of the cornea. Results suggest that these two sources of deforming force counteract each other and contribute to astigmatism in perpendicular directions.

1 Introduction

A finite element model of the eye was developed to investigate whether such a model might be helpful in predicting changes in the corneal curvature after cataract surgery. Cornea surgeons have observed that changes in cornea curvature often follow cataract surgery and alter pre-operative astigmatism. Further, they have found that the orientation of the astigmatism is related to the position of the surgical incision(s). For patients with pre-existing astigmatism, the astigmatism can be reduced or increased, depending on incision placement. Cornea surgeons have produced tables based on empirical observations of surgical results that allow them to predict the cornea curvature change that will result from a given incision [1]. However, a clear mechanical understanding of the causes of the observed changes does not exist.

Related work includes a study by Pinsky and Datye [2] that constructed a finite element model of the eye to examine the effects of radial keratotomy. Partial thickness corneal incisions were modeled on one quarter of the cornea; horizontal and vertical corneal symmetry was assumed. The work presented here expands on this earlier work by modeling the full cornea and the rest of the globe without making assumptions about symmetry that prevent the consideration of irregularities such as astigmatism. Another difference is the placement and depth of the modeled incision. This work models an incision along the periphery of the

J. Duncan and G. Gerig (Eds.): MICCAI 2005, LNCS 3750, pp. 591–598, 2005.

cornea that might be used for cataract or anterior segment surgery instead of the radial incisions used in radial keratotomy.

Other models of radial keratotomy have been developed by Vito, et al [3], Wray, et al[4], and Sawusch, et al [5]. Related work also includes a model of the phototherapeutic keratectomy procedure by Katsube, et al [6] and a simulation of eye trauma using a finite element model that was constructed by Uchio, et al [7].

Investigations into the material properties of the cornea provide a basis for the development of biomechanical models. Such work includes an analysis of cornea strain distribution by Shin, et al [8] and a micro-structural analysis of the cornea by Johnson [9].

The construction of the finite element mode used in this work is described in section 2, along with the simulated incision and application of deforming forces. Model deformation results are described in section 3 and discussed in light of the available patient data. Finally, section 4 presents conclusions and planned future work.

2 Finite Element Model

The finite element eye model in this study was designed to focus on the structural integrity of the cornea and sclera, the structures that form the outer shell of the eye. Initially, a geometric eye model was developed based on the female Visible Human image set, using anatomical image slices with 0.33 mm thickness. However, experience showed that the image resolution and clarity was not sufficient to adequately capture the small, detailed structures of the eye. A smoother, more appropriate model was subsequently developed using an analytically generated eye model based on the known geometry of the eye. This type of model has the further advantage of providing automatic generation of eye models to represent patients with a variety of eye and cornea geometry.

The model generation algorithm accepts as input the radii of curvature for the cornea and the larger eye globe, as well as the number and thickness of the layers that form the outer shell of the eye. The algorithm produces as output a finite element mesh composed of quadratic hexahedral elements. Quadratic hexahedra provide excellent representation of the eye's smooth curved surface geometry with a relatively small number of mesh nodes and elements. Each quadratic hexahedral elements had 27 nodes, as shown in Fig. 1. The eye mesh

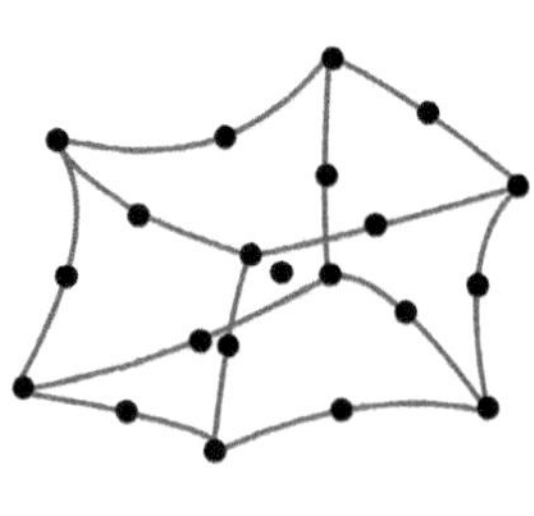

Fig. 1. Illustration of the structure of a quadratic hexahedral element. Each edge interpolates 3 nodes, resulting in a quadratic curve. The midpoint of each face and the center of the element also have nodes that support quadratic interpolation across all three spatial dimensions.

shown in Fig. 2 contains only 6804 nodes and 812 elements. Hexahedral elements also provide excellent numerical properties for finite element analysis [10].

The eye model is generated using two superimposed spherical coordinate systems. The model shown in Fig. 2 has realistic eye geometry, with a globe radius of 11.5 mm and a cornea radius of 7.8 mm. A linear elastic material model was used for the entire eye, but the stiffness and thickness of the different layers of the cornea varied. For the model in Fig. 2, the corneal layers were represented as shown in Table 1.

Mesh elements were created in layers to form concentric spherical shells. Each node was provided with both spherical coordinates (θ, ϕ, r) and Cartesian coordinates (x, y, z). A custom meshing pattern was developed to connect the cornea mesh and the globe mesh so that the eye model consisted of one continuous finite element mesh. For this model, the interior of the eye was assumed to have homogeneous material properties.

A linear elastic material model was applied to the eye model. The thick stroma layers of the cornea are composed predominantly of collagen and water. These layers account for much of the cornea's strength, and were assigned a Young's modulus 160 kPa, consistent with published stiffness values [11], and a Poisson's ratio of 0.49 to indicate near incompressibility. The shell of the globe was assigned the same material properties, while the interior of the eye and thinner layers of the cornea were assigned the same Poisson's ratio but were

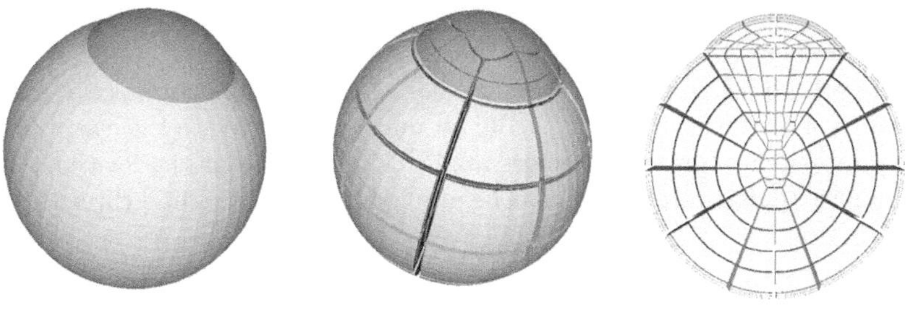

Fig. 2. Left: Exterior view of an eye model. Center: View showing divisions between the quadratic hexahedral elements that compose the finite element mesh. Right: Interior view of the structure of the volumetric mesh.

Table 1. Eye model layers and thicknesses

Name	Thickness (mm)
Epithelium	0.05
Bowman's membrane	0.012
Stroma (anterior)	0.25
Stroma (posterior)	0.25
Descemet's membrane	0.01
Endothelium	0.005

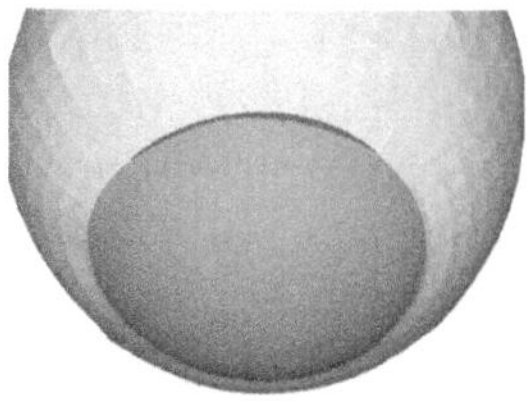

Fig. 3. To model an incision along the top edge of the cornea, connections between adjacent elements were removed through all of the corneal layers. Connections between the elements that compose the homogeneous interior of the eye were left intact. The black curve along the top corneal border indicates the placement of the cut.

given a Young's modulus an order of magnitude smaller. This choice of material properties was designed to capture the difference between the relatively tough outer shell of the eye and the interior of the eye that is filled with a much softer vitreous material.

To examine the effects of surgical incisions, a cut in the initial eye mesh was made, as shown in Fig. 3. The 9.5mm incision was made along the top border of the cornea and represents the incision made in an extra-capsular cataract extraction procedure. The incision alone does not cause post-operative astigmatism, but forces acting on an incised cornea cause it to deform differently than an intact cornea would. Therefore, two types of forces were defined to simulate the stresses to which corneas are ordinarily subjected.

The first set of forces represented intra-ocular pressure. In this case, a uniform force was applied across the cornea in the direction normal to the cornea surface at each point. The normal range for intra-ocular pressure is 10-21 mm Hg. For this experiment a pressure of 10 mm Hg was applied, which is equal to 1.33 kPa distributed over the surface area of the cornea.

The second set of forces were muscular. The superior, inferior, lateral, and medial recti eye muscles are the strongest muscles attached to the eye, and these were approximated by force vectors applied tangentially at the locations where those muscles insert on the globe. The applied muscle forces had three times the

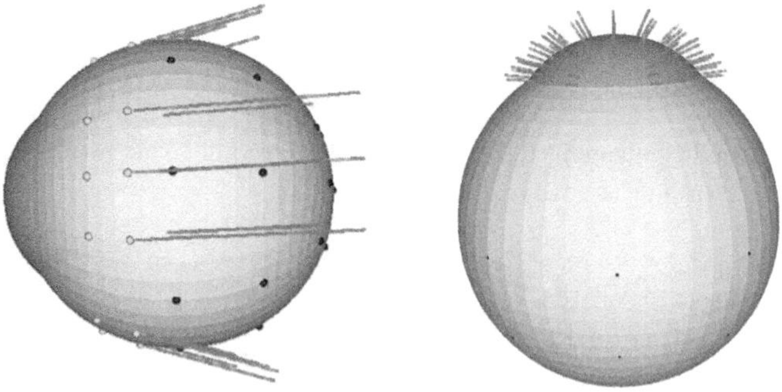

Fig. 4. Illustration of two sets of forces applied to the eye. For both sets of boundary conditions, nodes on the posterior portion of the eye remained fixed. These are marked with black dots. Left: Eye model with muscle forces applied tangential to the globe. Right: Eye model with intra-ocular pressure forces applied normal to the cornea.

magnitude of the intra-ocular pressure, but were applied to a smaller area. The force from each muscle was applied to a narrow patch located approximately 6.5 mm from the edge of the cornea. Fig. 4 illustrates both the muscle and intra-ocular force vectors. To maintain stability and prevent model translation or rotation under the application of these forces, the nodes on the posterior surface of the globe were assigned fixed positions.

The application of forces to the incised cornea model produced a deformed corneal surface, but further analysis was required to quantify the shape change. The shape change was analyzed by performing a least-squares fit of quadratic polynomial curves to the mesh nodes lying along the horizontal and vertical meridians of the deformed corneas. The radius of curvature of the quadratic curves was computed at the center point of the cornea, and then the radius of curvature was converted to diopters, a measure of refractive power. This allowed direct comparison between the model results and published patient data. Results are presented in the following section.

3 Results

Visualization of the height maps of the original and deformed corneas produced by the two sets of boundary conditions is provided in Fig. 5. Corresponding numerical results are shown in Table 2.

The results show that for an incision along the top border of the cornea model, muscle forces led to stretching and flattening of the cornea along the horizontal meridian. Forces from intra-ocular pressure led to stretching and flattening along the vertical meridian. This indicates that the two types of forces tend to counteract each other in terms of causing astigmatism.

Merriam showed that for the type of cornea incision modeled in this experiment, one month after surgery patients had an average of +1.6 diopters change in the vertical meridian (steepening) and -1.4 diopters change in the horizontal

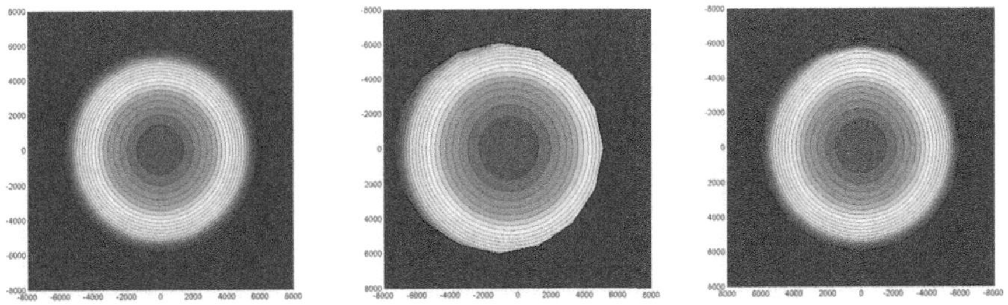

Fig. 5. Left: Contours of original, spherical cornea's height map Center: Contours of cornea model deformed by muscle forces, showing evidence of flattening in the horizontal direction Right: Contours of cornea model deformed by intra-ocular pressure, showing evidence of flattening in the vertical direction, but less pronounced than the flattening caused the muscle forces.

Table 2. Numerical results for the finite element model's cornea curvature across the horizontal and vertical meridians, given muscle force boundary conditions and intra-ocular pressure boundary conditions

	Vertical Axis Radius of Curvature (mm)	Vertical Axis Diopters	Horizontal Axis Radius of Curvature (mm)	Horizontal Axis Diopters
Original Cornea	7.80	43.27	7.80	43.27
Deformed by muscle forces	7.64	44.18	7.72	43.72
Deformed by intra-ocular pressure	7.89	42.76	7.59	44.47

meridian (flattening). However, five years after surgery patients exhibited astigmatism in the reverse direction, with an average of -0.7 diopters change in the vertical meridian and +0.6 diopters change in the horizontal meridian compared to their pre-operative condition [1]. This is likely because the vision change in first weeks after surgery is heavily influenced by tissue swelling and the healing response, whereas the long term vision change may be due to permanent structural changes in the cornea.

The finite element model results indicate that the long-term astigmatism observed in the patient population is consistent with the model deformation caused by forces from intra-ocular pressure. However this preliminary result requires further investigation, as not all of the factors influencing the cornea shape were represented in the initial finite element model. In particular, the effects of swelling and healing may influence the final visual result. In the healing process, scar tissue is formed that has different mechanical properties than normal cornea tissue. This scar tissue begins to form while the eye is still swollen from the surgical trauma. Therefore the final, healed geometry of the eye may depend on a patient's degree of swelling, rate of healing, and scar formation process as well as the forces exerted by intra-ocular pressure and eye muscles.

4 Conclusions and Future Work

In conclusion, this work has shown that the long-term astigmatism observed in the patient population is qualitatively similar to the model deformation caused by forces from intra-ocular pressure. However, extensive future work is needed to produce and validate a biomechanical model that could be used to help predict surgical outcomes.

Future work may expand on the current work in the following ways:

- Apply an oriented fiber tissue model to cornea.
  The corneal stroma is known to be composed of oriented bundles of

collagen [12]. The direction of collagen fibrils at a given point on the cornea is related to that point's distance from the center of the cornea and angle from the horizontal and vertical axes. A finite element oriented fiber material model requires that each element possess a vector that defines the direction of the fibers. Although an isotropic material model was assumed for this initial eye model, the use of spherical coordinate systems in the mesh construction will facilitate the future implementation of an oriented fiber material model for the cornea.

- Augment the finite element model with a time-dependent simulation of the healing response.
  By locally varying the cornea's material properties over time to account for swelling and scar formation, and then running the model over a number of simulated months, the impact of the healing process could be examined. A time-dependent simulation would also allow the influence of constant intra-ocular pressure versus the intermittent application of muscle forces to be investigated.

- Experiment with individualized eye models.
  By generating a variety of eye models with different corneal thickness, different degrees and orientations of pre-existing astigmatism, different levels of intra-ocular pressure, and different levels of muscle strength, the model generated deformations could be compared to existing data on patient surgical outcomes. This would assist in the development and validation of an individualizable, predictive cataract surgery model. Additionally, the effect of incision placement and size can be examined for the different eye models to see if surgeons' ability to reduce pre-existing astigmatism with carefully placed incisions can be accurately replicated by the model.

References

1. Merriam, J., Zheng, L., Merriam, J., Zaider, M.: The effect of incisions for cataract on corneal curvature. Ophthalmology **110** (2003) 1807–1813
2. Pinsky, P., Datye, D.: A microstructurally based finite element model of the incised human cornea. Journal of Biomechanics **24** (1991) 907–992
3. Vito, R.P., Shin, T.J., McCarey, B.E.: A mechanical model of the cornea: the effects of physiological and surgical factors on radial keratotomy surgery. Refract Corneal Surg **5** (1989) 82–88
4. Wray, W., Best, E., Cheng, L.: A mechanical model for radial keratotomy: toward a predictive capability. Journal of Biomechanical Engineering **116** (1994) 56–61
5. Sawusch, M., McDonnell, P.: Computer modeling of wound gape following radial keratotomy. Refractive Corneal Surgery **8** (1992) 143–145
6. Katsube, N., Wang, R., Okuma, E., Roberts, C.: Biomechanical response of the cornea to phototherapeutic keratectomy when treated as a fluid-filled porous material. Journal of Refractive Surgery **18** (2002) 593–597
7. Uchio, E., Ohno, S., Kudoh, J., Aoki, K., Kisielewicz, L.: Simulation model of an eyeball based on finite element analysis on a supercomputer. British Journal of Ophthalmology **83** (1999) 1106–1111

8. Shin, T., Vito, R., Johnson, L., McCarey, B.: The distribution of strain in the human cornea. Journal of Biomechanics **30** (1997) 497–503
9. Johnson, L.: The Mechanical and Microstructural Analysis of the Human Cornea. Dissertation, School of Mechanical Engineering, Georgia Institute of Technology (1998)
10. Benzley, S.E., Perry, E., Merkley, K., Clark, B., Sjaardama, G.: A comparison of all hexagonal and all tetrahedral finite element meshes for elastic and elasto-plastic analysis. Proceedings, 4th International Meshing Roundtable (1995) 179–191
11. Forster, W., Kasprzak, H., von Bally, G.: Measurement of elastic modulus of the central bovine cornea by means of holographic interferometry. Part II. Results. Optom Vis Science **71** (1994) 27–32
12. Hollman, K., Emelianov, S., Neiss, J., Jotyan, G., Spooner, G., Juhasz, T., Kurtz, R., O'Donnell, M.: Strain imaging of corneal tissue with an ultrasound elasticity microscope. Cornea **21** (2002) 68–73
13. Aghamohammadzadeh, H., Newton, R., Meek, K.: X-ray scattering used to map the preferred collagen orientation in the human cornea and limbus. Structure (Camb) **12** (2004) 249–256
14. Hjortdal, J.: Regional elastic performance of the human cornea. Journal of Biomechanics **29** (1996) 831–942
15. Sagar, M., Bullivant, D., Mallinson, G., Hunter, P.: A virtual environment and model of the eye for surgical simulation. International Conference on Computer Graphics and Interactive Techniques, Proceedings of the 21st annual conference on Computer graphics and interactive techniques (1994) 205–212

Characterization of Viscoelastic Soft Tissue Properties from *In vivo* Animal Experiments and Inverse FE Parameter Estimation

Jung Kim[1] and Mandayam A. Srinivasan[2]

[1] Dept. of Mechanical Engineering,
Korea Advanced Institute of Science and Technology, Korea
[2] The Touch Lab, Dept of Mechanical Engineering,
Massachusetts Institute of Technology, USA
jungkim@kaist.ac.kr, srini@mit.edu

Abstract. Soft tissue characterization and modeling based on living tissues has been investigated in order to provide a more realistic behavior in a virtual reality based surgical simulation. In this paper, we characterize the nonlinear viscoelastic properties of intra-abdominal organs using the data from *in vivo* animal experiments and inverse FE parameter estimation algorithm. In the assumptions of quasi-linear-viscoelastic theory, we estimated the viscoelastic and hyperelastic material parameters to provide a physically based simulation of tissue deformations. To calibrate the parameters to the experimental results, we developed a three dimensional FE model to simulate the forces at the indenter and an optimization program that updates new parameters and runs the simulation iteratively. We can successfully reduce the time and computation resources by decoupling the viscoelastic part and nonlinear elastic part in a tissue model. The comparison between simulation and experimental behavior of pig intra abdominal soft tissue are presented to provide a validness of the tissue model using our approach.

1 Introduction

Soft tissue characterization and modeling has been investigated in order to understand mechanisms of traumatic injury. For example, Farshad et al. [1] characterized the material parameters of pig kidney based on uniaxial tension tests on ex vivo samples. They were mainly interested in a tissue behavior under high speed or impact loading conditions, which occur in accidents, so their measurements were mainly ex vivo measurements. Recent developments in medical instruments have motivated the tissue characterization under the lower speed loading conditions and using the data from in vivo measurements which are expected to provide the properties of living tissues. Davies et al. [2] developed a two dimensional mathematical model for pig spleen tissue from uniform compression tests using a large-area indenter. They solved the nonlinear constrained boundary value problems numerically with an exponential stress-strain law and a finite element model (FEM). By varying the model size, they showed that the forces measured at the indenter were insensitive to the size of the model. Miller [3] developed a three-dimensional, hyperelastic, viscoelastic

J. Duncan and G. Gerig (Eds.): MICCAI 2005, LNCS 3750, pp. 599 – 606, 2005.

constitutive model for abdominal organ tissues. The model was developed from a strain-energy function with time dependent constants.

Although *in vivo* experiments can provide the data in a living state and they are essential to develop soft tissue models for surgical simulation or rehearsal, the characterization of soft tissue properties has not been successful. Because the target organs have non-uniform cross-sectional area and non-uniform strain across any given cross section. An analytic solution based on the boundary value problem was not a good candidate, given the complexity of the material behavior, the organ geometry, and the three-dimensional deformation imposed on the surface. To circumvent these difficulties, inverse finite element estimation has been investigated recently. This method estimates unknown material parameters for a selected material law by minimizing the least-squares difference between predictions of a finite element model and experimental responses. In this paper, we estimated viscoelastic material properties of soft tissue by using the *in vivo* animal experimental data and a FE tool to provide a model for medical simulation or off-line analysis.

2 *In vivo* Animal Experiments

We measured pig's liver and kidney under open surgical conditions to measure mechanical properties *in vivo* at the Harvard Center for Minimally Invasive Surgery in collaboration with surgeons from the Massachusetts General Hospital (MGH). A total of 10 pigs were used in these experiments. The pigs were first put under general anesthesia and placed on the surgical table. A midline incision was then made at its abdominal region and dissection carried out on the anatomical structures to expose the organs. The indentation stimuli were delivered using the haptic interface device, Phantom Premium-T 1.5 (SensAble Technologies, www.sensable.com) that was programmed to perform as a mechanical stimulator. Reaction forces were measured using a six-axis force transducer, Nano 17 (ATI Industrial Automation) that was attached to the tip of the Phantom. The transducer has a force resolution of 0.781 mN along each of the three orthogonal axes when connected to a 16-bit A/D converter. The indenter was a 2 mm diameter flat-tipped cylindrical probe that was fixed to the tip of the Phantom with the force transducer mounted in-between to accurately sense the reaction forces.

3 Estimation of Soft Tissue Properties

We used the quasi-linear viscoelasticity (QLV) framework proposed by Fung [5]. This approach assumes material behavior can be decoupled into two effects: a time-independent elastic response, and a linear viscoelastic stress relaxation response. These models can be determined separately from the experiments. The stresses in the tissues, which may be linear or nonlinear, are linearly superposed with respect to time.

The three-dimensional constitutive relationship in the framework of QLV is given by,

$$S(t) = G(t)S^{e}(0) + \int_{0}^{t} G(t-\tau)\frac{\partial S^{e}(E(\lambda))}{\partial \tau} d\tau \tag{1}$$

where S(t) is the second Piola-Kirchhoff stress tensor and G(t) is called the reduced relaxation function. $S^e(E(\lambda))$ is called the pure elastic response of the material and can be nonlinear or linear. The reduced relaxation function G(t) is a scalar function of time and can be often expressed by the Prony series,

$$G(t) = G_0\left(1 - \sum_{i=1}^{N} \overline{g}_i^P\left(1 - \exp\left(-\frac{t}{\tau_i}\right)\right)\right)$$
$$G_0 = G(0) \tag{2}$$

where $\overline{g}_i^P$ are the Prony series parameters.

For the nonlinear elastic response, we have used an incompressible hyperelastic material representation, which is commonly used for elastomer modeling. The material properties of a hyperelastic material can be determined by a strain energy function W. Ideally, W is defined with only as many parameters as are required in order to make a FE model. There are many specific material models that could be used, depending on how to approximate the strain energy function. The strain energy function of the three-dimensional incompressible Mooney–Rivlin model is given by

$$W = C_{10}(I_1 - 3) + C_{01}(I_2 - 3) \tag{3}$$

where C_{10}, C_{01} are material parameters (having unit of stress) and I_1, I_2 are principal invariants. Since the analytical solution considering the above material law and experimental conditions is very difficult, the Finite Element Method (FEM) has been widely used in simulation. Through modeling of indentation experiments with the QLV approach, the final outcome of the FE simulation can be simply expressed as,

$$Fs = FEM\_SIMULATION(p_i)$$
$$p_i = [\tau_i, \overline{g}_i^P, C_{ij}] \tag{4}$$

where F_s is the simulated force and p_i is the material parameter containing the viscoelasticity and nonlinear elasticity. For example, the number of the estimated parameters for the Mooney-Rivlin model is two. The goal of the characterization is to determine these parameters for a proposed material law by minimizing the errors between the simulated and the associated experimental measurements. This process is also called the inverse calculation because it is the opposite of an ordinary simulation (that is, solving for forces or displacements given material parameters and boundary conditions).

Instead of estimating all required parameters in one step, we separated the characterization process into two stages. In the first step the viscoelastic parameters were determined from the normalized force responses against ramp-and-hold indentation from the experiments. With the viscoelastic parameters estimated in the first stage, the inverse FEM parameter estimation method was used to determine the remaining elastic parameters.. This separation of parameters is also similar to the work by Kauer *et al.*[6]. However, they fixed the time constants of the stress relaxation

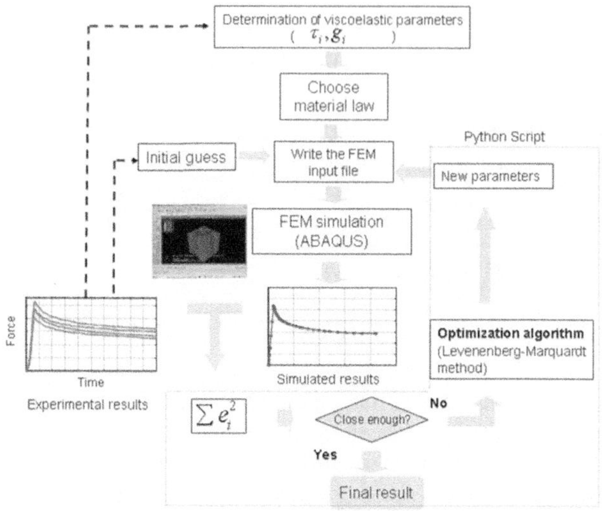

Fig. 1. Flow chart for the developed parameter estimation algorithm

(0.1s, 1s, 10s, and 100s), and fit their magnitudes, then determined the rest of the parameters using an inverse FEM calculation. In our work, the parameters in the viscoelastic model were estimated directly from the normalized force-displacement data in the experiments. The overall procedures of the characterization are illustrated in Fig. 1.

3.1 Determination of Viscoelastic Parameters

In this section we develop a three-dimensional linear viscoelastic model of the soft tissue based on the force-displacement experiment data. The simplest lumped parameter model that can capture the viscoelastic behavior of a solid is the three parameter linear solid model whose transfer function may be written as

$$\frac{F(s)}{\delta(s)} = F_{ss} \prod_{i=1}^{n} \left(\frac{1+\alpha_i \quad \tau_i s}{1+\tau_i s} \right) \tag{5}$$

where $F(s)$ and $\delta(s)$ are the Laplace transformed force and displacement variables, F_{ss} is the steady state value of the force response. τ is the relaxation time constant and α is the ratio of the initial response of the system to a step in displacement to the steady state value (α >1). Incidentally, this model has the similar to the Kelvin model. The point indenter is a good choice for model parameter estimation since it is the closest approximation of a punch on an elastic half space. From linear elastostatics we know that the total force, P, required to indent a frictionless circular cylindrical punch, of radius 'a', into an isotropic elastic halfspace, by a distance D is given by

$$P = \frac{8aG(G+3K)}{4G+3K}D \tag{6}$$

where G is the rigidity modulus, a is the diameter of the indenter and K is the bulk modulus.

From the correspondence principle and the incompressibility assumption, the above equation can be simplified,

$$P(s) = 8as\overline{G}(s)D(s) \tag{7}$$

From the above equations, the step response rigidity modulus may be written as,

$$\overline{G}(s) = \frac{F_{ss}}{8as}\prod_{i=1}^{2}\left(\frac{1+\alpha_i\tau_i s}{1+\tau_i s}\right) \tag{8}$$

Using the above model and the experimental data, we can find $g_{i,}\tau_i$ by using lsqnonlin.m, which is a built-in function for the nonlinear curve fitting in MATLAB. This approach allows the rigidity modulus to be expressed as a Prony series expansion in the time domain. Table 1 lists the computed Prony series parameters of the selected experiments.

3.2 Estimation of Nonlinear Elastic Parameters

In our application, the compared quantities are the simulated forces from the FEM simulation and the associated experimental forces at the indenter. Therefore, we can minimize a nonlinear sum of squares given by

$$\begin{aligned}\vec{E} &= \sum_{i}^{m}(\vec{F}_s(t_i)-\vec{F}_e(t_i))\cdot(\vec{F}_s(t_i)-\vec{F}_e(t_i)) \\ t_i &= (t_1,t_2\ldots t_m)\end{aligned} \tag{9}$$

where Fe, Fs, t_i, m are measured forces, simulated forces, time and the total number of data points, respectively. Among several optimization algorithms that could be used, we adopt the nonlinear least square optimization known as the Marquardt-Levenberg algorithm.

Although the Levenberg-Marqudt has been used successfully in finite strain applications [7], the entire process is computationally expensive. The FEM simulation, in which a few hours per run, is repeated as many times as necessary until

Table 1. Prony series parameters from the normalized force data

Organ	Depth (mm)	τ_1 (sec)	τ_2 (sec)	g_1	g_2	$\sum\varepsilon^2$
Liver	6	1.537	6.090	0.2866	0.2022	0.0754
Kidney	5	0.741	6.171	0.2054	0.2725	0.0653
Kidney	4	0.747	6.021	0.2305	0.2105	0.0867

the simulated results match the experimental results. The Jacobian vector is calculated at each iteration but this requires perturbing one parameter, running the entire FEM simulation, and measuring the effect of the perturbation. To construct the vector, this must be repeated for each parameter. Thus, for five free parameters, the FE model must be solved six times per iteration (the sixth solution is the reference to which the perturbations are compared). The entire characterization process takes several iterations to converge so the computational time is very large and hence it is better to reduce the number of parameters as much as possible as in our approach. It was this computational expense that led us to identify the viscoelastic parameters before undertaking the inverse FEM simulation. This allowed us to iterate using only two (Mooney-Rivlin) free parameters. Fig. 2 shows the developed model in ABAQUS. In our experiments, the deformation field appeared to be insensitive to the organ geometry. This made sense, since our indentations were small (millimeters) compared to the organs (centimeters). Accordingly, we simplified our analysis by modeling a subdomain of the organ. The size and the mesh density of the model are carefully adjusted to ensure a well-conditioned solution. Nonlinearities from both the material model and from large geometric deformation were allowed.

The contact between the indenter and tissues was modeled with a contact mechanics module in ABAQUS and the non-uniform element density over the model was used to improve accuracy of the contact region. We implemented the Levenberg-Marquardt algorithm with the Python language, which is a way to control the inputs and outputs of ABAQUS.

With the approximate initial values from the ABAQUS evaluation function, we used our Python code to iterate the FE model and update the parameters automatically. The parameters reached convergence with four or five iterations. Table 2 presents the initial parameters and converged parameters for both hyperelastic material models. With a good guess from a priori knowledge of the parameters, the parameters converged with three or four iterations in most of cases. Fig. 3 shows the predicted forces from the FE simulation with the estimated parameters and experimental forces for the pig liver and kidney. The force responses of the hyperelastic model in ABAQUS match the experimental data well.

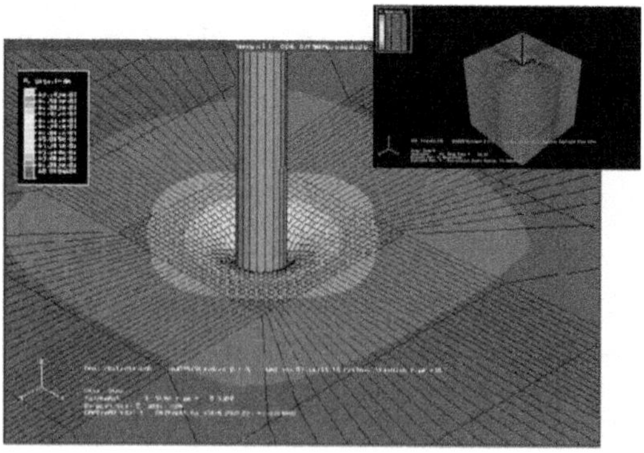

Fig. 2. FEM simulation of the experiment developed with ABAQUS. The upper right shows the shape of sub-domain region for the simulation.

Table 2. Initial and estimated parameters in the Mooney-Rivlin model

Condition		Initial parameters		Iteration Number	Final parameters		$\sum \varepsilon^2$
Organ	Indentation	C10 (Pa)	C01(Pa)		C10(Pa)	C01(Pa)	
Liver	6mm	83.18	84.76	3	322.96	161.47	0.0028
Kidney	5 mm	682.31	700.02	2	868.66	467.11	0.0031

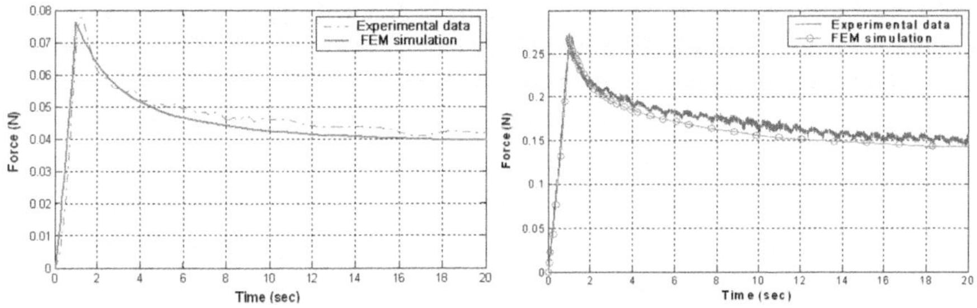

Fig. 3. Force responses of the model prediction and the experiments. (Left) liver with 5mm indentation. (Right) kidney with a 6mm indentation. The responses in (b) shows this noisy signal.

4 Concluding Remarks

In this paper, we have characterized the mechanical properties of intra-abdominal organs from the *in vivo* animal experiments. To calibrate the parameters to the experimental results, we developed a three dimensional FE model to simulate the forces at the indenter and an optimization program that updates new parameters and runs the simulation iteratively. Key assumptions in our approach are that the organs are incompressible, homogenous, and isotropic, and that the deformations we imposed were small compared to the size of the organ. With these limitations in mind, the material models presented in this study offer two basic uses in a VR-based medical simulation. First, they can be used directly in the simulator to compute visual deformations and interaction forces that are displayed in real time. Second, the mathematical models presented here can be used as a standard for the evaluation of new real time algorithms for computing deformation.

References

[1] M. Farshad, M. Barbezat, P. Flueler, F. Shmidlin, P. Graber, and P. Niederer, "Material Characterization of the Pig Kidney in Relation with the Biomechanical Analysis of Rental Trauma," *Journal of Biomechanics*, vol. 32, pp. 411-425, 1999.

[2] P. J. Davis, F. J. Carter, D. G. Loxburgh, and A. Cuschieri, "Mathematical Model for Keyhole Surgery Simulation: spleen capsule as an elastic membrane," *Journal of Theoretical Medicine*, vol. 1, pp. 247-262, 1999.

[3] K. Miller, "Constitutive Modeling of Abdominal Organs," *Journal of Biomechanics*, vol. 33, pp. 367-373, 1999.

[4] B. K. Tay, S. De, N. Stylopoulos, D. W. Rattner, and M. A. Srinivasan, "*In vivo* Force Response of Intra-abdominal Soft Tissue for the Simulation of Laparoscopic Procedures," presented at Proceedings of the MMVR Conference, 2002.

[5] Y. C. Fung, *Biomechanics: Mechanical Properties of Living Tissues*. New York: Springer-Verlag, 1993.

[6] M. Kauer, V. Vuskovic, J. Dual, G. Szekely, and M. Bajka, "Inverse Finite Element Characterization of Soft Tissue," presented at Medical Image Computing and Computer-Assisted Intervention - MICCAI 2001, 2001.

[7] P. Seshaiyer and J. D. Humphrey, "A Sub-Domain Inverse Finite Element Characterization of Hyperelastic Membranes Including Soft Tissues," *Journal of Biomechanical Engineering, Transaction of the ASME*, vol. 125, pp. 363-371, 2003.

A Fast-Marching Approach to Cardiac Electrophysiology Simulation for XMR Interventional Imaging

M. Sermesant[1], Y. Coudière[2], V. Moreau-Villéger[3], K.S. Rhode[1], D.L.G. Hill[4,*], and R.S. Razavi[1]

[1] Division of Imaging Sciences, King's College London, 5th floor Thomas Guy House, Guy's Hospital, London, UK
[2] Jean Leray Mathematics Laboratory, Nantes University, France
[3] Epidaure Research Project, INRIA, Sophia Antipolis, France
[4] Centre for Medical Image Computing, University College London, UK
derek.hill@ucl.ac.uk

Abstract. Cardiac ablation procedures are becoming more routine to treat arrhythmias. The development of electrophysiological models will allow investigation of treatment strategies. However, current models are computationally expensive and often too complex to be adjusted with current clinical data. In this paper, we have proposed a fast algorithm to solve Eikonal-based models on triangular meshes. These models can be used to extract hidden parameters of the cardiac function from clinical data in a very short time, thus could be used during interventions. We propose a first approach to estimate these parameters, and have tested it on synthetic and real data derived using XMR imaging. We demonstrated a qualitative matching between the estimated parameter and XMR data. This novel approach opens up possibilities to directly integrate modelling in the interventional room.

1 Introduction

The treatment of cardiac arrhythmias has changed considerably in the last fifteen years. Radio-frequency cardiac ablation techniques are becoming widely available as an alternative treatment to drug therapy. These are carried out under x-ray fluoroscopic guidance, with specialised catheters for making invasive recordings of the electrical activity in the heart, and even reconstruct the chamber geometry (CARTO from Biosense, EnSite from ESI).

These procedures can be highly effective with minimal side effects, but in some groups of patients have unsatisfactory success rates, are often very long, and can involve high x-ray radiation dose to both patient and staff. Moreover, serious side effects can arise if the lesions extend beyond the target area. There is a need for substantial innovation in order to reliably achieve successful results in an acceptable time, with lower radiation dose and reduced risk of accidental damage to adjacent structures.

* Corresponding author.

J. Duncan and G. Gerig (Eds.): MICCAI 2005, LNCS 3750, pp. 607–615, 2005.

The aim of this research work is to design models of the cardiac electrical activity that are suited for clinical use and to propose methods to combine these models with interventional data in order to better estimate the patient cardiac function and help in the guidance of procedures.

1.1 Electrophysiology Models

Modelling the electrophysiology of the cell is an active research area since the seminal work of Hodgkin and Huxley [1]. The precise modelling of the myocardium involves a cell membrane model embedded into a set of partial differential equations (PDE) modelling a continuum. We can divide these models into three categories, from the more complex to the simpler (numerically):

- Biophysical models: semi-linear evolution PDE + ionic models. Up to fifty equations for ion concentrations and channels (Luo-Rudy, Noble)
- Phenomenological models: semi-linear evolution PDE + mathematical simplification of biophysical models. Reducing to two equations representing the intra- and extra-cellular potentials (bi-domain, mono-domain)
- Eikonal models: one static non-linear PDE for the depolarisation time derived from the previous models (Eikonal-Curvature, Eikonal-Diffusion)

Solutions of the evolution PDE are very computationally demanding, due to the space scale of the electrical propagation front being much smaller than the size of the ventricles. The motion of the front governed by the Eikonal equation is observed at a much larger scale, resulting in much faster computations.

For our interventional purpose, and as parameter adjustment often requires several simulations, we want to design a very fast model. Moreover, clinical data currently available is mainly on depolarisation times. For these reasons we chose to base the presented work on the Eikonal models. Even if these models are not able to precisely simulate the whole range of cardiac pathologies, they open up possibilities for fast estimation, filtering, interpolation and extrapolation. The long-term goal is to build up a hierarchy of models where a more complex model could be used in pathological areas.

1.2 Clinical Measures

XMR suites are a new type of clinical facility combining in the same room a MR scanner and a mobile cardiac x-ray set. The patient can be easily moved between the two systems using a specially modified sliding MR table top that docks with and transfers patients to a specially modified x-ray table. Techniques have been designed to register the two imaging spaces [2]. Therefore it is possible to combine patient anatomy with electrophysiology recordings.

2 A Fast Electrophysiology Model

The classical Eikonal equation is:

$$c\|\nabla T\| = 1 \tag{1}$$

where T is the depolarisation time and c is the local propagation speed.

However, the propagation in an excitable medium like the myocardium depends on the curvature of the propagating front. It can be explained physically by the fact that if a convex front is propagating outward, the excitation of the neighbours is more spread out, so the excitation is slower than for a planar wave. Two different formulations have been proposed to introduce this effect. Both are based on asymptotic development of the solution around the activation front given by the Nagumo equation: $\partial_t u = D\Delta u + kf(u)$, where u is the action potential. f and k describe the cell membrane, they refer to the ionic reactions in the cell. D is the volumetric electrical conductivity of the tissue i.e. the transmission of the electrical wave from cell to cell. In the case of cardiac pathology, the conductivity and the ion channel mediated change of polarisation of the cardiac cells can be both involved.

The two resulting formulations are the Eikonal-Curvature equation [3]:

$$c\sqrt{kD}\|\nabla T\| - D\kappa(T) = 1 \tag{2}$$

with $\kappa(T) = \|\nabla T\|\text{div}\left(\frac{\nabla T}{\|\nabla T\|}\right)$, and the Eikonal-Diffusion equation [4]:

$$c\sqrt{kD}\|\nabla T\| - D\Delta T = 1 \tag{3}$$

c is a constant depending only on the function f.

2.1 Fast-Marching Approach

Different numerical approaches have been proposed to solve these equations. A temporal evolution term and finite differences have been applied to Eq. 2 [3]: $c\sqrt{kD}\|\nabla T\| - D\kappa(T) = \partial_t T$, and an evolution term and finite elements to the Eq. 3 [4]: $\partial_t T + c\sqrt{kD}\|\nabla T\| - D\Delta T = 1$.

A time dependant PDE like these needs up to thousands of iterations, each of which might be a linear (or non-linear) system to solve. Furthermore, additional stability conditions constrain the computations. The static solving of Eikonal equations 2 and 3, first proposed by [5] with a Newton's method, requires to solve only one non-linear system of equations.

For sake of efficiency, our approach is also to directly solve the static equations 2 and 3, but takes advantage of the Fast-Marching Method (FMM) [6] to solve the non-linear system. FMM are numerical algorithms for solving Eq. 1 on a Cartesian grid in $O(MlogM)$ steps ($O(M^2)$ for a Newton's method), where M stands for the number of grid points. Consistent upwind discretisations of the gradient are used that select the correct viscosity solution, and leads to a causality relationship between the unknowns: the solution at a grid point depends only on the smaller adjacent points, and the unknown can be computed from point to point in an ascending manner.

We evaluate a first guess T_0 for T by solving the Eq. 1 with the FMM, and then compute the curvature effect from T_0 to correct the equation and re-evaluate T. The iterative process is: $c\|T^{k+1}\| = 1 + F(T^k)$, where $F(T^k) = \kappa(T^k)$ for Eq. 2 and $F(T^k) = \Delta T^k$ for Eq. 3. The curvature term being only a small perturbation of the equation, the sequence (T^k) hopefully converges quickly. Then its limit is a solution of the discretised equation.

2.2 Unstructured Grids Implementation

The complexity of the heart geometry is difficult to describe with structured grids. Moreover, most of the 3D medical data is in the form of triangulated surfaces or point clouds. It is thus important to be able to deal with this kind of domain. This is why we implemented our algorithm on triangulations.

The FMM has been extended to unstructured grids, with criteria on the triangles to compute the narrow band values [7]. We implemented Eq. 3 using using P1 Lagrange Finite Elements to compute the Laplacian. Experimental evidence suggests no flux on the myocardium surface, so we use Neumann boundary conditions. We integrate this in the stiffness matrix K: $K_{ij} = \int \nabla\phi_i \nabla\phi_j$ coming from an integration by parts of the Laplacian in the variational formulation, with ϕ_i and ϕ_j the P1 Lagrange shape functions.

We compute the curvature flow for Eq. 2 with the formula proposed in [8]. We adapted the edge-based formula into a triangle-based formula, faster for the neighbourhood iterators we are using, and to cope with the presence of holes in the mesh. The curvature flow at point i is then:

$$\kappa(T) \approx \|\nabla T\|_i \frac{\sum_{n\in\mathcal{N}_i} W^i_j(T_j - T_i) + W^i_k(T_k - T_i)}{\sum_{n\in\mathcal{N}_i} meas(n)}$$

with $\mathcal{N}_i$ the triangle neighbour set incident to i; j and k the two other vertices of triangle n (and α_j, α_k the corresponding angles); $\|\nabla T\|_i$ the pointwise mass-lumped Galerkin approximation of the gradient in i; and $W^i_j = cotan(\alpha_k)/(2\|\nabla T\|_n)$; and $meas(n)$ the area of n.

Our C++ implementation using the sorted containers of the Standard Template Library and precomputed neighbouring iterators makes it possible to compute the FMM and these terms in less than a second for a 13 000 nodes mesh.

2.3 Validation of the Algorithm: Convergence and Precision

The numerical approach has been tested on Eq. 2 with $c = 1$ and $\alpha = 0.002$, on a family of unstructured meshes with up to 13092 nodes. Since we study the effect of curvature, the front is initially a circle of radius $r_0 = 0.1$ in the square $[-1, 1] \times [-1, -1]$. As a consequence, the solution is expected to be mainly dependent on $r = \sqrt{x^2 + y^2}$ so that its curvature $\kappa = 1/r$ varies from $1/r_0 = 10$ down to 1.

The computation of numerical solutions to Eq. 2 introduces errors when approximating the differential terms by differences on a mesh of nodes, and also when solving the resulting non-linear discrete problem.

We investigated numerically:

1. the algorithmic convergence of the sequence of approximation T^k towards a limit, expected to be the solution T_N of the discrete problem on a given mesh with N nodes, Fig. 1 (Left);
2. the mesh convergence of the solution T_N as $N \to \infty$, Fig. 1 (Right).

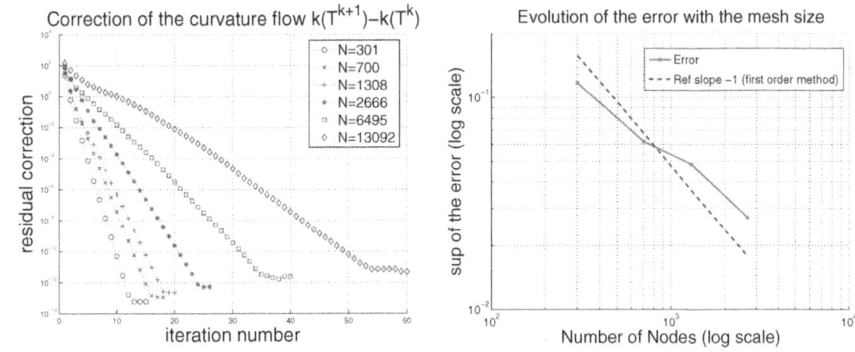

Fig. 1. (Left) Convergence of the algorithm for different mesh sizes. (Right) Evolution of the error with the mesh size.

Concerning point 1, the sequence T^k seems to converge, as shown in Fig. 1 Left. The number of iterations necessary for the residual correction $\|T^{k+1} - T^k\|_\infty$ to be of order 10^{-10} increase slowly as N, but remains reasonable: about 50 iterations on a 13 092 nodes mesh, which means that 50 FMM solutions has been successively computed. Our FMM iterative algorithm looks like a good replacement for a Newton's method.

Concerning point 2, a reference solution is constructed on the finer mesh, and compared to the solutions on coarser meshes. As expected from the first order upwind differences used to discretise the gradient, the error decreases as $1/N$ (ie as $h^{\frac{1}{2}}$ in 2D, standard for such methods). Of course higher order methods exist to discretise the gradient in an upwind manner. But, on unstructured meshes, they are not usually compatible with a Fast-Marching type algorithm.

3 Local Apparent Conductivity Estimation

Depolarization times on the endocardium are difficult to interpret due to the influence of the geometry and the curvature. The idea is to estimate hidden parameters using the proposed model and the clinical measurements in order to help diagnosis and therapy planning from electrophysiology study. A first step is to locate differences in local conductivity. In this section, we present a method to estimate this parameter using the fast Eikonal-Curvature model presented in the previous section (it could also be applied to the Eikonal-Diffusion).

Such parameters could eventually be estimated from the measured data using a signal processing approach. The model based method has the advantage of allowing the use of the model in a predictive way, once adjusted to the data. This can be very useful to test therapies and plan interventions. Moreover, it can be extended to partial observations: we aim to model the whole volumetric myocardium, but we will still have only access to surface data.

Estimating the parameters of a model from patient specific data is part of the field of data assimilation. Existing methods are generally based on the minimisation of the quadratic error between the model and the data: $\mathcal{C}(\mathbf{P}) = \sum_i (T_i^m - T_i^s(\mathbf{P}))^2$, where T_i^m is the measured depolarisation time at vertex i and $T_i^s(\mathbf{P})$ is the depolarisation time at vertex i computed with the set of parameters $\mathbf{P}$. The minimisation is either sequential like in Kalman filtering based methods or global like in adjoint methods.

The time introduced in Eq. 3 or 2 to solve the Eikonal equation is an artificial time, therefore the sequential methods are not the natural framework to solve this problem. Moreover sequential methods involve the updating of all the variables and of a covariance matrix of the same size, involving additional computational costs. The adjoint methods propose a precise method to compute the gradient of $\mathcal{C}$ but the numerical scheme proposed, alternating a fast marching step and the computation of diffusion/curvature term, implies that the adjoint methods are not directly applicable to this problem.

The adaptation of one of these methods to the proposed discrete model is still work in progress. As a first approach, we proposed to adjust the conductivity parameter D by iterating the two following steps:

- convergence of the Eq. 2 using presented algorithm
- local adjustment by multiplying D by $1 + \varepsilon$ or $1 - \varepsilon$ depending on the sign of the difference between the measured and simulated depolarisation times

We expect this parameter to be different (smaller) in pathological regions.

3.1 Synthetic Data

We simulated on a triangulated sphere different propagation conditions to test the estimation procedure. On this normalised test, $c_0 = 1$, $k = 1$, $D_0 = 0.01$. We defined three different zones: one excitation zone for the initialisation, one zone where $D = 2D_0$, and one zone where $D = D_0/2$. We simulated the propagation and stored the depolarisation times. We then started the data assimilation procedure with $D = D_0$.

After convergence of this procedure, we obtain a mean error of 2.95×10^{-3} and a maximum error of 8.46×10^{-3} on the depolarisation times which are between 0 and 31 (arbitrary units). We were thus able to detect very precisely the areas with different conductivity and these conductivities were well estimated (cf Fig. 2).

3.2 XMR Interventional Data

XMR registration makes it possible to integrate in a same coordinate space the electrophysiology measurements and the patient anatomy. This opens up possibilities to obtain very rich data to validate the estimation procedure, as MR can give spatial information on the location of the pathology.

We used measurements from the Ensite system (Endocardial Solutions), which is a non-contact invasive catheter based device for recording the electrical activity of the heart (reconstructed on 256 points). Due to the tangential aspect of the fibre orientations, we believe that the 3D aspect of the propagation

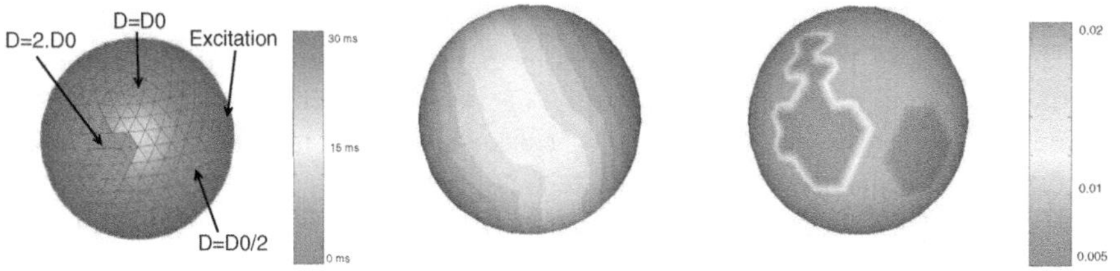

Fig. 2. (Left) Simulation of different conduction zones with D twice the normal value (left zone) and half the normal value (right hexagonal zone). (Middle) Resulting isochrones with the Eikonal-Curvature equation. The excitation zone is on the right side of the sphere. (Right) Estimated D with the parameter estimation procedure.

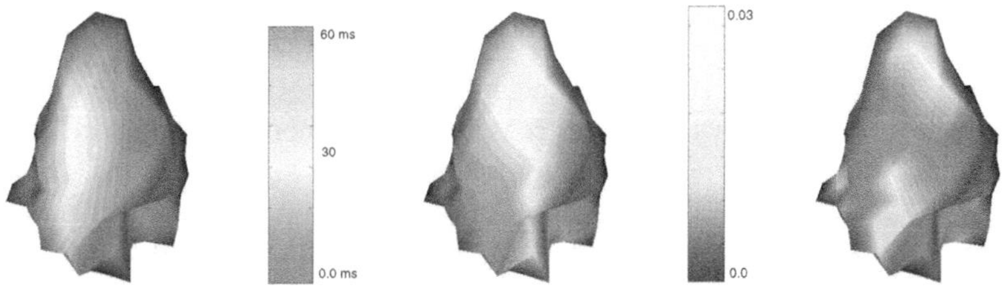

Fig. 3. (Left) Initial propagation with standard parameters. (Middle) Resulting isochrones with adjusted the Eikonal-Curvature equation . (Right) Estimated D with the parameter estimation procedure. Mesh: 256 nodes.

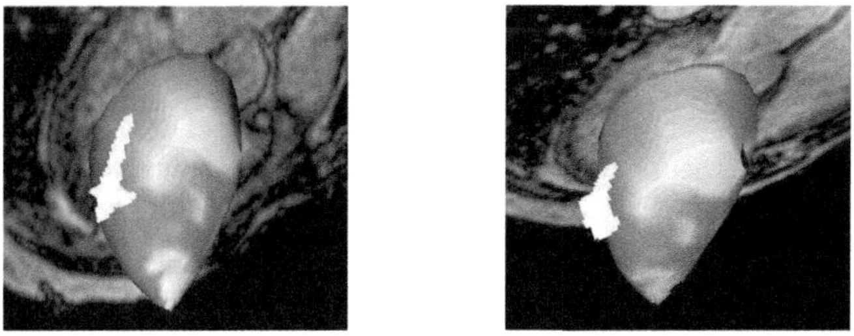

Fig. 4. Matching between the conductivity estimated with the described procedure and a scar segmented in a late enhancement MR image (white voxels). The complete XMR registration involves non-rigid deformation, this is why the shape of the basket is different between Fig. 3 and Fig. 4.

does not interfere too much with the surface endocardial recordings. This data is from a patient with a left bundle branch block, so the initialisation does not come from the Purkinje network, but through the septum. From these recordings, we initialise the depolarisation in the model. We then adjusted the local conductivity. We obtain a mean error of 7.75×10^{-1} ms and a maximum error of 9.75 ms on the depolarisation times which are between 0 and 66 ms.

The XMR registration makes it possible to locate these electrophysiology measurements in the MR coordinate space. This patient had multiple scars in the myocardium, leading to a left bundle branch block and poor cardiac function. Using late enhancement MR, some of these scars were manually segmented by an expert. The local apparent conductivity estimation procedure can then be compared with the scars locations. Precise comparison is still work in progress, but the first results obtained compare qualitatively well with the segmented scar. We can see in Fig. 4 that the segmented scar corresponds to a lower apparent conductivity zone (blue).

The mean value of the adjusted local apparent conductivity is 0.0149 and the maximum value is 0.0309.

4 Conclusion

We presented in this article a new algorithm to achieve fast simulations of electrophysiology, along with a procedure to adjust the model parameters from interventional data. This algorithm has been validated on analytical solutions and the procedure has been tested on synthetic and real data. It was used to estimate the local apparent conductivity from interventional data, and the first results obtained are very encouraging. Having such a model opens up possibilities for real-time filtering and interpolation of electrophysiology recordings. Moreover, hidden parameter estimation is of great use for a better evaluation of the extent of the pathology and for planning of the therapy . An excellent example application is the planning of bi-ventricular pacing therapy for treatment of heart failure. A model with accurate information on the local conductivity would allow a better placement of the pacing leads and thus man improve of the 50-60% success rate of the procedure.

This simulation part could be improved by using higher order schemes for the FMM and the curvature term, and the improvement of the implementation in case of obtuse angles in the triangulation. The current implementation does not treat these cases separately, but the numerical schemes should be different. Also, including the fibre orientations, which is rather straightforward in this formulation, could give more reliable results. We also plan to study more sophisticated estimation procedures, to achieve a precise and robust adjustment. In particular, we want to study the possibility to adapt a sequential method, like unscented Kalman filtering, or adjoint methods to this parameter estimation problem.

References

1. Hodgkin, A., Huxley, A.: A quantitative description of membrane current and its application to conduction and excitation in nerve. J. of Physio. **177** (1952) 500–544
2. Rhode, K., Hill, D., Edwards, P., Hipwell, J., Rueckert, D., Sanchez-Ortiz, G., Hegde, S., Rahunathan, V., Razavi, R.: Registration and tracking to integrate X-ray and MR images in an XMR facility. IEEE Trans. on Med. Imaging **22** (2003)
3. Keener, J., Sneyd, J.: Mathematical Physiology. Springer (1998)

4. Franzone, P.C., Guerri, L., Rovida, S.: Wavefront propagation in activation model of the anisotropic cardiac tissue. J. Math. Biol. (1990)
5. Tomlinson, K., Hunter, P., Pullan, A.: A FEM for an eikonal equation model of myocardial excitation wavefront propagation. SIAM J. Appl. Math. (2002)
6. Sethian, J.: Level Set Methods and Fast Marching Methods. CUP (1999)
7. Kimmel, R., Sethian, J.: Computing geodesic paths on manifolds. Proceedings of National Academy of Sciences **95** (1998) 8431–8435
8. Barth, T., Sethian, J.: Numerical schemes for the Hamilton-Jacobi and Level Set equations on triangulated domains. J. of Computational Physics **145** (1998) 1–40

An Inverse Problem Approach to the Estimation of Volume Change

Martin Schweiger[1], Oscar Camara-Rey[2], William R. Crum[2], Emma Lewis[2], Julia Schnabel[2], Simon R. Arridge[1], Derek L.G. Hill[2], and Nick Fox[3]

[1] Department of Computer Science, University College London
[2] Centre for Medical Image Computing, University College London
[3] Dementia Research Centre, Institute of Neurology, University College London

Abstract. We present a new technique for determining structure-by-structure volume changes, using an inverse problem approach. Given a pre-labelled brain and a series of images at different time-points, we generate finite element meshes from the image data, with volume change modelled by means of an unknown coefficient of expansion on a per-structure basis. We can then determine the volume change in each structure of interest using inverse problem optimization techniques. The proposed method has been tested with simulated and clinical data. Results suggest that the presented technique can be seen as an alternative for volume change estimation.

1 Introduction

There are a wide number of clinical applications where it is desirable to localize structural change from serial imaging, such as dementia, tumour growth and multiple sclerosis. Several approaches have been proposed to estimate such volume changes [1,2,3]. The most powerful make use of serial imaging in conjunction with image registration techniques such as the BBSI [1], the SIENA [2] or the VCM [3]. These techniques are mostly based on a voxel-by-voxel analysis, while clinical interest is normally in structure-by-structure changes.

We propose a new technique for determining structure-by-structure volume changes, using an inverse problem approach. Given a pre-labelled brain, and a series of images at different time-points, we generate finite element meshes from the image data, with volume change modelled by means of an unknown coefficient of expansion on a per-structure basis. The inverse problem then consists of recovering the coefficients of expansion for each structure which would result in the observed volume changes in the mesh. Therefore, the algorithm directly solves for the unknown volume changes in anatomically relevant structures, rather than using an arbitrary regular voxel array. This approach in due course will enable us to incorporate more anatomical and histological information about the disease.

The method has been applied to the recovery of synthetic deformations simulated by an elasticity forward model, to test its robustness in the presence of background noise and local perturbations. Furthermore, it has been applied to 9 pairs of Alzheimer's disease patient images to identify the rate of brain volume change.

J. Duncan and G. Gerig (Eds.): MICCAI 2005, LNCS 3750, pp. 616–623, 2005.

2 Inverse Problem

2.1 Finite Element Deformation Model

We use a thermoelastic model of soft tissue deformation to simulate the change in brain structure caused by degenerative diseases such as Alzheimer's disease. Thermoelasticity is a convenient way of inducing structural volume change but it should be noted that the thermal expansion coefficient in this model does not have a physical meaning beyond introducing an initial stress term that leads to a volume displacement field. This avoids the need of more accurate models of tissue thermal distributions such as the bioheat equation [4].

The deformation model employs a linear elastic finite element method [5]. Each element of the generated tetrahedral meshes is assigned a set of elastic material properties represented by the elasticity matrix D. The finite element solver is based on the TOAST package [6] which is freely available[1]. In this paper we consider isotropic elastic deformations, where D is symmetric and can be expressed in terms of two parameters, usually Young's modulus E and Poisson's ratio ν. The elastic coefficients are assumed time-invariant. The deformation of the mesh is induced by assigning an isotropic thermal expansion coefficient $\alpha^{(i)}$ to each element i, and simulating a global temperature change ΔT. The resulting isotropic thermal expansion enters the description of elastic deformation in the form of an initial element strain $\varepsilon_0^{(i)} = \{\ \alpha^{(i)}\ \Delta T,\ \alpha^{(i)}\ \Delta T,\ \alpha^{(i)}\ \Delta T,\ 0,\ 0,\ 0\ \}$, where the relation between stresses σ and strains ε is given by

$$\sigma^{(i)} = \mathsf{D}^{(i)}(\varepsilon^{(i)} - \varepsilon_0^{(i)}) + \sigma_0^{(i)} \tag{1}$$

Assembling all element contributions of the mesh leads to the linear system

$$\mathsf{K}\mathbf{u} + \mathbf{f} + \mathbf{f}' = \mathbf{r}, \qquad K_{ij} = \int_V \mathsf{B}_i^T \mathsf{D} \mathsf{B}_j dV \tag{2}$$

with stiffness matrix K. In an n-noded element, B is the $6\times 3n$ strain displacement matrix $\mathsf{B} = \{\mathsf{B}_i\}$ with

$$\mathsf{B}_i = \left\{ \begin{matrix} \frac{\partial N_i}{\partial x} & 0 & 0 \\ 0 & \frac{\partial N_i}{\partial y} & 0 \\ 0 & 0 & \frac{\partial N_i}{\partial z} \\ \frac{\partial N_i}{\partial y} & \frac{\partial N_i}{\partial x} & 0 \\ 0 & \frac{\partial N_i}{\partial z} & \frac{\partial N_i}{\partial y} \\ \frac{\partial N_i}{\partial z} & 0 & \frac{\partial N_i}{\partial x} \end{matrix} \right\}, \qquad \mathbf{f}' = \int_V \mathsf{B}^T \mathsf{D} \varepsilon_0 dV, \tag{3}$$

given nodal shape functions N_i. $\mathbf{f}'$ contains the volume forces arising from the initial thermal strain, $\mathbf{f}$ combines all other surface and volume force terms, $\mathbf{r}$ defines explicit displacements, and $\mathbf{u}$ is the vector of nodal displacements.

[1] `http://www.medphys.ucl.ac.uk/~martins/toast/index.html`

2.2 Inverse Model

We formulate the inverse problem of coefficient reconstruction as follows:

> Given two meshes corresponding to a baseline state and a distorted target state, e.g. obtained from segmented patient images at two stages of disease, recover the coefficients of expansion $\alpha^{(i)}$, $i = 1 \dots m$ in a suitable basis of dimension m that, applied to the baseline state, minimise an error norm of difference between the transformed baseline state and the target state.

In this paper we consider an objective function ψ that defines the square sum of nodal displacements $\mathbf{a}_i \to \bar{\mathbf{a}}_i$ between two states,

$$\psi = \sum_i |\mathbf{a}_i - \bar{\mathbf{a}}_i|^2. \tag{4}$$

If the mesh representations of the two states are not structurally equivalent, a suitable nodal interpolation of the displacement field must be applied. Given the mesh discretisation, the distribution of coefficients of expansion $\alpha(\mathbf{r})$ can now be represented in the element basis $\alpha^{(i)}$ of the mesh. For the purpose of reconstruction we restrict the search space by the additional assumption that the expansion coefficients be homogeneous or piecewise homogeneous within each of a set of anatomical structures of the brain. The inverse problem thus reduces to finding one coefficient of expansion for each segmented region or subregion. Let m be the number of regions, and n the number of mesh nodes. To recover $\alpha = \{\alpha^{(i)}\} \in \mathbb{R}^m$, we employ an iterative Levenberg-Marquardt solver,

$$\alpha_{k+1} = \alpha_k + (\mathsf{J}_k^T \mathsf{J}_k + \eta \mathsf{I})^{-1}(\mathsf{J}_k^T(\mathbf{a}_k - \mathbf{a}_{\text{tgt}})), \tag{5}$$

where $\mathbf{a}_k$ and $\mathbf{a}_{\text{tgt}}$ are the nodal positions of the deformed and the target mesh, respectively, and $\mathsf{J} \in \mathbb{R}^{n \times m}$ is the Jacobian matrix $J_{ij} = \frac{\partial u_i}{\partial \alpha_j}$, and η is a trust-region control parameter. Because m is small, J can be calculated by explicit perturbation of the region coefficients.

3 Experiments and Results

We obtained the labelled reference images identifying brain tissue types of the baseline MR image with the FAST algorithm [7]. From the labelled reference image we generated a surface mesh of the whole brain with the marching cubes algorithm [8]. Volume finite element meshes were then obtained using the NETGEN mesh generation software[2].

In this paper we present two initial tests of reconstruction of the coefficients of expansion: In the first test, synthetic target images are generated by a forward model of thermoelastic deformation, given distributions of the elastic and

[2] `http://www.hpfem.jku.at/netgen/`

thermal coefficients in the volume domain. The reconstruction algorithm is then applied to recover region thermal coefficients from the mesh deformation. The performance of the reconstruction algorithm in the presence of random background noise and localised perturbations is investigated. In the second test, the reconstruction is applied to pairs of clinical MR images obtained from AD patients at a 12-month interval. Comparison of the true changes with model predictions from the reconstructed thermal coefficients gives an indication of the fidelity of the reconstruction when applied to realistic structural change.

3.1 Simulated Deformation Recovery

A finite element brain mesh consisting of 163765 nodes and 868404 4-noded tetrahedral elements, segmented into 5 regions of background, CSF, grey and white matter and hippocampi was generated from MR data. To obtain the deformed target image, piecewise constant elastic and thermal coefficients were applied to each of the regions. The region coefficients are shown in Table 1.

An axial cross section of the target distribution of thermal coefficient α is shown in Fig. 1a). In addition to the homogeneous region coefficients, deformations were generated from two further sets of coefficients, by adding random Gaussian background noise (standard deviation $\sigma = 0.03$) to the coefficients throughout the domain (Fig. 1b), and by including a localised perturbation of $\alpha = -0.3$ in the grey matter compartment of a frontal lobe (Fig. 1c).

Using the linear elasticity forward model, nodal displacements were calculated for each of the three parameter distributions. The surface of the mesh was assumed to coincide with the inner surface of the skull, and Dirichlet boundary conditions were introduced using a Payne-Irons ("big spring") method to suppress the displacements of boundary nodes. The nodal displacements served as the target data for the inverse solver. For this simulation, the reconstruction assumes correct region boundaries of the baseline mesh, and correct elastic coefficients E and ν. The initial estimate of the thermal coefficients α is zero for all regions. The reconstruction results for the region α-values are compared to the target values in the left graph of Fig 2. The imposed boundary condition of fixing the mesh surface imposes a constraint of constant mesh volume on the reconstruction, leading to a non-uniqueness which allows to recover α subject to

Table 1. Elastic material properties (Young's modulus $E \times 10^3 NM^{-2}$ and Poisson's ratio ν) and target coefficients of expansion (α) used for simulating deformation

region	E	ν	α
background	1	0.45	0.000
CSF	1	0.45	0.300
grey matter	8	0.45	-0.050
white matter	4	0.45	0.030
hippocampi	1	0.45	-0.1

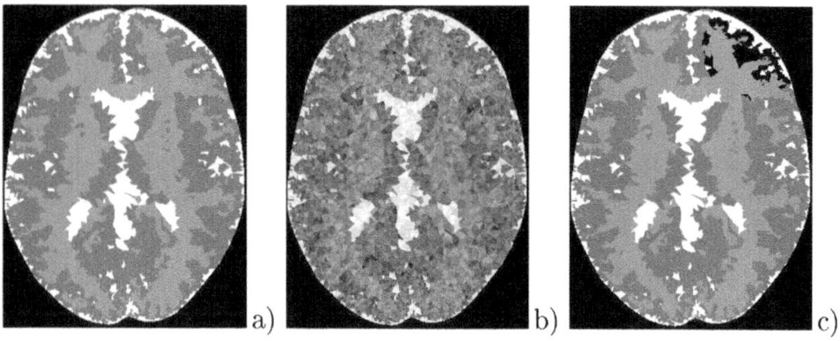

Fig. 1. Axial cross sections of target thermal coefficient distributions. a) piecewise constant region coefficients, b) added random Gaussian background noise, c) added localised grey matter perturbation.

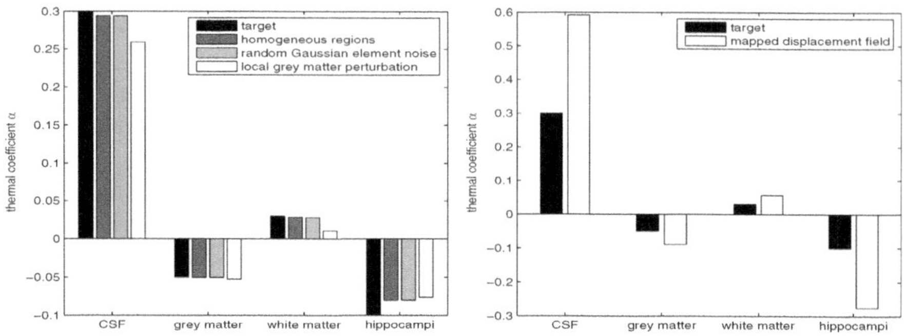

Fig. 2. Left: Reconstructed region thermal coefficients for the 3 distributions shown in Fig. 1. Right: reconstructed coefficients after mapping the displacement field onto a coarse mesh.

an arbitrary global additive term. We take this into account by normalising all results to a value of $\alpha = 0$ for the background region.

We find that the reconstruction of homogeneous region parameters provides good quantitative results, and that the addition of Gaussian random noise does not affect the recovered values significantly. The application of a localised perturbation of α has a more significant effect on the recovered region values, because the target distribution is now no longer in the support of the region basis. It is interesting to note that mostly the CSF and white matter regions are affected, but not the grey matter region where the local perturbation was applied.

A further test was performed to investigate the effect of an imperfect knowledge of the region boundaries on the parameter reconstruction, by mapping the nodal displacements calculated for the piecewise homogeneous α-distribution (case a) onto a coarser mesh consisting of 10749 nodes and 52297 tetrahedra. The parameter reconstruction was then performed on the coarse mesh, using the interpolated displacement field. The reconstructed region coefficients are shown in the right graph of Fig. 2. Due to the misalignment of region boundaries, the target distribution is no longer in the solution space, leading to a degraded quantitative reconstruction. However, the qualitative expansion trends in all regions are still recovered.

3.2 Clinical Data

From 9 pairs of Alzheimer MRI images taken at a 12-month interval the corresponding baseline and deformed meshes are generated by using mesh warping techniques [9]. This leads to pairs of meshes with conforming structure and known volumetric differences. In future applications, this method can be replaced by direct mapping of displacement fields between non-conforming meshes. The generated meshes have between 79505 and 138916 elements. Label information is mapped from the reference image into the mesh through a rasterization procedure [10] which computes fractional element labels. To reduce the discretisation error of mapping region boundaries into the mesh, additional boundary regions containing mixed-label elements were introduced, leading to a total of 15 coefficients to be recovered.

Each brain grey-level image at each time-point was registered to the reference image using a 9 degrees of freedom registration[3] with Normalised Mutual Information as the image similarity measure. Non-rigid fluid registration [11], run at half image resolution was applied. Fluid registration has the advantage for mesh warping purposes that provides diffeomorphic transformations (i.e. they do not fold or tear). After mesh warping based on fluid registrations, we have observed that the geometric quality of the meshes is only slightly reduced (the mean±STD aspect ratio[4] was (a) before mesh warping = 0.67±0.06 (b) after mesh warping = 0.66±0.06), but it does not furnish critical elements (aspect ratio < 0).

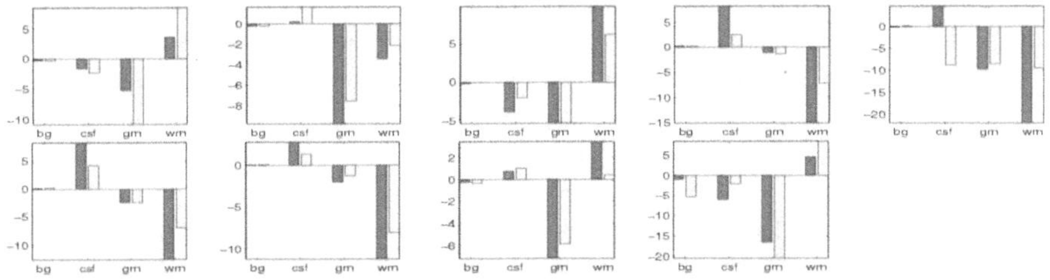

Fig. 3. Comparison between observed and reconstructed volume changes of 4 regions (background, CSF, grey and white matter) in 9 cases

After generating the conforming baseline and target mesh pairs for the 9 cases, the inverse Levenberg-Marquardt solver described in Section 2.2 was used

[3] `http://www.image-registration.com`

[4] The aspect ratio is defined as the ratio between the longest edge and the radius of the inscribed circle in a tetrahedron, being 1 in the case of optimal quality.

to recover the coefficients of expansion in the 15 generated regions which minimise the nodal displacement between the deformed baseline mesh and the target mesh. In all cases, the reconstructions were started from an initial value $\alpha = 0$ in all regions. The element volume changes introduced as a result of the reconstructed deformation were then collected into the 4 segmented regions, using the partial volume information from each element.

Figure 3 shows a comparison of volume changes between baseline and target (dark bars) and between baseline and reconstruction (bright bars) for all 9 cases. It can be seen that the reconstructed deformations predict the trend of volume change correctly in the majority of cases, although the absolute values are not always agreeing well. The results show that the thermoelastic deformation model has a potential to describe the types of structure change seen in AD, but that a further subdivision of the anatomical structure may be required to provide a sufficiently large search space for accurate representation of the deformation in the basis of the inverse solver.

4 Discussion and Conclusion

The method of recovering coefficients of expansion from a baseline and a deformed mesh has been shown to converge robustly in simulated data generated from piecewise homogeneous region parameters even in the presence of random zero-mean background noise and localised parameter perturbations. Where deformations were applied that could not be represented in the low-dimensional basis of homogeneous region coefficients, a qualitative recovery of trends within the regions is still feasible, but the quantitation of region parameters deteriorates. In that case, the convergence of the inverse solver could be improved by further subdivision of the segmented regions and increasing the dimension of the parameter solution space, for example by a segmentation into anatomical sub-regions using information from manually segmented atlases that separate structures likely to undergo structural changes in the course of disease. This will maintain an anatomical interpretation of the deformation coefficients and allow to easily distinguish between specific patterns of different types of dementia.

The proposed technique has also been applied to a set of 9 pairs of images from AD patients. Despite the restriction to a low-dimensional solution space of 15 regions the reconstruction results show good qualitative agreement of region volume change when compared with target data in the majority of cases. As with the simulated data set, further improvement can be expected by increasing the dimension of the search space. One strategy of parameter space refinement that retains the correspondance with anatomical features would be a subdivision of tissue types into separate lobes of the brain.

The results presented in this paper indicate that a region-based approach of structure change can be seen as a feasible alternative to other volume change estimation techniques. By representing the coefficients of deformation in a basis that is directly associated with the underlying anatomical structure, the recovered expansion parameters can be interpreted more immediately than in a voxel-based technique in terms of anatomical change, such as grey-matter volume loss. A further subdivision of the basis representation into regions of interest may be suitable to recover disease-specific parameters and so aid in the diagnosis of dementia. Future work will also be focused on a rigorous validation of the presented technique, by comparing its performance with classical volume change measurement methods such as the BBSI or the VCM.

Acknowledgments

The authors acknowledge grant support from the Engineering and Physical Sciences Research Council, grants GR/N148/01 and GR/S48837/02, and from the Medical Research Council.

References

1. Freeborough, P.A., Fox, N.C.: The boundary shift integral: an accurate and robust measure of cerebral volume changes from registered repeat MRI, IEEE Transactions on Medical Imaging, **16** (5) (1997) 623–629
2. Smith, S.M., De Stefano, N., Jenkinson, M., Matthews, P.M.: Normalized accurate measurement of longitudinal brain change, Journal of Computer Assisted Tomography, **25** (3) (2001) 466–475
3. Fox, N.C., Crum, W.R., Scahill, R.I., Stevens, J.M., Janssen, J.C., Rossor, M.N.: Imaging of onset and progression of Alzheimer's disease with voxel-compression mapping of serial magnetic resonance images, Lancet, **358** (9277) (2001) 201–205
4. Durkee, J.W, Antich, P.P.: Exact solutions to the multi-region time-dependent bioheat equation with transient heat sources and boundary conditions, Phys. Med. Biol, **36** (3) (1991) 345–368
5. Zienkiewicz, O.C., Taylor, R.L.: The Finite Element Method. 4th edn. McGraw-Hill, London (1987)
6. Schweiger, M., Arridge, S.R.: Image reconstruction in optical tomography using local basis functions. Journal of Electronic Imaging **12** (2003) 583–593
7. Zhang, Y., Brady, M., Smith, S.: Segmentation of brain MR images through a hidden Markov random field model and the expectation maximization algorithm, IEEE Transactions on Medical Imaging, **20** (1) (2001) 45–57
8. Lorensen, W.E., Cline, H.E.: Marching cube, a high resolution 3D surface reconstruction algorithm, Proceedings of SIGGRAPH 1987, **21** (1987) 163–169
9. Castellano-Smith, A.D., Hartkens, T., Schnabel, J.A., Hose D.R., Liu, H. , Hall, W.A., Truwit, C.L., Hawkes, D.J., Hill, D.L.G.: A registration based mesh construction technique for finite element models of brains. Proceedings of SPIE Medical Imaging 2002, volume 4683, 538–549
10. Sermesant, M., Forest, C., Pennec, X., Delingette, H., Ayache, N.: Deformable biomechanical models: Application to 4D cardiac image analysis, Medical Image Analysis, **7** (4) (2003) 475–488
11. Crum, W.R., Rueckert, D., Jenkinson, M., Kennedy, D., Smith, S.M.: A Framework For Detailed Objective Comparison of Non-Rigid Registration Algorithms in Neuroimaging, Proceedings of MICCAI 2004, LNCS 3216, 679–686

A Velocity-Dependent Model for Needle Insertion in Soft Tissue*

Jessica R. Crouch[1], Chad M. Schneider[2], Josh Wainer[2], and Allison M. Okamura[2]

[1] Computer Science Dept., Old Dominion University, VA, USA
jrcrouch@odu.edu
[2] Engineering Research Center for Computer Integrated Surgical Systems & Technology, Johns Hopkins University, Baltimore, MD, USA
aokamura@jhu.edu

Abstract. Models that predict the soft tissue deformation caused by needle insertion could improve the accuracy of procedures such as brachytherapy and needle biopsy. Prior work on needle insertion modeling has focused on static deformation; the experiments presented here show that dynamic effects such as relaxation are important. An experimental setup is described for recording and measuring the deformation that occurs with needle insertion into a soft tissue phantom. Analysis of the collected data demonstrates the time- and velocity-dependent nature of the deformation. Deformation during insertion is shown to be well represented using a velocity-dependent force function with a linear elastic finite element model. The model's accuracy is limited to the period during needle motion, indicating that a viscoelastic tissue model may be required to capture tissue relaxation after the needle stops.

1 Introduction

An important source of error in needle insertion procedures such as brachytherapy and needle biopsy is the soft tissue deformation that occurs as a needle is inserted. The guidance accuracy provided by a pre-operative planning image is limited by the difference between the location of a tissue target pre-operatively and its location intra-operatively, when the target and surrounding tissues are deformed by needle insertion forces. Needle placement errors due to tissue deformation have been documented for breast biopsy [1] and prostate brachytherapy seed placement [2] [3]. If the deformation caused by needle insertion could be accurately predicted, and the needle placement could be accurately controlled, the effectiveness of needle-based procedures would be improved.

Various needle insertion simulators have employed heuristic models of tissue stiffness supported by user studies but not experimental measurements of tissue deformation [4] [5]. An impediment to the development of more realistic and

* This work was supported by NSF grants EIA-0312551 and EEC-9731478, and Whitaker Foundation grant RG-02-911. The authors thank Darius Burschka for assistance with the stereo-vision system and Gregory Hager for use of his cameras.

J. Duncan and G. Gerig (Eds.): MICCAI 2005, LNCS 3750, pp. 624–632, 2005.

carefully validated deformable tissue models is the scarcity of data about soft tissue mechanical properties. Very limited data is available for prostate and other soft pelvic and abdominal organs. Especially lacking from the literature are experiments investigating the dynamic response of living soft tissue to interaction with needles and other surgical instruments. The instrument-tissue experiments that have been reported are limited to force recordings and do not include tissue deformation data [6] [7]. Factors making the design of such experiments challenging include acquisition speed limits for 3D imaging modalities and the difficulty of accurately extracting point displacements from soft tissue images.

Lacking force and deformation data for real tissues, prior work by DiMaio and Salcudean [8] relied on data from needle insertions into a soft tissue phantom for the development of an insertion simulation based on an elastostatic material model. Our work also relies on phantom data, but differs in that it focuses on the dynamic effects of needle insertion. Other related work includes the 2D prostate needle insertion simulation developed by Alterovitz, et al. [9], and the Truth Cube developed by Kerdok, et al. [10]. Our tissue phantom's design was inspired by the Truth Cube, a silicone gel volume with embedded fiducials whose displacements were tracked to estimate the gel's properties in compression tests.

2 Experiment Design

An 18 gauge diamond-tip brachytherapy needle was inserted at a constant velocity into a tissue phantom impregnated with a grid of tiny fiducials for each experiment trial. Needle forces were recorded for insertion velocities from 3 to 21 mm/s. The phantom deformation was monitored by optically tracking the fiducial displacements. The experiment hardware included a specially constructed tissue phantom, a device that precisely controlled needle motion, a force/torque sensor, and calibrated stereo video cameras for recording fiducial motion.

2.1 Tissue Phantom

The tissue phantom was made of GE RTV-6166, the same transparent, homogeneous silicone gel used for the Truth Cube [10]. An experienced brachytherapy surgeon selected this gel as providing more realistic resistance to a needle than alternative soft plastic and porcine gelatin materials.

The phantom was constructed by pouring gel into an acrylic box in 8 mm layers, placing it in a vacuum chamber to remove air bubbles, and then dropping a row of 0.8 mm fiducials onto the surface as the gel began to set. Subsequent layers were added before curing completed so that boundaries did not form between layers. The needle was inserted perpendicular to the plane of the layers, so variations in stiffness caused by the layer construction would have caused periodic irregularities in the force data corresponding to the layer width. Layer effects were deemed negligible because such irregularities were not detected.

The fiducials' small size minimizes their influence on the material properties of the phantom tissue. Kerdok performed indentation tests on samples of RTV-6166 with and without implanted fiducials and reported that there was no discernible change in its material properties even when using fiducials that had nearly twice the diameter of the ones used in our work [10].

2.2 Needle Insertion Device

The needle was inserted using an encoded Maxon A-max 22 DC motor connected to a translational stage via a capstan drive. Constant velocity during insertion was maintained using a proportional-derivative controller for the needle stage position. A 6-axis force/torque sensor (Nano-17 from ATI Industrial Automation) was mounted at the needle base. Needle forces, position, and velocity were recorded at 500 Hz. The phantom was attached to the needle insertion device as shown in Fig. 1 so that the needle was aligned with the plane of fiducials.

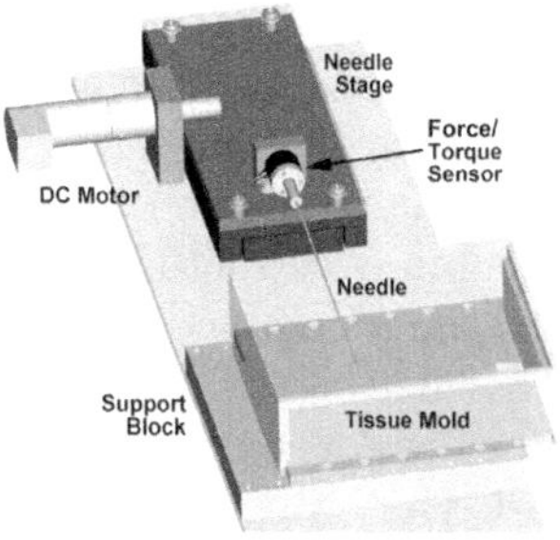

Fig. 1. Tissue phantom was 113 mm × 135 mm × 30 mm; the fiducial grid has 5 mm × 8 mm spacing

2.3 Fiducial and Needle Tracking

Insertions were recorded by two Sony DFW-X700 digital cameras at 7.5Hz and 640 × 480 resolution. A 9 × 9 grid of fiducials was tracked by convolving each captured image with a rotationally symmetric Laplacian of Gaussian (LoG) kernel that was width matched to the fiducials. The maximum match near each fiducial was tagged as the fiducial's center. Tracking results are shown in Fig. 2.

The needle trajectory was found by convolving one image from each trial with a LoG kernel that was width matched to the needle diameter, selecting the peak match points, and performing a least squares fit of a line to the match point coordinates. Needle tip tracking was performed using images that were masked to include only the portion of the image near the needle trajectory. Tracking was accomplished by computing difference images between successive video frames. The needle's stripes caused bright bands in the difference images when the needle was shifted; the leading band indicated the needle tip position.

2.4 3D Reconstruction and Error Estimation

The fiducial and needle tracking algorithms provide pairs of corresponding image coordinates from the right and left camera views. From these, 3D coordinates

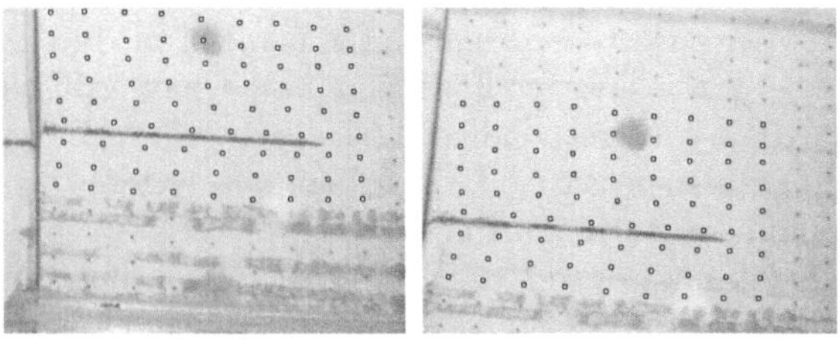

Fig. 2. Both camera views are shown with tracked fiducials marked by black circles. Untracked peripheral fiducials appear fainter. The fiducials and needle are clearly visible because the transparent gel is backlit.

were computed using a standard computer vision algorithm that relies on stereo camera calibration parameters [11]. The error present in the 3D coordinates can be attributed to uncertainty in the camera calibration and to limitations in point tracking accuracy. This error can be estimated by examining the coordinates computed for the needle tip. Since the needle path is known to be a straight line (there is no needle bending, as verified by visual and force data inspection), the deviation of the 3D tip coordinates from a line is an indication of the error. To investigate this, a least squares line fit was performed for the 3D needle tip coordinates of nine trials. The mean distance between the tip coordinates and the line was 0.73 mm with a standard deviation of 1.23 mm. The largest component of the error was along the camera's viewing direction, with a mean of 0.65 mm and standard deviation of 1.10 mm in that direction.

3 Force and Deformation Data

3.1 Insertion Force

Needle forces were recorded for three insertions at each of the following velocities: 3, 6, 9, 12, 15, 18, and 21 mm/s. Fig. 3 shows total needle force versus insertion depth for all trials, demonstrating a velocity-dependent effect. Fig. 4 graphs the slopes of the curves in Fig. 3 vs. insertion velocity. As shown, a good approximation to the force function is provided by a scaled and shifted log function.

3.2 Force Decay

A gradual reduction in force after the needle halts was another dynamic effect observed. Fig. 5 shows the force decaying for 500 seconds after the needle halts. The decay can be analyzed using the following time dependent function:

$$f_i = (1 - \alpha_i) * f_{i-1} \tag{1}$$

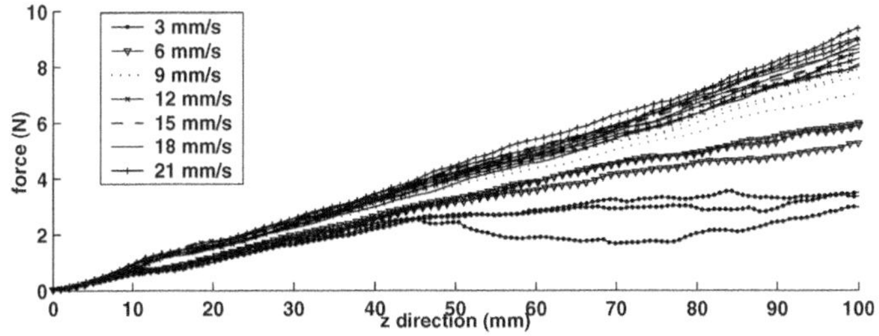

Fig. 3. Total needle force vs. needle insertion depth for different insertion velocities

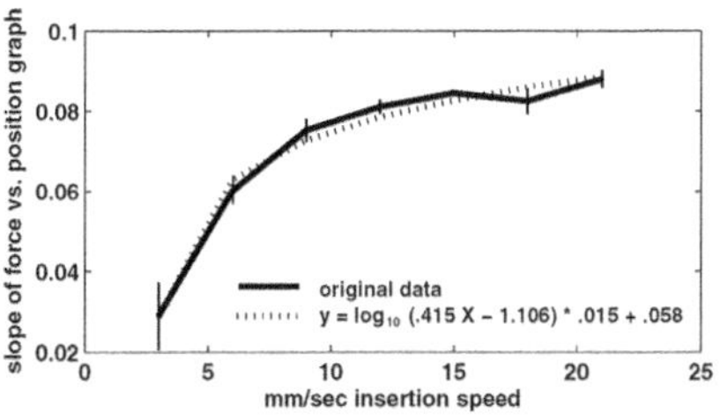

Fig. 4. Slope of force vs. position for different insertion speeds is shown by the solid line. The observed slope data is averaged across three trials for each speed, and standard deviations are shown. The dotted line shows the best fit scaled and shifted log function.

α_i represents the fraction of force that dissipates each time step. The α_i values in Fig. 5 were computed for the recorded force data. The shape of the α curves suggested a good fit might be obtained using Gaussian functions. Thus, the following function models α:

$$\alpha(f) = h_\alpha * G(f, \sigma, \mu) \quad \text{where} \qquad \begin{aligned} \sigma &= (c_1 * max(f)) + c_2 \\ \mu &= (c_3 * max(f)) + c_4 \\ h &= c_5 * \sigma \\ G(x, \sigma, \mu) &= \frac{1}{\sigma\sqrt{2\pi}} e^{\frac{-(x-\mu)^2}{2\sigma^2}} \quad \text{(Gaussian eqn.)} \end{aligned} \tag{2}$$

f is the needle force. Optimizing this model to fit the recorded data yielded constant values: $c_1 = 0.1267$ $\quad c_2 = 0.7613$ $\quad c_3 = 0.8171$ $\quad c_4 = 0.8194$ $\quad c_5 = 2.15$. The force decay model with these constants is shown in Fig. 6. The difference between recorded forces and model forces was at all points less than 0.5 N.

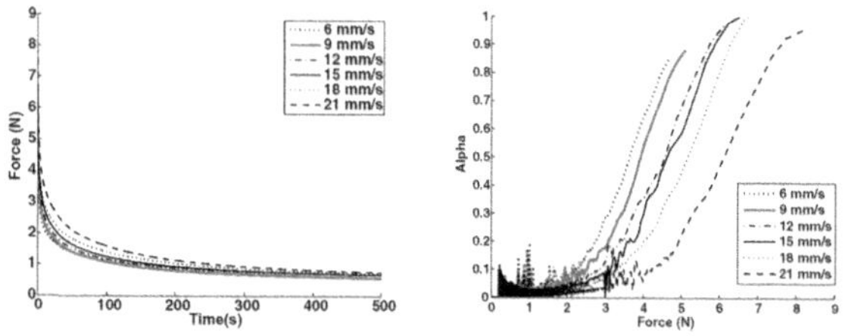

Fig. 5. Left: 500 sec. of recorded needle force, showing force decay after needle halts. Right: α parameter computed for the recorded needle force data

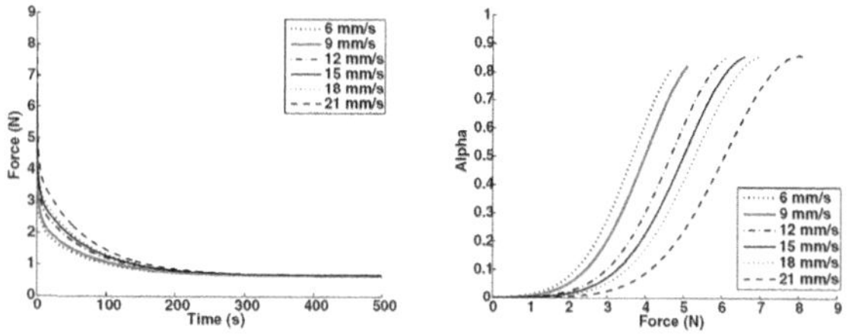

Fig. 6. Left: 500 sec. of model generated needle force, showing force decay after needle halts. Right: α parameter computed for the model generated force data

3.3 Needle Shaft Force Distribution

The simplest force distribution is a constant force level defined by the slope of the appropriate curve from Fig. 3. To investigate the validity of this simple model, shaft force constants defined by the equation in Fig. 4 were integrated along the length of the needle shaft for trials at different insertion speeds. The results of the integration shown in Fig. 7 closely match the measured needle forces, supporting a generally flat force distribution model.

To further examine the distribution of needle force, an optimization approach was applied in conjunction with a finite element model. Using the recorded experiment data, the fidelity of a needle model can be judged based on the accuracy with which it predicts fiducial motion. For the optimization, needle force models were represented by piecewise cubic splines. Two spline segments were allocated for 3 mm near the tip, and one segment was allocated to each 10 mm along the rest of the needle shaft. The spline functions represented the force magnitude; consistent with the data recorded from the force/torque sensor, the force direction was assumed to be the insertion direction.

The finite element model shown in Fig. 8 was constructed with Femlab (COMSOL, Inc.). A linear elastic material model was applied, with a Young's modulus of 14.9 kPa based on the work by Kerdok [10], and a Poisson's ratio of 0.49 to indicate near incompressibility. Fixed boundary conditions were applied to the phantom sides held stationary by the acrylic casing. Given a force distribution, finite element analysis yielded the deformation and fiducial displacements, as shown in Fig. 9.

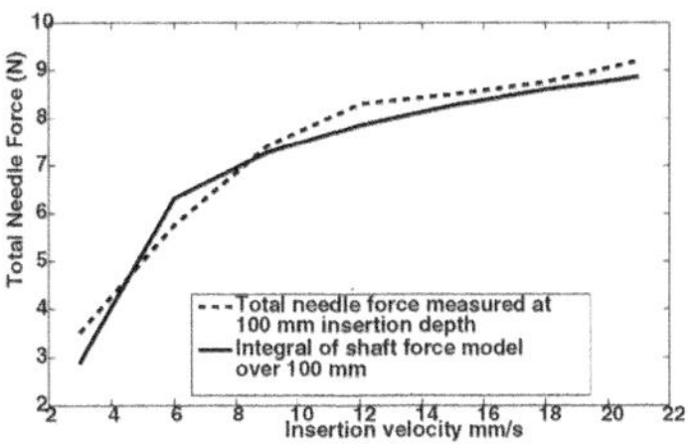

Fig. 7. Force vs. needle insertion velocity at 100 mm needle insertion integrated constant model force across all insertion

A quasi-Newton optimization method was applied to the force distribution with the objective of minimizing the error in the predicted fiducial displacements. A portion of the optimization results are shown in Fig. 10. Though noisy, the optimized distributions indicate relatively constant force along the needle shaft followed by a dip and pronounced peak at the tip. The force peak is required to overcome the material's resistance to cutting/crack propagation. The dip may be due to a snap-back effect that occurs as compressed tissue at the tip fractures and relaxes. The mean error in the predicted fiducial motion was 0.31 mm, with a standard deviation of 0.21 mm. Optimization was performed over a period of two weeks using a PC workstation with two 3.2 GHz Intel Xeon processors.

Based on these results, the following time and velocity-dependent function for needle force was constructed to fit the experiment data:

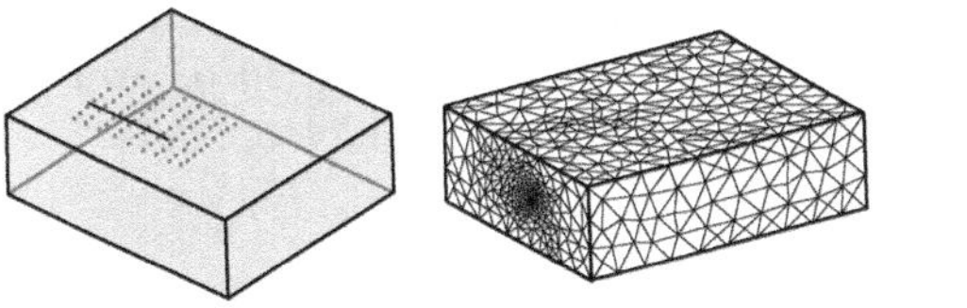

Fig. 8. Femlab phantom tissue model and tetrahedral mesh with higher resolution around the needle

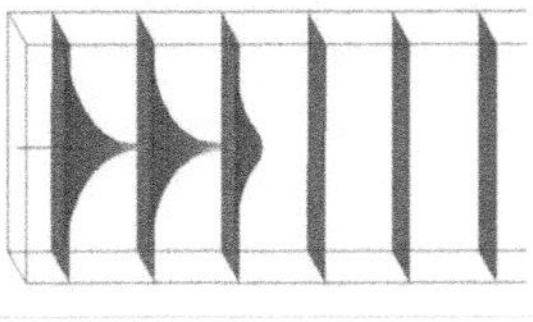

Fig. 9. Slices through the deformed finite element model

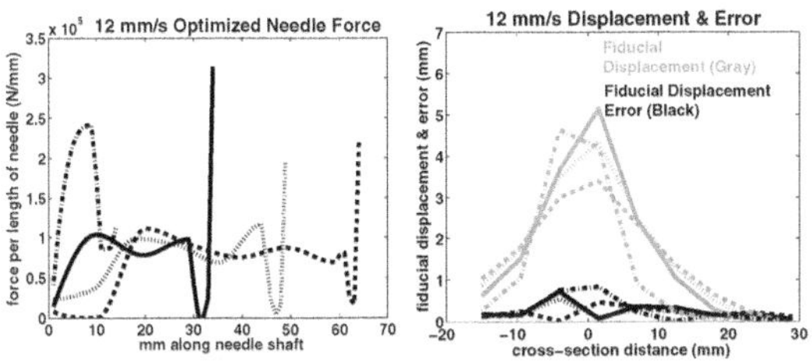

Fig. 10. Left: optimized distributions for 4 time points during insertion at 12 mm/s. Right: deformation in a slice perpendicular to the needle. In gray, the magnitude of recorded fiducial displacements; in black, the displacement prediction error.

$$f_i(x,v) = \begin{cases} 2 * shaftForce & \text{if } v > 0, x < 1 \\ 0.5 * shaftForce & \text{if } v > 0, 1 \leq x < 2 \\ shaftForce & \text{if } v > 0, x \geq 2 \\ f_{i-1} * (1 - \alpha_i * \Delta t) & \text{if } v = 0 \end{cases} \quad (3)$$

where $shaftForce = \log(0.415 * v - 1.106) * 0.015 + 0.058$ (see Fig.4)

Here x is distance from the needle tip, v is insertion velocity, i is time step index, α_i is defined by Eqn. 2, and Δt is time step length. f_i defines the force magnitude applied in the direction of needle insertion. Constants in Eqn. 3 will vary depending on the selection of needle and material.
The needle force function was constructed to satisfy these observations:

- The needle force depends on insertion velocity, as shown in Figs. 3 and 4.
- The majority of the needle force is evenly distributed along the shaft because: (1) for constant velocity insertion the force increases at a nearly constant rate (see Fig. 3) and (2) assuming a flat force distribution results in a total needle force that closely matches the measured force (see Fig. 7).
- Optimization indicated a force peak at the tip preceded by a small force dip.
- When the needle halts, the force decays according to Eqns. 1 and 2.

4 Results

Force profiles were generated by the model given in Eqn. 3 and were applied to the Femlab 3D finite element model. Some of the force profiles generated and cross-sections of the corresponding fiducial displacements are shown in Fig. 11. The results indicate this model produces an excellent approximation to the forces and deformations recorded in the experiment during the active insertion phase. When the needle halts, the model produces force relaxation that closely match the decay in needle force recorded in the experiment (see Fig. 4). However, the deformation produced by the model in the relaxation phase does not match the recorded deformation as well. As shown in Fig. 11, the recorded deformation decayed more quickly than the recorded force after the needle stopped.

5 Conclusions and Future Work

Through experimental observation and FEM modeling, this work has shown that a static linear elastic tissue model combined with a dynamic force function can accurately model forces and deformations during insertion at varying speeds. However, the accuracy of the model diminishes during the relaxation phase after the needle halts because real and phantom soft tissues are viscoelastic [12]. A viscoelastic model, to be considered in future work, might account for differing rates of force and deformation decay, consistent with the results shown Fig. 11.

It is not ideal that phantoms are used rather than in vivo tissues, but this is necessary for repeatability and validation. Thus, future work may include tests on real tissues, using a modified experimental setup. By using bi-plane x-ray

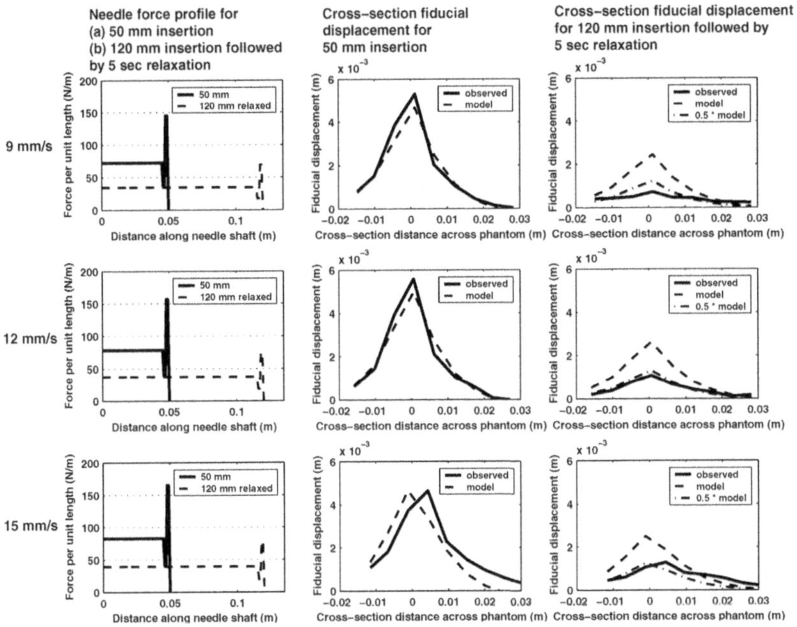

Fig. 11. Column 1: model force profile for 50 mm insertion without relaxation and 120 mm insertion with 5 sec. relaxation. Column 2: model and experiment displacements for 50 mm insertion. Column 3: model and experiment displacements for 120 mm insertion with 5 sec. relaxation; 0.5 times model displacements is also shown.

to track radio-opaque fiducials or tissue features, the experimental methodology could be applied to non-transparent tissue samples. The effect of perfusion will likely impact on a tissue's dynamic response [13]. Further experiments should include many repetitions to allow statistical measures of model accuracy.

References

1. Deurloo, E., Gilhuijs, K., Kool, L., Muller, S.: Displacement of breast tissue and needle deviations during stereotactic procedures. Invest. Rad. **36** (2001) 347–353
2. Roberson, P.L., Narayana, V., McShan, D.L., et al: Source placement error for permanent implant of the prostate. Medical Physics **24** (1997) 251–257
3. Nath, S., Chen, Z., Yue, N., Trumpore, S., Peschel, R.: Dosimetric effects of needle divergence in prostate seed implant using 125I and 103Pd radioactive seeds. Medical Physics (2000) 1058–1066
4. Xuan, J., Wang, Y., Sesterhenn, I., Mou, J., Mun, S.: 3-D model supported prostate biopsy simulation and evaluation. MICCAI **1496** (1998) 358–367
5. Gorman, P., Krummel, T., Webster, R., Smith, M., Hutchens, D.: A prototype haptic lumbar puncture. Proc of Medicine Meets Virtual Reality (2000) 106–109
6. Brouwer, I., Ustin, J., Bentley, L., et al: Measuring in vivo animal soft tissue properties for haptic modeling in surgical simulation. Medicine Meets Virtual Reality (2001) 69–74

7. Okamura, A.M., Simone, C., O'Leary, M.D.: Force modeling for needle insertion into soft tissue. IEEE Transactions on Biomedical Engineering (2004) 1707–1716
8. DiMaio, S.P., Salcudean, S.E.: Needle insertion modelling and simulation. IEEE Trans on Robotics and Automation: Special Issue on Medical Robotics (2003)
9. Alterovitz, R., Pouliot, J., Taschereau, R., Hsu, I., Goldberg, K.: Needle insertion and radioactive seed implantation in human tissues: Simulation and sensitivity analysis. Proc. IEEE Intl Conference on Robotics and Automation (2003)
10. Kerdok, A.E., Cotin, S.M., Ottensmeyer, M.P., Galea, A., Howe, R.D., Dawson, S.L.: Truth cube: Establishing physical standards for real time soft tissue simulation. Medical Image Analysis **7** (2003) 283–291
11. Forsyth, D., Ponce, J.: Computer Vision, A Modern Approach. Prentice Hall, Upper Saddle River, New Jersey (2003)
12. Fung, Y.C.: Biomechanics: Mechanical Properties of Living Tissues. Springer, New York (1993)
13. Ottensmeyer, M.P., Kerdok, A.E., Howe, R.D., Dawson, S.L.: The effects of testing environment on the viscoelastic properties of soft tissues. Second International Symposium on Medical Simulation (2004) 9–18

Material Properties Estimation of Layered Soft Tissue Based on MR Observation and Iterative FE Simulation

Mitsunori Tada[1,2], Noritaka Nagai[3], and Takashi Maeno[3]

[1] Digital Human Research Center,
National Institute of Advanced Industrial Science and Technology,
2-41-6, Aomi, Koto-ku, Tokyo 135-0064, Japan
m.tada@aist.go.jp
[2] CREST, Japan Science and Technology Agency
[3] Keio University

Abstract. In order to calculate deformation of soft tissue under arbitrary loading conditions, we have to take both non-linear material characteristics and subcutaneous structures into considerations. The estimation method of material properties presented in this paper accounts for these issues. It employs a compression test inside MRI in order to visualize deformation of hypodermic layered structure of living tissue, and an FE model of the compressed tissue in which non-linear material model is assigned. The FE analysis is iterated with updated material constant until the difference between the displacement field observed from MR images and calculated by FEM is minimized. The presented method has been applied to a 3-layered silicon rubber phantom. The results show the excellent performance of our method. The accuracy of the estimation is better than 15 %, and the reproducibility of the deformation is better than 0.4 mm even for an FE analysis with different boundary condition.

1 Introduction

The rapid progress in computational power and algorithm enable us to carry out finite element (FE) analysis of massive mechanical structures. This technique is being applied to the structural simulation of human body that lead to successful stress/strain analysis of hard tissue such as bone.

In surgical training system and computer assisted diagnosis system, precise FE analysis of soft tissue is required in order to predict the response of the tissue under arbitrary loading conditions. Mechanical characterization of living soft tissue is thus one of the key technologies in such medical systems.

Many methodologies have been proposed for estimating mechanical properties of living soft tissue. One intuitive method is to indent the surface of the tissue [1,2]. Material property is then obtained from the relation between the indentation depth and the reaction force. Although this method is simple and applicable to the entire surface of human body, they have two fatal disadvantages. They cannot take large deformation and subcutaneous structure into considerations as is obvious from the principle.

J. Duncan and G. Gerig (Eds.): MICCAI 2005, LNCS 3750, pp. 633–640, 2005.

Recent progress in diagnostic imaging modalities allows us to develop new elasticity imaging techniques. Magnetic resonance elastography (MRE) is one of the promising method [3,4]. It visualizes strain waves that propagate within soft tissue by using MRI. We can estimate distribution of the stiffness even for a subcutaneous tissue since the wavelength visualized by MRE is proportional to the stiffness. However, several problems arise when applying this technique to a practical application. Damping and reflection of the strain waves cause artifacts in MR image, and thus they lead to error in the stiffness estimation.

Quasi-static MRE is another elasticity imaging method [5]. It employs a constitutive equation of linear elasticity to reconstruct the stiffness distribution from the strain field visualized also by MRI. It was found, however, that in this method, since the constitutive equation assumes small deformation, non-linear characteristics of soft tissue caused by large deformation cannot be taken into accounts.

In order to calculate deformation of soft tissue under arbitrary loading conditions, we have to take both non-linear material characteristics and subcutaneous structures into considerations. The estimation method of material properties presented in this paper accounts for these issues. It employs a compression test inside MRI in order to visualize deformation of hypodermic layered structure of living tissue, and an FE model of the compressed tissue in which non-linear material model is assigned. The FE analysis is iterated with updated material constant until the difference between the displacement field observed from MR images and calculated by FEM is minimized.

Different from similar approaches presented in the literature [6], we employ an MR-compatible optical force sensor [7] in order to determine the strict boundary conditions for the FE analysis. Furthermore, the extended Kalman filter used in the iterative optimization help us to achieve fast convergence to the final estimate. The presented method has been applied to a 3-layered silicon rubber phantom. The results show the excellent performance of our method. The accuracy of the estimation is better than 15 %, and the reproducibility of the deformation is better than 0.4 mm even for an FE analysis with different boundary condition.

2 Method and Implementation

2.1 Method Overview

Our method for material properties estimation involves four steps.

MR compression test: Compress the tissue inside MRI in order to visualize deformation of the subcutaneous structure. The reaction force is simultaneously measured by using an MR-compatible force sensor [7].

MR image processing: Extract the displacement field within the tissue by applying an image registration technique to the obtained MR images.

FE mesh generation: Generate a finite element model of the subcutaneous structure from the pre-compression MR image. The same boundary conditions as the MR compression test are given to the FE model.

Iterative FE analysis: Assign the initial estimate of the material constant to the model, and repeat the FE analysis with updated material constant until the difference between the displacement field observed from MR images and calculated by FEM is minimized (see Section 2.2 for detail).

This method has distinct advantages over the conventional approaches [1,2,3,4,5]. Firstly, both non-linear characteristics and subcutaneous structure are incorporated at a time. Secondly and equally important for medical applications, the reproducibility of the FE analysis in which the estimated material properties are assigned is guaranteed, since they are determined so that the result of the FE analysis is adapted to the observed deformation.

2.2 Implementation of the Iterative FE Analysis

To be precise, the iterative FE analysis is a minimization process of a disparity function D defined by Equation (1),

$$D(\boldsymbol{m}) = \sum_i \left(d_i^{MRI} - d_i^{FEM}(\boldsymbol{m})\right)^2 \tag{1}$$

where, $\boldsymbol{m}$ is the material constant, d_i^{MRI} is the observed displacement, $d_i^{FEM}(\boldsymbol{m})$ is the calculated displacement when the material constant is $\boldsymbol{m}$, and i is an index of the corresponding point between the MR image and the FE model.

An extended Kalman filter (EKF) is employed for the minimization of the disparity function. In the case of this implementation, the measurement equation of the EKF is the FE analysis itself, and material constant $\boldsymbol{m}$ does not change during the time update phase of the EKF (a steady condition is given to the state equation). Functional capability of this Kalman filter is therefore equivalent to that of non-linear optimization algorithms such as Levenberg-Marquadt method.

As formulated in Equation (2), Kalman gain $\boldsymbol{K}_k$ at step k is calculated from the error covariance $\boldsymbol{P}_{k-1}$, the measurement noise covariance $\boldsymbol{R}_k$ and the measurement jacobian $\boldsymbol{H}_k$.

$$\boldsymbol{K}_k = \boldsymbol{P}_{k-1}\boldsymbol{H}_k^T\left(\boldsymbol{H}_k\boldsymbol{P}_{k-1}\boldsymbol{H}_k^T + \boldsymbol{R}_k\right)^{-1} \tag{2}$$

The measurement jacobian $\boldsymbol{H}_k$ is approximated by a numerical difference of the forward FE analyses as given by Equation (3),

$$H_{ij} = \frac{\partial d_i}{\partial m_j} = \frac{d_i^{FEM}(\boldsymbol{m} + \boldsymbol{dm}) - d_i^{FEM}(\boldsymbol{m})}{dm_j} \tag{3}$$

where $\boldsymbol{dm}$ is the minute increment of the material constant that have dm_j at the j-th element and 0 at the rests. Thus, if $\boldsymbol{m}$ contains n variables, $n+1$ times FE analyses are required in total to compute the measurement jacobian. The time update and the measurement update process of the EKF is iterated until the disparity function $D(\boldsymbol{m})$ is minimized. This procedure is implemented on the commercial FE solver, MSC Marc2003, by using a programming language Python.

3 Material Model

3.1 Silicon Rubber Phantom

The estimation method given in Section 2 is applied to a 3-layered silicon rubber phantom. The dimension of this phantom is 12 mm in both width and height, and 70 mm in depth. It has the same 3-layered structure along the longitudinal direction. Thus, mechanical behavior at the center section of this phantom is given by a two-dimensional plane strain model, if the boundary conditions are also identical along this direction.

The material constant of each layer is estimated by a uni-axial compression test for reference, and by the proposed method for validation. The detail description of the uni-axial compression test is given in Section 4.1. The results of the estimation by the presented method are given in Section 4.2 to 4.4.

3.2 Material Model

To deal with non-linear characteristics of the silicon rubber, first-term Ogden model is employed [8]. It is one type of a hyperelastic model widely used in the analysis of rubber-like material and soft tissue [9]. As shown in Equation (4), the nominal stress σ is formulated by a function of the nominal strain ε and two material constants, μ and α, in the case of a uni-axial compression/tension.

$$\sigma = \mu\left((\varepsilon+1)^{\alpha-1} - (\varepsilon+1)^{-\frac{\alpha}{2}-1}\right) \tag{4}$$

Shown in Fig. 1 is the relation between the nominal strain ε and the normalized nominal stress σ/E (nominal stress divided by the Young's modulus E) for different α. As is obvious from this figure, the stress-strain curves are almost identical when the strain is within the range of -0.5 to 0.25 that shows the redundancy between the two material parameters. This redundancy inhibits us

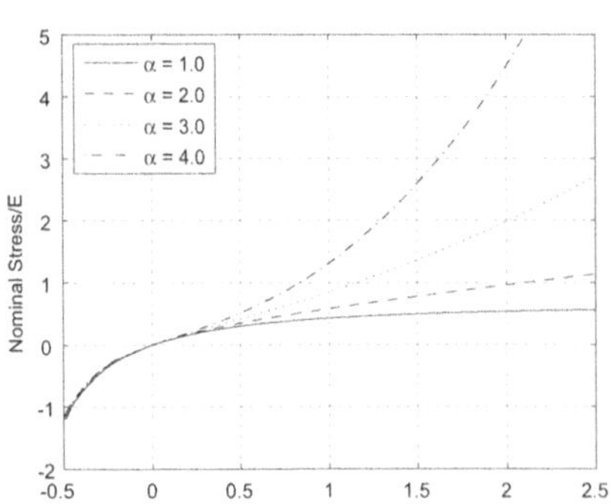

Fig. 1. Stress-strain diagrams of the first-term ogden model for different α

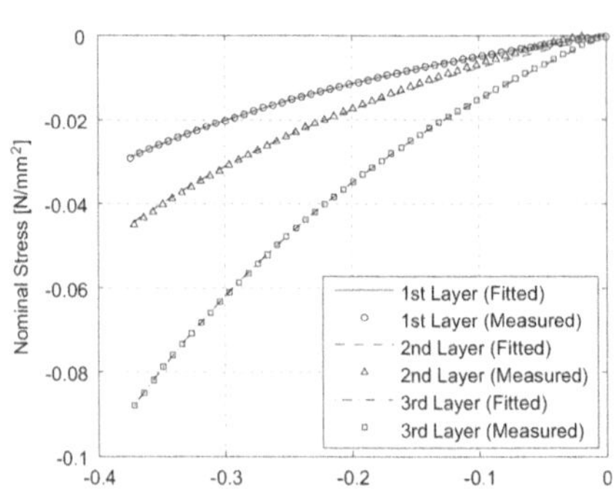

Fig. 2. Stress-strain diagrams of the silicon rubber in each layer

from estimating them uniquely by a compression test. The material constant α is therefore fixed to 1.4 referring to the conventional solution [10]. The material model used in this research is finally given by Equation (5).

$$\sigma = \mu \left((\varepsilon + 1)^{0.4} - (\varepsilon + 1)^{-1.7} \right) \quad (5)$$

The simplified Ogden model contains only one material constant to be estimated. The material constant $\boldsymbol{m}$ in Equation (1) is thus given by $(\mu_{1st}, \mu_{2nd}, \mu_{3rd})^T$, where subscript means the position of the rubber in the layered structure.

4 Experiment

4.1 Uni-axial Compression Test

Three cylindrical silicon rubbers that have 8 mm in height and diameter are prepared for the uni-axial compression test. Each rubber has the same material property as each layer of the phantom. Both end surfaces of the cylindrical rubbers are lubed by a silicon oil to achieve ideal uni-axial compression. They are compressed by a linear stage with the indentation speed of 0.1 mm/sec until the indentation depth becomes 3.0 mm.

Figure. 2 shows the stress-strain diagrams of the cylindrical rubbers. The material constant μ is identified by fitting Equation (5) to each diagram. The results of the identification are shown in the second column of Table 1.

4.2 MR Compression Test

Shown in Fig. 3-(a) and (b) are the MR images of the center section during the compression test with a flat indenter and a cylindrical indenter, respectively.

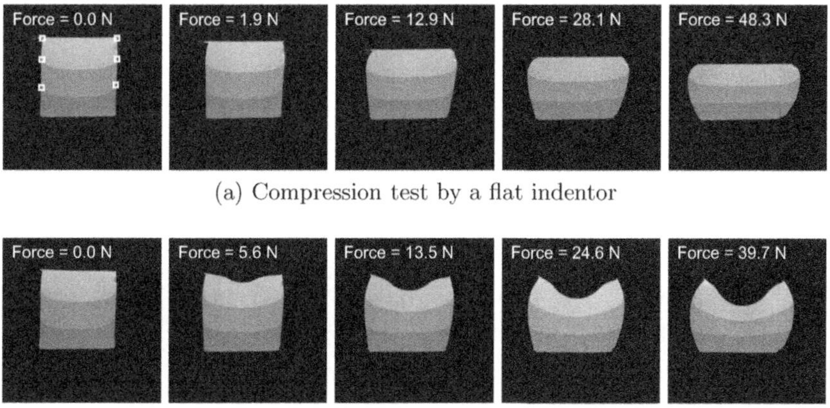

(a) Compression test by a flat indentor

(b) Compression test by a cylindrical indentor

Fig. 3. Results of the MR compression test

All images have a resolution of 256 × 256 pixels and a pixel size of 0.098 × 0.098 mm. They are obtained with the Varian Unity INOVA, 4.7 Tesla scanner for experimental purpose. The imaging sequence is Spin Echo with TE = 19 msec and TR = 500 msec. An MR-compatible optical force sensor is employed for the reaction force measurement. The rated force and the accuracy of this sensor is 60 N and 1.0 %, respectively. As can be seen in Fig. 3, the reaction force as well as the deformation of the subsurface structure are clearly obtained.

The bottom face of the phantom is glued to the base, and the indenters have the same profile along the longitudinal direction. Mechanical behavior of the center section is thus given by a two-dimensional plane strain model.

4.3 Estimation Results

Coarse and fine FE models consist of 133 and 1870 plane strain triangular elements are prepared for the estimation. The same boundary conditions as the MR compression test with the flat indenter are given to these models. Nodal displacements are measured at the boundary of the layers (square-marked 6 points in the first column of Fig. 3-(a)) by manual operations. Since there are 4 successive im-

Table 1. Result of the material constants estimation

	Uni-axial compression test	Our method	
		Coarse model	Fine model
μ_{1st}	0.0212 N/mm^2	0.0229 N/mm^2	0.0227 N/mm^2
Error in μ_{1st}	—	8.0 %	7.1 %
μ_{2nd}	0.0356 N/mm^2	0.0447 N/mm^2	0.0405 N/mm^2
Error in μ_{2nd}	—	25.6 %	13.8 %
μ_{3rd}	0.0654 N/mm^2	0.0370 N/mm^2	0.0593 N/mm^2
Error in μ_{3rd}	—	43.4 %	9.3 %
Error in displacement (mean)	—	0.17 mm	0.17 mm
Error in displacement (max.)	—	0.34 mm	0.38 mm

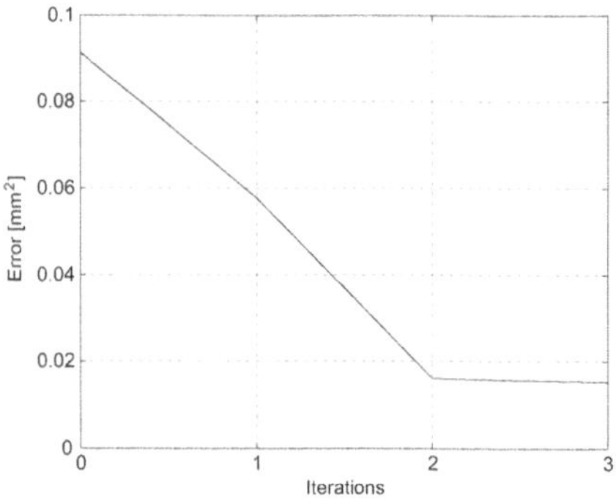

Fig. 4. Transition of the disparity function during the iteration (fine model)

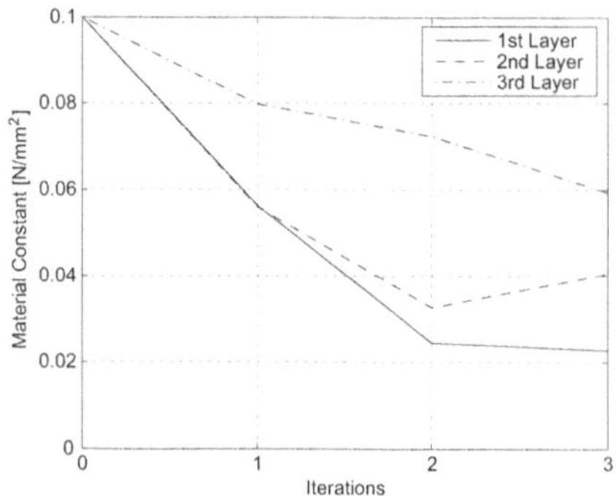

Fig. 5. Transition of the material constants during the iteration (fine model)

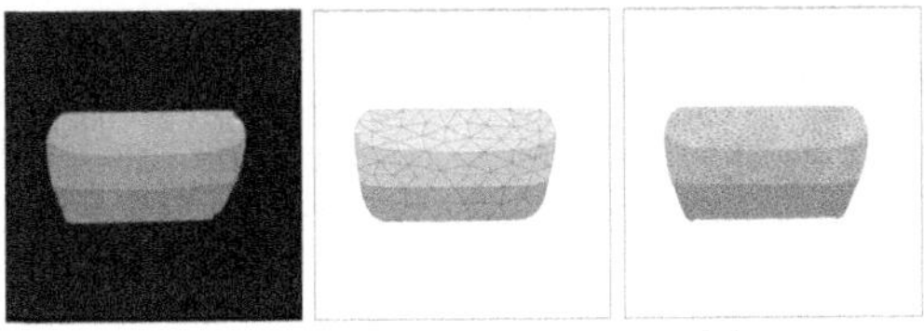

(a) MR image (b) Coarse (c) Fine

Fig. 6. Result of the iterative FEM analysis

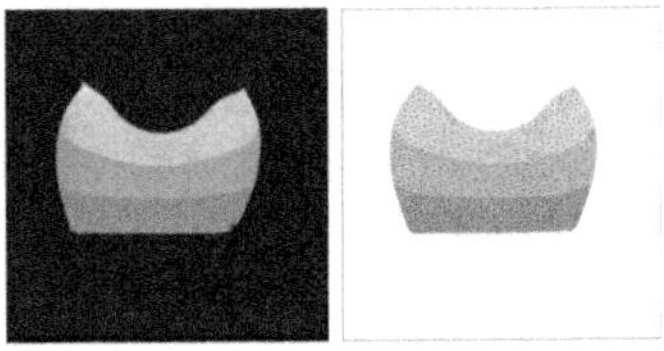

(a) MR image (b) FE analysis

Fig. 7. Reproducibility Test

ages (the second to the fifth column of Fig. 3-(a)), total 24 displacement data are used for the estimation of material properties. The material constant $\boldsymbol{m}$ is initially set to $(0.1, 0.1, 0.1)^T$. Note that the initial values are about 1.5 to 4.0 times greater than the material constant identified by the uni-axial compression test.

The iterative FE analysis terminate after 4 iterations with the coarse model and 3 iterations with the fine model. Transition of the disparity function and the material constants are shown in Fig. 4 and Fig. 5, respectively. The results of the estimations are shown in the third and the fourth column of Table 1. It should be remarked that the errors in the material constants estimated with the coarse model are greater than that with the fine model, whereas the errors in the displacement are almost identical in both models.

Figure 6 shows the observed MR image and the result of the FE analysis with the final estimates. There are better correspondences in the whole profile of the phantom between Fig. 6-(a) and (c), while there are correspondences only in the reference points between (a) and (b). This is the causal explanation of the phenomenon described in the previous paragraph. These results suggest that better estimates can be achieved, 1) if the FE model is finer, and 2) if there are enough reference points to be compared even in the coarse model.

4.4 Reproducibility Test

In order to validate the estimated material constants, FE simulation of the compression test with a cylindrical indenter is carried out. Figure 7 shows the observed MR image and the result of the simulation with the estimated material constants in the fourth column of Table 1. Better correspondences in the whole profile of the phantom can be confirmed. The mean and the maximum error in the displacement reproducibility are 0.22 mm and 0.35 mm that are almost identical to the results in Section 4.3.

The results of these experiments show the capability of our method that can incorporate both non-linear characteristics and subsurface layered structure of soft tissue. As mentioned in the previous section, the accuracy of the estimation can be improved by using finer model with enough reference points.

5 Conclusion

A new estimation method of material properties was presented in this paper. Since this method employs MR observation and iterative FE simulation, it can incorporate both non-linear material characteristics and hypodermic layered structure of living soft tissue. The excellent performance of our method was shown by carrying out estimation for a 3-layered silicon rubber phantom. This warrants future works on the noninvasive material properties estimation of real soft tissue.

References

1. J.F.M.Manschot, A.J.M.Brakkee: The measurement and modeling of the mechanical properties of human skin in vivo–i. the measurement. Journal of Biomechanics **19** (1986) 511–515
2. A.Z.Hajian, R.D.Howe: Identification of the mechanical impedance at the human finger tip. Journal of Biomechanical Engineering **119** (1997) 109–114
3. R.Muthupillai, D.J.Lomas, P.J.A., R.L.Ehman: Magnetic resonance elastography by direct visualization of propagation acoustic strain waves. Science **269** (1995) 1854–1857
4. J.Bishop, G.Poole, M., D.B.Plewes: Magnetic resonance imaging of shear wave propagation in excised tissue. Journal of Magnetic Resonance Imaging **8** (1998) 1257–1265
5. T.L.Chenevert, A.R.Skovoroda, M., S.Y.Emelianov: Elasticity reconstructive imaging by means of stimulated echo mri. Magnetic Resonance in Medicine **39** (1998) 382–490
6. G.Soza, R.Grosso, C.G., P.Hastreiter: Estimating mechanical brain tissue properties with simulation and registration. In: Proceeding of the 7th International Conference on Medical Image Computing and Computer Assisted Intervention. Volume 2. (2004) 276–283
7. M.Tada, T.Kanade: An MR-compatible optical force sensor for human function modeling. In: Proceeding of the 7th International Conference on Medical Image Computing and Computer Assisted Intervention. Volume 2. (2004) 129–136
8. R.W.Ogden: Large deformation isotropic elasticity – on the correlation of the theory and experiment for incompressible rubberlike solids. In: Proceedings of the Royal Society of London. (1972) 567–583
9. J.Z.Wu, R.G.Dong, W., A.W.Schopper: Modeling of time-dependent force response of fingertip to dynamic loading. Journal of Biomechanics **36** (2003) 383–392
10. O.H.Yeoh: On the ogden strain-energy function. Rubber Chemistry and Technology **70** (1996) 175–182

Simulating Vascular Systems in Arbitrary Anatomies

Dominik Szczerba and Gábor Székely

Computer Vision Lab, ETH, CH-8092 Zürich, Switzerland

Abstract. Better physiological understanding of principles regulating vascular formation and growth is mandatory to their efficient modeling for the purpose of physiologically oriented medical applications like training simulation or preoperative planning. We have already reported on the implementation of a visually oriented modeling framework allowing to study various physiological aspects of the vascular systems on a macroscopic scale. In this work we describe our progress in this field including (i) extension of the presented model to three dimensions, (ii) addition of established mathematical approaches to modeling angiogenesis and (iii) embedding the structures in arbitrary anatomical elements represented by finite element meshes.

1 Introduction

As pointed out in our previous work [1], the vascular systems do not simply influence organ appearance as part of their surface texture, but also behave like physical objects with certain mechanical properties. In particular, they will deform along with the hosting tissue and lead to bleeding when cut through. The ultimate goal is to provide a tool which, given a 3D representation of a given tissue/organ and an intuitive set of physiologically meaningful parameters, will generate vascular structures in an arbitrary anatomical region. Such systems are not expected to carry only geometrical information but also provide data on mechanical properties of the vascular system and the related blood flow.

In the previous work we have proposed a macroscopic model allowing to generate various vascular systems with high graphical fidelity for simulation purposes. The presented model included the formation of a primitive capillary plexus prior to maturation of the vascular system and treated its later development as a dynamic growth controlled by biophysical factors. This way the remodeling of the vascular system could be described, and full information on biophysical properties and hemodynamic conditions in the system could be provided at any time. The model, successful in generating a diversity of visually appealing vascular structures suffers, however, from a fundamental limitation. Whereas various geometrical constraints on the growth process can be imposed *a priori*, the domains to be vascularized are basically addressed as *continuum* and represented analytically. Such treatment is very convenient and widely used in developing and investigating mathematical modeling methods. Their implementation for real-life applications over complex domains represented in discrete forms is, however, not straightforward and needs special attention. The goals of the present work therefore are:

J. Duncan and G. Gerig (Eds.): MICCAI 2005, LNCS 3750, pp. 641–648, 2005.

- the full extension of the existing framework to three dimensions;
- the integration of the established mathematical modeling of angiogenesis with our previous simulation framework with the emphasis on visually realistic appearance;
- the embedding of such vascular networks in real-life anatomical objects defined by finite element meshes.

In practice, these objectives will be strongly inter-dependent. In order to solve differential equations governing the vessel formation one needs to provide a discretization scheme and proceed by finding the solution numerically. This is to be performed on a mesh, with the simplest one to use being an isotropic Cartesian grid. Offering significant implementational simplicity, which is advantageous from the algorithmic point of view, such meshes do not, however, provide the desired flexibility to efficiently map complex anatomical domains. Because of irregularity and high unpredictability, modeling such a diverse range of anatomical geometries is only possible through unstructured meshes. Such meshes are also convenient for modeling elastic properties of the tissue and organs.

Vascular structures are subject to computer modeling for a longer time now. A detailed overview of the available literature is given in our previous work [1] and will not be repeated here. The approaches discussed there include fractal self-similar constructs, functional macroscopic pipelines and continuous mathematical models. Still another group of approaches, not discussed previously, is based on optimization principles of theoretical physiology, which is well exemplified by the recent work by M. Georg *et.al.* [2]. Their model is initialized by a simple sub-optimal tree filling of the entire organ at a given resolution. It then becomes subject to optimization, mainly intra-vascular volume minimization, which is one of the major principles driving vascular system development as discussed in the literature. As compared to another popular optimization-based method, namely Constrained Constructive Optimization (CCO) [3], this new algorithm can also implement topological changes, which are essential to the optimization process. The generated structures presented by the authors prove to be similar to real experimental data acquired from corrosion casts, with the emerging symmetry explained in terms of global optimality. The fundamental difference to our approach is in that (1) we explicitly address capillary networks supplied by higher order vessels and (2) we model blood vessel formation by relying exclusively on local interactions, without enforcing any global optima. Our approach is well justified in cases of malignant tumors, where the vascular systems are known to be often unstable, leaky or otherwise sub-optimal.

One of the inspirations to continue our previous work is a recent proposition of a non-lattice mathematical model of angiogenesis [4]. Whereas established mathematical models to date restrict endothelial cell movements to 4 discrete directions on an isotropic Cartesian grid, the authors of that work propose to depart from a fixed lattice and adopt the governing equations for arbitrary (continuous) directions. They still, however, use very simple geometrical domains (squares) and provide biochemical agents only in form of analytically prescribed profiles. As described in the next section, we will adopt their topological freedom to model endothelial cell motility but with significant differences in the discretization scheme and representation of the underlying biochemical factors.

2 The Model

The formation of blood vessels during angiogenesis in general - healthy or cancerous - is a process where capillary sprouts depart from pre-existing parent vessels in response to externally supplied chemical stimuli. By means of endothelial cell proliferation and migration the sprouts then organize themselves into a branched, connected network structure. In this work we tend to focus specifically on tumor induced angiogenesis, which involve cancerous solid tumor cells secreting a number of biochemicals collectively known as growth factors. The general formalism can, however, also be applied to healthy anatomies if global functional optimality is not the primary focus of investigation. This is the case e.g. in early vascular development stages with only preliminary capillary beds present. Moreover, the remodeling procedure introduced in our previous work can readily be applied to the structures generated here. The preliminary capillary plexus does not necessarily require blood flow to form. Once the blood enters the freshly formed vessels it inflates the elastic walls. Regions of high stress disproportions, where the capillaries started to sprout from the parent vessels are remodeled first. Inflating vessels will not only change their initial distribution of radii but also adjust the bifurcation angles. The optimal bifurcation design discussed so often in the literature may arise from local conditions determined by e.g. the elastic properties of the walls forming the initial tripod. In a completely different modeling approach, involving cells as opposed to pipes used here, we have demonstrated that local variations in the shear stress rebuild a uniform distributions of tissue pillars into a set of non-symmetric bifurcations [5] observed *in vivo*. Even thought the resulting structure is not guaranteed to be optimal, the initial symmetry is broken and the bifurcations and micro-vessels emerge as a result of a simulation instead of being composed *a priori* out of basic structural elements as pipes or tripod. Therefore, instead of presumptively imposing optimality rules on the sprouting and bifurcating capillaries we start our modeling from the widely accepted assumption that the initial response of the endothelial cells to the angiogenic growth factors is due to chemotaxis, enforcing the cell migration towards the tumor or ischemic cell. Once secreted, the growth factors diffuse into the surrounding tissue and the extracellular matrix, establishing a certain concentration gradient between the chemical source and the parent vessels. As the endothelial cells migrate through the extracellular matrix in response to this gradient there is some uptake and binding of the growth factors by the cells [6]. Therefore, it can be modeled by a diffusion equation with a natural decay term:

$$\frac{\partial c}{\partial t} = S_c + D_i \nabla^2 c - \theta_0 c \, , \tag{1}$$

with c being the chemical concentration, S_c its source, D the diffusion coefficient and θ decay rate. Once the initial distribution of the growth agents due to secretion by the malignant or ischemic cells has been established, endothelial cells start to respond to the stimulus by sprouting, eventually modifying the initial growth factor concentration by cellular bindings. Partial differential equations governing the endothelial density evolution are derived from a general form of transport equation and can be written in the following form:

$$\frac{\partial n}{\partial t} = D_0 \nabla \cdot (f_0(c) \nabla n) - D_c \nabla \cdot (f_c(c) n \nabla c) \quad (2)$$

$$\frac{\partial c}{\partial t} = -\theta_1 n c \quad (3)$$

with n the endothelial cell density and D_i, θ_i positive constants.

A similar set of partial differential equations with respect to cellular density evolution was first postulated by [7]. Below is the interpretation of these equations needed for their adaptation to our simulation framework, as well as discussion of the main difference to our modeling approach. The first term in Equation 2, *chemokinesis*, is the random displacement of the endothelial cells with the transition probability modulated by the concentration of the chemical stimuli. In a specific case of constant growth factor concentration this reduces to the classical diffusion equation with the diffusion constant D_0, in a general case of non-constant concentrations, however, this term allows to selectively change random motility of the migrating cells. In particular, it is reasonable to assume that as the cells approach the angiogenic source they will become more motile and more chaotic in their migration. In our model we address this issue taking a simple linear form of f_0. The second term in the same equation is known in literature as *chemotaxis*. It is the advective term in the general transport equation with the difference in that the advection velocity is replaced by another vector field, namely the gradient of the (scalar) growth factor concentration. This is well justified from experimental observations, as it is widely known that the endothelial cells tend to "climb up" the gradients of biochemical growth stimuli [8]. Similar to Anderson and Chaplain, we take the chemotactic amplitude $f_c(c)$ as a receptor-kinetic function of the form $f_c(c) \sim 1/c$. This represents an intuitive assumption of decreased cellular sensitivity with the increased chemical stimulus. The second equation (Equation 3) models the biochemical growth factors concentration by linear uptake functions due to degradation through cellular bindings. We make two important simplifications in our modeling, namely that the concentration of the growth factor does not change throughout the vessel growth process (i.e. Equation 3 is not solved) and that the haptotactic response due to fibronectin, present in the original formulation, is neglected. Inclusion of these components in the transport equation appears to be crucial to obtain physiologically normalizable models, in the first implementation, however, with the emphasis on real-life modeling of the underlying arbitrary hosting tissue, we did not find them mandatory for providing a realistic network coverage of the domain of interest. This could, however, be integrated in the next version of the framework to increase the physiological correctness of the model.

Anderson and Chaplain proceed by discretizing the partial differential equations on an isotropic Cartesian grid and either modeling the endothelial cell density (the *continuous* model) or by introducing transition probabilities and displacing the endothelial sprouting tips explicitly (the *discrete* model). Instead, we follow the way sketched for simple geometries in [4] and depart from fixed vascular topology, which allows us to flexibly handle arbitrary finite element meshes.

A detailed description of an example method to generate unstructured tetrahedral meshes out of surfaces (extracted by e.g. segmentation of magnetic resonance imaging of real anatomical objects) can be found in [9]. Here we proceed by interpreting the governing equations in terms of a given mesh. We start by discretizing the ∇ operator needed for establishing the initial chemotactic gradient as well as for diffusive transport of the growth factors. In case of tetrahedral meshes a natural choice of discretization is the *finite volume* scheme. The transport phenomena described by Equation 1 and Equation 2 in such a nomenclature take the following general form:

$$\int_V (\frac{\partial \phi}{\partial t}) dV + D_c \oint_A f_c(c) n\vec{n} \cdot \nabla c \, dA = D_0 \oint_A f_0(c)\vec{n} \cdot \nabla n \, dA + \int_V S_c \, dV \ . \quad (4)$$

with ϕ a general scalar field, V denoting the control volume, A control volume surface, $\boldsymbol{n}$ the surface normal vectors (not to be confused with n scalar) and S_c the growth factor sources (e.g. secretion by tumor or ischemic cells). We linearize these equations and express their discretized versions using the control volume central values in order to facilitate the iterative solution procedure:

$$C_i \phi_i + C_{i,j} \phi_{i,j} = S_i^{\phi} \ , \quad (5)$$

with the Einstein summation over the control element's direct (i) and indirect (i, j) neighbors. $\phi_i, \phi_{i,j}$ correspond to the scalar field's cell centered values, and S^{ϕ} is determined by the boundary conditions. Derivation of the coefficient matrix C is nontrivial and will not be presented here.

By proceeding with the Eulerian formulation used so far, we would have to solve this kind of equations three times: to establish the initial concentration gradients ($\phi = c$), and to solve the transport equation terms ($\phi = n$ and $\phi = c$). Instead, we solve it only once, for the initial steady-state equilibrium of c (Equation 1), and change our formulation of Equation 2 to Lagrangian dynamics of sprouting vessel tips. Such a continuous approach, as opposed to a discrete Eulerian treatment, is particularly beneficial in case of finite element meshes, as the generated vascular structures are limited by neither the underlying mesh resolution nor the topology. In addition, the resulting structure can straightforwardly be converted to a flow network required to solve the Hagen-Poiseuille's flow equations, as described in our previous paper [1]. Therefore, by realizing that the diffusive term in the transport equation is responsible for random motility of the endothelial cells (modulated by f_0), and that the advective term effectively displaces the cells towards the regions of higher chemical concentration, we arrive at the following equation of a sprouting tip motion:

$$\frac{d\vec{r}}{dt} \equiv \vec{v_{tot}} = d_1(c)\vec{v_0} + d_2(c)\vec{v_c} + d_3(c)\vec{v_i}, \quad (6)$$

with dr being the net displacement of the sprouting tip due to the following contributions:

- diffusive motility $\vec{v_0}$ in a random direction (e.g. picking a random point on a sphere),
- directed motility $\vec{v_c}$ in the direction of a local growth factor's gradient (estimated e.g. using the Gauss theorem),
- inertial motility $\vec{v_i}$ enforcing a certain resistance of the sprouting tip to rapidly change the currently followed direction.

The functions $d_i(c)$ regulate the relative importance of the three contributions to the net displacement and depend on the local growth factor concentrations in the same way as the previously discussed coefficients D_i. We additionally introduce a function $\beta(c)$ regulating bifurcation probability at the sprouting tip and allow for fusion of colliding vessels (anastomosis). In addition, once a vessel reaches a minimal diameter (corresponding to a capillary), it is no more bifurcating (as it would lead to further decrease in diameter, which is not observed in reality). As stated in section 1 - and opposed to our previous approach - we do not anymore attempt to provide optimal bifurcation angles nor diameters *a priori*, instead we simply chose a random deviation from the followed direction within $[0, \pi)$. Even if such a selection may seem arbitrary, these angles are strongly influenced by chemotaxis, and practically anyway limited to forward directions.

3 Results

The model described in the preceding sections was tested with a finite element volumetric mesh of an early development stage of a uterine polyp model presented in [10]. A few interior elements in the structure's head were picked and marked as actively dividing cells, which will be continuously secreting angiogenic growth factors and regulating the endothelial response. Because there is an uptake of these chemicals in the extracellular matrix, as discussed before, a steady state concentration gradient will form after some iterations. Now the vessels are allowed to start sprouting, with the bifurcation probability and random motility increasing and the chemotactic sensitivity decreasing with the concentration of the growth factor. Such separation between the initial and the growth phase is not unrealistic since it is very likely that the sprouting begins only when a certain triggering threshold in the local concentration is reached. The input surface mesh along with the output vascular network, with the initial growth starting from the base of the polyp, is shown in Figure 1. The steady state distribution of the growth factors is visualized on the surface (leftmost) and inside (middle) of the model. Note the chaotic nature of the resulting vessels (right) as compared to the results presented in the

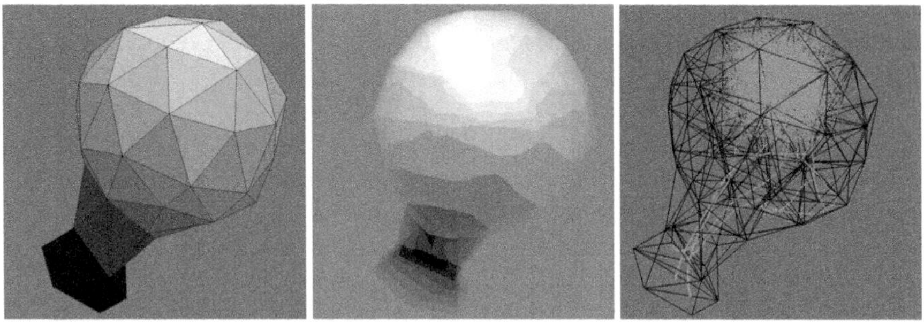

Fig. 1. Simulation results of the vascular growth model described in the text. Left: input mesh with the surface triangles color-coded according to the growth factor concentration on the surface. Middle: volumetric "see-through" visualization of the growth factor concentration inside the model. Right: generated vascular structure and wire-frame of the input mesh.

previous work [1]. As expected - and as observed in real tumors - the blood vessels become gradually very chaotic as they approach the cancerous epicenter. This is achieved in the simulation by letting the random motility and the bifurcation probability increase rapidly as the tumor is approached. At the same time the vessel tip inertia as well as the ability to reorient itself along the local gradient is continuously quenched. This results in approximately parallel vessels along the polyp's neck and ends with a dense "brush" in the epicenter. The full procedure leading to the results presented above, including mesh generation, establishment of the initial gradients and generation of the vessels, took approximately 10 minutes on a PC with Pentium4/3.0GHz and 1GB RAM. Calculation of flow conditions in the generated network and the according oxygen penetration of the tissue took another 10 minutes.

These results demonstrate the model's ability to deal with realistic conditions encountered in early development stages of small vascular tumors and at the same time providing realistic visualization along with necessary bio-physical information required by surgical training simulations. Moreover, as indicated before, the meshes used for the discretization purposes were designed with the possible tissue elastic deformation in mind. It is straight-forward now to mechanically deform the vessels together with the hosting tissue using e.g. a simple and fast mass-spring modeling. In addition, using the flow network model described in our previous work, we can readily provide the flow conditions at any location of interest and use this information for e.g. visualization of bleeding when a surgeon cuts in the tissue during a virtual training session. Together with the real-time elastic deformation this provides reasonably realistic environment for virtual-reality based medical training.

4 Outlook

The presented simulation takes into account basic experimental knowledge of the growing process, namely endothelial cell proliferation and migration, and their modulated response to changes in local growth factor concentrations. Achieved results correspond well to both experimental findings and to the established mathematical models of angiogenesis. In addition, the key components of the previously introduced model - the flow network and stress driven remodeling - can readily be applied. The network coverage is, however, provided under the quasi-static assumption of a steady development state of the tumor and the underlying chemical factors. While the mechanical deformation of the resulting structure can be easily applied, further increase of realism can only be achieved by simultaneous simulation of the vascular growth and the tumor development. This would allow to study both the mechanical interplay between developing structures (e.g. deformation due to stretching and strains) as well as their coupled biochemical dependence. Such modeling is already under way and will soon be integrated into the presented framework.

We are aware that in case of healthy anatomies the generated structures may be suboptimal in the sense of a network coverage, building material or diffusive exchange. The enforcement of such an optimum based exclusively on local interactions will require much better understanding of short-range mechanisms acting on the cellular level, but is an attractive vision for the ultimate explanation of the origins of natural self-symmetry and functional optimality.

References

[1] Szczerba, D., Székely, G.: Macroscopic modeling of vascular systems. In: Medical Image Computing and Computer-Assisted Intervention - MICCAI 2002. Volume 2489 of Lecture Notes in Computer Science., LNCS Springer (2002) 284–292

[2] Georg, M., Hahn, H., Preusser, T., Peitgen, H.O.: Global constructive optimization of vascular systems. Submitted to IEEE transactions on Medical Imaging (2004)

[3] Schreiner, W., Neumann, M., Neumann, F., Roedler, S., End, A., Buxbaum, P., Muller, M., Spieckermann, P.: The branching angles in computer-generated optimized models of arterial trees. J. Gen. Physiol. **103** (1994) 975–989

[4] Plank, M.J., Sleeman, B.D.: Lattice and non-lattice models of tumour angiogenesis. Bulletin of Mathematical Biology **66(6)** (2004) 1785–1819

[5] Szczerba, D., Székely, G.: Computational model of flow-tissue interactions in intussusceptive angiogenesis. Journal of Theoretical Biology **234** (2005) 87–97

[6] Ausprunk, D.H., Folkman, J.: Migration and proliferation of endothelial cells in preformed and newly formed blood vessels during tumor angiogenesis. Microvascular Research (1977)

[7] Anderson, A., Chaplain, M.: Continuous and discrete mathematical models of tumor-induced angiogenesis. Bulletin of Mathematical Biology **60** (1998) 857–899

[8] Terranova, V., DiFlorio, R., Lyall, R., Hic, S., Friesel, R., Maciag, T.: Human endothelial cells are chemotactic to endothelial cell growth factor and heparin. J. Cell Biol. **101** (1985) 2330–2334

[9] Szczerba, D., Székely, G.: A computational model of micro-vascular growth. In: Simulation of Multiphysics Multiscale Systems, ICCS 2005: 5th International Conference on Computational Science , Atlanta. Volume 3516 of Lecture Notes in Computer Science., Springer-Verlag (2005) 17–24

[10] Sierra, R., Bajka, M., Székely, G.: Pathology growth model based on particles. In Ellis, R.E., Peters, T.M., eds.: Procs. of the Sixth International Conference on Medical Image Computing and Computer-Assisted Intervention. Volume 1., Springer (2003) 25–32

Physiological System Identification with the Kalman Filter in Diffuse Optical Tomography

Solomon Gilbert Diamond[1], Theodore J. Huppert[1], Ville Kolehmainen[3], Maria Angela Franceschini[1], Jari P. Kaipio[3], Simon R. Arridge[2], and David A. Boas[1]

[1] Massachusetts General Hospital, Martinos Center for Biomedical Imaging*, Charlestown MA 02129, USA
sdiamond@nmr.mgh.harvard.edu
http://www.nmr.mgh.harvard.edu/PMI
[2] Department of Computer Science, University College London, London, UK
[3] Department of Applied Physics, University of Kuopio, Kuopio, Finland

Abstract. Diffuse optical tomography (DOT) is a noninvasive imaging technology that is sensitive to local concentration changes in oxy- and deoxyhemoglobin. When applied to functional neuroimaging, DOT measures hemodynamics in the scalp and brain that reflect competing metabolic demands and cardiovascular dynamics. Separating the effects of systemic cardiovascular regulation from the local dynamics is vitally important in DOT analysis. In this paper, we use auxiliary physiological measurements such as blood pressure and heart rate within a Kalman filter framework to model physiological components in DOT. We validate the method on data from a human subject with simulated local hemodynamic responses added to the baseline physiology. The proposed method significantly improved estimates of the local hemodynamics in this test case. Cardiovascular dynamics also affect the blood oxygen dependent (BOLD) signal in functional magnetic resonance imaging (fMRI). This Kalman filter framework for DOT may be adapted for BOLD fMRI analysis and multimodal studies.

1 Introduction

Diffuse optical tomography (DOT) is a noninvasive imaging technology that uses near infrared (IR) light to image biological tissue. The dominant chromophores in this spectrum are oxyhemoglobin (HbO), deoxyhemoglobin (HbR), lipids and water. The basis of DOT is *in vivo* near infrared spectroscopy of these dominant chromophores in the tissue. Tomographic images in DOT are constructed by simultaneously measuring from many local regions that cover a larger volume of tissue. The in-plane resolution limit of DOT increases rapidly with depth because biological tissue is a highly scattering medium for near infrared light. This diffuse property of the light also limits the penetration depth in adult human

* This research was funded by NIH T32-CA09502, P41-RR14075, R01-EB001954 and the MIND Institute.

J. Duncan and G. Gerig (Eds.): MICCAI 2005, LNCS 3750, pp. 649–656, 2005.

brain imaging to about 3 cm, which is sufficient to study most of the cerebral cortex. See Gibson et al. for a complete description of DOT [1]. Clinical and research applications of DOT arise due to is its specificity to the physiologically relevant chromophores HbO and HbR. Potential clinical and research applications for DOT abound in brain injury, degenerative neurovascular diseases and in cognitive neuroscience. Other research areas for DOT include fetal and neonatal monitoring and breast cancer detection. DOT is particularly suitable for *in situ* monitoring and multi-modal imaging [2].

The dynamics measured with DOT in the functional neuroimaging application are caused by local changes in blood volume and oxygenation in the scalp and in the brain. Due to the physical constraints of noninvasive imaging with DOT, the scalp and brain effects are combined in the measurements. The measured hemodynamics are caused by blood pressure regulation, cerebral blood flow autoregulation, local vasomotion and the vascular response to neuronal activity. Complexity arises because of interactions between these factors. The primary aim of DOT functional neuroimaging is to separate the stimulus related brain function signal from the background physiology related signal. The main problem is that the latter of these two is much stronger. A method to help resolve the physiological components in DOT is to include noninvasive auxiliary physiological measurements in the analysis. Many instruments can be used during DOT experiments. Examples are the blood pressure monitor, pulse oximeter, electrocardiogram (ECG), chest band respirometer, spirometer and capnograph. A further complexity of DOT analysis is that even when auxiliary physiology is included in the analysis, their effects do not appear to be stationary in time or space. We commonly observe that signal dynamics that are correlated with respiration, for example, will vary significantly in amplitude and relative phase angle at different measurement locations even when breathing rate and depth are held constant. The present objective is to separate the physiological components of DOT with a dynamical model.

State-space estimation has previously been applied to DOT without physiological regressors [3]. Prince et al. [4] fit the amplitude and phase angle of three non-stationary sinusoids to DOT time-series data using the Kalman filter. While supporting the principle of using the Kalman filter in DOT analysis, the three-sinusoid model does not allow for the most commonly used event related experimental designs nor can it use readily available physiological measurements such as blood pressure as a regressor. Zhang et al. used principal component analysis (PCA) to reduce the background physiological variance in functional neuroimaging experiments [5]. Anecdotal evidence was presented that certain principal components correlate with blood pressure and respiratory dynamics. This observation of statistically uncorrelated blood pressure and respiratory dynamics contradicts known respiratory interactions in blood pressure regulation [6]. Due to physiological interactions, the orthogonal projections in PCA are more likely to be mixtures of physiological effects. Standard linear regression methods in fMRI analysis [7] accept multiple regressors that could easily include auxiliary physiological measurements but will not accommodate temporal non-stationarity of the linear models. Dynamical system identification for fMRI is at the forefront of new analysis methods [8]. These advances in fMRI have not extended to DOT thus far mainly because the DOT inverse problem is typically ill posed and requires a more complicated physical model. In this paper, we present a framework that employs the Kalman filter for dynamical modeling of the physiological components of DOT.

2 Methods

The Kalman filter is a recursive solution to discrete linear filtering and prediction problems [9]. The objective of the Kalman filter is to estimate the time-varying states of a discrete-time process that is described by stochastic equations for updating the states and measurements over time. There are many ways to model the same physical system within the generality of the Kalman filter. Our proposed Kalman filter model of the DOT system begins by naming the constants in table 1 and naming the model variables in table 2. The respective sizes of each variable are indicated with a parenthetical subscript notation and those that vary with time are indicated.

The inputs $\mathbf{u}$ in the DOT model are the Boolean stimulus time vector and time-series physiological measurements such as blood pressure and heart rate variability. The states $\mathbf{x}$ in the DOT model are the discrete finite impulse response (FIR) functions that are convolved with the inputs to yield local concen-

Table 1. Length constant names

n_u	inputs (regressors)	n_w	wavelengths
n_d	source-detector pairs	n_c	chromophores
n_s	voxels	n_g	spatial basis functions
n_r	regression time points	n_h	temporal basis functions
n_x	states ($n_x = n_u n_c n_g n_h$)	n_y	measurements ($n_y = n_w n_d$)
n_z	auxiliary states ($n_z = n_u n_c n_g n_r$)	n_k	total time points

Table 2. Variable names and sizes

$k(t)$	time index	$\mathbf{u}_{(n_u,1)}(t)$	input vector
$\mathbf{x}_{(n_x,1)}(t)$	state vector	$\mathbf{V}_{(n_x,n_x)}(t)$	state covariance
$\mathbf{w}_{(n_x,1)}(t)$	process noise	$\mathbf{Q}_{(n_x,n_x)}$	process noise covariance
$\mathbf{z}_{(n_z,1)}(t)$	auxiliary state vector	$\mathbf{y}_{(n_y,1)}(t)$	measurement vector
$\mathbf{v}_{(n_y,1)}(t)$	measurement noise	$\mathbf{R}_{(n_y,n_y)}$	meas. noise covariance
$\mathbf{A}_{(n_x,n_x)}$	state update model	$\mathbf{B}_{(n_z,n_z)}$	auxiliary update model
$\mathbf{C}_{(n_z,n_u)}$	auxiliary input model	$\mathbf{D}_{(n_y,n_x)}(t)$	measurement model
$\mathbf{K}_{(n_x,n_y)}(t)$	Kalman gain matrix	$\mathbf{S}_{(n_y,n_u n_y)}$	summing matrix
$\mathbf{U}_{(n_u n_c n_g,n_z)}(t)$	input matrix	$\mathbf{M}_{(n_u n_c n_g,n_z)}$	input mask matrix
$\mathbf{L}_{(n_u n_y,n_u n_w n_s)}$	pathlength matrix	$\mathbf{L}_{0(n_w n_d,n_w n_s)}$	pathlength submatrix
$\mathbf{G}_{(n_u n_w n_s,n_u n_w n_g)}$	spatial basis set	$\mathbf{G}_{0(n_s,n_g)}$	spatial basis submatrix
$\mathbf{E}_{(n_u n_w n_g,n_u n_c n_g)}$	extinction matrix	$\mathbf{E}_{0(n_w,n_c)}$	extinction submatrix
$\mathbf{H}_{(n_z,n_x)}$	temporal basis set	$\mathbf{H}_{0(n_r,n_h)}$	temporal basis submatrix

tration changes in HbO and HbR. In order to perform this convolution within a Kalman filter framework, it is convenient to define auxiliary states $\mathbf{z}$ that merely store a regression length n_r of most recent inputs. The measurements $\mathbf{y}$ are the time-series of changes in optical density (ΔOD) for each source-detector pair and wavelength. This discrete-time process can be described as

$$\mathbf{x}_k = \mathbf{A}\mathbf{x}_{k-1} + \mathbf{w}_{k-1} \quad (1)$$

$$\mathbf{z}_k = \mathbf{B}\mathbf{z}_{k-1} + \mathbf{C}\mathbf{u}_k \quad (2)$$

$$\mathbf{y}_k = \mathbf{D}(\mathbf{z}_k)\mathbf{x}_k + \mathbf{v}_k \ . \quad (3)$$

In order to include a physical model for the DOT inverse problem, the model elements $\mathbf{A}$, $\mathbf{B}$, $\mathbf{C}$ and $\mathbf{D}$ are defined as

$$\mathbf{A} = \mathbf{I}_{(n_x)} \quad (4)$$

$$\mathbf{B} = \mathbf{I}_{(n_u n_c n_g)} \otimes \begin{bmatrix} \mathbf{0}_{(1,n_r-1)} & 0 \\ \mathbf{I}_{(n_r-1)} & \mathbf{0}_{(n_r-1,1)} \end{bmatrix} \quad (5)$$

$$\mathbf{C} = \mathbf{I}_{(n_u)} \otimes \mathbf{1}_{(n_c n_g,1)} \otimes \begin{bmatrix} 1 \ \mathbf{0}_{(n_r-1,1)} \end{bmatrix} \quad (6)$$

$$\mathbf{S} = \mathbf{1}_{(1,n_u)} \otimes \mathbf{I}_{(n_y)} \quad (7)$$

$$\mathbf{L} = \mathbf{I}_{(n_u)} \otimes \mathbf{L}_0 \quad (8)$$

$$\mathbf{G} = \mathbf{I}_{(n_u n_w)} \otimes \mathbf{G}_0 \quad (9)$$

$$\mathbf{E} = \mathbf{I}_{(n_u)} \otimes \mathbf{E}_0 \otimes \mathbf{I}_{(n_g)} \quad (10)$$

$$\mathbf{M} = \mathbf{I}_{(n_u n_c n_g)} \otimes \mathbf{1}_{(1,n_r)} \quad (11)$$

$$\mathbf{H} = \mathbf{I}_{(n_u n_c n_g)} \otimes \mathbf{H}_0 \quad (12)$$

$$\mathbf{U}(\mathbf{z}_k) = \mathbf{1}_{(n_u n_c n_g,1)}\mathbf{z}_k^T \odot \mathbf{M} \quad (13)$$

$$\mathbf{D}(\mathbf{z}_k) = \mathbf{SLGEU}(\mathbf{z_k})\mathbf{H} \ , \quad (14)$$

where T is the transpose operator, $\otimes$ is the Kronecker tensor product, $\odot$ is term-by-term array multiplication, $\mathbf{I}$ is the identity matrix, $\mathbf{1}$ is a matrix of ones, $\mathbf{0}$ is a matrix of zeros and matrix sizes are indicated with parenthetical subscripts. The submatrix $\mathbf{L}_0$ is a block diagonal matrix formed from meassurement by voxel average effective pathlengths for each wavelength as described by [10]. The columns of $\mathbf{G}_0$ contain a set of spatial basis functions that can be used to reduce the number of states and/or impose spatial smoothing of the state estimates. Known optical extinction coefficients are contained in the wavelength by chromophore submatrix $\mathbf{E}_0$. The columns of $\mathbf{H}_0$ contain temporal basis functions to reduce the number of states and/or impose temporal smoothing.

The Kalman filter is a recursive solution to the state estimation problem for the discrete-time process described by equations 1, 2 and 3. The recursions require initialization of the state estimate $\hat{\mathbf{x}}_0$ and estimated state covariance $\hat{\mathbf{V}}_0$ and then proceed with the following prediction-correction algorithm

$$\hat{\mathbf{x}}_{k|k-1} = \mathbf{A}\hat{\mathbf{x}}_{k-1|k-1} \quad (15)$$

$$\mathbf{z}_{k|k-1} = \mathbf{B}\mathbf{z}_{k-1|k-1} + \mathbf{C}\mathbf{u}_k \quad (16)$$

$$\hat{\mathbf{V}}_{k|k-1} = \mathbf{A}_t \hat{\mathbf{V}}_{k-1|k-1} \mathbf{A}^T + \mathbf{Q} \tag{17}$$

$$\mathbf{U}_k = \mathbf{1}_{(n_u n_c n_g, 1)} \mathbf{z}_{k|k-1}^T \odot \mathbf{M} \tag{18}$$

$$\mathbf{D}_k = \mathbf{SLGEU}_k \mathbf{H} \tag{19}$$

$$\mathbf{K}_k = \hat{\mathbf{V}}_{k|k-1} \mathbf{D}_k^T \left(\mathbf{D}_k \hat{\mathbf{V}}_{k|k-1} \mathbf{D}_k^T + \mathbf{R} \right)^{-1} \tag{20}$$

$$\hat{\mathbf{x}}_{k|k} = \hat{\mathbf{x}}_{k|k-1} + \mathbf{K}_t \left(\mathbf{y}_k - \mathbf{D}_k \hat{\mathbf{x}}_{k|k-1} \right) \tag{21}$$

$$\mathbf{z}_{k|k} = \mathbf{z}_{k|k-1} \tag{22}$$

$$\hat{\mathbf{V}}_{k|k} = \hat{\mathbf{V}}_{k|k-1} - \mathbf{K}_k \mathbf{D}_k \hat{\mathbf{V}}_{k|k-1} \,. \tag{23}$$

We designed an experiment to test the basic functionality of this proposed method. We combine real DOT data with a simulated functional response and then analyze the result with static deconvolution and the proposed Kalman filter method. This experiment allows us to compare the estimated responses with the "true" response. Only a single trial is examined so the results are mainly illustrative. Data was collected from a human subject who was instructed to sit quietly and breath freely. Measurements were taken with a continuous wave DOT instrument [11] then demodulated and down sampled to 1 Hz. The measurements were high pass filtered in a forward then reverse direction with a 6th order IIR Butterworth filter with a cutoff frequency of 0.05 Hz and zero phase distortion. This filtering removes slow physiology that is sufficiently outside the frequency range of interest for the hemodynamic response that it can be ignored. Short-term variability including the respiratory sinus arrhythmia, Mayer waves and vasomotion remain after filtering. The photon fluence $\Phi(t, \lambda)$ was then converted to a change in optical density ΔOD

$$\Delta \mathrm{OD}(t, \lambda) = \ln \left(\frac{\Phi(t, \lambda)}{\Phi_0(\lambda)} \right) \,, \tag{24}$$

where Φ_0 is average detected photon fluence, $\Delta\mathrm{OD}(t, \lambda)$ are measurements $\mathbf{y}$ as a function of time t and wavelength λ. The three model inputs contained in $\mathbf{u}$ were the Boolean stimulus time vector, the blood pressure (BP) and heart rate variability (HRV) with normalized variances.

Data from only a single source fiber and three detector locations were included in the analysis. The three detectors were arranged about 2 cm apart in a row and the source was placed 3 cm away from the center detector and equidistant from the other two. Three voxels defined the tissue volume under the optical probes. Voxel 1 represented the scalp and was common to all the detectors. Voxels 2 and 3 represented two regions of the brain located under the scalp voxel. A simulated functional response was added into the baseline hemodynamics in voxel 2. The stimulus paradigm was event related with a 12 to 18 second inter-stimulus interval over the 300 second trial. The model used to simulate the hemodynamics was one period of a raised cosine with a delay and amplitude set differently for the HbO and HbR functional responses. The simulated waveforms can be seen in the results figures.

The pathlength submatrix $\mathbf{L}_0$ was computed with a diffusion approximation to the transport equation for a semi-infinite medium [10]. An identity matrix was used for the spatial basis set $\mathbf{G}_0$ and a normalized Gaussian function was used for the temporal basis set $\mathbf{H}_0$. The standard deviation for the Gaussian function was fixed at 1.5 seconds and the means were separated by 1.5 seconds over the regression time. The same temporal basis set was used for the static deconvolution. The state update noise covariance $\mathbf{Q}$ only contained nonzero terms on the diagonal elements. Diagonal terms related to the functional response were set to 3×10^{-6} and those related to BP and HRV were set to 10^{-5}. This imbalance in state update noise caused the functional response model to evolve more slowly than the systemic physiological models. The measurement noise covariance matrix $\mathbf{R}$ was set to an identity scaled by 10^{-3}. These variances act as regularization and were adjusted to stabilize the estimation scheme.

3 Results

The state estimates from the Kalman filter were propagated through the forward model to calculate the component of the measurements that relates to each input. An example result of this signal separation for the 890 nm measurement from detector 1 is shown in figure 1. The functional response to the stimulus only accounts for 2.8% of the variance in the measurement whereas BP and HRV account for 11.3% and 77.9% respectively. The sum of the modeled components accounts for over 99.9% of the variance in the measurement.

The results of the static deconvolution analysis to recover the functional hemodynamic response is shown in figure 2. The functional responses are clearly present in the estimates but are distorted by large physiological noise artifacts. Compared to the true hemodynamics, the HbO estimate resulted in $R^2 = 0.78$, which is reasonably good considering that the physiological noise dominates the measurement. For the smaller HbR signal, $R^2 = 0.57$ with the true hemodynam-

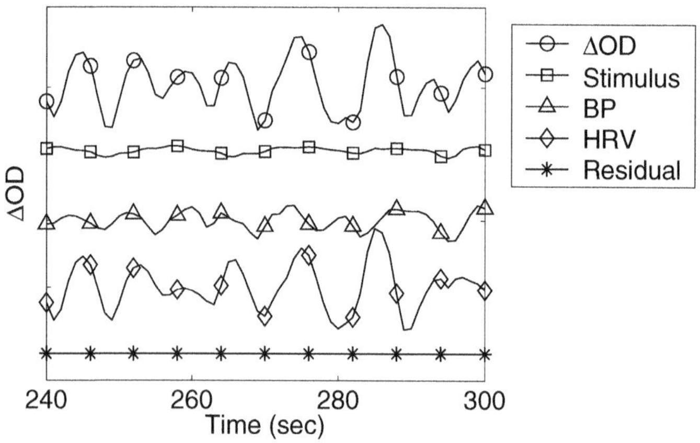

Fig. 1. Separating a ΔOD measurement into components related to each model input. The scale for each component of ΔOD was shifted for visual comparison.

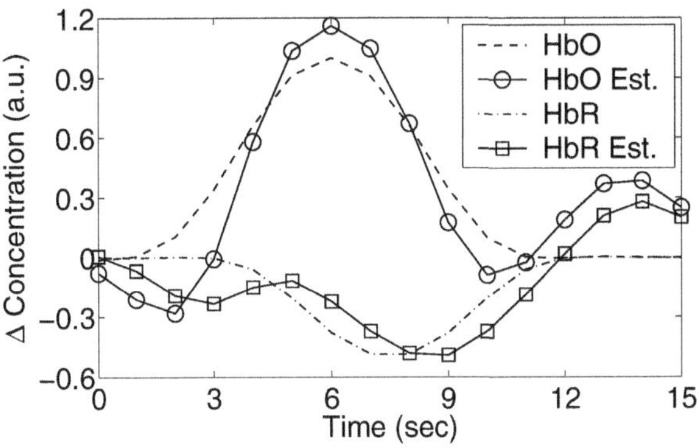

Fig. 2. Result for deconvolution of functional response from hemodynamics in voxel 2

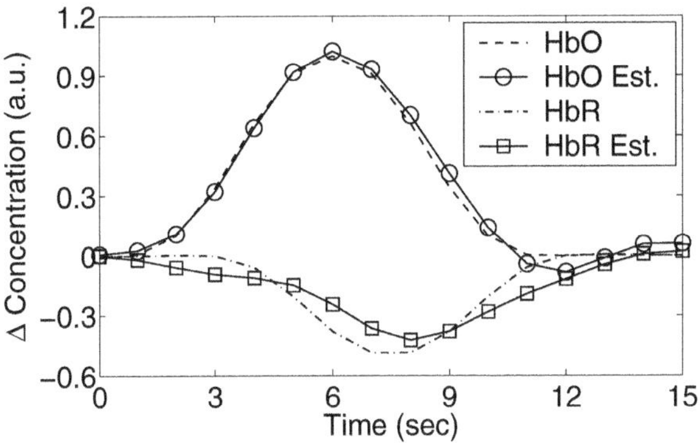

Fig. 3. Result for proposed Kalman filter estimate functional response in voxel 2

ics, indicating that the physiological noise artifacts are of comparable magnitude to the actual response.

The result for the Kalman filter was taken to be the last state estimate computed during a forward pass through the data. This result, shown in figure 3, appears to be a significant improvement over the deconvolution approach. The HbO estimate improved to $R^2 = 0.99$ and the HbR estimate jumped to $R^2 = 0.89$. There is some lag in the Kalman filter result which may have been caused by only using a forward pass through the data.

4 Discussion

We successfully implemented the Kalman filter for system identification in DOT. Based on the preliminary results described, the proposed analysis framework may help to improve estimates of functional hemodynamics in DOT neuroimaging. This result is potentially significant because improved hemodynamic estimates could make a broader range of brain activation paradigms possible with DOT.

The ability to separate signals into physiological components may also reveal new information about the local regulatory physiology and may be useful in identifying certain vascular pathologies. Unlike the prior work with the Kalman filter for DOT, the present formulation has the flexibility to be applied to any experimental design and for problems of reasonably large spatial and temporal dimension. The proposed Kalman filter formulation may also be useful for other imaging modalities such as fMRI, MEG and EEG or when multiple modalities are combined with a single state-space model of the underlying physiology.

References

1. A.P. Gibson, J.H., Arridge, S.: Recent advances in diffuse optical imaging. Phys. Med. Biol. **50** (2005) R1–R43
2. Strangman, G., Culver, J., Thompson, J., Boas, D.: A quantitative comparison of simultaneous bold fMRI and NIRS recordings during functional brain activation. NeuroImage **17** (2002) 719–731
3. Kolehmainen, V., Prince, S., Arridge, S., Kaipio, J.: State-estimation approach to the nonstationary optical tomography problem. J. Opt. Soc. Am. A **20** (2003) 876–889
4. Prince, S., Kolehmainen, V., Kaipio, J., Franceschini, M., Boas, D., Arridge, S.: Time-series estimation of biological factors in optical diffusion tomography. Phys. Med. Biol. **48** (2003) 1491–1504
5. Zhang, Y., Brooks, D., Franceschini, M., Boas, D.: Eigenvector-based spatial filtering for reduction of physiological interference in diffuse optical imaging. Journal of Biomedical Optics **10** (2005) 011014–1–11
6. Cohen, M.A., Taylor, J.A.: Short-term cardiovascular oscillations in man: measuring and modelling the physiologies. Journal of Physiology **542.3** (2002) 669–683
7. Frackowiak, R., Friston, K., Frith, C., Dolan, R., Price, C., Zeki, S., Ashburner, J., Penny, W., eds.: Human Brain Function. 2nd edn. Academic Press (2003)
8. Roche, A., Pinel, P., Dehaene, S., Poline, J.: Solving incrementally the fitting and detection problems in fMRI time series. Medical Image Computing and Computer-Assisted Intervention (MICCAI'04), Part 2, Lecture Notes in Computer Science **3217** (2004) 719–726
9. Kalman, R.: A new approach to linear filtering and prediction problems. Trans. of the ASME–Journal of Basic Engineering **82** (1960) 35–45
10. Arridge, S., Cope, M., Delpy, D.: The theoretical basis for the determination of optical pathlengths in tissue: temporal and frequency analysis. Phys. Med. Biol. **37** (1992) 1531–1560
11. Franceschini, M., Fantini, S., Thompson, J., Culver, J., Boas, D.: Hemodynamic evoked response of the sensorimotor cortex measured non-invasively with near-infrared optical imaging. Psychophysiology **40** (2003) 548–560

Brain Surface Parameterization Using Riemann Surface Structure

Yalin Wang[1], Xianfeng Gu[2], Kiralee M. Hayashi[3], Tony F. Chan[1], Paul M. Thompson[3], and Shing-Tung Yau[4]

[1] Mathematics Department, UCLA, Los Angeles, CA 90095, USA
[2] Comp. Sci. Department, SUNY at Stony Brook, Stony Brook, NY 11794, USA
[3] Lab. of Neuro Imaging, UCLA School of Medicine, Los Angeles, CA 90095, USA
[4] Department of Mathematics, Harvard University, Cambridge, MA 02138, USA
{ylwang, chan}@math.ucla.edu, gu@cs.sunysb.edu,
{khayashi, thompson}@loni.ucla.edu, yau@math.harvard.edu

Abstract. We develop a general approach that uses holomorphic 1-forms to parameterize anatomical surfaces with complex (possibly branching) topology. Rather than evolve the surface geometry to a plane or sphere, we instead use the fact that all orientable surfaces are Riemann surfaces and admit conformal structures, which induce special curvilinear coordinate systems on the surfaces. Based on Riemann surface structure, we can then canonically partition the surface into patches. Each of these patches can be conformally mapped to a parallelogram. The resulting surface subdivision and the parameterizations of the components are intrinsic and stable. To illustrate the technique, we computed conformal structures for several types of anatomical surfaces in MRI scans of the brain, including the cortex, hippocampus, and lateral ventricles. We found that the resulting parameterizations were consistent across subjects, even for branching structures such as the ventricles, which are otherwise difficult to parameterize. Compared with other variational approaches based on surface inflation, our technique works on surfaces with arbitrary complexity while guaranteeing minimal distortion in the parameterization. It also offers a way to explicitly match landmark curves in anatomical surfaces such as the cortex, providing a surface-based framework to compare anatomy statistically and to generate grids on surfaces for PDE-based signal processing.

1 Introduction

In brain imaging research, parameterization of various types of anatomical surface models in magnetic resonance imaging (MRI) scans of the brain involves computing a smooth (differentiable) one-to-one mapping of regular 2D coordinate grids onto the 3D surfaces, so that numerical quantities can be computed easily from the resulting models [1,2]. Even so, it is often difficult to smoothly deform a complex 3D surface to a sphere or 2D plane without substantial angular or area distortion. Here we present a new method to parameterize brain surfaces based on their Riemann surface structure. By contrast with variational

J. Duncan and G. Gerig (Eds.): MICCAI 2005, LNCS 3750, pp. 657–665, 2005.

approaches based on surface inflation, our method can parameterize surfaces with arbitrary complexity including branching surfaces not topologically homeomorphic to a sphere (higher-genus objects) while formally guaranteeing minimal distortion.

1.1 Previous Work

Brain surface parameterization has been studied intensively. Schwartz et al. [3], and Timsari and Leahy [4] compute quasi-isometric flat maps of the cerebral cortex. Hurdal and Stephenson [5] report a discrete mapping approach that uses circle packings to produce "flattened" images of cortical surfaces on the sphere, the Euclidean plane, and the hyperbolic plane. Angenent et al. [6] represent the Laplace-Beltrami operator as a linear system and implement a finite element approximation for parameterizing brain surfaces via conformal mapping. Gu et al. [7] propose a method to find a unique conformal mapping between any two genus zero manifolds by minimizing the harmonic energy of the map.

1.2 Theoretical Background and Definitions

We begin with some formal definitions that will help to formulate the parameterization problem(for further reading, please refer to [8]). For a manifold M with an atlas $\mathcal{A} = \{U_\alpha, \phi_\alpha\}$, if all chart transition functions $\phi_{\alpha\beta} = \phi_\beta \circ \phi_\alpha^{-1} : \phi_\alpha(U_\alpha \cap U_\beta) \to \phi_\beta(U_\alpha \cap U_\beta)$ are holomorphic, $\mathcal{A}$ is a conformal atlas for M. A chart $\{U'_\alpha, \phi'_\alpha\}$ is *compatible* with an atlas $\mathcal{A}$, if the union $\mathcal{A} \cup \{U'_\alpha, \phi'_\alpha\}$ is still a conformal atlas. Each conformal compatible equivalence class is a conformal structure. A 2-manifold with a conformal structure is called a *Riemann surface.* It has been proven that all metric orientable surfaces are Riemann surfaces.

Holomorphic and meromorphic functions and differential forms can be generalized to Riemann surfaces by using the notion of conformal structure. For example, a *holomorphic one-form* ω is a complex differential form, such that in each local frame $z_\alpha = (u_\alpha, v_\alpha)$, the parametric representation is $\omega = f(z_\alpha)dz_\alpha$, where $f(z_\alpha)$ is a holomorphic function. On a different chart $\{U_\beta, \phi_\beta\}$, $\omega = f(z_\alpha(z_\beta))\frac{dz_\alpha}{dz_\beta}dz_\beta$. For a genus g closed surface, all holomorphic one-forms form a real $2g$ dimensional linear space.

At a *zero point* $p \in M$ of a holomorphic one-form ω, any local parametric representation $\omega = f(z_\alpha)dz_\alpha, f|_p = 0$. According to the Riemann-Roch theorem, in general there are $2g - 2$ zero points for a holomorphic one-form defined on a surface of genus g.

A holomorphic one-form induces a special system of curves on a surface, the so-called *conformal net.* A curve $\gamma \subset M$ is called a horizontal trajectory of ω, if $\omega^2(d\gamma) \geq 0$; similarly, γ is a vertical trajectory if $\omega^2(d\gamma) < 0$. The horizontal and vertical trajectories form a web on the surface. The trajectories that connect zero points, or a zero point with the boundary are called *critical trajectories.* The critical horizontal trajectories form a graph, which is called the *critical graph.* In general, the behavior of a trajectory may be very complicated, it may have infinite length and may be dense on the surface. If the critical graph is finite, then all the horizontal trajectories are finite. The critical graph partitions the surface into a set of non-overlapping patches that jointly cover the surface, and each patch is either a topological disk or a topological cylinder. Each patch $\Omega \subset M$ can be mapped to the complex plane using the following formulae. Suppose we pick a base point $p_0 \in \Omega$, and any path γ that connects p_0 to p. Then if we define $\phi(p) = \int_\gamma \omega$, the map ϕ is conformal, and $\phi(\Omega)$ is a parallelogram. We say ϕ is the conformal parameterization of M induced by ω. ϕ maps the vertical and the horizontal trajectories to iso-u and iso-v curves respectively on the parameter plane. The structure of the critical graph and the parameterizations of the patches are determined by the conformal structure of the surface. If two surfaces share similar topologies and geometries, they can support consistent critical graphs and segmentations (i.e. surface partitions), and the parameterizations are consistent as well. Therefore, by matching their parameter domains, the entire surfaces can be directly matched in 3D. This generalizes prior work in medical imaging that has matched surfaces by computing a smooth bijection to a single canonical surface, such as a sphere or disk.

This paper takes the advantage of conformal structures of surfaces, consistently segments them and parameterizes the patches using a holomorphic 1-form. We call this process - i.e., finding a critical graph and partitioning the surface into conformally parameterized patches - the *holomorphic flow segmentation*. This parameterization and partitioning of the surface is completely determined by the surface geometry and the choice of the holomorphic 1-form. (Note that this differs from the typical meaning of segmentation in medical imaging, and is concerned with the segmentation, or partitioning, of a general surface, rather than classification of voxels in an image). Computing holomorphic 1-forms is equivalent to solving elliptic differential equations on surfaces, and in general, elliptic differential operators are stable. Therefore the resulting surface segmentations and parameterizations are intrinsic and stable, and are applicable for matching noisy surfaces derived from medical images.

2 Holomorphic Flow Segmentation

To compute the holomorphic flow segmentation of a surface, first we compute the conformal structure of the surface; then we select one holomorphic differential form, and locate the zero points on it. By tracing horizontal trajectories through the zero points, the critical graph can be constructed and the surface is divided into several patches. Each patch can then be conformally mapped to a planar parallelogram by integrating the holomorphic differential form.

In our work, surfaces are represented as triangular meshes, namely piecewise polygonal surfaces.The computations with differential forms are based on solving elliptic partial differential equations on surfaces using the finite element method.

2.1 Conformal Structures Computation

A method to compute the conformal structure of a surface was introduced in [9]. Suppose M is a closed genus $g > 0$ surface with a conformal atlas $\mathcal{A}$. The conformal structure $\mathcal{A}$ induces holomorphic 1-forms; all holomorphic 1-forms form a linear space $\Omega(M)$ of dimension $2g$ which is isomorphic to the first cohomology group of the surface $H^1(M, \mathcal{R})$. The set of holomorphic one-forms determines the conformal structure.

2.2 Canonical Conformal Parameterization Computation

Given a Riemann surface M, there are infinitely many holomorphic 1-forms, but each of them can be expressed as a linear combination of the basis elements. We define a canonical conformal parameterization as any linear combination of the set of holomorphic basis functions ω_i, $i = 1, ..., g$. They satisfy $\int_{\varsigma_i} \omega_j = \delta_i^j$, where $\zeta_i, i = 1, ...n$ are homology bases and δ_i^j is the Kronecker symbol. Then we compute a *canonical conformal parameterization* $\omega = \sum_{i=1}^{n} \omega_i$.

2.3 Zero Points Location

For surface with genus $g > 1$, any holomorphic 1-form ω has $2g - 2$ zero points. The horizontal trajectories through the zero points will partition the surface into several patches. Each patch is either a topological disk or a cylinder, and can be conformally parameterized by ω using $\phi(p) = \int_\gamma \omega$.

Estimating the Conformal Factor. Suppose we already have a global conformal parameterization, induced by a holomorphic 1-form ω. Then we can estimate the conformal factor at each vertex, using the following formulae: $\lambda(v) = \frac{1}{n} \sum_{[u,v] \in K_1} \frac{|\omega([u,v])|^2}{|r(u)-r(v)|^2}, u, v \in K_0$, where n is the valence of vertex v.

Locating Zero Points. We find the cluster of vertices with relatively small conformal factors (the lowest $5 - 6\%$). These are candidates for zero points. We cluster all the candidates using the metric on the surface. For each cluster, we pick the vertex that is closest to the center of gravity of the cluster, using the surface metric to define geodesic distances.

2.4 Holomorphic Flow Segmentation

Tracing Horizontal Trajectories. Once the zero points are located, the horizontal trajectories through them can be traced. First we choose a neighborhood U_v of a vertex v representing a zero point, U_v is a set of neighboring faces of v, then we map it to the parameter plane by integrating ω. Suppose a vertex $w \in U_v$, and a path composed by a sequence of edges on the mesh is γ, then the parameter location of w is $\phi(w) = \int_\gamma \omega$.

The map $\phi(w)$ is a piecewise linear map. Then the horizontal trajectory is mapped to the horizontal line $y = 0$ in the plane. We slice $\phi(U_v)$ using the line $y = 0$ by edge splitting operations. Suppose the boundary of $\phi(U_v)$ intersects $y = 0$ at a point v', then we choose a neighborhood of v' and repeat the process. Each time we extend the horizontal trajectory and encounter edges intersecting the trajectory, we insert new vertices at the intersection points, until the trajectory reaches another zero point or the boundary of the mesh. We repeat the tracing process until each zero point connects 4 horizontal trajectories.

Critical Graph. Given a surface M and a holomorphic 1-form ω on M, we define the graph $G(M, \omega) = \{V, E, F\}$, as the critical graph of ω. Here V is the set of zero points of ω, E is the set of horizontal trajectories connecting zero points or the boundary segments of M, and F is the set of surface patches segmented by E.

Given two surfaces with similar topologies and geometries, by choosing appropriate holomorphic 1-forms, we can obtain isomorphic critical graphs, which will be used for patch-matching described in the next section.

3 Experimental Results

We tested our algorithm on various anatomic surfaces extracted from 3D MRI scans of the brain to illustrate the approach.

Figure 1 (a)-(d) shows experimental results for a hippocampal surface, a structure in the medial temporal lobe of the brain. The original surface is shown in (a). (b) shows the conformal mapping of (a) to a sphere with a variational method introduced in [7]. Since the shape of hippocampal surface is not quite similar to a sphere, lots of distortion has been introduced. In our method, we leave two holes on the front and back of the hippocampal surface, representing its anterior junction with the amygdala, and its posterior limit as it turns into the white matter of the fornix. It can be logically represented as an open boundary genus one surface, a cylinder (note that spherical harmonic representations would also be possible, if the ends were closed). The computed conformal structure is shown in (c). Then we can conformally map the hippocampus to a rectangle (d). Since the surface of rectangle is similar to the one of hippocampus, the detailed surface information is well preserved in (d). Compared with other spherical parameterization methods (e.g. (b)), which may have high-valence nodes and dense tiles at the poles of the spherical coordinate system, our parameterization can represent the surface with minimal distortion.

Shape analysis of the lateral ventricles is of great interest in the study of psychiatric illnesses, including schizophrenia, and in degenerative diseases such as Alzheimer's disease. These structures are often enlarged in disease and can provide sensitive measures of disease progression. We can optimize the conformal parameterization by topology modification. For the lateral ventricle surface in each brain hemisphere, we introduce five cuts. Since these cutting positions are at the end of the frontal, occipital, and temporal horns of the ventricles, they can potentially be located automatically. The second row in Figure 1 shows 5 cuts introduced on three subjects ventricular surfaces. After the cutting, the surfaces become open boundary genus 4 surfaces.

Figure 1 (e)-(g) show parameterizations of the lateral ventricles of the brain. (e) shows the results of parameterizing a ventricular surface for a 65-year-old patient with HIV/AIDS (note the disease-related enlargement), (f) the results for the ventricular model of a 21-year-old control subject, and (g) the results for a 28-year-old control subject. The surfaces are initially generated by using an unsupervised tissue classifier to isolate a binary map of the cerebrospinal fluid in

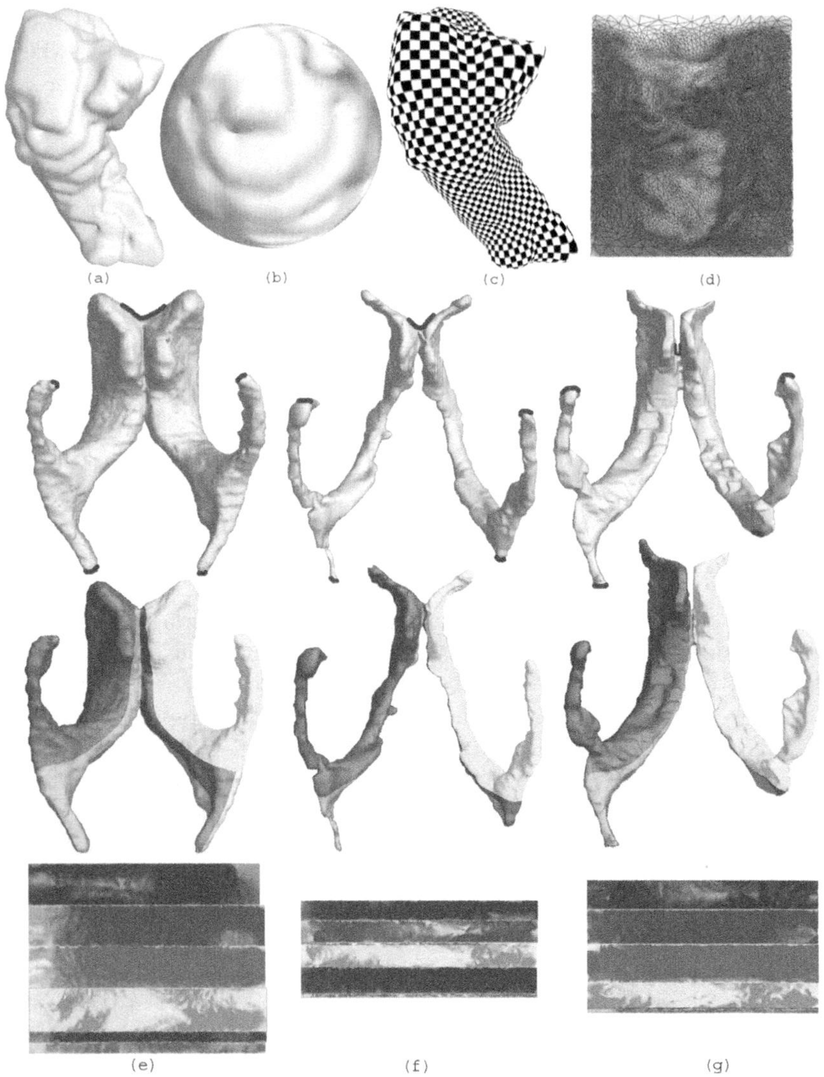

Fig. 1. Illustrates surface parameterization results for the hippocampal surface and the lateral ventricles. (a) is the original hippocampal surface; (b) the result of inflation of surface (a) to a sphere; (c) the computed conformal structure; and (d) the rectangle that (a) is conformally mapped to. The second row shows how 5 cuts are introduced; they convert the lateral ventricle surface into a genus 4 surface. (e)-(g) show models parameterized using holomorphic 1-forms, for a 65-year- old subject with HIV/AIDS, a healthy 21-year-old subject and a second healthy 28-year-old subject, respectively. The computed holomorphic flow segmentations and their associated sets of rectangular parameter domains are shown (the texture mapped into the parameter domain here simply corresponds to the intensity of the surface rendering, which is based on the surface normals).

the MR image, and tiling the surface of the largest connected component inside the brain. Based on the computed conformal structure, we can partition the surface into 6 patches. Each patch can be conformally mapped to a rectangle. Although the three brain ventricle shapes are very different, the segmentation results are consistent in that the surfaces are partitioned into patches with the same relative arrangement and connectivity. Thus our method provides a way for direct surface matching between any two ventricles.

For the surface of the cerebral cortex, our algorithm also provides a way to perform surface matching, while explicitly matching sulcal curves or other landmarks lying in the surface. Note that typically two surfaces can be matched by using a landmark-driven flow in their parameter spaces. An alternative approach is to supplement the critical graph with curved landmarks that can then

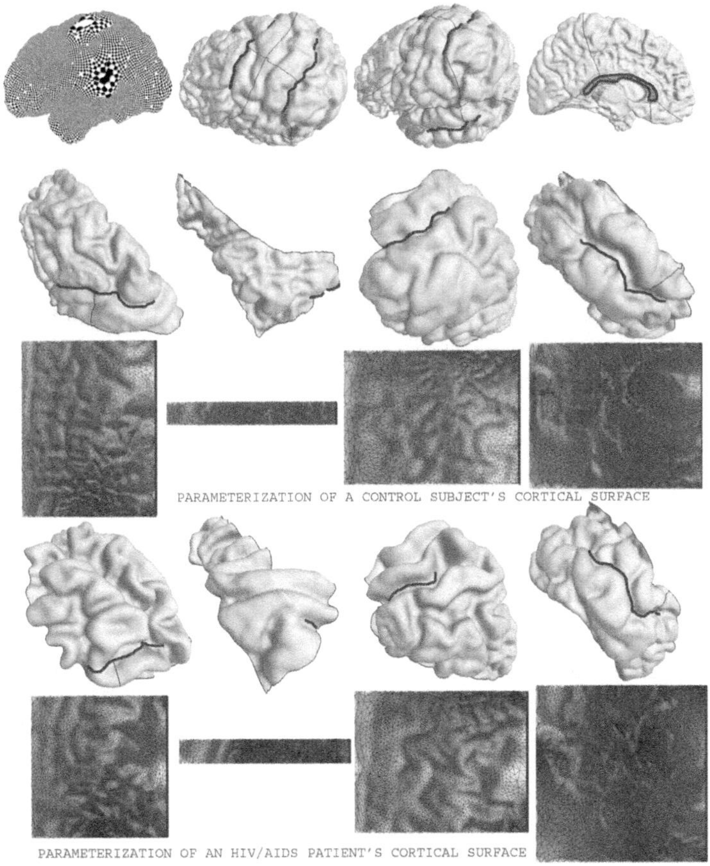

Fig. 2. Illustrates the parameterization of cortical surfaces using the holomorphic 1-form approach. The thick lines are landmark curves, including several major sulci lying in the cortical surface. These sulcal curves are always mapped to a boundary in the parameter space images.

be forced to lie on the boundaries of rectangles in the parameter space. This has the advantage that conformal grids are still available on both surfaces, as is a correspondence field between the two conformal grids. Figure 2 shows the results for the cortical surfaces of two left hemispheres. As shown in the first row, we selected four major landmark curves, for the purpose of illustrating the approach (thick lines show the precental and postcentral sulci, and the superior temporal sulcus, and the perimeter of the corpus callosum at the midsagittal plane). By cutting the surface along the landmark curves, we obtain a genus 3 open boundary surface. There are therefore two zero points (observable as a large white region and black region in the conformal grid; an illustration of the conformal structure is shown in the first panel the first row). We show cortical surfaces from two different subjects in Figure 2 (these are extracted using a deformable surface approach, but are subsequently reparameterized using holomorphic 1-forms). The second and fourth rows show the segmented patches for each cortical surface. The rectangles that these patches conformally map to are shown on the third and fifth row, respectively. Since the landmark curves lie on the boundaries of the surface patches, they can be forced to lie on an iso-parameter curve and can be constrained to map to rectangle boundaries in the parameter domain. Although the two cortex surfaces are different, the selected sulcal curves are mapped to the rectangle boundaries in the parameter domain. This method therefore provides a way to warp between two anatomical surfaces while exactly matching an arbitrary number of landmark curves lying in the surfaces. This is applicable to tracking brain growth or degeneration in serial scans, and composite maps of the cortex can be made by invoking the consistent parameterizations. Lamecker et al's work [10] has the similar motivation as ours for the cortex case, which is to partition a surface into canonical patches and parameterize the patches with minimal distortion. However, our partition method is based on intrinsic Riemann surface structure and theirs is based on shortest paths along lines of high curvature. Thus our method is global and more stable.

4 Conclusion and Future Work

In this paper, we presented a brain surface parameterization method that invokes the Riemann surface structure to generate conformal grids on surfaces of arbitrary complexity (including branching topologies). We tested our algorithm on the hippocampus, lateral ventricle surfaces and on surface models of the cerebral cortex. The grid generation algorithm is intrinsic (i.e. does not depend on any initial choice of surface coordinates) and is stable, as shown by grids induced on ventricles of various shapes and sizes. Compared with other work conformally mapping brain surfaces to sphere, our work may introduce less distortion and may be especially convenient for other post-processing work such as surface registration and landmark matching. Our future work include automatic location of cutting positions and more experiments on disease assessment.

References

1. Thompson, P., et al. Nature **404** (2000) 190–193
2. Thompson, P., et al. In: Human Brain Mapping. Volume 9. (2000) 81–92
3. Schwartz, E., et al. IEEE PAMI **11** (1989) 1005–1008
4. Timsari, B., Leahy, R. In Hanson, K., ed.: Proc. SPIE, Medical Imaging. Volume 3979. (2000) 698–708
5. Hurdal, M.K., Stephenson, K. NeuroImage **23** (2004) S119–S128
6. Angenent, S., et al. MICCAI (1999) 271–278
7. Gu, X., et al. IEEE TMI **23** (2004) 949–958
8. Schoen, R., Yau, S.T.: Lectures on Harmonic Maps. International Press (1997)
9. Gu, X., Yau, S.T. Communication of Information and Systems **2** (2002) 121–146
10. Lamecker, H., et al. In: MICCAI, Springer (2002) 422–427

Automated Surface Matching Using Mutual Information Applied to Riemann Surface Structures

Yalin Wang[1], Ming-Chang Chiang[2], and Paul M. Thompson[2]

[1] Mathematics Department, UCLA, Los Angeles, CA 90095, USA
[2] Lab. of Neuro Imaging, UCLA School of Medicine, Los Angeles, CA 90095, USA
ylwang@math.ucla.edu, mcchiang@ucla.edu, thompson@loni.ucla.edu

Abstract. Many medical imaging applications require the computation of dense correspondence vector fields that match one surface with another. To avoid the need for a large set of manually-defined landmarks to constrain these surface correspondences, we developed an algorithm to automate the matching of surface features. It extends the mutual information method to automatically match general 3D surfaces (including surfaces with a branching topology). First, we use holomorphic 1-forms to induce consistent conformal grids on both surfaces. High genus surfaces are mapped to a set of rectangles in the Euclidean plane, and closed genus-zero surfaces are mapped to the sphere. Mutual information is used as a cost functional to drive a fluid flow in the parameter domain that optimally aligns stable geometric features (mean curvature and the conformal factor) in the 2D parameter domains. A diffeomorphic surface-to-surface mapping is then recovered that matches anatomy in 3D. We also present a spectral method that ensures that the grids induced on the target surface remain conformal when pulled through the correspondence field. Using the chain rule, we express the gradient of the mutual information between surfaces in the conformal basis of the source surface. This finite-dimensional linear space generates all conformal reparameterizations of the surface. We apply the method to hippocampal surface registration, a key step in subcortical shape analysis in Alzheimer's disease and schizophrenia.

1 Introduction

In computational anatomy, surface-based computations are used to statistically combine or compare 3D anatomical models across subjects, or map functional imaging parameters onto anatomical surfaces. When comparing data on two anatomical surfaces, a correspondence field must be computed to register one surface nonlinearly onto the other. Multiple surfaces can be registered nonlinearly to construct a mean shape for a group of subjects, and deformation mappings can encode shape variations around the mean. This type of deformable surface registration has been used to detect developmental and disease effects on

J. Duncan and G. Gerig (Eds.): MICCAI 2005, LNCS 3750, pp. 666–674, 2005.

brain structures such as the corpus callosum and basal ganglia [1], the hippocampus [2], and the cortex [3]. Nonlinear matching of brain surfaces can also be used to track the progression of neurodegenerative disorders such as Alzheimer's disease [2], to measure brain growth in development [1], and to reveal directional biases in gyral pattern variability [4].

Surface registration has numerous applications, but a direct mapping between two 3D surfaces is challenging to compute. Often, higher order correspondences must be enforced between specific anatomical points, curved landmarks, or subregions lying within the two surfaces. This is often achieved by first mapping each of the 3D surfaces to canonical parameter spaces such as a sphere [5,6] or a planar domain [7]. A flow, computed in the parameter space of the two surfaces [1,8], then induces a correspondence field in 3D. This flow can be constrained using anatomic landmark points or curves, or by constraining the mapping of surface regions represented implicitly using level sets [7]. Feature correspondence between two surfaces can be optimized by using the L^2-norm to measure differences in convexity [5]. Artificial neural networks can rule out or favor certain types of feature matches [9]. Finally, correspondences may be determined by using a minimum description length (MDL) principle, based on the compactness of the covariance of the resulting shape model [10]. Anatomically homologous points can then be forced to match across a dataset. Thodberg [11] identified problems with early MDL approaches and extended them to an MDL appearance model, when performing unsupervised image segmentation.

By the Riemann uniformization theorem, all surfaces can be conformally embedded in a sphere, a plane or a hyperbolic space. The resulting embeddings form special groups. Using holomorphic 1-forms and critical graphs, global conformal parameterization [12] can be used to conformally map any high genus surface (i.e., a surface with branching topology) to a set of rectangular domains in the Euclidean plane. In this paper, we use conformal parameterizations to help match arbitrary 3D anatomical surfaces. Mutual information is used to drive a diffeomorphic fluid flow that is adjusted to find appropriate surface correspondences in the parameter domain. We chose the mean curvature and the conformal factor of the surfaces as the differential geometric features to be aligned in this study as they are intrinsic and stable. These choices are illustrative - any scalar fields defined on the surfaces could be matched, e.g. cortical thickness maps, functional imaging signals or metabolic data. Since conformal mapping and fluid registration techniques generate diffeomorphic mappings, the 3D shape correspondence established by composing these mappings is also diffeomorphic (i.e., provides smooth one-to-one correspondences).

2 Theoretical Background and Definitions

Due to space limitations, here we list some formal definitions that help describe our approach, without detailed explanation. For further reading, please refer to [13] and [14].

2.1 Surface Parameterization with Riemann Surface Structure

An *atlas* is a collection of consistent coordinate charts on a manifold, where transition functions between overlapping coordinate charts are smooth. We treat R^2 as isomorphic to the complex plane. Let S be a surface in $\mathbb{R}^3$ with an atlas $\{(U_\alpha, z_\alpha)\}$, where (U_α, z_α) is a chart, and $z_\alpha : U_\alpha \to \mathbb{C}$ maps an open set $U_\alpha \subset S$ to the complex plane $\mathbb{C}$. An atlas is called *conformal* if **(1).** each chart (U_α, z_α) is a conformal chart. Namely, on each chart, the first fundamental form can be formulated as $ds^2 = \lambda(z_\alpha)^2 dz_\alpha d\bar{z_\alpha}$; **(2).** the transition maps $z_\beta \circ z_\alpha^{-1} : z_\alpha(U_\alpha \cap U_\beta) \to z_\beta(U_\alpha \cap U_\beta)$ are holomorphic.

A chart is *compatible* with a given conformal atlas if adding it to the atlas again yields a conformal atlas. A *conformal structure* (*Riemann surface structure*) is obtained by adding all compatible charts to a conformal atlas. A *Riemann surface* is a surface with a conformal structure. It has been proven that all metric orientable surfaces are Riemann Surfaces.

One coordinate chart in the conformal structure introduces a *conformal parameterization* between a surface patch and the image plane. The conformal parameterization is angle-preserving and intrinsic to the geometry.

The surface conformal structure induces special curvilinear coordinate system on the surfaces. Based on a global conformal structure, a critical graph can be recovered that connects zero points in the conformal structure and partitions a surface into patches. Each of these patches can be conformally mapped to a parallelogram by integrating a holomorphic 1-form defined on the surface. Figure 1(a)-(c) show an example of the conformal parameterization of a lateral ventricle surface of a 65-year-old HIV/AIDS patient. The conformal structure of

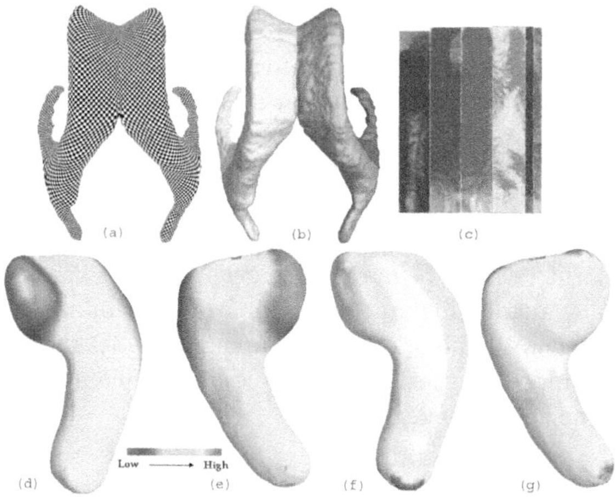

Fig. 1. Illustrates conformal surface parameterization. (a) - (c) illustrate conformal parameterizations of ventricular surfaces in the brain for a 65-year-old HIV/AIDS patient. (d)-(g) show the computed conformal factor and mean curvature on a hippocampal surface, (d)-(e) are two views of the hippocampal surface, colored according to conformal factor; (f)-(g) are two views of the hippocampal surface, colored according to mean curvature.

the ventricular surface is shown in (a). (b) shows a partition of the ventricular surface, where each segment is labeled by a unique color. (c) shows the parameterization domain, where each rectangle is the image, in the parameterization domain, of a surface component in (b).

For a Riemann surface S with genus $g > 0$, all holomorphic 1-forms on S form a complex g-dimensional vector space ($2g$ real dimensions), denoted by $\Omega^1(S)$. The conformal structure of a higher genus surface can always be represented in terms of a holomorphic one-form basis, which is a set of $2g$ functions $\omega_i : K_1 \rightarrow R^2, i = 1, 2 \cdots, 2g$. Any holomorphic one-form ω is a linear combination of these functions. The quality of a global conformal parameterization for a high genus surface is fundamentally determined by the choice of the holomorphic 1-form.

2.2 Conformal Representation of a General Surface

For a general surface S, we can compute conformal coordinates (u, v) to parameterize S. Based on these coordinates, one can derive scalar fields including the conformal factor, $\lambda(u, v)$, and mean curvature, $H(u, v)$, of the surface position vector $S(u, v)$: $\frac{\partial S}{\partial u} \times \frac{\partial S}{\partial v} = \lambda(u, v) n(u, v)$, and $H(u, v) = |\frac{1}{\lambda^2(u,v)}(\frac{\partial^2}{\partial u^2} + \frac{\partial^2}{\partial v^2}) r(u, v)|$. From the theorem [15], we can regard the tuple (λ, H) as the conformal representation of $S(u, v)$.

Clearly, various fields of scalars or tuples could be used to represent surfaces in the parameter domain. Because the conformal structure is intrinsic and independent of the data resolution and triangulation, we use the conformal representation, $\lambda(u, v)$ and $H(u, v)$, to represent the 3D surfaces. This representation is stable and computationally efficient. Figure 1 (d)-(g) shows the conformal factor((d) and (e)), and mean curvature((f) and (g)), indexed in color on a hippocampal surface.

2.3 Mutual Information (MI) for Surface Registration

We now describe the mutual information functional used to drive the scalar fields $\lambda(u, v)$ and $H(u, v)$ into correspondence, effectively using the equivalent of a 2D image registration in the surface parameter space (i.e., in conformal coordinates). Let I_1 and I_2 be the target and the deforming template images respectively, and $I_1, I_2 : R^2 \rightarrow R$. Let $\Omega \subset R^2$ be the common parameter domain of both surfaces (if both are rectangular, the target parameter domain is first matched to the source parameter domain using a 2D diagonal matrix). Also, let u be a deformation vector field on Ω. The MI of the scalar fields (treated as 2D images) between the two surfaces is defined by $I(u) = \int_{R^2} p_u(i_1, i_2) log \frac{p_u(i_1, i_2)}{p(i_1) p_u(i_2)} di_1 di_2$. where $p(i_1) = P(I_1(x) = i_1)$, $p_u(i_2) = P(I_2(x - u) = i_2)$ and $p_u(i_1, i_2) = P(I_1(x)) = i_1$ and $I_2(x - u) = i_2$.

We adopted the framework of D'Agostino et al. [16] to maximize MI with viscous fluid regularization. Briefly, the deforming template image was treated as embedded in a compressible viscous fluid governed by Navier-Stokes equation for conservation of momentum [17], simplified to a linear PDE:

$$Lv = \mu \nabla^2 v + (\lambda + \mu) \nabla (\nabla \cdot v) + F(x, u) = 0 \quad (1)$$

Here v is the deformation velocity, and μ and λ are the viscosity constants. Following [16], we take the first variation of $I(u)$ with respect to u, and use the Parzen window method [18] to estimate the joint probability density function (pdf) $p_u(i_1, i_2)$.

3 The Surface Mutual Information Method for an Arbitrary Genus Surface

To match two high genus surfaces (i.e., surfaces with the same branching topology), we apply our surface mutual information method piecewise. First, we compute conformal representations of the two surfaces based on a global conformal parameterization. [1] These conformal representations are aligned with mutual information driven flows, while enforcing constraints to guarantee that the vector-valued flow is continuous at the patch boundaries. [2] When the chain rule is used, we can further optimize the mutual information matching results by optimizing the underlying global conformal parameterization.

Let S_1 and S_2 be two surfaces we want to match and the conformal parameterization of S_1 is τ_1, conformal parameterization for S_2 is τ_2, $\tau_1(S_1)$ and $\tau_2(S_2)$ are rectangles in R^2. Instead of finding the mapping ϕ from S_1 to S_2 directly, we can use mutual information method to find a diffeomorphism $\tau : D_1 \to D_2$, such that: $\tau_2^{-1} \circ \tau \circ \tau_1 = \phi$. Then the map ϕ can be obtained from $\phi = \tau_1 \circ \tau \circ \tau_2^{-1}$. Because τ_1, τ and τ_2 are all diffeomorphisms, ϕ is also a diffeomorphism.

3.1 Mutual Information Contained in Maps Between High Genus Surfaces

A global conformal parameterization for a high genus surface can be obtained by integrating a holomorphic one-form ω. Suppose $\{\omega_i, i = 1, 2, \cdots, 2g\}$ is a holomorphic 1-form basis, where an arbitrary holomorphic 1-form has the formula

[1] Several variational or PDE-based methods have been proposed to match surfaces represented by parametric meshes [5], level sets, or both [7]. Gu et al. [19] found a unique conformal mapping between any two genus zero manifolds by minimizing the harmonic energy of the map. Gu and Vemuri [20] also matched genus-zero closed 3D shapes by first conformally mapping them to a canonical domain and aligning their 2D representations over the class of diffeomorphisms.

[2] The mutual information method [14] measures the statistical dependence of the voxel intensities between two images. Parameters of a registration transform can be tuned so that MI is maximal when the two images are optimally aligned. The MI method has been successful for rigid [21] and non-rigid [22,23] image registration. Here, we generalize it to match 3D surfaces. For MI to work, a monotonic mapping in grayscales between images is not required, so images from different modalities can be registered [24]. Hermosillo et al. [25] adopted linear elasticity theory to regularize the variational maximization of MI. D'Agostino et al. [16] extended this approach to a viscous fluid scheme allowing large local deformations, while maintaining smooth, one-to-one topology [17].

$\omega = \sum_{i=1}^{2g} \lambda_i \omega_i$. Assuming the target surface's parameterization is fixed, the mutual information between it and the source surface's parameterization is denoted $E(\omega)$, which is a function of the linear combination of coefficients λ_i. A necessary condition for the optimal holomorphic 1-form is, $\frac{\partial E}{\partial \lambda_i} = 0, i = 1, 2, \cdots, 2g$. If the Hessian matrix $(\frac{\partial^2 E}{\partial \lambda_i \partial \lambda_j})$ is positive definite, then E will reach the minimum. If the Hessian matrix is negative definite, E will be maximized.

Our surface mutual information method depends on the selection of holomorphic 1-form ω. To match surfaces optimally, we find the holomorphic 1-form that maximizes the mutual information metric. Suppose a holomorphic function $\omega = \sum_{i=1}^{2g} \lambda_i \omega_i$, our goal is to find a set of coefficients $\lambda_i, i = 1, ..., 2g$ that maximize the mutual information, E_{MI}. We solve this optimization problem numerically as follows:

$$dE_{MI} = (\frac{dE_{MI}}{du}, \frac{dE_{MI}}{dv}) \begin{pmatrix} \frac{du}{d\lambda_1} & \frac{du}{d\lambda_2} & \cdots & \frac{du}{d\lambda_{2g}} \\ \frac{dv}{d\lambda_1} & \frac{dv}{d\lambda_2} & \cdots & \frac{dv}{d\lambda_{2g}} \end{pmatrix} \begin{pmatrix} d\lambda_1 \\ d\lambda_2 \\ \cdots \\ d\lambda_{2g} \end{pmatrix} \tag{2}$$

where (u, v) is the conformal coordinate.

Once we compute $\frac{dE_{MI}}{d\lambda_i}, i = 1, 2, ..., 2g$, we can use steepest descent to optimize the resulting mutual information. A complete description of the surface mutual information method follows.

Algorithm 1. *Surface MI Method (for surfaces of arbitrary genus)*
Input (mesh M^1, M^2,step length δt, MI difference threshold δE),
Output($t : M^1 \to M^2$) where t minimizes the surface mutual information.

1. *Compute global conformal parameterization of two surfaces, $\omega^j = \sum_{i=1}^{2g} s_i \omega_i$, $j = 1, 2; i = 1, 2, ..., 2g$, where g is the surface genus number of two surfaces M^1 and M^2, and $s_i^j, j = 1, 2, i = 1, 2, ..., 2g$ are the coefficients of a linear combination of holomorphic function basis elements. The steps include computing the homology basis, cohomology basis, harmonic one-form basis and holomorphic one-form basis.*
2. *Compute holomorphic flow segmentation of the target surface, M^2, from the global conformal parameterization, ω^2, which conformally maps the 3D surface to a set of rectangles in the Euclidean plane.*
3. *Compute 2D conformal representation for the target surface, $\lambda^2(u, v)$ and $H^2(u, v)$, where (u, v) is the conformal coordinate;*
4. *Compute holomorphic flow segmentation of the source surface, M^1, and 2D conformal representation $\lambda^1(u, v)$ and $H^1(u, v)$;*
5. *Apply the mutual information method to optimize the correspondence between two surfaces, $t : (\lambda^1(u, v), H^1(u, v)) \to (\lambda^2(u, v), H^2(u, v)), j = 1, 2$ and $H^j(u, v), j = 1, 2$; and compute mutual information E_{MI}^0;*
6. *Compute derivative Dt.*
7. *Update the global conformal parameterization of source surface, M^1, by changing the coefficients $s^1(v) = Dt(v)\delta t$.*
8. *Compute mutual information E, with steps 3, 4, 5.*
9. *If $E_{MI} - E_{MI}^0 < \delta E$, return t. Otherwise, assign E to E_0 and repeat steps 6 through 9.*

Currently, we use the following numerical scheme in step 6:

1. Compute dE_{MI}/du and dE_{MI}/dv, $du/ds_i, i = 1, 2, ..., 2g$;
2. Compute $dv/ds_i, i = 1, 2, ..., 2g$;
3. Compute $Dt = dE_{MI}/ds_i, i = 1, 2, ..., 2g$ with Equation 2.

4 Experimental Results

To make the results easier to illustrate, we chose to encode the profile of surface features using a compound scalar function $C(u, v) = 8\lambda(u, v) + H(u, v)$, where $\lambda(u, v)$ is conformal factor and $H(u, v)$ the mean curvature. Several examples are shown matching hippocampal surfaces in 3D. This type of deformable surface registration can help track developmental and degenerative changes in the brain, and can create average shape models with appropriate boundary correspondences. In the experiments, the velocity field v in Equation 1 was computed iteratively by convolution of the force field with a filter kernel derived by Bro-Nielsen and Gramkow [26]. The viscosity coefficients λ and μ were set to 0.9 and 6.0 respectively. The deformation field in the parameter domain (u) was obtained from v by Euler integration over time, and the deformed template image was regridded when the Jacobian determinant of the deformation mapping at any point in $x - u$ was smaller than 0.5 [17]. At each step, the joint pdf was updated and the MI re-computed. Iterations were stopped when MI was no longer monotonically increasing or when the number of iterations reached 350. The Parzen parameter h was set to 10 for smoothing the joint pdf. Figure 2 (a) shows the matching fields for several pairs of surfaces, establishing correspondences between distinctive features. Here geometric features on 3D hippocampal surface, conformal factor and mean curvature, were conformally flattened to a 2D square. In the 2D parameter domain, data from a healthy control subject was registered to data from several Alzheimer's disease patients. Each mapping can be used to obtain a reparameterization of the 3D surface of the control subject, by convecting the original 3D coordinates along with the flow. Importantly, in Figure 2 (a), some consistent 3D geometric features are identifiable in the 2D parameter domain; bright area (arrows) correspond to high curvature features in the hippocampal head.

Although validation on a larger sample is required, we illustrate the approach on left hippocampal surface data from one healthy control subject and five patients with Alzheimer's disease. We register the control subject's surface to each patient, generating a set of deformation mappings. Figure 2 (b)-(e) show the correspondences as a 3D vector field map connecting corresponding points on two surfaces being registered. (d) and (e) are a part of surface before and after the registration. After reparameterization, a leftward shift in the vertical isocurves adds a larger tangential component to the vector field. Even so, the deformed grid structure remains close to conformal. The lengths of the difference vectors are reduced after the MI based alignment; a formal validation study in a larger sample is now underway.

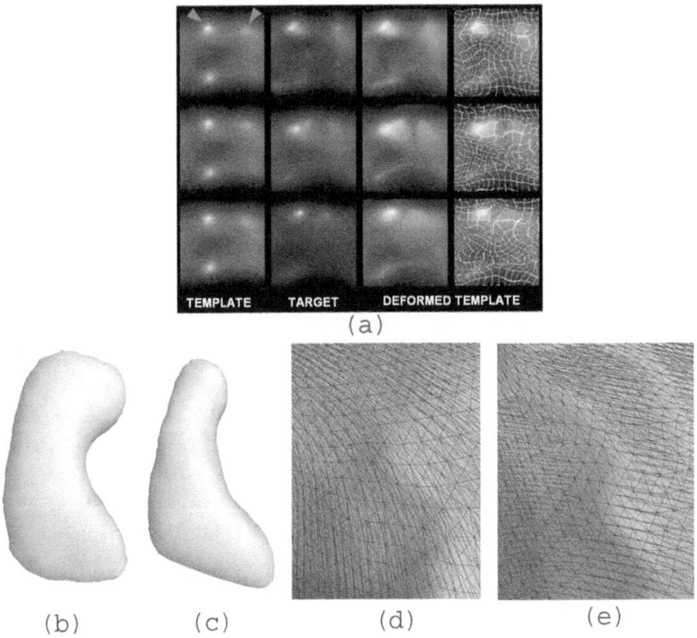

Fig. 2. (a) Geometric features on 3D hippocampal surfaces (the conformal factor and mean curvature) were computed and compound scalar fields were conformally flattened to a 2D square. In the 2D parameter domain, data from a healthy control subject (the template, leftmost column) was registered to data from several Alzheimer's disease patients (target images, second column). The deformed template images are shown in the third and fourth (gridded) columns. (b)-(c) show the two 3D hippocampal surfaces being matched, for (b) a control subject and (c) an Alzheimer's disease patient. We flow the surface from (b) to (c). (d)-(e) show the 3D vector displacement map, connecting corresponding points on the two surfaces, (d) before and (e) after reparameterization of the source surface using a fluid flow in the parameter domain. These 3D vector fields store information on geometrical feature correspondences between the surfaces.

5 Conclusions and Future Work

We extended the mutual information method to match general surfaces. This has many applications in medical imaging. Future work will validate the matching of hippocampal surfaces in shape analysis applications in degenerative diseases, as well as building statistical shape models to detect the anatomical effects of disease, aging, and development. The hippocampus is used as a specific example, but the method is general and is applicable in principle to other brain surfaces such as the cortex. Whether or not our new method provides a more relevant correspondences than those afforded by other criteria (minimum description length, neural nets, or hand landmarking) requires careful validation for each application. Because different correspondence principles produce different shape models, we plan to compare them in future for detecting group differences in brain structure.

References

1. Thompson, P., et al. Nature **404** (2000) 190–193
2. Csernansky, J., et al. Proc. Natl. Acad. Sci. **95** (1998) 11406–11411
3. Thompson, P., et al. In: Human Brain Mapping. Volume 9. (2000) 81–92
4. Kindlmann, G., et al. In: Proc. IEEE EMBS, San Francisco, CA (2004)
5. Fischl, B., et al. In: Human Brain Mapping. Volume 8. (1999) 272–284
6. Bakircioglu, M., et al. In: SPIE Medical Imaging. Volume 3661. (1999) 710–715
7. Leow, A., et al. NeuroImage **24** (2005) 910–927
8. Davatzikos, C. J. Comp. Assisted Tomography **20** (1996) 656–665
9. Pitiot, A., et al. In: IPMI. (2003) 25–37
10. Davis, R., et al. In: IEEE TMI. Volume 21. (2002) 525–537
11. Thodberg, H. In: IPMI. (2003) 51–62
12. Gu, X., Yau, S. Communication of Information and Systems **2** (2002) 121–146
13. Schoen, R., Yau, S.T.: Lectures on Harmonic Maps. International Press (1997)
14. Wells, W., et al. Medical Image Analysis **1** (1996) 35–51
15. Gu, X., et al. Communication of Information and Systems **3** (2005) 171–182
16. D'Agostino, E., et al. Medical Image Analysis **7** (2003) 565–575
17. Christensen, G., et al. IEEE TIP **5** (1996) 1435–1447
18. Parzen, E. The annals of mathematical statistics **33** (1962) 1065–1076
19. Gu, X., et al. IEEE TMI **23** (2004) 949–958
20. Gu, X., Vemuri, B. In: MICCAI. (2004) 771–780
21. West, J., et al. Journal of Computer Assisted Tomography **21** (1997) 554–566
22. Meyer, C., et al. Medical Image Analysis **1** (1997) 195–206
23. Rueckert, D., et al. IEEE TMI **18** (1999) 712–721
24. Kim, B., et al. NeuroImage **5** (1997) 31–40
25. Hermosillo, G. PhD thesis, Universitè de Nice (INRIA-ROBOTVIS), Sophia Antipolis, France (2002)
26. Bro-Nielsen, M., Gramkow, C. In: Visualization in Biomedical Computing (VBC'96). Volume 1131., Springer (1996) 267–276

Optimization of Brain Conformal Mapping with Landmarks

Yalin Wang[1], Lok Ming Lui[1], Tony F. Chan[1], and Paul M. Thompson[2]

Mathematics Department, UCLA, Los Angeles, CA 90095, USA
Lab. of Neuro Imaging, UCLA School of Medicine, Los Angeles, CA 90095, USA
{ylwang, malmlui, chan}@math.ucla.edu, thompson@loni.ucla.edu

Abstract. To compare and integrate brain data, data from multiple subjects are typically mapped into a canonical space. One method to do this is to conformally map cortical surfaces to the sphere. It is well known that any genus zero Riemann surface can be conformally mapped to a sphere. Therefore, conformal mapping offers a convenient method to parameterize cortical surfaces without angular distortion, generating an orthogonal grid on the cortex that locally preserves the metric. To compare cortical surfaces more effectively, it is advantageous to adjust the conformal parameterizations to match consistent anatomical features across subjects. This matching of cortical patterns improves the alignment of data across subjects, although it is more challenging to create a consistent conformal (orthogonal) parameterization of anatomy across subjects when landmarks are constrained to lie at specific locations in the spherical parameter space. Here we propose a new method, based on a new energy functional, to optimize the conformal parameterization of cortical surfaces by using landmarks. Experimental results on a dataset of 40 brain hemispheres showed that the landmark mismatch energy can be greatly reduced while effectively preserving conformality. The key advantage of this conformal parameterization approach is that any local adjustments of the mapping to match landmarks do not affect the conformality of the mapping significantly. We also examined how the parameterization changes with different weighting factors. As expected, the landmark matching error can be reduced if it is more heavily penalized, but conformality is progressively reduced.

1 Introduction

An effective way to analyze and compare brain data from multiple subjects is to map them into a canonical space while retaining the original geometric information as far as possible. Surface-based approaches often map cortical surface data to a parameter domain such as a sphere, providing a common coordinate system for data integration [1,2]. One method is to map the cortical surface conformally to the sphere. Any genus zero Riemann surfaces can be mapped conformally to a sphere, without angular distortion. Therefore, conformal mapping offers a convenient way to parameterize the genus zero cortical surfaces of the brain. To compare cortical surfaces more effectively, it is desirable to adjust the conformal parameterizations to match specific anatomical features on the cortical surfaces

J. Duncan and G. Gerig (Eds.): MICCAI 2005, LNCS 3750, pp. 675–683, 2005.

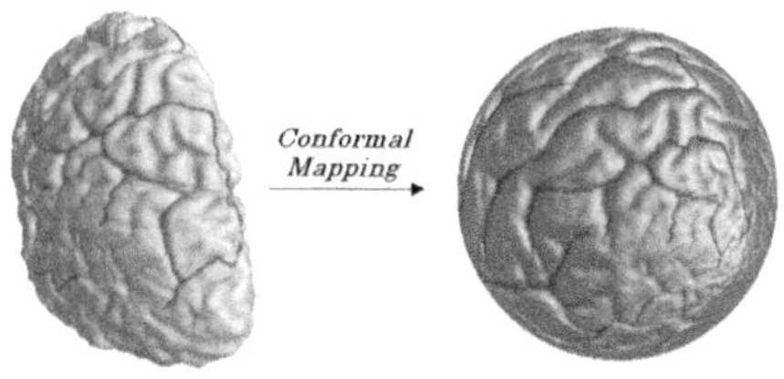

Fig. 1. Manually labeled landmarks on the brain surface. The original surface is on the left. The result of mapping it conformally to a sphere is on the right.

as far as possible (such as sulcal/gyral landmarks in the form of landmark points or 3D curves lying in the surface). Here we refer to these anatomical features as landmarks. Some examples of landmarks are shown in Figure 1.

1.1 Previous Work

Several research groups have reported work on brain surface conformal mapping. Hurdal and Stephenson [3] reported a discrete mapping approach that uses circle packing to produce "flattened" images of cortical surfaces on the sphere, the Euclidean plane, or the hyperbolic plane. They obtained maps that are quasi-conformal approximations to classical conformal maps. Haker et al. [4] implemented a finite element approximation for parameterizing brain surfaces via conformal mappings. They represented the Laplace-Beltrami operator as a linear system and solved it for parameterizing brain surfaces via conformal mapping. Gu et al. [5] proposed a method to find a unique conformal mapping between any two genus zero manifolds by minimizing the harmonic energy of the map. They demonstrated this method by conformally mapping the cortical surface to a sphere.

Optimization of surface diffeomorphisms by landmark matching has been studied intensively. Gu et al. [5] proposed to optimize the conformal parametrization by composing an optimal Möbius transformation so that it minimizes the landmark mismatch energy. The resulting parameterization remains conformal. Glaunés et al. [6] proposed to generate large deformation diffeomorphisms of the sphere onto itself, given the displacements of a finite set of template landmarks. The diffeomorphism obtained can match the geometric features exactly but it is, in general, not a conformal mapping. Leow et al. [7] proposed a level set based approach for matching different types of features, including points and 2D or 3D curves represented as implicit functions. Cortical surfaces were flattened to the unit square. Nine sulcal curves were chosen and were represented by the intersection of two level set functions, and used to constrain the warp of one cortical surface onto another. The resulting transformation was interpolated using a large deformation momentum formulation in the cortical parameter space, generalizing an elastic approach for cortical matching developed in Thompson et al. [8]. Duygu et al. [9] proposed a more automated mapping technique that results in good sulcal alignment across subjects, by combining parametric relaxation, iterative closest point registration and inverse stereographic projection.

1.2 Basic Idea

In this paper, we propose a new method to adjust conformal parameterizations of the cortical surface so that they match consistent anatomical features across subjects. This matching of cortical patterns improves the alignment of data across subjects, e.g., when integrating functional imaging data across subjects, measuring brain changes, or making statistical comparisons in cortical anatomy [10].

Our new method, which is based on a new energy functional, optimizes the conformal parameterization of cortical surfaces by using landmarks. This is done by minimizing the compound energy functional $E_{new} = E_{harmonic} + \lambda E_{landmark}$, where $E_{harmonic}$ is the harmonic energy of the parameterization and $E_{landmark}$ is the landmark mismatch energy. We prove theoretically that our proposed E_{new} is guaranteed to be decreasing and study the rate of changes of $E_{harmonic}$ and $E_{landmark}$. Experimental results show that our algorithm can considerably reduce the landmark mismatch energy while effectively retaining the conformality property. Based on these findings, we argue that the conformal mapping provides an attractive framework to help analyze anatomical shape, and to statistically combine or compare 3D anatomical models across subjects.

2 Algorithm

2.1 Combined Energy Definition

A diffeomorphism $f : M \to N$ is a *conformal mapping* if it preserves the first fundamental form up to a scaling factor (the conformal factor). Mathematically, this means that $ds_M^2 = \lambda f^*(ds_N^2)$, where ds_M^2 and ds_N^2 are the first fundamental form on M and N, respectively and λ is the conformal factor. For a diffeomorphism between two genus zero surfaces, a map is conformal if it minimizes the harmonic energy[1] ,$E_{harmonic}$ [1]. Based on this fact, we can compute the conformal mapping by a variational approach, which minimizes the harmonic energy.

Here we propose a new algorithm that optimizes the conformal parameterization using discrete landmarks. This algorithm optimizes the landmark mismatch energy over all degrees of freedom in the reparameterization group. The map obtained can considerably reduce the landmark mismatch energy while retaining conformality as far as possible.

Suppose C_1 and C_2 are two cortical surfaces we want to compare. We let $f_1 : C_1 \to S^2$ be the conformal parameterization of C_1 mapping it onto S^2. We manually label the landmarks on the two cortical surfaces as discrete point sets, as shown in Figure 1. We denote them as $\{p_i \in C_1\}$, $\{q_i \in C_2\}$, with p_i matching q_i. We proceed to compute a map $f_2 : C_2 \to S^2$ from C_2 to S^2, which minimizes the harmonic energy as well as minimizing the so-called landmark mismatch energy. The landmark mismatch energy measures the Euclidean distance between

[1] We adapted the harmonic energy computation in [5].

the corresponding landmarks. Alternatively, landmark errors could be computed as geodesic distances with respect to the original surfaces, rather than on the sphere; here we chose to perform distance computations on the sphere. Using our algorithm, the computed map should effectively preserve the conformal property and match the geometric features on the original structures as far as possible.

Let $h : C_2 \to S^2$ be any homeomorphism from C_2 onto S^2. We define the landmark mismatch energy of h as, $E_{landmark}(h) = 1/2 \sum_{i=1}^{n} ||h(q_i)) - f_1(p_i)||^2$. where the norm represents distance on the sphere. By minimizing this energy functional, the Euclidean distance between the corresponding landmarks on the sphere is minimized.

To optimize the conformal parameterization, we propose to find $f_2 : C_2 \to S^2$ which minimizes the following new energy functional (instead of the harmonic energy functional), $E_{new}(f_2) = E_{harmonic}(f_2) + \lambda E_{landmark}(f_2)$, where λ is a weighting factor (Lagrange multiplier) that balances the two penalty functionals. It controls how much landmark mismatch we want to tolerate. When $\lambda = 0$, the new energy functional is just the harmonic energy. When λ is large, the landmark mismatch energy can be greatly reduced. But more conformality will be lost (here we regard deviations from conformality to be quantified by the harmonic energy).

Now, let K represent the simplicial realization (triangulation) of the brain surface C_2, let u, v denote the vertices, and $[u, v]$ denote the edge spanned by u, v. Our new energy functional can be written as:

$$
\begin{aligned}
E_{new}(f_2) =& 1/2 \sum_{[u,v]\in K} k_{u,v}||f_2(u) - f_2(v)||^2 + \lambda/2 \sum_{i=1}^{n} ||f_2(q_i) - f_1(p_i)||^2 \\
=& 1/2 \sum_{[u,v]\in K} k_{u,v}||f_2(u) - f_2(v)||^2 + \lambda/2 \sum_{u\in K} ||f_2(u) - L(u))||^2 \chi_M(u)
\end{aligned}
$$

where $M = \{q_1, ..., q_n\}$; $L(q_i) = p_i$ if $u = q_i \in M$ and $L(u) = (1, 0, 0)$ otherwise. The first part of the energy functional is defined as in [5]. Note that by minimizing this energy, we may give up some conformality but the landmark mismatch energy is progressively reduced.

2.2 Optimization of Combined Energy

We next formulate a technique to optimize our energy functional. Suppose we would like to compute a mapping f_2 that minimizes the energy $E_{new}(f_2)$. This can be solved easily by steepest descent.

Definition 3.1: Suppose $f \in C^{PL}$, where C^{PL} represent a vector space consists of all piecewise linear functions defined on K. We define the Laplacian as follows: $\Delta f(u) = \sum_{[u,v]\in K} k_{u,v}(f(u) - f(v)) + \lambda \sum_{u\in K}(f_2(u) - L(u))\chi_M(u)$.

Definition 3.2: Suppose $\vec{f} \in C^{PL}$, $\vec{f} = (f_0, f_1, f_2)$, where the f_i are piecewise linear. Define the Laplacian of $\vec{f}$ as $\Delta \vec{f} = (\Delta f_0(u), \Delta f_1(u), \Delta f_2(u))$.

Now, we know that $f_2 = (f_{20}, f_{21}, f_{22})$ minimizes $E_{new}(f_2)$ if and only if the tangential component of $\Delta f_2(u) = (\Delta f_{20}(u), \Delta f_{21}(u), \Delta f_{22}(u))$ vanishes. That is $\Delta(f_2) = \Delta(f_2)^{\perp}$.

In other words, we should have $P_{\vec{n}} \Delta f_2(u) = \Delta f_2(u) - (\Delta f_2(u) \cdot \vec{n})\vec{n} = 0$. We use a steepest descent algorithm to compute $f_2 : C_2 \to S^2$: $\frac{df_2}{dt} = -P_{\vec{n}} \Delta f_2(t)$.

Algorithm 1. *Algorithm to Optimize the Combined Energy E_{new}*
Input (mesh K, step length δt, energy difference threshold δE), output($f_2 : C_2 \to S^2$), which minimizes E. The computer algorithm proceeds as follows:

1. *Given a Gauss map $I : C_2 \to S^2$. Let $f_2 = I$, compute $E_0 = E_{new}(I)$*
2. *For each vertex $v \in K$, compute $P_{\vec{n}} \Delta f_2(v)$*
3. *Update $f_2(v)$ by $\delta f_2(v) = -P_{\vec{n}} \Delta f_2(v) \delta t$*
4. *Compute energy E_{new}*
5. *If $E_{new} - E_0 < \delta E$, return f_2. Otherwise, assign E to E_0. Repeat steps 2 to 5.*

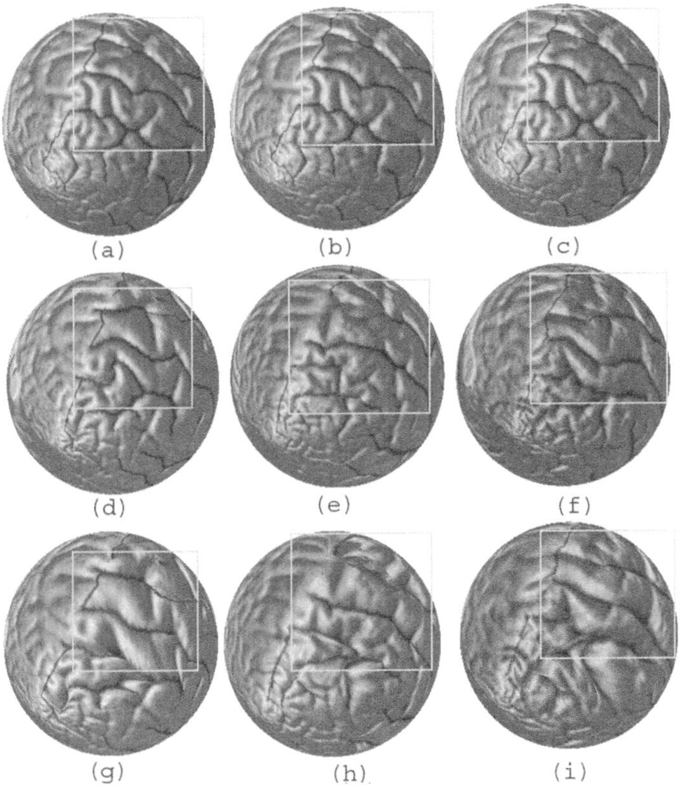

Fig. 2. In (a), the cortical surface C_1 (the control) is mapped conformally ($\lambda = 0$) to the sphere. In (d), another cortical surface C_2 is mapped conformally to the sphere. Note that the sulcal landmarks appear very different from those in (a) (see landmarks in the green square). In (g), the cortical surface C_2 is mapped to the sphere using our algorithm (with $\lambda = 3$). Note that the landmarks now closely resemble those in (a) (see landmarks in the green square). (b) and (c) shows the same cortical surface (the control) as in (a). In (e) and (f), two other cortical surfaces are mapped to the spheres. The landmarks again appears very differently. In (h) and (i), the cortical surfaces are mapped to the spheres using our algorithm. The landmarks now closely resemble those of the control.

3 Experimental Results

In our experiment, we tested our algorithm on a set of left hemisphere cortical surfaces generated from brain MRI scans of 40 healthy adult subjects, aged 27.5+/-7.4SD years (16 males, 24 females), scanned at 1.5 T (on a GE Signa scanner). Data and cortical surface landmarks were those generated in a prior paper, Thompson et al. [10] where the extraction and sulcal landmarking procedures are fully detailed. Using this set of 40 hemispheric surfaces, we mapped all surfaces conformally to the sphere and minimized the compound energy matching all subjects to a randomly selected individual subject (alternatively, the surfaces could have been aligned to an average template of curves on the sphere). An important advantage of this approach is that the local adjustments of the mapping to match landmarks do not greatly affect the conformality of the mapping. In Figure 2(a), the cortical surface C_1 (a control subject) is mapped conformally ($\lambda = 0$) to the sphere. In (d), another cortical surface C_2 is mapped conformally to the sphere. Note that the sulcal landmarks appear very different from those in (a) (see landmarks in the green square). This means that the geometric features are not well aligned on the sphere unless a further feature-based deformation is applied. In Figure 2(g), we map the cortical surface C_2 to the sphere with our algorithm, while minimizing the compound energy. This time, the landmarks closely resemble those in (a) (see landmarks in the green square).

In Figure 3, statistics of the angle difference are illustrated. Note that under a conformal mapping, angles between edges on the initial cortical surface should be preserved when these edges are mapped to the sphere. Any differences in angles can be evaluated to determine departures from conformality. Figure 3(a) shows the histogram of the angle difference using the conformal mapping, i.e. after running the algorithm using the conformal energy term only. Figure 2(b) shows the histogram of the angle difference using the compound functional that also penalizes landmark mismatch. Despite the fact that inclusion of landmarks requires more complex mappings, the angular relationships between edges on

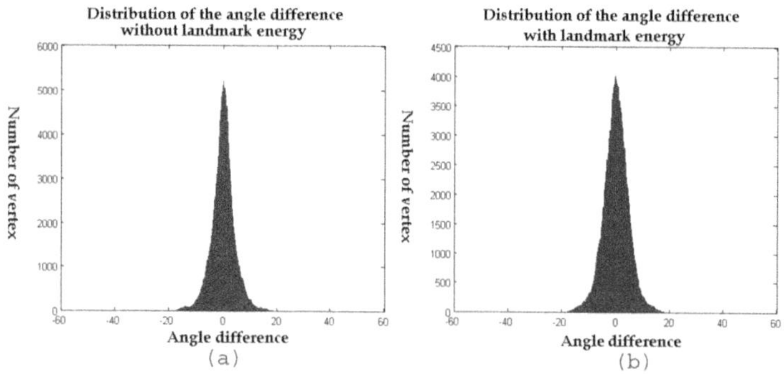

Fig. 3. Histogram (a) shows the statistics of the angle difference using the conformal mapping. Histogram (b) shows the statistics of the angle difference using our algorithm ($\lambda = 3$). It is observed that the angle is well-preserved.

Table 1. Numerical data from our experiment. The landmark mismatch energy is greatly reduced while the harmonic energy is only slightly increased. The table also illustrates how the results differ with different values of λ. The landmark mismatch error can be reduced by increasing λ, but conformality will increasingly be lost.

	$\lambda = 3$	$\lambda = 6$	$\lambda = 10$
$E_{harmonic}$ of the initial (conformal) parameterization:	100.6	100.6	100.6
$\lambda E_{landmark}$ of the initial (conformal) parameterization:	81.2	162.4	270.7
Initial compound energy $(E_{harmonic} + \lambda E_{landmark})$:	181.8	263.0	371.3
Final $E_{harmonic}$	109.1 ($\nearrow$ 8.45%)	111.9 ($\nearrow$ 11.2%)	123.0 ($\nearrow$ 22.2%)
Final $\lambda E_{landmark}$	11.2 ($\searrow$ 86.2%)	13.7 ($\searrow$ 91.6%)	15.6($\searrow$ 95.8%)
Final compound energy $(E_{harmonic} + \lambda E_{landmark})$	120.3 ($\searrow$ 33.8%)	125.6($\searrow$ 52.2%)	138.6 ($\searrow$ 62.7%)

the source surface and their images on the sphere are clearly well preserved even after landmark constraints are enforced.

We also tested with other parameter λ with different values. Table 1 shows numerical data from the experiment. From the Table, we observe that the landmark mismatch energy is greatly reduced while the harmonic energy is only slightly increased. The table also illustrates how the results differ with different values of λ. We observe that the landmark mismatch error can be reduced by increasing λ, but conformality is increasingly lost.

4 Conclusion and Future Work

In conclusion, we have developed a new algorithm to compute a map from the cortical surface of the brain to a sphere, which can effectively retain the original geometry by minimizing the landmark mismatch error across different subjects. The development of adjustable landmark weights may be beneficial in computational anatomy. In some applications, such as tracking brain change in an individual over time, in serial images, it makes most sense to place a high priority on landmark correspondence. In other applications, such as the integration of functional brain imaging data across subjects, functional anatomy is not so tightly linked to sulcal landmarks, so it may help to trade landmark error to increase the regularity of the mappings. In the future, we will study the numerical parameters of our algorithm in details to determine how the weighting factor λ affects the signal to noise for different neuroimaging applications. We will also compare our algorithm with other existing counterpart quantitatively. Furthermore, more analysis will be done to examine how well the alignment of the sulci/gyri is, such as averaging the maps.

References

1. Drury, H., et al. In: Brain Warping. Academic Press (1999) 337–363
2. Fischl, B., et al. In: Human Brain Mapping. Volume 8. (1999) 272–284
3. Hurdal, M.K., Stephenson, K. NeuroImage **23** (2004) S119–S128
4. Haker, S., et al. IEEE TVCG **6** (2000) 181–189
5. Gu, X., et al. IEEE TMI **23** (2004) 949–958
6. Glaunès, J., et al. J. Maths. Imaging and Vision **20** (2004) 179–200
7. Leow, A., et al. NeuroImage **24** (2005) 910–927
8. Thompson, P., et al. Human Brain Mapping **9** (2000) 81–92
9. Tosun, D., et al. Med. Image Anal. **8** (2004) 295–309
10. Thompson, P., et al. NeuroImage **23** (2004) S2–S18

Appendix

A Energy Is Decreasing

Claim : With our algorithm, the energy is strictly decreasing.
Proof : Our energy (in continuous form) can be written as: $E(u) = 1/2 \int ||\nabla u||^2 + \lambda \int \delta_E ||(u-v)||^2$ where v is the conformal mapping from the control cortical surface to the sphere. Now,
$\frac{d}{dt}|_{t=0} E(u+tw) = \int \nabla u \cdot \nabla w + \lambda \int \delta_E (u-v) \cdot w = \int \Delta u w + \lambda \int \delta_E (u-v) \cdot w$
In our algorithm, the direction w is taken as: $w = -\Delta u - \lambda \delta_E (u-v)$. Substituting this into the above equation, we have $\frac{d}{dt}|_{t=0} E(u+tw) = -\int (\nabla u - (\lambda) \int \delta_E ||u - v||)^2 < 0$. Therefore, the overall energy of the mapping is strictly decreasing, as the iterations proceed.

B Rate of Changes in $E_{harmonic}$ and $E_{landmark}$

To explain why our algorithm can effectively preserve conformalilty while greatly reducing the landmark mismatch energy, we can look at the rate of change of $E_{harmonic}$ and $E_{landmark}$. Note that the initial map u we get is almost conformal. Thus, initially Δu is very small.
Claim : With our algorithm, the rate of change of $E_{harmonic}(u)$ is $\mathcal{O}(||\Delta u||_\infty)$ and the rate of change of $E_{landmark}$ is $\lambda^2 E_{landmark}(u) + \mathcal{O}(||\Delta u||_\infty)$. Here the norm is the supremum norm over the surface.
Proof : Recall that in our algorithm, the direction w is taken as: $w = -\Delta u - \lambda \delta_E (u-v)$. Now, the rates of change are:

$$
\begin{aligned}
E_{harmonic} &= |\frac{d}{dt}|_{t=0} E_{harmonic}(u+tw)| = |\int \nabla u \cdot \nabla w| = |\int \Delta u \cdot w| \\
&= |\int ||\Delta u||^2 + \int \delta_E \Delta u \cdot (u-v)| \leq ||\Delta u||_\infty^2 + 8\lambda\pi ||\Delta u||_\infty = \mathcal{O}(||\Delta u||_\infty) \\
E_{landmark} &= |\frac{d}{dt}|_{t=0} E_{landmark}(u+tw)| = |\int (\lambda \delta_E)^2 (u-v) \cdot w + \int \delta_E (u-v) \cdot \Delta u| \\
&\leq \lambda^2 E_{landmark}(u) + 8\pi ||\Delta u||_\infty = \lambda^2 E_{landmark}(u) + \mathcal{O}(||\Delta u||_\infty)
\end{aligned}
$$

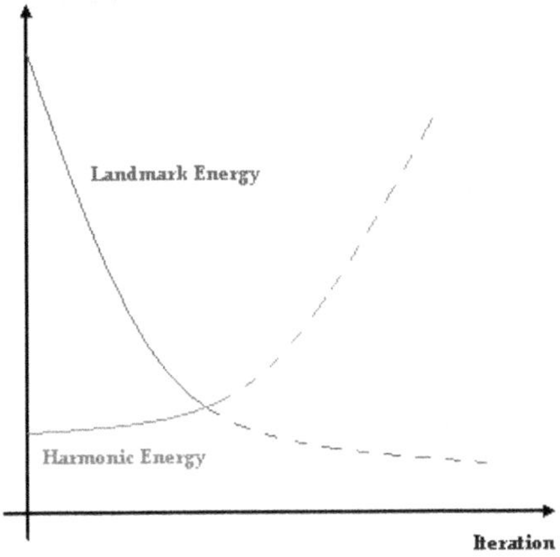

Fig. 4. This figure shows how the harmonic energy and landmark energy change, as the number of iterations increases, using our steepest descent algorithm. Initially, the rate of change of the harmonic energy is small while the rate of change of landmark energy is comparatively large. Note that a Lagrange multiplier governs the weighting of the two energies, so a compromise can be achieved between errors in landmark correspondence and deviations from conformality.

Since initially the map is almost conformal and Δu is very small, the change in harmonic energy is very small. Conversely, initially the landmark energy is comparatively large. Since the rate of change of $E_{landmark}$ is $\lambda^2 E_{landmark}(u) + \mathcal{O}(||\Delta u||_\infty)$, the change in landmark energy is more significant (see Figure 4 for an illustration).

A New Method for SPECT Quantification of Targeted Radiotracers Uptake in the Myocardium

Shimin Li, Lawrence W. Dobrucki, Albert J. Sinusas, and Yi-Hwa Liu

Section of cardiovascular Medicine, Department of Internal Medicine,
Yale University School of Medicine, New Haven, CT, USA
Shimin.li@yale.edu

Abstract. We developed a new method for absolute quantification of targeted radiotracers uptake in the myocardium using hybrid SPECT/CT and an external reference point source. A segmentation algorithm based on the level set was developed to determine the endocardial edges from CT, which were subsequently applied to the physically co-registered SPECT. A 3-D Gaussian fitting method was applied for quantification of the external point source. The total targeted radiotracer activity in the myocardium was normalized to that in the point source to calculate the absolute uptake of targeted radiotracer in the myocardium. Preliminary validation was performed in rats with ischemia-induced angiogenesis. The quantified in vivo radiotracer uptake was compared to the postmortem tissue radioactive well-counting of the myocardium. Our methods worked well for identification of the endocardial edges. Quantification of the focal uptake was consistent with the well-counting data. Our methods may have the potential of providing precise absolute quantification of targeted radiotracer uptake in the myocardium.

1 Introduction

Recently substantial research was directed toward the developments of targeted molecular imaging agents [1] for the cardiovascular system and radiotracer based imaging techniques for noninvasive visualization of the molecular processes in the myocardium. Radio-labeled agents targeted at the molecular processes often result in focal "hotspot" images, which are distinctly different from the perfusion images conventionally acquired in nuclear cardiology. Because the changes in the myocardial uptake of these targeted radiotracers are generally small, precisely tracking these subtle changes requires a sophisticated quantitative method to assess the absolute hotspot uptake in the myocardium. However, quantification of myocardial uptake of targeted radiotracers has not been extensively investigated previously in part due to the background activity in the cardiac images. Quantification of hotspot focal uptake in the myocardium from single photon emission computerized tomography (SPECT) presents another challenge due to the effects of image resolution, background activity [2, 3], object size, shape and voxel size in SPECT images [4]. Other confounding factors such as photon attenuation and the partial volume effect may also cause errors in quantification of absolute hotspot tracer uptake [5] in the myocardium. On the other hand, it is difficult to obtain anatomical information from focal hotspot SPECT

J. Duncan and G. Gerig (Eds.): MICCAI 2005, LNCS 3750, pp. 684–691, 2005.

images and thus reference images such as ^{201}Tl or CT images are needed to identify the position and orientation of the heart. Currently, quantitative approaches are not available for serial evaluation of changes in the uptake of these targeted radiotracers. Previous studies in quantification of targeted cardiac images are mostly derived only from visual analysis. Recently, we developed a stochastic approach [6] for quantification of focal uptake from cardiac SPECT/CT images using a ^{99m}Tc/^{201}Tl dual-isotope SPECT imaging protocol in which ^{201}Tl SPECT was used as the reference perfusion image. However, quantification of the targeted radiotracer uptake using two isotopes may require assumptions of the reciprocal relation between the ^{99m}Tc and ^{201}Tl images which may not be true due to the cross-talk between the two tracers on board. Using CT image to replace ^{201}Tl image as the reference image may potentially address this issue.

In this paper, we introduce a new level-set-based SPECT/CT segmentation and quantification approach for absolute quantification of myocardial uptake of radiotracers targeted at the molecular processes such as angiogenesis. Absolute myocardial uptake is quantified from SPECT images with the support of co-registered SPECT/CT images in identification of the left ventricular (LV) myocardium.

2 Methods

2.1 The Level Set Approach for Image Segmentation

The level set method, developed previously by Osher and Sethian [7, 8], is a numerical approach for tracking the evolution of the surfaces. Let $\Gamma(t)$ denote a time-dependent closed $(n\text{-}1)$-dimensional hyper-surface which evolves in its normal direction. Instead of maneuvering the hyper-surface directly, the desired hyper-surface is embedded in the zero level set of a higher n-dimensional function $\phi(x,t)$, which can be described as:

$$\Gamma(t) = \{x \mid \phi(x,t) = 0\}, \tag{1}$$

The value of ϕ at point x is defined by:

$$\phi(x,t) = \pm d\ , \tag{2}$$

where d is the shortest distance from x to the desired hyper-surface $\Gamma(t)$. The sign is determined by either the point x lying outside (+d) or inside (-d) the hyper-surface $\Gamma(t)$. The level-set function is evolved under the control of the differential equation:

$$\frac{\partial \phi(x,t)}{\partial \tau} + F\left|\nabla \phi(x,t)\right| = 0\ , \tag{3}$$

where $|\nabla \phi|$ is the norm of the gradient of the level set function ϕ. The speed term F in Equation 3 to be defined in the next section depends on the feature of the image segmented and the intrinsic geometrical property of the surface (eg. curvature of the surface). Given $\phi(x,t)= 0$, the evolving surface can be obtained by extracting the zero level-set as expressed in Equation 1. For details of the level set methods, the reader can refer to [9].

2.2 The Cavity Separation

In vivo cardiac CT images have very low contrast and ambiguous boundaries due to the cardiac motion. Segmentation of the myocardium from the in vivo CT images is challenging. Instead of segmenting the myocardium, we segment the cavity from the in vivo CT images because of the complex shape of the myocardium. We also rescale the CT images to enhance the intensity in the LV regions. Let I_C denote the rescaled CT image. The speed term used in Equation 3 can be formulated as [9]:

$$F = (\alpha - \beta \cdot \kappa) \cdot g_{I_C} - \gamma \frac{\nabla g_{I_C} \cdot \nabla \varphi}{|\nabla \varphi|}, \tag{4}$$

where $g_{I_C} = \frac{1}{1+|\nabla(G_\sigma * I_C)|}$ and $\kappa = \nabla \cdot \frac{\nabla \phi}{|\nabla \phi|}$. The expression $G_\sigma * I_C$ denotes the rescaled CT images convolved with a Gaussian smoothing filter of which the characteristic width is denoted as σ. We use the Gaussian filter to reduce the noise of the edges and facilitate the edge detection for the anatomical structures of the LV. κ is a curvature-based geometric smoothing term. The last term $\frac{\nabla g_{I_C} \cdot \nabla \phi}{|\nabla \phi|}$ in Equation 4 is used to direct the curve to the boundaries of the LV cavity. The scalars α, β and γ are the parameters used to weigh the relative influence of each of the terms on the movement of the edges.

Proper initialization is critical for the level set algorithm. A seed region with one or more pixels needs to be manually introduced into the cavity volume. Ultimately, the cavity volume is updated iteratively with the speed term F until it reaches the endocardial edges.

2.3 Point Source Extraction

In order to calculate the total counts of the external reference point source, the volume of the reference point source needs to be extracted from the SPECT images. A 3-D Gaussian fitting is incorporated into the point source extraction. Total counts of the external point source fitted as a 3-D elliptical Gaussian shape are integrated from the center of the volume to 2 standard deviation (SD) outward in the 3-D space to acquire 97.5% of the counts in the elliptical shape. The 3-D Gaussian function of the point source can be formulated as

$$P(x, y, z) = A \cdot \exp^{-\frac{1}{2}(X-X_n)^T M (X-X_n)}, \tag{5}$$

Where $X = (x, y, z)^T$ denote the spatial coordinates, $X_n = (x_n, y_n, z_n)^T$ denote the spatial coordinates of the center of the point source, A is the height of the Gaussian shape, and $M = \begin{pmatrix} \frac{1}{\sigma_x^2} & 0 & 0 \\ 0 & \frac{1}{\sigma_y^2} & 0 \\ 0 & 0 & \frac{1}{\sigma_z^2} \end{pmatrix}$. The variance of the Gaussian in different directions

(σ_x, σ_y, σ_z) are not necessarily the same. The parameters of the point source distribution can be estimated by a gradient-expansion algorithm [10] to compute a non-linear least squares with the seven parameters shown above.

To locate the point source in the SPECT images, a seed is manually introduced into the region of the point source. The initial center of the point source can be defined by the position of maximal value pixel in the finite region around the seed. After the parameter estimation, the count of the point source can be collected from the 3-D elliptical volume with the estimated standard deviations.

2.4 Quantification of Targeted Radiotracer Uptake from SPECT Images

The signed distance map as described in Section 2.1 can be generated with incorporation of the LV cavity volume obtained from the CT images. In the signed distance map, pixel values represent the shortest signed distance of the points from the contour. Consequently, the myocardial volume is obtained by integrating all the pixels within an assumed myocardial thickness. The myocardium determined by CT can be applied to the targeted radiotracer SPECT images (see Fig. 1(c)) thanks to the co-registration of the SPECT and CT images.

The point source filled with ^{99m}Tc was used as a known reference to quantify absolute uptake of the targeted radiotracers in the LV myocardium. The boundary between the left ventricular and left atrial myocardium was determined manually and was located approximately one half of the whole LV length as evidenced by the CT images. Targeted radiotracer uptake in the LV myocardium was normalized to the total counts of the external point source of which the volume was determined by the method described in Section 2.3. Relative radiotracer uptake was calculated as a summation of pixels values in the segmented LV myocardium volume. The resulted relative radiotracer uptake was in turn weighted by the known dose of the external point source to obtain absolute radiotracer uptake. The total absolute radiotracer uptake is calculated by

$$\text{Targeted radiotracer uptake} = \frac{\iint \zeta(v)dv}{\iint \theta(u)du} \cdot c\,, \tag{6}$$

where $\zeta(v)$ denotes the targeted activity in the LV myocardium volume v, $\theta(u)$ denotes the targeted activity in point source volume u, and c represents the known radioactivity (μCi) in the point source.

3 Rat Experiments

3.1 Surgical and Imaging Preparation

Rats weighting 200-250 gm were used in our preliminary validation for the methods. The rats were anesthetized with isoflurane and the hearts was exposed via a limited left anterolateral thoracotomy. The left anterior descending coronary artery was ligated at 7 mm distal to the origin. The coronary occlusion was subsequently released after 45 minutes resulting in non-transmural infarction and the chest was closed in layers. One week following myocardial infarction, the rats were anesthetized with isoflurane and positioned in a hybrid microSPECT/CT imaging system (XSPECT Gamma Medica, Northridge, CA) for microCT and microSPECT imaging. A point source filled with 32 μCi ^{99m}Tc was placed under the imaging table and near the rat. A ^{99m}Tc-labeled radiotracer (4~5 mCi) targeted at the αvβ3 integrin (NC100692, GE Healthcare), a marker of angiogenesis, was injected into the rats. The rats were also injected with an intravascular vascular contrast agent (Fenestra VC, Alerion Biomedical, San Diego, CA) to visually separate the myocardium from LV cavity.

3.2 Image Acquisitions and Reconstructions

Non-gated CT projections were acquired for 15 minutes. A total of 512 projections were acquired. The CT images were reconstructed using the filtered back-projection algorithm. The matrix size of CT images was 512×512×512 voxels. The voxel size of CT reconstruction was 0.1557 mm cubic.

After CT imaging, SPECT images were acquired using the same dual-head microSPECT/CT camera with pinholes collimators (1 mm aperture) for 35 minutes, with a 20% energy window symmetrically centered at 140 keV photopeak of ^{99m}Tc. Eighty-two projections were acquired for each head in a 180^0 circular orbit. The SPECT images were also reconstructed using the filtered back-projection algorithm. The matrix size of SPECT images was 82x82x82 voxels, with voxel size of 1.524 mmx1.524 mmx1.524 mm. CT and SPECT images were fused to obtain co-registered SPECT/CT images. All fused images had an image matrix size of 256x256x256 voxels, with voxel size of 0.3114 mmx0.3114 mmx0.3114 mm.

3.3 CT Image Segmentation and SPECT Image Quantification

The level set image segmentation method was applied to the CT images to determine the endocardial edges and the resulted edges were subsequently applied to the SPECT images to calculate the focal radiotracer uptake in the LV myocardium as described in Section 2.

3.4 Tissue Well-Counting

Rats were sacrificed after SPECT/CT imaging. The heart was extracted from the chest and was sliced for tissue well-counting measurements of the radioactivity in the LV myocardium. The well-counting data was corrected for decay based on the time interval between the SPECT imaging and well-counting.

4 Results

Fig.1(a) illustrates the in vivo CT images for one rat. The cavity of the left ventricle determined using the level set method is shown in Fig. 1(b) in red and the myocardium between the endocardial and epicardial edges is shown in green. The thickness of the myocardium shown in Fig.1(b) was seven pixels (~ 2.2 mm). The LV edges were subsequently applied to the targeted SPECT images as shown in Fig. 1(c) to integrate the total photon counts in the targeted regions in the LV myocardium. The

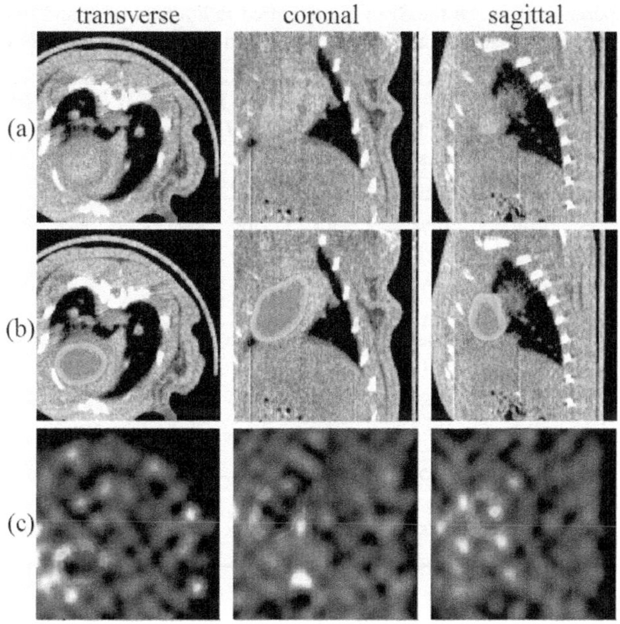

Fig. 1. (a) In vivo CT images, (b) In vivo CT images with LV cavity (in red) and myocardium (in green) superimposed, (c) In vivo SPECT images superimposed with the LV myocardial edges from (b). The myocardial thickness is 7 pixels width in this illustration.

integrated tracer counts were normalized to that in the point source to calculate the absolute radiotracer dose in the LV myocardium as described in Section 2.4. Point source dose (μCi) was calculated using the method described in Section 2.3. Because only one point source was used in our experiments, the absolute dose in the point source was decay corrected for each rat.

Table 1 shows the well-counting dose and SPECT quantified doses with 7 different wall thicknesses assumed in our segmentation method. The ratio shown in Table 1 was calculated as the SPECT dose divided by the true well-counting dose. The well-counting data was also corrected in the same way based on the time interval between the SPECT imaging and well-counting. As seen in Table 1, the ratio is linearly increased as a function of the assumed LV myocardium thickness. The positive linearity is expected because a thicker LV thickness assumed should reflect higher integrated counts from the myocardium. Notice that the SPECT quantified dose using seven-pixel thickness (~ 2.2 mm) resulted in the smallest error as compared to the other thicknesses used. The true thickness of rat myocardium is approximately 1~1.5mm. By taking into account the intrinsic pinhole SPECT resolution (~1 mm) and low-pass filtering effect on SPECT images, the myocardial thickness assumed in SPECT images needs to be at least 2 times image resolution to compensate for the partial volume effect. This may explain that the assumed seven-pixel thickness resulted in a better estimation of the uptake of the targeted radiotracer.

Table 1. Comparisons between the SPECT quantified radiotracer dose and true well-counting dose in 7 different thicknesses assumed for the left ventricular myocardium of rat

Rat #	Well counting dose (μCi)	D= 4 pixels SPECT dose (μCi)	D= 4 pixels Ratio	D= 5 pixels SPECT dose (μCi)	D= 5 pixels Ratio	D= 6 pixels SPECT dose (μCi)	D= 6 pixels Ratio
1	1.93	0.76	0.39	1.08	0.56	1.56	0.81
2	1.56	0.75	0.48	1.09	0.70	1.53	0.98

D= 7 pixels SPECT dose (μCi)	D= 7 pixels Ratio	D= 8 pixels SPECT dose (μCi)	D= 8 pixels Ratio	D= 9 pixels SPECT dose (μCi)	D= 9 pixels Ratio	D= 10 pixels SPECT dose (μCi)	D= 10 pixels Ratio
1.91	0.99	2.56	1.33	3.17	1.65	3.93	2.03
1.94	1.24	2.52	1.62	3.11	1.99	3.82	2.45

5 Discussion and Conclusion

We have derived an image segmentation method using the level set scheme to identify the LV cavity in CT images and developed a SPECT quantification approach for assessment of absolute targeted radiotracer uptake in the LV myocardium. A hybrid microSPECT/CT imaging system was used for imaging. The methods were evaluated using an in vivo rat model and a radiotracer targeted at angiogenesis. The validity of the results was demonstrated in 2 rats with 7 different myocardium thicknesses assumed in our methods. The linearity of SPECT quantified radiotracer uptake with respect to the thickness confirmed that the results of absolute radiotracer uptake quantification in our rat data were quite promising. Using the 7-pixel wall thickness in consideration of image resolution and the partial volume effect, the resulted SPECT quantified dose was comparable to the true dose obtained from the well-counting data.

While the preliminary results presented herein are encouraging, we did not apply photon attenuation and scatter corrections to the SPECT images in this animal validation. We believe that the estimation of absolute quantification of targeted radiotracer uptake in the LV myocardium can be further improved when these corrections are incorporated. Also, the level sets used in the myocardium segmentation may be affected by the complicated parameter settings and the initial placement of seed region in the cavity. Thus, further validation of our methods in adjusting those settings is warranted.

Acknowledgments

This work was supported in part by the National Institutes of Health (NIH) under Grants R21-EB001774 and R01-HL65662. The authors would like to thank Xiao-Yu Hu, MD and Patti Cavaliere for their assistance in the animal preparation and surgery. The authors also acknowledge that the NC100692 was provided by GE Healthcare.

References

1. Okada R.D., Johnson G., et al.: 99mTc-HL91: "hot spot" detection of ischemic myocardium in vivo by gamma camera imaging. Circulation, 97: 2557-66, 1998.
2. Kessler R.M., et al.: Analysis of emission tomographic scan data: limitations imposed by resolution and background. J Comput Assit Tomogr, 8:514:522, 1984.
3. Kojima A., Matsumoto M., et al.: Effect of spatial resolution on SPECT quantification values. J Nucl Med, 30:508-514, 1989.
4. King M.A., Long D.T., Brill A.B.: SPECT volume quantitation: influence of spatial resolution, source size and shape, and voxel size. Med. Phys, 18:1016-1024, 1991.
5. Da Silva A.J., Tang H.R., Wong K.H., et al.: Absolute in vivo quantitation of myocardial activity. IEEE Trans. Nucl Sci, 47:1093-1098, 2000.
6. Liu Y.H., Li S., Bourke B., Weyman C., Sinusas A.J.: A stochastic approach for quantification of hotspot focal uptake from cardiac SPECT imaging: a canine validation. J Nucl Cardiol, 12:S73,2005.
7. Osher S., Sethian J.: Fronts propagating with curvature dependent speed:algorithms based on the Hamilton–Jacobi formulation. J. Comp. Phys, 79:12–49, 1988.
8. Malladi R., Sethian J., Vemuri B.: Shape modeling with front propagation: A level set approach. IEEE Trans. PAMI, 17(2):158-175, 1995.
9. Caselles V., Kimmel R., Sapiro G.: Geodesic Active Contours. Int'l J. Comp. Vision, 22(1):61–79, 1997.
10. Marquardt D W.: An Algorithm for Least-Squares Estimation of Nonlinear Parameters. J. Soc. Indust. Appl. Math. 11:431-41, 1963.

Tracking and Analysis of Cine-Delayed Enhancement MR

Thomas O'Donnell[1], Engin Dikici[1], Randolph Setser[2], and Richard D. White[2]

[1] Siemens Corporate Research, 755 College Road East, Princeton, NJ 08540
[2] Cleveland Clinic Foundation, Division of Radiology, 9500 Euclid Ave., Cleveland, OH, 44195
tom.odonnell@siemens.com

Abstract. Cine-DEMR is a new cardiac imaging technique which combines aspects of Cine and Delayed Enhancement MR. Like Cine, it displays the heart beating over time allowing for the detection of motion abnormalities. Like DEMR, non-viable (dead) tissues appear with increased signal intensity (it has been shown that the extent of non-viable tissue in the left ventricle (LV) of the heart is a direct indicator of patient survival rate). We present a technique for tracking the myocardial borders in this modality and classifying myocardial pixels as viable or non-viable. Tracking is performed using an affine deformed template of borders manually drawn on the first phase of the series and refined using an ASM-like approach. Classification employs a Support Vector Machine trained on DEMR data. We applied our technique on 75 images culled from 5 patient data sets.

1 Introduction

Cine-Delayed Enhancement Magnetic Resonance imaging (Cine-DEMR) is a novel imaging technique targeted to the left ventricle of the heart which combines the advantages of both Cine MR and Delayed Enhancement MR (DEMR). Like Cine imaging, Cine-DEMR recovers the motion of the heart over the cardiac cycle - the detection of motion abnormalities such as hypokinesis in Cine is a well established indicator of cardiac health [Schwartzman]. Like DEMR images, non-viable (dead) myocardial tissue appears bright in Cine-DEMR images, allowing the amount of non-viable myocardium to be quantified - the extent of non-viable tissue in DEMR is directly correlated with improved cardiac function after revascularization therapy (e.g. coronary bypass surgery) [Kim NEJM]. Thus, Cine-DEMR unites morphology (Cine) with function (DEMR). Figure 1 shows sample images from a Cine-DEMR study and compares them to Cine and DEMR images.

Cine-DEMR has advantages over the combination of separate Cine and DEMR acquisitions. First, it decreases scanning time by replacing two acquisitions with one – no small benefit given the costs of imaging. Second, it supplants the mental integration of the two sequences with a perfectly fused simultaneous visualization. Third, it avoids potential mis-registration of the two separate sequences. Cine and DEMR are typically acquired minutes apart. During that time the patient may have moved, or chest positions may be at variance due to differing breath intakes. The

J. Duncan and G. Gerig (Eds.): MICCAI 2005, LNCS 3750, pp. 692 – 700, 2005.

resulting images may describe regions millimeters apart. Fourth, the optimal phase for evaluating scar (non-viable) tissue may not be end-diastole (the phase in which DEMR is typically acquired). Fifth, due to motion of the myocardium normal to the imaging plane as the heart contracts, the scar may appear and disappear. With Cine-DEMR, the phase which best describes the scar is much more likely to be imaged simply because more than one phase is acquired. Finally, in cases where the scar does not completely cover the wall (is not transmural), it is easier to see how the healthy portion moves as compared to Cine because the two regions can be distinguished.

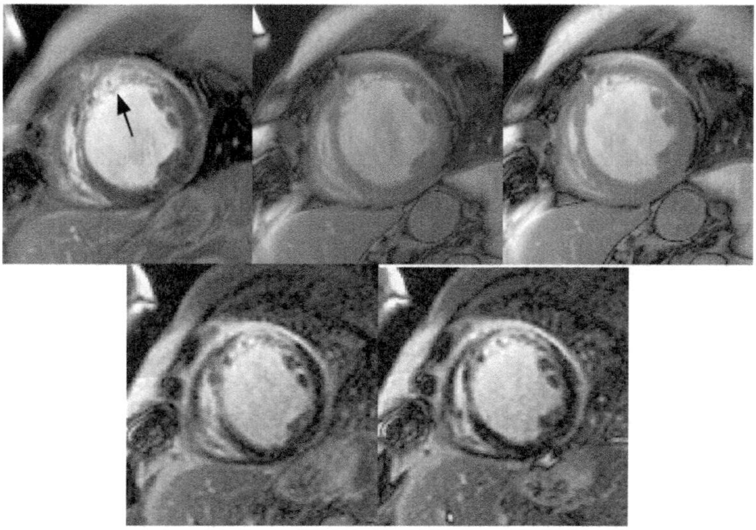

Fig. 1. Top Left: A DEMR image showing non-viable regions with increased signal intensity (denoted by arrow) (Note: DEMR images are single phase). Top Middle and Right: End-diastolic and end-systolic images from a mid-ventricular short-axis Cine acquisition. Bottom: Images from a 15 phase Cine-DEMR study. End-diastole is on the left, end-systole on the right.

The above benefits, however, come at a cost. Cine-DEMR has both decreased spatial and temporal resolution compared to the individual sequences. Nevertheless, preliminary studies in which clinicians analyzed Cine-DEMR, Cine, and DEMR images of the same individual have shown showed a strong correlation in the categorization of tissues [Setser]. And, work is currently being done to improve the temporal resolution via parallel imaging and/or segmented K-space schemes [Setser].

The ultimate goal of our work is the quantification of myocardial scar in Cine-DEMR images. By quantification we mean the identification and measurement of dead myocardial tissue. This implies a two part analysis scheme. First, the myocardium must be defined via the delineation of its borders. Then, those myocardial tissues must be classified as viable or non-viable.

The first part of the scheme, the delineation of the myocardium, is quite challenging. Compared to the same task in Cine MR, it is harder since the myocardial borders may be completely missing. That is, the signal of the myocardium may be the same as that of the bloodpool in non-viable regions. And, since the scar may appear and disappear due to thru plane motion we cannot guarantee that the same intensity pattern will be present over the cycle. Compared to the task in DEMR, it is also difficult. Previous quantification schemes for DEMR [Dikici] assumed the existence of a Cine study so that the true morphology could be referenced. With the advent of Cine-DEMR there may not be a separate Cine study.

Thus, to simplify the delineation task, we assume the existence of a manually drawn contour on the first frame and track the borders over the cycle using this starting point. Briefly, we register this first frame to each of the subsequent (target) frames, copy the endo and epi contours over and fit them to the edges in the target frame using affine transforms. To refine the fit, we take an active shape model approach by attempting to match the radial intensity profiles in the target image to those in the first frame. A spline is then fit to the individual contour points to smooth them. For the second part of the scheme, the classification of the tissues, we rely on a Support Vector Machine (SVM) [Cristianini] which has been trained to recognize non-viable tissue in DEMR images.

The remainder of this paper is as follows. In Section 2 we describe related work. In Section 3 we provide a more detailed description of our algorithms. In Section 4 we show results on the tracking and analysis of Cine-DEMR studies from 5 patients with 15 frames each for a total of 75 images. Discussion of these results are presented in Section 5 and finally, in Section 6 we submit our conclusions.

2 Related Work

While both Cine and Delayed Enhancement MR have become standard protocol for assessment of cardiac viability when using MR [Schwartzman], Cine-DEMR is new enough that, to our knowledge, no work has been published on its automatic or semi-automatic analysis.

Dikici et. al. [Dikici], segmented *static DEMR* on a slice by slice basis using a standard Cine image set as a morphology reference. The employment of an affine deformed template for the tracking of the myocardium was done by [Sun] which bares resemblance to our initial tracking scheme. Our refinement of the tracking uses an active shape model [Cootes] approach similar to that of [Mitchell], however, it is not "trained" on a set of images. Rather, we simply use the first frame of the series as a comparison.

Regarding the classification of myocardial tissues using DEMR, Noble et. al., registered Cine and DEMR image sets in 3D in order to detect hibernating (dormant but not dead) myocardium [Noble]. As well, there are several semi-automatic segmentation techniques for classifying DEMR published in the literature [Kim]. Some of these studies have defined a threshold for non-viable pixels as >2*std dev of the signal intensity of remote, viable myocardium (which was defined manually) [Kim]; other studies have used 3*std dev as the threshold [Fieno]. We employ a Support Vector Machine to classify tissues and in this regard are similar to El-Naqa et. al., in their work on mammogram analysis [El-Naqa] and Dikici et. al.,[Dikici] in their work on the heart.

3 Materials and Methods

3.1 Segmentation of the Myocardium

Let $\overline{C}_n$ represent a vector of Cine-DEMR images with n consecutive phases describing one spatial slice of the heart. Let $S_1(r)$ represent a contour manually drawn on phase 1.

3.1.1 Localization of the LV in Phases $2..n$

The approximate position of the LV in phases $k = 2..n$ is found through a non-rigid registration of C_1 with C_k, $k = 2..n$. This results in a series of deformation fields D_k such that

$$C_1(\vec{x}) \mapsto C_{k,}(D_k(\vec{x})),\ k = 2..n$$

These deformation fields are then applied to $S_1(r)$, $r: 0 \rightarrow 1$, to arrive at

$$S_{localized_k}(r) = D_k(S_1(r)),\ k = 2..n$$

The centroid of $S_{localized_i}(r)$,

$$\vec{x}_{center_k} = \int_{S_{localized_k}} S_{localized_k}(r)dr$$

is the position from which we start our search for the LV in $C_k, k = 2..n$. This deformation is too imprecise for any other inferences. The resulting contour is too deformed to serve as a starting point for the next step of the procedure. Rather, we simply copy over C_1 to C_k and center it on $\vec{x}_{center_k}$ resulting in $S_k'(r)$.

3.1.2 Affine Transformation of Contours

We deform $S_k'(r)$ to fit the image C_k by applying an affine deformation composed of 5 parameters: translation in the x and y dimensions $\vec{\tau}_k$, shearing parameters s_{q_k} and s_{m_k} in $H_k(s_{q_k}, s_{m_k}) = \begin{pmatrix} 1 & s_{q_k} \\ s_{m_k} & 1 \end{pmatrix}$, and a scaling parameter ω_k. The translation is bound by the distance of 10 pixels, the shearing bound by ±*60* degrees and scaling by ±*%20*.

The affine parameters are adjusted to minimize an energy term made up of the components: E_1, E_2, and E_3 such that:

$$S_k''(r) = \underset{\tau_k, s_{q_k}, s_{m_k}, \omega_k}{ArgMax} \begin{bmatrix} W_1 \int E_1(\omega_k H(s_{q_k}, s_{m_k}) S'_{k_{endo}}(r) + \tau_k) dr + \\ W_2 \int E_2(\omega_k H(s_{q_k}, s_{m_k}) S_{k_{epi}}(r) + \tau_k) dr + W_3 \oint E_3(\omega_k H(s_{q_k}, s_{m_k}) S'_{k:epi}(r) + \tau_k) dr \end{bmatrix}$$

The resulting contour $S_k''(r)$ serves as a starting point for a local refinement process.

3.1.3 Local Refinement of the Tracking

Over the course of the cardiac cycle, the shape of the LV deforms in a non-rigid manner. The affine transformation from the previous section is capable of describing this only to a limited extent. However, it does provide a good basis from which to begin a less constrained search. Therefore, we apply an ASM-like approach to refining $S_k''(r)$.

Essentially, we determine the signatures of radial profiles in the neighborhoods of the inner and outer contours of $S_1(r)$. We then locally deform $S_k''(r)$ such that the signature of its profiles in the neighborhoods of the inner and outer contours match those of $S_1(r)$.

3.1.4 Profile Calculation

We sample both inner and outer contours in j radial directions yielding profiles $\vec{p}_{kj_{endo}}(\rho)$ and $\vec{p}_{kj_{epi}}(\rho)$, $k = 1..n$. The radial directions are centered at the centroid, $\vec{\mu}_k$, of $S_{1_{epi}}(r)$ or $S_{k_{epi}}''(r)$ (depending on k). Note: $\vec{\mu}_k$ may be different from $\vec{x}_{center_k}$ due to the affine transformation in Section 3.1.2). The rays intersect $S_1(r)$ or $S_k''(r)$ (depending on k) at $\vec{q}_{kj_{endo}}$ and $\vec{q}_{kj_{epi}}$.

For a particular image k (we drop the k subscript here for clarity), profile $\vec{p}_j(\rho)$ (whether for the inner contour $\vec{p}_{j_{endo}}(\rho)$ or outer contour $\vec{p}_{j_{epi}}(\rho)$) is a linear function of ρ, $-\frac{\kappa}{2} \le \rho \le \frac{\kappa}{2}$ centered at $\vec{q}_j$.

$$\vec{p}_j(\rho) = ((\mu_x + rad_j - \frac{\kappa}{2} + \rho) Cos\phi_j, (\mu_y + rad_j - \frac{\kappa}{2} + \rho) Sin\phi_j)$$

where $rad_j = \sqrt{(\vec{\mu} - \vec{q}_j)^2}$, $\vec{\mu} = (\mu_x, \mu_y)$, and κ is the length of the profile.

The energy ε_{data} for matching the profiles is expressed as a function of the offset $\vec{\upsilon}_{kj}$ from $\vec{q}_{kj}$ (returning to the k subscript),

$$\varepsilon_{data}(\vec{\upsilon}_{kj}) = \int_{-\frac{\kappa}{2}}^{\frac{\kappa}{2}} ((C_k(\vec{p}_{kj}(\rho) + \vec{\upsilon}_{kj}) - C_1(\vec{p}_{1j}(\rho)))^2) d\rho$$

This energy is minimal where the profile in image C_k is offset by $\vec{\upsilon}_{kj}$ best matches the profile in image C_1.

3.1.5 Refining the Contours

For the outer contour, the optimal offset is determined simply by minimizing $\varepsilon_{data}(\vec{\upsilon}_{kj_{epi}})$ with respect to $\vec{\upsilon}_{kj_{epi}}$,

$$\vec{\upsilon}_{kj_{epi}} = \underset{\vec{\upsilon}'_{kj_{epi}}}{ArgMin}\, \varepsilon(\vec{\upsilon}'_{kj_{epi}})$$

For each $s''_{k_{epi}}(r)$, a cubic spline is fit to the points $(\vec{q}_{kj_{epi}} + \vec{\upsilon}_{kj_{epi}})$, for all j, to form the final outer contour, $F_{k_{epi}}(r)$.

The fitting of the inner contour is less stable and requires a smoothing coefficient. This coefficient represents a tethering of the inner contour to the fixed outer contour with a spring which limits its deformation. For a given image, $k = 2..n$ (we drop the k subscript here for clarity),

$$\gamma(\vec{\upsilon}_{j_{endo}}) = 1 + \frac{\left| dist(\vec{q}'_{j_{epi}} - \vec{q}_{j_{endo}}) - dist(\vec{q}'_{j_{epi}} - (\vec{q}_{j_{endo}} + \vec{\upsilon}_{j_{endo}})) \right|}{dist(\vec{q}'_{j_{epi}} - \vec{q}_{j_{endo}})}$$

Where $\vec{q}'_{j_{epi}}$ is the intersection in the radial direction with the final outer contour $F_{k_{epi}}(r)$. Therefore, the optimal offset for the inner contour is determined by minimizing with respect to $\vec{\upsilon}_{kj_{endo}}$ (returning to the k subscript),

$$\vec{\upsilon}_{kj_{endo}} = \underset{\vec{\upsilon}'_{kj_{endo}}}{ArgMin}(\gamma(\vec{\upsilon}'_{kj_{endo}})\varepsilon(\vec{\upsilon}'_{kj_{endo}}))$$

Similarly, a cubic spline is fit to the points $(\vec{q}_{kj_{endo}} + \vec{\upsilon}_{kj_{endo}})$ to form the final contour $F_{k_{endo}}(r)$.

3.2 Classification of Tissues

We employ an SVM to classify the myocardial pixels once the borders have been detected. For our kernel function of the SVM we use a Gaussian radial basis function of the form:

$$k(\bar{\phi}(\vec{x}), \bar{\phi}(\vec{x}')) = e^{-\left\|\bar{\phi}(x) - \bar{\phi}(x')\right\|^2 / 2\sigma^2}$$

where $\bar{\phi}$ is the vector of features. The feature vector $\bar{\phi}$ is made up of three components: First, the intensity of a pixel, relative to the average myocardial intensity. Second, the standard deviation of the relative pixel intensities with respect to its next neighbors. Finally, the "myocardial contrast" defined as the ratio of the mean myocardial intensity and the mean image intensity of the image. Training was performed on static DEMR images due to the lack of available Cine-DEMR examples. To determine σ in our kernel as well as K, a compromise between maximizing the margin and minimizing the number of training set errors, we employed the "leave-one-out strategy".

3.3 Acquisition Protocol

Cine-DEMR imaging is based on inversion recovery, single-shot, balanced steady state free precession (bSSFP) imaging [Chung]. Each image frame of the ECG-triggered cine series is acquired during a separate RR-interval using a constant inversion time. Image frames are acquired every other heart beat to allow magnetization recovery. To create a cine series, the trigger delay is varied between image frames, resulting in a series of single-shot images, each from a different phase of the cardiac cycle.

Cine-DE images were acquired using a 1.5T MRI scanner (Magnetom Sonata, Siemens Medical Solutions, Erlangen, Germany), using the following typical acquisition parameters: flip angle 50°, repetition time 2.5 ms, echo time 1.1 ms, bandwidth 1090 Hz/pixel, field-of-view 380 mm, rectangular field-of-view 75%, acquisition matrix 192 x 115 (frequency, phase). By default, 15 image frames are acquired in each CINE-DE series, with a variable temporal spacing to cover the cardiac cycle. Images are acquired during a single breath-hold, approximately 10-20 minutes after intravenous injection of 40 ml of 0.5 mmol/ml gadopentetate dimeglumine (Magnevist, Berlex Imaging, Wayne NJ).

4 Results

We validated our study by comparing our automated results with ground truth provided by an expert. Three phases (frames 5, 10, and 15) from each patient were collected for a total of 15 images. An expert different from the one providing ground truth supplied the initial segmentation to initialize the tracking (frame 1). Figure 2 (Left) shows an example frame.

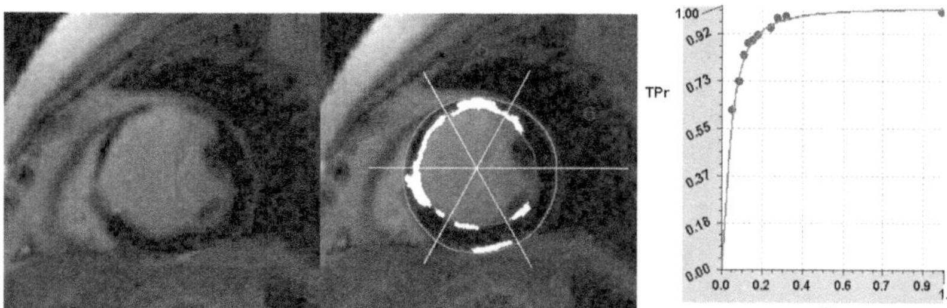

Fig. 2. Left: An example Cine-DEMR image. Middle: the tracking/classification protocol applied to the example image. The white pixels represent those found to be non-viable. Right: The ROC curve describing the results of our experiments. 96.80% of the area is under the curve.

For the segmentation, 32 radial directions were used for the profiles. Both the inner and outer profiles had length $\kappa = 5$ pixels and the search space for matching the profiles was 3 square pixels. The tracking of the myocardial borders had an average error of 2.1 pixels over all images. Regarding the classification of pixels as viable or non-viable, appropriate SVM parameters were found to be $\sigma = 0.01$ and $K = 20$. Our experiments had a sensitivity of 80.76%, specificity 96.54% with 96.80% of the area covered under the ROC (see Figure 2 (Right)). The general correctness rate was 93.46%.

5 Discussion

The tracking of the myocardial borders was performed from the first phase to every other phase ($1 \rightarrow n$) rather than from one phase to the next ($n \rightarrow n+1$). This approach was taken because the profile signatures in phase 1 were guaranteed to be correct (having been based on manually drawn contours) and were a better basis for matching. We initially attempted a consecutive frame ($n \rightarrow n+1$) approach but found that a slight drift over the series resulted in poorer segmentations. Our scheme depends on the general appearance of the myocardium staying constant over the cardiac cycle. As mentioned in the introduction, this may not always be the case due to through plane motion. Therefore, we are currently investigating a Kalman filter approach to this tracking.

As described in Section 3.1.5, the refinement of the endocardial and endocardial contours is treated differently in the tracking. The endocardial border generally deforms much less significantly than the endocardial border over the cardiac cycle. Because the endocardial border is subject to such variability, we found that without the smoothing effect of tethering to the epicardium, the endocardial segmentation was far too jagged to appear natural. This tethering had a strong impact particularly when the tissue was very damaged. In these cases the myocardium was bright enough to be indistinguishable from the blood pool so there was little influence from the data energy ε_{data}. In these cases, the dead tissue moves very little since it is, in fact, dead. Therefore reliance on the tethering influence yielded good results.

Finally, as mentioned in the introduction, Cine-DEMR and DEMR have different resolutions and thus appear slightly dissimilar from one another. Our training set for the classification of the myocardial tissues was based on standard DEMR datasets since we had few Cine-DEMR datasets on which to train the SVM. We attribute our relatively low sensitivity in our results to the fact that the training set and testing sets do not come from the same population.

6 Conclusions

We have presented preliminary findings on the tracking and classification of a new MR imaging sequence Cine-DEMR. In the future we hope to develop methods for the segmentation of the first phase of these series thereby creating a fully automatic quantification procedure.

References

[Cootes] T. Cootes and C. Taylor, "Statistical Models of Appearance for Computer Vision" October 26, 2001, pp 37-43, available at www.isbe.man.ac.uk.

[Cristianini] Cristianini N, Shawe-Taylor J. An Introduction to Support Vector Machines and other kernel-based learning methods. Cambridge University Press 2000.

[El-Naqa] El-Naqa I,, Yongyi Yang, Miles N. Wernick, Nikolas P. Galatsanos, and Robert Nishikawa, "Support Vector Machine Learning for Detection of Microcalcififcations in Mammograms", IEEE ICIP, Rochester, NY, September 2002

[Fieno] Fieno DS, Kim RJ,et.al.,. Contrast enhanced MRI of myocardium at risk: distinction between reversible and irreversible injury throughout infarct healing. 2000;36:1985-1991.

[Kim] R.J. Kim, D.S. Fieno, et. al., "Relationship of MRI Delayed Contrast Enhancement to Irreversible Injury, Infarct Age, and Contractile Function", Circulation 1999; 100: 1992-2002.

[Dikici] Engin Dikici, T. O'Donnell. et. al.,., "Quantification of Delayed Enhancement Images", Proceedings of MICCAI 2004.

[Schwartzman] Schwartzman PR., White RD. Magnetic Resonance Imaging. In: Topol EJ, ed. Textbook of Cardiovascular Medicine, 2nd edition. Philadelphia: Lippincott-Raven, 2002.

[Kim NEJM] Kim RJ, Wu E, Rafael A, Chen EL, Parker MA, Simonetti O, Klocke FJ, Bonow RO, Judd RM. The Use of Contrast-Enhanced Magnetic Resonance Imaging to Identify Reversible Myocardial Dysfunction. N Engl J Med 2000; 343:1445-53.

[Setser] Setser RM, Chung YC, Kim JK, Stillman AE, Simonetti OP, Weaver JA, White RD. Cine Delayed Enhancement Imaging of the Heart. J Cardiovascular Magn Reson 2002; 7(1): 298-299 (Abstract).

[Chung] Chung YC, Vargas J, Simonetti O. Infarct imaging in a single heart beat. J Cardiovasc. Magn Reson 2002; 4: 12 (Abstract)

[Mitchell] S.C. Mitchell, J.G. Bosch, et. al., "3D Active Appearance Models: Segmentation of Cardiac MR and Ultrasound images." IEEE TMI vol. 20(9), 2002

[Noble] Noble N., Hill, D.. et. al., "The Automatic Identification of Hibernating Myocardium", MICCAI 2004, pgs. 890-898.

[Sun] Sun, Y, Jolly, MP. Moura J, "Contrast Invariant Registration of Cardiac and Renal MR Perfusion Images", MICCAI04 905-910.

Characterizing Vascular Connectivity from microCT Images

Marcel Jackowski[1], Xenophon Papademetris[1,2], Lawrence W. Dobrucki[1,3], Albert J. Sinusas[1,3], and Lawrence H. Staib[1,2]

[1] Departments of Diagnostic Radiology
[2] Biomedical Engineering
[3] Medicine (Cardiology), Yale University, New Haven CT 06520

Abstract. X-ray microCT (computed tomography) has become a valuable tool in the analysis of vascular architecture in small animals. Because of its high resolution, a detailed assessment of blood vessel physiology and pathology is possible. Vascular measurement from noninvasive imaging is important for the study and quantification of vessel disease and can aid in diagnosis, as well as measure disease progression and response to therapy. The analysis of tracked vessel trajectories enables the derivation of vessel connectivity information, lengths between vessel junctions as well as level of ramification, contributing to a quantitative analysis of vessel architecture. In this paper, we introduce a new vessel tracking methodology based on wave propagation in oriented domains. Vessel orientation and vessel likelihood are estimated based on an eigenanalysis of gray-level Hessian matrices computed at multiple scales. An anisotropic wavefront then propagates through this vector field with a speed modulated by the maximum vesselness response at each location. Putative vessel trajectories can be found by tracing the characteristics of the propagation solution between different points. We present preliminary results from both synthetic and mouse microCT image data.

1 Introduction

Methods for the quantification of vascular structure are crucial in a number of domains. While 3D localization and visualization are important, the power of vascular imaging methods lies in quantitative analysis including characterizing and measuring connectivity, level of ramification, segment length as well as cross-sectional area and volume. A particularly important application is the study of changes that occur in response to angiogenic therapy which has tremendous potential for treatment in vessel disease and would benefit from non-invasive methods for quantitative evaluation of vasculature growth and remodeling.

X-ray microCT imaging combined with perfused contrast agents provides a robust methodology for evaluation of intact vascular networks [4]. However, the ability to extract and quantify vessels, especially those of smaller diameter, is limited by noise, contrast and extraneous features, such as bone. In CT using contrast agents, vessels appear as relatively bright; in magnetic resonance

J. Duncan and G. Gerig (Eds.): MICCAI 2005, LNCS 3750, pp. 701–708, 2005.

angiography (MRA), they may be dark or bright depending on the technique. They are curved structures of varying width with greatest width at the aorta, generally decreasing in diameter with branching and greater distance from the aorta. The geometry is quite complex making 3D imaging a necessity (2D serial section analysis is only of limited use).

Techniques for filtering curved structures have been applied to vessel images [15,9,6,11], especially using multiscale techniques. In these methods, the Hessian of the gray level intensities is computed at multiple scales. The eigenstructure of the Hessian is determined in order to characterize the local structure (linear, planar or no structure) and if linear, the orientation of the vessel. Methods have been developed for vessel segmentation using thresholding [15], active contours [11], model-based methods [9,8], expectation maximization [1] as well as level set-based approaches [12,3]. Lorigo *et al.* [12] applied a novel level-set segmentation formulated specifically for 3D curves. Vessel segmentation, however, is prone to errors and may result in discontinuous segments and inclusion of extraneous features, such as bone. Work on tracing vessel trajectories has also been attempted before. Olabarriaga *et al.* find a minimum cost path through a vesselness image using bidirectional search [14]. Flasque *et al.* [5] track vessels from MRA using a model-based approach, tracking centerlines using a search strategy. Deschamps and Cohen presented a minimal-path method based on the Fast Marching algorithm applied to vessel centerline extraction for virtual endoscopy [2]. Lin [10] also investigated extracting minimal paths using an anisotropic version of the Fast Marching method that incorporates orientation and was applied to MRA and fluorescence images.

In this paper, we also focus on extracting vessel trajectories. Our approach is similar to that of Lin [10], by using an anisotropic wavefront evolution method, and like Descoteaux [3], we also make use of Frangi's vesselness measure. While we are interested in finding the size of extracted vessels, which can be obtained by the vesselness response across scales, we do not use level sets to explicitly reconstruct vessel boundaries. Levels sets for explicit surface reconstruction can easily bleed out into regions with similar vessel intensities. They also have difficulty extracting finer-scale vessels and may result in disconnected vessel segments. In the next section, we describe our vessel tracing approach using a static anisotropic wavefront propagation method combined with a multiscale vessel analysis.

2 Approach

In this section, we briefly describe the multiscale vessel localization procedure and how to obtain the vessel likelihood measure [6]. Then we describe the wave propagation equation that will drive the front evolution using information from the Hessian matrix as well as the maximum vessel likelihood response across different scales. Finally, we describe how to extract vessel trajectories by tracing the characteristics of the front evolution PDE. An anisotropic version of the static front evolution method is used to build a cost map which will be minimum for pathways in highly oriented structures and with high vesselness measure.

2.1 Vessel Filtering

One way to account for the varying size of vessels is by multiscale analysis. It allows us to detect structures of different sizes according to the scale at which they give maximal response. In order to enhance blood vessels at a particular scale σ, Frangi [6] designed the filter $V(x, \sigma)$, which is a nonlinear combination of the eigenvalues of the Hessian matrix $\mathcal{H}$ computed at each voxel of the image. This vesselness measure has given reasonable results in the segmentation of blood vessels by other investigators [3] and is also employed here. The scale corresponds to the vessel radius in pixels.

The filter V provides a likelihood value for a structure having a tubular shape. At each scale σ, the image is first convolved by a 3-D Gaussian with standard deviation equal to that scale in pixels and then the vesselness measure is computed as:

$$V(x,\sigma) = \begin{cases} 0, & \text{if } \lambda_2 > 0 \text{ or } \lambda_3 > 0 \\ \left(1 - \exp\left(-\frac{R_A^2}{2\alpha^2}\right)\right) \exp\left(-\frac{R_B^2}{2\beta^2}\right) \left(1 - \exp\left(-\frac{S^2}{2c^2}\right)\right), & \text{otherwise} \end{cases} \tag{1}$$

where $R_A = \frac{|\lambda_2|}{|\lambda_3|}$, $R_B = \frac{|\lambda_1|}{\sqrt{|\lambda_2 \lambda_3|}}$, $S = \sqrt{\lambda_1^2 + \lambda_2^2 + \lambda_3^2}$ and the eigenvalues are ordered according to their magnitudes as $|\lambda_1| \leq |\lambda_2| \leq |\lambda_3|$. Since the vessels are bright against a darker background in microCT images, the eigenvalues are negative. The quantities R_A, R_B and S are designed to punish cross-sectional asymmetry, blobness and low energy, respectively. The parameters α, β and c are used to tune the sensitivity of the filter to deviations from perfect tubular structures. This measure will yield maximum response at the center of vessels and close to zero outside them. The filter V is applied at different scales in order to detect vessels with different scales. We vary σ from σ_{min} to σ_{max}, and compute the maximum vessel likelihood across all chosen radii:

$$V_{\text{max}}(x) = \max_{\sigma_{\text{min}} \leq \sigma \leq \sigma_{\text{max}}} V(x, \sigma). \tag{2}$$

2.2 Front Evolution

Once the maximum response V_{max} is computed for all points in the domain, not only will we have a vessel likelihood map but also a map containing the corresponding Hessian matrix $\mathcal{H}_{\text{max}}$ at the maximum scale. From the eigenanalysis of $\mathcal{H}_{\text{max}}$, the eigenvector $\boldsymbol{u} = \boldsymbol{u}_1$ which corresponds to the smallest eigenvalue will represent the vessel orientation. In our implementation, we will propagate a wavefront through the vector field defined by $\boldsymbol{u}$. The front will move fastest in regions where its normal vector $\boldsymbol{n} = \frac{\nabla T}{\|\nabla T\|}$ lines up with the vector field and in regions with a high vesselness measure. T represents the time of arrival of the front at each location. Such evolution can be modeled by the following static anisotropic evolution equation:

$$\|\nabla T\| \, V_{\text{max}}(x) \, F(x, \boldsymbol{n}) = 1, \quad F(x, \boldsymbol{n}) = \exp(\{\boldsymbol{n} \cdot \boldsymbol{u}\}^2). \tag{3}$$

This propagation equation will evolve a wavefront driven by the directionality of the vector field $\boldsymbol{u}$ but will stop its evolution near the boundary with non-vessel structures, since $V_{\max}$ will be close to zero in these regions. Since the Hessian matrix is indefinite [10], not all eigenvalues have the same sign. Hence, $\mathcal{H}_{\max}$ may not represent an ellipsoid at all times. Instead of using the full Hessian as an ellipsoidal speed profile, we resort to driving our wavefront according to the colinearity between the front normal $\boldsymbol{n}$ and $\boldsymbol{u}$.

Equations such as (3) cannot be correctly solved by isotropic propagation methods, such as the Fast Marching Method. Hence, we employ an iterative approach combined with a Lax-Friedrichs (LF) discretization of our propagation equation. A nonlinear Gauss-Seidel updating scheme is used to solve the equation in terms of neighboring grid points. No minimization is required when updating an arrival time, and thus it becomes very easy to implement.

In order to track vessel segments, we seed the evolution at a point inside the vessel, and let the propagation take place. When the evolution has converged to a solution, it will represent a cost map which can be used to find a minimal cost path representing the vessel trajectory.

2.3 Vessel Tracking

Minimum-cost trajectories are determined by the characteristic curves of the respective partial differential equation [13,7]. In our propagation model, the gradient ∇T of the solution will not point to the minimum-cost path, since our equation is anisotropic and the speed profile is not circular. One must explicitly calculate the appropriate characteristic directions of the obtained arrival times solution at every point.

A generic first-order PDE with m independent variables can be written as:

$$H(x_i, T, p_i) = 0, \text{ where } p_i = \partial T/\partial x_i, \; i = 1, ..., m \tag{4}$$

where T is a function of each of the independent variables x_i. In our case, T represents the arrival times of the wavefront. The characteristic vector $\boldsymbol{a}$ can be obtained via Charpit's equations [13] and is defined as $a_i = \partial H/\partial p_i$. Our wavefront evolution equation (3) can be written in generic form by discarding its dependence on location x:

$$H = \sqrt{p_1^2 + p_2^2 + p_3^2}\, V_{\max}\; F(p_1, p_2, p_3) - 1 = 0 \tag{5}$$

By differentiating H with respect to p_1, p_2 and p_3, we find the characteristic vector $\boldsymbol{a}$. Because the speed function F is a function of the gradient ∇T, the characteristic vector $\boldsymbol{a}$ does not necessarily coincide with the gradient. Therefore, one must integrate $\frac{dX}{dt} = -\boldsymbol{a}$ instead of $\frac{dX}{dt} = -\nabla T$ to obtain the minimum-cost path, X.

3 Experimental Results

In order to evaluate our vessel tracing method, we first applied it on a synthetic dataset obtained from the Laboratory of Mathematics in Imaging at Harvard

University [9]. Figure 1a depicts the Y-junction vessel model which contains 2 segments of different radii (1 and 3 pixels). They have Gaussian intensity profiles with a maximum intensity value of 100 at their centerlines. Fig. 1b shows the corresponding ridges (centerlines) from the model. The centerlines are assumed to be the true trajectories. We investigated how close the resulting trajectories were to the true centerlines, with and without noise. Gaussian noise with $\sigma^2 = 10, 20, 40$ was added to the original image. The maximum vesselness measure $V_{\max}$ and the respective Hessian $\mathcal{H}_{\max}$ were then computed at two different scales, 1 and 3 pixels to match the exact model dimensions (Fig. 1c-e). Parameters α, β and c were set to 0.5, 0.5 and half the maximum Frobenius norm of the Hessian matrices, respectively, according to [6]. Next, we employed our wave propagation technique by first selecting a seed point for propagation (see cross-hairs in Fig. 1a). After propagation reached convergence, we traced the centerlines from the extreme points of the two branches (Figs. 1f-h) and compared the results to the true trajectories (Fig. 1b).

As can be seen in Figs. 1f-h, the technique is robust enough to recover the trajectories embedded in very noisy backgrounds. This is partly due to the Gaussian

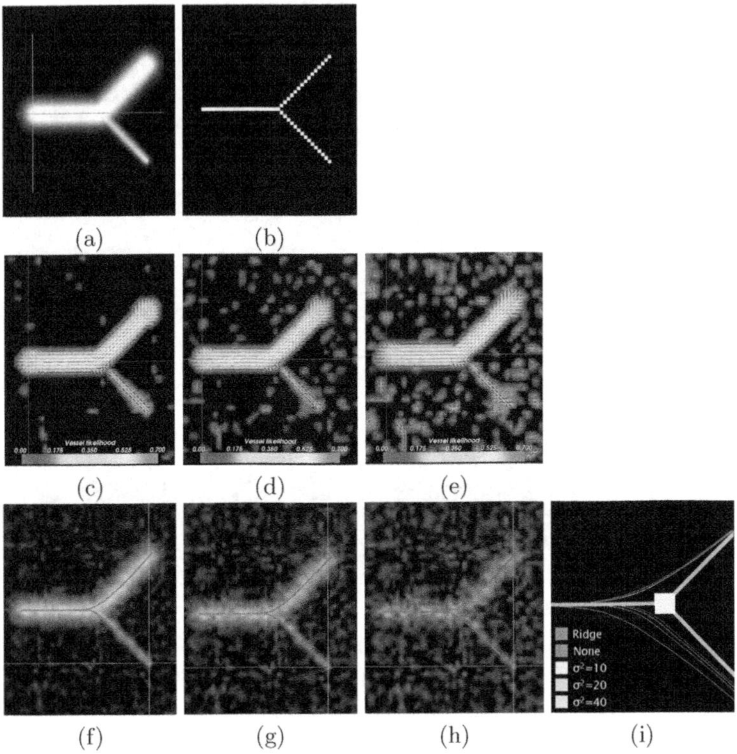

Fig. 1. (a) Synthetic dataset. (b) Corresponding centerlines. Second row: Vector field $\boldsymbol{u}$ at different noise levels; (c) $\sigma^2 = 10$, (d) $\sigma^2 = 20$, (e) $\sigma^2 = 40$. Third row: Resulting trajectories at different noise levels. (i) Close-up at branching point.

smoothing that is applied at each scale when determining the maximum vesselness response. Figure 1i shows a close-up view of the branching point in the model. The maximum disparities between the centerline (shown in gray) and the resulting trajectories were found to be at the center of the branching point (shown as a white square in Fig. 1i). This is because our speed term does not currently follow the ridges of the vessels, only their directionality. Therefore, the minimum-cost trajectory may not pass exactly through the true center of the intersection. For the larger branch (3 pixels in radius), the maximum error averaged ≈ 1 voxel, with and without added noise (no-noise trajectory shown in red). The largest error was obtained for the smaller size branch, as large levels of noise destroyed a lot of its structure and subsequent smoothing altered its final

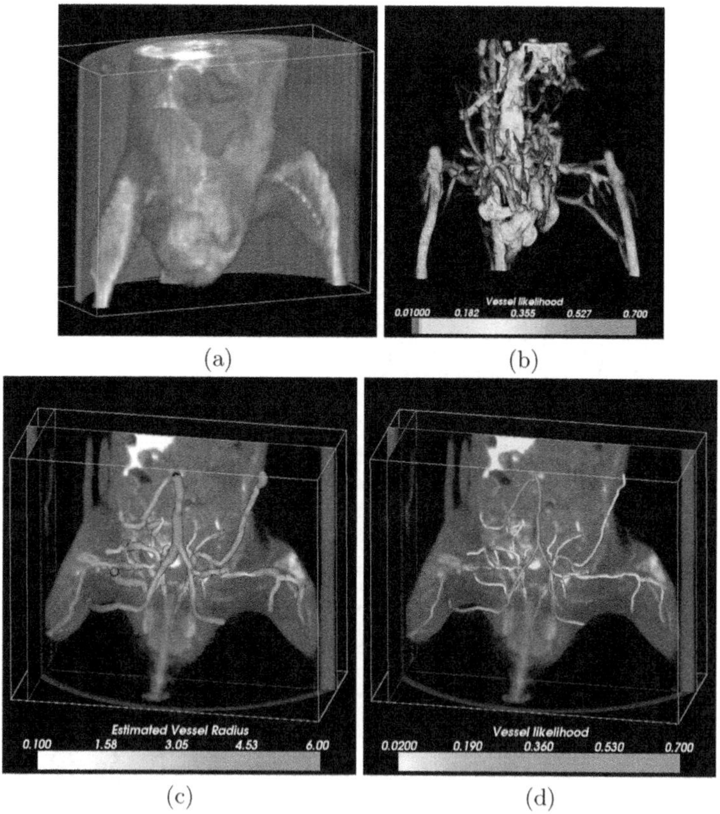

Fig. 2. (a) Volume rendering of the CT dataset depicting the lower body of a mouse. (b) Three-dimensional view of the vector field $\boldsymbol{u}$ colored by the vesselness measure. Both bones and vessels can be seen. (c) Reconstruction of the major vessels connecting to the aorta shown with volume rendering. Vessels are colored according to their estimated size. (d) Reconstructed vessels colored according to their maximum vesselness measure. Vessels located in the inferior half of the volume were partially obscured for better spatial perception.

shape. A maximum error of ≈ 1.7 voxels resulted at $\sigma^2 = 40$. The corresponding errors for no-noise was 0.79 voxels, with noise $\sigma^2 = 10$ was 0.92, $\sigma^2 = 20$ was 1.13 and $\sigma^2 = 40$ reached 1.73 voxels. Despite the discrepancies from the true centerline, the technique presented here allows for fine vessel extraction in the presence of significant noise, and will not result in disconnected structures, as may occur with other level set-based techniques.

To evaluate our method on a real image, an ex-vivo mouse microCT dataset using barium-sulfate contrast was acquired at a resolution of $50 \times 50 \times 100$ μm. (Figure 2a). After cropping, the resulting image size was $291 \times 131 \times 226$. A mean curvature-based smoothing was first applied to eliminate undesired background noise while preserving edge information. Multiscale analysis was performed in 10 uniformly sampled Gaussian scales ranging from 0.5 to 5 voxels. The maximum vesselness measure and the corresponding Hessian $\mathcal{H}_{\max}$ was computed at each location. Figure 2b shows the vector field $\boldsymbol{u}$ after diagonalizing $\mathcal{H}_{\max}$. The vector field is colored according to the vesselness measure at each point. Both vessels and bones can be seen. A seed point was placed inside the aorta and a wavefront was propagated in the vector field $\boldsymbol{u}$. In order to initialize tracking, 45 points were selected manually by picking the center of vessels at different planes. Vessel trajectories were then traced back into the aorta. Estimates of radius and vesselness measures were calculated at every point on the trajectories.

Figure 2c shows the resulting trajectories as tubular structures and colored according to their estimated radius. Because a discrete number of scales were employed, tubes representing the vessels did not change in size continuously. With a more continuous scaling, better radii estimates can be determined. Radii were determined by the scale in which the vesselness measure was maximum. Figure 2d shows the extracted vessels colored according to their maximum vesselness measure.

4 Conclusions

An anisotropic front propagation method was described for determining vascular pathways in mouse microCT images. Using multiscale analysis, the maximum vesselness measure was computed at every point and the corresponding Hessian matrix was recorded. A wavefront was propagated in the vector field defined by the smallest eigenvector of the Hessian matrix. The propagation speed was defined by the colinearity between front normal and the smallest eigenvector of the Hessian. The front stopped at regions of very low vesselness. Using the characteristic vector of the propagation solution, the technique was able to recover trajectories in both synthetic and real microCT data.

Results on mouse CT datasets were presented where major vessels were recovered and reconstructed. Vessel trajectories were fit with tubular structures with a radius corresponding to the scale in which they were detected. Further investigation will be done on new forms of the evolution PDE for tracking the ridges. We will also fit ellipses instead of circles for the vessel reconstruction by using the eigenvalue magnitudes from the Hessian matrix. In addition, we will investigate an automated approach for initializing the vessel tracing which will enable us to reconstruct the entire vessel tree and allow for its quantification with minimum manual intervention. Features such as connectivity, level of ramification, segment length as well as cross-sectional area and volume can then be calculated. These measures may ultimately improve quantitative diagnosis and allow the measurement of change due to disease or therapy.

References

1. A. Chung and J. A. Noble. Statistical 3D vessel segmentation using a Rician distribution. In *MICCAI*, pages 82–89. LNCS 1679, Springer, 1999.
2. D. Deschamps and L. D. Cohen. Fast extraction of minimal paths in 3d images and applications to virtual endoscopy. *Medical Image Analysis*, 5(4), Dec 2001.
3. M. Descoteaux. A multi-scale geometric flow for segmenting vasculature in MRI: Theory and validation. Master's thesis, School of Computer Science, McGill University, Montréal, June 2004.
4. C. L. Duvall, W. R. Taylor, D. Weiss, and R. E. Guldberg. Quantitative microcomputed tomography analysis of collateral vessel development after ischemic injury. *Am. J. Physiol. Heart. Circ. Physiol.*, 287(1):H302–310, 2004.
5. N. Flasque, M. Desvignes, J. Constans, and M. Revenu. Acquisition, segmentation and tracking of the cerebral vascular tree on 3D magnetic resonance angiography images. *Medical Image Analysis*, 5(3):173–183, Sep 2001.
6. A. F. Frangi, W. J. Niessen, K. L. Vincken, and M. A. Viergever. Multiscale vessel enhancement filtering. In *MICCAI*, pages 130–137. LNCS 1496, Springer, 1998.
7. F. John. *Partial Differential Equations*, volume 1. Springer, 4th edition, 1982.
8. K. Krissian, R. Kikinis, and C. Westin. Algorithms for extracting vessel centerlines. Technical Report 0003, Department of Radiology, Brigham and Women's Hospital, Harvard Medical School, Laboratory of Mathematics in Imaging, September 2004.
9. K. Krissian, G. Malandain, N. Ayache, R. Vaillant, and Y. Trousset. Model-based detection of tubular structures in 3D images. *Comp. Vision and Image Understanding*, 80(2):130–171, 2000.
10. Q. Lin. *Enhancement, Extraction and Visualization of 3D Volume Data.* PhD thesis, Dept. of Electrical Engineering, Linköping University, Sweden, 2003.
11. C. Lorenz, I.-C. Carlsen, T. M. Buzug, C. Fassnacht, and J. Weese. A multi-scale line f ilter with automatic scale selection based on the Hessian matrix for medical image segmentation. In *Scale-Space Theories in Computer Vision*, pages 152–163. LNCS 1252, Springer, 1997.
12. L. M. Lorigo, O. D. Faugeras, W. E. Grimson, R. Keriven, R. Kikinis, A. Nabavi, and C. F. Westin. CURVES: curve evolution for vessel segmentation. *Medical Image Analysis*, 5(3):195–206, Sep 2001.
13. J. Ockendon, S. Howison, A. Lacey, and A. Movchan. *Applied Partial Differential Equations.* Oxford University Press, revised edition, 2003.
14. S. D. Olabarriaga, M. Breeuwer, and W. J. Niessen. Minimum cost path algorithm for coronary artery central axis tracking in CT images. In R. E. Ellis and T.M. Peters, editors, *MICCAI*, pages 687–694, Berlin, 2003. LNCS 2879, Sprin ger.
15. Y. Sato, S. Nakajima, N. Shiraga, H. Atsumi, S. Yoshida, T. Koller, G. Gerig, and R. Kikinis. Three-dimensional multi-scale line filter for segmentation and visualization of curvilinear structures in medical images. *Medical Image Analysis*, 2(2):143–168, 1998.

Shape Modeling Using Automatic Landmarking

Jun Xie and Pheng-Ann Heng

Department of Computer Science and Engineering
and
Shun Hing Institute of Advanced Engineering,
Chinese University of Hong Kong, Shatin, Hong Kong
{jxie, pheng}@cse.cuhk.edu.hk

Abstract. This paper describes a novel approach to automatically recover accurate correspondence over various shapes. In order to detect the features points with the capability in capturing the characteristics of an individual shape, we propose to calculate the skeletal representation for the shape curve through the medial axis transform. Employing this shape descriptor, mathematical landmarks are automatically identified based on the local feature size function, which embodies the geometric and topological information of the boundary. Before matching the resulting landmarks, shape correspondence is first approached by matching the major components of the shape curves using skeleton features. This helps in keeping the consecutive order and reducing the search space during the matching process. Point matching is then performed within each pair of corresponding components by solving a consecutive assignment problem. The effectiveness of this approach is demonstrated through experimental results on several different training sets of biomedical object shapes.

1 Introduction

Deformable models in medical imaging have a variety of applications including anatomical registration, segmentation and morphological analysis. Since shape information is a crucial visual cue for human perception, one of the most promising class of deformable models, the statistical model of shape [1], has been proposed to capture the patterns of variation in the shapes and spatial relationships in a class of objects. In this approach, a shape is commonly described by locating a finite number of points, the landmarks, on the boundary. Landmarks are well-defined points which are supposedly homologous from one instance to the next.

Although manual landmarking is an intuitive way to obtain those discernable points in practice, it is subjective and labor intensive and studies have shown that the precision of manual landmarking drifts with time and the accuracy varies among the landmarkers. There are also some semi-automatic and automatic landmarking approaches [2]. The mathematical landmarks are located according to some mathematical or geometric properties such as curvature, angel and arc length. One of the problem with curvature-defined landmarks is that in some applications (e.g. biological imaging), these points are not always born out clearly or uniquely by the individual shape, and in this case the landmarks must be inferred from a more global context.

Davies *et al.* [3] proposed to use the Minimum Description Length (MDL), as a quantitative measure of "simpleness", to achieve a dense correspondence across a set of

J. Duncan and G. Gerig (Eds.): MICCAI 2005, LNCS 3750, pp. 709–716, 2005.

shapes. However, like other global shape correspondence methods [4], the MDL-based approach constructs a very complicated and highly nonlinear cost function. Belongie *et al.* [5] introduced a shape matching scheme using roughly uniform samplings. Based on the proposed descriptor, this approach has produced encouraging results on a wide variety of data sets [6]. However, as shown by many researchers (e.g. [3]), the equally space landmarks can result in poor models, which indicates unit-length sampling cannot capture the shape's crucial characteristics if the sampling is not dense enough. Another weakness of this approach is the absence of any consecutive constraint. This leads to more erroneous matches. Recently, a continuity constraint was incorporated into the shape context matching scheme by Thayananthan [7] and the cost function was optimized using a dynamic programming.

In this paper, we present a simple and fast algorithm to obtain shape correspondence via an automatic landmarking scheme. Given a shape, we first re-sample the shape curve in an optimal way based on the Medial Axis Transform (MAT) proposed by Blum [8]. Landmarks along the shape curve are located using the Local Feature Size (LFS) function, which is determined by the geometric and topological features around the curve points. The major contribution of the paper is a fast and robust approach to match those non-uniformly samplings. It consists of two steps. First, the characteristic points on the medial axis are matched. This leads to an initial correspondence of different major components of the shapes. Then point correspondences are obtained within each pair of corresponding curve segments.

2 Optimal Shape Sampling

2.1 Medial Axis Transform

Let $F(u) = (x(u), y(u))$ be a smooth curve representing a shape. A point is on the medial axis (or skeleton) of the shape if it is equidistant from two or more points on the shape curve as shown in Fig. 1(a).

There are three kinds of points on a medial axis, including the endings, the midpoints and the junctions. In the continuous case, the distinction between an ending, a

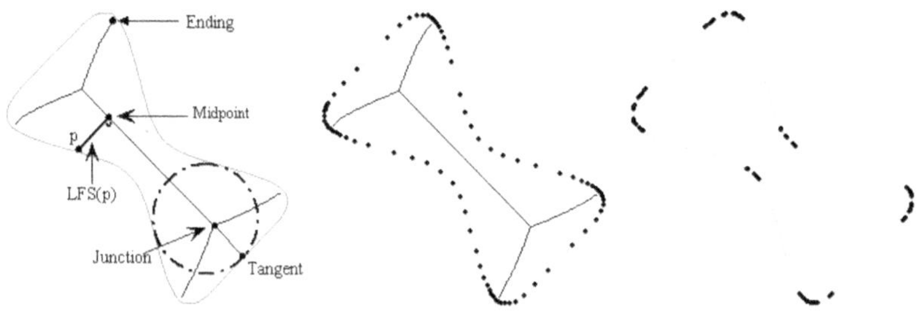

Fig. 1. An illustration of the shape sampling rule. (Left) A curve (light) and its medial axis (heavy). The circle indicates a maximal disk. (Middle) The sampling result using the γ-sampling rule. There are totally 85 samples with $\gamma = 0.4$. (Right) The sampling result using curvature maxima (top 85 points).

midpoint and a junction of the skeleton follows from the number of times a disc centered at the point intersects the skeleton. The endings and midpoints are equidistant from exactly two boundary points while the junctions are equidistant from three or more points on the boundary. The maximal disk associated with the singular medial location osculates the object's boundary, meaning that the curvature radius (CR) of the boundary at the location of tangency is equal to the radius of the maximal disk. The two involutes necessarily converge at this location of tangency.

Based on the medial axis directly, many approaches [9,10] have been developed for shape matching. However, comparing shapes via exact matching of medial axes is not trivial since the internal structure of medial axis may change greatly due to minute deformation or occlusion of shape curves as shown in Fig. 3.

2.2 Shape Sampling

Given a shape, we seek a method to sample the shape curve with a compact set of points, which can characterize the inherent feature of this shape uniquely. In other words, this set of samplings can lead to only one possible smoothed curve, the original shape. Our sampling condition is based on a geometric length scale, local feature size, which was first proposed by Ruppert [11] for mesh generation. The local feature size for a shape F is a continuous function: $LFS : F \rightarrow R^2$ defined as distance of $p \in F$ to the medial axis of F, see Fig. 1(a). Because it is defined on the medial axis, the local feature size function is dominated by both the geometric features (e.g. curvature and orientation) and the topological features (e.g. symmetry and width).

Using this detail descriptor, we sample a curve under the following γ-sampling condition. Let $S \in R^2$ be a set of points on a shape F. Set S is defined as a γ-sample of F if for each point $p \in F$, there is a sample point $q \in S$ so that $||p - q|| \leq \gamma LFS(q)$. This condition makes sampling density vary with the local feature size on the curve, so that areas of less detail will be sampled less densely. Two sampling results using γ-sampling condition and curvature maxima are shown in Fig. 1(b) and Fig. 1(c), respectively. We can see that γ-sampling can produce a more representative and full descriptor for the shape than the curvature maxima based sampling method.

It has been observed that for $\gamma \geq 1$, the sample set may produce more than one curve that is the polygonal reconstruction of a smooth curve γ-sampled by S. This indicates the sampling is not dense enough for the unique reconstruction of the original shape. In this case, there are some small features on the shape that are sampled inadequately. Therefore, such a undersampling will block the success of point distribution based shape matching. On the other hand, for considerably smaller γ (e.g. $\gamma < 1$), Amenta [12] and Dey [13] have shown that there is only one possible reconstruction of the curve. Typically, in our approach, $\gamma = 1/3$ gives a good performance for all experiments.

3 Shape Correspondence

After the optimal sampling process, each shape is represented by a set of sampling points $S = \{s_1, s_2, ..., s_n\}$, $s_i \in R^2$. Because our sampling rule is an adaptive strategy based on the medial axis, the number of resulting samplings at each shape may not equal. Given two shapes and their sampling sets, S_1 and S_2, we wish to match one point in S_1 to another point in S_2, in an optimal scheme. One way to achieve this purpose is to check all possible matchings of the two sets of points and choose the assignment with maximal similarity as the result [5]. However, this is computationally expensive and prone to produce erroneous matches. It would be desirable to obtain a good correspondence in the first step. We thus propose the following two-stage matching scheme.

3.1 Initial Matching

In the first step, we match the two shapes using only the topological principle points on the medial axis. The skeleton is a nice shape descriptor because it captures the notion of parts and components, while the skeleton's principle points are important features to describe the topological information embedded in the skeleton.

We assume that different shapes of a certain object usually compose of the similar significant components. Because each ending on the medial axis generally locates in a major component or part of the shape, these endings have a good capability in indexing the major parts. On the other hand, we observe that the junctions and midpoints on medial axis are too sensitive to the changes of the shape curve. Therefore, we choose only the endings for the coarse matching. A point on the medial axis can be identified as an ending if there is only one skeleton point in its eight neighbors.

To match two sets of endings, we use the shape context matching method [5]. Given a set of samplings $S = \{s_i\}_{i=1}^{L}$ of a shape F and the endings $E = \{e_k\}_{k=1}^{K}$ of its medial axis, the shape context of each ending $e_k \in E$ is a log-polar histogram h_k, which records the relative locations of the sampling points referring to e_k.

The optimal matching of two sets of endings is achieved by minimizing the total matching cost $\sum_1^K C(k, \pi_k)$, where π_k is the index of correspondence of e_k and $C(k, \pi_k)$ denotes the cost of matching e_k with e_{π_k}, measured using the χ^2 statistic of their shape contexts. When the two sets of endings have difference sizes, dummy points will be added to each set. The resulting square cost matrix is then input to an assignment problem (AP) and the optimal matching between the two sets of endings is obtained by solving this AP problem using the algorithm in [14].

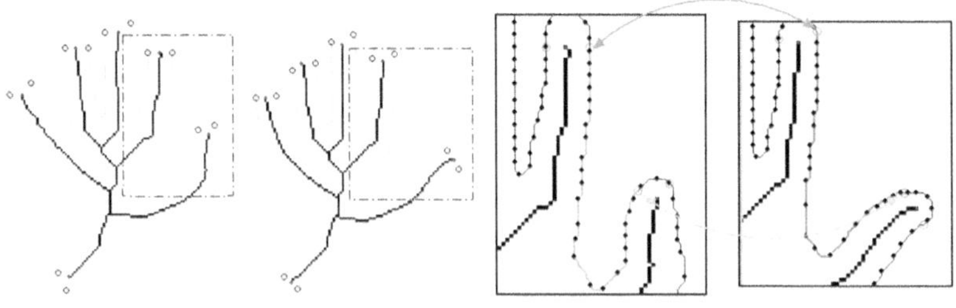

(a) (b) (c)

Fig. 2. An example of ending matching. (a) and (b) are two shapes of a hand. Because the two shapes have the same significant components, the ending correspondence is very intuitive. (c) A pair of corresponding segments in (a) and (b). The two arcs direct the corresponding ending tangents.

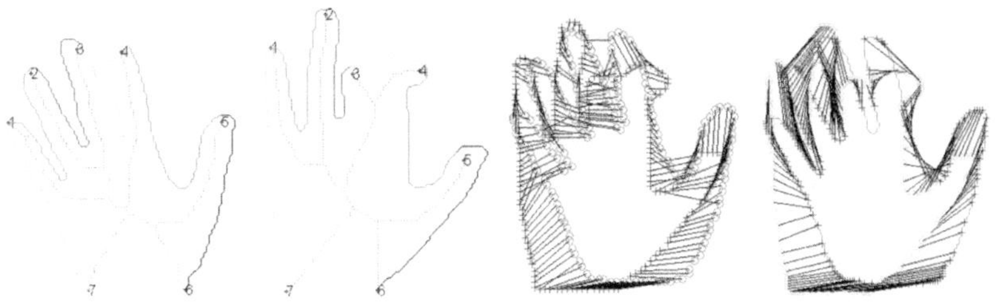

(a) (b) (c) (d)

Fig. 3. An example of shape matching. (a) and (b) are two hand outlines with corresponding segments. The same colors indicate the corresponding segments. The point matching results of the shape context method and our method are shown in (c) and (d), respectively.

Recall that each point on the medial axis has two or more tangents on the shape. Particularly, each ending has exactly two tangents. We can imagine the ending tangents as hinges between a sequence of segments of the shape curve. Each segment consists of an opened curve and two ending tangents (see Fig. 2).

To find the point correspondence across two shapes, we want to match these segments first. This can be done easily with the matching of the medial axis endings. Consider a pair of corresponding endings of two shapes. There are only two possible mapping of their ending tangents from one shape to another. For an ending tangent t_i on the first shape, we choose as its correspondence the candidate t_j on the second shape with the smaller matching cost $C(t_i, t_j)$. Because each segment of the shape can be identified by two neighboring ending tangents, the correspondence of ending tangents on the two shapes leads to a unique matching of these segments. See Fig. 3(a-b) for an example of the initial matching result.

3.2 Point Correspondence Within Segments

After obtaining the segment correspondence, the point correspondence problem can be restricted to searching the optimal matching within only each pair of corresponding segments. This provides a significant gain to increasing the robustness of shape matching, for the mismatch from one component to others is avoided. Moreover, this matching strategy can improve the speed of the matching process greatly since, for each point on one shape, only several points on the corresponding segment will be considered.

Now, we consider the point correspondence problem within a pair of corresponding segments. Recall each segment has two terminals, i.e. two ending tangents. Given two segments $\Gamma_1=\{t_{11}, s_{11}, \cdots, s_{1i}, \cdots, s_{1m}, t_{12}\}$ and $\Gamma_2=\{t_{21}, s_{21}, \cdots, s_{2j}, \cdots, s_{2n}, t_{22}\}$, we want to find the best match across the two sets of points. Without loss of generality, we suppose the points on each segment are in the following order $t_{11} < s_{11} < \cdots < s_{1i} < \cdots < s_{1m} < t_{12}$, $t_{21} < s_{21} < \cdots < s_{2j} < \cdots < s_{2n} < t_{22}$ and $m \leq n$. Because those samplings are selected in an optimal way, all of them are useful for describing the input shapes. Therefore, we wish to find the largest match between the pair of segments. In other words, we want to find $min(n, m)$ pairs of corresponding points across the two segments.

Note that the points on each segment are arranged in a string order. We constrain our method to preserve this ordering in the matching. Meanwhile, since Γ_1 and Γ_2 are corresponding segments, their terminals should also be corresponding to each other, i.e. $t_{11} \leftrightarrow t_{21}$ and $t_{12} \leftrightarrow t_{22}$. Fig.2(c) gives an illustration of this matching problem, which we define as Consecutive Assignment Problem (CAP). This problem can be solved by the following optimal combination scheme.

Because Γ_1 contains fewer samplings than Γ_2 ($m \leq n$), for each sampling $s_{1i} \in \Gamma_1$, we need to find one sampling from Γ_2. Thus, finding one-to-one point matching between two segments is equivalent to removing $(n - m)$ samplings from Γ_2 so that the remaining set of samplings on Γ_2 have the same size as that on Γ_1. Because each set of samplings is in a string order and the terminals of the two strings are already matched, there is a unique matching between the two sets of samplings. To measure the similarity of points, the shape context of each point is calculated using all the samplings obtained through the re-sample process introduced in previous sections. The point correspondence is found by minimizing the sum of cost $\sum_{i=1}^{m} C(i, \pi_i)$.

The search space for this consecutive assignment problem is $C_n^{(n-m)}$, which is much smaller than that for the assignment problem in [5]. Moreover, the points to be considered in this step are restricted in the curve segment. Therefore, the number of points in this case is only a small set of the total samplings of the whole shape. Those greatly improve the matching speed. A matching example of two outlines of a hand is shown in Fig. 3.

4 Experiments

To demonstrate the performance of our approach for statistical shape modeling, we apply it on several training sets of biomedical objects. For an object, each shape in the training set is matched to all others with the minimal sum of matching cost, which is defined as the difference of each pair of shapes. The shape with the minimal total difference is selected to find the overall correspondence of the whole set, by selecting the same corresponding points among the matching results of it with other shapes.

Fig. 4 shows two of our experimental results. The hand training set contains 15 hand outlines extracted from the Jochen Triesch Static Hand Posture Database [15] and the

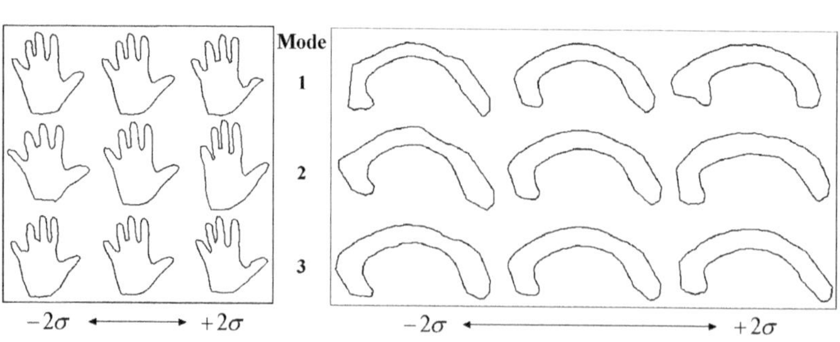

Fig. 4. Two models automatically generated using the proposed approach

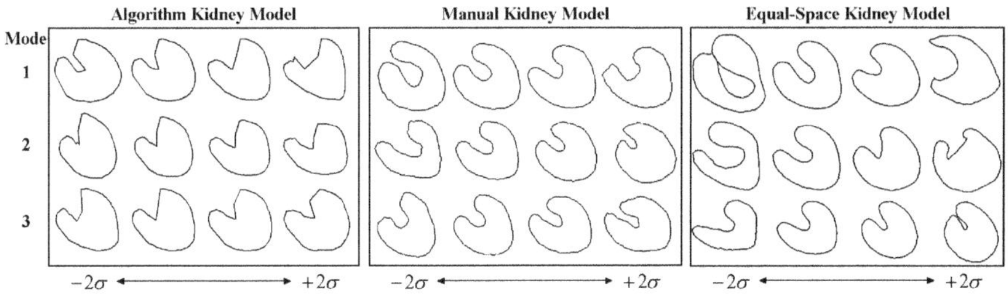

Fig. 5. Three kidney models generated using the proposed method, manual landmarks and even-space samplings

Table 1. Evaluation of The Three Kidney Models

Kidney Model	Number of Points	Variance			
		Mode 1	Mode 2	Mode 3	Total
Automatic Landmarking	81	46.89	34.92	13.08	94.89
Manual Landmarking	54	60.13	34.91	14.58	109.62
Even-space Sampling	81	172.86	35.44	30.82	239.12

callosum set contains 14 callosum shapes extracted from 14 MRI brain slices. Using the proposed automatic landmarking algorithm, we obtained 128 landmarks on each shape for the hand data set and 112 for the callosum data set. Each three rows of the two experiments show the first three modes of each model varied by $\pm 2\sigma$, where σ refers to the standard deviation along principal directions.

To evaluate our method quantitatively, we compared the automatic model (Fig. 5) with those built using manual landmarkers and equally spaced samplings, in terms of variance of the three largest modes of the models. The training data is the kidney data set from [16] which contains 20 2D left kidney shapes from different patients. The quanlity results in Table 1 show that the automatically generated model has the smallest variances in all three principal directions.

5 Conclusions

In this paper we have presented a novel approach for automatic landmarking of shapes. To capture the crucial characteristic of a shape, we sample the shape curve based on the local geometric and topological features. Then the shape correspondence is obtained through a two-stage matching approach, which stands for the major contribution of this paper. The course mapping of the skeleton endings provides an initial correspondence of the major components of the shapes, yet allows the following local point matching so that the computation complex is considerably reduced. Meanwhile, because the consecutive enforcement included in the point matching process, our approach enables better correspondences. We evaluated the proposed approach using the statistical shape modeling on various shapes of biomedical objects and the results are excellent in terms of both compact and speed.

Acknowledgments

The work described in this paper was supported by a grant (Project No. CUHK4223/04E) from the Research Grants Council of the Hong Kong Special Administrative Region, China and CUHK Shun Hing Institute of Advanced Engineering.

References

1. T. Cootes, C. Taylor, D. Cooper, and J. Graham, "Active shape models-their training and application," *Computer Vision and Image Understanding*, vol. 61, pp. 38–59, 1995.
2. F. Mokhtarian and R. Suomela, "Robust image corner detection through curvature scale space," *IEEE Trans. Pattern Anal. Machine Intell.*, vol. 20, no. 12, pp. 1376–1381, 1998.
3. R. Davies, C. Twining, T. Cootes, J. Waterton, and C. Taylor, "A minimum description length approach to statistical shape modeling," *IEEE Trans. Med. Imag.*, vol. 21, no. 5, pp. 525–537, 2002.
4. A. Hill, C. Taylor, and A. Brett, "A framework for automatic landmark identification using a new method of nonrigid correspondence," *IEEE Trans. Pattern Anal. Machine Intell.*, vol. 22, no. 3, pp. 241–251, 2000.
5. S. Belongie, J. Malik, and J. Puzicha, "Matching shapes," in *Proc. IEEE Int. Conf. on Computer Vision*, Vancouver, Canada, 2001, pp. 454–463.
6. ——, "Shape matching and object recognition using shape contexts," *IEEE Trans. Pattern Anal. Machine Intell.*, vol. 24, pp. 509–522, 2002.
7. A. Thayananthan, B. Stenger, P. H. S. Torr, and R. Cipolla, "Shape context and chamfer matching in cluttered scenes," in *Proc. IEEE Computer Vision and Pattern Recognition*, vol. I, Madison, USA, June 2003, pp. 127–133.
8. H. Blum, "A transformation for extracting new descriptors of shape," in *Proc. Models for the Perception of Speech and Visual Form*, W. Wathen-Dunn, Ed. Cambridge, MA: MIT Press, Nov. 1967, pp. 362–380.
9. D. Sharvit, J. Chan, H. Tek, and B. B. Kimia, "Symmetry-based indexing of image databases," *Journal of Visual Communication and Image Representation*, vol. 9, no. 4, pp. 366–380, Dec. 1998.
10. T. B. Sebastian, P. N. Klein, and B. B. Kimia, "Recognition of shapes by editing shock graphs," in *Proc. IEEE Int. Conf. on Computer Vision*, 2001, pp. 755–762.
11. J. Ruppert, "A new and simple algorithm for quality 2-dimensional mesh generation," in *Proc. ACM-SIAM Symposium on Discrete algorithms*, 1993, pp. 83–92.
12. D. E. N. Amenta, M. Bern, "The crust and the β-skeleton: Combinatorial curve reconstruction," *Graphical Models and Image Processing*, vol. 60, no. 2, pp. 125–135, 1998.
13. T. Dey, J. Giesen, S. Goswami, J. Hudson, R. Wenger, and W. Zhao, "Undersampling and oversampling in sample based shape modeling," in *Proc. IEEE Visualization*, vol. I, San Diego, California, Oct. 2001, pp. 83–90.
14. R. Jonker and A. Volgenant, "A shortest augmenting path algorithm for dense and sparse linear assignment problems," *Computing*, vol. 38, no. 4, pp. 325–340, 1987.
15. J. Triesch and C. Malsburg, "A system for person-independent hand posture recognition against complex backgrounds," *IEEE Trans. Pattern Anal. Machine Intell.*, vol. 23, no. 12, pp. 1449–1453, 2001.
16. J. Xie, Y. Jiang, and H. Tsui, "Segmentation of kidney from ultrasound images based on texture and shape priors," *IEEE Trans. Med. Imag.*, vol. 24, no. 1, pp. 45–57, Jan. 2005.

A Computer-Aided Design System for Revision of Segmentation Errors

Marcel Jackowski[1] and Ardeshir Goshtasby[2]

[1] Yale School of Medicine, Diagnostic Radiology Dept., New Haven, CT 06520
[2] Computer Science & Eng. Dept., Wright State University, Dayton, OH 45435

Abstract. Automatic image segmentation methods often involve errors, requiring the assistance of the user to correct them. In this paper, a computer-aided design system is introduced for correcting such errors. The proposed system approximates each 3-D region by a parametric surface. Region voxels are first parametrized spherically using a coarse-to-fine subdivision method. By using the voxel positions and their parameter coordinates, control points of a rational Gaussian surface are determined through a least-squares method to approximate the region. Finally, this surface is overlaid with the volumetric image and by locally pulling or pushing it with the mouse while viewing image information, the surface is revised as needed. Typically, a few minutes are sufficient to correct errors in a region.

1 Introduction

Image segmentation is the process of partitioning an image into meaningful parts. The objective is to extract objects or their parts in an image. Difficulties arise when noise is present in the image or when properties within objects vary. The problem is worsened when their boundaries become blurred or when boundary information is absent, owing to different tissues having similar properties. These variations, which are often unpredictable, make it impossible to develop an automatic method that can segment all images correctly. At the present, the best one can hope for is to have a method that can correctly delineate most parts of an object of interest, and in areas where it makes a mistake, allow the user to interactively correct the errors.

Various user-guided and interactive segmentation methods have been developed. A popular method described by Falcão, Mortensen, Udupa, and others [6,1,10] is known as "live-wire." In this method, the user selects a number of points on the region boundary, and the program automatically finds optimal boundary segments between consecutive points by minimizing a cost function based on the image gradient information. Minimum-cost segment paths are calculated in real time, allowing the user to interactively snap each segment to the intended boundary to constrain the search space for the optimum solution and improve speed. An extension of it known as "live-lane" was later devised [5] where the optimization process is restricted to a small area around the image

J. Duncan and G. Gerig (Eds.): MICCAI 2005, LNCS 3750, pp. 717–724, 2005.

edges, called a "lane." More recently, Falcão and Bergo introduced a full volumetric interactive segmentation approach based on Image Foresting Transforms (IFT) [4]. The IFT is Dijkstra's shortest-path algorithm modified to handle multiple sources using more general cost functions. Seed points are added or removed interactively as needed and cost graphs are pruned in real time, thereby allowing revision of the segmentation result.

An interactive segmentation method based on a genetic algorithm was described by Cagnoni *et al.* [2]. In this method, the boundary contour of a region of interest is manually drawn in one of the slices. The boundary contour is then considered an initial contour in the subsequent slice and the contour is refined by a genetic algorithm using image information.

Energy-minimizing models or "snakes" have also been used for segmentation as well as revision of regions [9]. Since some points in a snake may trap in local minima during the optimization process, the globally optimal solution can be missed. To avoid this, often the user is required to intervene and either move some of the snake's points that are thought to have converged to local minima or guide the snake to the optimal position by interactively controlling the external forces. The Insight Registration and Segmentation Toolkit (ITK) initiative provides a semi-automated segmentaion tool based on watersheds where the user can hand-select regions of interest [12]. A survey of interactive segmentation methods providing different levels of user control is given by Olabarriaga and Smeulders [11].

The new idea introduced in this paper is to use the capabilities of a computer-aided design system to quickly and easily refine the result of a 3-D segmentation, just like editing a 3-D geometric model. We assume that a volumetric image has been segmented and regions of interest have been extracted. A region is composed of connected voxels that represent the bounding surface of an object, which we call a *digital shape*. Under these assumptions, we first describe the parametric surface that will be used to represent a given digital shape. Next, we show how to parametrize the shape voxels and optimally determine the control points of the approximating surface. Then we describe the segmentation refinement process, involving interactive free-form surface deformations. Finally, we present experimental results by the proposed method.

2 Approach

2.1 Surface Approximation

Since voxels in a digital shape usually do not form a regular grid, we use a rational Gaussian (RaG) surface [7] to represent the shape. The standard deviation of Gaussians in a RaG surface may be used to control the smoothness of the created surface. Given a set of (control) points $\mathbf{V}_i = \{(x_i, y_i, z_i) : i = 1, \ldots, n\}$ and their parameter coordinates $\{(u_i, v_i) : i = 1, \ldots, n\}$, the RaG surface approximating the control points is defined by $\mathbf{P}(u, v) = \sum_{i=1}^{n} \mathbf{V}_i g_i(u, v)$, where $u, v \in [0, 1]$ and $g_i(u, v)$ is the ith blending function of the surface given by

$$g_i(u,v) = \frac{G_i(u,v)}{\sum_{j=1}^{n} G_j(u,v)}. \tag{1}$$

$G_i(u,v)$ is the Gaussian centered at (u_i, v_i) in the parameter space. The parameter coordinates determine the adjacency relation between the points. The standard deviation of all Gaussians are set to the same value σ and controlled globally.

When the shape under consideration is closed and has a spherical topology, the parameter coordinates at the shape voxels can be determined by mapping the voxels to a sphere. Assuming that $\phi \in [-\pi/2, \pi/2]$ and $\theta \in [0, 2\pi]$ represent the spherical coordinates of voxels of a digital shape, we will use $u = (\phi + \frac{\pi}{2})/\pi$ and $v = \theta/2\pi$ in the equation of the RaG surface approximating the shape. In the following sections, we show how to spherically parametrize voxels in a closed digital shape and approximate the shape by a RaG surface using the least squares method.

2.2 Shape Parametrization

To approximate the digital shape with a RaG surface, one must first find the parameter coordinates of the shape voxels. Here we employ a coarse-to-fine subdivision method described in [8]. Initially, the given digital shape and a unit sphere are simultaneously approximated by two octahedra. The process involves placing a regular octahedron at the center of gravity of the shape and extending its axes until they intersect the shape (see Fig. 1a). By establishing the correspondence between the triangles in the shape approximation and triangles in the sphere approximation (Fig. 1b), parameters of the shape control points are determined. In the case of irregular shapes, the center of the octahedron is taken as the midpoint of the major axis segment inside the shape.

The projection of each triangular facet onto the shape determines a digital patch. The triangles obtained by the octahedral subdivision are further subdivided into smaller facets in a recursive manner [8]. This process continues until

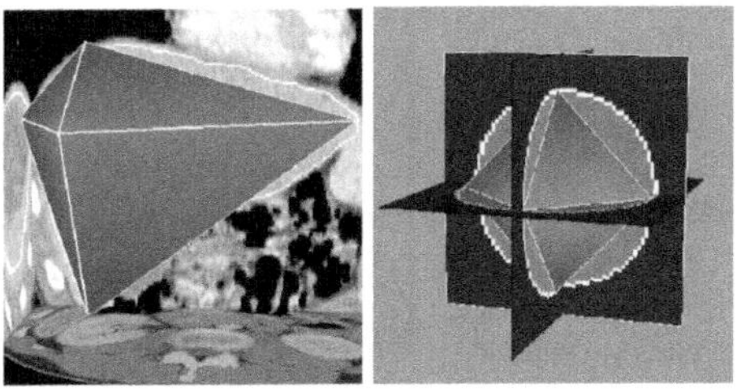

(a) (b)

Fig. 1. (a) Approximation of a digital shape by an octahedron. (b) Approximation of a sphere by an octahedron. Parameter coordinates of octahedral vertices in the sphere are assigned to the octahedral vertices in the shape.

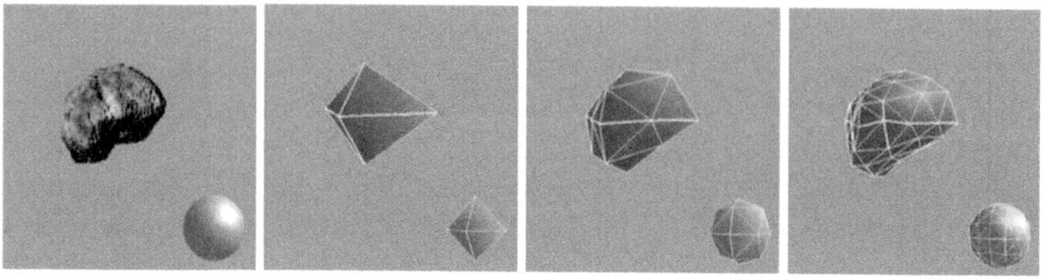

(a) (b) (c) (d)

Fig. 2. (a) A digital shape and a unit sphere in the lower right corner. (b-d) Three simultaneous subdivisions of a digital shape and the reference sphere.

the distance between each triangular facet and its associating patch falls below a prescribed tolerance. Whenever a triangle in the shape approximation is subdivided, the corresponding triangle in the sphere approximation is subdivided also. Hence, there always exists a one-to-one correspondence between triangles in the shape approximation and triangles in the sphere approximation. By knowing the parameters of mesh vertices in the sphere, we will know the parameters of corresponding mesh vertices in the shape. The process is graphically shown in Fig. 2. By using the vertices of the triangular mesh as the control points of a RaG surface and the parameters at mesh vertices as its nodes, a smooth parametric surface can be obtained to approximate the shape. Note, however, that the surface obtained in this manner will only approximate the mesh vertices and will not necessarily pass through the vertices. In the next section, we show how to improve the shape recovery process by determining the control points of a RaG surface that interpolates the mesh vertices.

2.3 Least-Squares Computation of the Control Points

Suppose a digital shape is available and the shape voxels are parametrized according to the procedure outlined in the preceding section. Also, suppose the shape is composed of N voxels: $\{\mathbf{P}_j : j = 1, \ldots, N\}$ with parameter coordinates $\{(u_j, v_j) : j = 1, \ldots, N\}$. We would like to determine a RaG surface with control points $\{\mathbf{V}_i : i = 1, \ldots, n\}$ that can approximate the shape points optimally in the least-squares sense. Let $\mathbf{P}_j = (X_j, Y_j, Z_j)$, $\mathbf{P}(u, v) = [x(u, v), y(u, v), z(u, v)]$, and $\mathbf{V}_i = (x_i, y_i, z_i)$. Then the sum of squared distances between the voxels and the approximating surface can be written as:

$$E^2 = \sum_{j=1}^{N} \{[x(u_j, v_j) - X_j]^2 + [y(u_j, v_j) - Y_j]^2 + [z(u_j, v_j) - Z_j]^2\} \tag{2}$$

$$= E_x^2 + E_y^2 + E_z^2. \tag{3}$$

Since the three components of the surface are independently defined, to minimize E^2, we minimize E_x^2, E_y^2, and E_z^2, separately. This involves determining the partial derivatives of E^2 with respect to each variable, setting the partial derivatives to zero and solving the obtained system of equations. For E_x^2, the following system of n linear equations are obtained:

$$E_x^2 = \sum_{j=1}^{N} g_k(u_j, v_j) \sum_{i=1}^{n} [x_i g_i(u_j, v_j) - X_j] = 0, \qquad k = 1, \ldots, n, \tag{4}$$

which can be solved for $x_i, i = 1, \ldots, n$. Components y_i and z_i are determined similarly. The standard deviation of all Gaussians is set to the same value σ and controlled globally. Since RaG basis functions monotonically decrease from a center point, if σ is not very large, these equations will have diagonally dominant matrices of coefficients, ensuring a solution. Note that the above process positions the n control points of a RaG surface so that the surface will approximate the N image voxels with the least sum of squared errors. n depends on the size and complexity of the shape being approximated (n is typically a few hundred). The smallest surface-fitting error will be obtained when the standard deviation of Gaussians matches the level of detail of the shape. This minimum error can be determined by a steepest-descent algorithm. However, since the given region is known to contain errors, finding the surface that is very close to the region may not be of particular interest. Currently, after the control points of an approximating surface are determined, the user is allowed to interactively vary the smoothness (standard deviation) of the surface and view the obtained surface as well as the associating RMSE. In this manner, the standard deviation of Gaussians is interactively selected to reproduce a desired level of detail in the constructed shape.

2.4 Shape Editing

Once the result of an automatic segmentation is represented by a free-form parametric surface, the surface can be revised to a desired geometry by appropriately moving its control points. In the system we have developed, an obtained surface is overlaid with the original volumetric image. Then by going through different image slices along one of the three orthogonal directions, the user visually observes the intersection of the surface with the image slices and verifies the correctness of the segmentation. When an error is observed, one or more control points are appropriately moved to correct it. As the control points are moved, the user will observe changes in the surface in real-time.

Figure 3a shows the surface approximating a brain tumor within the original volumetric image. By picking the surface at a point near where the error occurred (shown by white arrow), a spherical attractor is activated and the control points (darker dots) falling inside the attractor are selected. By changing the radius of action, different numbers of control points are selected. Each point is translated in the appropriate direction by connecting it to the center of the attractor and by using the amount proportional to the cosine of the angle between that direction and the direction of motion of the mouse. Only those control points falling inside the hemisphere with positive cosines are moved. This avoids the movement of control points with negative cosines in the opposing direction. It also ensures that

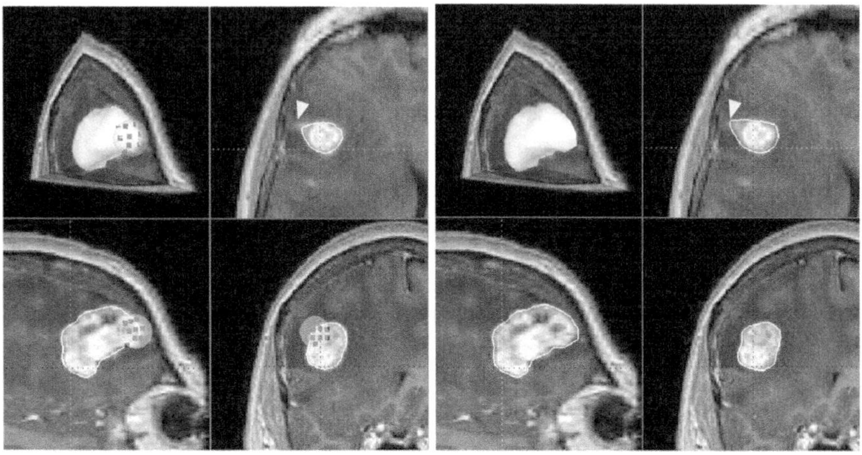

(a) (b)

Fig. 3. (a) Overlaying of the approximated tumor surface and the volumetric image. Dots show the selected control points during surface editing. The upper-left window shows the 3-D view of the image volume with all three orthogonal slices. Arrow points to the revision area. (b) The tumor after necessary modifications. This is the final result in parametric form.

discontinuities will not occur between points that are moved and points that are not. Fig. 3b shows the resulting surface after revision. Surface revision can be performed gradually and repeatedly while observing the image information. The sensitivity of the surface to the motion of the mouse can be changed by increasing or decreasing the weights assigned to the control points.

3 Results

Examples of the proposed segmentation revision method are shown in Fig. 4. The first column shows the original images, the second column shows the initial segmentation results, and the third column shows the results after the necessary revisions. Both the ventricular blood pool (Fig. 4, first row) and the brain tumor (Fig. 4, second row) were initially segmented by applying a smoothing operation and an optimal intensity thresholding method. At the optimal threshold value, a small change in threshold value will change the segmentation result minimally. This threshold value corresponds to the intensity at object boundaries where intensities change sharply. Therefore, a slight error in estimation of the threshold value will not change the segmentation result drastically. The liver (Fig. 4, third row) was segmented by a 3-D Canny [3] edge detector. Weak edges were removed by interactively varying the gradient threshold value and observing the resulting edges. In these figures, results of the initial segmentation are shown after RaG surface fitting by the least-squares method. RaG surfaces were then interactively

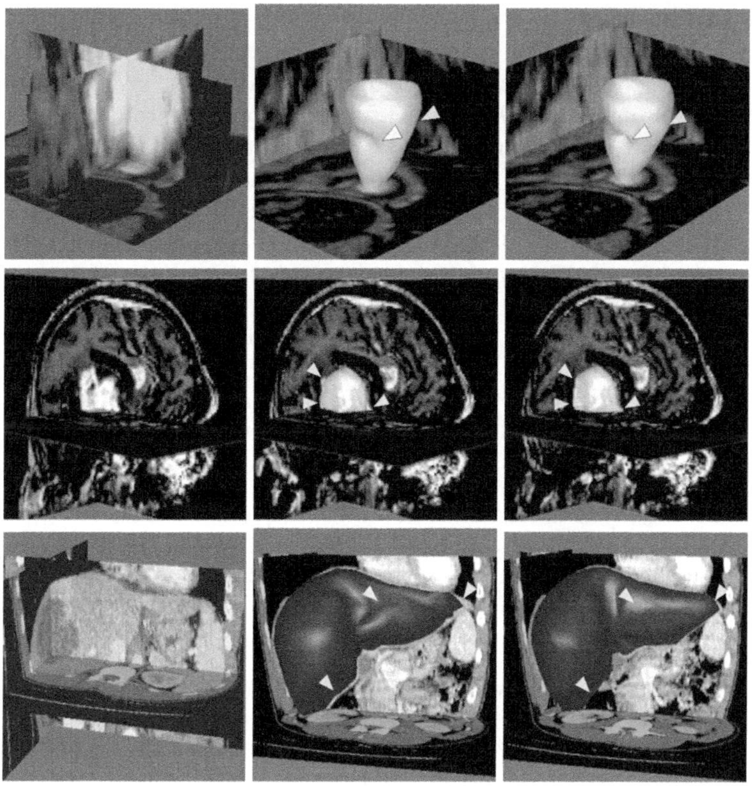

Fig. 4. First row: A short-axis cardiac MR image and segmentation of the left ventricular cavity. Second row: An MR brain image and segmentation of the tumor. Third row: An abdominal CT image and segmentation of the liver. The first column shows the original images, the middle column shows the initial segmentation results, and the right column shows the results after the necessary modifications (white arrows).

revised as needed while viewing the overlaid surface and volumetric image. Final segmentation results are shown in the third column of Fig. 4.

Approximation of the initial regions by triangular meshes took from 10 to 30 seconds and approximation of the regions with RaG surfaces by the least-squares method took from 40 to 60 seconds. Interactive revision of the initial surfaces to obtain the final surfaces took from 1 to 2 minutes. All these times are measured on an SGI Octane computer with R10000 processor. Although the time to subdivide a region into a triangular mesh and the time to fit a RaG surface to a volumetric region are fixed for a given region, the time needed to revise an initial surface to a desired one depends on the speed of the user and the severity of errors in the initial segmentation. The final result of a segmentation obtained by the proposed system is thus user-dependent. Since users have different experiences in image interpretation, results obtained by different users may differ.

4 Conclusions

In this paper, the idea of using a computer-aided design system to refine the result of an automatically determined segmentation was introduced. In the proposed system, a RaG surface is fitted to voxels covering a 3-D region by the least-squares method. The surface and the original volumetric image are then overlaid and the surface is interactively revised until the desired segmentation is achieved. Because a 3-D shape is represented by a parametric surface, the surface may be sent to a computer-aided manufacturing system for construction of an actual 3-D model of the shape. The proposed system provides tools with which a user can modify a segmentation result freely. There are no limitations in shape, size, or complexity of a region except that it should have a spherical topology.

References

1. W. Barrett and E. Mortensen. Fast, accurate, and reproducible live-wire boundary extraction. *Proc. Visualization in Biomedical Computing*, 1996.
2. S. Cagnoni, A. B. Dobrzeniecki, R. Ploi, and J. C. Yanch. Genetic algorithm-based interactive segmentation of 3-d medical images. *Image and Vision Computing*, 17:881–895, 1999.
3. J. Canny. A computational approach to edge detection. *IEEE Trans. Pattern Analysis and Machine Intelligence*, 8(6):679–698, 1986.
4. A. X. Falcão and Felipe P. G. Bergo. Interactive volume segmentation with differential image foresting transforms. *IEEE Trans. Medical Imaging*, 23(9):1100–1108, 2004.
5. A. X. Falcão and J. K. Udupa. A 3-d generalization of user-steered live-wire segmentation. *Medical Image Analysis*, 4:389–402, 2000.
6. A. X. Falcão, J. K. Udupa, S. Samarasekera, S. Sharma, B. E. Hirsch, and R. A. Lotufo. User-steered image segmentation paradigms: live-wire and live-lane. *Graphical Models and Image Processing*, 60(4):233–260, 1998.
7. A. Goshtasby. Design and recovery of 2-d and 3-d shapes using rational gaussian curves and surfaces. *Intl. Journal of Computer Vision*, 10(3):233–256, 1993.
8. M. Jackowski, M. Satter, and A. Goshtasby. Approximating digital 3-d shapes by rational gaussian surfaces. *IEEE Trans. Visualization and Computer Graphics*, 9(1):56–69, 2003.
9. A. Kass, A. Witkin, , and D. Terzopoulos. Snakes: Active contour models. *Intl. Journal of Computer Vision*, 1:321–331, 1987.
10. E. N. Mortensen, B. S. Morse, W. A. Barrett, and J. K. Udupa. Adaptive boundary detection using live-wire two-dimensional dynamic programming. *IEEE Proc. Computers in Cardiology*, pages 635–638, 1992.
11. S. D. Olabarriaga and A. W. M. Smeulders. Interaction in the segmentation of medical images: A survey. *Medical Image Analysis*, 5:127–142, 2001.
12. T. S. Yoo, M. J. Ackerman, W. E. Lorensen, W. Schroeder, V. Chalana, S. Aylward, D. Metaxes, and R. Whitaker. Engineering and Algorithm Design for an Image Processing API: A Technical Report on ITK - The Insight Toolkit. In *Proc. of Medicine Meets Virtual Reality*, pages 586–592, 2002.

Statistical Modeling of Shape and Appearance Using the Continuous Medial Representation

Paul A. Yushkevich, Hui Zhang, and James C. Gee

Department of Radiology, University of Pennsylvania

Abstract. We describe a novel approach to combining shape and appearance features in the statistical analysis of structures in medical images. The continuous medial representation is used to relate these two types of features meaningfully. The representation imposes a shape-based coordinate system on structure interiors, in a way that uses the boundary normal as one of the coordinate axes, while providing an onto and nearly one-to-one parametrization. This coordinate system is used to sample image intensities in the context of shape. The approach is illustrated by the principal components analysis of the shape and appearance of the hippocampus in T1-weighted MRI from a schizophrenia study.

1 Introduction

In medical image analysis, it is typical to describe anatomical structures in terms of either shape or appearance. Combining these two classes of descriptors is challenging because appearance features are local measurements of certain tissue properties (e.g., T1 relaxation) that are sampled on a lattice, while shape features are derived from geometric loci (e.g., boundaries) that are modeled by meshes or parametric manifolds. The importance of combining shape and appearance features in the statistical analysis of anatomical structures is underscored by the wide use of Active Shape and Active Appearance models (ASM/AAM) [4,5].

In this paper, we demonstrate how the continuous medial representation (*cm-rep*) [13] can be used to co-analyze shape and appearance. Specifically, we focus on the unique way in which *cm-reps* impose a common shape-based coordinate system on anatomical structures in a population. This coordinate system extends the boundary parametrization $\mathbf{y}(u^1, u^2)$ onto the entire volumetric region enclosed by the boundary, in a way that (1) is depth-based, i.e., it preserves coordinates u^1 and u^2 along vectors normal to the boundary, and (2) is onto and, except at a codimension 1 set of points, one-to-one. The first property is akin to ASMs, which use fixed-length intensity profiles normal to the boundary to associate shape features with appearance features. The second property is analogous to AAMs. Hence, our method combines two attractive, but mutually exclusive, properties of ASMs and AAMs. However, it does so at the cost of representational accuracy, as *cm-rep* models are restricted to a class of shapes with non-branching skeletons. In [13], we estimated the accuracy with which *cm-reps* can describe the hippocampus. In this paper, we illustrate how *cm-reps* can be used to study the variability in hippocampal shape and appearance.

J. Duncan and G. Gerig (Eds.): MICCAI 2005, LNCS 3750, pp. 725–732, 2005.

2 Methods and Experimental Results

2.1 Modeling Anatomical Structures with *CM-Reps*

In the first approximation, the *cm-rep* approach is the continuous analog of the Pizer et al. *m-rep* method [11]. Anatomical structures are modeled by inverting the process of skeletonization: the skeleton of a structure is defined explicitly and the boundary is derived from the skeleton analytically. In our method, the skeleton is described parametrically as a combination of a *medial manifold* and a positive-valued *radial scalar field* given at each point on this manifold (the modeling of branching skeletons as a set of connected medial manifolds is the subject of ongoing research). The radial scalar field is in turn derived from a *radial conductance scalar field* by solving a Poisson PDE. This step is necessary to conform to the equality constraints imposed on the radial scalar field by the medial geometry. The medial manifold and the radial conductance scalar field are defined using basis functions whose coefficients can be varied in order to apply deformations to the model. Actual anatomical structures are represented by fitting a template to characteristic images in a Bayesian estimation framework. In the following paragraphs, we describe our approach in greater detail. However, for a complete treatment of the subject, we refer the reader to [13].

A *cm-rep* model is defined uniquely by two sequences of coefficients: a vector-valued sequence $\mathbf{w}_1, \ldots, \mathbf{w}_N$ in $\mathbb{R}^3$ and a real-valued sequence $\omega_1, \ldots, \omega_M$. These coefficients are used together with a sequence of orthogonal twice-differentiable basis functions $f_i(u^1, u^2)$ on a regular domain $\Omega \in \mathbb{R}^2$ to define the medial manifold $\mathbf{x}$ and the radial conductance scalar field ρ as

$$\mathbf{x}(u^1, u^2) = \sum_{i=0}^{N} \mathbf{w}_i f_i(u^1, u^2) \; ; \qquad \rho(u^1, u^2) = \sum_{i=0}^{M} \omega_i f_i(u^1, u^2) \; . \tag{1}$$

Currently, we use the real components of the Fourier basis to define functions f_i, but we expect that in the future a wavelet basis will prove to be better suited for Bayesian estimation of the coefficients.

The radial scalar field R is derived from the medial manifold $\mathbf{x}$ and the radial conductance field ρ by solving the following variant of the Poisson PDE:

$$\triangle_{\mathbf{x}} R^2 = \rho ; \qquad ||\mathrm{grad}_{\mathbf{x}} R|| = 1 \text{ on } \partial\Omega , \tag{2}$$

where $\triangle_{\mathbf{x}}$ and $\mathrm{grad}_{\mathbf{x}}$ denote, respectively, the Laplace-Beltrami operator and the Riemannian gradient on the manifold $\mathbf{x}$. These operators are intrinsic manifold generalizations of the Laplacian and gradient operators in $\mathbb{R}^n$. Despite the unusual non-linear boundary condition, the PDE carries many desirable properties, such as uniqueness (which we can prove formally), existence and stability (which are supported by empirical evidence), invariance under similarity transforms applied to $\mathbf{x}$, etc. We solve this PDE numerically using Newton's method in the Finite Differences framework.

The boundary surface $\mathbf{y}$ associated with a *cm-rep* model is generated analytically from the medial manifold and the radial field. This surface is naturally partitioned into two halves, $\mathbf{y}^+$ and $\mathbf{y}^-$, one on each side of the medial manifold:

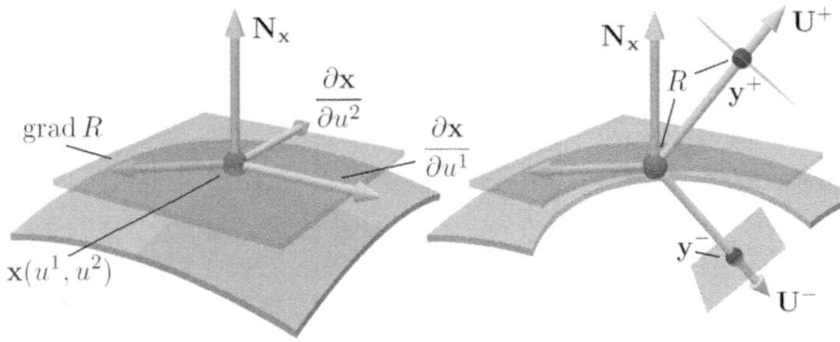

Fig. 1. The local geometry of a point on the medial manifold

$$\mathbf{y}^{\pm} = \mathbf{x} + R\,\mathbf{U}^{\pm}\,, \quad \text{where} \quad \mathbf{U}^{\pm} = -\text{grad}_{\mathbf{x}} R \pm \sqrt{1 - ||\text{grad}_{\mathbf{x}} R||^2}\,\mathbf{N_x}\,, \tag{3}$$

and $\mathbf{N_x}$ is the unit normal to the medial manifold. This expression is essentially the inverse of Blum's Medial Axis Transform [1] in 3-D. It describes two points of tangency between the sphere of radius R centered at $\mathbf{x}$ and the boundary surface. Unit vectors $\mathbf{U}^{\pm}$ are orthogonal to the boundary surface at $\mathbf{y}^{\pm}$. Fig. 1 illustrates the medial-boundary relationship described by (3).

It is easy to verify from the boundary condition in (2) that boundary halves $\mathbf{y}^+$ and $\mathbf{y}^-$ coincide along $\partial\Omega$. This coincidence is a form of an equality constraint imposed by the medial geometry on functions $\mathbf{x}$ and R. If, instead of deriving R using the PDE (2), we had modeled R explicitly as a weighted sum of basis functions, we would be presented with a severely overconstrained problem, as the number of places where the constraint holds would be infinite (all of $\partial\Omega$), while the number of coefficients defining $\mathbf{x}$ and R would be finite. In addition to this equality constraint, there are certain inequality constraints that the coefficients $\mathbf{w}_i$ and ω_i must satisfy in order to ensure that $\mathbf{y}^+$ and $\mathbf{y}^-$ form a smooth closed surface. These are handled in the course of Bayesian estimation.

The three stages of *cm-rep* construction are illustrated in Fig. 2: the first panel shows the medial manifold and the radial conductance field, the second panel plots the radial field, and the third panel shows the boundary surface. Note that the medial manifold has corners; this is an undesirable side effect of using the unit square as the domain Ω. We are working to extend our method to arbitrary domains in $\mathbb{R}^2$.

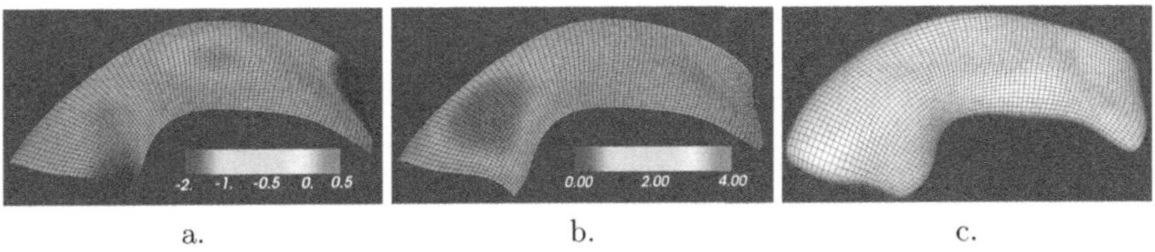

Fig. 2. The three steps of constructing a *cm-rep*. **a.** A medial manifold $\mathbf{x}$ with the radial conductance function ρ. **b.** The radial function R computed by solving the Poisson equation (2) on the manifold. **c.** Boundary surface $\mathbf{y}$ computed using (3).

The basic ideas behind *cm-rep* deformable modeling are derived from the discrete m-rep methodology [11], which is based on pattern theory [10]. First, a template *cm-rep* is generated. Currently that is done in an *ad hoc* manner, but in the future we plan to study optimal template selection, perhaps adapting techniques developed for m-reps [12]. The deformable template is fitted to instances of the anatomical structure by minimizing the posterior probability of the coefficients $\{\mathbf{w}_i\}$ and $\{\omega_i\}$, given data in the form of a binary characteristic image of the structure. In a classical Bayesian estimation framework, the posterior probability is factored into a likelihood term, which measures the match between the *cm-rep* boundary/interior and the binary image, and a prior term. We use volumetric overlap (which can be computed efficiently using the *cm-rep* interior parametrization, Sec. 2.2) and boundary-based match metrics to compute the likelihood. Penalty prior terms are used to enforce the inequality constraints on $\{\mathbf{w}_i\}$ and $\{\omega_i\}$ 'softly'. In addition, a regularization prior is used to minimize the distortion in area element on the medial manifold, thus providing a rudimentary correspondence between instances.

The deforming *cm-rep* template can only assume shapes for which the skeleton is a single manifold. This clearly limits the representational ability of the model. However, in practice, it appears that many anatomical structures can be modeled with *cm-reps* fairly accurately. Indeed, Styner [12] proved that certain subcortical structures can be represented using single-figure discrete m-reps with sub-voxel error. To evaluate the representational ability of *cm-reps* in a similar manner, we fitted the hippocampus template to 174 (87 right, 87 left) segmentations of the hippocampus from a MRI schizophrenia study [3]. The segmentation was computed using the Joshi et al. [9] algorithm for large deformation diffeomorphic registration with manually placed anatomic landmarks. This approach is used extensively in brain morphometry [6] and was shown to be more accurate and reliable than manual segmentation [8]. The data in the form of boundary meshes was graciously provided by Profs. Guido Gerig (UNC Depts. of Comp. Sci. and Psychiatry) and Sarang Joshi (UNC Dept. of Rad. Onc.).

The results of the fitting are illustrated in Fig. 3. The fit was computed in a multi-resolution procedure where the number of basis functions and coefficients was gradually increased. At the highest resolution, $8 \times 12 \times (3+1)$ coefficients were used. After the fitting, we computed the average of several goodness-of-fit scores over the entire data set. These include mean squared distance from the

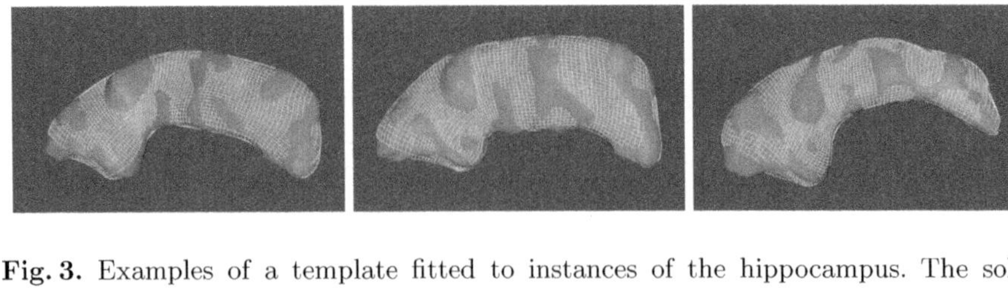

Fig. 3. Examples of a template fitted to instances of the hippocampus. The solid blue surface is the boundary of the subject hippocampus, and the white mesh is the boundary of the fitted *cm-rep* template.

cm-rep boundary to the hippocampus boundary (0.201 mm), maximum distance from *cm-rep* to the hippocampus (1.576 mm), maximum distance from the hippocampus to the *cm-rep* (2.558 mm) and volume overlap between the *cm-rep* and the hippocampus (91.3%). These error scores are slightly worse than the *m-rep* results (avg. model-to-hippo. distance of 0.17 mm.) [12] that were computed on the same images, but using a different manual segmentation. The *m-rep* model does not enforce strict conformance to medial geometry, so we expect it to fit somewhat better than *cm-reps*.

2.2 CM-Rep Interior Parametrization

One advantage of *cm-reps* over discrete *m-reps* and boundary shape shape representations is the ability to impose, with ease, a shape-based coordinate system on the *cm-rep* interior, i.e, the region of space enclosed by the *cm-rep* boundary. For 'valid' *cm-reps*, the interior is homeomorphic to a unit ball. The vectors $\mathbf{U}^{\pm}(u^1, u^2)$ with tails at $\mathbf{x}(u^1, u^2)$ span the *cm-rep* interior. We can use these properties to define a shape-based coordinate system that consists of the coordinates $(u^1, u^2) \in \Omega$ and a scalar $\xi \in [-1, 1]$ that describes a point's location with respect to the medial axis and the boundary. Formally, we define a mapping from $\Omega \times [-1, 1]$ onto the *cm-rep* interior:

$$\mathbf{z}(u^1, u^2, \xi) = \mathbf{x}(u^1, u^2) + |\xi| R(u^1, u^2)\ \mathbf{U}^{\text{sign}\xi}(u^1, u^2) \tag{4}$$

Under this parametrization, points on the medial manifold have $\xi = 0$ and points on the boundary have $\xi = \pm 1$. If Q is some point on the boundary, then all points along the inward boundary normal vector with tail at Q have the same first two coordinate values as Q, due to the fact that the vectors $\mathbf{U}^{\pm}$ are orthogonal to the *cm-rep* boundary. The distance from a point on the *cm-rep* interior to the nearest point on the *cm-rep* boundary is equal to $(1 - |\xi|)R(u^1, u^2)$.

Thus, we have parameterized the entire object interior, in a way that, roughly speaking, associates each interior point with the nearest point on the boundary. This type of interior parametrization is consistent with the way that the ASM [4] samples image intensities inside objects using profiles that extend in the normal direction from the boundary. Unlike ASM, but like AAM [5], our parametrization is onto. It is also one-to-one, with the exception of a codimension 1 set of points whose coordinates $(u^1, u^2) \in \partial\Omega$. For these points, $z(u^1, u^2, \xi) = z(u^1, u^2, -\xi)$. Thus, we may say that our coordinate system combines the best of ASM and AAM: the preservation of boundary normal direction and (nearly) one-to-one and onto parametrization.

When *cm-reps* are fitted to anatomical objects in medical images, we are able to use this coordinate system to sample image intensities. This ability is illustrated in Figs. 4 and 5a. Here, a *cm-rep* has been fitted to the hippocampus in a T1 image (Fig. 4a.). The values of u^1, u^2 and ξ coordinates of on the *cm-rep* interior are shown using color maps in Figs. 4b-d. Fig. 5a shows the image intensities mapped back to the u^1, u^2 and ξ space. This mapping of image intensities associates shape features with intensity features, and is a unique way of establishing across-subject correspondences between intensities on the basis of geometry.

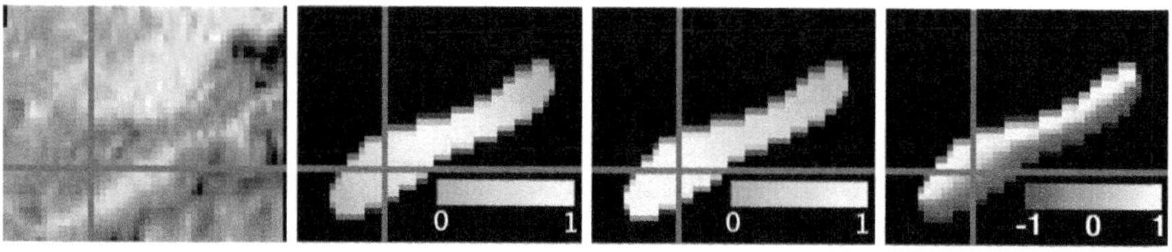

a. b. c. d.

Fig. 4. The shape-based coordinate system induced by a *cm-rep*. **a.** A slice through the hippocampus in a T1 weighted MRI, to which a *cm-rep* template has been fitted. **b, c.** The values of the coordinates u^1, u^2, which span the medial manifold, plotted at each point in the hippocampus using a color map. **d.** The values of the ξ coordinate, which goes from the medial manifold to the boundary.

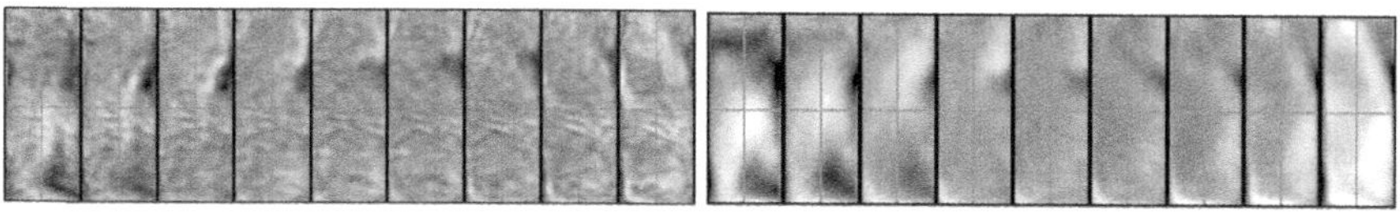

a. b.

Fig. 5. a. MRI intensities of the hippocampus in Fig 4a, sampled on a lattice in the shape-based coordinate system. The slices are taken as ξ goes from -1 to 1, and the axes are along the u^1 and u^2 coordinates. Sampling used cubic interpolation. **b.** The PCA mean of the hippocampal image intensities in the shape-based coordinate system. The CSF adjacent to the hippocampus can be seen near the edges; this illustrates the error in the initial segmentation combined with the error in *cm-rep* fitting.

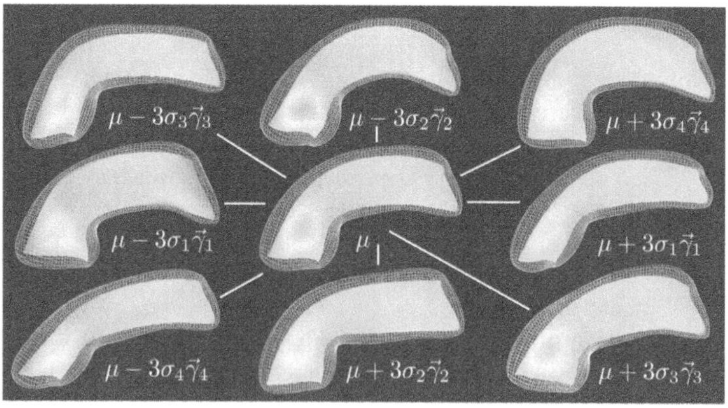

Fig. 6. Four principal modes of variability in the left hippocampus shape. The eigenvalues corresponding to these modes are 2.57, 2.28, 1.81 and 0.96, the total spectrum is 11.38, so the modes shown here represent 66.8% of total variability. The color map represents the radius function.

2.3 Statistical Modeling

To show how *cm-reps* would be used for shape characterization, we performed principal component analysis (PCA) on the shape and appearance features of *cm-reps* fitted to the hippocampus data. The shape features were computed by taking the values of the coefficients $\{\mathbf{w}_i\}, \{\omega_i\}$ after aligning the *cm-reps* using the Generalized Procrustes method [7]. The appearance features were sampled on a regular lattice in the u^1, u^2, ξ space. Fig. 6 shows the mean shape and principal modes of shape variability, and Fig. 5b shows the mean intensity pattern. Our PCA did not take into account the fact that some linear combinations of the *cm-rep* parameters that PCA generates can violate one of the inequality constraints mentioned above. However, no invalid *cm-reps* were generated by staying within 2.8 standard deviations from the mean in the first 10 principal modes. This indicates that valid and invalid *cm-reps* are well separated in feature space.

3 Discussion and Conclusions

We have presented *cm-reps*: a shape representation that models the continuous geometric relationship between the boundaries and skeletons of objects. The ability to impose a coordinate system on the interior of structures in a way that preserves two of the three coordinates along boundary normals and is nearly one-to-one and onto is the strength of the representation. The lossy nature of the representation, which is a potential weakness, was evaluated for the hippocampus, and the average representational error was found to be relatively small. The utility of *cm-reps* for the statistical analysis of shape and appearance was demonstrated by applying PCA to the *cm-reps* of the hippocampus. In the future, we plan to address the problem of *cm-rep* correspondence more directly and to use the *cm-rep* PCA as a component in an algorithm for the segmentation the hippocampus in structural MRI. We also intend to use *cm-reps* for structure-oriented fMRI analysis.

Other approaches to depth-based parametrization of interiors of anatomical structures have appeared in the recent literature. These methods typically employ distance transforms or skeletonization algorithms to assign a depth-based coordinate system to objects. For instance, Bouix et al. [2] find the dominant medial surface in the hippocampus and flatten it to form a reference space. The advantage of our method is that it is model-based, so a consistent shape-based coordinate system is given by construction, while methods such as [2] require pruning of skeletal branches and registration to find a common coordinate frame.

Acknowledgement

This work was supported by the NIH grant NS045839. We thank Prof. Charles L. Epstein, Prof. Jean Gallier and Marcelo Siqueira (Penn) for insightful discussions. We are indebted to Profs. Guido Gerig, Stephen M. Pizer, Sarang Joshi, and Martin Styner (UNC) for providing data and inspiration for this work.

References

1. H. Blum and R.N. Nagel. Shape description using weighted symmetric axis features. *Pattern Recognition*, 10(3):167–180, 1978.
2. Sylvain Bouix, Jens C Pruessner, D. Louis Collins, and Kaleem Siddiqi. Hippocampal shape analysis using medial surfaces. *Neuroimage*, 25(4):1077–89, May 2005.
3. M. H. Chakos, S. A. Schobel, H. Gu, G. Gerig, D. Bradford, C. Charles, and J. A. Lieberman. Duration of illness and treatment effects on hippocampal volume in male patients with schizophrenia. *Br J Psychiatry*, 186(1):26–31, 2005.
4. T. F. Cootes, C. J. Taylor, D. H. Cooper, and J. Graham. Active shape models – their training and application. *Computer Vision and Image Understanding*, 61(1):38–59, 1995.
5. T.F. Cootes, G.J. Edwards, and C.J. Taylor. Active appearance models. In *European Conference on Computer Vision*, volume 2, pages 484–498, Freiburg, Germany, June 1998.
6. J. Csernansky, S. Joshi, L. Wang, J. Haller, M. Gado, J. Miller, U. Grenander, and M. Miller. Hippocampal morphometry in schizophrenia via high dimensional brain mapping. In *Proc. National Academy of Sciences*, volume 95, pages 11406–11411, 1998.
7. J.C. Gower. Generalized procrustes analysis. *Psychometrika*, 40:33–51, 1975.
8. J.W. Haller, A. Banerjee, G.E. Christensen, M. Gado, S. Joshi, M.I. Miller, Y.I. Sheline, M.W. Vannier, and J.G. Csernansky. Three-dimensional hippocampal MR morphometry by high-dimensional transformation of a neuroanatomic atlas. *Radiology*, 202:504–510, 1997.
9. S. Joshi, U. Grenander, and M. Miller. On the geometry and shape of brain sub-manifolds. *IEEE Transactions on Pattern Analysis and Machine Intelligence*, 11:1317–1343, 1997.
10. D. Mumford. Pattern theory: a unifying perspective. In D. C. Knill and W. Richards, editors, *Perception as Bayesian Inference*, pages 25–62. Cambridge Universiry Press, 1996.
11. S. M. Pizer, P. T. Fletcher, S. Joshi, A. Thall, J. Z. Chen, Y. Fridman, D. S. Fritsch, A. G. Gash, J. M. Glotzer, M. R. Jiroutek, C. Lu, K. E. Muller, G. Tracton, P. Yushkevich, and E. L. Chaney. Deformable m-reps for 3D medical image segmentation. *International Journal of Computer Vision*, 55(2):85–106, Nov 2003.
12. M. Styner, G. Gerig, S. Joshi, and S.M. Pizer. Automatic and robust computation of 3D medial models incorporating object variability. *International Journal of Computer Vision*, 55(2):107–122, November 2003.
13. P.A. Yushkevich, H. Zhang, and J.C. Gee. Parametric medial shape representation in 3-D via the Poisson partial differential equation with non-linear boundary conditions. In G.E. Christensen and M. Sonka, editors, *Information Processing in Medical Imaging*, pages 162–173, 2005.

Vertebral Shape: Automatic Measurement with Dynamically Sequenced Active Appearance Models

M.G. Roberts, T.F. Cootes, and J.E. Adams

Department of Imaging Science and Biomedical Engineering,
University of Manchester,
Manchester, M13 9PL, UK
martin.roberts@manchester.ac.uk

Abstract. The shape and appearance of vertebrae on lateral dual x-ray absorptiometry (DXA) scans were statistically modelled. The spine was modelled by a sequence of overlapping triplets of vertebrae, using Active Appearance Models (AAMs). To automate vertebral morphometry, the sequence of trained models was matched to previously unseen scans. The dataset includes a significant number of pathologies. A new dynamic ordering algorithm was assessed for the model fitting sequence, using the best quality of fit achieved by multiple sub-model candidates. The accuracy of the search was improved by dynamically imposing the best quality candidate first. The results confirm the feasibility of substantially automating vertebral morphometry measurements even with fractures or noisy images.

1 Introduction

1.1 Context – Osteoporosis and Vertebral Fracture

Osteoporosis is a progressive skeletal disease characterized by a reduction in bone mass, resulting in an increased risk of fractures. Vertebral fractures are the most common, and their presence significantly increases the risk of further vertebral and non-vertebral fractures [7]. The accurate identification of prevalent vertebral fractures is therefore clinically important. However there is no precise definition of exactly what constitutes a vertebral fracture, though a variety of methods of describing them have been developed [1]. These include semi-quantitative methods involving some subjective judgement by an expert radiologist, and fully quantitative morphometric methods. The latter require the manual annotation of six (or more) points on each vertebra. This annotation is time consuming, and subtle shape information is lost in the reduction of shape to 6 points.

Our ultimate aim is to define more reliable quantitative fracture classification methods based on a complete definition of the vertebra's shape. The first step must therefore be to achieve a reliable automatic segmentation. Some success in automatically locating vertebrae has been reported by several authors [8,9,6,3]. The purpose of this study was firstly to assess the feasibility of using an Active

J. Duncan and G. Gerig (Eds.): MICCAI 2005, LNCS 3750, pp. 733–740, 2005.

Appearance Model (AAM) [11] approach to a challenging dataset, including fractured vertebrae, and noisy images. A second aim was to improve the accuracy and robustness of the techniques by improving the sequence in which vertebral locations are determined.

2 Materials and Methods

2.1 Data – DXA Images

Assessment for vertebral fracture is traditionally carried out using spinal radiographs. This study used dual x-ray absorptiometry (DXA) images however. Despite the images being noisier and of lower resolution, DXA has several advantages, such as a substantially lower radiation dose, and a lack of projective effects. Figure 1a shows a typical DXA scan with some endplate fractures, and Figure 1b shows the solution superimposed. The models cover the lumbar starting at L4 and continuing up the thorax up to vertebra T7.

The DXA images used were obtained from two previous studies [8,4], obtained from a Hologic (Bedford, MA) QDR2000plus scanner and a QDR4500A scanner respectively. Pixel dimensions are 1.0mm and 0.5mm respectively. The combined dataset of 202 images contains 173 fractures in total, and many images are very noisy due to an inherent bias towards obese patients in the clodronate study (second dataset). The images were manually annotated using an in-house tool, by one of the authors (MGR), with supervision by an experienced radiologist

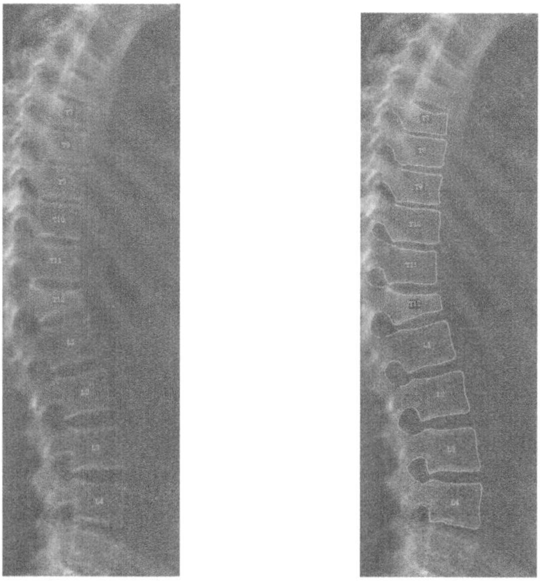

Fig. 1. Lateral DXA image of a spine displaying some symptoms of osteoporosis (e.g. T12 fracture). a) shows the raw image; b) shows the model solution superimposed.

(JEA). Each vertebral contour uses between 32 to 40 points around the vertebral body (32 points for T10 and above), with 8 further points around the pedicles for L4 to T10.

2.2 Statistical Models in Medical Imaging

Many problems in medical image interpretation require an automated system to interpret images. These images may provide noisy data, and typically complex structure. Model based methods offer solutions to these difficulties, by enforcing strong priors learned from a set of annotated training images. A widespread such current approach is the Active Appearance Model (AAM) [11].

One fundamental problem is that under-training of the model means that it may be insufficiently adaptable on a local level, especially when pathologies are present. In previous work [9] we showed that this problem could at least be mitigated by using multiple sub-models. The sub-structures were linked by partially overlapping them, and using the constrained form of the AAM [10].

2.3 Combining Multiple Sub-models

In [9] we demonstrated this approach on Smyth's original dataset [8] of predominantly normal spines. We modelled the spine by using a sequence of overlapping triplets of vertebrae. In this paper we improve the robustness and generality of the algorithm by developing a dynamic sequencing method for the order in which the sub-models are fit.

The sequence of sub-model solutions were combined in [9] as follows, using a fixed ordering starting by going up the lumbar. Each vertebra is fit using the triplet sub-model in which it is central (Figure 2). Note that subsequent iterations do not update any point positions which have already been determined, unless the point is in the central vertebra of the triplet. When a triplet model has been fit it provides part of the initialisation (via the overlapping vertebrae) for subsequent iterations which fit its neighbours. Furthermore constraints are applied [10] so that overlapping vertebrae cannot be moved far from the provisional positions determined previously. This feed-forward of constraints is further aided by re-fitting the global shape model to the solution so far. This is used to initialise a starting solution for vertebrae not yet fit, and relatively low constraint weights are attached to this global prior. Thus information in the global shape model is still used in guiding the solution, but the global shape constraints are downweighted, which allows their violation to a degree if the image evidence locally supports such a solution.

Our approach differs somewhat from that of Davatzikos *et al* [2], who propose a hierarchical Active Shape Model based on a wavelet decomposition of the shape contours, in which local regions of the wavelet transform space are decoupled when applying the shape model constraints. In [2] coarse global constraints continue to apply in a strict sense. However, in the case of vertebral morphometry, certain pathologies of the spine such as scoliosis may cause even coarse aspects of the shape model to be violated, as whole vertebrae can be laterally

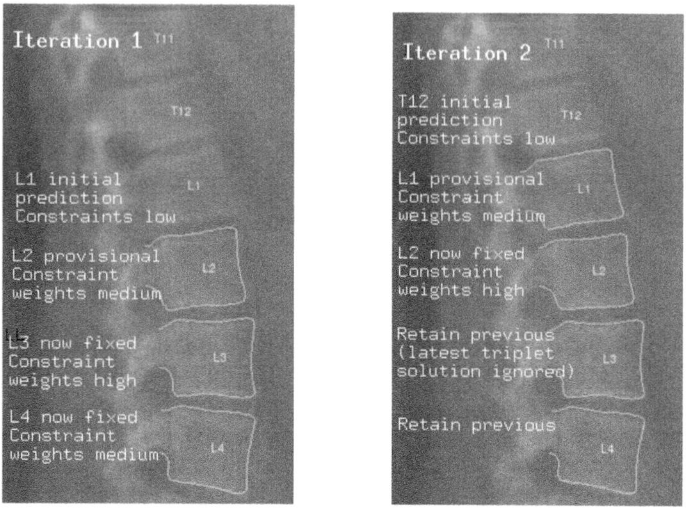

Fig. 2. An illustration of the first two iterations (static fit ordering) combining vertebral triplet sub-models. a) shows the result of fitting the first triplet containing L4/L3/L2. b) indicates the next iteration which fits L3/L2/L1. The second iteration resets L2 and provides an initialisation of L1, and an updated prediction for T12 via the global shape model.

shifted outside the region captured in the training set. Therefore we use multiple overlapping AAMs instead, which allows a wider range of pathologies to be adequately fitted. Furthermore there may be some advantages in decomposing the image search process, as well as the application of shape constraints.

2.4 Dynamic Sub-model Sequence Ordering Algorithm

If one sub-model fit fails, then this can misalign the starting solution for subsequent iterations. In such a case it would be better to adapt the sequence dynamically by comparing the fit quality of several candidate sub-models. Picking the best fitting model as the one to impose at this iteration will tend to defer noisier or poorly fitting regions until they have been better constrained by their neighbours.

In this new approach a subset of N active candidate sub-models is maintained. Each such candidate is provisionally fitted, then the submodel with the best quality of fit (see next section) is imposed into the overall solution, and removed from the candidate list. A new candidate sub-model to replace the one just imposed is added at the end of each iteration by searching from the latest best candidate to locate its nearest remaining neighbour[1]. As with the static ordering, the global shape model is then fitted to the subset of all points determined so far, and used to predict an initial solution for all points which have not yet formed part of any imposed sub-model solution. These iterations continue

[1] "Remaining" means that the submodel has never been in the candidate list.

until all sub-models have either been fitted and imposed already, or are now in the set of candidates. When no more candidates can be added the remaining $N-1$ sub-models are fitted (best quality first) and the search concludes. It is to be noted that all candidates in the active subset are re-fitted at each iteration, as they will generally have a slightly different initialisation and altered shape constraints as a consequence of imposing the last accepted candidate. We used a set of 3 candidate sub-models, starting with the top, bottom and middle of the spine.

2.5 Quality of Fit Measure

The quality of fit measure used to pick the best candidate sub-model is based on the scaled residual sum of squares S, which is calculated as:

$$S = \sum_{i=1}^{n} \frac{r_i^2}{\hat{\sigma}_i^2} \tag{1}$$

where r_i is the grey level residual at point i, and $\hat{\sigma}_i$ is its estimated standard deviation. However, when comparing different sub-models with different numbers of points it is not meaningful to directly compare values of S. Instead we pick the best fitting sub-model, in the sense of having the lowest probability of obtaining a residual sum of squares any better (i.e. lower) than that achieved. So S is mapped to a value z on a standard Gaussian approximating the theoretically χ^2 distribution of S, but with further scaling parameters α and β for its overall mean and variance. These scaling parameters are necessary because the set $\hat{\sigma}_i$ are underestimated, as they are calculated at model creation by refitting the model to the training set, and do not account for model inadequacies in fitting to unseen images. To more accurately model the true distribution of S, the boosting parameters α and β in mean and variance due to model inadequacy are derived by running a preliminary set of randomised train/test set partitions. The final standardised Gaussian z-value used is then:

$$z = \frac{S - \alpha n}{\alpha\sqrt{2n\beta}} \tag{2}$$

The quality measure is obtained by just negating this, as picking the highest value of $-z$ is equivalent to choosing the candidate with the lowest probability of obtaining a residual sum of squares any better than that achieved.

2.6 Experiments

Leave-8-out tests were performed over the 202 images. When the algorithm is run interactively in an associated prototype clinical tool, the clinician initialises the solution by clicking on 3 points. These are the bottom of L4, top of T12 and top of T7. The global shape model fit to these 3 points is used as the starting solution. On each experiment the 3-point initialisation was simulated by using the known equivalent marked points and adding random offsets to them. These were zero-mean Gaussian errors with SD of 1mm in the y-direction (along the spine) and 3mm in the x-direction. Twenty replications (i.e. random initialisations) of each image were performed. The AAMs sampled the gradient along profiles spanning 6mm either side of the shape, with the overall sample renormalised onto the sample cdf.

3 Results

The accuracy of the search was characterised by calculating the absolute point-to-line distance error for each point on the vertebral body. The error is the distance from each located point to the nearest point (in the same vertebra) on the smooth bezier spline passing through the manually annotated points.

3.1 Optimal Sub-models

We assessed the effect of the size of structures used for the sub-models. As well as triplets, we tried using individual vertebra models, and a central vertebra with the neighbouring half-vertebrae. Scaling up the structure size, we assessed the use of quintets (5 vertebrae). Space does not permit the inclusion of full results. In summary, structures smaller than triplets were found to be too unconstrained and therefore unreliable. Triplets performed slightly better than quintets on fractured vertebrae, but there was little difference between triplets and quintets on normal vertebrae. We concluded that triplets are the optimal sub-structure to model.

3.2 Dynamic vs Static Ordering

The overall mean point accuracies are 0.79, 1.03, and 0.92 mm for the dynamically ordered, statically ordered, and global model approaches respectively. Table 1 compares results for static and dynamic sub-model ordering, but decomposing the data into points within normal or fractured vertebrae. Each row gives the mean, median and 75th percentiles, and the percentage of point errors in excess of 2mm. The threshold of 2mm would be around 2SDs of manual precision, and can be viewed as a fairly stringent point failure indicator. The Eastell morphometric method [5] was used to determine fracture status.

Comparing the dynamic and static ordering results in table 1, there is an improvement by using the new dynamic ordering method, but this is mainly

Table 1. Search Accuracy Percentiles by Fracture Status

	Normal				Fractured			
Model Fit Strategy	Mean Acc	Median Acc	75%ile Acc	%ge errors over 2mm	Mean Acc	Median Acc	75%ile Acc	%ge errors over 2mm
Dynamic	0.70	0.50	0.92	4.96%	1.23	0.70	1.41	16.22%
Static	0.88	0.55	1.04	7.54%	1.80	0.83	1.79	22.21%
Global	0.84	0.62	1.12	7.12%	1.37	0.84	1.63	18.17%

evident in the tails of the error distribution. Although there is little difference in median accuracy, the reduction in extent of the error tails leads to an overall mean improvement of 0.24mm, rising to 0.57mm for fractures. The symmetric (in probability) 98% confidence interval of the mean improvement (derived by bootstrap resampling) is [0.143,0.385].

4 Discussion

The previously observed accuracy improvement [9] of around 0.4mm between the statically ordered triplet approach and a global model disappears with a larger training set. A similar effect was noted in [2] comparing a standard and an hierarchical ASM. But the mean difference between the dynamic sub-model approach and a single global model is statistically significant (using a 98% bootstrap confidence interval on the mean difference). So there does appear to be a real improvement from the heuristic of first imposing the better fitting regions, and then using the constraints implied by them in subsequent (partial) searches. Further gains might possibly be derived from increasing the size of the candidate subset N, but this would of course increase the computation time of the algorithm.

With the new dynamic ordering method the mean location accuracy of 0.7 mm for normal (i.e. not fractured) vertebrae is comparable to typical manual precision. Over 95% of points in normal vertebrae are located to within 2mm. The performance on fractured vertebrae worsens, but remains quite respectable, and the mean of 1.23mm is still comparable with manual precision on fractures. Fractured vertebrae present a more challenging problem, as the variation is much greater for pathological cases than for normals, and also when a vertebral end-plate collapses a remnant of the stronger outer ring of cortical bone can provide a weaker outer edge to further confuse the search algorithm.

Nevertheless around 84% of points in fractured vertebrae are located to within 2mm with the dynamic method. The remaining 16% in the tail of the distribution are due to a combination of under-training of the models, and false local minima. In the former case the problem is that the shape model cannot fit to some of the more extreme fractures. In the latter case, there appear to be problems with local minima where the top of a vertebra is erroneously fit to the bottom of the vertebra above (or vice versa). Fractured vertebrae may be prone to this failure mode, as the true edge of a collapsed vertebral body may well be further from the starting solution than the opposite side of its neighbour. It may ultimately prove necessary to search using multiple initialisations to segment pathological cases more reliably - for example by using a normal and a fractured candidate. However even here our framework could still be used, as multiple candidates of the same sub-model can essentially be treated in the same way as multiple different sub-models.

The accuracy is better than other comparable cited figures in the literature [8,9,6,3]. For example de Bruijne *et al* [3] obtained a mean point-to-contour accuracy of 1.4mm on lumbar radiographs using shape particle filtering, whereas we achieve a mean accuracy of 0.8mm, even though DXA images are typically noisier than radiographs and have poorer resolution, and we also include the mid-thorax which has more soft-tissue clutter and a greater probability of fracture.

Our latest results confirm the feasibility of substantially automating vertebral morphometry measurements even with fractures or noisy images. However some work remains on extending the models and search process to cope with the more severe fractures. Furthermore the sub-model approach offers scope for greater gains on radiographic images, which have significant local variation in projective effects, which could be compensated for by varing the affine pose of the sub-models.

References

1. Guermazi A, Mohr A, Grigorian M, Taouli B, and Genant HK. Identification of vertebral fractures in osteoporosis. *Seminars in Musculoskeletal Radiology*, 6(3):241–252, 2002.
2. Davatzikos C and Tao. Hierachical active shape models: Using the wavelet transform. *IEEE Trans. Med. Imag.*, 22(3):414–423, 2003.
3. de Bruijne M and Nielsen M. Image segmentation by shape particle filtering. In *International Conference on Pattern Recognition*, pages 722–725. IEEE Computer Society Press, 2004.
4. McCloskey E, Selby P, de Takats D, and et al. Effects of clodronate on vertebral fracture risk in osteoporosis: a 1-year interim analysis. *Bone*, 28(3):310–5, 2001.
5. R Eastell, SL Cedel, HW Wahner, BL Riggs, and LJ Melton. Classification of vertebral fractures. *J Bone Miner Res*, 6(3):207–215, 1991.
6. B. Howe, A. Gururajan, H. Sari-Sarraf, and R. Long. Hierarchical segmentation of cervical and lumbar vertebrae using a customized generalized hough transform and extensions to active appearance models. In *Proc IEEE 6th SSIAI*, pages 182–186, 2004.
7. Melton LJ III, Atkinson EJ, Cooper C, O'Fallon WM, and Riggs BL. Vertebral fractures predict subsequent fractures. *Osteoporosis Int*, 10:214–221, 1999.
8. Smyth PP, Taylor CJ, and Adams JE. Vertebral shape: automatic measurement with active shape models. *Radiology*, 211:571–578, 1999.
9. M.G. Roberts, T.F. Cootes, and J.E. Adams. Linking sequences of active appearance sub-models via constraints: an application in automated vertebral morphometry. In *14th British Machine Vision Conference*, pages 349–358, 2003.
10. Cootes TF and Taylor CJ. Constrained active appearance models. In *8th International Conference on Computer Vision*, volume 1, pages 748–754. IEEE Computer Society Press, July 2001.
11. Cootes TF, Edwards GJ, and Taylor CJ. Active appearance models. In Burkhardt H and Neumann B, editors, *5th European Conference on Computer Vision*, volume 2, pages 484–498. Springer (Berlin), 1998.

Geodesic Active Contours with Adaptive Neighboring Influence

Huafeng Liu[1,2], Yunmei Chen[3], Hon Pong Ho[2], and Pengcheng Shi[2]

[1] State Key Laboratory of Modern Optical Instrumentation, Zhejiang University, Hangzhou, China
[2] Department of Electrical and Electronic Engineering, Hong Kong University of Science and Technology, Hong Kong
[3] Department of Mathematics, University of Florida, Gainesville, USA

Abstract. While geometric deformable models have brought tremendous impacts on shape representation and analysis in medical image analysis, some of the remaining problems include the handling of boundary leakage and the lack of global understanding of boundaries. We present a modification to the geodesic active contour framework such that influence from local neighbors of a front point is explicitly incorporated, and it is thus capable of robustly dealing with the boundary leakage problem. The fundamental power of this strategy rests with the local integration of evolution forces for each front point within its local influence domain, which is adaptively determined by the local level set geometry and image/prior information. Due to the combined effects of internal and external constraints on a point and the interactions with those of its neighbors, our method allows stable boundary detection when the edge information is noisy and possibly discontinuous (e.g. gaps in the boundaries) while maintaining the abilities to handle topological changes, thanks to the level set implementation. The algorithm has been implemented using the meshfree particle domain representation, and experimental results on synthetic and real images demonstrate its superior performance.

1 Introduction

Shape recovery has been one of the most active research areas in medical image analysis because of its practical importance and theoretical challenges. Over the last two decades, various parametric and geometric deformable models have gained much popularity [4,7]. Geodesic active contours have been proposed [1] to connect classical parametric *snakes* based on energy minimization to geometric active contours based on the theory of curve evolution [8], and thus maintain the desirable properties of allowing topological changes during the curve evolution process. Nevertheless, these geometric snakes still have certain drawbacks, i.e. they face difficulties in handling weak edges/gap problems [1,10] where the evolving contour cannot stick to the object boundary and would simply leak through the gaps, they are very sensitive to local minima in noisy images [11].

In order to overcome these problems, considerable progress has already been made through the use of additional force (or energy) terms. An extra stopping

J. Duncan and G. Gerig (Eds.): MICCAI 2005, LNCS 3750, pp. 741–748, 2005.

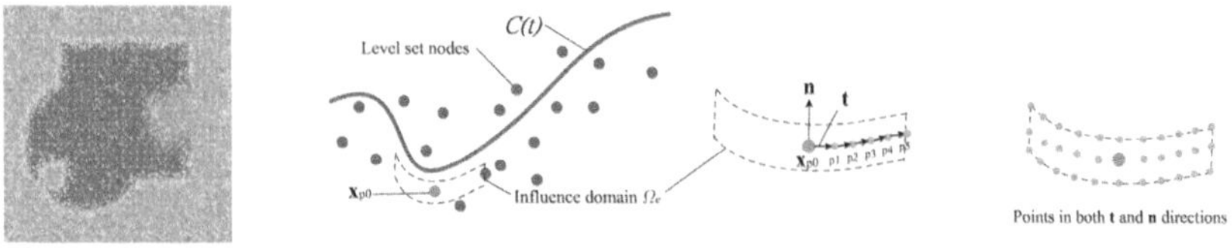

Fig. 1. 1st: adaptive point-based domain representation; 2nd: influence domain (and the associated other points) of the red point; 3rd: closeup which illustrates the generation of neighboring points in the tangent direction (we generate the points p_n through $\mathbf{x}_{p_n} = \mathbf{x}_{p_{(n-1)}} + \frac{t_{scale}}{|\kappa|}\mathbf{t}$, with κ the curvature and $\mathbf{t}$ the tangent vector of point $p_{(n-1)}$); 4th: generated neighboring points in both normal and tangent directions (and thus the influence domain) for the red point.

term for pulling back the contour if it passes the boundary was investigated in [1], although this formulation is still susceptible to boundary leakage problem. A weighted area functional force has been introduced to help the snake be more robust with respect to small gap problem [10]. Diffused external data forces, such as the gradient vector flow (GVF), have also been adopted to deal with the leakage problem and noisy data [12]. And boundary and region information has been integrated under a curve-based minimization framework [9]. These later approaches own the benefits provided by external force potential field in achieving a larger capture range and robustness against the boundary leakage problem [9,12]. More recently, a region-aided geometric snake, which integrates gradient flow forces with region vector flow forces obtained through the diffusion of the region segmentation map, has been developed and implemented within level set platform [11]. These integrated forces give another way to be more robust toward weak edges. Similar region-based strategies have been explored by other works as well [2].

We realize that the boundary leakage problem can be more readily solved if the behavior of individual curve point is constrained by local edge information of itself and that of its neighboring points. These inter-point relationships act as *diffused* local internal energy, which would make the snakes less sensitive to noisy or broken edges. Thus, our aim is to develop a robust segmentation framework that imposes adaptive local inter-point constraints into geodesic active contours. Instead of using additional external forces, we make use of the image data at the adaptively determined local support domain around each point of interest, which effectively enlarges the capture range of each point to have a better local understanding of the image information within its local neighborhood. In other words, we modify the image forces on each point of the geodesic contour in a way such that it is capable of providing sufficient information to define a desired segmentation which is robust against boundary leakage and noise impact. One key issue is the proper determination of the local neighborhood of each curve point such that the integration of information can be performed. In this paper, we present a numerical implementation of the strategy on the meshfree particle representation of the evolution domain, where the local neighbor is adaptively selected based on image data and curve geometry.

2 Methodology

2.1 Geodesic Active Contours (GACs)

Let us consider an active contour $C(s)$ parameterized by $s \in [0,1]$. It has been known that the problem of boundary detection can be casted into the problem of minimizing the curve length in Riemannian space $min \int_0^1 g(|\nabla I(C(s))|)|C'(s)|ds$, where $g(.)$ is a strictly decreasing edge-function such that $g(0) = 1$ and $lim_{x->\infty}$ $g(x) = 0$ [1]. Now we represent the evolving contour C implicitly as the zero level set of a scalar Lipschitz function ϕ: $C(t) = \{x|\phi(x,t) = 0\}$. The corresponding energy over the image domain Ω in terms of level set function ϕ becomes:

$$E(\phi) = \int_{\Omega} g(|\nabla I(x)|)|\nabla H(\phi(x))|dx \tag{1}$$

where $H(x)$ is the Heaviside function, that is $H(x) = 1$ if $x >= 0$, and $H(x) = 0$ if $x < 0$, and let $\delta_{\varepsilon}(x) = H'(x)$ be the Dirac measure. Then, the length of zero level set is given by $\int_{\Omega} |\nabla H(\phi(x))| = \int_{\Omega} \delta_{\varepsilon}(\phi)|\nabla \phi(x)|$. The energy can be rewritten:

$$E(\phi) = \int_{\Omega} \delta_{\varepsilon}(\phi) g(|\nabla I(x)|)|\nabla \phi(x)|dx \tag{2}$$

The minimization process can be achieved by solving the Euler-Lagrange equation, obtained by minimizing Eqn. (2) with respect to ϕ and parameterizing the descent directions by an artificial time t:

$$\frac{\partial \phi}{\partial t} = \delta_{\varepsilon}(\phi) div \left(g(|\nabla I(x)|) \frac{\nabla \phi}{|\nabla \phi|} \right) \tag{3}$$

We reach the following equations by expanding the divergence term and replacing $\delta_{\varepsilon}(\phi)$ by $\nabla \phi$ [13]:

$$\frac{\partial \phi}{\partial t} = g(|\nabla I(x)|)|\nabla \phi| div \left(\frac{\nabla \phi}{|\nabla \phi|} \right) + \nabla g(|\nabla I(x)|). \nabla \phi \tag{4}$$

where $\frac{\nabla \phi}{|\nabla \phi|}$ denotes the unit normal vector. The divergence of the unit normal vector $div \left(\frac{\nabla \phi}{|\nabla \phi|} \right)$ represents the curvature of the current point.

2.2 GACs with Adaptive Neighboring Influence (GAC-ANI)

The main idea in the GAC-ANI formulation is that centered at each front point, there is an *influence domain* Ω_e which contains points that have effects on the evolution of the concerned front point. Hence, each front point moves under the influence of two forces: the typical data force provided by image information such as GVF, and the *neighborhood force* due to the interaction of the point with other points in the influence domain. With proper formulation of the neighboring interactions, front points at the weak edges or gaps will be dominated by the neighborhood force such that the front would be discouraged from leaking through the boundary. For front points with good data force, their movement is still mostly controlled by image information and thus would stick to the object boundary exhibited in the image. Due to the combined effects of data constraints and interactions with the neighboring points, GAC-ANI exhibits robustness against boundary leakage while maintaining the desired geometrical characteristics of GACs.

While there could be many ways to incorporate the inter-point relationship into the GAC-ANI formulation, one simple way of enforcing neighborhood influence is to replace the edge function $g(x)$ in Equation (2) by $G(x) = \int_{\Omega_e} \mathbf{N} g(y)dy$, where $\mathbf{N}$ is a shape function that assigns proper weights to each point within the influence domain. In this sense, the evolution force on point x is now constrained by the image data at the point itself and at the other points within its influence domain. The modified objective function of GAC-ANI now becomes:

$$E(\phi) = \int_{\Omega} \delta_{\varepsilon}(\phi) \left(\int_{\Omega_e} \mathbf{N} g(y)dy \right) | \bigtriangledown \phi(x)|dx = \int_{\Omega} \delta_{\varepsilon}(\phi) G(x) | \bigtriangledown \phi(x)|dx \quad (5)$$

The evolution equation related to the Euler-Lagrange equation for Eqn. (5) is:

$$\frac{d}{d\tau} E(\phi + \tau\Phi)|_{\tau=0} = 0 \quad (6)$$

Now, let us take care of the left hand side of the equation:

$$\frac{d}{d\tau} \int_{\Omega} \delta_{\varepsilon}(\phi + \tau\Phi) G(x) | \bigtriangledown \phi + \tau \bigtriangledown \Phi|dx = - \int_{\Omega} \delta_{\varepsilon}(\phi) div \left(G(x) \frac{\bigtriangledown \phi}{|\bigtriangledown \phi|} \right) \Phi dx (7)$$

Finally, the following Euler-Lagrange equation can be achieved:

$$\delta_{\varepsilon}(\phi) div \left(G(x) \frac{\bigtriangledown \phi}{|\bigtriangledown \phi|} \right) = 0 \quad (8)$$

It is common to expand the divergence term to obtain the alternative equation:

$$\delta_{\varepsilon}(\phi) G(x) div \left(\frac{\bigtriangledown \phi}{|\bigtriangledown \phi|} \right) + \delta_{\varepsilon}(\phi) \bigtriangledown G(x). \frac{\bigtriangledown \phi}{|\bigtriangledown \phi|} = 0 \quad (9)$$

where $\bigtriangledown G = \int_{\Omega_e} \bigtriangledown \mathbf{N} g(y)dy$. The steady state solution of the above equation results in the GAC-ANI formulation in level set representation, where a standard rescaling can be made through replacing $\delta_{\varepsilon}(\phi)$ by $|\bigtriangledown \phi|$ [13]:

$$\frac{\partial \phi}{\partial t} = G(x) | \bigtriangledown \phi| div \left(\frac{\bigtriangledown \phi}{|\bigtriangledown \phi|} \right) + \bigtriangledown G(x). \bigtriangledown \phi \quad (10)$$

Discussions. It should be noted that the most attractive property of the above GAC-ANI formulation is that the influence domain Ω_e controls the trade-off between a parametric snake and a geodesic snake at the front point.

Consider the case where the size of the local influence domain is approaching zero, e.g. the level set value of the point is mainly determined by itself. Hence, Eqn. (10) goes back to the standard geodesic active contours. On the other hand, if we enlarge the influence domain to cover the entire curve, the integration is then taken over the whole contour. Perceptually, the behavior of all curve points are now inter-related, and we effectively have a parametric deformable model instead. In practice, influence domains of different sizes generate different G and $\bigtriangledown G$, which in turn are suitable for different situations. For example, large influence domains are effective in robust segmentation of noisy images or object with broken edges. On the other hand, small influence domains are needed for object boundaries with many fine details. Schemes to adaptively determine the sizes of the influence domains will be discussed in the following section.

2.3 Numerical Implementations of GAC-ANI

We have implemented the GAC-ANI on the evolution domain represented by adaptively distributed meshfree particles [3]. Here, we want to point out that any numerical implementations such as traditional finite difference schemes can also be used for GAC-ANI without any fundamental algorithmic modifications.

Let $\phi(\mathbf{x}, t = 0) = \pm d$, where $\pm d$ is the signed distance to the interface. The level set updating procedures on the meshfree particle domain are:

1. *Initialization:* Initialize $\phi(\cdot, 0)$ to be the signed distance function.
2. *Domain Representation:* We adopt an adaptive point distribution scheme to represent the domain by meshfree particles (see Fig. 1 for an example). The point distribution is adaptive towards both local level set geometry and image gradient, and it allows extremely convenient enhancement/reduction of curve precision by simply putting more/fewer points on the computation domain. A detailed discussion of this scheme can be found in [3]. Then, find all the points in the narrow band of the current zero level set.
3. *Influence Domain Generation:* Generate a proper influence domain for each point within the narrow band (see detailed discussion later).
4. *Shape Function Construction:* Here, we use the concept of moving least squares (MLS) to construct the shape functions. It is assumed the current active point $\mathbf{x}$ with its neighboring nodes $\mathbf{x}_I$, $I = 1, 2, ..., n$ are given in the influence domain. Following the work in [5], the MLS-derived shape function is $N_I(\mathbf{x}) = \sum_j^m p_j(\mathbf{x})(\mathbf{A}^{-1}(\mathbf{x})\mathbf{B}(\mathbf{x}))_{jI} = \mathbf{p}^T\mathbf{A}^{-1}\mathbf{B}_I$, with $\mathbf{A}(\mathbf{x}) = \sum_I w(\mathbf{x} - \mathbf{x}_I)\mathbf{p}(\mathbf{x}_I)\mathbf{p}^T(\mathbf{x}_I)$, $\mathbf{B}_I = w(\mathbf{x} - \mathbf{x}_I)\mathbf{p}(\mathbf{x}_I)$, $\mathbf{B}(\mathbf{x}) = [\mathbf{B}_1, \mathbf{B}_2, ..., \mathbf{B}_n]$. $\mathbf{p}(\mathbf{x})$ is polynomial basis functions, and $w(\mathbf{x} - \mathbf{x}_I)$ is the weighting function.
5. *Evaluation of Integrals:* To update level set function of Equation (10), matrices G and $\bigtriangledown G$ need to be calculated. That is, one needs to integrate over the influence domain. This can be carried out through numerical techniques which approximate a continuous integral over Ω_e into a discrete sum:

$\int_{\Omega_e} f(\xi) = \sum_{l=1}^{n_q} w_l f(\xi_l)$, where n_q is number of quadrature points, ξ_l is the coordinates of sampling point l, and w_l is the corresponding weighting factor. Here, we use the Gaussian quadrature technique which is the most commonly used integration scheme in meshfree particle methods [6].

6. *Updating Procedure:* Update level set function ϕ using Equation (10).
7. *Reinitialization:* Re-initialize $\phi(\cdot, t+1)$ to be the signed distance function of its zero level set.
8. *Convergence Test:* Set proper convergence criterion to test whether the zero level set reaches object boundary. If no, go back to step 2.

Influence Domain Determination. In the level set formulation based on distance measure, there is an entire family of isocontours of different level set values (although only one of which is the zero level set). For each data point in the narrow band, or a node, its all important influence domain Ω_e is determined by a data-driven local operation. And the geometry of the resulting influence domain adapts to the isocontour segment to which it belongs (see Fig. 1 for an illustration).

First, we calculate the image gradient magnitude $|\bigtriangledown I(\mathbf{x}_{nb})|$ within the narrowband and normalize them to $[0, 1]$, where $\mathbf{x}_{nb}$ is the narrow band node points set. Starting with an arbitrary narrow band point $\mathbf{x}_{nb(i)}$ (the red point in Fig. 1), let $\mathbf{x}_i = \mathbf{x}_{nb(i)}$ and tag it as *active*. We then compute the normal vector $\mathbf{n}$, the tangent vector $\mathbf{t}$, and curvature κ of the *active* point. Adding a tangent virtual node along the *tangent direction* use $\mathbf{x}_i = \mathbf{x}_i + \frac{t_{scale}}{|\kappa|}\mathbf{t}$ (adding the opposite point by $\mathbf{x}_i = \mathbf{x}_i - \frac{tscale}{|\kappa|}\mathbf{t}$), where t_{scale} is the tangential scale factor. This way, the higher the curvature, the closer the added point will be to the *active* point, which will in turn guarantee that fine shape details will be preserved. We then tag the new added point as *active* point. This process is executed iteratively until the number of added points has reached a specified limit, which is determined by $\frac{tot_{scale}}{exp(|\bigtriangledown I(\mathbf{x}_{nb(i)})|)}$, where tot_{scale} is another scale factor. This entire procedure implies that for low image gradient node, many virtual points will be added in the tangent direction (large Ω_e dimension size in the tangent direction). Of course for high image gradient node, there will be few virtual points added and the Ω_e dimension size in the tangent direction will be small. In the same fashion, virtual nodes in *normal direction* can be added using a similar scheme by $\mathbf{x}_i \pm n_{scale}|\bigtriangledown I(\mathbf{x}_i)|\mathbf{n}$ where n_{scale} is the normal direction scale factor.

3 Experiments and Results

In Fig. 2, comparison is made between traditional GAC and GAC-ANI on their ability to deal with boundary gaps. The test object contains a big blurred area on the right boundary and a small blurred area on the lower left boundary. Clearly, the traditional GAC curve keeps shrinking and leaks through the broken edges, while GAC-ANI does not suffer from such leakage problem and converges to the true boundary since the neighborhood point information offers useful

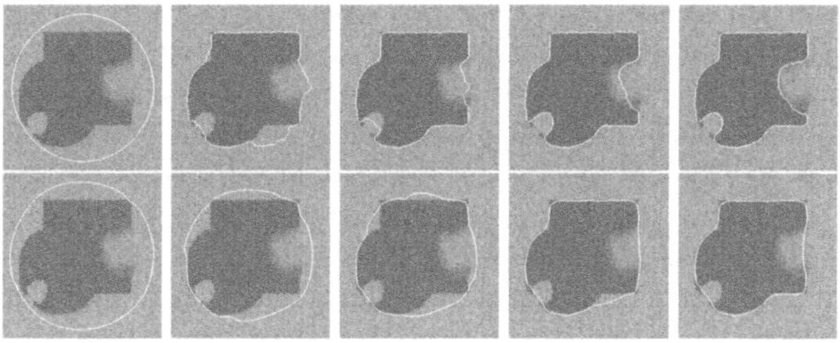

Fig. 2. Segmentation of noisy synthetic image with boundary occlusion: traditional level set implemented on finite difference grid (top); GAC-ANI on adaptive point cloud.

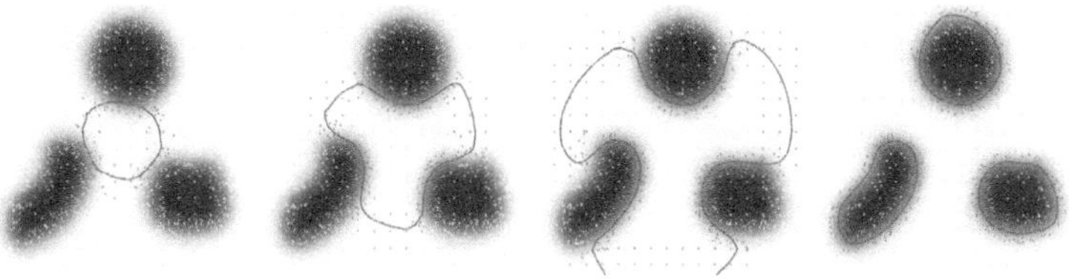

Fig. 3. The ability of the GAC-ANI to handle topological changes

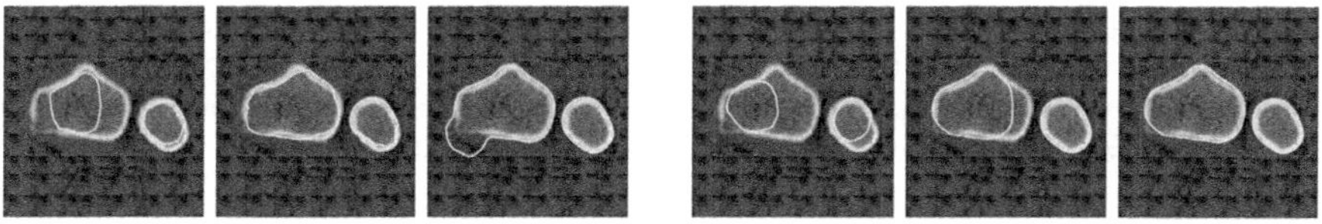

Fig. 4. Segmentation process on the bone CT image: GAC (left) and GAC-ANI (right)

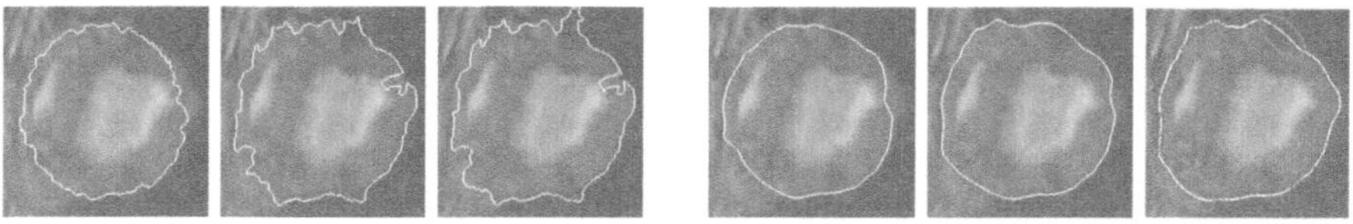

Fig. 5. Epicardial segmentation process on canine MRI image: traditional GAC (left three) and GAC-ANI (right three). The red circles highlight the ill-defined boundary areas (upper-right: image void caused by implanted marker; lower-left: weak contrast between myocardium and background tussue) where neighboring influence is dominant.

expanded view on the image boundaries. Each contour point of the GAC-ANI belonging to the blurred area is adaptively assigned large influence domain and thus detects the boundary properly, while front point elsewhere is determined to have very small influence domain and thus behaves just like the traditional level set point. In Fig. 3, starting from a single front, GAC-ANI manages to split and capture all the boundaries of three objects, just like a traditional GAC. During the segmentation process, as the front moves, the nodes in the narrow band are adaptively constructed depending on local image (red points) and geometry (cyan points). Finally, we show the segmentation results on several real medical images. In the bone CT image segmentation (Fig. 4), the low-left corner of the big bone has a relatively weak edge. While the traditional GAC leaks through the edge (left figures), GAC-ANI properly stops at that part of the edge (right figures). In the difficult task of epicardial segmentation from the canine cardiac MRI image (Fig. 5), the ill-defined epicardium from its background and the void caused by implanted imaging-opaque markers make the traditional GAC fail to produce appropriate definition of the boundary, while the proposed GAC-ANI yields proper, smooth segmentation result.

Acknowledgement. This work is supported in part by the 973 Program of China (2003CB716104), by the HKRGC-CERG HKUST6252/04E, by the NSF of China(60403040).

References

1. V. Caselles, R. Kimmel, and G. Sapiro. Geodesic active contours. *International Journal of Computer Vision*, 22(1):61–79, 1997.
2. T. Chan and L. Vese. Active contours without edges. *IEEE Transactions on Image Processing*, 10(2):266–277, 2001.
3. H. Ho, Y. Chen, H. Liu, and P. Shi. Level set active contours on unstructured point cloud. In *IEEE Computer Vision and Pattern Recognition*, 2005.
4. M. Kass, A. Witkin, and D. Terzopoulos. SNAKES: Active contour models. *International Journal of Computer Vision*, 1:321–332, January 1988.
5. P. Lancaster and K. Salkauskas. Surface generated by moving least squares methods. *Mathematics of Computation*, 37(155):141–158, 1981.
6. H. Liu and P. Shi. Meshfree representation and computation: Applications to cardiac motion analysis. In *Information Processing in Medical Imaging*, pages 560–572, Ambleside, U.K, July 2003.
7. R. Malladi, J.A. Sethian, and B.C. Vemuri. Shape modeling with front propagation: A level set approach. *IEEE Transactions on Pattern Analysis and Machine Intelligence*, 17(2):158–175, 1995.
8. S. Osher and J.A. Sethian. Fronts propagating with curvature-dependent speed: Algorithms based on hamilton-jacobi formulations. *Journal of Computational Physics*, 79:12–49, 1988.
9. N. Paragios and R. Deriche. Coupled geodesic active regions for image segmentation: a level set apporach. In *Proceedings of the Europe Conference on Computer Vision*, pages 224–240, 2000.
10. K. Siddiqi, Y. Lauziere, A. Tannenbaum, and S. Zucker. Area and length-minimizing flows for shape segmentation. *IEEE Transactions on Image Processing*, 7:433–443, 1998.
11. X. Xie and M. Mirmehdi. RAGS: Region-aided geometric snake. *IEEE Transactions on Image Processing*, 13(5):640–652, May 2004.
12. C. Xu and J. Prince. Generalized gradient vector flow external forces for active contours. *Signal Processing*, 71(2):131–139, 1998.
13. H. Zhao, T. Chan, B. Merriman, and S. Osher. A variational level set approach to multiphase motion. *Journal of Computational Physics*, 127:179–185, 1996.

A Construction of an Averaged Representation of Human Cortical Gyri Using Non-linear Principal Component Analysis

G. Lohmann[1], D.Y. von Cramon[1], and A.C.F. Colchester[2]

[1] Max-Planck-Institute for Human Cognitive and Brain Sciences, Leipzig, Germany
[2] University of Kent at Canterbury, UK

Abstract. Because of the complex shape of human cortical gyri and great variation between individuals, development of effective representation schemes which allow establishment of correspondence between individuals, extraction of average structure of a population, and co-registration has proved very difficult. We introduce an approach which extracts line representations of gyri at different depths from high resolution MRI, labels main gyri semi-automatically, and extracts a template from a population using non-linear principal component analysis. The method has been tested on data from 96 healthy human volunteers. The model captures the most salient shape features of all major cortical gyri, and can be used for inter-subject registration, for investigating regionalized inter-subject variability, and for inter-hemispheric comparisons.

1 Introduction

The idea of constructing a model brain is not new. Perhaps the most well-known example is the Talairach brain atlas. While this atlas constituted a tremendous step forward because for the first time a generally accepted coordinate system was introduced, it also soon became clear that a number of problems still remain to be solved. In particular, the Talairach atlas [1] is based on one single brain so that it does not account for inter-individual anatomical variations. For this reason, more representative brain templates have been introduced [2]. Probabilistic atlases detailing anatomical structures were targeted by the ICBM consortium [3]. These templates provide presence probability maps of different structures. Transfer of labels between atlas and new subject requires co-registration of a T1-weighted MRI scan, that is already linked to the atlas labels, to the same type of MRI obtained in the new subject. Voxel-based co-registration of highly variable structures such as cortical sulci and gyri is imperfect. Averaging co-registered scans tends to blur the boundaries even of major sulci and gyri and generally does not allow accurate transfer of labels from atlas to subject. For example, a sulcus label from the atlas will frequently overlie a gyrus and vice versa.

An alternative and promising approach is to extract gyri by data-driven segmentation followed by object-based matching between subjects. Surface-based

J. Duncan and G. Gerig (Eds.): MICCAI 2005, LNCS 3750, pp. 749–756, 2005.

methods analyse cortical curvature and use geodesic distance metrics to define boundaries [4]. However, manual selection of neighbouring sulcus-pairs was required to initiate segmentation of a gyrus, and did not resolve the difficulties of substantial inter-subject variation whereby a significant number of the gyri in one individual seem to have no clear matching gyri in another. In preliminary experiments we found a voxel-based method for extracting gyral cores [5] to be more robust and we based our approach on this.

Our framework allows matching of the important gyri across subjects. In addition to supporting automated labelling, the gyral representation should allow inter-subject registration and may be used for quantitative studies of inter-subject variability and inter-hemispheric differences.

2 Data and Pre-processing

Our input data consisted of 96 T1-weighted MRI brain data of healthy human volunteers acquired on a 3-Tesla magnetic resonance scanner (Bruker Medspec 300) using a MDEFT pulse sequence [6]. The within-plane spatial resolution was set to $1 \times 1mm$, the between plane resolution was approximately $1.5mm$. All data sets were rotated and shifted into a standard stereotactic coordinate system with the origin residing halfway between CA and CP [1]. At the same time, the data sets were resampled so that isotropic voxels of size $1 \times 1 \times 1mm^3$ resulted. After resampling, each data set consisted of 160 image slices that contained 160×200 voxels covering the entire brain. We restricted our attention to the large primary gyri that can be identified in almost all healthy individuals on the lateral aspect of hemispheres. Secondary, and particularly tertiary, cortical folds have a high degree of inter-subject variability so that it is unrealistic to derive a valid model for them.

3 Methods

In our algorithm, cortical folds are represented as 3D polygonal lines so that folds extracted from a group of individuals form a cloud of such lines. The central idea of our approach is to subject such data clouds to non-linear principal component analysis so that a principal curve for each major gyrus results. A principal curve captures the most salient shape features of a data cloud. Our gyral model is a collection of such principal curves. In the following, we will present this sequence of processing steps in more detail.

3.1 Representation of Gyri Using 3D Polygonal Lines

The initial steps for automatically extracting the polygonal line representation of gyral cores are similar to those described in [5]. In the current work, we extend this approach to include extraction of the deep white matter surface, which smoothly connects the fundi of the major sulci, and we express the depth of gyri as a proportion of the distance between the outer (closed) and inner (opened) white matter surfaces. The rationale behind this approach is that various regions of the brain show marked differences in the depth of the cortical foldings. For example, pre-frontal sulci are generally more shallow than parietal sulci. A relative measure of depth as introduced here allows us to incorporate all major folds into a common framework so that regional differences in sulcal depth play a lesser role.

The algorithm consists of the following steps (fig. 1):

1. White matter segmentation.
2. Extraction of a superficial white matter surface (corresponding to the arachnoid surface overlying the superficial grey matter) by 3D morphological closing of the segmented white matter [7], using a spherical 12 mm radius structuring element.
3. Extraction of the deep white matter surface using a morphological opening with a 8 mm diameter spherical structuring element.
4. 3D distance transform to define the depth from the closed white matter surface [8].
5. 3D distance transform to define the distance from the opened white matter surface.

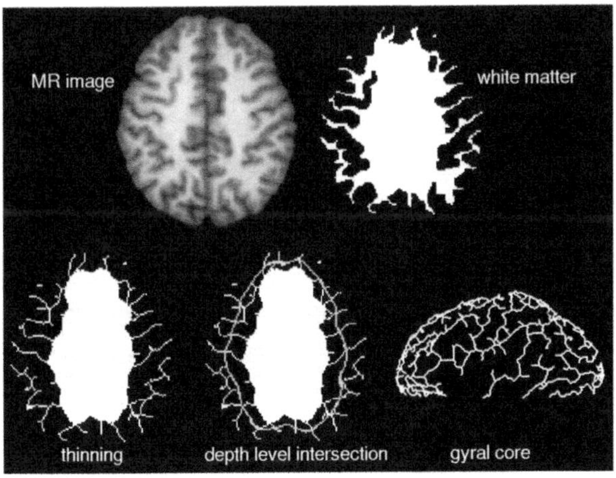

Fig. 1. The processing chain for obtaining the gyral core graph

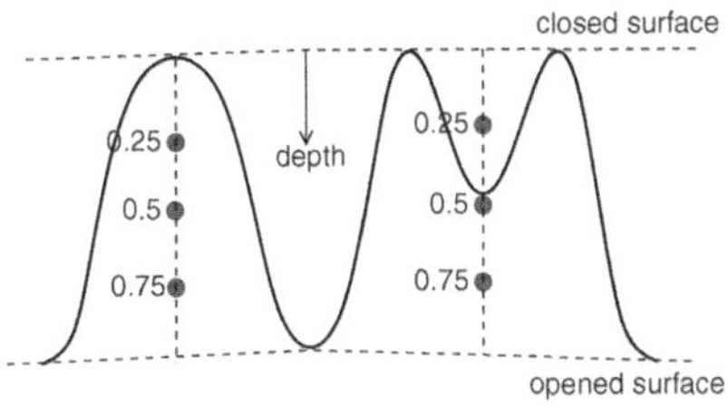

Fig. 2. Definition of relative depth

6. Calculation of relative depth of any point as the ratio of the distance from the superficial surface to the sum of the two distances (to superficial and deep surfaces) (fig. 2).
7. Extraction of the gyri via a top-hat transformation (the white matter image minus the result of a 3D morphological opening).
8. 3D topological thinning of the gyri [9],[10].
9. Extraction of the intersections of the thinned gyri at a series of relative depths, to form "gyral cores".
10. Representation of the intersection as an undirected graph. The nodes in the graph correspond to voxels. Any two nodes are linked by an arc if their corresponding voxels are 26-connected.

We call our representation the *"core graph"*. A path within the core graph is called a *"gyral core"*. In the following, we will discuss some specific gyral cores that are of interest because of their interindividual consistency.

3.2 Anatomical Labelling of Gyral Cores

At the 0.95 depth level, gyri appear geometrically simple. They are smoother and less convoluted than at more shallow depth levels. This makes their identification much easier. Therefore, we initially attach anatomical labels only to gyral cores at the deepest depth level. These labels are then subsequently propagated upwards to all other levels of depth. We selected gyri which show high consistency across subjects to form the basis of the labelling scheme. These included the precentral, postcentral, middle frontal, parietal, inferior temporal, and superior temporal gyri (fig. 3). At the deepest relative depth levels, it was clear that the superior temporal gyral core was continuous with the opercular gyral bank

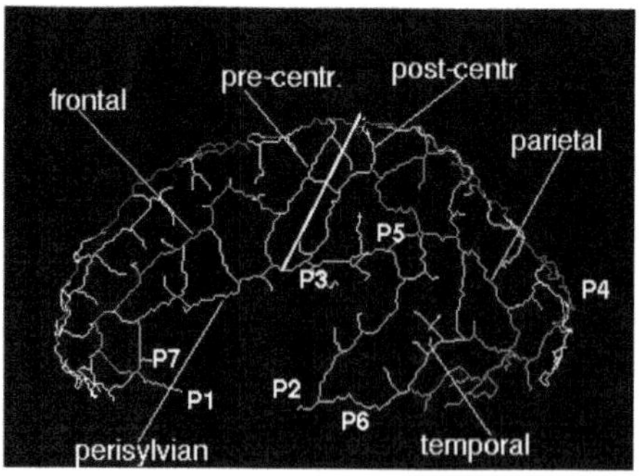

Fig. 3. Illustration of the gyral labelling procedure. Anchor points P1 and P2 mark the endpoints of the perisylvian core. The perisylvian core is defined as the shortest path in the core graph connecting P1 and P2. Other anchor points and the shortest paths between them are used for identifying other gyri. To identify the pre- and postcentral gyri, we additionally impose the constraint that the two gyri must be roughly parallel.

above the circular sulcus of the insula, so we named this continuous gyral core perisylvian (fig. 3).

We devised a semi-automatic algorithm for labelling the above named gyral cores. For each of these six types of gyral cores we have devised a set of heuristic rules to be used in the identification process. Dijkstra's algorithm for finding shortest paths in graphs is one of the key elements of our method. For instance, to identify the perisylvian core, we first identify the two anchor points P1 and P2 that mark the anterior and posterior ends of this core. We then apply Dijkstra's algorithm for finding the shortest path in the core graph that connects P1 to P2. P1 is defined as the most ventral point whose y-coordinate in the stereotactic Talairach system is less than -10. P2 is defined by a similar rationale.

Once the core graph of a data set is anatomically labelled at the deepest depth level, we can propagate its anatomical labels upwards to the next higher depth level, and so on, until the graph is labelled at all depths. This process is not very exact However, for the purpose of generating a generic model that is representative of 96 individuals, it is not essential to obtain a highly accurate labelling in each case.

3.3 Principal Curves

We have applied the anatomical labelling to all 96 data sets. In order to extract a generic gyral model from these data, we integrated the labelled gyral cores from all subjects into one data set using a common coordinate frame. We then extracted principal curves from this combined data set in order to reveal the generic structure of the data.

Principal curves are defined to be polygons which pass through the center of an n-dimensional data cloud. The data cloud is assumed to have an elongated shape so that a polygonal line can be considered to represent its most salient shape features. Its mathematical formulation is the following [11].

Let $X = \{x_1, ..., x_n\}, x_i \in R^n$ be a set of data points. A curve f is called a *principal curve* of length L for X if f minimizes

$$\Delta(f) \;=\; E[\,\inf_t ||X - f(t)||^2]$$

the expected squared distance between X and the curve, over all curves of length less than or equal to L. In [11], a suboptimal algorithm for learning principal curves from training data X is described. The algorithm starts with a straight line segment that is iteratively refined as new vertices are added. With each addition of a new vertex, the resulting polygon achieves a more precise representation of the data. Figure 4 illustrates this process. For a more detailed description of the algorithm see [11].

This process was performed for each of the six anatomical labels and for each of the eight depth strata separately. More precisely, we extracted each of the six different type of anatomical labels from the combined data set in each depth level separately, and applied the principal curve extraction method described in [11].

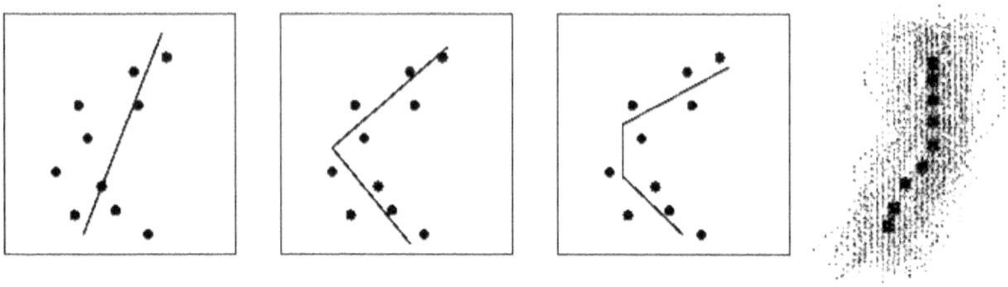

Fig. 4. Illustration of the principal curve algorithm [11]. In the first iteration step, a straight line segment is placed such that it runs through the center of gravity of points projecting to it. In subsequent iterations, the shape representation is refined by adding more vertices. The rightmost image shows a principal curve running through the data cloud representing a post-central gyrus.

4 Results

We have applied the method for gyral core identification to all 96 data sets. In table 1, a list of the identification rates is given. Note that some types of gyral cores could be located in almost every data set while others were less robustly identified. The main reason for failure are topological interruptions of the gyral stalks because the algorithm relies on finding paths in the gyral graph. A disconnected gyral stalk produces a gap in the graph structure so that a 26-connected path from one anchor point to the next does not exist. In cases where the automatic identification failed, it was supplied manually. In some regions – especially in the anterior part of the middle frontal gyrus – the gyral core was only partially identifiable.

The resulting non-linear PCAs from eight depth levels were assembled into one output set to create the averaged representation of human cortical gyri (fig. 5). Note that the most shallow level of the representation is more convoluted than the deepest level (fig.5c,d). Furthermore, an inter-hemispheric difference emerges in the vicinity of the planum temporale. This region is connected to language processing, and it is well known that the left-hemispheric planum temporale is larger than the right [12].

Table 1. Identification accuracy of the gyral labelling. The numbers represent the absolute number of cases (out of a total of 96 data sets) in which the identification was successful. In some cases, gyral cores could be only partially identified (see text).

Frontal, left	94
Frontal, right	94
Pre- and postcentral, left	92
Pre- and postcentral, right	89

Perisylvian, left	96
Perisylvian, right	96
Temporal, left	91
Temporal, right	95
Parietal, left:	95
Parietal, right:	95

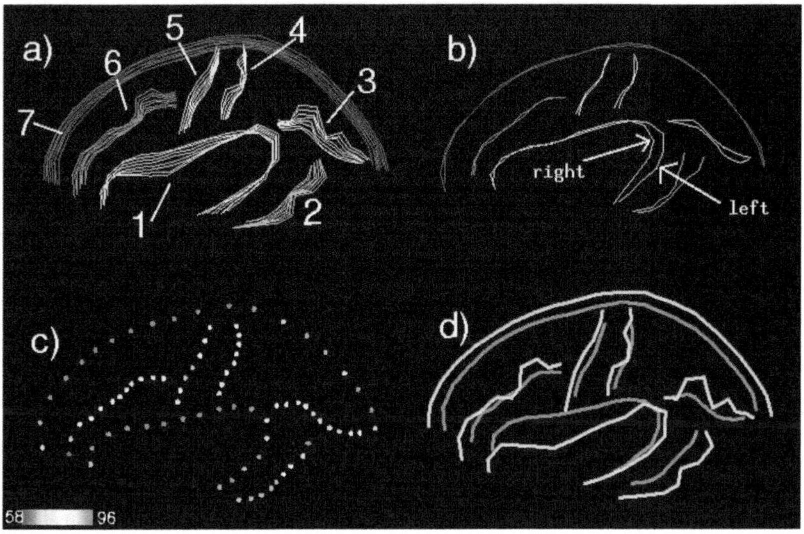

Fig. 5. The gyral model. 5a): the left hemisphere of the model in all its depth levels, 1:perisylvian, 2: inferior temporal, 3:parietal, 4:postcentral, 5:precentral, 6:frontal, 7:dorsal rim. 5b): an inter-hemispheric comparison where the right hemispheric model is flipped around the x-axis and superimposed onto the left hemisphere. The arrows indicate a region of inter-hemispheric differences in the vicinity of the planum temporale. 5c): the degree to which the model is representative of the population from which it was derived. Each node in the model graph has a label that indicates how many of the 96 inidividual labelled core graphs have a node of the same label within a 6 mm neighbourhood around the model node. Note that some segments of the model graph represent the data better than others. The anterior part of the middle frontal gyrus has low values indicating a high degree of inter-individual variability. Fig. 5d compares the deepest depth level of the model (red) with the most shallow level (green). Note that the gyri at the shallow level are more convoluted than at the deepest level.

5 Discussion

We have presented a method of constructing an averaged representation of human cortical gyri from a large population of individuals. We restrict the study to the gyri which are known from qualitative study of our data and from anatomical texts to be the most consistent. The method is based on measuring relative depth based on the deep white matter surface, on extraction of gyral cores which are 1-D structures in 3-D space at specific relative depths, and applying non-linear principal component analysis to the point sets to extract an average representation of the gyri. The model represents even quite subtle features of the cortical folding; for example, inter-hemispheric differences around the planum temporale are preserved. By comparing different strata of depth within the model, it is evident that the cortical gyri generally become smoother and less convoluted with depth. However, this appears not to hold for the precentral gyrus. The model also highlights areas of high inter-individual variability such as the anterior part of the middle frontal gyrus.

In addition to allowing study of gyral variability across individuals and between hemispheres, the representation provides a framework which can be used for future work on non-rigid registration.

References

1. Talairach, P. Tournoux, J.: Co-planar Stereotaxic Atlas of the Human Brain: 3-Dimensional Proportional System - an Approach to Cerebral Imaging. Thieme Medical Publishers, New York (1988)
2. Evans, D.L. Collins, S.R. Mills, E.D. Brown, R.L. Kelly, T.M. Peters, A.C.: 3d statistical neuroanatomical models from 305 mri volumes. In: Proc. IEEE-Nuclear Science Symposium and Medical Imaging Conference. (1993) 1813–1817
3. J.Mazziotta, A.Toga, A.Evans, M.Fox, J.Lancaster, K.Zilles, et al.: A probabilistic atlas and reference system for the human brain: International consortium for brain mapping (ICBM). Philosophical Trans. of the Royal Society: Biological Sciences **356** (2001) 1293–1322
4. Cachia, J.F. Mangin, D. Riviere, F. Kherif, N. Boddaert, A.Andrade, D. Papadopoulos-Orfanos, J.B. Poline, I. Bloch, M. Zilbovicius, P. Sonigo, F. Brunelle, J. Regis, A.: A primal sketch of the cortex mean curvature: A morphogenesis based approach to study the variability of the folding patterns. IEEE Transactions on Medical Imaging **22** (2003) 754–765
5. G. Lohmann: Extracting line representations of sulcal and gyral patterns in MR images of the human brain. IEEE Transactions on Medical Imaging **17** (1998) 1040–1048
6. Norris, D.: Reduced power multi-slice MDEFT imaging. J. Magn. Reson. Imaging **11** (2000) 445–451
7. Maragos, R.W. Schafer, P.: Morphological systems for multidimensional signal processing. Proc. of the IEEE **78** (1990) 690–709
8. Borgefors, G.: On digital distance transformations in three dimensions. Computer Vision, Graphics, and Image Processing: Image Inderstanding **64** (1996) 368–376
9. Tsao, K.S. Fu, Y.: A parallel thinning algorithm for 3D pictures. Computer Graphics Image Proc. **17** (1981) 315–331
10. A.Manzanera,T.Bernard,F.Preteux,B.Longuet: nD skeletonization: a unified mathematical framework. Journal of Electronic Engineering **11** (2002) 25–37
11. Kégl, B.: Learning and design of principal curves. IEEE Transactions on Pattern Analysis and Machine Intelligence **22** (2000) 281–297
12. Jancke, H. Steinmetz, L.: Auditory lateralization and planum temporale asymmetry. Neuroreport **5** (1993) 169–172

Efficient Kernel Density Estimation of Shape and Intensity Priors for Level Set Segmentation

Mikael Rousson and Daniel Cremers

Department of Imaging and Visualization,
Siemens Corporate Research, Princeton, NJ
{mikael.rousson, daniel.cremers}@siemens.com

Abstract. We propose a nonlinear statistical shape model for level set segmentation which can be efficiently implemented. Given a set of training shapes, we perform a kernel density estimation in the low dimensional subspace spanned by the training shapes. In this way, we are able to combine an accurate model of the statistical shape distribution with efficient optimization in a finite-dimensional subspace. In a Bayesian inference framework, we integrate the nonlinear shape model with a nonparametric intensity model and a set of pose parameters which are estimated in a more direct data-driven manner than in previously proposed level set methods. Quantitative results show superior performance (regarding runtime and segmentation accuracy) of the proposed nonparametric shape prior over existing approaches.

1 Introduction

Originally proposed in [5,11] as a means to propagate interfaces in time, the level set method has become increasingly popular as a framework for image segmentation. The key idea is to represent an interface $\Gamma \subset \Omega$ in the image domain $\Omega \subset \mathbb{R}^3$ implicitly as the zero level set of an embedding function $\phi : \mathbb{R}^3 \rightarrow \Omega$:

$$\Gamma = \{x \in \Omega \mid \phi(x) = 0\}, \tag{1}$$

and to evolve Γ by propagating the embedding function ϕ according to an appropriate partial differential equation. The first applications of this level set formalism for the purpose of image segmentation were proposed in [1,10,7]. Two key advantages over explicit interface propagation are the independence of a particular parameterization and the fact that the implicitly represented boundary Γ can undergo topological changes such as splitting or merging. This makes the framework well-suited for the segmentation of several objects or multiply-connected objects.

When segmenting medical images, one commonly has to deal with noise, missing or misleading image information. For certain imaging modalities such as ultrasound or CT, the structures of interest do not differ much from their background in terms of their intensity distribution — see Figure 1. Therefore they can no longer be accurately segmented based on the image information

J. Duncan and G. Gerig (Eds.): MICCAI 2005, LNCS 3750, pp. 757–764, 2005.

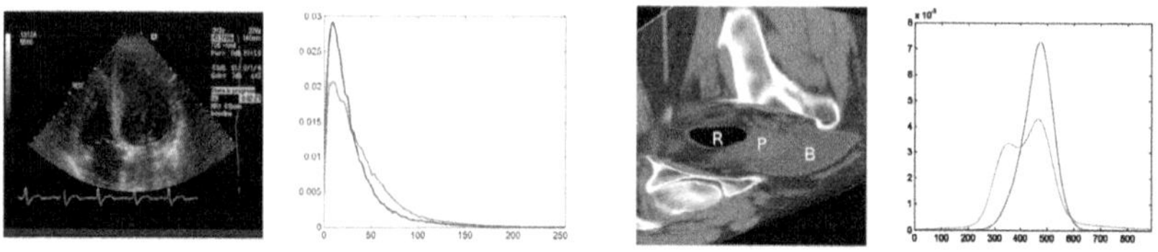

Cardiac ultrasound Histograms Prostate CT Histograms

Fig. 1. Segmentation challenges and estimated intensity distributions. The two curves on the right correspond to the empirical probability of intensities inside and outside the left ventricle (for the ultrasound image) and the prostate (for the CT image). The region-based segmentation of these structures is a challenging problem, because objects and background have similar histograms. Our segmentation scheme optimally exploits the estimated probabilistic intensity models.

alone. In recent years, researchers have therefore proposed to enhance the level set method with statistical shape priors. Given a set of training shapes, one can impose information about which segmentations are *a priori* more or less likely. Such prior shape information was shown to drastically improve segmentation results in the presence of noise or occlusion [9,16,3,14,4,6]. Most of these approaches are based on the assumption that the training shapes, encoded by their signed distance function, form a Gaussian distribution. This has two drawbacks: Firstly, the space of signed distance functions is not a linear space, therefore, the mean shape and linear combinations of eigenmodes are typically no longer signed distance functions. Secondly, even if the space were a linear space, it is not clear why the given set of sample shapes should be distributed according to a Gaussian density. In fact, as we will demonstrate in this work, they are generally not Gaussian distributed. Recently, it was proposed to use nonparametric density estimation in the space of level set functions [3] in order to model nonlinear[1] distributions of training shapes. While this resolves the above problems, one sacrifices the efficiency of working in a low-dimensional subspace (formed by the first few eigenmodes) to a problem of infinite-dimensional optimization.

In the present paper, we propose a framework for knowledge-driven level set segmentation which integrates three contributions: Firstly, we propose a statistical shape prior which combines the efficiency of low-dimensional PCA-based methods with the accuracy of nonparametric statistical shape models. The key idea is to perform kernel density estimation in a linear subspace which is sufficiently large to embed all training data. Secondly, we propose to estimate pose and translation parameters in a more data-driven manner. Thirdly, we optimally exploit the intensity information in the image by using probabilistic intensity models given by kernel density estimates of previously observed intensity distributions.

[1] The term *nonlinear* refers to the fact that the manifold of permissible shapes is not merely a linear subspace.

2 Level Set Segmentation as Bayesian Inference

The goal of level set segmentation can be formulated as the estimation of the optimal embedding function $\phi\colon \Omega \to \mathbb{R}$ given an image $I\colon \Omega \to \mathbb{R}$. In the Bayesian framework, this can be computed by maximizing the posterior distribution

$$\mathcal{P}(\phi \,|\, I) \propto \mathcal{P}(I \,|\, \phi)\, \mathcal{P}(\phi). \tag{2}$$

The maximization of (2) results in a problem of infinite-dimensional optimization. Given a set of training shapes encoded by their signed distance functions $\{\phi_i\}_{i=1..N}$, Tsai et al. [16] proposed to reduce the segmentation problem to one of finite-dimensional optimization by constraining the optimization problem to the finite-dimensional subspace spanned by the training shapes.

In this paper, we make use of this compact representation of the embedding function. Given the distance d on the space of signed distance functions defined by: $d^2(\phi_1, \phi_2) = \int_\Omega (\phi_1(x) - \phi_2(x))^2\, dx$, we align the set of training shapes with respect to translation and rotation. Subsequently, we constrain the level set function ϕ to a parametric representation of the form:

$$\phi_{\boldsymbol{\alpha},h,\theta}(x) = \phi_0(R_\theta x + h) + \sum_{i=1}^{n} \alpha_i\, \psi_i(R_\theta x + h), \tag{3}$$

where $\phi_0(x) = \frac{1}{N}\sum_{i=1}^{N} \phi_i(x)$ represents the mean shape, $\{\psi_i(x)\}_{i=1..n}$ are the eigenmodes of the distribution, and $n < N$ is the dimension of the subspace spanned by the N training shapes. The parameter vector $\boldsymbol{\alpha} = (\alpha_1, \ldots, \alpha_n)$ models shape deformations, while the parameters $h \in \mathbb{R}^3$ and $\theta \in [0, 2\pi]^3$ model translation and rotation of the respective shape.[2]

The infinite-dimensional Bayesian inference problem in (2) is therefore reduced to a finite-dimensional one where the conditional probability

$$\mathcal{P}(\boldsymbol{\alpha},\, h,\, \theta \,|\, I) \propto \mathcal{P}(I \,|\, \boldsymbol{\alpha},\, h,\, \theta)\, \mathcal{P}(\boldsymbol{\alpha},\, h,\, \theta), \tag{4}$$

is optimized with respect to the shape parameters $\boldsymbol{\alpha}$, and the transformation parameters h and θ. In the following, we will assume a uniform prior on these transformation parameters, i.e. $\mathcal{P}(\boldsymbol{\alpha}, h, \theta) = \mathcal{P}(\boldsymbol{\alpha})$. In the next section, we will discuss three solutions to model this shape prior.

3 An Efficient Nonparametric Statistical Shape Model

Given a set of aligned training shapes $\{\phi_i\}_{i=1..N}$, we can represent each of them by their corresponding shape vector $\{\boldsymbol{\alpha}_i\}_{i=1..N}$. In this notation, the goal of statistical shape learning is to infer a statistical distribution $\mathcal{P}(\boldsymbol{\alpha})$ from these

[2] In our applications, where the scale of objects is known, a generalization to larger transformations groups (e.g. similarity or affine) did not appear useful.

sample shapes. Two solutions which have been proposed are based on the assumptions that the training shapes can be approximated by a **uniform distribution** [16,14]: $\mathcal{P}(\boldsymbol{\alpha}) = \text{const.}$, or by a **Gaussian distribution** [9]:

$$\mathcal{P}(\boldsymbol{\alpha}) \propto \exp\left(-\boldsymbol{\alpha}^\top \Sigma^{-1} \boldsymbol{\alpha}\right), \quad \text{where } \Sigma = \frac{1}{N} \sum_i \boldsymbol{\alpha}_i \boldsymbol{\alpha}_i^\top. \tag{5}$$

In the present paper, we propose to make use of nonparametric density estimation [13] to approximate the shape distribution within the linear subspace. We model the shape distribution by the **kernel density estimate**:

$$\mathcal{P}(\boldsymbol{\alpha}) = \frac{1}{N\sigma} \sum_{i=1}^{N} K\left(\frac{\boldsymbol{\alpha} - \boldsymbol{\alpha}_i}{\sigma}\right), \quad \text{where } K(u) = \frac{1}{\sqrt{2\pi}} \exp\left(-\frac{u^2}{2}\right). \tag{6}$$

There exist various methods to automatically estimate appropriate values for the width σ of the kernel function, ranging from k-th nearest neighbor estimates to cross-validation and bootstrapping. In this work, we simply set σ to be the average nearest neighbor distance: $\sigma^2 = \frac{1}{N} \sum_{i=1}^{N} \min_{j \neq i} |\boldsymbol{\alpha}_i - \boldsymbol{\alpha}_j|^2$.

In the context of level set based image segmentation, the kernel density estimator (6) has two advantages over the uniform and Gaussian distributions:

- The assumptions of uniform distribution or Gaussian distribution are generally not fulfilled. The kernel density estimator, on the other hand, is known to approximate arbitrary distributions. Under mild assumptions, it was shown to converge to the true distribution in the limit of infinite sample size. We refer to [15] for a proof.
- The space of signed distance functions is known to not be a linear space. Therefore, neither the mean shape ϕ_0 nor a linear combination of eigenmodes as in (3) will in general be a signed distance function. As a consequence, the functions $\phi(x)$ favored by the uniform or the Gaussian distribution cannot be expected to be signed distance functions. The kernel density estimator (6), on the other hand, favors shape vector α which are in the vicinity of the sample shape vectors α_i. By construction, these vector correspond to signed distance functions. In fact: **In the limit of infinite sample size, the distribution inferred by the kernel density estimator (6) converges towards a distribution on the manifold of signed distance functions.**

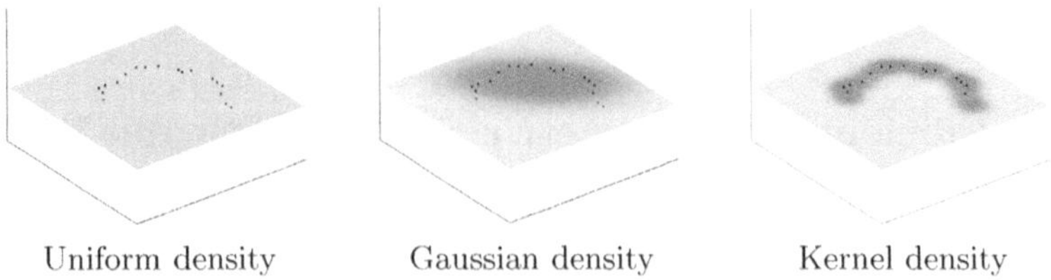

Fig. 2. Schematic plots of different density estimates within a subspace. Darker shading indicates areas of high probability density for the respective models. The kernel density estimator adapts to the training data more flexibly since it does not rely on specific assumptions about the shape of the distribution.

Figure 2 shows schematic plots of the three methods for a set of sample data spanning a two-dimensional subspace in $\mathbb{R}^3$. The kernel density estimator clearly captures the distribution most accurately.

In analogy to the shape learning, we make use of kernel density estimation to learn the conditional probability for the intensity function I in (4) from examples. A similar precomputation of intensity distributions by means of mixture models was proposed in [12]. Given a set of presegmented training images, the kernel density estimate of the intensity distributions p_{in} and p_{out} of object and background are given by the corresponding smoothed intensity histograms. This has two advantages: Firstly, the kernel density estimator does not rely on specific assumptions about the shape of the distribution. Figure 1 shows that the intensity distributions for ultrasound and CT images are not well approximated by Gaussian or Laplacian models. Secondly, in contrast to the joint estimation of intensity distributions (cf. [2,8]), this simplifies the segmentation process which no longer requires an updating of intensity models. Moreover, we found the segmentation process to be more robust to initialization in numerous experiments.

4 Energy Formulation and Minimization

Maximizing the posterior probability in (2), or equivalently minimizing its negative logarithm, will generate the most probable segmentation of a given image. With the nonparametric models for shape and intensity introduced above, this leads to an energy of the form

$$E(\boldsymbol{\alpha}, h, \theta) = -\log \mathcal{P}(I|\boldsymbol{\alpha}, h, \theta) - \log \mathcal{P}(\boldsymbol{\alpha}), \tag{7}$$

The nonparametric intensity model permits to express the first term and equation (6) gives exactly the second one. With the Heaviside step function H and the short hand $H_\phi = H(\phi_{\boldsymbol{\alpha},h,\theta}(x))$, we end up with:

$$E(\boldsymbol{\alpha}, h, \theta) = -\int_\Omega H_\phi \log p_{in}(I) + (1-H_\phi) \log p_{out}(I) dx - \log\left(\frac{1}{N\sigma} \sum_{i=1}^{N} K\left(\frac{\boldsymbol{\alpha}-\boldsymbol{\alpha}_i}{\sigma}\right)\right),$$

With $e(x) = \left[\log \frac{p_{out}(I(x))}{p_{in}(I(x))}\right]$, $K_i = K\left(\frac{\boldsymbol{\alpha}-\boldsymbol{\alpha}_i}{\sigma}\right)$, and $\boldsymbol{\psi} = (\psi_1, \ldots, \psi_n)$, we obtain the following system of coupled gradient descent equations:

$$\begin{cases} \dfrac{d\boldsymbol{\alpha}}{dt} = \displaystyle\int_\Omega \delta(\phi_{\boldsymbol{\alpha},h,\theta}(x))\, \boldsymbol{\psi}(R_\theta x + h)\, e(x)\, dx + \frac{1}{\sigma^2} \frac{\sum_{i=1}^N (\boldsymbol{\alpha}_i - \boldsymbol{\alpha}) K_i}{\sum_{i=1}^N K_i}, \\ \dfrac{dh}{dt} = \displaystyle\int_\Omega \delta(\phi_{\boldsymbol{\alpha},h,\theta}(x))\, \nabla \phi_{\boldsymbol{\alpha},h,\theta}(x)\, e(x)\, dx, \\ \dfrac{d\theta}{dt} = \displaystyle\int_\Omega \delta(\phi_{\boldsymbol{\alpha},h,\theta}(x))\, (\nabla \phi_{\boldsymbol{\alpha},h,\theta}(x) \cdot \nabla_\theta R x)\, e(x)\, dx. \end{cases} \tag{8}$$

In applications, we solve these equations by initializing the shape $\boldsymbol{\alpha}$ with the mean shape ($\boldsymbol{\alpha} = 0$) and the transformation parameters h and θ with some

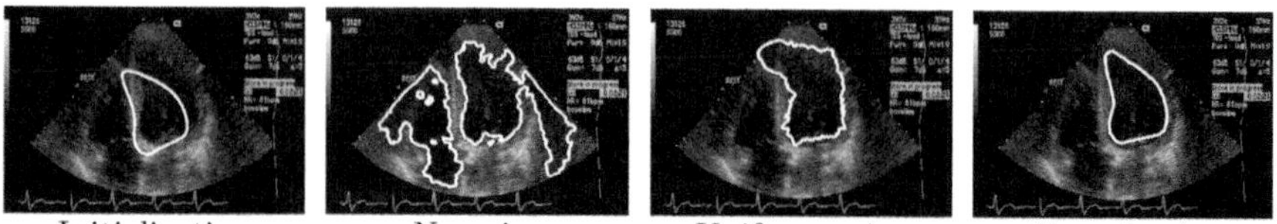
Initialization No prior Uniform prior Kernel prior

Fig. 3. Model Comparison. Level set segmentations obtained without prior, with a uniform prior in the subspace and with a kernel prior in the subspace. In contrast to the uniform prior, the nonparametric prior accurately constrains the segmentation to a submanifold of familiar shapes (90% correctly classified, 2.7% false positives).

reasonable estimates. Subsequently, we discretize the above partial differential equations by a standard finite difference scheme.

Note that in all equations, the Dirac delta function δ appears as factor inside the integrals over the image domain Ω. This allows to restrict all computations to a narrow band around the zero crossing of ϕ. While the evolution of translation and pose parameters h and θ are merely driven by the data term $e(x)$, the shape vector $\boldsymbol{\alpha}$ is additionally drawn towards each training shape with a strength that decays exponentially with the distance to the respective shape.

5 Experimental Results and Validation

Heart Segmentation from Ultrasound Images

Figure 3 shows experimental results obtained for the segmentation of the left ventricle in 2D cardiac ultrasound sequences, using shape priors constructed from a set of 21 manually segmented training images. In contrast to the segmentation with uniform prior (top row), the nonparametric statistical shape prior allows to accurately constrain the segmentation (bottom row). This becomes particularly apparent in areas where the data term is too weak. As a quantitative evaluation we computed the percentage of correctly classified object pixels and that of misclassified ones. During energy minimization, the percentage of correctly classified pixels increases from 56% to 90% while the percentage of false positives decreases from 27% to 2.7% by using the kernel prior. Using the uniform prior, we attain 92% correctly classified, yet the percentage of false positives increases to 42%: Merely constraining the boundary evolution to the linear subspace spanned by the training shapes is insufficient to provide for accurate segmentation results.

Prostate Segmentation from 3D CT Images

We built a nonparametric 3D shape model of the prostate using 12 manually extracted prostates (with seminal vesicles) collected from two different patients. In contrast to existing work, we subsequently used a single shape model for the segmentation of images from different patients.

We employed a leave-one-out strategy by removing the image of interest from the training phase. Figure 5 shows 2D cuts of a few results obtained using this strategy. With a one-click initialization inside the organ, the algorithm lead to a

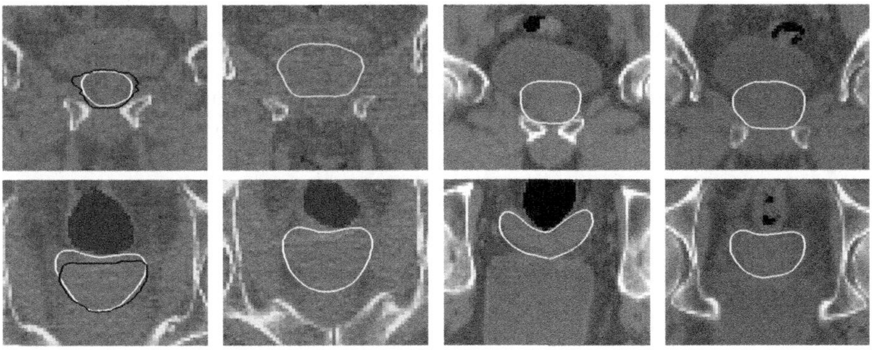

Fig. 4. Prostate segmentation for 2 patients with the same shape model. Each column shows coronal and axial slices of the same segmentation, for the first patient (left two columns) and the second one (last two). The first column also shows the manual segmentation (black contour).

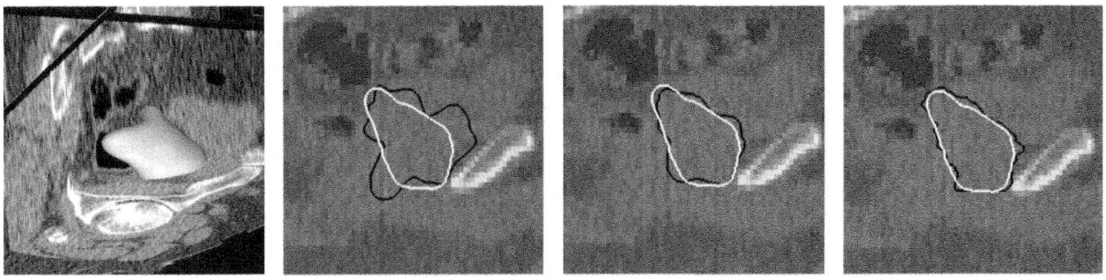

Fig. 5. Comparison of the segmentations obtained with the kernel prior (white) and with alternative approaches (black).

steady-state solution in less than 20 seconds. We obtained 86% successfully classified organ voxels and 11% mis-classified organ voxels. This compares favorably to the intra-patients results reported in [6]. Figure 4 provides qualitative comparisons to the manual segmentation, as well as to the segmentations obtained with uniform and Gaussian approximations of the shape distribution.

6 Conclusion

We proposed an efficient and accurate statistical shape prior for level set segmentation which is based on nonparametric density estimation in the linear subspace spanned by the level set surfaces of a set of training shapes. In addition, our segmentation scheme integrates nonparametric estimates of intensity distributions and efficient optimization of pose and translation parameters. We reported quantitative evaluation of segmentation accuracy and speed for cardiac ultrasound images and for 3D CT images of the prostate. These indicate that the proposed nonparametric shape prior outperforms previously proposed shape priors for level set segmentation.

Acknowledgments

We thank Christophe Chefd'hotel for fruitful discussions. We thank Marie-Pierre Jolly for providing us with image and training data for the ultrasound sequences.

References

1. V. Caselles, F. Catté, T. Coll, and F. Dibos. A geometric model for active contours in image processing. *Numer. Math.*, 66:1–31, 1993.
2. T.F. Chan and L.A. Vese. Active contours without edges. *IEEE Trans. Image Processing*, 10(2):266–277, 2001.
3. D. Cremers, S. J. Osher, and S. Soatto. Kernel density estimation and intrinsic alignment for knowledge-driven segmentation: Teaching level sets to walk. In *Pattern Recognition*, volume 3175 of *LNCS*, pages 36–44. Springer, 2004.
4. E.B. Dam, P.T. Fletcher, S. Pizer, G. Tracton, and J. Rosenman. Prostate shape modeling based on principal geodesic analysis bootstrapping. In *MICCAI*, volume 2217 of *LNCS*, pages 1008–1016, September 2004.
5. A. Dervieux and F. Thomasset. A finite element method for the simulation of Raleigh-Taylor instability. *Springer Lect. Notes in Math.*, 771:145–158, 1979.
6. D. Freedman, R.J. Radke, T. Zhang, Y. Jeong, D.M. Lovelock, and G.T. Chen. Model-based segmentation of medical imagery by matching distributions. *IEEE Trans Med Imaging*, 24(3):281–292, March 2005.
7. S. Kichenassamy, A. Kumar, P. J. Olver, A. Tannenbaum, and A. J. Yezzi. Gradient flows and geometric active contour models. In *Proc. IEEE Intl. Conf. on Comp. Vis.*, pages 810–815, Boston, USA, 1995.
8. J. Kim, J. W. Fisher, A. Yezzi, M. Cetin, and A. Willsky. Nonparametric methods for image segmentation using information theory and curve evolution. In *Int. Conf. on Image Processing*, volume 3, pages 797–800, 2002.
9. M. Leventon, W. Grimson, and O. Faugeras. Statistical shape influence in geodesic active contours. In *CVPR*, volume 1, pages 316–323, Hilton Head Island, SC, 2000.
10. R. Malladi, J. A. Sethian, and B. C. Vemuri. A topology independent shape modeling scheme. In *SPIE Conference on Geometric Methods in Computer Vision II*, volume 2031, pages 246–258, 1994.
11. S. J. Osher and J. A. Sethian. Fronts propagation with curvature dependent speed: Algorithms based on Hamilton–Jacobi formulations. *J. of Comp. Phys.*, 79:12–49, 1988.
12. N. Paragios and R. Deriche. Geodesic active regions and level set methods for supervised texture segmentation. *Int. J. of Computer Vision*, 46(3):223–247, 2002.
13. F. Rosenblatt. Remarks on some nonparametric estimates of a density function. *Annals of Mathematical Statistics*, 27:832–837, 1956.
14. M. Rousson, N. Paragios, and R. Deriche. Implicit active shape models for 3d segmentation in MRI imaging. In *MICCAI*, pages 209–216, 2004.
15. B. W. Silverman. *Density estimation for statistics and data analysis.* Chapman and Hall, London, 1992.
16. A. Tsai, A. J. Yezzi, and A. S. Willsky. A shape-based approach to the segmentation of medical imagery using level sets. *IEEE Trans. on Medical Imaging*, 22(2):137–154, 2003.

Corpus Callosum Subdivision Based on a Probabilistic Model of Inter-hemispheric Connectivity

Martin A. Styner[1,2], Ipek Oguz[1], Rachel Gimpel Smith[2], Carissa Cascio[2], and Matthieu Jomier[1]

[1] Dept. of Computer Science, Univ. of North Carolina, Chapel Hill NC 27599, USA
[2] Dept. of Psychiatry, Univ. of North Carolina, Chapel Hill NC 27599, USA

Abstract. Statistical shape analysis has become of increasing interest to the neuroimaging community due to its potential to locate morphological changes. In this paper, we present the a novel combination of shape analysis and Diffusion Tensor Image (DTI) Tractography to the computation of a probabilistic, model based corpus callosum (CC) subdivision. The probabilistic subdivision is based on the distances of arc-length parameterized corpus callosum contour points to trans-callosal DTI fibers associated with an automatic lobe subdivision. Our proposed subdivision method is automatic and reproducible. Its results are more stable than the Witelson subdivision scheme or other commonly applied schemes based on the CC bounding box. We present the application of our subdivision method to a small scale study of regional CC area growth in healthy subjects from age 2 to 4 years.

1 Introduction

Quantitative morphologic assessment of individual brain structures is often based on global volume and area measurements, which are intuitive features as they may explain atrophy or dilation due to illness. On the other hand, structural changes at specific locations are not sufficiently reflected in volume and area measurements. Shape analysis has thus become of increasing interest to the neuroimaging community. In this paper, shape analysis is employed to compute a probabilistic subdivision model of the Corpus Callosum(CC).

The corpus callosum is the major commisural pathway between the hemispheres and plays an integral role in relaying sensory, motor and cognitive information from homologous region in the two hemispheres. It has been a structure of much interest in neuroimaging studies of normal development [1], schizophrenia [2], autism, bipolar and unipolar disorder. In-vivo assessment of the commisural pathways through the CC is difficult, but can be approximated using Diffusion Tensor Imaging (DTI) and Tractography [3,4,5] (see Figure 1).

The computation of regional volumes and areas based on subdivision schemes of anatomical structures is quite common in neuroimaging. Most common subdivision protocols are executed manually by relabeling an already segmented

J. Duncan and G. Gerig (Eds.): MICCAI 2005, LNCS 3750, pp. 765–772, 2005.

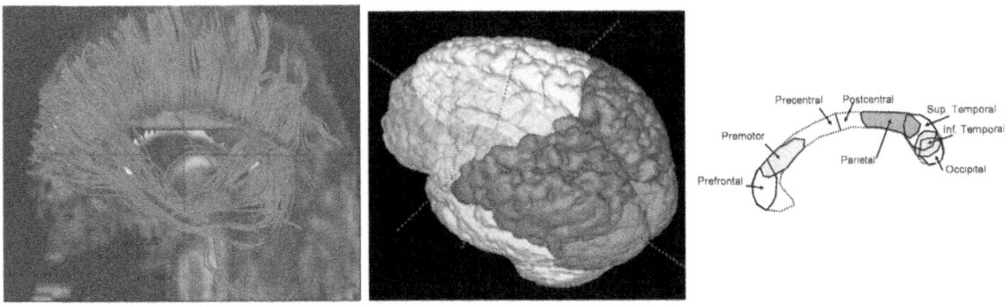

Fig. 1. Left: Visualization of interhemispheric, trans-callosal DTI Fibers. Middle: Result of an automatic lobe subdivision. Right: Schematic subdivision based on neurohistological studies [6].

structure into subregions. These methods are time-consuming, not reproducible and subjective. Further, they are often based on the structure's bounding box and are thus likely to mix different parts of the structure into the same subdivision due to the non-convex shape of most anatomical structures. Subdivision schemes can also be categorized into hard and probabilistic subdivisions. A hard subdivision assigns a single regional label for every image element. A probabilistic subdivision on the other hand assigns multiple labels with individual probabilistic weights for each element.

The currently most widely applied subdivision scheme for the CC was originally proposed by Witelson [6] and is motivated by neurohistological studies. It has been adapted in many studies [7,2]. The Witelson based subdivisions use somewhat arbitrarily defined hard subdivision boundaries and is often still applied manually, even though automatic and probabilistic methods exist[8]. To our knowledge probabilistic subdivision methods in combination with fiber connectivity information have not been proposed before.

In this paper we propose a novel model based probabilistic subdivision scheme of the CC. The subdivision model described in section 2.1 is computed as the average model of a training population of automatic cortical lobe subdivisions propagated via inter-hemispheric, trans-callosal DTI fibers. The subdivision model is then applied to a small study of CC area growth in healthy children.

2 Methods

Subjects and Image Acquisition: There are 2 mutually exclusive sets of subjects used in this paper: one for the computation of the subdivision model and one for the small study on normal growth. The subdivision model was built from 5 different subjects of a larger database of healthy (2 cases), autistic (2) and developmentally delayed children (1) at age of 2 years (2) and 4 years (3). The growth study was computed on 3 additional healthy subjects with scans at age 2 and age 4. All subjects were scanned on the same GE 1.5 Tesla Sigma Advantage MR system. The structural MRI (sMRI) dataset was acquired using a 3D IR Prepped SPGR protocol with a 256x256x124 image matrix at 0.9375x0.9375x1.5mm resolution. The DTI dataset was acquired using a 12 direction, 4 repetition DTI sequence with a 128x128x30 image matrix at 1.875x1.875x4.2mm resolution.

Corpus Callosum Segmentation: Our automatic segmentation of the CC from the sMRI data is an extension of Kelemen's 2D Fourier descriptor based Active Shape Model [9]. The shape model is described with complex Fourier descriptors up to degree 11. It was derived from a large, mixed population of adult controls, schizophrenics, pediatric controls and autistics. Based on a prior automatic tissue segmentation [10] the initial values for position, scale and grayscale normalization were computed automatically. From these initial values, the CC segmentation is performed in 2 steps: first within a larger search region (6 mm along each profile) using a fully constrained model deformation, then secondly within a small search region (1 mm along each profile) using an unconstrained deformation. Each step is computed until convergence. We applied this method so far to over 150 pediatric cases with less than 2% cases that needed manual interaction in the segmentation process.

Correspondence via Fourier Descriptors (arc-length parametrization): The segmentation procedure yields Fourier coefficients with an inherent correspondence based on its arc-length parametrization. The start-point for the arc-length parametrization is given by the first order ellipse. The fourier descriptor were then uniformly sampled into a single polygon curve (100 points, spacing along curve is about 0.75mm).

Alignment and Scale: Alignment of the CC contours is achieved using the Procrustes[11] alignment method without scaling. We chose the iteratively computed average CC as the template of the Procrustes alignment. In the longitudinal study presented in this paper the CC contours were analyzed in their original scale and thus no scaling normalization was performed.

Model based subdivision: Our novel CC subdivision method is based on a prior subdivision model (described below in section 2.1). The subdivision model consists of 4 probabilistic maps that assign to each contour point $C(x)$ the probabilities $p_i(x)$ to belong to any of the 4 connectivity based subdivisions S_i. These probabilities are assigned to the contour points of each individual CC contour using the contour correspondence of the Fourier Descriptors. Our model subdivides thus not the full cross-section of the CC, but rather only its contour. The subdivision probabilities for the whole CC cross section are determined by closest point correspondence to the contour. This closest point operation results in the probabilistic area maps for the CC cross-section(see Figure 4). From the probabilistic area maps, the area values of the 4 regions are computed by simple summation. The computation of these probabilistic areas is automatic and reproducible.

2.1 Subdivision Model

The subdivision model was built from 5 pediatric cases combining fiber tract information from DTI data, and cortical lobe subdivision and shape information from T1w sMRI data. In summary we first compute for each case its lobe subdivision and the CC segmentation. Then the lobe subdivision is used for the computation of the interhemispheric lobar DTI fiber tracts. The next step computes a distance-weighted probabilistic subdivision of each case's CC contour from the location of all tracts. The resulting probabilistic subdivisions are averaged to produce the final CC subdivision model.

During several steps of the model computation, the results of the previous steps is transformed from DTI to sMRI coordinate space or vice-versa. This transformation was computed using a fully affine registration of the sMRI image to the $B0$ DTI image based on normalized mutual information [12].

In the first step of the model computation, we employ a fluid registration [13] to propagate the lobe parcellation from a single template to all sMRI images. The lobe subdivisions were then controlled by experts. Only in few cases manual corrections are necessary. The result of the lobe subdivision is a set of separate left and right hemispheric lobes: frontal, parietal, occipital and temporal lobe. As a next step, the CC is segmented using the Fourier Descriptor Active Shape Model.

The lobe subdivision and the CC segmentation serve as automatic selection regions for the source (lobes) and target (CC) of the DTI fiber tract computation. This results in 4 sets of fibers that originate in each of the lobes, pass through the CC and end up in the corresponding lobe of the other hemisphere. The fibers from the occipital and temporal lobes are joined as their fiber tracts are highly overlapping. The limiting factor for a higher degree of lobar subdivision is the moderate resolution of the DTI datasets employed in this study. The fibers of the frontal lobe are further subdivided using an interactive 3D DTI tract clustering and manipulation tool called FiberViewer, which was developed at our lab. This fiber subdivision creates two fiber sets, one with fibers that are anteriorly oriented (anterior-frontal fibers) and one with fibers that are superiorly oriented (posterior-frontal fibers). A reconstruction of the 4 sets of fibers computed for a sample case is visualized in Figure 2. The fiber sets are quite overlapping and thus we chose to describe the model as a probabilistic subdivision, which is clearly better suited than a hard subdivision.

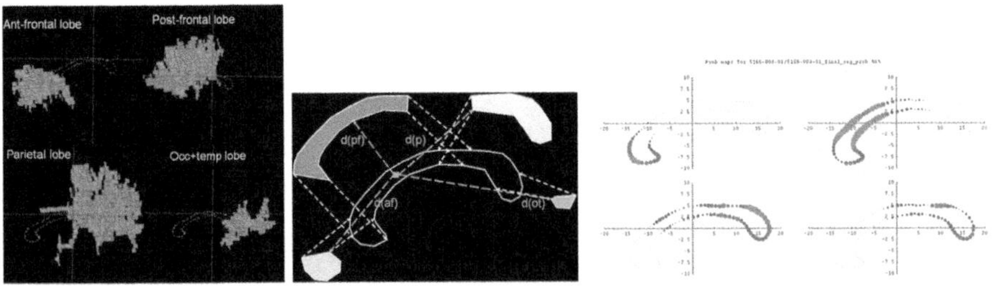

Fig. 2. Subdivision model computation. Left: Reconstruction of the fiber sets associated with each lobe in DTI coordinate space. Middle: Schematic visualization of the probability computation. Right: Sample CC contour probability map plotting disks of radii relative to the corresponding probability at each contour point.

The 4 probabilistic subdivisions $p_i(x)$ of the CC contour are computed using the closest distances $d_i(x) = \text{dist}(C(x), f(i))$ of every contour point $C(x)$ to the reconstructed 4 fiber sets $f(i)$: $p_i(x) = (\text{maxdist} - d_i^2(x))/\sum_{i=0}^{4}(\text{maxdist} - d_i^2(x))$ where maxdist represents the maximal possible distance predetermined at the average length of the CC. The computation of the probabilities is schematically shown in Figure 2 along with the result of the probabilistic contour subdivision of a sample case. The contour subdivision is shown for each lobe separately plotting at each CC contour point disks with radii relative to the corresponding probability. The final probabilistic subdivision model is computed by linearly averaging the probabilities for each CC contour point across the training population.

3 Results

Probabilistic CC subdivision model: The contour probability maps of all 5 cases in the training population show a high similarity across all cases (see Figure 3A) and so does the final subdivision model(see Figure 3C). The largest variabil-

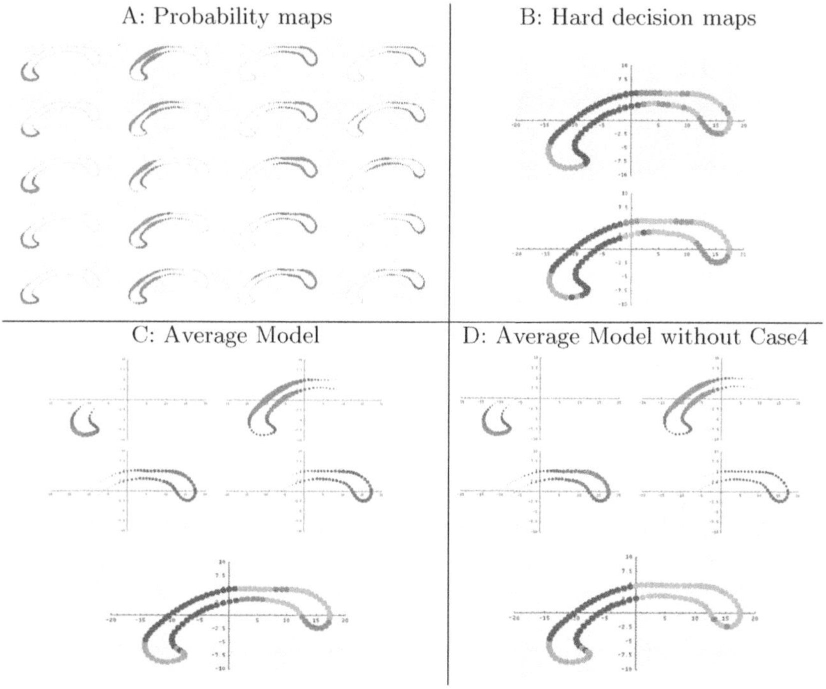

Fig. 3. Results of the subdivision model computation. A: Contour probability maps for all training cases. B: Hard decision maps for 2 selected training cases(cyan:anterior-frontal, purple:posterior-frontal, brown:parietal, red:occipital-temporal lobe). C: Probabilistic and hard decision map of the final subdivision model. D: Probabilistic and hard decision map of the subdivision model excluding a single training case.

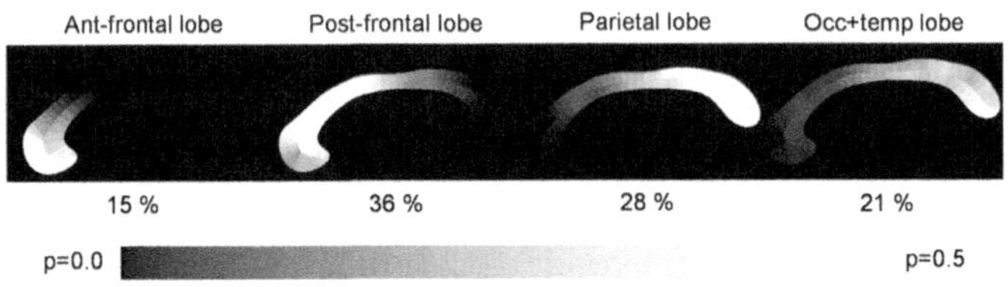

Fig. 4. Probabilistic area maps for a sample case. Each region is annotated with the respective probabilistic area percentage relative to the overall area.

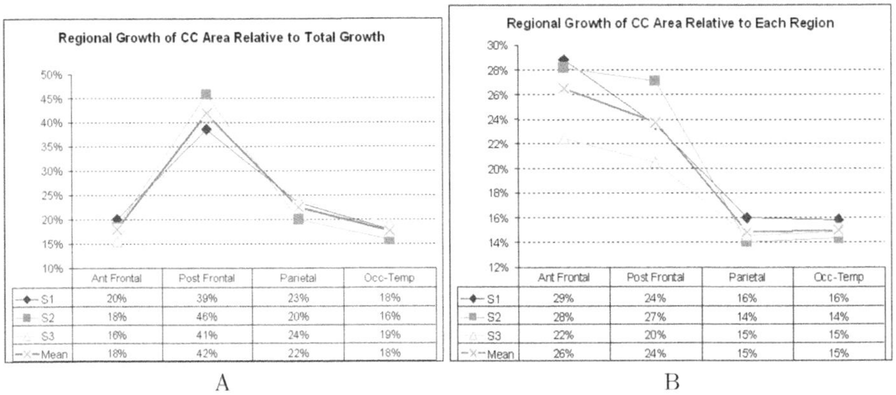

	Ant Frontal	Post Frontal	Parietal	Occ-Temp
S1	20%	39%	23%	18%
S2	18%	46%	20%	16%
S3	16%	41%	24%	19%
Mean	18%	42%	22%	18%

	Ant Frontal	Post Frontal	Parietal	Occ-Temp
S1	29%	24%	16%	16%
S2	28%	27%	14%	14%
S3	22%	20%	15%	15%
Mean	26%	24%	15%	15%

Fig. 5. Relative growth curves of CC subdivision regions. Data from 3 healthy subjects along mean curves from age 2 to age 4. A: Regional growth relative to the overall CC growth. B: Regional growth relative to the size of the corresponding region at age 2.

ity seems to be present in the occipital-temporal lobe section. Alternatively to the probability maps, we also computed the hard decision maps by associating each contour point with a single region based on the highest probability. The high decision variability between the 2 selected cases shown in Figure 3B clearly illustrates the main drawback of a hard decision map for the training cases. A similarly high variability is also present in a single leave-one-out experiment of a hard subdivision model computed from the final probability maps as shown in Figures 3C and D.

The result of the final subdivision model applied to a sample CC contour is shown in Figure 4. The occipital-temporal lobe region clearly shows a low probability in a relatively large region, which remains low even in the posterior-most sections of the CC. The resulting probabilistic area is relatively large (21% for the shown sample case). In contrast, a hard decision model as illustrated in Figures 3C would compute a much lower area value and would thus highly underestimate the CC area associated with the occiptal-temporal lobe fibers.

Application of the model to a study of CC growth: In order to illustrate the potential of the subdivision model, we applied it to a small study of CC growth in 3 healthy children of age 2 to 4. We applied the model after CC segmentation and computed the probabilistic area sum for the 4 regions. Figure 5 shows the resulting regional area growth A) relative to the overall CC growth and B) relative to the regional area of corresponding CC region at age 2. The first shows the largest growth in the posterior-frontal lobe region and the smallest growth in the anterior-frontal lobe region. As the posterior-frontal region is overall the largest region and the anterior-frontal region is the smallest region, this growth curve plot can be misleading. The second plot captures the local growth more intuitively, as it shows the regional growth relative to the overall regional size. In this plot one can clearly see that the main growth is happening in the frontal lobe regions with the anterior-frontal lobe region experiencing the largest relative growth from age 2 to age 4 at 26%.

4 Discussion and Conclusion

We present in this paper a novel method for the computation of a probabilistic subdivision model of an anatomical structure. The subdivision is not based on commonly applied arbitrarily subdivision boundaries based on the bounding box. Rather the subdivision is computed from probabilistic maps based on the distance to trans-callosal DTI fibers associated with a lobe subdivision.

Even though our CC subdivision model is based directly on DTI fiber connectivity information, the individual CC subdivisions are based on the geometric correspondence of the boundary to the subdivision model. On one hand, this scheme allows us to apply the subdivision model to retrospective CC data that lack an appropriate DTI dataset. On the other, if an appropriate DTI dataset is given, then we could directly compute the subdivision from the DTI fibers. For our present clinical studies either without DTI data or only with low-resolution DTI data the choice of a probabilistic subdivision model is the optimal method. In our future studies we are planning to recompute this subdivision model for a higher resolution data and investigate the direct computation of the CC subdivision from the DTI fibers.

The regions in our subdivision model are quite similar to those of the Witelson subdivision model [6], which is motivated by neurohistological studies. In contrast to the Witelson method is more stable due to the probabilistic nature of the subdivision and has been directly computed from connectivity information.

We are currently using the subdivision model to study regional CC growth in a large neurodevelopmental study of autistic, developmentally delayed and healthy subjects from age 2 to 4. For a subset of this study additional relatively low-resolution DTI data is also available and we plan to use the model to study regional histograms of DTI properties such as Geodesic Anisotropy. We further plan to employ the model for the computation of regionally cumulative shape measurements, such as the mean distance between the mean contours of two populations in every CC subdivision region.

The results of the small scale study of callosal growth from year 2 to 4 is quite preliminary due to the low number of subjects. The high similarity of the results in all cases is though suggesting that the frontal lobe regions experience a larger growth than those of the posterior lobes in that stage of healthy development.

Acknowledgment. We are thankful to Sean Ho for the original corpus callosum segmentation software. We would further like to thank Daniel Rueckert for the affine registration tools and Sarang Joshi for the fluid registration program. This research is supported by the UNC Neurodevelopmental Disorders Research Center HD 03110.

References

1. Thompson, P., Giedd, J., Woods, R., MacDonald, D., Evans, A., Toga, A.: Growth patterns in the developing brain detected by using continuum mechanical tensor maps. Nature **6774** (2000) 190–3
2. Keshavan, M., Diwadkar, V., Harenski, K., Rosenberg, D., Sweeney, J., Pettegrew, J.: Abnormalities of the corpus callosum in first episode, treatment naive schizophrenia. J Neurol Neurosurg Psychiatry **6** (2002) 757–60
3. Fillard, P., Gilmore, J., Lin, W., Piven, J., Gerig, G.: Quantitative analysis of white matter fiber properties along geodesic paths. In: MICCAI. Number 2879 in Lecture Notes in Computer Science (2003) 16–23
4. Xu, D., Mori, S., Solaiyappan, M., van Zijl, P., Davatzikos, C.: A framework for callosal fiber distribution analysis. NeuroImage **17** (2002) 11311143
5. Gee, J., Zhang, H., Dubb, A., Avants, B., Yushkevich, P., Duda, J.: Anatomy-based visualizations of diffusion tensor images of brain white matter. In: Visualization and Image Processing of Tensor Fields. (2005)
6. Witelson, S.: Hand and sex differences in the isthmus and genu of the human corpus callosum. a postmortem morphological study. Brain **3** (1989) 799–835
7. Narr, K., Thompson, P., Sharma, T., Moussai, J., Cannestra, A., Toga, A.: Mapping morphology of the corpus callosum in schizophrenia. Cereb Cortex **1** (2000) 40–9
8. Bermudez P, Z.R.: Sexual dimorphism in the corpus callosum: methodological considerations in mri morphometry. Neuroimage **13** (2001) 1121–30
9. Székely, G., Kelemen, A., Brechbühler, C., Gerig, G.: Segmentation of 2-D and 3-D objects from MRI volume data using constrained elastic deformations of flexible Fourier contour and surface models. Medical Image Analysis **1** (1996) 19–34
10. Van Leemput, K., Maes, F., Vandermeulen, D., Suetens, P.: Automated model-based tissue classication of mr images of the brain. IEEE Transactions on Medical Imaging **18** (1999) 897–908
11. Bookstein, F.: Shape and the Information in Medical Images: A Decade of the Morphometric Synthesis. Comp. Vision and Image Under. **66** (1997) 97–118
12. Rueckert, D., Frangi, A.F., Schnabel, J.A.: Automatic construction of 3d statistical deformation models of the brain using non-rigid registration. IEEE Transactions on Medical Imaging **8** (2003) 1014–1025
13. Joshi, S., Davis, B., Jomier, M., Gerig, G.: Unbiased diffeomorphic atlas construction for computational anatomy. NeuroImage **23** (2004) S151–S160

Random Walks for Interactive Organ Segmentation in Two and Three Dimensions: Implementation and Validation

Leo Grady[1], Thomas Schiwietz[1], Shmuel Aharon[1], and Rüdiger Westermann[2]

[1] Department of Imaging and Visualization, Siemens Corporate Research, 755 College Rd. East, Princeton, NJ, USA
[2] Technische Universität München, Lehrstuhl für Informatik 15, Boltzmannstrasse 3, 85748 Garching, Germany

Abstract. A new approach to interactive segmentation based on random walks was recently introduced that shows promise for allowing physicians more flexibility to segment arbitrary objects in an image. This report has two goals: To introduce a novel computational method for applying the random walker algorithm in 2D/3D using the Graphics Processing Unit (GPU) and to provide quantitative validation studies of this algorithm relative to different targets, imaging modalities and interaction strategies.

1 Introduction

A general-purpose, automatic, segmentation engine for medical images is extremely challenging due to the drastic changes in image data as a result of pathology and changes in radiologist preference. Therefore, efforts have continued toward providing *interactive* tools that allow a physician to quickly obtain an image/volume segmentation meeting their specific goals and criteria. Recently, a promising new interactive approach was introduced that uses random walks to define segmentation boundaries given user-placed seeds indicating K objects [1] (for arbitrary K). It was shown in [1] that this random walks algorithm is robust to weak boundaries and image noise. With the theory developed in [1], the current work introduces a faster, GPU-based, method of computation and offers a quantitative validation of the segmentations produced by this method.

The major computational hurdle of the random walker algorithm in [1] is the solution to a sparse system of equations for which a generic conjugate-gradients approach is employed. Although achieving reasonable speeds for moderately sized images (four seconds for a 256×256 2D image), the size of modern medical volumes requires a more efficient implementation to achieve an interactive speed. Therefore, we introduce a GPU-based implementation that offers over an order of magnitude speed increase for the processing of 2D and 3D datasets.

Validation of a general-purpose, interactive segmentation tool is difficult. Since this tool will provide an arbitrary segmentation with enough user interaction (i.e., if the user seeds every pixel), the main concerns are: 1) How sensitive

J. Duncan and G. Gerig (Eds.): MICCAI 2005, LNCS 3750, pp. 773–780, 2005.

are the results to exact seed placement? 2) How sensitive are the results to the quantity of seeds placed? 3) How much time, both user and computer, is required to perform a segmentation? 4) What is the subjective quality of the segmentations across different imaging modalities and different segmentation targets? These are the four questions that we address in the validation section.

The major interactive techniques for general-purpose organ segmentation are graph cuts, intelligent scissors and level sets. Graph cuts [2] treat the image as a graph where each pixel is associated with a node and a lattice edge structure is imposed, weighted to reflect intensity changes. Although performing well in many situations, there are a few concerns associated with this technique. For example, if a small number of seeds are used, the algorithm will often return the smallest cut as the cut that minimally separates the seeds from the rest of the image. Therefore, a user often has to continue placing seeds in order to overcome this "small cut" problem. Additionally, the K-way graph cuts problem is NP-Hard, requiring use of a heuristic to obtain a solution. The intelligent scissors algorithm [3] again views the image as a graph and employs Dijsktra's algorithm to compute the shortest path between user-defined points, treating this path as the object boundary. Unfortunately, a low-contrast or noisy boundary may require the specification of many points and the algorithm is inapplicable to 3D boundaries. Although the family of active contours and level sets is large [4] a user is generally asked to place a contour near the desired boundary and the algorithm evolves the boundary to a local energy minimum. The main problems with level set methods are difficulty of implementation (often requiring specification of several free parameters) and difficulty in fixing an incorrect solution, especially if the desired contour does not correspond to a local energy minimum.

This paper is organized as follows: In Section 2 we review the random walker algorithm and Section 3 details our novel GPU implementation in 2D/3D. Section 4 provides the results of our validation studies with respect to the questions raised above. Section 5 follows with a conclusion.

2 Random Walks for Image Segmentation

In this section we review the random walker image segmentation algorithm introduced in [1]. In the case of two labels, we determine the label for a non-seed pixel by asking: Given a random walker starting at this pixel, what is the probability that the random walker will reach a foreground seed before it reaches a background seed? If this probability is above one-half, then we assign this pixel to the foreground and if it is below one-half, we assign this pixel to the background. If more than two labels are used, the pixel is assigned the label for which a random walker is most likely to reach first. In [1], a Gaussian weighting function was used to represent the image structure as random walker biases (i.e., edge weights). This function has a single free parameter (representing the only free parameter in the algorithm), β, that was set to $\beta = 1500$ for all 2D experiments and $\beta = 4000$ for all 3D experiments.

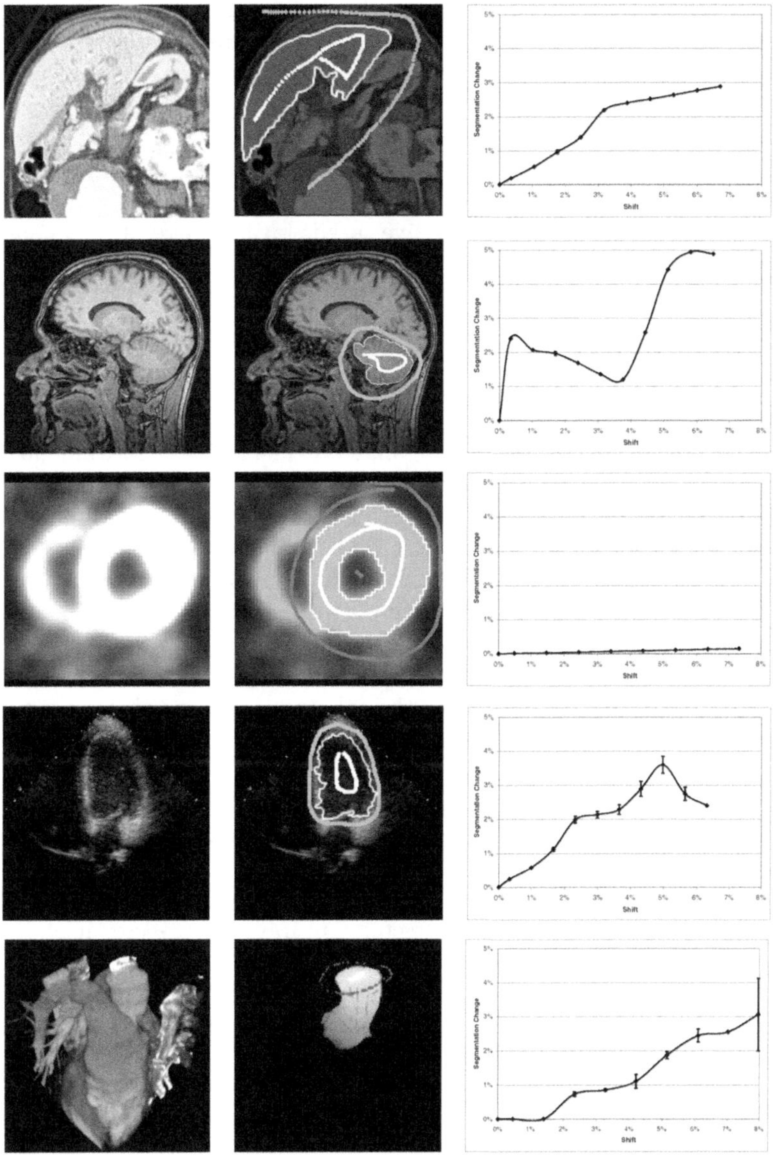

Fig. 1. Sensitivity analysis of segmentation to random shifts of seed placement in direction and magnitude over 1,000 trials. Left: Original 2D datasets from each of the four major imaging modalities and a 3D (CT) dataset. Middle: Foreground and background seeds are given by the gray markers. The white line represents the initial segmentation boundary (in 2D datasets). Right: Experimental results. The x-axis represents the ratio of the shift measured in pixels to the horiztonal image resolution. The y-axis represents the ratio of the pixels that switched label to the number of pixels originally labeled foreground. The plotted line represents the mean, with error bar indicating one standard error of the mean.

The equivalence between the random walker problem and the Dirichlet problem from potential theory was exploited in [1] to transform the computation of the random walker probabilities into the solution to system of linear equations. Although the system is sparse, symmetric and positive definite, allowing application of fast solvers like conjugate gradients, interactive speeds were not achieved for high-resolution images in [1]. For this reason, we present in the next section a GPU-based method that the solves the linear system (i.e., calculates the random walker probabilities) at interactive speeds for higher-resolution images and volumes.

3 GPU Implementation

Commodity graphics cards have been successfully used in recent years to enhance the speed of computation for image segmentation algorithms [5,6]. The computation of the random walker algorithm fits perfectly with the GPU in three respects: 1) All necessary linear algebra operators are computed extremely fast due to the inherit parallelism of the GPU and efficient caching, 2) Since a GPU processes four channels (RGBA), each channel may be used to represent a set of probabilities, allowing four labels to be solved simultaneously, 3) The segmentation may be continuously updated on the screen for the benefit of the user. An additional benefit of simultaneously solving the system of equations for multiple labels is that one may stop the computation when three of the four labels have converged and simply subtract the converged probabilities from unity to obtain the probabilities for the unconverged label.

Either a 2D or 3D dataset may be processed using the GPU. However, the limited size of the on-board memory of today's GPUs (256MB) constrains us to images with a resolution of 1024×1024 or volumes of resolution $128 \times 128 \times 128$. The implementation of a conjugate gradients method requires only two non-trivial operations: a sparse-matrix vector multiply and a vector inner product. The sparse-matrix vector multiply is described below and the vector inner product is described by Bolz *et al.* [7] and Krüger *et al.* [8]. Each row of the 2D-Laplacian matrix represents one pixel and the four values on the sub-diagonals indicate the weights of that pixel to each of its neighbors. Since the diagonal contains redundant information (i.e., the diagonal entry equals the negative sum of the off-diagonals), we can represent the Laplacian matrix as a 2D, four-channels, texture with size equal to the number of pixels in the image. The matrix-vector multiplication is therefore executed by multiplying the four channels of a given pixel (row) by the values of the four neighboring pixels of the vector. The diagonal value of the matrix is retrieved by summing and negating the four channel values. This value is then multiplied by the corresponding vector pixel. The five multiplication values are then summed together to provide the current output vector element results.

The Laplacian matrix for a 3D lattice has six sub-diagonals. However, due to matrix symmetry, one need only store three out of six sub-diagonals. The other three sub-diagonals can be retrieved by sampling neighboring matrix entries. In

2D and 3D a matrix-vector operation requires one rendering pass only. In 3D we put all slices of a volume in one 2D flat texture side-by-side. Operations on a flat texture have proven to be much faster than on a stack of slices (textures) [9].

4 Validation

The original exposition of the random walker technique demonstrated that the algorithm is capable of finding weak (i.e., low-contrast or no-contrast) boundaries, behaving robustly to noise and giving good quality results. However, since a user may achieve an arbitrary segmentation with the placement of enough seeds, a strict error measure is practically meaningless. An ideal interactive segmentation algorithm would not require an excess of seeds or require user precision to carefully choose the seed locations. An additional criterion is obviously speed of computation and user time. Therefore, in this section we provide a quantitative validation of the algorithm by studying the following questions: 1) How sensitive are the results to exact seed placement? 2) How sensitive are the results to the quantity of seeds placed? 3) How much time, both user and computer, is required to perform a segmentation? We examine the first two questions with a 2D example from each of the major imaging modalities of MR, CT, PET and Ultrasound as well as a 3D (CT) volume. The third question is addressed by applying the algorithm to a range of targets in images of differing image modalities. For simplicity, all of these experiments were conducted on a lattice with a 4-connected topology using a two-label scenario. However, these results should extend to the multilabel setting since the probabilities for each label are computed by effectively viewing the label as the foreground opposed to the background of all of the other labels.

Obviously, the segmentation obtained with the random walker algorithm will depend on the location of the seeds. If this were not true, no seeds would need to be placed. However, a small difference in the placement of the seeds within the same object should not result in a significant change in the computed segmentation. Ideally, the user should be free from a requirement that the seeds are drawn very carefully or placed in prescribed locations. We performed five experiments in seed placement using a 2D example from each of the four imaging modalities described above and a 3D (CT) dataset. For each of these seed placements, the locations of the foreground seeds were shifted (as a group) in a random direction with random magnitude. Although no range of magnitudes was pre-established, we rejected any perturbation that would have moved foreground seeds into the background. After the seed placements were perturbed, the segmentation was recomputed and the change in pixel labeling was reported as the ratio of pixels that switched labels to the number of pixels originally labeled as foreground. The original images, initial segmentations and experimental results of the perturbation studies are shown in Figure 1.

As one might expect, a greater magnitude shift produces a greater change in the segmentation. However, the algorithm does appear to be stable in the traditional sense that a small change in input (i.e., seed placement) produces a small change in output (i.e., the segmentation). In fact, perturbations within the original object all produced changes in the segmentation under 5%. However, image content does influence the segmentation response to seed perturbation, as may be seen by comparing the plots in Figure 1. For example, the low-contrast boundary of the cerebellum in this particular MR image results in a greater sensitivity to seed location than the more straightforward cardiac PET image, although all segmentations remain within 5% of the original. Therefore, we conclude that a user need not be very accurate in placing seeds, since a small deviation will not be expected to make a large difference in the results.

A second important question is: How many seeds does a user need to place in order to achieve the desired segmentation? If many seeds are required, the algorithm has little to offer over a purely manual segmentation. As above, we have used a foreground/background scenario for simplicity. We used following design in examining this question quantitatively: We start with the initial segmentations of Figure 1, filling the object with foreground seeds and the background with background seeds. Then, we shrink the two seed groups by applying a morphological erosion operation to each group and track the change in the segmentation as the number of seeds are reduced. Figure 2 illustrates the change in segmentation as the number of seeds are reduced. As desired, small reductions in the numbers of seeds preserve the object boundaries almost exactly. In fact, it is only after the number of seeds has dropped dramatically, to less than 50% of the

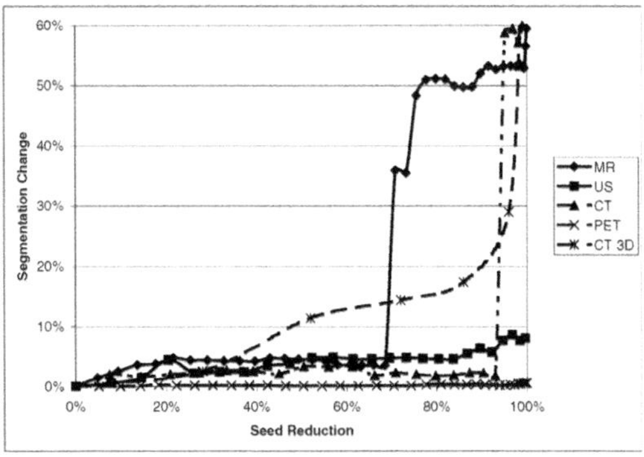

Fig. 2. Sensitivity analysis of segmentation to the numbers of seeds used. For each image in 1, we initially filled the inside of the initial segmentation with foreground seeds and the outside with background seeds. Then, we performed morphological erosion until the seeds were entirely removed and tracked the change in segmentation after each erosion step. The x-axis indicates the percentage of seeds remaining (with respect to the initial seeding) and the y-axis represents the ratio of the number of seeds that changed label to the total number of foreground seeds. Since this experiment was deterministic, the resulting value is simply reported after each erosion operation. Seed reductions of 50% or more are seen to produce only minor changes in the resulting segmentation. Note that the 100% value is not actually reported — the experiment was terminated when erosion would have removed the final seed.

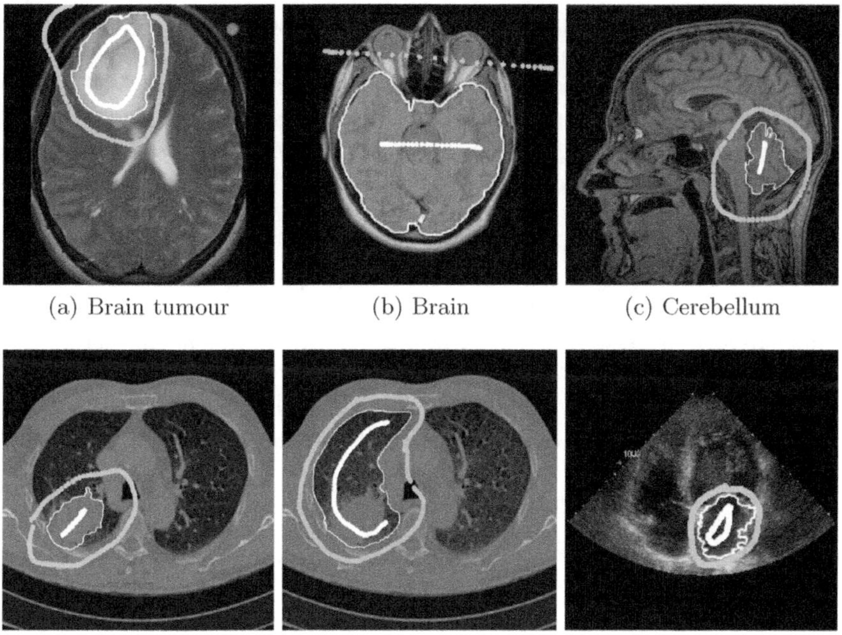

(a) Brain tumour (b) Brain (c) Cerebellum

(d) Lung tumour (e) Lung with tumour (f) Left atrium

Fig. 3. User and computer time for image segmentations. User time indicates the estimated time taken to place seeds. Computer time is given with both a CPU and GPU implementation. a) User: 2s, CPU: 10s, GPU: 0.7s, b) User: 2s, CPU: 6s, GPU: 1.5s, c) User: 2s, CPU: 83s, GPU: 0.3s, d) User: 3s, CPU: 3s, GPU: 0.9s, e) User: 5s, CPU: 23s, GPU: 1.3s, f) User: 4s, CPU: 3s, GPU: 0.8s.

original, that the effects of reduced seeds are noticeable. Therefore, we conclude that only a fraction of the seeds necessary to specify a manual segmentation are required to produce a nearly identical segmentation.

The time required by a user to obtain a desired segmentation (with editing) is more crucial than the computation time. Figure 3 shows the results of segmenting several different targets in different imaging modalities. The caption details the total user time required to place the seeds (including edits) and the computation time on the CPU and GPU. The experiments were performed on a Pentium 4 with 2.8 GHz and a ATI Radeon X800 XT graphics card. User time ranged from 2–5s, CPU computation time from 3–83s and GPU time from 0.3–1.5s. As a comparison, we note that segmenting the 3D volume of Figure 1 required 35s for the CPU, 1s for the GPU and 5s of user time to place seeds.

5 Conclusion

Anatomical differences between patients and the patient pathology often prevent a fully automatic algorithm from producing high-quality segmentations without user interaction. The random walker method presented in [1] has proven a useful tool for general-purpose, interactive segmentation.

Since a diligent user could achieve an arbitrary segmentation by placing enough seeds, it is important to validate this technique using metrics that measure the speed and ease of use for a naive user. Our experiments above examined how sensitive the segmentation is to seed placement and how many seeds are needed to obtain a quality segmentation. Furthermore, we have presented a simple method for reducing the computation time of the random walker algorithm by over an order of magnitude on commodity graphics hardware and measured the total time required for a user to obtain a desired segmentation. Our experiments support the statement that the random walker algorithm allows a user to quickly obtain a desired segmentation without concern for placing an excess of seeds, placing them very carefully or in a prescribed pattern. Ultimately, we believe that these qualities will lead to the widespread use of the random walker segmentation algorithm in varied applications.

References

1. Grady, L., Funka-Lea, G.: Multi-label image segmentation for medical applications based on graph-theoretic electrical potentials. In Šonka, M., Kakadiaris, I.A., Kybic, J., eds.: ECCV 2004 Workshops CVAMIA and MMBIA. LNCS3117, Prague, Czech Republic, Springer (2004) 230–245
2. Boykov, Y., Jolly, M.P.: *Interactive graph cuts* for optimal boundary & region segmentation of objects in N-D images. In: International Conference on Computer Vision. Volume I. (2001) 105–112
3. Mortensen, E., Barrett, W.: Interactive segmentation with intelligent scissors. Graphical Models in Image Processing **60** (1998) 349–384
4. Sethian, J.A.: Level Set Methods and Fast Marching Methods. Cambridge Monograph on Applied and Computational Mathematics. Cambridge University Press (1999)
5. Lefohn, A.E., Cates, J.E., Whitaker, R.T.: Interactive, GPU-based level sets for 3D segmentation. In: Medical Image Computing and Computer Assisted Intervention (MICCAI). (2003) 564–572
6. Sherbondy, A., Houston, M., Napel, S.: Fast volume segmentation with simultaneous visualization using programmable graphics hardware. In: IEEE Visualization 2003, Seattle, WA, IEEE (2003) 171–176
7. Bolz, J., Farmer, I., Grinspun, E., Schröder, P.: Sparse matrix solvers on the GPU: Conjugate gradients and multigrid. In: ACM Transactions on Graphics. Volume 22 of SIGGRAPH. (2003) 917–924
8. Krüger, J., Westermann, R.: Linear algebra operators for GPU implementation of numerical algorithms. In: ACM Transactions on Graphics. Volume 22 of SIGGRAPH. (2003) 908–916
9. Harris, M.J.: Real-time cloud simulation and rendering. Technical Report TR03-040, University of North Carolina (2003)

Robust Pulmonary Nodule Segmentation in CT: Improving Performance for Juxtapleural Cases

K. Okada[1], V. Ramesh[1], A. Krishnan[2], M. Singh[1], and U. Akdemir[1]

[1] Real-Time Vision & Modeling Dept., Siemens Corporate Research, Princeton, USA
[2] CAD Program, Siemens Medical Solutions, Malvern, USA

Abstract. Two novel methods are proposed for robust segmentation of pulmonary nodules in CT images. The proposed solutions locate and segment a nodule in a semi-automatic fashion with a marker indicating the target. The solutions are motivated for handling the difficulty to segment juxtapleural, or wall-attached, nodules by using only local information without a global lung segmentation. They are realized as extensions of the recently proposed robust Gaussian fitting approach. Algorithms based on i) 3D morphological opening with anisotropic structuring element and ii) extended mean shift with a Gaussian repelling prior are presented. They are empirically compared against the robust Gaussian fitting solution by using a large clinical high-resolution CT dataset. The results show 8% increase, resulting in 95% correct segmentation rate for the dataset.

1 Introduction

Pulmonary nodule segmentation is one of the major goals of the computer-aided diagnosis with the chest CT data (chest CAD [1,2,3]). A semi-automatic robust segmentation solution is required for realizing reliable volumetric measurement of nodules [4,5], as an integral part of lung cancer screening and management.

Intensity-based segmentation solutions, such as local density maximum algorithm [6], have been successfully applied to the nodule segmentation problem. Although such solutions can be effective for solitary nodules, they cannot separate noduels from juxtaposed surrounding structures, such as walls and vessels, due to their similar intensity. Recently, to address this issue, more sophisticated approaches have been proposed to incorporate nodule-specific geometrical constraints [7,8]. However, *juxtapleural*, or wall-attached, nodules still remain as a challenge because they can grossly violate such geometrical assumption and also appear frequently in practice. Another source of problem is rib bones which appear with high intensity values in CT. Such high-intensity regions near a given marker can bias the semi-automatic nodule center estimator. Robust segmentation of the juxtapleural cases can be addressed in two approaches: a) global lung or rib segmentation [6,9,10,11] and b) local non-target removal or avoidance [4]. The former can be effective but also computationally complex and dependent on the accuracy of the whole-lung segmentation. The latter is more efficient than the former but more difficult to achieve high performance due to the limited amount of information available for the non-target structures.

J. Duncan and G. Gerig (Eds.): MICCAI 2005, LNCS 3750, pp. 781–789, 2005.

Addressing the above issue of the juxtapleural cases, this article proposes two novel 3D nodule segmentation solutions based on the local non-target removal and avoidance approach. The local analysis-based approach is preferred to the global one in the semi-automatic CAD context due to its efficiency. The first solution detects and removes the lung wall region within an input sub-volume by using 3D binary morphological opening operation. Similar approaches have been proposed [9,4], however our solution employs data-driven ellipsoidal 3D structuring element unlike others. The second solution is based on an extended mean shift framework incorporating a repeller (negative) prior which pushes the convergence away from a specific data point. This prior-constrained mean shift is used for correctly detecting the nodule center despite the presence of rib bones, thereby improving the segmentation accuracy without an explicit removal of the walls and ribs. Both proposed solutions are realized as extensions of the robust anisotropic Gaussian fitting solution [8], which is employed for deriving the ellipsoidal structuring element and the repeller prior.

This article is organized as follows. Section 2 summarizes the robust Gaussian fitting solution. Section 3 introduces the proposed solutions for handling the juxtapleural nodules. Section 4 presents the results of our performance validation with a large clinical CT dataset. Section 5 presents our conclusive remarks.

2 Robust Anisotropic Gaussian Fitting

This section summarizes the robust anisotropic Gaussian fitting algorithms proposed previously as a solution to the semi-automatic (one-click) 3D nodule segmentation problem [8,12]. The one-click segmentation assumes that we are given a marker $\mathbf{x}_p$ indicating a rough location of the target nodule. Such marker can be provided from the radiologist's readings by eye-appraisal or the outcome of automatic nodule detection system [13,14]. For computational efficiency, the algorithm is usually applied to a sub-volume $V(\mathbf{x})$ centered at the marker and extracted from the 12-bit CT volume data $I(\mathbf{x}) : \mathcal{R}^3_+ \rightarrow \mathcal{R}_+$.

The algorithm results in a Gaussian function which fits the local intensity distribution of the target nodule best: $I(\mathbf{x}) \simeq \alpha \times \Phi(\mathbf{x};\mathbf{u},\mathbf{\Sigma})|_{\mathbf{x}\in\mathcal{S}}$ where $\Phi(\mathbf{x};\mathbf{u},\mathbf{\Sigma}) = |2\pi\mathbf{\Sigma}|^{-1/2}\exp(-1/2(\mathbf{x}-\mathbf{u})^t\mathbf{\Sigma}^{-1}(\mathbf{x}-\mathbf{u}))$ is the anisotropic 3D Gaussian function. α is a positive magnitude factor. $\mathcal{S}$ is a local neighborhood forming a basin of attraction of the target. $\mathbf{u}$ is the fitted Gaussian mean indicating the estimated nodule center. $\mathbf{\Sigma}$ is the fitted Gaussian covariance matrix indicating the nodule's anisotropic spread. The nodule's 3D boundary is approximated by the 35% confidence ellipsoid of the fitted Gaussian, determined empirically.

The algorithm performs a multiscale analysis by considering a Gaussian scale-space of the input sub-volume. The Gaussian scale-space $L(\mathbf{x};h)$ is a solution of the diffusion equation $\partial_h L = \frac{1}{2}\nabla^2 L$ with an initialization $L(\mathbf{x};0) = I(\mathbf{x})$. Such a scale-space is defined by a convolution of $I(\mathbf{x})$ with a Gaussian kernel $K_H(\mathbf{x})$ with a bandwidth matrix $\mathbf{H}$: $L(\mathbf{x};h) = I(\mathbf{x}) * K_H(\mathbf{x};\mathbf{H} = h\mathbf{I})$. The algorithm considers a Gaussian scale-space constructed over a set of densely sampled discrete *analysis scales* $\{h_k|k = 1,..,K\}$. At each analysis scale, a fixed-scale robust analysis is performed for fitting an anisotropic Gaussian function in each scale space image. Given a set of estimated Gaussians, the most stable estimate across the scales determines the final outcome.

The fixed-scale analysis performs a robust Gaussian fitting with scale-space mean shift, a convergent weighted mean shift defined in the Gaussian scale-space,

$$\mathbf{m}(\mathbf{x}; \mathbf{H}_k) = \frac{\int \mathbf{x}' K_H(\mathbf{x}-\mathbf{x}'; \mathbf{H}_k) I(\mathbf{x}') d\mathbf{x}'}{\int K_H(\mathbf{x}-\mathbf{x}'; \mathbf{H}_k) I(\mathbf{x}') d\mathbf{x}'} - \mathbf{x} = h_k \frac{\nabla L(\mathbf{x}; h_k)}{L(\mathbf{x}; h_k)} \quad (1)$$

Gaussian mean $\mathbf{u}$ as the nodule center is estimated by the convergence of the majority of initial seeds sampled around $\mathbf{x}_p$. A set of new seeds are sampled around the estimated mean $\mathbf{u}$. The mean shift procedures are then performed from each seed. Gaussian covariance is estimated by a constrained least-squares solution of a linear system with unknown $\mathbf{\Sigma}$, constructed with mean shift vectors *only* along the convergent trajectories. The linear system can also be constructed with the response-normalized scale-space Hessian [12].

The multiscale analysis, given a set of Gaussians estimated at the analysis scales $\{(\mathbf{u}_k, \mathbf{\Sigma}_k)\}$, is realized by finding the most stable estimate among others using a divergence-based stability test. For this purpose, the algorithm employs the Jensen Shannon divergence (JSD) of three neighboring Gaussians computed at each analysis scale. Assuming the normal form of distributions, JSD can be expressed in the following simple form [15],

$$JSD(k) = \frac{1}{2}\log \frac{|\frac{1}{3}\sum_{i=k-1}^{k+1} \mathbf{\Sigma}_i|}{\sqrt[3]{\prod_{i=k-1}^{k+1} |\mathbf{\Sigma}_i|}} + \frac{1}{2}\sum_{i=k-1}^{k+1} (\mathbf{u}_i - \mathbf{u})^t (\sum_{i=k-1}^{k+1} \mathbf{\Sigma}_i)^{-1} (\mathbf{u}_i - \mathbf{u}) \quad (2)$$

where $\mathbf{u} = \frac{1}{2}\sum_{k-1}^{k+1} \mathbf{u}_i$. The minimization of a JSD profile across the scales h_k results in the most-stable-over-scales estimate $(\mathbf{u}^*, \mathbf{\Sigma}^*)$ [12].

The robustness is due to two aspects of this algorithm. First, the fixed-scale Gaussian fitting solution performs robust model fitting with the outlier removal using the scale-space mean shift convergence analysis. This helps to mitigate the problem of juxtaposed neighboring structures. Second, the usage of the stability-based scale selection robustifies the fitting process even for intensity distributions that do not follow the Gaussian assumption well. This facilitates the effectiveness of the solution for segmenting clinically significant but technically challenging ground-glass nodules [8,16].

3 Segmentation for Juxtapleural Cases

Two proposed solutions described below extends the above robust Gaussian fitting solution for handling not only the solitary but also the juxtapleural cases. Both solutions first execute the robust Gaussian fitting. The resulting fitted Gaussian undergoes a goodness-of-fit test, analyzing chi-square errors between the data and fitted model, as well as a linear DC bias [8]. Only when the initial fitting results fail to pass the test, either of the following two solutions is invoked.

Our pilot study resulted in following two empirical observations. First, the most of gross segmentation failures which can be detected by the goodness-of-fit test are due to the juxtapleural cases. Second, the initial fitted Gaussians for such failures tend to approximate the wall and rib structures. Exploiting these observations, we develop the segmentation solutions which employ the initial fitted Gaussian as an input to their process.

3.1 Wall Removal by 3D Morphological Opening

The input sub-volumes of the juxtapleural failure cases contain lung wall regions. Such wall regions appear typically as a large connected region with CT values higher than surrounding pulmonary parenchyma. The juxtapleural nodule will appear as a nodular structure partially embedded into the wall. The first solution explicitly removes the wall regions from the sub-volume using the morphological operation. Then the robust Gaussian fit is performed again on the wall-removed data, resulting in an improved segmentation of the target nodule. The algorithm consists of the following steps.

Wall Removal: Given the input $(V(\mathbf{x}), \mathbf{x}_p)$ and a fitted Gaussian $(\mathbf{u}^*, \mathbf{\Sigma}^*)$ failing the goodness-of-fit test, remove wall regions in $V(\mathbf{x})$, resulting in $V_r(\mathbf{x})$.
1. Binarize the input sub-volume $V(\mathbf{x})$ with an intensity threshold th_1, resulting in a binarized sub-volume $B_o(\mathbf{x})$.
2. Compute the average diameter d_{ave} of the ellipsoid defined by $\mathbf{\Sigma}^*$.
3. Initialize a 3D structuring element: $\mathbf{E} = \mathbf{\Sigma}^*$ if $d_{ave} > th_2$, otherwise $\mathbf{E}$ is set to a 3D ball with a fixed radius r_b.
4. Perform 3D binary morphological opening, resulting in smoothed volume $B_s(\mathbf{x})$ retaining only the large wall region: $B_s(\mathbf{x}) = [B_o(\mathbf{x}) \ominus \mathbf{E}] \oplus \mathbf{E}$.
5. Perform a wall removal by masking $V(\mathbf{x})$ with the negative of $B_s(\mathbf{x})$: $V_r(\mathbf{x}) = V(\mathbf{x}) \times \mathrm{NOT}[B_s(\mathbf{x})]$

Nodule Segmentation: Perform the robust Gaussian fitting algorithm on $V_r(\mathbf{x})$ with $\mathbf{x}_p$, providing an improved nodule segmentation $(\mathbf{u}_{wr}, \mathbf{\Sigma}_{wr})$.

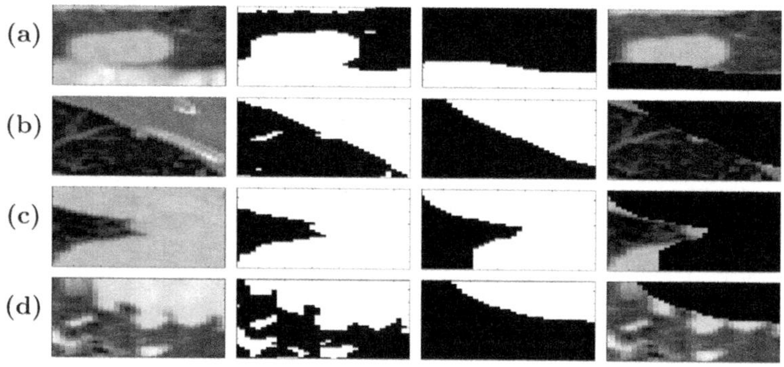

Fig. 1. Examples of the 3D morphological opening results shown in 2D cross-section images. From left to right column: input sub-volume $V(\mathbf{x})$, binarized sub-volume $B_o(\mathbf{x})$, smoothed sub-volume $B_s(\mathbf{x})$, wall-removed sub-volume $V_r(\mathbf{x})$.

This algorithm utilizes a data-dependent ellipsoidal structuring element estimated for each data unlike the similar approach with a disc-like element [7]. Our experimental results later show that this algorithm effectively reduces the segmentation failures due to the juxtapleural cases. Figure 1 illustrates some examples of the morphological opening applied to the real CT data. It shows that the operation effectively removes the walls with large (1a), small (1b), heavily-embedded (1c), and irregular (1d) nodules. Note that this was achieved without using a set of structuring elements of different sizes.

3.2 Mean Shift Constrained by Gaussian Repelling Prior

The second solution is proposed for detecting the nodule center correctly without an explicit removal of the walls and ribs despite the presence of rib bones.

The prior-constrained mean shift incorporates a spatial prior information to the data-driven mean shift analysis. Suppose that the robust Gaussian fitting is performed on the sub-volume $V(\mathbf{x})$, resulting in the nodule center and spread estimate $(\mathbf{u}^*, \mathbf{\Sigma}^*)$. This fitted Gaussian can be interpreted as the normal probability distribution $Q(\mathbf{x})$ indicating a likelihood of $\mathbf{x}$ being the estimated center,

$$Q(\mathbf{x}) = \mathcal{N}(\mathbf{x}; \mathbf{u}^*, \mathbf{\Sigma}^*) = |2\pi\mathbf{\Sigma}^*|^{-1/2} \exp(-\frac{1}{2}(\mathbf{x} - \mathbf{u}^*)^t \mathbf{\Sigma}^{*-1}(\mathbf{x} - \mathbf{u}^*)) \quad (3)$$

Suppose next that this estimate *failed* the goodness-of-fit test. This indicates that the estimated location $\mathbf{u}^*$ is *not* at the center of the target nodule and that the estimated spread $\mathbf{\Sigma}^*$ roughly expresses the extent of the (rib/wall) structure which *falsely* attracted the mean shift convergence away from the true nodule center. Our main idea here is to re-estimate the nodule center with the constrained mean shift whose convergence is biased by the knowledge of $Q(\mathbf{x})$ so as to pushes the convergence away from the failed estimate $\mathbf{u}^*$.

To incorporate such a repelling (negative) prior, we consider resampling, or associating weights to, available data $I(\mathbf{x})$ to denote the notion that some data points are more likely to occur than others. We define such prior-induced positive weights by a negative of Q($\mathbf{x}$),

$$w_Q(\mathbf{x}) = 1 - |2\pi\mathbf{\Sigma}^*|^{1/2} Q(\mathbf{x}) \quad (4)$$

Incorporating the negative prior leads to the following resampled scale-space $\tilde{L}(\mathbf{x}; h)$ expressed in the discretized data space,

$$\tilde{L}(\mathbf{x}; h) = \sum_{i=1}^{N} w_Q(\mathbf{x}_i) I(\mathbf{x}_i) K_h(\mathbf{x} - \mathbf{x}_i) \quad (5)$$

We call the mean shift $\mathbf{m}_r(\mathbf{x}; h, Q)$ that is convergent to a mode in $\tilde{L}(\mathbf{x}; h)$ negative prior-constrained scale-space mean shift. It is defined by,

$$\mathbf{m}_r(\mathbf{x}; h, Q) = \frac{\sum_i \mathbf{x}_i K_h(\mathbf{x} - \mathbf{x}_i) I(\mathbf{x}_i) w_Q(\mathbf{x}_i)}{\sum_i K_h(\mathbf{x} - \mathbf{x}_i) I(\mathbf{x}_i) w_Q(\mathbf{x}_i)} - \mathbf{x} \quad (6)$$

Its convergence property is maintained because $w_Q(\mathbf{x}_i) \geq 0 \, \forall \mathbf{x}_i$.

A new Gaussian fitting solution is constructed by replacing the original scale-space mean shift (1) by this prior-constrained mean shift (6) in the robust fitting algorithm described in Section 2. Given an initial Gaussian $(\mathbf{u}^*, \mathbf{\Sigma}^*)$ failing the goodness-of-fit test, this new solution with $\mathbf{m}_r(\mathbf{x}; h, Q)$ is executed on the original data $V(\mathbf{x})$, resulting in an improved segmentation with $(\mathbf{u}_{ms}, \mathbf{\Sigma}_{ms})$.

4 Experimental Results

We compare the segmentation results of the two proposed methods against the baseline robust Gaussian fitting solution. We use a clinical HRCT dataset, consisting of 39 patients with 1312 nodules whose size ranges from 1 mm to 30 mm in diameter. The markers are provided by certified radiologists' eye-appraisal.

Table 1. Segmentation performance of the robust Gaussian fitting solution. GOF: the goodness-of-fit test. TP: accepted correct estimates. FN: rejected correct estimates. TN: rejected false estimates. FP: accepted false estimates.

Classif.	**# Cases (%)**	**GOF**	**# Cases (%)**
Correct	1156 (88.1)	**TP**	1095 (83.5)
		FN	61 (4.6)
Failure	156 (11.9)	**TN**	123 (9.4)
		FP	33 (2.5)

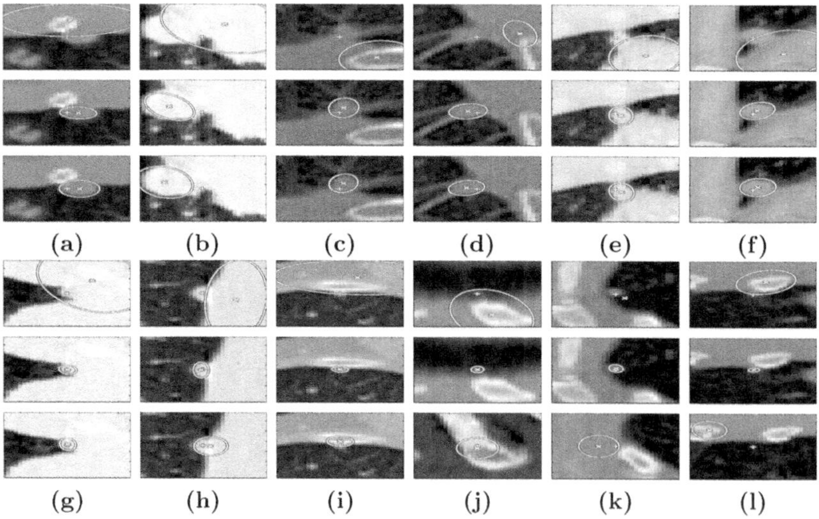

Fig. 2. Twelve examples of the 3D nodule segmentation results. 1st and 4th rows: $(\mathbf{u}^*, \mathbf{\Sigma}^*)$ by the robust Gaussian fitting of Section 2, 2nd and 5th rows: $(\mathbf{u}_{wr}, \mathbf{\Sigma}_{wr})$ by the morphological opening of Section 3.1, 3rd and 6th rows: $(\mathbf{u}_{ms}, \mathbf{\Sigma}_{ms})$ by the prior-constrained mean shift of Section 3.2.

$V(\mathbf{x})$ is set to 33x33x33 in voxels centered at the markers. The correct/failure classification of the segmentation results are given by the agreement of experts by eye-appraisal. The implementation of the systems follows the parameter settings in [8] with an additional 2-layer Gaussian pyramid for handling larger nodules. For the morphological opening, we set $th_1 = 500$ for the normalized intensity $I(\mathbf{x}) \in [0, 4095]$, $r_b = 14$, and $th_2 = 16.6$ in voxels, determined empirically. The prior-constrained mean shift does not have a free parameters to be tuned.

Table 1 summarizes the quantitative performance of the segmentation by the baseline robust Gaussian fitting solution. Together with the goodness-of-fit test, 88.1% and 9.4% resulted as true positives (TP) and negatives (TN). Among the 123 true negative cases, 108 were visually confirmed to be juxtapleural cases. The proposed nodule segmentation systems are tested with the 123 TN cases.

Figure 2 shows some illustrative examples. Both methods successfully segmented the difficult juxtapleural cases that failed initially: large (2a-b), irregular (2c-d), and heavily-embedded (2e-h). The morphological opening-based solution (WallRemove: WR) segmented the small nodules better than the negative prior-constrained mean shift solution (MeanShift: MS) as shown in (2i-l). Incorporating more negative priors in MS by iterating the whole procedure can improve some failure cases that are surrounded by multiple distractors (2l).

The quantitative performance comparison is summarized in table 2. The results indicate that WR (71.5%) performs better than MS (34.1%), especially for the small juxtapleural cases. WR thus improves the overall segmentation performance from 88.1% to 94.8%. Although MS's improvement was much lower than that of WR, there are some cases in which MS performs better than WR, as shown in Figure 3. When the nodules are attached to, or influenced by, non-

Table 2. Quantitative comparison of the two proposed segmentation solutions

Classif.	MeanShift	WallRemove
Correct	42 (34.1)	88 (71.5)
Failure	81 (65.9)	35 (28.5)
Tot. Corr.	1198 (91.3)	1239 (94.8)

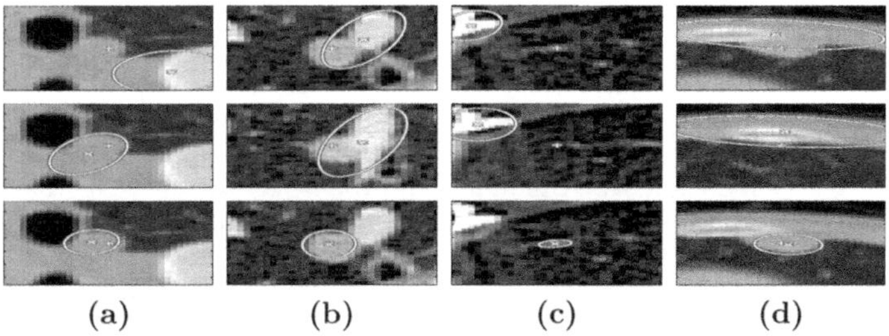

Fig. 3. Four example cases where the prior-constrained mean shift-based solution works better than the solution with wall removal using the morphological opening. From top to bottom row: initial fitted Gaussian $(\mathbf{u}^*, \mathbf{\Sigma}^*)$, after morphological opening $(\mathbf{u}_{wr}, \mathbf{\Sigma}_{wr})$, with prior-constrained mean shift $(\mathbf{u}_{ms}, \mathbf{\Sigma}_{ms})$.

wall structures (3a-c), the morphological opening cannot be effective thus MS performs better. There are also several cases where a very large nodule was attached to a thin part of lung wall (3d). Such a case will result in over-estimation of the structuring element thus a failure of the wall removal.

5 Conclusions

We proposed two novel 3D nodule segmentation solutions which improve performance for the difficult juxtapleural cases. The morphological opening-based (WR) and prior-constrained mean shift-based (MS) solutions, extended from the robust Gaussian fitting approach, are evaluated with a large clinical CT dataset. The validation results show that i) they can effectively segment the juxtapleural cases, ii) WR performs better than MS for the small juxtapleural cases, and iii) MS performs better than WR for the cases attached to non-wall structures. Toward our goal of the volumetric measurement of nodules, the accuracy by our methods is limited due to the ellipsoidal boundary approximation. However, further improvement of segmentation quality is possible by incorporating a non-parametric segmentation with a Gaussian prior derived by using the proposed methods [17]. Developing such an accurate non-parametric system together with the proposed solutions remains our future work.

References

1. Reeves, A.P., Kostis, W.J.: Computer-aided diagnosis of small pulmonary nodules. Seminars in Ultrasound, CT, and MRI **21** (2000) 116–128
2. van Ginneken, B., ter Harr Romeny, B.M., Viergever, M.A.: Computer-aided diagnosis in chest radiography: A survey. IEEE Trans. Med. Imag. **20** (2001) 1228–1241
3. Ko, J.P., Naidich, D.P.: Computer-aided diagnosis and the evaluation of lung disease. J. Thorac Imag. **19** (2004) 136–155
4. Ko, J.P., et al.: Small pulmonary nodules: Volume measurement at chest CT - phantom study. Radiology **228** (2003) 864–870
5. Wormanns, D., et al.: Volumetric measurements of pulmonary nodules at multi-row detector CT : in vivo reproducibility. Eur. Radiol. **14** (2004) 86–92
6. Zhao, B., et al.: Two-dimensional multi-criterion segmentation of pulmonary nodules on helical CT images. IEEE Trans. Med. Imag. **22** (2003) 1259–1274
7. Kostis, W.J., Reeves, A.P., Yankelevitz, D.F., Henschke, C.I.: Three-dimensional segmentation and growth-rate estimation of small pulmonary nodules in helical CT images. IEEE Trans. Med. Imag. **22** (2003) 1259–1274
8. Okada, K., Comaniciu, D., Krishnan, A.: Robust anisotropic Gaussian fitting for volumetric characterization of pulmonary nodules in multislice CT. IEEE Trans. Med. Imag. **24** (2005) 409–423
9. Armato, S., et al.: Computerized detection of pulmonary nodules on CT scans. RadioGraphics **19** (1999) 1303–1311
10. Wang, P., O'Dell, W.: Automated detection of juxta-pleural lung nodules in chest CT using lung contour corrected by anatomic landmarks. In: AAPM. (2004)
11. Shen, H., Liang, L., Shao, M., Qing, S.: Tracing based segmentation for the labeling of individual rib structures in chest CT volume data. In: MICCAI. (2004)

12. Okada, K., Comaniciu, D., Krishnan, A.: Scale selection for anisotropic scale-space: Application to volumetric tumor characterization. In: IEEE Conf. Comput. Vision and Pat. Recog. (2004)
13. Lee, Y., Hara, T., Fujita, H., Itoh, S., Ishigaki, T.: Automated detection of pulmonary nodules in helical CT images based on an improved template-matching technique. IEEE Trans. Med. Imag. **20** (2001) 595–604
14. Novak, C., Shen, H., Odry, B., Ko, J., Naidich, D.: System for automatic detection of lung nodules exhibiting growth. In: SPIE Med. Imag. (2004)
15. Comaniciu, D.: An algorithm for data-driven bandwidth selection. IEEE Trans. Pat. Anal. Mach. Intell. **25** (2003) 281–288
16. Henschke, C.I., et al.: CT screening for lung cancer: frequency and significance of part-solid and non-solid nodules. AJR Am. J. Roentgenol. **178** (2002) 1053–1057
17. Okada, K., Comaniciu, D., Krishnan, A.: Robust 3D segmentation of pulmonary nodules in multislice CT images. In: MICCAI, Saint Malo (2004)

Tissue Classification of Noisy MR Brain Images Using Constrained GMM

Amit Ruf[1], Hayit Greenspan[1], and Jacob Goldberger[2]

[1] Department of Biomedical Engineering, Tel-Aviv University, Israel
[2] School of Engineering, Bar-Ilan University, Israel

Abstract. We present an automated algorithm for tissue segmentation of noisy, low contrast magnetic resonance (MR) images of the brain. We use a mixture model composed of a large number of Gaussians, with each brain tissue represented by a large number of the Gaussian components in order to capture the complex tissue spatial layout. The intensity of a tissue is considered a global feature and is incorporated into the model through parameter tying of all the related Gaussians. The EM algorithm is utilized to learn the parameter-tied Gaussian mixture model. A new initialization method is applied to guarantee the convergence of the EM algorithm to the global maximum likelihood. Segmentation of the brain image is achieved by the affiliation of each voxel to a selected tissue class. The presented algorithm is used to segment 3D, T1–weighted, simulated and real MR images of the brain into three different tissues, under varying noise conditions. Quantitative results are presented and compared with state–of–the–art results reported in the literature.

1 Introduction

MRI images contain various noise artifacts, such as intra-tissue noise, inter-tissue intensity contrast reduction, partial-volume effects and others [1]. Reviews on methods for brain image segmentation (e.g., [2]) present the degradation in the quality of segmentation algorithms due to such noise, and recent publications can be found addressing various aspects of these concerns (e.g. [3]). Due to the artifacts present, classical voxel-wise based classification methods, such as Mixture of Gaussians modeling (e.g., [4]), may give unrealistic results, with tissue class regions appearing granular, fragmented, or violating anatomical constraints. Incorporating statistical spatial information via a statistical atlas [5], provides a means for improving the segmentation results. The co-registration of the input image and the atlas, a computationally intensive procedure, is critical in this scenario. Another conventional method to improve segmentation smoothness and immunity to noise is by using a Hidden Markov Random Field (HMRF), thus modeling neighboring voxels interactions [6,7].

This paper describes a robust, unsupervised and parametric method for the tissue segmentation of 3D MR brain images with a high degree of noise. The

J. Duncan and G. Gerig (Eds.): MICCAI 2005, LNCS 3750, pp. 790–797, 2005.

number of tissues is assumed given. Each tissue is modeled with multiple four-dimensional Gaussians, where each Gaussian represents a localized region (3 spatial features) and the intensity characteristic per region (T1 intensity feature). The incorporation of the spatial information within the feature space is novel, as well as the use of a large number of Gaussians per brain tissue in order to capture the complicated spatial layout of the individual tissues. Note that models to-date use a single Gaussian per tissue type (e.g. [4]). An elaborate initialization scheme is suggested to link the set of Gaussians per tissue type, such that each Gaussian in the set has similar intensity characteristics with minimal overlapping spatial supports. The hypothesis is that all the Gaussians within the same class represent the same physical tissue with the same mean intensity and the same intensity covariance. It is assumed that the intensity inhomogeneity effect has been dealt with in a pre-processing phase. A detailed description of the proposed algorithm is provided in Sect.2. Experimental results are presented in Sect.3. The algorithm is validated on simulated brain as well as real brain volumes.

2 The CGMM Segmentation Framework

Given a brain volume, a 4-dim. feature vector is extracted for each voxel v. The main feature is the voxel intensity, denoted by v^I. In order to include spatial information, the (x, y, z) position is appended to the feature vector. We use the notation $v^{xyz} = (v^x, v^y, v^z)$ for the three spatial features. Denote the set of the feature vectors by $\{v_t \,|\, t = 1, ..., T\}$ where T is the number of voxels in the image. In order to capture the complex spatial layout, we model the image using a mixture of many Gaussians: $f(v_t|\theta) = \sum_{i=1}^{n} \alpha_i f_i(v_t|\mu_i, \Sigma_i)$ such that n is the number of components in the mixture model, μ_i and Σ_i are the mean and the covariance of the i-th Gaussian component f_i, and α_i is the i-th mixture coefficient. The spatial shape of the tissues is highly non-convex. However, since we use a mixture of many components, each Gaussian component is modeling a small local region. Hence, the implicit convexity assumption induced by the Gaussian distribution is reasonable (and is empirically justified in the next section).

The intra variability of the intensity feature within a tissue (bias) is mainly due to artifacts of the MRI imaging process and once eliminated (via bias-correction schemes) is significantly less than the inter-variability among different tissues. It is therefore sufficient to model the intensity variability within a tissue by a single Gaussian (in the intensity feature). To incorporate this insight into the model, we further assume that each Gaussian is linked to a single tissue and all the Gaussians related to the same tissue share the same intensity parameters.

Technically, this linkage is defined via a grouping function. In addition to the GMM parameter set θ, we define a parameter π which is a grouping function $\pi : \{1, ..., n\} \rightarrow \{1, ..., k\}$ from the set of Gaussians to the set of tissues. We assume that the number of tissues is known and the grouping function is learned in the initialization step. The intensity feature should be roughly uniform in each Gaussian component spatial support, thus, its spatial and intensity features are assumed uncorrelated. These assumptions impose the following structure on the mean and variance of the Gaussian components:

$$\mu_i = \begin{pmatrix} \mu_i^{\mathrm{xyz}} \\ \\ \mu_{\pi(i)}^{\mathrm{I}} \end{pmatrix} \qquad \Sigma_i = \begin{pmatrix} \Sigma_i^{\mathrm{xyz}} & 0 \\ \\ 0 & \Sigma_{\pi(i)}^{\mathrm{I}} \end{pmatrix} \qquad i = 1, ..., n \qquad (1)$$

where $\pi(i)$ is the tissue linked to the i-th Gaussian component and μ_j^{I} and Σ_j^{I} are the mean and variance parameters of all the Gaussian components that are linked to the j-th tissue. We term the GMM model with the additional constraints Constrained-GMM (CGMM). The main advantage of the CGMM is the ability to combine in a tractable way, a local description of the spatial layout of a tissue with a global description of the tissue's intensity.

2.1 Model Initialization

We present a novel semi-supervised top-down initialization method that utilizes our knowledge about the number of tissues of interest. The initialization is a dual step procedure. In the first step K-means clustering is done based only on the intensity feature in order to extract a rough segmentation into 6 tissue classes (WM, GM, CSF, WM+GM, WM+CSF, GM+CSF) where combination of classes is due to partial volume effects. We assume the WM voxels to be of highest intensity, and the CSF voxels to be of lowest intensity. Voxels that belong to the four other classes are labeled as GM voxels. This rough but important initial clustering determines an initial group of voxels that belong to each tissue. We use this segmentation to calculate the approximate position of the Gaussians in each tissue. The next step is a top-down procedure. We iteratively split regions until we obtain convex regions that are suitable for Gaussian modeling. Each iteration of the spatial region splitting algorithm involves three steps: 1) A connected–components (CC) algorithm is used to define distinct regions which should be modeled by one or more Gaussians. Regions with less voxels than a user defined threshold are deleted and their voxels are marked as background noise, thus avoiding redundant Gaussians caused by noise; 2) Each region is encircled with the smallest ellipsoid possible[1]. If the volume inside the ellipsoid, that is *not* part of the region, is higher than a user defined threshold and the ellipsoid volume supports more voxels than the defined threshold value of minimum voxels per a region, the region is marked for further splitting; 3) A marked region is further split using K-means on the spatial features, into two distinct (not necessarily connected) subregions. The splitting algorithm iteratively proceeds as long as at least one region is marked for partitioning. Once the regions are determined, each region is modeled with a single Gaussian. The Gaussian's spatial parameters are estimated using the spatial features of the voxels supported by the region, while the intensity parameters is estimated using all the voxels supported by all the regions of the same tissue. Thus, Gaussians from the same tissue receive the same initial intensity parameter. Furthermore, each Gaussian is tagged with a label which indicates its tissue affiliation. Overall, the initialization process determines and fixes the grouping function π.

[1] Using the GBT® (Geometric Boundary Toolbox).

Figure 1(a)-(e) illustrates the steps of the initialization process as applied to a 2D synthetic image with two tissues. A similar process is performed in 3D using a 3D ellipsoid instead of a 2D convex polygon for the convexity measure.

2.2 Parameter Learning for the Constrained GMM

Following initialization, an iterative maximum-likelihood (ML) learning process is conducted. Gaussians with the same tissue–label are constrained to have the same intensity parameters throughout. A modification of the standard (EM) algorithm for learning GMM is required, as shown in the following equations. The expectation step of the EM algorithm for the CGMM model is (same as the unconstrained version):

$$w_{it} = p(i|v_t) = \frac{\alpha_i f_i(v_t|\mu_i, \Sigma_i)}{\sum_{l=1}^{n} \alpha_l f_l(v_t|\mu_l, \Sigma_l)} \qquad i = 1, ..., n \qquad t = 1, ..., T \qquad (2)$$

We shall use the abbreviations:

$$n_i = \sum_{t=1}^{T} w_{it} \quad , \quad k_j = \sum_{i \in \pi^{-1}(j)} n_i \qquad j = 1, ..., k \qquad i = 1, ..., n \qquad (3)$$

such that n_i is the expected number of voxels that are related to the i-th Gaussian component and k_j is the expected number of voxels that are related to the j-th tissue. The maximization in the M-step is done given the constraint on the intensity parameters.

$$\alpha_i = \frac{n_i}{n} \qquad i = 1, ..., n \qquad j = 1, ..., k \qquad (4)$$

$$\mu_i^{\mathrm{xyz}} = \frac{1}{n_i} \sum_{t=1}^{T} w_{it} v_t^{\mathrm{xyz}} \qquad \Sigma_i^{\mathrm{xyz}} = \frac{1}{n_i} \sum_{t=1}^{T} w_{it} \left(v_t^{\mathrm{xyz}} - \mu_i^{\mathrm{xyz}}\right) \left(v_t^{\mathrm{xyz}} - \mu_i^{\mathrm{xyz}}\right)^{\top}$$

$$\mu_j^{\mathrm{I}} = \frac{1}{k_j} \sum_{i \in \pi^{-1}(j)} \sum_{t=1}^{T} w_{it} v_t^{I} \qquad \Sigma_j^{\mathrm{I}} = \frac{1}{k_j} \sum_{i \in \pi^{-1}(j)} \sum_{t=1}^{T} w_{it} \left(v_t^{\mathrm{I}} - \mu_j^{\mathrm{I}}\right)^2$$

The grouping function π that links between the Gaussian components and the tissues is not altered by the EM iterations. Therefore, the affiliation of a Gaussian component to a tissue remains unchanged. However, since the learning is performed simultaneously on all the tissues, voxels can move between tissues during the iterations.

Figure 1(f) shows the CGMM model obtained for the synthetic image shown in Fig.1(a) after seven EM iterations (following the top-down initialization). A 2σ spatial projection of the region-of-support for each Gaussian in the model is shown (where different shades of gray represent the two distinct tissues present).

If the representation phase is a transition from voxels to clusters (Gaussians) in feature space, the segmentation process can be thought of as forming a linkage

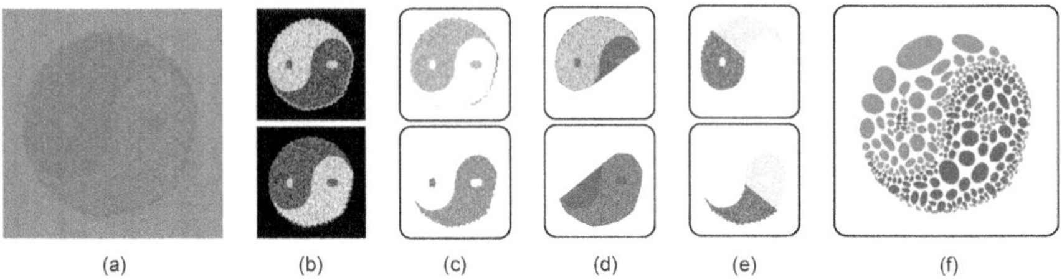

Fig. 1. Illustration of the Initialization process on a 2D synthetic image: (a) Input image; (b) Segmentation into two groups using the intensity feature only; (c) Connected–components (CC) algorithm; (d) CC (region) is encircled with a convex polygon; (e) CC is clustered into two regions based on spatial features only; (f) Gaussian mixture modeling (seven EM iterations).

back from the feature space to the raw input domain. Each voxel is linked to the most probable Gaussian cluster, i.e. to the component of the model that maximizes the a-posteriori probability. The current model uses multiple Gaussians per tissue. Thus we need to sum over the posterior probabilities of all the identical tissue Gaussians to get the posterior probability of each voxel to originate from a specific tissue:

$$\text{tissue-label}_t = \arg\max_{j\in\{1,...,k\}} \sum_{i\in\pi^{-1}(j)} \alpha_i f_i(v_t|\mu_i, \Sigma_i) \qquad t = 1, ..., T \qquad (5)$$

such that tissue-label$_t \in \{1, ...k\}$ is one of the tissues. The linkage of each voxel to a tissue label provides the final segmentation map.

3 Experiments and Results

In the following we present a set of experiments to validate the proposed framework. We used a severely noised normal T1 MR brain data set from the BrainWEB simulator repository [2] as well as 15 real normal T1 MR brain data sets from the Center for Morphometric Analysis at Massachusetts General Hospital repository [3] (hereon termed IBSR). An important pre-processing step is used to extract the brain region as well as to correct any intensity inhomogeneity (bias) present within the images. A variety of techniques are known in the literature. We use the algorithm proposed by Van-Leemput [6] as implemented in the EMS software package [4]. Next we applied our initialization step followed by EM iterations for CGMM. In our experiments a threshold of 250 voxels per region (Gaussian) is used in the initialization stage. In the first experiment we demon-

[2] http://www.bic.mni.mcgill.ca/brainweb/
[3] http://www.cma.mgh.harvard.edu/ibsr/
[4] http://www.medicalimagecomputing.com/EMS/

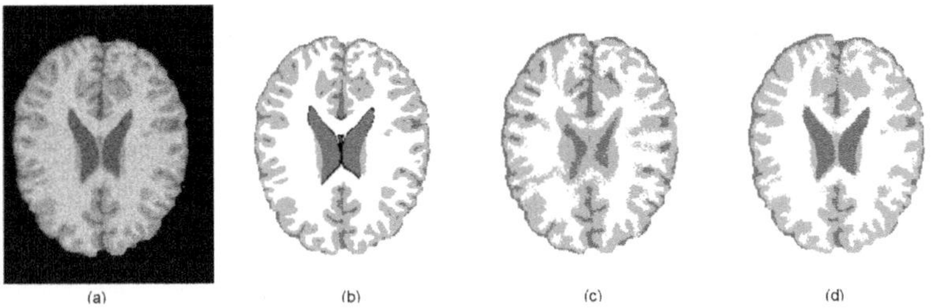

Fig. 2. (a) Slice number 95 from the BrainWEB normal brain simulator; (b) Ground-truth; (c) GMM-Without constraints; (d) CGMM-With constraints.

strate the performance of the CGMM framework as compared with regular EM-based modeling and segmentation. Figure 2 shows slice number 95 taken from the BrainWEB normal simulated brain volume, contaminated with 9% thermal noise artifact (relative to the white matter intensity). The Gaussian parameters were once learned using EM-based modeling (without intensity constraints) and once learned using the CGMM framework (with intensity constraints). Figure 2(c) shows the final segmentation using regular EM-based modeling. The segmentation result is noticeably distorted due to the high noise present. The segmentation results of the CGMM framework are shown in Fig.2(d). A considerable improvement in the segmentation results can be seen. In the next set of experiments, a comparison is conducted with the well-known EM-based segmentation algorithm of Van-Leemput (hereon termed KVL) [6] implemented by the EMS software package. In the KVL implementation the statistic brain atlas of the SPM99[5] was normalized to the target brain volume. The EMS algorithm was setup to use the HMRF option as well as intensity inhomogeneity correction with 3D polynomial of order 4. Experiments were conducted on the simulated normal MR brain volume with very high thermal noise artifacts as well as on 15 real MR brain volumes from the IBSR. In the CGMM implementation, we used the EMS to remove any intensity inhomogeneity effects from the original real MR brain volumes as well as to extract only the brain tissues from the head volume.

We choose to compare the CGMM and the KVL algorithm with the volumetric overlap metric (the volumetric overlap metric is not claimed to be the best metric for medical image comparisons, but it is widely used). which was also used by [6]. This metric is used to quantitatively measure the overlap between the automatic segmentation and the ground truth for each tissue and every algorithm. Denote by V_{ae}^k the number of voxels that are assigned to tissue k by both the ground truth and the automated algorithm. Similarly, let V_a^k and V_e^k denote the number of voxels assigned to tissue k by the algorithm and the ground truth, respectively. The overlap between the algorithm and the ground truth for tissue k is measured as: $2V_{ae}^k / \left(V_a^k + V_e^k\right)$. This metric attains the value of one if both segmentations are in full agreement and zero if there is no overlap at all.

[5] http://www.fil.ion.ucl.ac.uk/spm/

Table 1. Average and Std volumetric overlap results for CGMM on 16 brain volumes

KVL			CGMM		
WM	GM	CSF	WM	GM	CSF
86.0 ± 2.0	78.9 ± 5.3	20.7 ± 16.6	85.9 ± 3.6	79.5 ± 5.7	26.0 ± 16.3

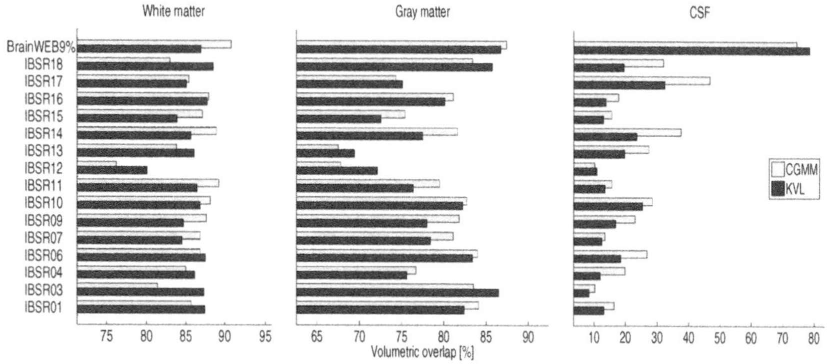

Fig. 3. Overlap metric of the CGMM algorithm (bright) and the KVL algorithm(dark) per each of the 16 volumes. Each graph shows a different tissue. The BrainWEB9% is a simulated volume, where all the rest are real brain volumes.

Figure 3 shows the segmentation results of the CGMM algorithm (bright) and the KVL algorithm (dark). The CGMM performance improvement over the KVL is shown in most of the volumes and in all of the tissue types. However, CGMM's gain over the KVL is especially evident within the CSF tissue since the volumetric overlap tend to be more sensitive to outliers when dealing with small objects. Table 1 shows that the average results of the CGMM are slightly better than KVL in gray matter and even more significant in CSF. Furthermore, Fig.4 shows the smoothness in the segmentation output. The strength of the CGMM framework is more clearly evident in its robustness to noise and smooth segmentation results in increased noise levels.

4 Discussion

We present a fully automated, parametric, unsupervised algorithm for tissue classification of extremely noisy and low contrast MR images of the brain. The tissues are assumed to have been cleaned (preprocessed) of any intensity inhomogeneity. The algorithm was tested on different real brain volumes as well as heavily noised simulated brain volume. Quantitative comparison with KVL state-of-the-art algorithm in the presence of extremely noised images was performed and has shown that the CGMM presents better visual results in presence of high noise as well as better quantitative results - especially in CSF segmentation. This result holds with increased noise up to 9%, a level that presents a challenge

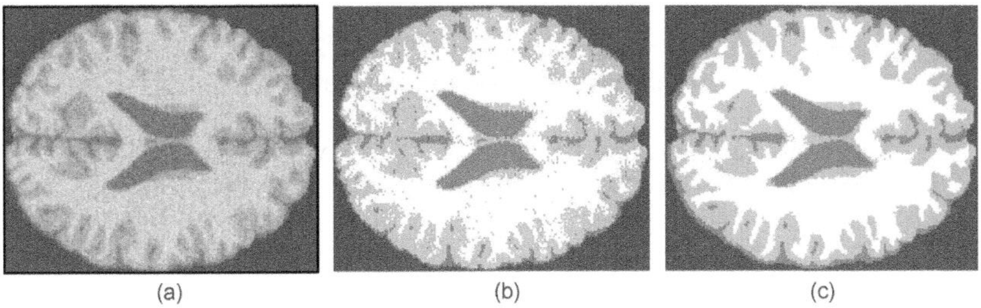

Fig. 4. Comparison of CGMM vs. KVL algorithm for segmentation of slice 95 from BrainWEB simulator with 9% noise level and no bias (a) Original image (b) KVL algorithm (c) CGMM algorithm

for most of the existing segmentation algorithms. The linkage of Gaussians has strong resemblance to using a HMRF model. The main difference is that the intensity information is linked adaptively and globally within the image, in contrast to a HMRF model that integrates information from the nearest neighbors only and in predetermined neighborhoods. These differences result in improved segmentation and decreased tissue region granularity in the presence of extreme noise. The CGMM is shown to provide a parametric framework good enough for segmentation without requiring a priori registration to a brain atlas, thus, it can be useful for abnormal brain segmentation, image registration as well as image retrieval. Currently we are working on an extension of the model to incorporate intensity inhomogeneities as well as to support multi-channel volumes.

References

1. Macovski, A.: Noise in MRI. Magn. Reson. Med. **36** (1996) 494–7
2. Pham, D.L., Xu, C., Prince, J.L.: Current methods in medical image segmentation. Annual Review of Biomedical Engineering **2** (2000) 315–337
3. Dugas-Phocion, G., Ballester, M.Á.G., Malandain, G., Lebrun, C., Ayache, N.: Improved em-based tissue segmentation and partial volume effect quantification in multi-sequence brain mri. In: MICCAI. (2004) 26–33
4. Kapur, T., Grimson, W.E., Wells, W.M., Kikinis, R.: Segmentation of brain tissue from magnetic resonance images. Med Image Anal. **1** (1996) 109–27
5. Prastawa, M., Gilmore, J., Lin, W., Gerig, G.: Automatic segmentation of neonatal brain mri. In: MICCAI. (2004) 10–17
6. Leemput, K.V., Maes, F., Vandermeulen, D., Suetens, P.: Automated model-based tissue classification of MR images of the brain. IEEE trans. on medical imaging **18** (1999) 897–908
7. Zhang, Y., Brady, M., Smith, S.: Segmentation of brain MR images through a hidden markov random field model and the expectation-maximization algorithm. IEEE trans. on medical imaging **20** (2001) 45–57

Automatic Left Atrium Segmentation by Cutting the Blood Pool at Narrowings

Matthias John and Norbert Rahn

Siemens Medical Solutions, Henkestrasse 127, 91052 Erlangen,Germany
{matthias.mj.john, norbert.rahn}@siemens.de

Abstract. This paper presents a method to extract heart structures from CTA and MRA data sets, in particular the left atrium. First, the segmented blood pool is subdivided at narrowings in small components. Second, these basic components are merged automatically so that they represent the different heart structures. The resulting cutting surfaces have a relatively small diameter compared to the diameter of the neighboring heart chambers. Both steps are controlled by only one fixed parameter. The method is fast and allows interactive post-processing by the user. Experiments on various data sets show the accuracy, robustness and repeatability of this approach.

1 Introduction

Atrial fibrillation is the most common heart arrhythmia and greatly increases the risk of stroke. This irregular heart rhythm originates in the atrial heart chambers. Over 2 million people are affected in the U.S. alone. One way to treat and cure atrial fibrillation is catheter ablation. First electrical signals in the heart muscle are mapped and localized. One successful approach to finally eliminate the atrial fibrillation is to isolate the pulmonary veins of the left atrium electrically from the rest of the heart by ablation. The dissimilarity of different left atrium shapes complicates the procedures. CT or MR imaging supports planning and intervention of these catheter ablations. After segmenting the left atrium and the pulmonary veins from the images the individual patient morphology can be visualized and the extracted boundary surface can be provided to electro-anatomical mapping systems.

CTA and MRA images are CT and MR images enhanced by contrast agent filled blood vessels and chambers. This provides higher image intensities for the blood pool than for surrounding tissues and helps to extract the left atrium voxels. Nevertheless, the left atrium segmentation is usually done manually or by segmentation tools that are not specific to this task, which yields segmentation times larger than 30 minutes. The reason for the absence of more specific automatic segmentation algorithms might be the complex and varying shape of the left atrium. (For instance position and number of the pulmonary veins can vary for different patients.) This is in contrast to the left ventricle, where a lot of segmentation approaches were suggested. Automatic methods for left ventricle segmentation are usually level-set methods [13], atlas-based methods or algorithms based on active shape models [3]. Active shape models are the most common approach for such segmentations. Recently, a shape model approach for the left atrium segmentation from CT images was proposed in [1].

J. Duncan and G. Gerig (Eds.): MICCAI 2005, LNCS 3750, pp. 798 – 805, 2005.

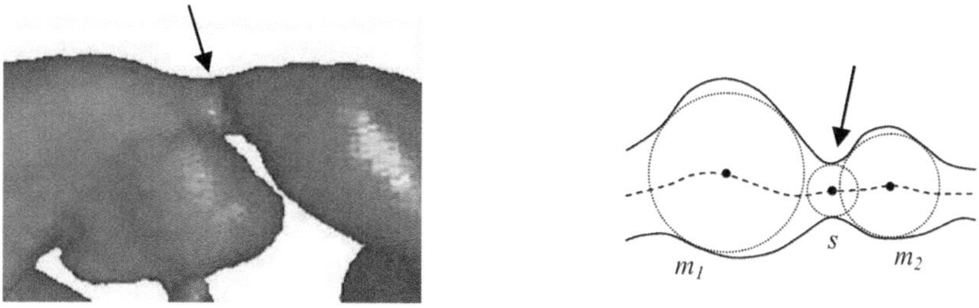

Fig. 1. Left: A narrowing and a possible cut. **Right:** Medial Axis (dashed line) of a two dimensional object (interior of the solid lines) and two locally maximal medial balls m_1, m_2 and the smallest medial ball s between m_1 and m_2. The ball s lies at the narrowing between m_1 and m_2.

In our method we make use of the fact that neighboring heart chambers can be separated with cuts at narrowings of the blood pool. The size of such a cutting surface is relatively small compared to the size of the neighboring heart chambers. We give an algorithmic formulation how to cut a blood pool at all narrowings. This subdivision into basic components is related to the medial axis transform which describes a volumetric object as a union of balls. The balls touch the surface of the object in at least two points, their center points build the medial axis (see Fig. 1). In this paper we associate with every locally maximal ball a basic component. If we follow the union of balls along the centers from a maximal ball to a neighboring maximal ball the radii first get smaller and then increase. At the smallest ball on this way we have a narrowing of the object, which is a possible cut. Because of this relation between our components and the medial axis transform we make use of a distance transformation algorithm [4] that helps to construct this data structure and gives information about the size of the basic components.

The merging of the basic components to build up the heart chambers is similar to the merging process used in watershed-transformation algorithms [11] and algorithms for surface reconstruction of geometric point sets [5]: In our setting two components are merged if the separating structure is large, so the difference to the size of the neighboring components is small. Observe that the common merging procedure for watershed-transformations in medical image segmentation handles every voxel as one element, whereas an element in our merging procedure is a basic component that usually consist of thousands of voxels. Furthermore the merging does not depend on the gray values but on the geometric structure of the object. Also for fast and efficient interactive post-processing by the user we adapt techniques originally developed for interactive watershed-transformations [7,8].

2 Method

Before we discuss the technical details of our segmentation method we want to give an intuition about its basic ideas. Figure 2 gives an overview of the whole method.

To decompose a segmented blood pool object into the different heart chambers and vessel structures it can be cut at narrowings. Figure 1 shows such a narrowing for a vessel which might be a possible cut. The problem is to find the right cuts

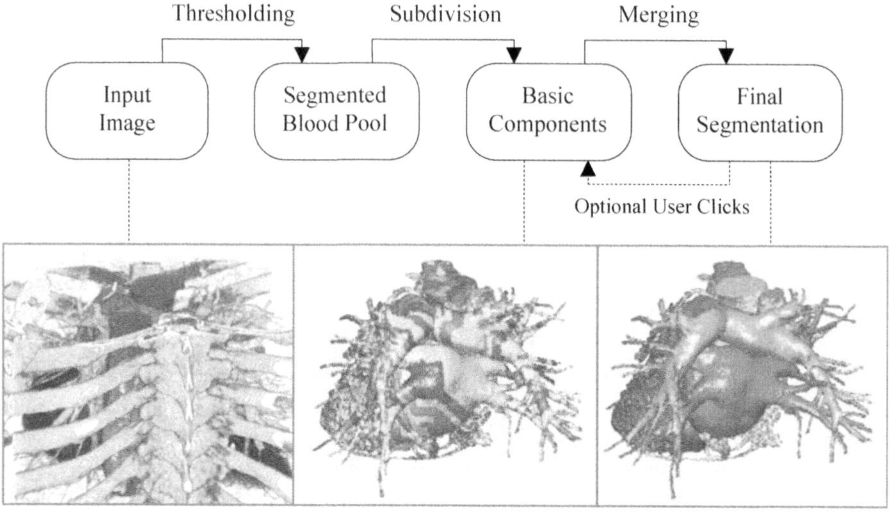

Fig. 2. Overview of the algorithm. Three steps of the algorithm are visualized in the images with a CTA data set. **Left:** A volume visualization of the complete data set. **Middle:** Subdivision of the blood pool into basic components. **Right:** Merged components that represent the heart chambers and vessels.

automatically. We can make the following observation: The diameter of the correct cuts is small compared to the diameter of the adjacent components.

The main idea of the algorithm is to subdivide the segmented blood pool object at all possible narrowings and merge the resulting basic components to get the heart structures. We start with the basic components and merge neighboring components if the diameter of a separating surface (i.e. the cut at the narrowing) is nearly as large as the diameter of the adjacent components. We end up with cuts with relatively small diameters compared to the adjacent components.

2.1 Segmenting the Blood Pool

The extraction of heart structures requires the extraction of the blood pool from the contrast enhanced CTA and MRA data sets. We use a simple threshold-based approach. With a given threshold we separate the blood pool voxels from other structures. This works fine with MRA data sets. With CTA data sets such a threshold also segments voxels that represent bone tissue. Fortunately, blood pool structures and bone structures only touch each other, but do not intersect deeply. Therefore, it is no problem to separate these structures by the subsequent steps of the algorithm (see Section 2.2 and 2.3).

For CTA data one can use a constant Hounsfield threshold for segmenting the blood pool. Alternatively, the algorithm can let the user pick a voxel inside the blood pool. A threshold can then be computed automatically from the local neighborhood of this seed point.

If we allow the algorithm to let the user select a voxel inside the blood pool, we can use region growing. This helps to eliminate a lot of bone tissue voxels at the beginning and speeds up the subsequent algorithm steps.

2.2 Computing Basic Components

In this section we will show how to subdivide a binary image into several components. Figure 3 gives an overview of this part of the algorithm.

The first step is to compute the distance transformation of the binary image. For each marked voxel (inside object) we compute its squared Euclidian distance to the closest unmarked voxel (outside object). So voxels deep inside the object get a high value, voxels close to the boundary of the object get a small value. Zero is assigned to all voxels outside the object. Several algorithms were proposed for this task, see [4] for an overview. We use the fast and exact method described in [12].

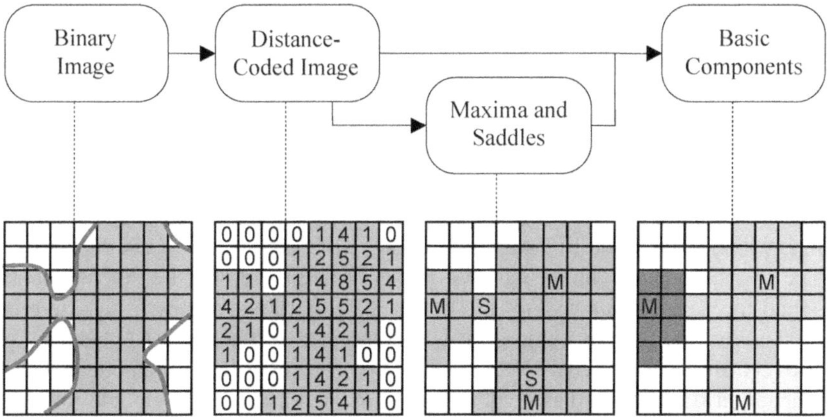

Fig. 3. Subdivision overview. The lower row shows a two dimensional example on a 2D grid. First, a distance transformation is computed. Then maxima and saddle points are extracted. Finally every object voxel is assigned to a maximum which results in the basic components.

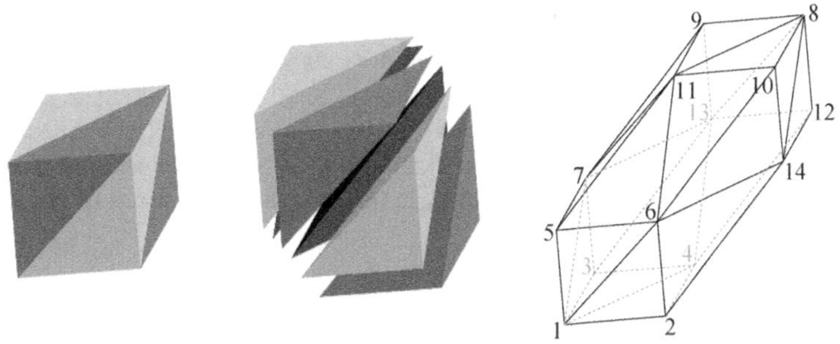

Fig. 4. Left: A Freudenthal subdivision of a cube. **Right:** The 14-neighborhood of a grid vertex of a regular cubic grid, if every grid cube is subdivided by the Freudenthal scheme.

In a second step we determine all voxels that are local maxima and saddle points of the distance transformation. A (local) maximum is a voxel, that has a larger value than all its neighboring voxels. A saddle (point) is a voxel that has (at least) two voxels with larger values in its neighborhood and a ring of voxels with smaller values that separates the two larger ones.

Both maxima and saddles lie on the medial axis of the object. Every maximum lies in the center of a basic component. Every saddle lies at the center of a separating surface between two neighboring basic components which is the cutting surface at a narrowing of the object. The other way around, every basic component contains a maximum and every separating surface between two basic components contains a saddle. So, determining these two types of voxels helps to compute the basic components.

It can happen, that two neighboring voxels have the same value. To simplify the handling of maxima and saddles we want to avoid this situation when comparing voxels. Solutions to such equality problems are discussed in [11]. We prefer a simple one: We define a fixed order over all voxels (only depending on the x-,y-, and z-coordinates). In the case of equal voxel values we compare the voxels with respect to this order.

In a third step we assign every voxel to a basic component. Each local maximum is the center of a basic component. To assign a voxel to a basic component, we follow the gradient of this voxel until we end up in a maximum. To be more precise we follow a line of voxels with increasing distance function values until we reach a maximum. We determine this line by computing for each voxel the neighboring voxel with the steepest ascent.

The whole computation of maxima, saddles and basic components depends on the choice of the local neighborhood. We use a 14-neighborhood, i.e. 14 neighbors are assigned to each voxel (see Figure 4). This neighborhood comes from a tetrahedral subdivision of the regular cubic grid, where the grid vertices are the center points of the voxels. If we take a voxel v, all voxels that are connected by an edge to v in the tetrahedral grid are defined as neighbors of v. We get a regular 14-neighborhood if we use the Freudenthal subdivision. This and other tetrahedral subdivisions are discussed in [2]. The computation of maxima and saddles can be done fast using lookup tables; such techniques are described in [6] in the context of multiresolution isosurface extraction. The advantage of the 14-neighborhood is the resulting regular grid and the relatively small number of neighbors compared to the standard 26-neighborhood. Furthermore, we have the following guarantees: Every basic component contains a maximum and the surface between two components contains a saddle. This is because the 14-neighborhood goes back to a tetrahedral subdivision, which directly extends the discrete samples of the volume space to the whole space R^3 by linear interpolation. So the maxima and saddles are critical points of a real continuous space and the guarantees described above come from the Morse theory of continuous spaces [10].

2.3 Merging of Basic Components

The granularity of the basic components is too large to represent real heart structures. Therefore we need to merge the basic components to build up larger structures. We start merging neighboring components m_1 and m_2 that have a separating surface s with a large diameter, i.e. if

$$\text{merging value}(m_1, m_2, s) = \min(\text{diam}(m_1), \text{diam}(m_2)) - \text{diam}(s) \quad (1)$$

is small. The diameter of a component is the Euclidian distance function value of its corresponding maximum. The diameter of a separating surface is the Euclidian distance function value of its corresponding saddle.

Merging two components means algorithmically: Deleting symbolically the corresponding saddle and the smaller maximum and rearranging the saddles that were incident to the smaller maximum. Observe that some of the other merging values can change in this step.

We merge all neighboring components with a merging value smaller than a given threshold. We start with the components with the smallest merging value and go on in increasing order.

After the merging process the resulting components are separated at narrowings which have a small diameter compared to the diameter of the adjacent regions. Their merging value is larger than the given merging threshold.

2.4 Interactive User Control

After the previous algorithm steps the user can mark voxels as positive (= has to be part of the final segmentation) and negative (= not part of the final segmentation). We assign these markers to the basic components corresponding to the marked voxels. Now we can restart the merging process of Section 2.3, but we forbid merging of different labeled components and force merging of components with the same label.

Because the merging is very fast and the basic component subdivision can be reused, marking voxels by the user gives the user immediately a result.

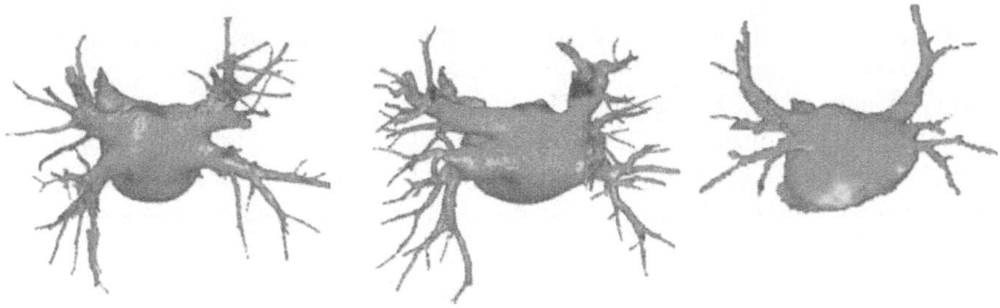

Fig. 5. Some results of the left atrium segmentation method. **Left, Middle:** CTA **Right:** MRA.

3 Experiments and Results

We applied our algorithm to 40 coronary CTA and 20 coronary MRA data sets from different manufacturers and clinics. The results were evaluated and discussed with electrophysiologists and radiologists. The goal of our study was to extract the left atrium with as little user interaction as possible. The user started the segmentation by selecting a voxel in the left atrium as a seed point. After the automatic segmentation procedure the user was able to mark additional voxels to interactively improve the result. The results were visualized either by a marching cubes isosurface [9] or by volume rendering.

All data sets had an in-slice resolution of 512 × 512 voxels, the number of slices varied from 40 to 500, and the voxel size varied from $0.318 \times 0.318 \times 0.4\ mm^3$ to $0.859 \times 0.859 \times 1.4\ mm^3$. The data sets included anomaly cases (more than two pulmonary veins on one side of the left atrium) and images with rather bad scan quality.

In all data sets we successfully extracted the left atrium with a merging threshold of 2.3 mm. On some of the data sets user interaction helped to improve the results, usually for images with poor quality. In all cases the algorithm was able to segment the left atrium including all pulmonary veins and the left atrial appendage. All neighboring structures like the left ventricle, the right atrium, and veins close to the pulmonary veins were excluded. Furthermore, the bone structures in the CTA images were eliminated correctly. The segmentation results were practically independent of the exact position of the users click into the left atrium. This is mainly due to the computation and merging of the basic components which only depends on the geometry of the blood pool. Noisy data sets did not much effected the merging results, because small components due to noise are merged in an early phase to larger and more robust components.

We tested the algorithm on a 2 GHz Pentium IV PC with 1 GB of RAM. The runtime of the algorithm depends on the number of blood pool voxels and varies between 5 (for small MRA data sets) and 45 seconds (for large CTA data sets). After the user added an additional marker the update of the segmentation took always less than a second, which made interactive post-processing with immediate feedback feasible.

4 Conclusions

To extract the left atrium from CTA and MRA images we suggest to cut the blood pool using geometric properties, i.e. to cut at narrowings that are small compared to their neighboring components. This approach gives correct results, which was tested on 40 CTA and 20 MRA data sets. The results are repeatable because of the stable method and the minimization of user interaction. The algorithm is fast, especially the merging procedure (that operates on the set of maxima and saddles which is much smaller than the number of all object voxels). The algorithm gives robust results even for noisy data sets.

To further evaluate the algorithm we will start a more detailed clinical evaluation. Besides supporting the intervention by visualizing the left atrium we will use the results for accurate 3D volume measurements and the support of electro-anatomical mapping systems. Possible future research directions are the automatic segmentation of other heart chambers and the automatic bone removal from CTA images.

References

1. Berg, J. v., Lorenz, C.: Accurate left atrium segmentation in multislice CT images using a shape model. Proc. SPIE Medical Imaging, San Diego, 2005.
2. Carr, H., Möller, T. Snoeyink, J.: Simplicial subdivisions and sampling artifacts. Proc. 11th IEEE Visualization, 99-106, 2001.
3. Cootes, T. F., Taylor, C. J.: Statistical models of appearance for medical image analysis and computer vision. Proc. SPIE Medical Imaging, San Diego, 2001.

4. Cuisenaire O.: Distance transformations: fast algorithms and applications to medical image processing. PhD thesis, Université catholique de Louvain (UCL), Belgium, 1999.
5. Giesen, J., John, M.: Surface reconstruction based on a dynamical system. Computer Graphics Forum, 21(3):363-371, 2002.
6. Gerstner, T., Pajorola, R.: Topology preserving and controlled topology simplifying multiresolution isosurface extraction. Proc. 10th IEEE Visualization , 259-266, 2000.
7. Kahn, H. K., Peitgen, H. O., IWT – Interactive watershed transform: A hierarchical method for efficient interactive and automated segmentation of multidimensional grayscale images. Proc. SPIE Medical Imaging, 5032:643-653, 2003.
8. Kuhnigk, J. M., Hahn, H. K., Hindennach, M., Dicken, V., Krass, S., Peitgen, H. O.: Lung lobe segmentation by anatomy-guided 3D watershed transform. Proc. SPIE Medical Imaging, 5032:1482-1490, 2003.
9. Lorensen, W., Cline, H.: Marching cubes: A high resolution 3D surface construction algorithm. Computer Graphics, 21(4): 163-169, 1987.
10. Milnor, J.: Morse Theory. Princeton University Press, New Jersey, 1963.
11. Roerdink, J. B. T. M., Meijster, A.: The watershed transform: Definitions, algorithms, and parallelization strategies, Fundamenta Informaticae, 41:187-228, 2000.
12. Saito, T., Toriwaki, J.: New algorithms for Euclidian distance transformation of an n-dimensional digitized picture with applications. Pattern Recognition, 27(11):1551-1565, 1994.
13. Sethian, J. A.. Level set methods and fast marching methods: Evolving interfaces in computational geometry, fluid mechanics, computer vision, and materials science. Cambridge University Press, 1999.

Automatic Vascular Tree Formation Using the Mahalanobis Distance

Julien Jomier, Vincent LeDigarcher, and Stephen R. Aylward

Computer-Aided Diagnosis and Display Lab, Department of Radiology,
The University of North Carolina at Chapel Hill, 27510 Chapel Hill, USA
{jomier, aylward}@unc.edu
vincent.ledigarcher@cpe.fr

Abstract. We present a novel technique for the automatic formation of vascular trees from segmented tubular structures. Our method combines a minimum spanning tree algorithm with a minimization criterion of the Mahalanobis distance. First, a multivariate class of connected junctions is defined using a set of trained vascular trees and their corresponding image volumes. Second, a minimum spanning tree algorithm forms the tree using the Mahalanobis distance of each connection from the "connected" class as a cost function. Our technique allows for the best combination of the discrimination criteria between connected and non-connected junctions and is also modality, organ and segmentation specific.

1 Introduction

Segmentation of vascular structures from volume images reflects several challenges. Among them, accuracy of centerline extraction as well as complex formation of the vascular trees have led to powerful algorithms.

Several segmentation techniques have shown high accuracy and robustness in extracting vascular structures from MR and CT datasets. In fact, the curve evolution algorithm [5] produces accurate vascular segmentations by combining the modified curvature diffusion equation (MCDE) with a level-set based technique. On the other hand, Aylward et al. [1] use a ridge traversal technique with width estimation to extract vascular centerline and estimated radius at each point along blood vessels. Both techniques have shown robustness to noise and high accuracy. However, most of the vascular segmentation algorithms do not form trees at the time of extraction but rather consider each blood vessel independently.

Being able to visualize the vascular tree is a real motivation. In fact, neurosurgeons and interventional radiologists must often occlude blood vessels during vascular procedures. The risk of stroke to the patient depends largely upon the collateral flow provided by other parts of the circulation. It is therefore important for the clinician to visualize vascular connections in order to make correct decisions about vessel occlusion. Moreover, in parenchymal organs, the identification of vascular territories is crucial for providing resection proposals as well as for preoperatively estimating resection volumes and patient outcome [4]. Some

J. Duncan and G. Gerig (Eds.): MICCAI 2005, LNCS 3750, pp. 806–812, 2005.

recent model-to-image registration methods also rely on a vascular network to perform a hierarchical registration strategy [2].

The most closely related work for tree creation has been done by Bullitt et al. [3]. They have shown that by using a combination of both linear distance and image intensity in suspected regions of connection, a tree can be formed with high accuracy. The combination of the distance and image intensity as a cost function for the minimum spanning tree algorithm is described by the following weighted equation: $4 \cdot I + d$, where I is the ratio of mean intensities along the centerline μ_c of a cylinder centered on the vessel junction (radius larger than that of the child) and on the surface of that same cylinder μ_e such that $I = \frac{\mu_e}{\mu_c}$.

Our method differs from the previous technique in that it combines multiple criteria for connection in an optimal way using a linear discriminant strategy. Moreover, by creating training classes, our algorithm can be made specific to a particular modality, organ and even extraction method.

2 Methods

Our method relies on the centerline representation of a blood vessel. In fact, each extracted blood vessel is defined as centerline points (x, y, z) with associated radius r. The tangent $\boldsymbol{t}$ and normal plane $(\boldsymbol{n_1}, \boldsymbol{n_2})$ are computed using finite differences.

2.1 Minimum Spanning Tree and Mahalanobis Distance

Our technique makes use of the minimum spanning tree algorithm based on Prim's method [6]. The main difficulty in forming such vascular tree lies in defining an effective cost function for the junctions and, even with a set of "good" criteria, it can be difficult to find an appropriate linear combination of these values. By definition, in a tree structure, a child can only have one parent. Moreover, a vascular network is usually formed of several trees and if those trees overlap, i.e portal and hepatic vascular systems in the liver, it is often the case where an automated algorithm has to make the choice between two (or more) parents.

Figure 1 shows an example of vascular configuration with two trees. In this case, vessel 5 can be connected to two parents and relies on the cost function to decide the best connection between C_{35} and C_{45}.

Our method provides an optimal way to combine the criteria defining junctions using the Mahalanobis distance. The Mahalanobis distance is a statistic value which measures the distance of a single data point from the sample mean or centroid in the space of the independent variables used to fit a multiple regression model. The Mahalanobis can be formulated as:

$$d_S(x, y) = \sqrt{(x - y)^t S^{-1} (x - y)} \tag{1}$$

where y is the corresponding mean from the class and S its covariance matrix.

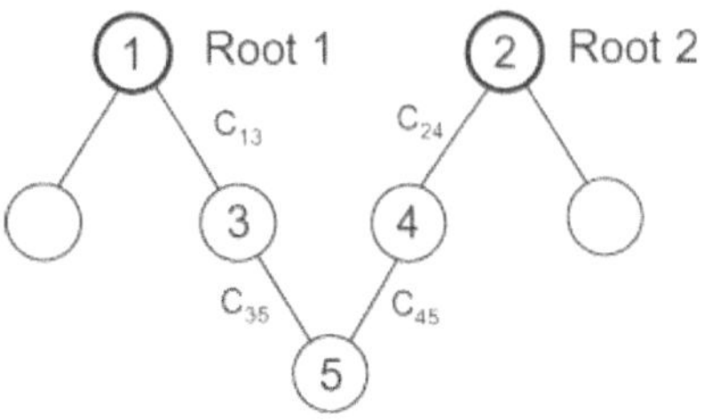

Fig. 1. Example of tree configuration. Vessel 5 should only have one parent. The choice is based on the minimum Mahalanobis distance between C_{35} and C_{45}.

We first define a multivariate class of connected junctions using five criteria:

1. **Distance** from the first point of the child vessel to the closest parent point.
2. **Angle** between the tangent direction of the parent point and the first point of the selected child.
3. **Ratio between the radius** of the parent point and the selected child.
4. **Difference between the radius** of the parent point and the selected child.
5. **Ridgeness**, defined as the mean of the ridgnesses rn at each point from the parent point and the first point of the selected child. rn is defined as follows: $rn = \|\boldsymbol{d} \cdot \mathbf{V_3}\| \cdot \frac{\lambda_2}{\lambda_1} \cdot (1 - \frac{\lambda_3}{\lambda_2}) \cdot \lambda_2$, where d is the direction of the vessel at that point; V_3 is the eigen vector corresponding to the minimum eigen value of the Hessian of the image intensities λ_1, λ_2 and λ_3 the corresponding decreasing set of eigen values.

For each connected junction in the training set, the five criterion values are computed and define the "connected" class. A minimum spanning tree algorithm is then performed using the Mahalanobis distance of the selected connection criteria and the previously defined class. One can notice that the criterion values do not have to be especially minimize - they can be maximized - as long as the class definition and the corresponding Mahalanobis distance are computed with the same criteria. Moreover, our algorithm does not rely on the number of criteria or the quality of the criterion used since the linear discrimination will select the "best" features.

One constraint of this approach is that the Mahalanobis assumes a normal distribution of the variables. However, some of our criteria, i.e the ridgeness, does not fulfill this assumption since the ridgeness is linearly proportional to the significance of a connection. In order to approximate a normal distribution we use the exponential value of the ridgeness centered on zero mean. For each ridgeness value we actually define two values: e^{-rn} and $-e^{-rn}$ in the class definition.

2.2 Robust Class Definition

The definition of the "connected" class requires a set of trained vascular trees and corresponding dataset volumes. Each trained vascular tree is formed manually by an expert. However, the high number of possible connections (100 to 300) and the quality of the segmentation makes this task difficult. Therefore, we perform a robust algorithm to remove any outliers left in the training set. First the multivariate class is computed using all the possible connections available. Second, the Mahalanobis distance of each connection is checked against the defined class. Outliers are removed if their Mahalanobis distance is more than 2σ from the mean distances.

3 Results

We have tested our algorithm on nine brain MR and nine liver CT datasets. CT volumes are contrast enhanced $1 \times 1 \times 3mm^3$ voxels and MRA volumes are time-of-flight data with $1 \times 1 \times 1mm^3$ voxels. The class of connected junctions for both organs are reported in figure 2. As one can see, the connection criteria may have large differences depending on the modality and the organ concerned. This shows the importance of having an organ and modality specific "connected" class. Moreover, the radius ratio in the brain connected cases is close to one and has a small standard deviation compared to the radius ratio obtained for the liver datasets. In fact the segmentation algorithm used [1] is less robust close to the branching regions. This is especially true for our liver datasets where the blood contrast tends to weaken around branch points.

To show that the class definition is reliable across datasets, we perform a leave-one-out analysis. For each organ, the "connected" class is defined using

Criterion	Mean (σ) brains	Mean (σ) livers
Distance	0.534 *(1.450)*	3.441 *(2.696)*
Tangent	-0.021 *(0.553)*	0.038 *(0.604)*
Radius difference	0.216 *(0.338)*	1.200 *(1.063)*
Radius ratio	1.038 *(0.273)*	1.701 *(0.996)*
Ridgeness	0.000 *(0.274)*	0.000 *(0.186)*

Fig. 2. Criteria for connected junctions for brain and liver datasets

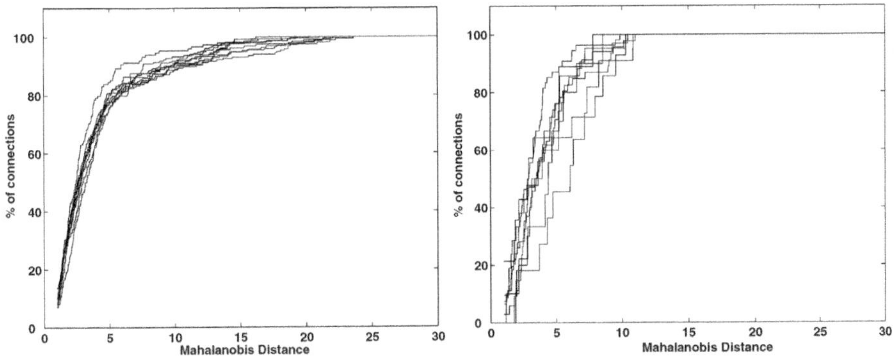

Fig. 3. Percentile of effective connections given a threshold for the Mahalanobis distance for nine brain MRI **(left)** and nine liver CT **(right)**.

eight vascular systems and the Mahalanobis distance is computed for each connection in the remaining vasculature. Figure 3 shows the percentile of accurate connections found given a threshold for the Mahalanobis distance. As one can see, (a) the curves are very similar meaning that the class definition and the Mahalanobis distance are reliable; (b) the thresholds to achieve 100% of connections are different for the brains and livers which strengthen the statement that an organ/modality specific class is necessary.

In the next paragraph we show that our algorithm is able to select junctions even for difficult cases in the brain and in the liver.

3.1 Difficult Cases

We found interesting to test the output of our algorithm in the only region of the human body where the vascular system forms a circle: the circle of Willis in the brain. In this particular case we test two junctions, $J2-3$ and $J2-1$, were the connection effectively exists as shown in figure 4. We trained our algorithm using the eight brain MR datasets previously presented and we computed the Mahalanobis distance for the two junctions. The results are shown in Figure 5.

As expected, the two junctions have similar Mahalanobis distances, therefore we can assume that they should be both connected (or not connected). The distance seems high compared to the class definition obtained during the

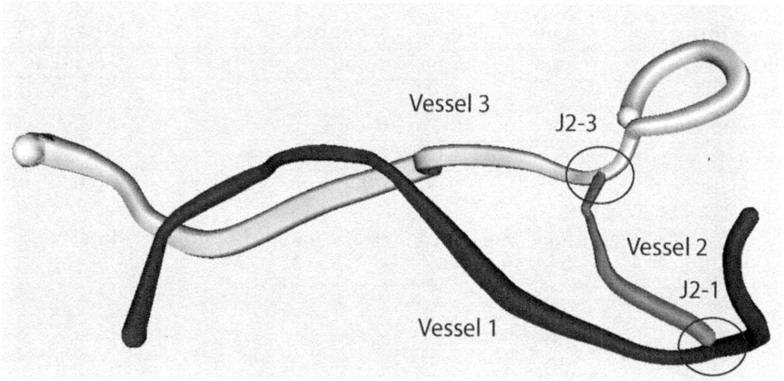

Fig. 4. Circle of Willis in the brain

Criterion	**J2-3**	**J2-1**
Distance	2.369	1.092
Tangent	0.334	-0.819
Radius difference	1.950	1.629
Radius ratio	1.864	2.256
Ridgeness	0.000	0.000
Mahalanobis distance	**30.169**	**34.342**

Fig. 5. Mahalanobis distance of the two junctions in the circle of Willis

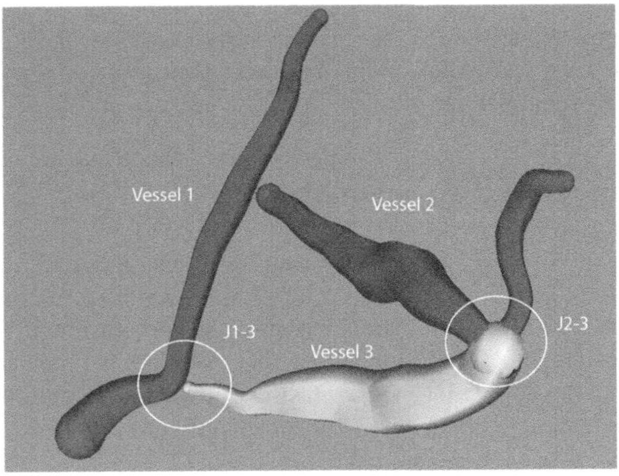

Fig. 6. Difficult case within the liver where the hepatic and portal venous systems overlap

Criterion	**J1-3**	**J2-3**
Distance	2.676	1.236
Tangent	-0.320	-0.769
Radius difference	1.006	1.692
Radius ratio	2.337	0.475
Ridgeness	0.001	0.316
Mahalanobis distance	**1.522**	**10.329**

Fig. 7. Mahalanobis distance of the two junctions in the liver. The distance is inversely proportional to the probability of connection.

training stage and will be in favor of a non connected function. This is due to the particularity of these junctions in the circle of Willis where the radius ratio and difference values are high compared to other connections in the brain. To test this hypothesis, we have trained and compared the junctions without the radius ratio and difference criteria and we obtained respectively $d_{J2-3} = 1.99$ and $d_{J2-1} = 2.25$.

We have also tested our method on a difficult case within the liver where the hepatic and portal venous systems overlap. Figure 6 shows the region of interest where the vessel 3 can be connected to either vessel 1 or vessel 2. In fact, due to a bad segmentation of vessel 3, a standard algorithm would make $J2-3$ the preferred connection over $J1-3$. However, the computed Mahalanobis distances, shown in figure 7, for both junctions are reporting $J1 - 3$ to be the selected connection and not $J2-3$. By looking at the image volume, and also the ridgeness values, $J1-3$ appears to be the real connection in this case as predicted by our algorithm. From the class definition shown in the previous section, one can see that the ratio between the radius of the child and the radius of the parent is not a high significant criterion ($\mu = 1.701, \sigma = 0.996$), therefore the linear discriminant will be less sensitive to this particular feature. Moreover, as one can notice, the value of the non-connected junction is close to the threshold defined in the previous section.

4 Discussion and Conclusions

We have presented a novel algorithm for automatic vascular tree formation based on the Mahalanobis distance. The main advantages of our algorithm are (a) the optimal combination of discrimination parameters and (b) the fact that the defined class from these criteria can be modality, organ and segmentation specific. We have also shown that the class definition is consistent among datasets based on the Mahalanobis distance measure and that our algorithm can detect real branching with high accuracy.

One of the weaknesses of our approach is that it relies on some information regarding the segmentation technique. If the segmentation predicts a radius far from the real radius, our method may fail. However, the other criteria, such as the tangent direction and the ridgeness can help in this case. We are currently working on extending our approach to include direction of the blood flow. This work has been developed using the Insight Toolkit [7].

This work is funded in part by the Whitaker Foundation (TF-04-0008) and the NIH-NIBIB (R01 EB000219).

References

1. Aylward, S., Bullitt, E.: Initialization, Noise, Singularities, and Scale in Height-Ridge Traversal for Tubular Object Centerline Extraction IEEE Transactions on Medical Imaging, Feb, 2002, Pages 61-75
2. Jomier J., Aylward S.: Rigid and Deformable Vasculature-to-Image Registration: A Hierarchical Approach. MICCAI 2004: 829-836
3. Bullitt, E., Aylward S., Liu A., Stone J., Mukherji S., Coffey C., Gerig G., Pizer SM.: 3D graph description of the intracerebral vasculature from segmented MRA and tests of accuracy by comparison with x-ray angiograms IPMI 99. Lecture Notes in Computer Science 1613:308-321
4. D. Selle, B. Preim, A. Schenk, and H.-O. Peitgen, Analysis of vasculature for liver surgical planning IEEE Trans. Med. Imaging., vol. 21,no. 11, pp. 13441357, Nov 2002.
5. Lorigo L., Faugeras O.,Grimson W.E.L.,Keriven R.,Kikinis R.,Nabavi A. and Westin C.-F.: Curves: Curve evolution for vessel segmentation. Medical Image Analysis, 5:195-206, 2001.
6. Aho A. V., Hopcroft J. E., Ullman J.: Data Structures and Algorithms. pp 237 Addison-Wesley Publishing Company, Lebanon, Indiana, U.S.A. 1982
7. L. Ibanez, W. Schroeder, L. Ng and J. Cates, The ITK Software Guide, published by Kitware Inc. ISBN: 1-930934-10-6

The Use of Unwrapped Phase in MR Image Segmentation: A Preliminary Study

Pierrick Bourgeat[1], Jurgen Fripp[1,3], Andrew Janke[2], Graham Galloway[2], Stuart Crozier[3], and Sébastien Ourselin[1]

[1] Autonomous Sytems Laboratory, BioMedIA Lab, CSIRO ICT Centre, Australia
{pierrick.bourgeat, jurgen.fripp, sebastien.ourselin}@csiro.au
[2] Centre for Magnetic Resonance, Queensland, Australia
{Andrew.Janke, gg}@cmr.uq.edu.au
[3] ITEE University of Queensland, Australia
stuart@itee.uq.edu.au

Abstract. This paper considers the problem of tissue classification in 3D MRI. More specifically, a new set of texture features, based on phase information, is used to perform the segmentation of the bones of the knee. The phase information provides a very good discrimination between the bone and the surrounding tissues, but is usually not used due to phase unwrapping problems. We present a method to extract textural information from the phase that does not require phase unwrapping. The textural information extracted from the magnitude and the phase can be combined to perform tissue classification, and used to initialise an active shape model, leading to a more precise segmentation.

1 Introduction

In MRI, the signal intensity, which is normally used for diagnostic purposes, depends upon spin density and relaxation time in order to enhance contrast between different type of tissues inside the body. However, intensity is only one part of the signal. The image acquisition is performed in the K-space [1], resulting in a complex signal, that can be decomposed as a magnitude, and a phase component as shown in Figure 1. Depending on the choice of the pulse sequence, the phase can represent different types of information:

- for angiography, the acquisition sequence is designed to purposefully sensitise the image to phase due to velocity of moving spins and emphasise the motion of blood.
- for conventional anatomical imaging methods, the images are usually displayed in magnitude mode and thus the phase information is not used. In this context the phase information is non-coherent dephasing caused by chemical shift and local magnetic susceptibility.

The latter effect is due to differing magnetic susceptibilities within the body and/or instrumental imperfections. Some imaging sequences are more sensitive

J. Duncan and G. Gerig (Eds.): MICCAI 2005, LNCS 3750, pp. 813–820, 2005.

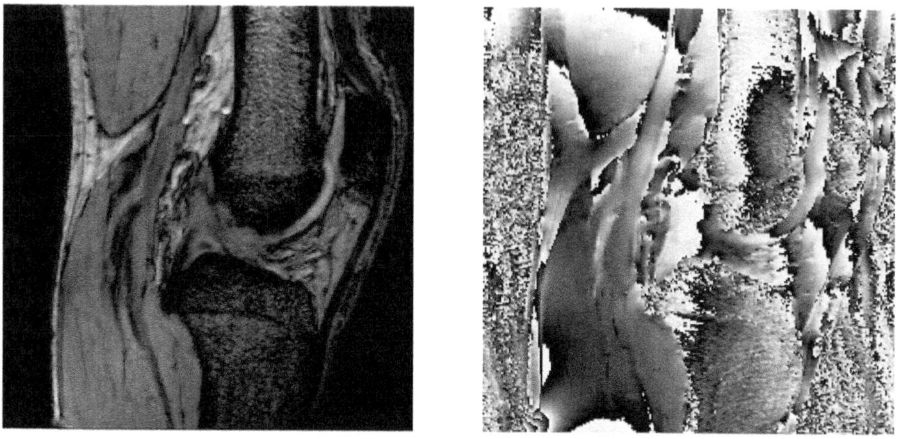

Fig. 1. Magnitude and phase image with $T_E = 10$ms. The wrapped phase image shows strong textural information in the bone and the background, compared to the relatively smooth areas in the cartilage and the muscles.

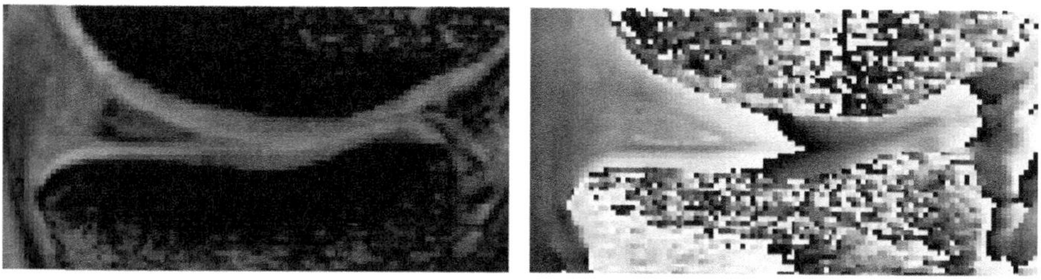

Fig. 2. Magnitude and phase image of the knee cartilage

to this effect than others, so the choice of the acquisition methods is very important. With a properly chosen sequence, the phase can give information about tissue interfaces. In the case of the articular cartilage, there is a large difference in magnetic susceptibility between the subchondral bone and the cartilage that creates a local magnetic gradient leading to loss of signal [2]. The study of the phase can give additional information on the cartilage/bone interface due to magnetic inhomogeneities caused by the local tissue transition. A closer look at the femur and tibia cartilage (Figure 2) shows that the magnitude is not efficient in separating the two cartilages. This is a common problem in cartilage segmentation, whereas the phase shows a strong black line between them. Unfortunately, phase is only defined within the interval $[0\ 2\pi[$, and phase unwrapping is required prior to processing [3][4]. Phase unwrapping is commonly used in MRI to perform the three points Dixon water/fat separation technique, and to reconstruct cardiovascular structures in phase contrast MRI, but the operation can be extremely time consuming, especially in 3D, and is prone to errors. Moreover, most algorithms can't handle the high level of noise that can be found in the background for example. As a result, only the magnitude of the complex MRI signal is used for clinical diagnostics. This results in the loss of information which is and can only be encoded in the phase of the signal. More information on phase acquisition can be found in Haacke et *al* [1].

This paper intends to demonstrate the potential benefit in including the phase information in segmentation algorithms. Since image processing algorithms have been mainly designed to work on magnitude images, the paper also presents the corresponding tools that have been developed to extract useful information from the complex image without the need of phase unwrapping.

2 Method

The images used in this paper where acquired on a Bruker Medspec 4T Whole-body MRI scanner with a specific knee coil. The acquisition was performed on a healthy patient with ($T_R/T_{E1}/T_{E2} = 45/10/20$ ms). The scans are made through the sagittal plane with a resolution of $0.5859 \times 0.5859 \times 1.5$ mm^3, and a size of $256 \times 256 \times 64$ pixels, which gives two complex images with two different T_E. Increasing the T_E increases the phase difference between the different type of tissues, but also increases the noise level in the magnitude image. As reminded by Ghiglia [3], it is important to note that phase is not a signal itself, but a property of a real signal, and should therefore be processed as such. A complex 3D image $I(x, y, z)$ can be expressed as :

$$I(x, y, z) = A(x, y, z) \times e^{j\varphi(x,y,z)}, \tag{1}$$

where $A(x, y, z)$ is the magnitude of the image, and $\varphi(x, y, z)$ the phase of the image. In areas of low intensity, such as the background, the signal does not contain enough information to produce an accurate measure of the phase, which is mainly composed of noise.

Reyes-Aldasoro and Bhalerao [5] presented a method based on texture analysis to perform 3D segmentation of the bone in MRI. They apply a subband filtering technique, similar to a Gabor decomposition, in the K-space in order to extract textural information from the different type of tissues, but this technique does not take full advantage of the information contained in the phase. The filter is set to select a region of the spatial and frequency domain. The amplitude of the output of the filter measures the signal energy within the selected region. This means that the output of the filter is strongly dependant on the local amplitude of the signal, and within the areas of low amplitude, the phase information will not be taken into account. We first introduced the idea to process the phase information separately from the amplitude information, without phase unwrapping, in the context of image segmentation in digital holography, where complex images are widely available [6]. Instead of applying a bank of Gabor on the complex image only, the same filters can be applied to the phase image after a normalisation step. In order to remove the sensitivity to amplitude variation, the complex image is divided by the amplitude, to generate a complex image $I_\varphi(x,y,z)$ of constant amplitude equal to 1, and therefore only composed of phase information :

$$I_\varphi(x,y,z) = \frac{I(x,y,z)}{A(x,y,z)} = e^{j\varphi(x,y,z)} = cos(\varphi(x,y,z)) + j.sin(\varphi(x,y,z)). \quad (2)$$

$I_\varphi(x,y,z)$ is a complex image that can be Fourier transformed and then filtered in order to extract phase information without phase unwrapping. Variations in the phase induce variations in the frequency of the signal, and therefore, a frequency analysis performed using Gabor filters on $I_\varphi(x,y,z)$ can extract usefull information about the phase. The same bank of Gabor filters can then be applied on both the amplitude image $A(x,y,z)$ and the phase image $I_\varphi(x,y,z)$, generating two different sets of features, containing different types of information.

3 Implementation

In 2D, the Gabor filters [7][8] are defined by their impulse response $h(x,y)$ such that:

$$h(x,y) = g(x,y)e^{j2\pi(Ux+Vy)}, \quad (3)$$

with:

$$g(x,y) = \frac{1}{2\pi\sigma_x\sigma_y} e^{-\frac{1}{2}\left[\left(\frac{x}{\sigma_x}\right)^2 + \left(\frac{y}{\sigma_y}\right)^2\right]}, \quad (4)$$

where $h(x,y)$ is a complex sinusoid of frequency (U,V) with a Gaussian envelop $g(x,y)$ of shape defined by (σ_x,σ_y). The Fourier transform of $h(x,y)$ is given by :

$$H(u,v) = G(u-U, v-V), \quad (5)$$

with

$$G(u,v) = e^{-2\pi^2\sigma_x\sigma_y(u^2+v^2)}, \quad (6)$$

the Fourier transform of $g(x,y)$. For our implementation, we used a bank of non symmetric Gabor filters with 5 scales and 6 orientations as presented in Figure 3. These parameters were chosen to obtain a good coverage of the frequency space. Because of the anisotropic nature of the images, most of the textural information is contained in the sagittal planes, so we opted for a two dimensional implementation of the Gabor filters. Each magnitude and phase image is Fourier transformed, and multiplied by each Gabor filter $H(u,v)$ corresponding to the different scales and orientations. A 3D Gaussian filter is then applied on the magnitude of the output of each filter to smooth the response across slices. It is important to preserve rotation invariance, since the knee can be in various positions, and more or less bent. Therefore, the magnitude of the output of the filters is summed across all orientations as shown in Figure 4, in order to obtain a set of features that is rotation invariant. Figure 5 presents the features obtained from the magnitude and the phase images with $T_E = 10$ ms. For each dataset, the magnitude of the image is low-pass filtered with the same 3D Gaussian filter to produce an additional feature for the classifier.

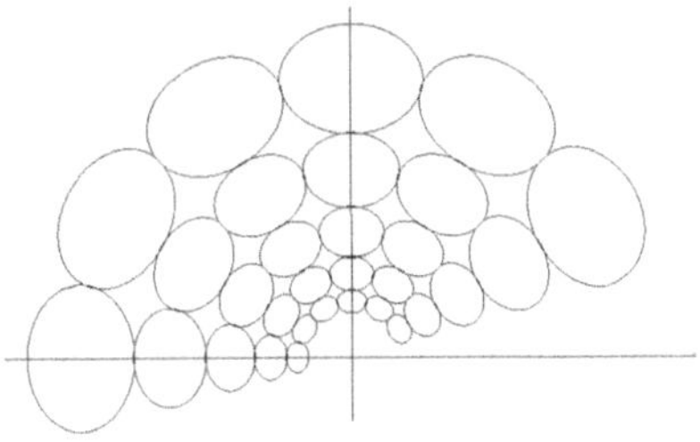

Fig. 3. Bank of Gabor filters, with the contour representing the half-peak magnitude of the filter response

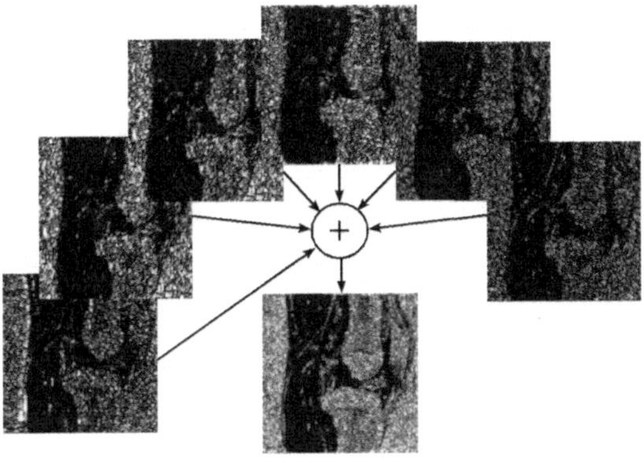

Fig. 4. Phase features at scale 5, all 6 orientations are summed together to produce a rotationally invariant feature

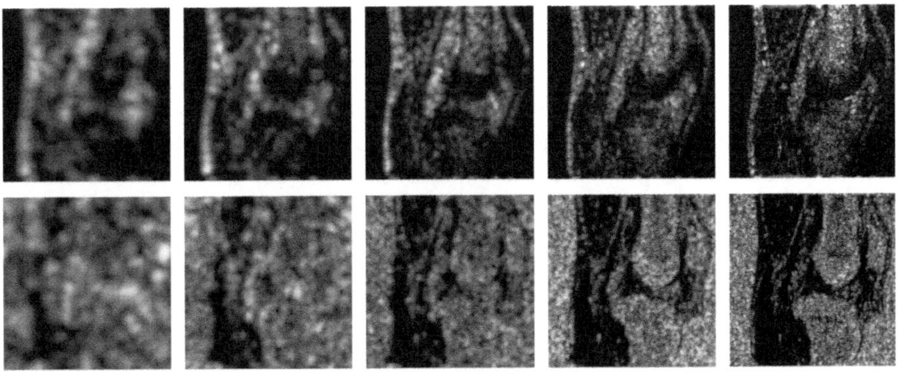

Fig. 5. Magnitude features (top row) and phase features (bottom row). The features represent a 5 levels decomposition, from low to high frequencies (presented left to right)

The feature images clearly show how the phase can be used to discriminate the bone from the other tissues, but are not of much utility for separating bone from background. On the other hand, the magnitude can discriminate between the bones and the background, so that the combination of the two sets of features can be used to effectively segment the bones. The pixels are classified using the SVM classifier [9]. The implementation relies on SVMLIB [10]. We use an RBF kernel, with the parameters (C, γ) optimised using a five fold cross validation.

4 Experimental Results and Discussion

A single slice, where the bones have been manually segmented, is used to train the classifier. In order to test the utility of phase for bone segmentation, the classifier was trained with three different sets of features :

- The first set of features is composed of the features extracted from the magnitude, and the low-pass filtered magnitude of the image for the two T_E values.
- The second set of features is composed of the features extracted from the phase, and the low-pass filtered magnitude of the image for the two T_E values.
- The third set of features is composed of the features extracted from the magnitude and the phase, and the low-pass filtered magnitude of the image for the two T_E values.

Since we are looking at segmenting large objects, a size filter is applied to the segmented image in order to remove small misclassified volumes. The sensitivity and specificity results after filtering are presented in Table 1. The phase by itself does not give good results as it produces a lot of misclassification in the background, since the bone and the background have a similar response. The magnitude produces better features than the phase, but there are misclassifications around the skin and the ligaments. The combination of the features extracted from the phase and the magnitude maintains the specificity around 97% but increases the sensitivity to 95%, and leads to a global misclassification rate of 3.3%. Moreover, only the combination of the features can successfully separate the four bones present in the image, the two other set of features merging the patella with the femur, and the fibula with the tibia. Slices of the segmented images for each type of feature are displayed in Figure 6, along with a 3D view

Table 1. Sensitivity, specificity, and global misclassification rate on the bone segmentation

	Magnitude	**Phase**	**Magnitude and Phase**
Sensitivity (%)	90.3	79.9	95.1
Specificity (%)	97.1	96.0	96.9
Misclassification rate (%)	3.8	6.3	3.3

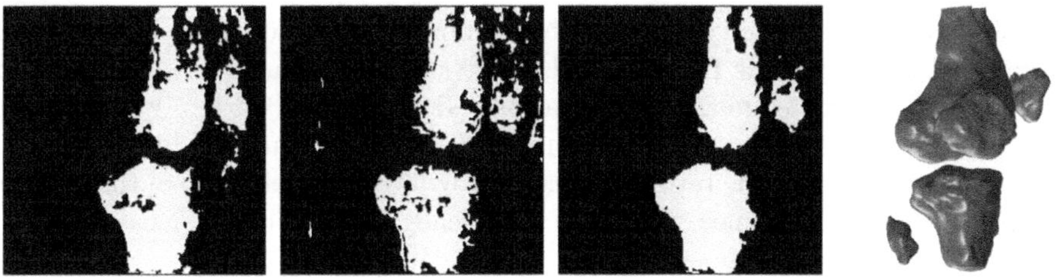

(a) (b) (c) (d)

Fig. 6. Segmentation results with (a) magnitude, (b) phase, (c) phase and magnitude, (d) phase and magnitude 3D view

of the segmented bones using the full set of features. On a 2.8GHz PC, with a C++ implementation of our technique, it took 6 minutes to generate the 22 features, 3 minutes to train the classifier, and 35 minutes to segment the image.

4.1 Discusion

The use of texture to perform segmentations rarely produces results of sufficient accuracy and robustness for medical image analysis. However, it can be used to automatically initialise other advanced segmentation algorithm such as active shape models [11]. Such models are highly dependent upon initialisation, with no accepted ways to initialise them, especially in 3D. The most promising approach relies on a registration of the resulting segmentation to an atlas (or statistical map) which is then used to initialise the active shape models.

To evaluate if the results are accurate enough to initialise a statistical shape model, the location of the centre of mass is measured for each bone in the segmented image, and compared to the manually segmented one. The distances are reported in Table 2. The largest difference is obtained for the patella with 2.8 mm. This difference can be explained by the high level of noise present in this area, produced by the different type of tissues (ligament, fat, skin) surrounding the patella which produce a lot of misclassification. Nevertheless, the position is sufficiently close to be used to initialise an active shape model.

Table 2. Distance to the centre of mass for each type of bone between the manually segmented mask, and the result of the segmentation using features extracted from the phase and the magnitude.

	Femur	**Tibia**	**Patella**	**Fibula**
Distance (in mm.)	0.69	1.07	2.8	1.72

5 Conclusion

In this paper, we have presented preliminary results on bone segmentation of the knee articulation using both phase and magnitude information. In most conventional anatomical imaging, the phase information is acquired, but is usually not used for diagnostic purposes. The phase image contains extra information that can be used in image segmentation. Gabor filters can easily extract this information, which is useful to discriminate bones from surrounding tissues. By using this technique, the future goal is to provide a complete map of the different type of tissues in the knee, and more specifically the cartilage, for use in clinical studies of osteoarthritis.

Acknowledgements

We would like to acknowledge Dr Katie McMahon and Mrs Martina Bryant for expertise in image acqusition and selection of imaging parameters.

References

1. Haacke, E., Brown, R., Thompson, M., Venkatesan, R.: Magnetic Resonance Imaging: Principles and Sequence Design. John Wiley & Sons, New York (1999)
2. Drapé, J., Pessis, E., Sarazin, L., Minoui, A., Godefroy, D., Chevrot, A.: MR imaging of articular cartilage. J. Radiology **79** (1998) 391–40
3. Ghiglia, D., Pritt, M.: Two-dimensional Phase Unwrapping: Theory Algorithms And Software. John Wiley & Sons, New York (1998)
4. Chavez, S., Xiang, Q., An, L.: Understanding phase maps in MRI: a new cutline phase unwrapping method. IEEE Trans. Medical Imaging **21** (2002) 966–977
5. Reyes-Aldasoro, C.C., Bhalerao, A.: Volumetric texture description and discriminant feature selection for MRI. In: IPMI'03, Ambleside, UK, Springer (2003)
6. Bourgeat, P., Meriaudeau, F., Gorria, P., Tobin, K., Truchetet, F.: Features extraction on complex images. In: ICIP'04, Singapore, IEEE (2004)
7. Bovik, A., Clark, M., Geisler, W.: Multichannel texture analysis using localized spatial filters. IEEE Trans. Pattern Analysis and Machine Intelligence **12** (1990) 55–73
8. Grigorescu, S., Petkov, N., Kruizinga, P.: Comparison of texture features based on Gabor filters. IEEE Trans. on Image Processing **11** (2002) 1160–1167
9. Vapnik, V.: The nature of statistical learning theory. Springer Verlag, New York (1995)
10. Chang, C.C., Lin, C.J.: LIBSVM: a library for support vector machines. (2001) Software available at `http://www.csie.ntu.edu.tw/~cjlin/libsvm`.
11. Cootes, T., Taylor, C., Cooper, D., Graham, J.: Active shape models - their training and application. Computer Vision and Image Undertanding **61** (1995) 38–59

2D and 3D Shape Based Segmentation Using Deformable Models

Ayman El-Baz[1], Seniha E. Yuksel[1], Hongjian Shi[1], Aly A. Farag[1], Mohamed A. El-Ghar[2], Tarek Eldiasty[2], and Mohamed A. Ghoneim[2]

[1] Computer Vision and Image Processing Laboratory, University of Louisville, Louisville, KY 40292
farag@cvip.louisville.edu
http://www.cvip.louisville.edu

[2] Mansoura University, Urology and Nephrology Center, Mansoura, Egypt

Abstract. A novel shape based segmentation approach is proposed by modifying the external energy component of a deformable model. The proposed external energy component depends not only on the gray level of the images but also on the shape information which is obtained from the signed distance maps of objects in a given data set. The gray level distribution and the signed distance map of the points inside and outside the object of interest are accurately estimated by modelling the empirical density function with a linear combination of discrete Gaussians (LCDG) with positive and negative components. Experimental results on the segmentation of the kidneys from low-contrast DCE-MRI and on the segmentation of the ventricles from brain MRI's show how the approach is accurate in segmenting 2-D and 3-D data sets. The 2D results for the kidney segmentation have been validated by a radiologist and the 3D results of the ventricle segmentation have been validated with a geometrical phantom.

1 Introduction

Both parametric deformable models and geometrical deformable models (level sets) are powerful methods and have been used widely for the segmentation problems; however, they both tend to fail in the case of noise, poor image resolution, diffused boundaries or occluded shapes, and they don't take advantage of the *a priori* models. Yet, especially in the area of medical imaging, organs have well constrained forms within a family of shapes [1]. Thus, additional constraints based on the shape of the objects are greatly needed besides the gray level information of these objects.

To allow shape driven segmentation, Leventon et.al. [2] used a shape prior whose variance is obtained thorough PCA, and used this shape prior to evolve the level sets to the maximum *a posteriori* shape. Chen et al. [3] defined an energy functional which basically minimizes an Euclidean distance between a given point and its shape prior. In [4], a representation of the segmenting curve was generated based on the pose and shape parameters of a training set, which were optimized using a region based energy functional. In [1,5] a shape prior and its variance

J. Duncan and G. Gerig (Eds.): MICCAI 2005, LNCS 3750, pp. 821–829, 2005.

obtained from training data are used to define a Gaussian distribution, which is then used in the external energy component of a level sets framework. In [6], a shape boundary prior was formed from the features of the boundary, and this boundary was used in a level set framework. Recently, Tsai et.al. [7] used a deterministic model to represent the desired shape as a linear combination of weighted signed 2D distance maps and estimated these weights by minimizing a mutual information based cost function. And Yang et.al. [8] described the shapes with a multidimensional Gaussian probability model of these weights.

Different from the previous studies, in our approach, instead of directly using the average image itself, we are estimating the density of the signed distance map inside and outside the object of interest of the registered training samples by our modified EM algorithm and use this estimated density in the external energy component of the proposed deformable model framework. This representation of shapes is invariant to rotation and translation, and it overcomes the deformable models' inability to stop in high noise or in the case of missing edges.

2 Proposed Deformable Models

In conventional deformable models, surfaces move in the direction that minimizes an energy function given as [9]:

$$E = E_{\text{int}} + E_{\text{ext}} = \int_{\tau \in T} \big(\xi_{\text{int}}\big(\phi(\tau)\big) + \xi_{\text{ext}}\big(\phi(\tau)\big)\big) d\tau \tag{1}$$

where $\xi_{\text{int}}\big(\phi(\tau)\big)$ and $\xi_{\text{ext}}\big(\phi(\tau)\big)$ denote the internal and external forces respectively.

Typical external forces designed in [9] lead a deformable model toward edges in a 2D/3D grayscale image. This and the other traditional external forces (e.g. based on lines or, edges, or the gradient vector flow) fail to make the deformable model closely approach an intricate boundary with concavities. Moreover, due to high computational complexity, the deformable models with such external energies are slow compared to the other segmentation techniques.

As a solution to these problems, we modify the external energy component of this energy formulation, and we formulate an energy function using the density estimations of two distributions: the signed distance map from shape models and the gray level distribution. The external energy component of our deformable models is formulated as:

$$\xi_{ext}\big(\phi(\tau)\big) = \begin{cases} -p_g(q|k)p_s(d|k) \text{ if } k = k^* \\ \;\;\, p_g(q|k)p_s(d|k) \text{ if } k \neq k^* \end{cases}$$

In this formulation, k is the region label with $k = 1, \ldots, K$, q is the gray level and d is the signed distance where $p_s(d|k)$ is the density that describes the signed distance map inside and outside the object, and $p_g(q|k)$ is the density estimation of the gray level. With this energy function, the stochastic external force for each control point $\phi(\tau)$ of the current deformable model evolves in a region k^*.

Specifically for the examples to be given in section 3, we assume that the empirical density comes from two classes, i.e. $k = 1, 2$. For the kidney segmentation problem, these classes are the kidney and the other tissues, and for the ventricle segmentation, the first class is the gray matter, white matter, fat and bones; while the second class is the CSF of the brain (inside and outside the ventricles).

2.1 Shape Model Construction

The signed distance map density $p_s(d|k)$ in the above mentioned external energy is calculated using a shape model, which is basically an average surface shape obtained from the images in the data set. The steps to construct this average surface shape is as follows:

1. Align the images in the data set using 2D/3D rigid registration based on Mutual Information [10].
2. Manually segment the objects of interest from the database.
3. Calculate the 2D/3D edge V that describes the boundary of the object for all the manually segmented N number of images obtained in Step 2.
4. From the N number of shapes calculated in Step 3, find the average 2D/3D shape V_m of the object by: $V_m = \frac{1}{N}\sum_{i=1}^{N} Vi.$
5. From the average shape, the distribution of the signed distance map inside and outside the 3D shape is calculated as follows: ($z = 0$ for 2D)

$$d(x, y, z) = \begin{cases} 0 & (x, y, z) \in V \\ S((x, y, z), V) & (x, y, z) \in R_V \\ -S((x, y, z), V) & Otherwise \end{cases} \tag{2}$$

   where R_v is the region lying inside the shape and $S((x, y, z), V)$ is the minimum Euclidean distance between the image location (x, y, z) and the curve V. This shape model is constructed only once throughout the whole algorithm.

The results of the average shape and signed distance calculations are shown for the kidney in Fig. 2, and the density estimation of this average shape is calculated using our modified EM approach which will be explained in Sec. 2.2.

2.2 Density Estimation

In this paper we will use our modified Expectation-Maximization algorithm that approximates an empirical probability density function of scalar data with a linear combination of discrete Gaussians (LCDG) with positive and negative components.

In the following, we describe this model to estimate the marginal density for the gray level distribution $p_g(q)$ in each region. The same approach is also used to estimate the density of the signed distances $p_s(d)$ in the given image.

Let $q \in \mathbf{Q} = \{0, 1, \ldots, Q-1\}$ denote the Q-ary gray level. The discrete Gaussian (DG) is defined as the discrete probability distribution $\Psi_\theta = (\psi(q|\theta) : q \in \mathbf{Q})$ on $\mathbf{Q}$ such that $\psi(q|\theta) = \Phi_\theta(q + 0.5) - \Phi_\theta(q - 0.5)$ for $q = 1, \ldots, Q-2$,

$\psi(0|\theta) = \Phi_\theta(0.5)$, $\psi(Q-1|\theta) = 1 - \Phi_\theta(Q-1.5)$ where $\Phi_\theta(q)$ is the cumulative Gaussian (normal) probability function with a shorthand notation $\theta = (\mu, \sigma^2)$ for its mean, μ, and variance, σ^2.

In contrast to a conventional mixture of Gaussians and/or other simple distributions, one per region, we closely approximate the empirical gray level distribution for the given image with a LCDG having C_p positive and C_n negative components:

$$p_{g:\mathbf{w},\mathbf{\Theta}}(q) = \sum_{r=1}^{C_\mathrm{p}} w_{\mathrm{p},r}\psi(q|\theta_{\mathrm{p},r}) - \sum_{l=1}^{C_\mathrm{n}} w_{\mathrm{n},l}\psi(q|\theta_{\mathrm{n},l}) \quad (3)$$

under the obvious restriction on the positive weights $\mathbf{w} = [w_{p,.}, w_{n,.}]$:

$$\sum_{r=1}^{C_\mathrm{p}} w_{\mathrm{p},r} - \sum_{l=1}^{C_\mathrm{n}} w_{\mathrm{n},l} = 1 \quad (4)$$

To estimate the parameters for the model shown in Eq. (4), we will use our modified EM algorithm that modified the conventional EM algorithm to take into account both positive and negative discrete Gaussian components. The details of the algorithm are shown in [11].

2.3 Stepwise Deformable Model Algorithm

For any given image, the proposed algorithm of segmenting the region k^* is as follows:

1. Register the given image to an average image using Mutual Information [10], where the average image is obtained by averaging the registered images of the database of Step 1 in Sec. 2. This step makes the algorithm invariant to scaling, rotation and translation.
2. Use the modified EM algorithm to estimate the density for signed distance map $p_s(d|k)$ inside and outside the object of interest from the average shape which was calculated *a priori*.
3. Calculate the normalized histogram for the given image/volume.
4. Use the modified EM algorithm to estimate the density for each class $p_g(q|k)$, k being the class number $k = 1...K$.
5. Initialize the control points $\phi(\tau)$ for the deformable model, and for each control point $\phi(\tau)$ on the current deformable model, calculate sign distances indicating exterior $(-)$ or interior $(+)$ positions of each of the eight nearest neighbors w.r.t. the contour.
6. Check the label $k = \mathbf{X}(\phi(\tau))$ for each control point:
   (a) If the point is assigned to the region $k = k^*$, then
      i. Estimate the region labels for its neighbors using Bayesian classifier such that they have the $(-)$ distance.
      ii. If some of these sites are also assigned to the class k^*, then move the control point to the neighboring position ensuring the minimum total energy (i.e., expand the contour).
      iii. Otherwise, do not move this point (the steady state).

(b) If the point is assigned to the region $k \neq k^*$, then
   i. Estimate the region labels for its neighbors using Bayesian classifier such that they have the (+) distance.
   ii. Move the control point to the neighboring position ensuring the minimum total energy (i.e. contract the contour)
7. If the iteration adds new control points, use the cubic spline interpolation of the whole surface and then smooth all its control points with a low pass filter.
8. Repeat steps 5, 6, and 7 until no positional changes occur in the control points.

3 Experimental Results

This section presents the results of our approach to segment the kidneys from the Dynamic Contrast-Enhanced MR images of the abdomen in 2D, and to segment the brain ventricles from MR images in 3D.

3.1 2D Results for the Kidney

In this study, Dynamic Contrast-Enhanced MRI (DCE-MRI), has been employed by a Signa Horizon GE 1.5T scanner using a contrast agent Gadolinium DTPA. In DCE-MRI, after the injection of a contrast agent Gd-DTPA, the abdomen is scanned rapidly and repeatedly resulting in high noise images because of the fast image acquisition. Moreover, the contrast of the kidney in the images changes continuously as the contrast agent perfuses into the kidney, resulting in very low contrast at some stages of the perfusion, necessitating the use of shape models in segmentation.

A typical DCE-MRI scan of a kidney is given in Fig. 1(a) with its empirical density (normalized histogram) shown in blue and the estimation of this density shown in red in Fig. 1(b). Figure 1(c) shows the positive and negative LCDG components used in our modified EM algorithm, and Fig. 1 (d) shows the estimated density for each class.

In Fig. 2(a) the average shape of a kidney obtained from 50 subjects is given with the signed distance map inside and outside the object as in Fig. 2(b). The density of this signed distance map is estimated with the same density estimation approach, the results of which are shown in Fig. 2(c), (d).

Finally, Fig. 3 shows the segmentation results of our approach compared to the segmentations by a radiologist.

3.2 3D Results for the Brain Ventricles

In the following part, we use the proposed segmentation approach on 3D data sets collected from 20 subjects to segment the lateral ventricles of the brain in MR images, and in the second part, we are evaluating the segmentation approach using the cone-beam CT scans of a mould ventricle phantom.

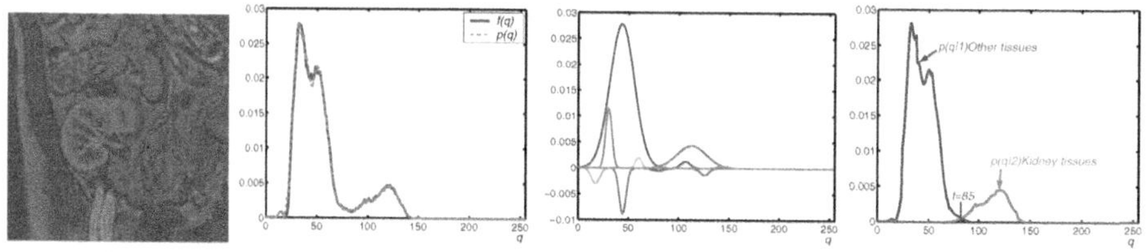

(a) (b) (c) (d)

Fig. 1. A typical MRI scan of a kidney (a), and its gray level density estimation with the Modified EM Algorithm: (b) LCG components of the density estimation, (c) The final estimated density $p_g(q)$ for the empirical density $f(q)$ of the kidney image, (d) The marginal density estimation for each class.

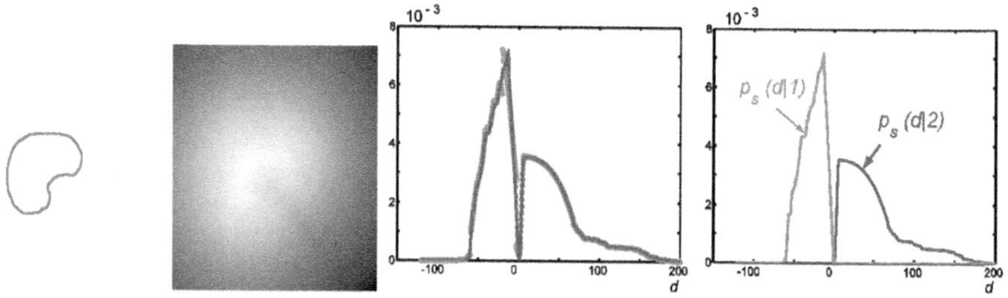

(a) (b) (c) (d)

Fig. 2. (a) An average shape for a certain cross-sections of the kidney. (b) The signed distance map of this shape. (c) Density estimation for the signed distance. (d) Marginal density estimations for each class.

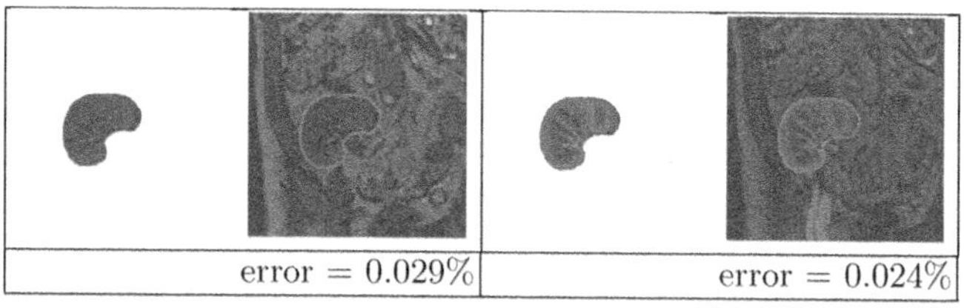

Fig. 3. Segmentation results (shown in red to the right) w.r.t. the radiologist's segmentation (to the left).

For ventricle segmentation from MRI, twenty data sets are not enough to get an accurate shape for the ventricles because the ventricles vibrate during the MRI or CT scans. Therefore, to cover all the shape variations of the brain ventricles for each subject, we performed finite element analysis on the motion of the real brain ventricles. For finite element analysis of the ventricle shape changes, assuming the cerebrospinal fluid (CSF) inside lateral ventricles is isotropic and linear elastic, we employed the linear elastic mechanical model. The Young's modulus of the CSF is 1000 Pascals and the Poisson ratio is 0.499 ([12]). For

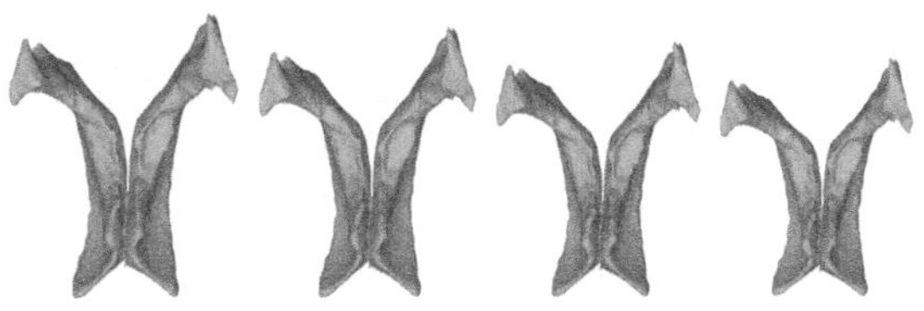

(a) (b) (c) (d)

Fig. 4. The four states of the real ventricles at t=0, 0.7, 0.9, 1.1 seconds (final) from left to right.

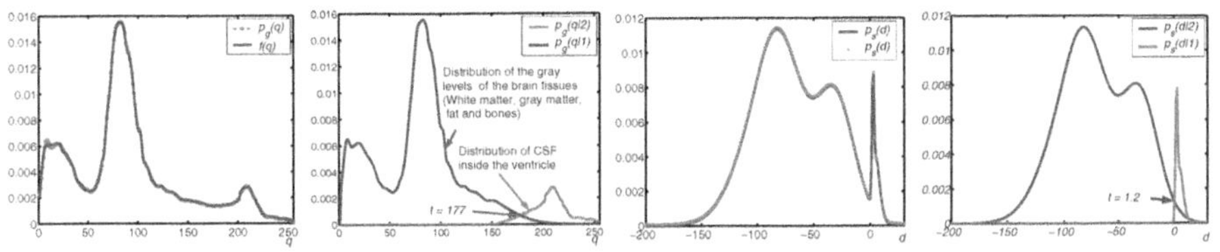

(a) (b) (c) (d)

Fig. 5. (a) Final density estimation for the mixed frequency gray level distribution, (b) The class model of gray level for each class, (c) Final density estimation for the sign map inside and outside the 3-D brain ventricle, (d) The final class model of signed distance map for each class.

adults, the pressure of the CSF under normal conditions ranges between 50 and 180 mmH_2O with a median pressure of 115 mmH_2O. Therefore, the uniform pressure of 115 mmH_2O is applied over the surfaces of the ventricles for each subject, and finite element analysis is performed to capture the variation of the ventricles. After finite element analysis, the 3D structure is re-sliced and 10 states of the ventricles are obtained resulting in 20 $subjects \times 10\ states = 200$ $datasets$. The four states of one subject's ventricles are shown in Fig. 4. Using the resulting 200 data sets for the ventricles, we followed our density estimation approach to estimate the density of the gray level distribution and the signed distance map inside and outside the ventricles. The results of density estimation using the proposed approach are shown in Fig. 5 and the segmentation results at different signal to ratios (SNR) (obtained by adding Gaussian noise with different variance) are shown in Fig. 6.

The hand segmentation of the radiologists may not always be accurate because of hand shaking. Therefore, to get accurate evaluation of our proposed approach, we used a mould ventricle phantom that resembles the geometrical structure of the real ventricles, scanned it with cone-beam CT, and used the scans for finite element simulation. Following the same procedure of the ventricle motion estimation, we captured all variations of the phantom ventricles. For the database obtained from the geometrical phantom, the inverse mapping method was used to get the same gray level distribution with the real ventricles; the gray level distribution of which was shown in Fig. 5(b). The final step of our algorithm is to estimate the pdf that describes the signed distance map inside

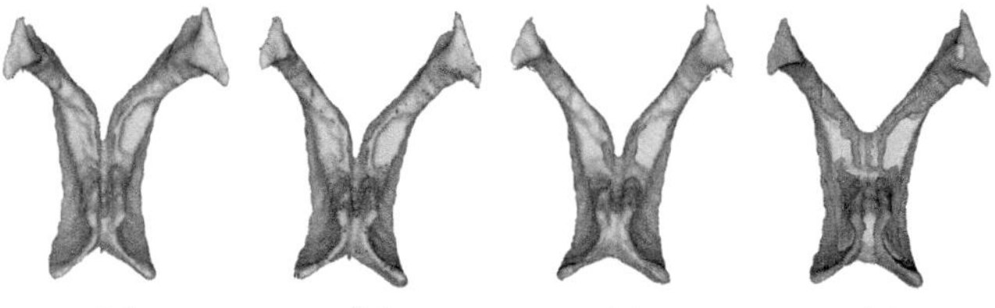

(a) (b) (c) (d)

Fig. 6. (a) Results of our segmentation approach at SNR = 28dB, $error$ = 0.01% (b)at SNR = 7.8dB, $error$ = 0.2% (c)at SNR = -1.9dB, $error$ = 2.8%. (d) Result of the segmentation errors using the conventional EM algorithm as a density estimator at SNR = 28dB, $error$ = 18.8%. The errors are shown in red.

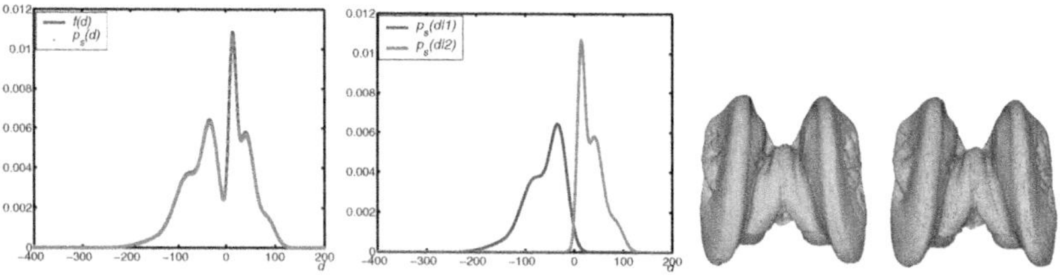

(a) (b) (c) (d)

Fig. 7. (a) Final density estimation for the signed distance map inside and outside the 3-D ventricle phantom, (b) The final class model of signed distance map for each class. Segmentation using our approach at different SNR (c) $SNR = 28dB$, $error = 0.008\%$, (d) $SNR = -1.9dB$, $error = 1.76\%$.

and outside the geometrical phantom; the results of our modified EM algorithm are shown in Fig. 7. Figure 7 (c – e) show the results of our segmentation for the geometrical phantom at different signal to noise ratios and the errors are calculated with respect to the ground truth from the phantom.

4 Conclusion

We have presented an approach for image segmentation which depends on both the intensity gray level and the shape information, and we have applied the algorithm on 2D and 3D images. Apart from the other shape based segmentation methods which calculate the mean and the variance and assume gaussian distribution, in our method, the mean and variance are all embedded into the estimated density, which is calculated using our modified EM algorithm. This algorithm is notably fast, and works both in 2D and 3D.

References

1. M. Rousson and N. Paragios, "Shape priors for level set representations," Proc. European Conf. on Computer Vision, Vol. 2351 of Lecture Notes in Computer Science, Springer, 2002.

2. M. Leventon, W. L. Grimson, and O. Faugeras, "Statistical shape influence in geodesic active contours," IEEE CVPR, 2000, pp. 1316–1324.
3. Y. Chen, S. Thiruvenkadam, H. Tagare, F. Huang, D. Wilson, "On the incorporation of shape priors into geometric active contours," IEEE VLSM, pp. 145–152, 2001.
4. A. Tsai, A.J. Yezzi, W.M. Wells et al., "Model-Based Curve Evolution Technique for Image Segmentation," IEEE CVPR, 2001, pp. 463–468.
5. N. Paragios, "A level set approach for shape-driven segmentation and tracking of the left ventricle," IEEE Trans. on Medical Imaging, vol. 22 , pp. 773–776 , 2003.
6. A. Litvin and W.C. Karl, "Levelset based segmentation using data driven shape prior on feature histograms," IEEE Workshop on Statistical Signal Processing, pp.166-169, 2003.
7. A. Tsai, W. Wells, C. Tempany, E. Grimson and A. Willsky, "Mutual Information in Coupled Multi-Shape Model for Medical Image Segmentation," Medical Image Analysis, Vol. 8, No.4, pp. 429–445, 2004.
8. J. Yang, and J. Duncan, "3D image segmentation of deformable objects with joint shape-intensity prior models using level sets," Medical Image Analysis, Vol. 8, pp. 285–294, 2004.
9. M. Kass, A. Witkin, and D. Terzopoulos, "Snakes: Active contour models," International Journal of Computer Vision, vol. 1, pp. 321–331, 1987.
10. P. Viola and W.M. Wells, "Alignment by maximization of mutual information," In Proc. 5th Int. Conf. Computer Vision, 1995, pp. 16–23.
11. A.A. Farag, A. El-Baz, and G. Gimel'farb "Density Estimation Using Modified Expectation Maximization for a linear combination of Gaussians, IEEE ICIP, 2004, Vol. I, pp. 194–197.
12. H. Takizawa, K. Sugiura, M. Baba et al., "Analysis of intracerebral hematoma shapes by numerical computer simulation using the finite element method," Neurol. Med. Chir., Vol. 34, pp. 65–69, 1994.

CT Hepatic Venography: 3D Vascular Segmentation for Preoperative Evaluation

Catalin Fetita[1], Olivier Lucidarme[2], Françoise Prêteux[1], and Philippe Grenier[2]

[1] ARTEMIS Project Unit, INT, Groupe des Ecoles des Télécommunications,
9 rue Charles Fourier, 91011 Evry Cedex, France
[2] Central Radiology Service, Pitié Salpêtrière Hospital,
47-83 boulevard de l'Hôpital, 75651 Paris Cedex 13

Abstract. Preventing complications during hepatic surgery in living-donor transplantation or in oncologic resections requires a careful preoperative analysis of the hepatic venous anatomy. Such an analysis relies on CT hepatic venography data, which enhances the vascular structure due to contrast medium injection. However, a 3D investigation of the enhanced vascular anatomy based on typical computer vision tools is ineffective because of the large amount of occlusive opacities to be removed. This paper proposes an automated 3D approach for the segmentation of the vascular structure in CT hepatic venography, providing the appropriate tools for such an investigation. The developed methodology relies on advanced topological and morphological operators applied in mono- and multiresolution filtering schemes. It allows to discriminate the opacified vessels from the bone structures and liver parenchyma regardless of noise presence or inter-patient variability in contrast medium dispersion. The proposed approach was demonstrated at different phases of hepatic perfusion and is currently under extensive validation in clinical routine.

1 Introduction

Liver surgery raises several challenges in terms of preoperative evaluation, both in the case of living-donor liver transplantation and oncologic resections. The key issue is to take into account the intrahepatic vessel anatomy specific to each patient in order to reduce surgical complications and/or planning a resection strategy [1,2]. The hepatic vascular system is composed of three hierarchical networks: portal tree, hepatic veins and hepatic arteries. Among them, the portal system defines the functional units of the liver while the hepatic veins are in charge with liver drainage. Their morphological analysis is thus mandatory at the preoperative stage in order to define virtual anatomical landmarks, a safety margin for resection, and the zone impacted by a vessel ligation. CT hepatic venography provides a vessel investigation modality based on MDCT data acquisition after injection of a contrast agent. The hepatic vasculature is progressively opacified and the different vascular systems irrigating the liver become visible. Developing computer vision tools for preoperative planning based on such data is still an active research area despite major advances in this field. Several virtual/augmented reality systems have been proposed for liver surgery planning,

J. Duncan and G. Gerig (Eds.): MICCAI 2005, LNCS 3750, pp. 830–837, 2005.

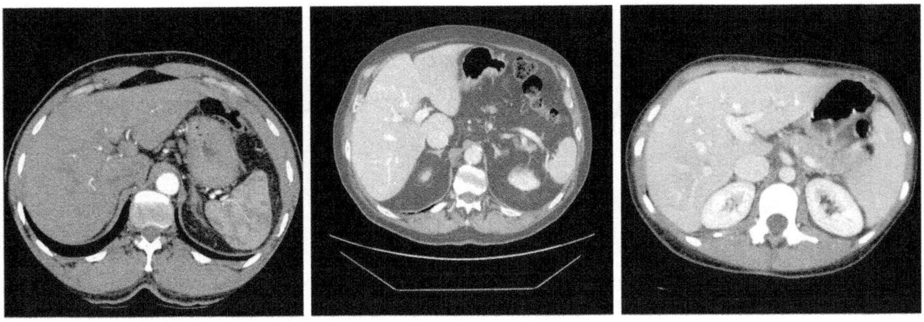

(a) Arterial phase. (b) Portal phase. (c) Venous phase.

Fig. 1. Some examples of CT hepatic venography axial images showing a strong noise, different levels of liver opacifying and vertebra-aorta artifact connections

relying on complex interaction interfaces [3,4,5,6] and different visualization and segmentation strategies [1,7,8,9]. Note that, solving the liver segmentation problems, generally requires excellent radiological data which is not always achievable in clinical routine. Strong noise, different levels of liver opacifying and partial volume effects resulting in bones-vessels artifact connections on CT images are the major difficulties to overcome (Fig. 1).

This paper addresses the issue of the automatic 3D segmentation of hepatic vessels in clinical CT hepatic venography and develops an original approach based on advanced topological and morphological operators combined in mono- and multiresolution filtering schemes. The proposed approach was applied to CT data acquired at different phases of liver perfusion (arterial, portal and venous, Fig. 1) in order to test its robustness with respect to anatomical variability.

The paper is organized as follows. Section 2 presents the multiresolution framework on which the segmentation approach relies, and introduces the 3D morphological operator involved. Section 3 describes and illustrates the developed segmentation strategy. Results are presented and discussed in Section 4.

2 A Multiresolution Segmentation Framework

In order to overcome the limitations related to the strong noise and to the variable level of liver opacifying, a multiresolution approach is used for vascular segmentation. Such an approach relies on a morphological operator, so-called *selective marking and depth constrained connection cost (SMDC-CC)*.

Defined on functions $f : X \subset \Re^n \rightarrow \Re$ of connected support $supp(f) = X$ and upper bounded, on any bounded subset of $supp(f)$, the SMDC-CC affects the local minima of f according to connectivity and morphometric criteria. While a complete mathematical definition of SMDC-CC can be found in [10], its intuitive interpretation will be given in the following. Let us imagine f as the surface of a relief. A point $x \in supp(f)$ is called *topographically connected* to a subset $Y \subset supp(f)$, if there is a descending path on f leading from x to Y. Computing

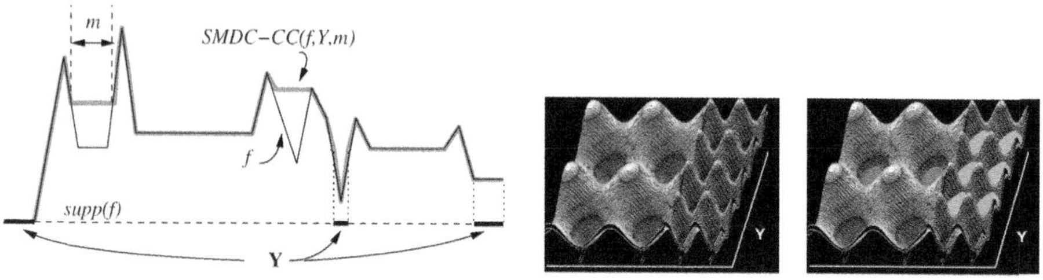

(a) 1-D example. (b) 2-D example (f left, $SMDC-CC$ right).

Fig. 2. SMDC-CC of f with respect to a Y subset, for a given SE size, m

SMDC-CC of f with respect to a non-empty subset $Y \subset supp(f)$ will result in "filling in", at constant level, all local minima of f topographically disconnected from Y. The "filling in" level is controlled by the size m of the structuring element (SE) associated with the SMDC-CC operator. If such a SE is a n-D ball, the "filling in" depth of a "valley" is given by the level at which the "valley" width becomes larger than m (Fig. 2).

By adjusting the m parameter, the SMDC-CC can be implemented in a multiresolution scheme, making it possible to segment structures of interest in a noisy environment. Such a scheme is visually described in Fig. 3, simulating the detection of the vascular structure in a liver-like, noisy environment (Fig. 3(a)). The reference Y subset is defined as the image border. The SMDC-CC is first applied on the negative data (Fig. 3(b)) with a small-size m to filter out the local minima corresponding to the noise (Fig. 3(c)). The small-size vasculature is not affected at this step due to the topographically connection with large caliber vessels. In a second step, by increasing the m size over the maximum vessel caliber, the SMDC-CC selects the desired structures (Fig. 3(d)). A histogram-based thresholding of the SMDC-CC difference (Fig. 3(e)) provides the vessel segmentation (Fig. 3(f)).

Note that the local maxima in the original data (white areas) which are situated at boundary and connected to Y (image border) were not segmented. This property will be useful for designing an additional vessels-bones discrimination approach in CT hepatic venography data, exploiting the described multiresolution framework.

3 An Automated Approach for CT Venography Segmentation

Looking back at the CT images from Fig. 1, we note that the real hepatic venography data raise additional challenges for vessel segmentation. Such challenges are related to the automated discrimination between the opacified vessels and the bone structures. Since density or morphological criteria are neither accurate nor robust for this purpose, the idea is to filter the original data in order to achieve the appropriate configuration for a SMDC-CC based segmentation

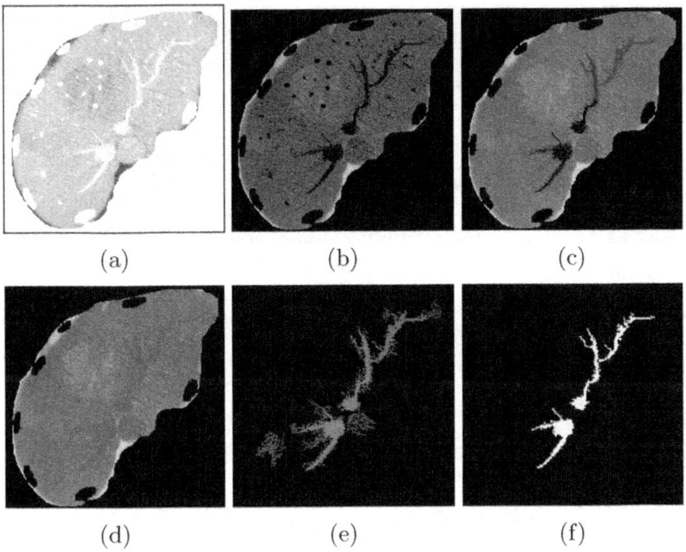

Fig. 3. SMDC-CC based multiresolution segmentation scheme: (a) original data, (b) negative data, (c) noise filtering with SMDC-CC of small-size m, (d) vessel selection with SMDC-CC of large-size m, leaving unaffected the "valleys" connected with the Y subset (image border), (e) difference (d)-(c), (f) adaptive thresholding of (e)

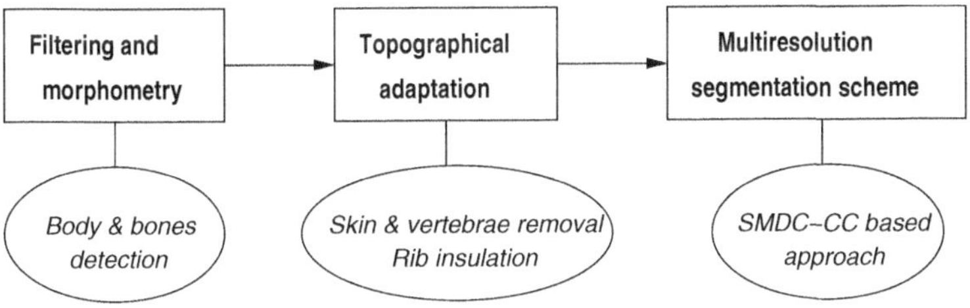

Fig. 4. Block diagram of the implemented segmentation approach

(Fig. 3(a)). More precisely, after the filtering step, the bones have to become topographically connected to the Y subset and disconnected from the opacified vessels. The latter condition need to be checked because of the presence of noise which, combined with partial volume effects, may produce on CT images an artifact connectivity between vertebrae and aorta (Fig. 1(b)).

Based on the previous considerations, the developed segmentation scheme consists of three modules, as illustrated in the block diagram from Fig. 4. The first module performs a morphological filtering for detecting the body and the bones, and extracting the parameters involved in the multiresolution segmentation scheme. The second module provides the topographical adaptation imposed by the multiresolution framework, by removing the skin and the vertebrae and insulating the ribs. The third module achieves the segmentation as discussed

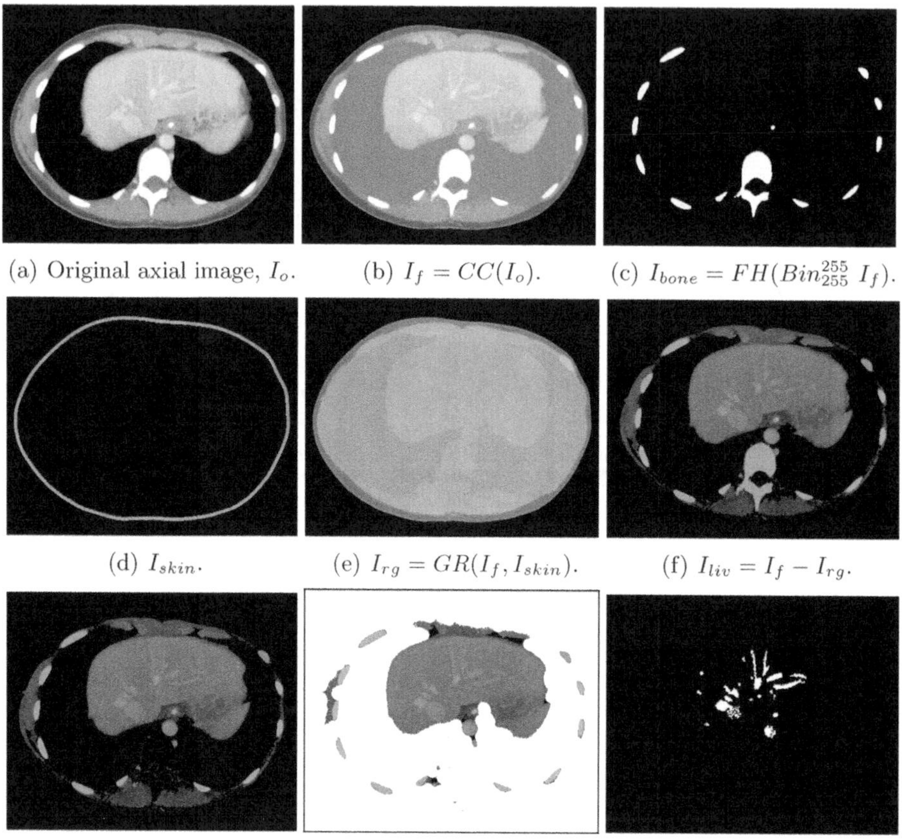

(a) Original axial image, I_o. (b) $I_f = CC(I_o)$. (c) $I_{bone} = FH(Bin_{255}^{255}\ I_f)$.

(d) I_{skin}. (e) $I_{rg} = GR(I_f, I_{skin})$. (f) $I_{liv} = I_f - I_{rg}$.

(g) I_{nv}. (h) I_{topo}. (i) $I_{seg} = MR(I_{topo})$.

Fig. 5. Stepwise illustration of the 3D segmentation algorithm presented in the Fig. 4 block diagram. The following notations were used: CC - connection cost with respect to borders, Bin_a^b - binarization between the thresholds a and b, $FH(.)$ - "fill holes" operator, $GR(I_1, I_2)$ - gray-level reconstruction of I_1 by I_2, and MR - multiresolution segmentation approach *cf.* §2.

in §2. The different steps of the segmentation approach are described in the following and illustrated in Fig. 5 at the level of an axial CT image (Fig. 5(a)).

A. *Filtering and morphometry*

1. The CT data is filtered by means of a *connection cost* (CC) operator [12] applied with respect to the volume borders (I_f, Fig. 5(b)). Such an operator performs like a SMDC-CC one, with $m = \infty$. It regularizes the noise, levels up the local minima and provides the threshold value for body detection.

2. The bone components and the highly opacified vessels are extracted by binarization followed by a 2D "fill holes" procedure (I_{bone}, Fig. 5(c)). The max-

imum axial size of the vertebrae, further denoted by VS, is computed along the volume data using a 2D distance map on I_{bone} with respect to the background.

B. Topographical adaptation

3. Based on the distance map computed with respect to the bone structures outside the body volume, an estimated of the minimal thickness of the skin and muscle tissues outside the rib cage is computed (I_{skin}, Fig. 5(d)). The body "background" (I_{rg}, Fig. 5(e)) is computed by means of a 3D gray-level reconstruction [11] of I_f by I_{skin}. The soft tissue outside the liver is then removed (I_{liv}, Fig. 5(f)) by subtracting from the body volume, I_f, its "background", I_{rg}.

4. The spine is detected from the bone data, I_{bone}, and removed from I_{liv} in order to prevent any artifact connection with aorta (I_{nv}, Fig. 5(g)). The procedure is based on 3D morphological opening of size $VS/2$ (removing the ribs and the other dense structures from I_{bone}) followed by a geodesic dilation with a small-size spherical structuring element (SE).

5. In order to achieve the configuration requested in §2, the ribs and the liver are insulated with maximum gray-level regions (I_{topo}, Fig. 5(h)) by means of 3D region growing with a spherical SE of radius $VS/2$, initiated at the volume lateral walls.

C. Multiresolution segmentation scheme

6. The multiresolution framework based on the SMDC-CC operator is applied to I_{topo} *cf.* §2 in order to achieve the vessel segmentation (I_{seg}, Fig. 5(i)). The reference subset Y is defined as the volume border, while the SE size is respectively set to $m = 2$, for noise removal, and to $m = VS$, for vascular selection.

4 Results and Discussion

The robustness of the developed vessel segmentation approach was tested on a CT hepatic venography database acquired in clinical routine in 10 patients at different phases of liver perfusion. No constraint was imposed on the acquisition protocol. MDCT data were provided by the Central Radiology Service of Pitié Salpêtrière Hospital in Paris which used either a Philips Brilliance40 or a General Electric LightSpeed scanner with collimations of 1.25, 2 and 2.5 millimeters and half overlapped or joint axial image reconstructions.

The segmentation results obtained on such a database were in good agreement with the analysis performed by an experienced radiologist on the native CT images. They demonstrate the robustness of the proposed methodology with respect to the anatomical variability and the liver opacifying degree. Fig. 6 illustrates some examples of 3D segmentation results for four patients at different perfusion phases. Note that such 3D segmentations must be interpreted with respect to the progression of the contrast bolus within the target vessels. When the degree of enhancement of a vessel decreases below some threshold, the vessel appears on the CT images as a collection of low-contrasted and disconnected small elements. Its components risk to be thus removed together with the overall noise during the multiresolution SMDC-CC based segmentation (Fig. 3(c)).

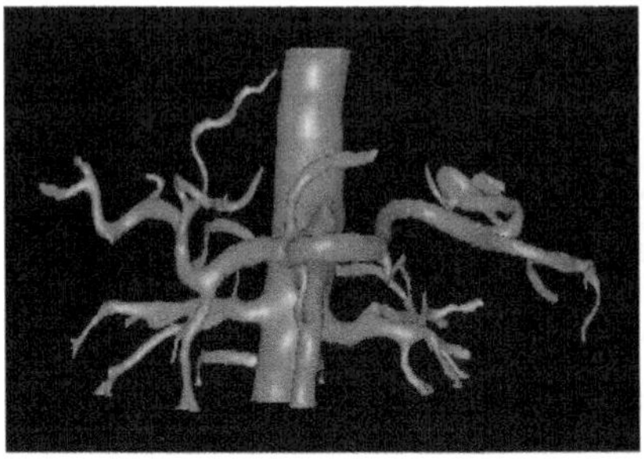

(a) Aorta and hepatic arteries at arterial phase.

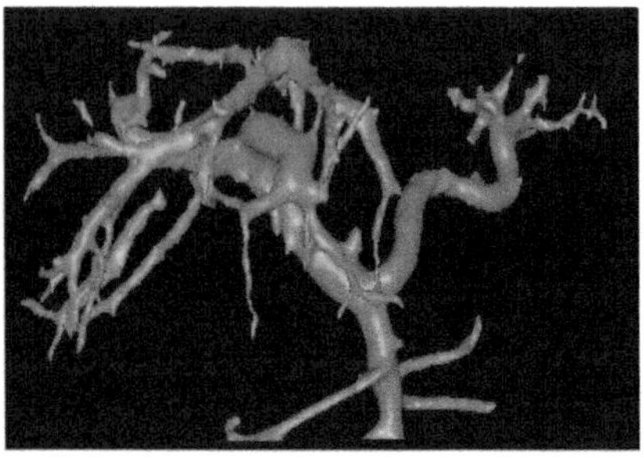

(b) Portal and hepatic veins at early portal phase.

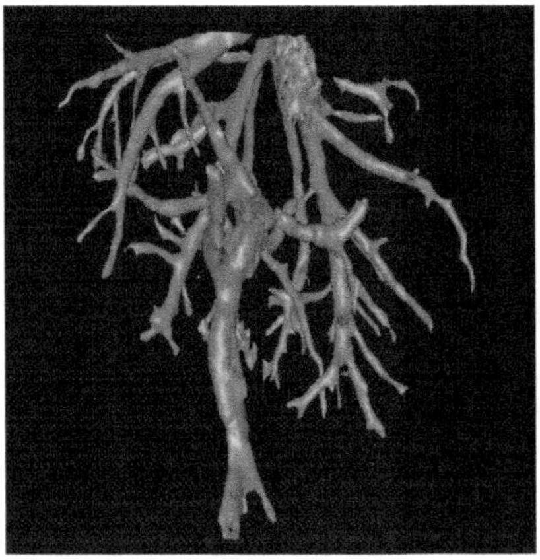

(c) Portal and hepatic veins at late portal phase.

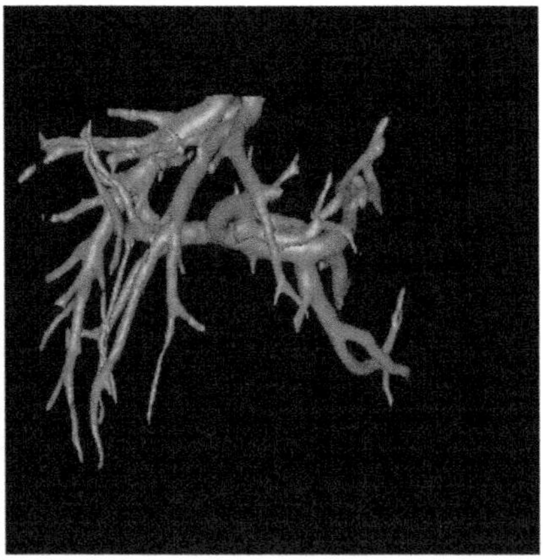

(d) Portal and hepatic veins at venous phase.

Fig. 6. Some results of 3D reconstructed hepatic vessels for different patients at different CT hepatic perfusion phases

In conclusion, the data acquisition triggering plays an important role in selecting the appropriate vessel enhancement. The analysis of portal and hepatic veins for preoperative purposes requires CT acquisitions at late portal phase which ensures the best contrast of such structures. Vessel topological analysis is possible after the 3D segmentation by means of a central axis-based description. In this respect, a central axis computation approach for tree-like structures and the related navigation/interaction tools have already been developed in the framework of pulmonary airways investigation. Their description is beyond the scope of this paper, but the interested reader could report to [13].

5 Conclusion

This paper addressed the issue of 3D segmentation of liver vessels from 3D CT hepatic venography data acquired in clinical routine with various protocols. It developed an original and automated 3D reconstruction methodology based on topological and morphological operators combined in a multiresolution scheme. Such an approach made it possible to overcome the limitations raised by the CT image variability in terms of liver opacifying degree and noise presence. Tested at different perfusion phases, the developed segmentation methodology is currently under extensive validation in a clinical framework of liver surgery planning.

References

1. Y. Onodera *et al.*, "Peripheral anatomic evaluation using 3D CT hepatic venography in donors: significance of peripheral venous visualization in living-donor transplantation", in *American Journal of Radiology*, **183**, pp. 1065 -1070, 2004.
2. H.-O. Peitgen *et al.*, "Risk analysis for liver surgery", *Matematica et Cultura 2000*, M. Emmer Ed., Springer, Milano, pp. 331-340, 2000.
3. D. Selle *et al.*, "Analysis of vasculature for liver surgical planning", in *IEEE Trans Med Imaging*, **21**(11), pp. 1344-1357, 2002.
4. B. Reitinger, A. Bornik, R. Beichel, G. Werkgartner, E. Sorantin, "Tools for Augmented Reality based Liver Resection Planning", *SPIE Medical Imaging 2004*, pp. 88-99, 2004.
5. H.-P. Meinzer, M. Thorn, C. Cardenas, "Computerized planning of liver surgery - an overview", *Computers & Graphics* **26**, pp. 569-576, 2002.
6. H. Bourquain *et al.*, "HepaVision2 - A software assistant for preoperative planning in living-related liver transplantation and oncologic liver surgery", *Proc. CARS 2002*, pp. 341-346, 2002.
7. P. Dokladal, C. Lohou, L. Perroton, G. Bertrand, "Liver blood vessel extraction by a 3D topological approach", *Proc. MICCAI*, **1679**, pp. 98-104, 1999.
8. E. K. Fishman, B. S. Kuszyk, D. G. Heath, L Gao, B. Cabral, "Surgical planning for liver resection", *IEEE Computer*, pp. 64-72, 1996.
9. L. Soler *et al.*, "Fully automatic anatomical, pathological, and functional segmentation from CT scans for hepatic surgery", *Computer Aided Surgery*, **6**(3), pp. 131-142, 2001.
10. C. Fetita, F. Preteux, C. Beigelman-Aubry, P. Grenier, "Pulmonary airways: 3D reconstruction from multi-slice CT and clinical investigation", *IEEE Transactions on Medical Imaging*, **23**(11), pp. 1353-1364, 2004.
11. L. Vincent, "Morphological gray scale reconstruction in image analysis: applications and efficient algorithms", *IEEE Trans on Image Processing*, **2**(2), pp. 176-201, 1993.
12. F. Prêteux, "On a distance function approach for gray-level mathematical morphology", in *Mathematical morphology in image processing*, M. Dekker ed., E. R. Dougherty, 1992.
13. D. Perchet, C. Fetita, L. Vial, F. Preteux, G. Caillibotte, G. Sbirlea-Apiou, M. Thiriet, "Virtual investigation of pulmonary airways in volumetric computed tomography", *Computer Animation & Virtual Worlds*, **15**(3-4), pp. 361-376, 2004.

Shape-Based Averaging for Combination of Multiple Segmentations

T. Rohlfing[1] and C.R. Maurer, Jr.[2]

[1] Neuroscience Program, SRI International, Menlo Park, CA, USA
torsten@synapse.sri.com
[2] Department of Neurosurgery, Stanford University, Stanford CA, USA
crmaurer@stanford.edu

Abstract. Combination of multiple segmentations has recently been introduced as an effective method to obtain segmentations that are more accurate than any of the individual input segmentations. This paper introduces a new way to combine multiple segmentations using a novel shape-based averaging method. Individual segmentations are combined based on the signed Euclidean distance maps of the labels in each input segmentation. Compared to label voting, the new combination method produces smoother, more regular output segmentations and avoids fragmentation of contiguous structures. Using publicly available segmented human brain MR images (IBSR database), we perform a quantitative comparison between shape-based averaging and label voting by combining random segmentations with controlled error magnitudes and known ground truth. Shape-based averaging generated combined segmentations that were closer to the ground truth than combinations from label voting for all numbers of input segmentations (up to ten). The relative advantage of shape-based averaging over voting was larger for fewer input segmentations, and larger for greater deviations of the input segmentations from the ground truth. We conclude that shape-based averaging improves the accuracy of combined segmentations, in particular when only a few input segmentations are available and when the quality of the input segmentations is low.

1 Introduction

Combination of multiple segmentations has recently been introduced as an effective method to obtain segmentations that are more accurate than any of the individual input segmentations [1,2,3,4]. Typically, such algorithms are based on local (i.e., voxel-wise) decision fusion schemes, such as voting, or on probability-theoretical combination of Bayesian classifiers that assign likelihoods to the possible output classes [5,6].

For classification of voxels in multi-dimensional images, this paper introduces a new way to combine multiple segmentations using a novel shape-based averaging method. Unlike many other classification problems, there is a natural distance relationship between the voxels of an n-dimensional image. We exploit this relationship to combine segmentations based on the signed Euclidean distance maps of the labels in each input segmentation. Compared to label voting, the new combination method produces smoother, more regular output segmentations, and it also produces segmentations that are closer to the ground truth as measured by the recognition rate.

J. Duncan and G. Gerig (Eds.): MICCAI 2005, LNCS 3750, pp. 838–845, 2005.

Our method is related to shape-based interpolation, which was introduced by Raya & Udupa [7] as a method for the interpolation of binary images. Grevera & Udupa [8] later extended the method to gray-level images by embedding an n-dimensional gray-level image into an $(n+1)$-dimensional binary image space. Our approach is similar in that we consider images with multiple classes of a segmentation. However, our approach is different insofar as it combines multiple such images on a common grid into one image, rather than resamples one image onto a new grid. In this sense, our method is a shape-based averaging method.

2 Methods

Let L be the number of classes in the segmentation. For simplicity, each class is identified with a number in the set $\Lambda = \{0, \ldots, L-1\}$, where class 0 without loss of generality represents the image background. For K different (input) segmentations of the same image, let $s_k(\mathbf{x}) \in \Lambda$ for $k = 1, \ldots, K$ be the class assigned to voxel $\mathbf{x}$ in segmentation k. We are particularly interested in atlas-based segmentations that are generated by mapping the coordinates of an image onto those of a segmented atlas image. For s_k, let the atlas image be A_k and the transformation $\mathbf{T}_k$, so that

$$s_k : \mathbf{x} \mapsto A_k(\mathbf{T}_k(\mathbf{x})) \in \Lambda. \tag{1}$$

2.1 Shape-Based Averaging of Segmentations

Let $d_{k,l}(\mathbf{x})$ be the signed Euclidean distance of the voxel at $\mathbf{x}$ from the nearest surface voxel with label l in segmentation k. The value of $d_{k,l}(\mathbf{x})$ is negative if $\mathbf{x}$ is inside structure l, positive if $\mathbf{x}$ is outside, zero if and only if $\mathbf{x}$ is a voxel on the surface of structure l in segmentation k. Note that in effect, we derive from each of the abstract-level classifications s_k a measurement-level classification $d_{k,*}$.

```
for all x do                          ▷ Loop over all voxels to initialize data structures
    S(x) ← L                                                 ▷ Set label to "undecided"
    D_min(x) ← ∞                             ▷ Initialize distance map as "far outside"
end for
for l = 0,...,L−1 do                                              ▷ Loop over all labels
    for all x do                                                  ▷ Loop over all voxels
        D ← Σ_k d_{k,l}(x)             ▷ Total signed distances for this voxel and label
        if D < D_min(x) then          ▷ Is new distance smaller than current minimum?
            S(x) ← l                                       ▷ Update combined label map
            D_min(x) ← D                               ▷ Update minimum total distance
        end if
    end for
end for
```

Fig. 1. Shape-based averaging algorithm. See text for details

Based on the distance maps of all structures in all input segmentations, we define the total distance of voxel $\mathbf{x}$ from label l as

$$D_l(\mathbf{x}) = \sum_{k=1}^{K} d_{k,l}(\mathbf{x}). \tag{2}$$

Note that since the number of segmentations K is constant, the total distance is directly proportional to the average distance. The combined segmentation $S(\mathbf{x})$ for voxel $\mathbf{x}$ is now determined by minimizing the total distance from the combined label (and, equivalently, the average distance) as

$$S(\mathbf{x}) = \arg\min_{l \in \Lambda} D_l(\mathbf{x}). \tag{3}$$

This can be iteratively computed using the algorithm in Fig. 1. Note that at any given time, due to the incremental nature of our algorithm, it requires space for three distance maps independent of the number of classes L: 1) the individual distance map $d_{k,l}$ for the current input segmentation k and class l, 2) the total distance map D_l over all segmentations for class l, and 3) the minimum total distance map $D_{\min}$ over all classes so far.

The main computational burden of our method stems from repeatedly computing the Euclidean distance transformation. We use an efficient algorithm by Maurer *et al.* [9] that computes the exact Euclidean distance in linear time $O(N)$, where N is the number of voxels in the image.

Examples of intermediate closest distance maps and corresponding label maps are illustrated in Fig. 2. For better graphical presentation, the images shown are from a simpler segmentation problem with a smaller number of less complex structures than there are in the human brain. As the algorithm iterates over all labels, areas that have been assigned to a label turn negative in the minimum total distance map (Fig. 2(b) and 2(c)), representing their location "inside" a structure. When all labels have been processed, the boundaries between structures are identified by the zero-level set in the final total distance map (Fig. 2(d)).

2.2 Label Voting

For comparison with our new method, we have implemented a standard segmentation combination scheme based on label voting. In atlas-based segmentation, labels need to be computed for non-grid locations in the atlas by interpolation. One interpolation technique that is applicable to label data and produces better results then nearest neighbor interpolation (NN) is partial volume (PV) interpolation, introduced by Maes *et al.* [10] for histogram generation in entropy-based image registration. Using PV interpolation, a vector of weights is returned as the classifier output, where each weight represents the relative share of one label. From these weights, we compute the combined segmentation for each voxel by sum fusion, i.e., by adding all weight vectors from the individual segmentations and selecting the class with the highest weight in the sum.

Note that by applying PV interpolation and sum fusion we effectively take advantage of the inherent sub-pixel resolution[1] of atlas-based segmentations. Other segmen-

[1] NB: sub-pixel *resolution* does not imply sub-pixel *accuracy*.

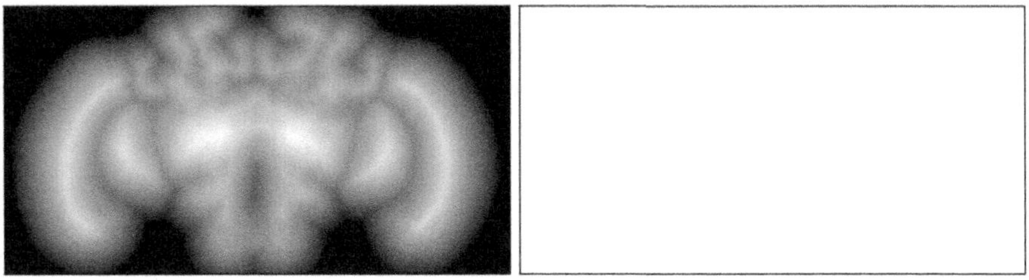

(a) $l = 0$ (background)

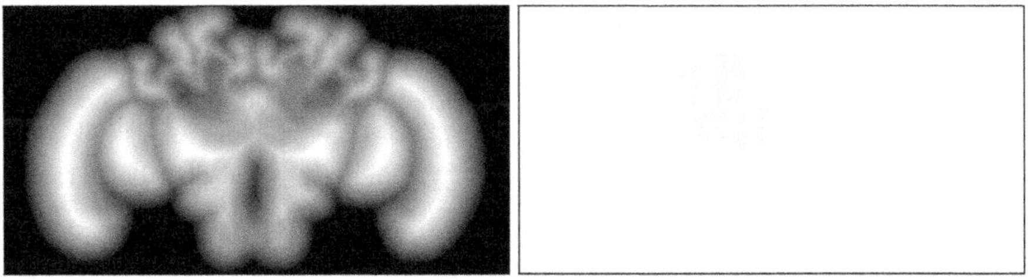

(b) $l \leq 2$

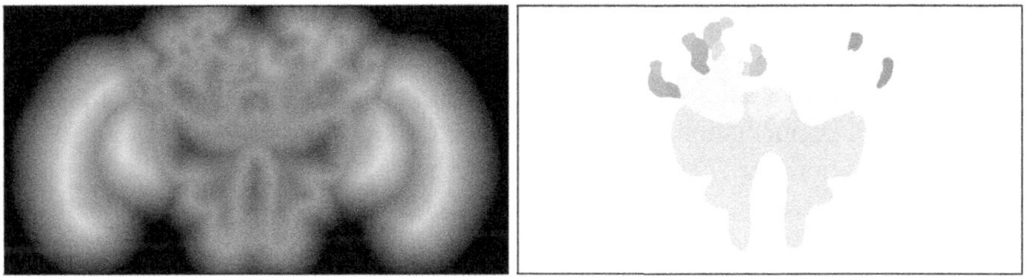

(c) $l \leq 11$

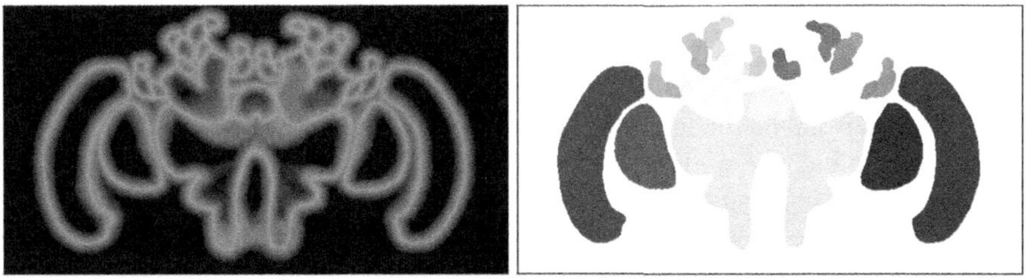

(d) $l \leq 22$ (final)

Fig. 2. Example of evolving minimum total distance maps $D_{\min}(\mathbf{x})$ (left image in each pair) and label maps $S(\mathbf{x})$ (right image in each pair). Brighter values in the distance maps correspond to positive values (i.e., outside of structures), darker values correspond to negative values (i.e., inside of structures). (a) Image background is canonically treated as an ordinary label. (b) First two non-background structures. (c) First 11 non-background structures. (d) Final combined segmentation (22 structures). For illustrative purposes, the images shown in this figure are from a different, simpler segmentation problem with a smaller number of less complex structures than there are in the human brain images used for quantitative evaluation in this paper.

tation methods, most notably manual segmentation, may not require label interpolation, in which case combination by sum fusion reduces to combination by vote fusion, i.e., counting of discrete votes for each label. The same is true for atlas-based segmentation when nearest (NN) is used instead of PV interpolation.

2.3 Evaluation

For quantitative evaluation of the combination method independent of the performance of a particular segmentation algorithm, we apply a strategy introduced by Rohlfing *et al.* [3]. This method evaluated classifier combination methods in atlas-based segmentation using segmentations with controlled error magnitudes and known ground truth. Based on the ground truth segmentation of an image, a random segmentation is generated by applying a nonrigid coordinate transformation of random magnitude. In particular, we apply B-spline free-form deformations (FFD) [11] with control point positions perturbed from the identity transformation by adding Gaussian-distributed random numbers. The choice of the FFD transformation model is motivated by its compact representation, as well as by the fact that it is also used in a popular nonrigid registration algorithm by Rueckert *et al.* [12].

A set of publicly available expert-segmented human brain MR images (T_1-weighted anatomical images) from ten subjects was obtained from the Internet Brain Segmentation Repository (IBSR; `http://www.cma.mgh.harvard.edu/ibsr/`). The corresponding segmentations with 43 anatomical structures provide the ground truths for the random segmentation evaluation outlined above (since we do not perform an actual segmentation, the anatomical MR images were not actually used in this study). All images had the same size, 256×256×128 voxels, with coronal slice orientation. The in-plane pixel size was either 0.9 mm or 1.0 mm. The slice spacing of all images was 1.5 mm.

For each image in our test set, twenty random segmentations were generated: ten with a standard deviation of the random perturbation of the FFD control points of $\sigma = 10$ mm, and another ten with $\sigma = 20$ mm. Note that larger values of σ correspond to larger magnitudes of the random FFDs, and thus to larger deviations of the random segmentations from the (undeformed) ground truth.

For each value of σ, we then computed combinations of two through ten of the respective random segmentations at that error level, once using shape-based averaging and once using label voting. The accuracy of each combined segmentation was then quantified by computing the recognition rate, i.e., the fraction of correctly labeled voxels as compared to the ground truth segmentation.

3 Results

Examples of combined segmentations using shape-based averaging and label voting are shown as 3-D renderings in Fig. 3. Shape-based averaging produced visually superior results. In particular, the inherent spatial continuity of the Euclidean distance maps avoided fragmentation of contiguous structures.

The recognition rates of combined human brain MR segmentations (simulated segmentations) using shape-based averaging and label voting are plotted in Fig. 4. Results

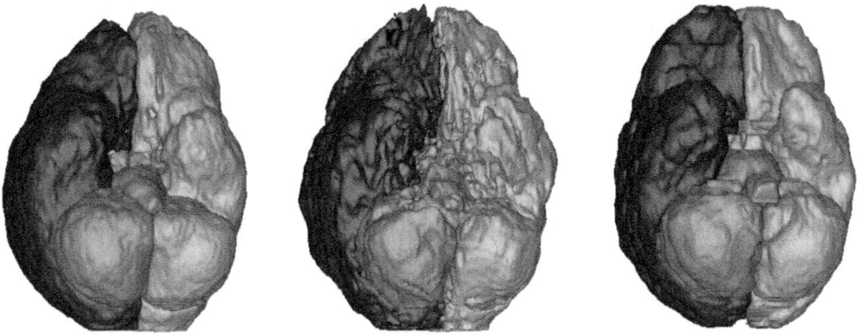

(a) (b) (c)

Fig. 3. Three-dimensional rendering of the inferior brain surface of the human brain MR data used for evaluation. (a) Shape-based averaging. (b) Label voting. (c) Ground truth. The renderings (a) and (b) are the result of averaging the same five simulated segmentations generated with FFD perturbation $\sigma = 20\,\text{mm}$.

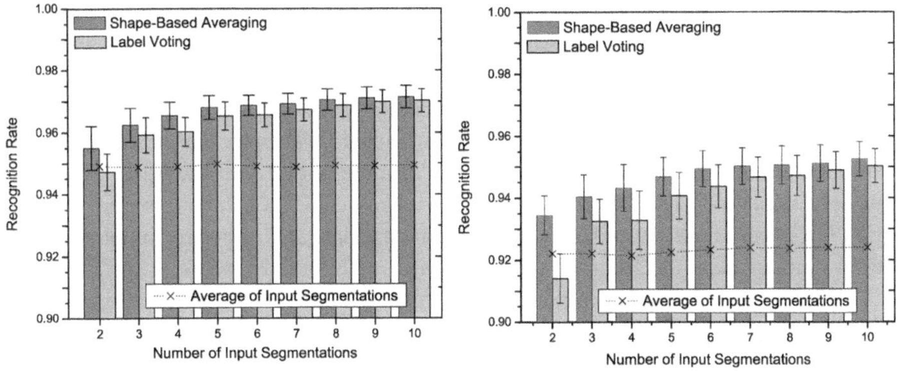

(a) $\sigma = 10\,\text{mm}$ (b) $\sigma = 20\,\text{mm}$

Fig. 4. Recognition rates of combined segmentations for shape-based averaging and label voting. (a) Input segmentations generated using random FFD with $\sigma = 10\,\text{mm}$. (b) Input segmentations generated using random FFD with $\sigma = 20\,\text{mm}$. In both graphs, the columns represent the mean recognition rates over ten subjects. The error bars represent the respective standard deviations. The dashed lines show the averaged recognition rates of the individual segmentations used as inputs for the combination methods.

using random deformations with $\sigma = 10\,\text{mm}$ are shown in Fig. 4(a), results using $\sigma = 20\,\text{mm}$ in Fig. 4(b).

Both segmentation combination methods generated outputs closer to the ground truth the more input segmentations were provided to them. Between the two combination methods, shape-based averaging clearly outperformed label voting in all cases. The relative advantage of shape-based averaging was larger for smaller numbers of input segmentations, and it was larger for greater deviations of the input segmentations from the ground truth ($\sigma = 20\,\mathrm{mm}$). The recognition rate of the combined segmentation using shape-based averaging improved consistently with added input segmentations, while label voting benefited less from even numbers of inputs than it did from odd numbers.

Note that combination of two segmentations by voting is not entirely reasonable as there is no way to decide the winning label in cases of disagreement. Therefore, the combined classification will fail wherever the two input segmentations disagree. As a result, the combination of only two segmentations by label voting has a worse recognition rate than the individual segmentations. Similarly, even numbers of input segmentations in general increase the likelihood of equal numbers of votes for more than one label in label voting. Neither is the case for shape-based averaging, which clearly improves recognition rates even for only two input segmentations, because each segmentation assigns a weight to every voxel based on its distance from the nearest structure boundary.

4 Discussion

This paper has introduced a method for shape-based averaging that can be applied to combine multiple segmentations of the same image. In a quantitative evaluation study using simulated segmentations, which makes it independent of the performance of any particular segmentation algorithm, we have demonstrated the superiority of our method to label voting. Applied to identical input segmentations, shape-based averaging generated combined segmentations that were substantially closer to the ground truth than those generated by label voting. The improvement achieved by shape-based averaging was larger for smaller number of input segmentations, and larger for input segmentations that deviate more from the ground truth.

While evaluation using randomly deformed ground truth segmentations borrows from concepts of atlas-based segmentations, our method is straight forward to apply to segmentations generated by arbitrary labeling methods. It works on as few as two segmentations, whereas label voting requires at least three and is prone to undecided voxels for small numbers of segmentations. These properties make our method potentially interesting for combination of multiple manual segmentations, where the number of available segmentations is typically small.

A potentially useful extension of our method is to use robust averaging rather than the arithmetic means of the individual distance functions as in the present paper (Eq. 3). This may improve the combination results in the presence of outliers, and ultimately also provide an effective way to address the problem of diversity [13] among the input segmentations.

Acknowledgments

The authors thank R. Menzel (Institute für Neurobiologie, Freie Universität Berlin, Berlin, Germany) and for R. Brandt (Mercury Computer Systems GmbH, Berlin, Germany) providing segmented bee brain microscopy images used for illustration in Fig. 2.

The normal MR brain data sets and their manual segmentations were provided by the Center for Morphometric Analysis at Massachusetts General Hospital and are available at `http://www.cma.mgh.harvard.edu/ibsr/`.

References

1. Rohlfing, T., Brandt, R., Menzel, R., Maurer, Jr., C.R.: Evaluation of atlas selection strategies for atlas-based image segmentation with application to confocal microscopy images of bee brains. NeuroImage **21** (2004) 1428–1442
2. Warfield, S.K., Zou, K.H., Wells, W.M.: Simultaneous truth and performance level estimation (STAPLE): An algorithm for the validation of image segmentation. IEEE Trans. Med. Imag. **23** (2004) 903–921
3. Rohlfing, T., Russakoff, D.B., Maurer, Jr., C.R.: Performance-based classifier combination in atlas-based image segmentation using expectation-maximization parameter estimation. IEEE Trans. Med. Imag. **23** (2004) 983–994
4. Rohlfing, T., Maurer, Jr., C.R.: Multi-classifier framework for atlas-based image segmentation. Pattern Recogn. Lett. (2005, in press)
5. Xu, L., Krzyzak, A., Suen, C.Y.: Methods of combining multiple classifiers and their applications to handwriting recognition. IEEE Trans. Syst. Man Cybern. **22** (1992) 418–435
6. Kittler, J., Hatef, M., Duin, R.P.W., Matas, J.: On combining classifiers. IEEE Trans. Pattern Anal. Machine Intell. **20** (1998) 226–239
7. Raya, S.P., Udupa, J.K.: Shape-based interpolation of multidimensional objects. IEEE Trans. Med. Imag. **9** (1990) 32–42
8. Grevera, G.J., Udupa, J.K.: Shape-based interpolation of multidimensional grey-level images. IEEE Trans. Med. Imag. **15** (1996) 881–892
9. Maurer, Jr., C.R., Qi, R., Raghavan, V.: A linear time algorithm for computing exact Euclidean distance transforms of binary images in arbitrary dimensions. IEEE Trans. Pattern Anal. Machine Intell. **25** (2003) 265–270
10. Maes, F., Collignon, A., Vandermeulen, D., Marchal, G., Suetens, P.: Multimodality image registration by maximisation of mutual information. IEEE Trans. Med. Imag. **16** (1997) 187–198
11. Sederberg, T.W., Parry, S.R.: Free-form deformation and solid geometric models. Comput. Graph. (ACM) **20** (1986) 151–160
12. Rueckert, D., Sonoda, L.I., Hayes, C., Hill, D.L.G., Leach, M.O., Hawkes, D.J.: Nonrigid registration using free-form deformations: Application to breast MR images. IEEE Trans. Med. Imag. **18** (1999) 712–721
13. Kuncheva, L.I.: Diversity in multiple classifier systems. Inform. Fusion **6** (2005) 3–4

Automatic Initialization Algorithm for Carotid Artery Segmentation in CTA Images

Martijn Sanderse[1], Henk A. Marquering[1], Emile A. Hendriks[2], Aad van der Lugt[3], and Johan H.C. Reiber[1]

[1] Dept. of Radiology, Div. of Image Processing, LUMC, Leiden, The Netherlands
{M.Sanderse, H.A.Marquering, J.H.C.Reiber}@lumc.nl
[2] ICT Group, Delft Univ. of Technology, Delft, The Netherlands
E.A.Hendriks@ewi.tudelft.nl
[3] Dept. Of Radiology, Erasmus Medical Center, Rotterdam, The Netherlands
A.vanderLugt@erasmusmc.nl

Abstract. Analysis of CT datasets is commonly time consuming because of the required manual interaction. We present a novel and fast automatic initialization algorithm to detect the carotid arteries providing a fully automated approach of the segmentation and centerline detection. First, the volume of interest (VOI) is estimated using a shoulder landmark. The carotid arteries are subsequently detected in axial slices of the VOI by applying a circular Hough transform. To select carotid arteries related signals in the Hough space, a 3-D, direction dependent hierarchical clustering is used. To allow a successful detection for a wide range of vessel diameters, a feedback architecture was introduced. The algorithm was designed and optimized using a training set of 20 patients and subsequently evaluated using 31 test datasets. The detection algorithm, including VOI estimation, correctly detects 88% of the carotid arteries. Even though not all carotid arteries have been correctly detected, the results are very promising.

1 Introduction

CT angiography images an anatomical region as a 3D volume. The axial source images can be used for visual inspection and to grade the severity of stenosis. However, this is a tedious job and it does not make full use of the advantages of 3D visualization. The 3D volume representation offers several post processing techniques such as Curved Planar Reformation (CPR) [1] to ease the evaluation of the artery. CPR resamples the dataset such that the centerline of an artery becomes a straight line. In current visualization workstations centerlines are not detected automatically, and user interaction is required to position several points inside the vessel [e.g. Vessel View; Siemens, Forchheim, Germany]. Several segmentation techniques and centerline detection algorithms can be used to segment the carotid arteries and detect their centerline [2,3,4,5]. However, all of these techniques need to be initialized manually by the specification of the start and end points of the artery segment.

J. Duncan and G. Gerig (Eds.): MICCAI 2005, LNCS 3750, pp. 846–853, 2005.

Here we present an Automatic iNITialization Algorithm (AnitA) to select the carotid arteries providing a fully automated approach of the segmentation of the carotid arteries and the detection of its centerline. This algorithm excludes any user interaction and therefore reduces the time required for the analysis of carotid arteries. The algorithm is designed to position a single initialization point in the common carotid arteries. This point can then be used by common segmentation algorithms, such as a wave front propagation segmentation algorithm [6]. Usually a full examination of the carotid arteries using CT images takes approximately 30 to 45 minutes. It is expected that a full automatic segmentation can reduce this time to 5 to 10 minutes.

There are only a few papers known that are concerned with the fully automatic detection of arteries. Cline et al. [7] have developed a method to automatically segment the coronary vessel tree with mathematical morphology operations. Lorenz [8] describes a heuristic approach for delineation of the cardiac volume, which includes the automatic detection of the descending aorta. Both methods are heuristic methods for different vessels and therefore not suitable to adapt to carotid artery detection.

To our knowledge no literature has been published that describes a fast and fully automated segmentation of a peripheral vessel (segment) in 3D datasets. Here we present a fast initialization algorithm that allows the fully automatic start of a the segmentation of the carotid arteries, which may be generally applicable to other vessels.

2 Methods

AnitA consist of two main steps. Because the lower part of the neck is best suited to detect the common carotid arteries, this area, or volume of interest (VOI) is estimated first. In the second step the common carotid arteries are detected in the VOI and the initialization point is selected for each carotid artery.

To automatically determine the VOI it is desirable to make use of distinct image features, or landmarks. A distinct (spatial) feature in CT images is the (vertical) position of the shoulders, which is close to the common carotid arteries. The shoulders are detected in Maximum Intensity Projections (MIPs) of the dataset on the coronal plane (xz-plane). The detection process starts at two positions: 6 cm left and right of the center of the MIP (figure 1). The closests pixels with bone intensities below these starting points are considered to be the shoulder landmark.

The VOI boundaries can be estimated based upon this position. First the VOI boundaries are manually determined in the training datasets. From the distances between these positions in single datasets, a general relation between VOI boundaries and landmarks is determined.

Because the common carotid arteries have a tubular shape and run near vertically, their appearance in horizontal slices approximates circles. The carotid arteries are detected in a number of steps, which are described below. First, small size contributions are removed by smoothing the image using a convolution with

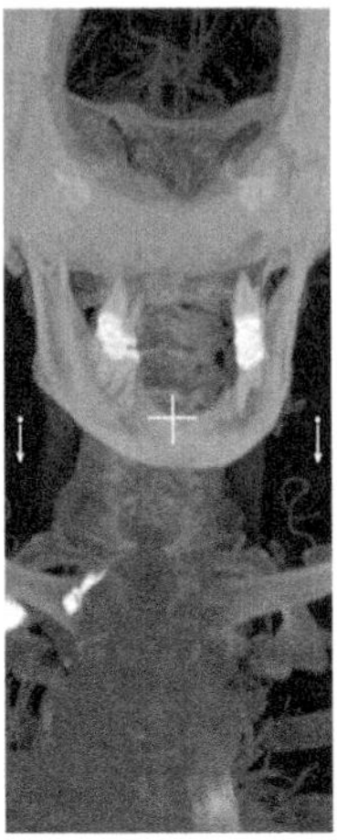

Fig. 1. Landmark detection starts next to the center of the MIP, and is then directed downwards

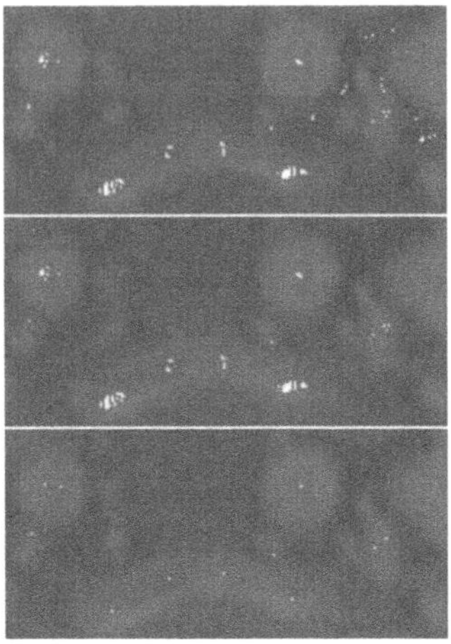

Fig. 2. Maxima (white dots) in a slice after thresholding Hough space (top), maxima reduced by threshold of values in corresponding position in original image (middle), and a second reduction by clustering and replacing the cluster with its center of gravity (bottom)

a Gaussian. In order to detect circles in the images, we need to extract the contour of the carotid arteries. Edges are detected by using a combination of the gradient magnitude and the Laplacian of the image in horizontal slices. Edges that are typical for the carotid arteries are selected by thresholding the gradient magnitude, excluding edges that are too sharp or too soft. The edge image is subsequently used to detect potential center points of the carotid arteries using the circular Hough transform. The Hough transform can be expressed as a convolution operation, using a circle with a radius r as the kernel:

$$H = E \otimes K_{Circle} \tag{1}$$

$$K_{Circle} = \begin{cases} 1, & \text{iff} \quad m^2 + n^2 = r^2 \\ 0, & \text{otherwise} \end{cases} \tag{2}$$

with H the Hough response, E the binary edge image, and K_{Circle} the circle kernel. The pixels that are most likely to be center points of a circle appear as maxima in the output image of the convolution operation. In order to be able to detect circles for a range of radii in one convolution operation, the kernel can be shaped like an annulus:

$$K_{Annulus} = \begin{cases} 1, & \text{iff} \quad r_{min}^2 < m^2 + n^2 < r_{max}^2 \\ 0, & \text{otherwise} \end{cases} \tag{3}$$

with $K_{Annulus}$ the annulus kernel, and r_{min} and r_{max} the minimum and maximum radius of the annulus [9]. To remove the contributions that are not related to the carotid arteries, only the local maxima are selected that have an intensity of at least 90% of the maximum intensity (figure 2). To reduce the number of maxima even further, the intensity in the original image at the corresponding positions is used to discard maxima that do not have an intensity value that is typical for contrast-enhanced blood. Because in a single slice multiple maxima per carotid artery are found, the number of maxima is finally reduced by clustering these maxima per slice. This can reduce the number of maxima per carotid artery to one, in a single slice. The clustering technique also reduces the number of non-carotid related maxima.

The procedure described above, produces a 3D volume with center points that are potentially related to the carotid arteries. To distinguish the carotid artery center points from other objects, we can make use of knowledge on the tubular shape and the running of the carotid arteries. This near vertical running of the common carotid arteries results in little deviation in horizontal position in subsequent axial slices. To exploit this anatomical property, a 3D clustering is applied in which a point is added to a cluster if the distance to the cluster is not larger than a given direction dependent distance. The distance between a cluster and a point is defined as the minimum distance between the point and any other point of the cluster and is calculated as

$$d = \sqrt{x^2 + y^2 + (\alpha \cdot z)^2}, \quad \text{with } 0 < \alpha < 1 \tag{4}$$

where α allows for larger deviation in the z-direction and consequently puts restrictions on the horizontal distance in the clustering. The two clusters containing the most Hough maxima are considered to contain the center points of the left and right common carotid artery.

A self test was introduced to value the results from the detection process based upon the number of center points per cluster. If the number of center points in one of the clusters was below a threshold, the detection process can be repeated using a different value for the annulus kernel. After the second run, the self test is used again to determine if the smaller radius range annulus provides a satisfying detection.

Finally, from each cluster the point with the highest intensity in Hough space is selected as the final initialization point.

3 Results

The estimation of the VOI and the detection of carotids were initially developed using a dataset of 20 patients. For the testing of the algorithm data from another 31 patients were used. This test set consisted of datas from 29 successive patients from one clinic, and two other datasets from two different clinics.

The shoulder landmarks were detected correctly on all test datasets. The VOI detector was constructed by comparing the data from the VOIs determined manually and the using the landmarks. The VOI detector based on the shoulder was constructed as follows:

$$VOI_{upper} = z_{shoulder} + d_{Vu} \quad (5)$$

$$VOI_{lower} = z_{shoulder} - d_{Vl} \quad (6)$$

with $z_{shoulder}$ the position of the shoulder landmark in the VOI, and d_{Vu} and d_{Vl} the average distance between upper and lower VOI boundaries and shoulder landmark. Table 1 and figure 3 show the results of the VOI estimation.

Because the carotid artery must be detected in a number of subsequent slices, the VOI does not have to be estimated perfectly accurate. However, it is important that the common carotid arteries are present in the bulk of the slices of the VOI. Therefore the VOIs are evaluated on the basis of the percentage of the slices in which the common carotid arteries are present. Taken the carotid artery detection in consideration, the VOI detection is considered successful if the common carotid arteries are present in at least 70% of the slices. For all steps of the carotid artery detection in the VOI, initially a range of values was used for each parameter to inspect which values gave the best performance. Because the optimal values of some parameters are dependent on the settings of other parameters, continuous tuning of the values of all parameters was done while developing the algorithm. Final values for all parameters can be found in Table 2.

On average the Hough transform resulted in 50 maxima for each slice. After removing contributions that do not have typical values for contrast enhanced blood in the original image in corresponding positions, on average 40 maxima

Table 1. VOI estimation results

	Number of test datasets
Total number of datasets tested	31
100% common carotid arteries present in slices	23
$\geq$ 70% common carotid arteries present in slices	30
$\geq$ 50% common carotid arteries present in slices	31

Table 2. Values of parameters for carotid arteries detection

Standard deviation Gaussian for smoothing	1.8 mm
Zero crossing margin in edge detector	10 HU/mm^2
Maximum gradient magnitude in edge detector	860 HU/mm
Minimum gradient magnitude in edge detector	172 HU/mm
Maximum clustering distance in 2D in maxima reduction	5.8 mm
Maximum cluster distance in 3D	5.8 mm
Factor to allow large cluster distance in z-direction α	0.001
First Hough transform annulus kernel radius-range	3.5 mm $< r <$ 4.5 mm
Second Hough transform annulus kernel radius-range	2.5 mm $< r <$ 3.5 mm

were present in each slice. After the reduction using the 2D clustering only 10 maxima were present on average in each slice. For the evaluation of the presented method, the carotid artery detection was performed on the test dataset. The algorithm provided 50 initialization points (25 datasets) that were considered accurate according to the self evaluation test. Of these 25 datasets, 16 were detected during the initial run and in 9 datasets the carotid arteries were detected in the second run. In 6 datasets, the self evaluation test decided that no accurate carotid artery detection was performed. Subsequently, the results of all test datasets were inspected visually. Initialization points that were classified as successful by the self test and proved to be correct by visual inspection were labeled true positive, see table 3. All true positive points were usable as initialization points according to expert opinion. In the training set all datasets were classified as successful by the self test. In the first run 37 initialization points were correctly positioned, after a second run, on three datasets, 39 initialization points were positioned correctly in total, resulting in a true positive percentage

Table 3. Results from carotid artery detection in estimated VOIs in test datasets

True positive	91%
True negative	67%
Unsuccessful datasets after re-run	21%

Table 4. Total numbers of correct and uncorrect detected initialization points in training and test sets

	# Correct init. points	# False init. points	Percentage
Training set (20 datasets)	39	1	97.5%
Test set (31 datasets)	51	11	82.3%
Total (51 datasets)	90	12	88.2%

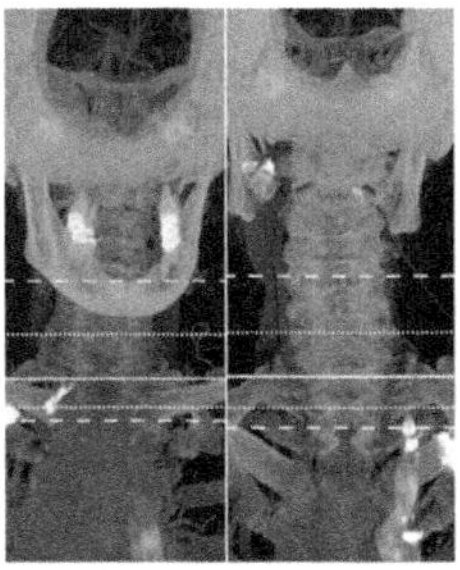

Fig. 3. Two VOI estimations, shoulder landmark in solid line, estimated VOI in dotted lines, manually selected VOI in dashed lines

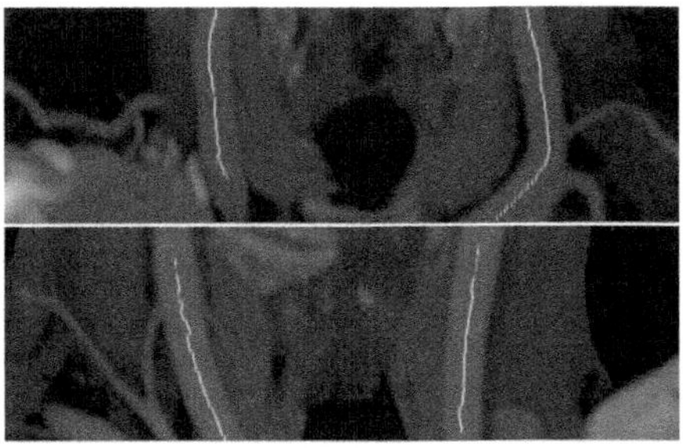

Fig. 4. Slab based MIPs of two VOIs, showing all center points found in the two largest clusters. They are positioned inside the carotid arteries.

of 97.5%. Table 4 shows the total numbers of correct and incorrect initialization points according to expert opinion. Figure 4 shows the detected centerpoints of the carotid arteries in slab based MIPs.

The average time necessary to detect the starting points in the datasets, including the time needed to read the data from hard disk is 120 sec. with a standard deviation of 20 sec., on a Pentium IV 2.5Ghz processor, with 1 GB of memory.

4 Discussion

We have presented a full automatic approach of detection the carotid arteries in CTA datasets using a VOI estimation and a Hough space based carotid artery detection. The shoulder landmark was detected correctly in all datasets, resulting in accurate VOI estimations using the average distance of shoulder and VOI boundaries.

While testing for the optimal radius for the Hough transform, most carotid arteries were detected using a radius of approximately 4 mm. In some datasets 4 mm was too large and a radius of around 3 mm gave correct results. It was not possible to detect carotid arteries using a Hough annulus kernel with a radius range that included both radii, because too many contributions from other structures in the Hough space were present. This was solved by introducing a feedback architecture using the self test allowing two runs with a different radius range. The self test was also used to grade the performance of the carotid artery detection. Currently this use of the test results in too many false negatives. Improvement of the self test is expected by incorporating a more advanced analysis of the shape and position of the cluster and anatomical knowledge.

The carotid artery detection was unsuccessful for a few datasets, because the intensity of the maxima related to the carotid arteries was smaller than required. Careful inspection of the various steps indicated that this can happen when parts of the contour are not detected. In some datasets the carotid arteries were detected, but in too few slices, resulting in a rejection by the self test classifier. Another cause for failure was the strong variation in the density of contrast material in CT images. In these cases, the intensities in other arteries and veins was significantly higher than was observed in the training set. As a result of this, in one dataset a jugular vein was detected instead of carotid arteries in the test set. It is expected that a full automatic segmentation can reduce analysis time of a single dataset from 30-45 minutes to 5-10 minutes. It has been shown that AnitA can detect the carotid arteries on average in 88%, therefore this approach can reduce the analysis time by a factor 3 on average.

5 Conclusions

Currently, a significant amount of time in the evaluation of arteries in CTA images is concerned with the manual interaction for the centerline detection. We have presented a novel approach for the full automatic detection of the carotid arteries. The implementation of such an automated detection results in a significant reduction of analysis time of the carotid arteries in CT-images.

The combination of the VOI estimator based on the shoulder landmark and a carotid artery detection based on a circular Hough transform and a hierarchical clustering algorithm has been proved to be successful on 31 test datasets. In 97% the VOI detection is correct, and in 88% the carotid artery detection in the estimated VOIs is correct. Even though not all carotid artery detections were successful, the results are very promising.

References

1. Kanitsar, A., Fleischmann, D., Wegenkittl, R., Felkel, P., Gröller, M.E.: Cpr: curved planar reformation. In: VIS '02: Proceedings of the conference on Visualization '02, Washington, DC, USA, IEEE Computer Society (2002) 37–44
2. Felkel, P., Wegenkittl, R., Kanitsar, A.: Vessel tracking in peripheral cta datasets – an overview. In: SCCG '01: Proceedings of the 17th Spring conference on Computer graphics, Washington, DC, USA, IEEE Computer Society (2001) 232
3. Kirbas, C., Quek, F.: A review of vessel extraction techniques and algorithms. ACM Comput. Surv. **36** (2004) 81–121
4. van Andl, H.A.F.G., Meijering, E.H.W., van der Lugt, A., Vrooman, H.A., Stokking, R.: Vampire: Improved method for automated center lumen line definition in atherosclerotic carotid arteries in cta data. In: MICCAI (1). (2004) 525–532
5. Koning, P.D.: Automated segmentation and analysis of vascular structures in magnetic resonance images. Magnetic Resonance Images **50** (2003) 1189–1198
6. Marquering, H.A., Dijkstra, J., Koning, P.J.D., Stoel, B.C., Reiber, J.H.: Towards quantitative analysis of coronary cta. The International Journal of Cardiovascular Imaging **21** (2005) 73–84
7. Cline, H.E., Thedens, D., Irarrazaval, P., Meyer, C., Hu, B., Nishimura, D., Ludke, S.: 3d mr coronary artery segmentation. Magnetic Resonance in Medicine **40** (1998) 697–702
8. Lorenz, C., Lessick, J., Lavi, G., Bülow, T., Renisch, S.: Fast automatic delineation of cardiac volume of interest in msct images. In: Medical Imaging 2004: Image Processing. Edited by Fitzpatrick, J. Michael; Sonka, Milan. Proceedings of the SPIE. Volume 5370. (2004) 456–466
9. Kerbyson, D., Atherton, T.: Circle detection using hough transform filters. In: Image Processing and its Applications, Fifth International Conference on. (1995) 370–374

Automated Nomenclature of Bronchial Branches Extracted from CT Images and Its Application to Biopsy Path Planning in Virtual Bronchoscopy*

Kensaku Mori[1], Sinya Ema[1], Takayuki Kitasaka[1], Yoshito Mekada[2], Ichiro Ide[1], Hiroshi Murase[1], Yasuhito Suenaga[1], Hirotsugu Takabatake[3], Masaki Mori[4], and Hiroshi Natori[5]

[1] Grad. School of Information Science, Nagoya University, Nagoya 464-8603, Japan
{kensaku, kitasaka, suenaga, ide, murase}@is.nagoya-u.ac.jp
[2] School of Life System Science and Technology, Chukyo University, Toyota 470-0393, Japan
[3] Minami Sanjo Hospital, Sapporo 060-0033, Japan
[4] Sapporo Kosei General Hospital, Sapporo 064-0063, Japan
[5] School of Medicine, Sapporo Medical Univerisity, Sapporo 060-8543, Japan

Abstract. We propose a novel anatomical labeling algorithm for bronchial branches extracted from CT images. This method utilizes multiple branching models for anatomical labeling. In the actual labeling process, the method selects the best candidate models at each branching point. Also a special labeling procedure is proposed for the right upper lobe. As an application of the automated nomenclature of bronchial branches, we utilized anatomical labeling results for assisting biopsy planning. When a user inputs a target point around suspicious regions on the display of a virtual bronchoscopy (VB) system, the path to the desired position is displayed as a sequence of anatomical names of branches. We applied the proposed method to 25 cases of CT images. The labeling accuracy was about 90%. Also the paths to desired positions were generated by using anatomical names in VB.

1 Introduction

Recent progress in 3-D medical imaging devices has enabled us to measure very precise volumetric data of the human body. Since these imaging devices output a lot of images, development of CAD systems is strongly expected to reduce medical doctors' load and to enable more accurate diagnosis. The bronchus is a very important organ in diagnosis of the lung. In the lung area, it is possible

* Parts of this research were supported by Grant-In-Aid for Scientific Research from the Ministry of Education, the 21st-Century COE program, a Grant-In-Aid for Scientific Research from the Ministry of Education, Culture, Sports, Science, and Technology, Japan Society for Promotion of Science, and a Grant-In-Aid for Cancer Research from the Ministry of Health and Welfare.

J. Duncan and G. Gerig (Eds.): MICCAI 2005, LNCS 3750, pp. 854–861, 2005.

to define dominant bronchial branches in each segmental lobe or subsegmental area. Bronchial branches connected to lesions are investigated when diagnosing diseases of the lung. Anatomical names of bronchial branches are systematically assigned based on branching patterns. When a medical doctor reviews chest CT images, bronchial branches connected to lesions are identified and their anatomical names are reported. In bronchoscopic examinations, such as transbronchial lung biopsy (TBLB), medical doctors identify appropriate paths for biopsy using the anatomical names on the paths. Automated nomenclature is one of the indispensable functions required in the CAD systems for the lung.

There are only a few reports on automated anatomical labeling of bronchial branches extracted from CT images [1,2,3]. Mori et al. proposed an automated anatomical labeling method where they prepared a branching model containing anatomical names before the labeling process[1]. This model consists of a set of information of each branch, such as running direction, anatomical name, parent branch name, child branch name. Graph representations of the bronchial branches were obtained by applying a thinning method to the bronchus regions. Automated nomenclature (anatomical labeling) process was sequentially performed from the center to the peripheral side by selecting the best fit branch from the model. However, this model is unable to handle variations in branching patterns. Kitaoka et al. proposed an automated labeling method using a graph matching algorithm[2]. It is still difficult to deal with branching pattern variations. The report from Ema et al. proposed a labeling method using multiple models of bronchial branches[3]. They divided the bronchus into four parts and prepared multiple models for each part. For each part, the best model was selected by calculating the evaluation values of fitting and actual labeling was then performed. However, since the model was selected by averaging the differences of the running directions between the models To solve these problems, we propose a new anatomical labeling algorithm that selects the best candidate models at each branching point in Section 2. Also a special labeling procedure is proposed from the right upper lobe. As an application of the automated nomenclature of bronchial branches, we utilize anatomical labeling results for assisting TBLB path planning in Section 4. When a user inputs a target point around suspicious regions on the display of a virtual bronchoscopy (VB) system[4], the path to the desired position is displayed as a sequence of anatomical names of branches. This function will greatly help a bronchoscopist. Experimental results and discussion are described in Sections 5 and 6.

2 Bronchial Branch Model

The bronchial model is a graph representation that shows the branching patterns of the bronchial branches in each lobe in the lung (RU: right upper lobe, RL: right middle and lower lobes, LU: left upper lobe, and LL: left lower lobe) (Fig. 1). The q-th model, M_q^p, for the lobe p is a set of attributions of branches v_i. The i-th branch has the following attribute information, E_i: branch number i, anatomical name N_i, pointer to parent branch t_i, running direction $\mathbf{d}_i$, pointer

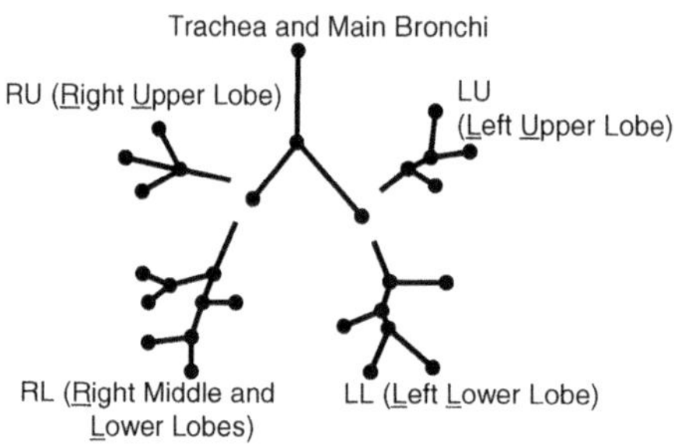

Fig. 1. Division of bronchial trees. A bronchial tree is divided into four lobes: RU, RL, LU, and LL.

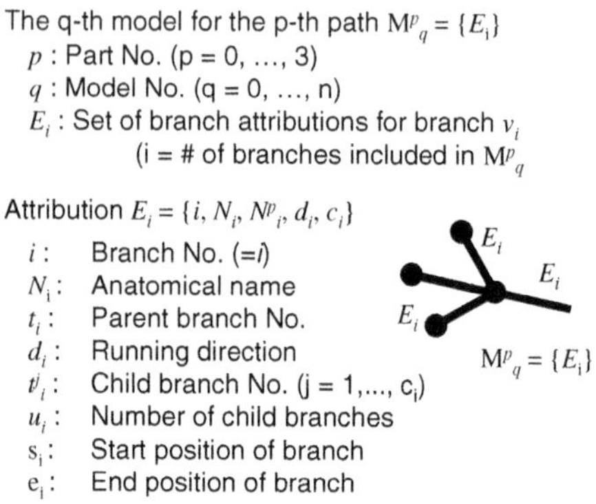

Fig. 2. Branch model structure

to child branches u_i^j $(j = 1, \ldots, c_i)$, number of child branches c_i, start point s_i, and end point e_i (Fig. 2). These models are prepared for each lobe (RU $(p = 0)$, RL $(p = 1)$, LU $(p = 2)$, and LL $(p = 3)$) by using hand-labeled bronchial branches extracted from multiple cases of CT images.

3 Automated Anatomical Labeling

The actual processing procedure consists of four parts: (a) extraction of bronchial regions and bronchial trees from CT image, (b) labeling of trachea and main bronchi, (c) labeling of the RU, and (d) labeling of remaining lobes (RL, LU, and LL). Bronchus regions and tree structres are extracted by using tree structure tracing algorithm presented in [5].

3.1 Labeling for RU

Temporal Labeling. Let B be the child branch of the right upper lobe bronchus (a child branch of the right main bronchus) and a model in the RU $M_q^0$is associated with B. A labeling process is sequentially performed from B to the peripheral branches by using model M_q^0 prepared for the RU and is saved as the temporal labeling results. Let B' be a branch in model M_q^0 that has the same anatomical name as B. Model M_q^0 is then rotated around the start point, B', so that the running direction of B' corresponds to that of B. For all possible combinations of one-to-one correspondence between the child branches of B and B', the sum of the inner products of running directions of the corresponding pairs is calculated. The combination that produces the minimum sum is considered as the best combination and then copy the anatomical name of B' to B and process child branches of B using a breadth-first search. Finally, the labeling results are obtained whose number is equal to the number of the models prepared for RU.

Model Selection. Using temporal labeling results, inappropriate models are removed from candidate models for the RU. First, three vectors are calculated that start from B and direct to the ends of the branches labeled as Rt.B^1, Rt.B^2, and Rt.B^3 using model M_q^0. These vectors are denoted as $\mathbf{U}_1$, $\mathbf{U}_2$, and $\mathbf{U}_3$. Also vectors are calculated on model M_q^0 as $\mathbf{V}_1$, $\mathbf{V}_2$, and $\mathbf{V}_3$ in the same way. If any of the inner products $\mathbf{V}_1 \cdot \mathbf{U}_1$, $\mathbf{V}_2 \cdot \mathbf{U}_2$, or $\mathbf{V}_3 \cdot \mathbf{U}_3$ is smaller than a given threshold value, the model M_q^0 is removed from the RU model candidates. This process is iterated for all models prepared for the RU.

Final Labeling. The labeling process is performed by using the remaining models. For each model, the model is deformed so that the model fits to the input tree structure and an average deformation angle is calculated. The final labeling is performed using the model whose average deformation angle is the smallest among the models. Anatomical names of the deformed model are assigned to the branches of the input tree structure [3].

3.2 Labeling for Remaining Parts

For each child branch of the main bronchi (except for the upper lobe bronchus, i.e. $p = 1, \ldots, 3$), the following steps are performed (Fig. 3).

1. An anatomical name is assigned to a child branch of a main bronchus (right or left main bronchus) and let it be O. The branch O and all candidate models associated with O are stored (for example, if O is left upper lobe bronchus, we associate all models of LU with O.) into a FIFO (first in first out) queue.
2. Branch O and a set of models, $\mathbf{M}^O$, associated with O are retrieved from the queue. If the queue is empty, the process is terminated.
3. If O does not have a child branch, return to Step 2. Otherwise, branches of O'_i are searched for whose anatomical names equal O's anatomical name in each model M_i^p contained in model set $\mathbf{M}^O$. If the number of child branches of O and O'_i differs, the model M_i^p is removed from model set $\mathbf{M}^O$. The removed model is not used for anatomical labeling of the descendant branches of O'_i.
4. Similarity is calculated between the descendent branches of O and each model M_i^p of model set $\mathbf{M}^O$. First, M_i^p is rotated around the start point of O'_i so that the running direction of O'_i equal the running direction of O. For all of possible combinations of one-to-one correspondence between child branches of O and O'_i, the sum of the inner products of the running directions of corresponding pairs is calculated. This sum of the inner products is considered similar between model M_i^p and the input tree structure.
5. From model set $\mathbf{M}^O$, the model, M_s^p, that has the smallest sum is selected and assigned the anatomical names of the child branches O'_s to the child branch of O.
6. The child branch names of O'_i and O'_s are compared for each model M_i^p of model set $\mathbf{M}^O$. If there is no branch, whose anatomical name is equal to that of O'_s, in the child branches of O'_i, model M_i^p is removed from $\mathbf{M}^O$.
7. The child branches of O and the model set $\mathbf{M}^O$ are stored into the queue.
8. Return to Step 2.

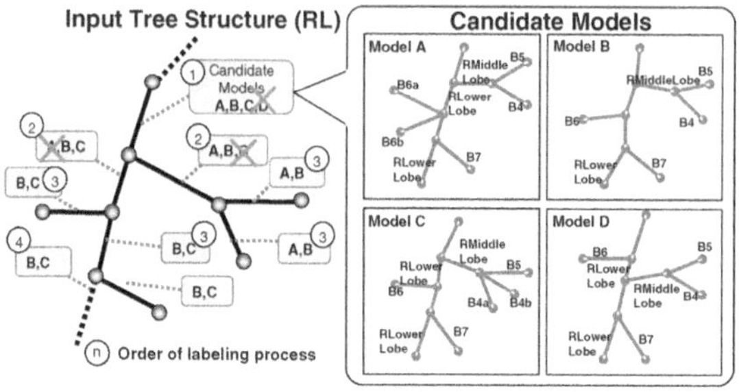

Fig. 3. Illustration of model selection

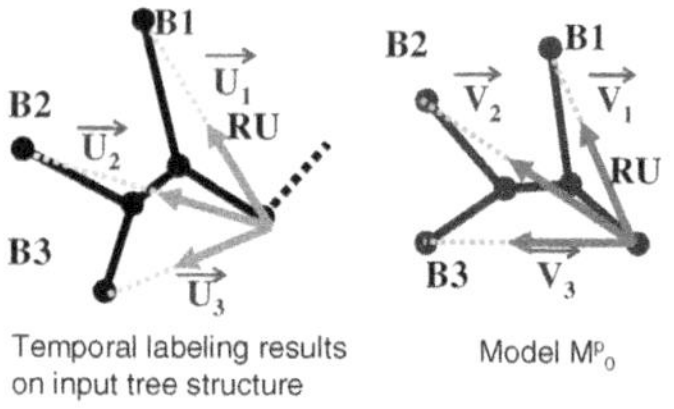

Fig. 4. Illustration of vectors $\mathbf{U}_1$, $\mathbf{U}_2$,$\mathbf{U}_3$, $\mathbf{V}_1$, $\mathbf{V}_2$, and $\mathbf{V}_3$

4 Path Generation for Biopsy Planning

We integrated the proposed labeling system into the VB system for assisting path planning for TBLB. A physician inputs a desired location on MPR (multi planner reconstruction) images or volume rendering images as end point $\mathbf{p}_e$. The start point is set as the start point of the trachea and a branch that is the closest to point $\mathbf{p}_e$ is located. In the tree structure of the bronchial branches extracted from CT images, each branch has the information of their path. The path is represented as a set of voxels. By finding the closest point to the specified point, it is possible to select the closest branch. Once the anatomical name of the selected branch is obtained, traverse up the tree structure up to the trachea. Anatomical names of branches existing on the traversed path are displayed on the VB views. Automated fly-through to the desired position is also possible with displaying the anatomical names of the branches on the path.

5 Experiments and Results

We applied the proposed method to bronchial branches extracted from twenty-five cases of chest CT images. For each case, a medical doctor assigned anatomical names to all of the branches. Bronchial branch models were constructed from

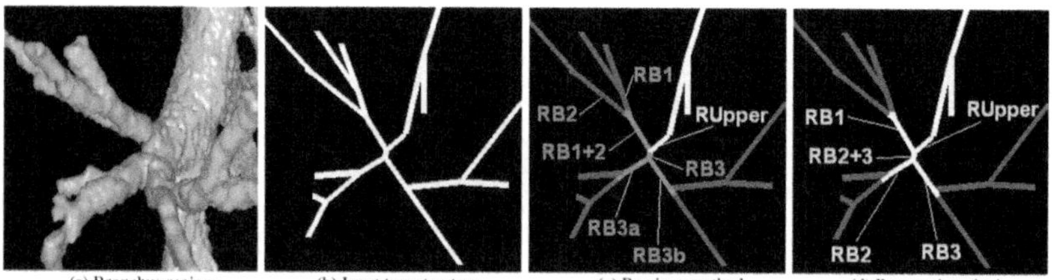

(a) Bronchus regions (b) Input tree structure (c) Previous method (d) Proposed method

Fig. 5. An example of partial view of bronchus region extracted from CT images (a), its tree structure (b), labeling results using previous (c) and proposed methods (d). Green characters mean correct labeling and red characters mean wrong labeling.

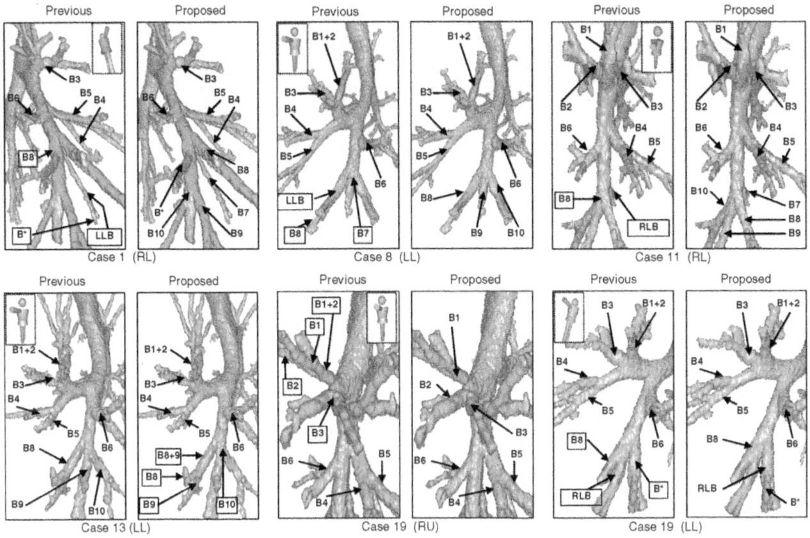

Fig. 6. Labeling results using proposed and previous [3] methods. Anatomical names surrounded by boxes show incorrect labeling.

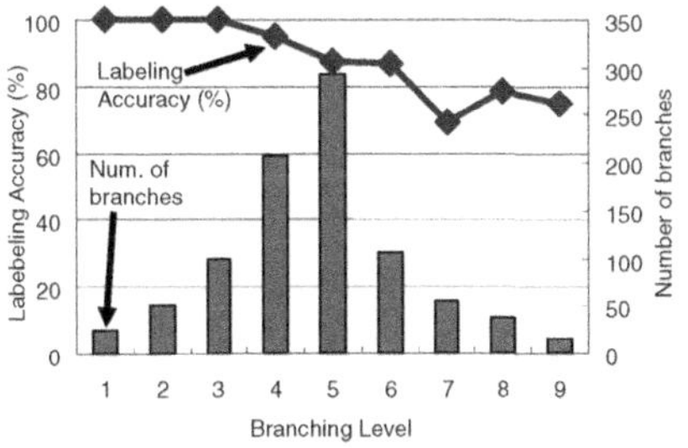

Fig. 7. Number of branches and labeling accuracy at each branching level

24 cases excluding the labeling target case (leave-out-method). We generated six models for the RU, eight models for RL, five models for LU, and six models for LL. We measured labeling accuracy of the proposed and previous methods. Image acquisition parameters of the CT images were: 512 × 512 pixels, 141 – 401 slices, 0.625 – 0.723 mm in pixel spacing, 1.0 – 2.5 mm in slice spacing, and 1.25 – 2.5 mm of X-ray collimation. All labeling results were evaluated by a medical doctor. Figure 5 shows an example of a partial view of the bronchus region extracted from CT images, its tree structure, and the labeling results using the proposed and previous methods. Table 1 lists the labeling accuracy at each part up to the segmental regions. We successfully assigned correct anatomical names to 799 out of the 888 branches using the proposed method, while 754 branches were assigned using the previous method. The proposed method was

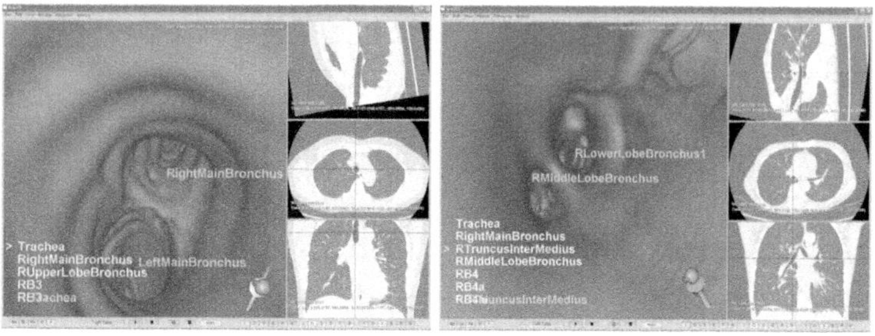

Fig. 8. Path generation for TBLB planning on VB. Anatomical names on the path are displayed on left side of VB view.

able to perform nomenclature on 90% of the branches extracted from CT images. Examples of anatomical labeling are shown in Fig. 6. Also we measured labeling accuracy at each branching level. Figure 7 shows the number of branches and the correct labeling rate.

We integrated the proposed labeling system into the VB system and tested automated path generation for TBLB path planning. Examples are presented in Fig. 8. In this figure, a user specifies suspicious shadows on slice images by a mouse click. The system automatically generated paths to the specified points and also displayed the paths by using anatomical names of the bronchial branches. These anatomical names are displayed on the left side of a VB view.

6 Discussion

From the results listed in Table 1, it is clear that the proposed method significantly improved labeling accuracy in comparison with the previous method. This is because the proposed method selected the appropriate models as branching level progressed. Also, the special model selection procedure for the RU contributed to increase labeling accuracy. Incorrect labeling was prevented by checking dominant regions of the Rt.B^1, Rt.B^2, and Rt.B^3 branches. In the labeling result of Case 11, the bronchus bifurcates in the order of Rt.B^6, Rt.B^7, Rt.B^8, Rt.B^9, Rt.B^{10}. The previous method selected the model having Rt.B^* branch and assigned the wrong names after Rt.B^7. The reason for the model mis-selection was the branching pattern and the running directions of branches after Rt.B^6 were very close to the input tree structure in the mis-selected model. The proposed method successfully assigned correct names to these branches because the method selected the best models branch by branch and removed inappropriate models from the model set. The special model selection technique worked well in Case 19, as shown in Fig. 6. In this case, the previous method selected the wrong model that assigned the name Rt.$B^{(1+2)}$ to branch Rt.B^1. However, in the proposed method, this model was removed by comparing the running directions of Rt.B^1, Rt.B^2, and Rt.B^3 of the model and those of the labeled tree.

Table 1. Labeling accuracy in segmental level

Part	Number of branches	Previous method[3]	Proposed method
Trachea and main bronchi	75	75 (100%)	75 (100%)
RU	124	106 (82.5%)	110 (88.7%)
RL	322	268 (83.2%)	291 (90.4%)
LU	183	159 (86.9%)	165 (90.2%)
LL	184	146 (79.3%)	158 (85.9%)
Total	888	754 (84.9%)	799 (90.0%)

The path for TBLB was automatically generated and described using a set of anatomical names in the proposed method. Also, a user was able to perform fly-through or automated fly-thorough checking anatomical names. Since accessibility to suspicious regions is discussed by using anatomical names of bronchial branches connected to it, it is very useful for medical doctors to see paths by their anatomical names. The automated anatomical labeling system proposed in this paper enabled us to implement function that makes VB systems intelligent.

This paper presented a novel anatomical labeling algorithm for bronchial branches extracted from CT images using multiple branching pattern models. The method presented here is another step towards createing truly intelligent computer aided diagnosis syetm. Annotations displayed on CT images will much assist a medical doctor to read images. Future work includes testing more cases, and improving model selection and removal.

References

1. K. Mori, J. Hasegawa, Y. Suenaga et al.: Automated Anatomical Labeling of the Bronchial Branch and Its Application to the Virtual Bronchoscopy System. IEEE Transactions on Medical Imaging, Vol 19, 2000.
2. H. Kitaoka, Y. Park, J. Tschirren et al.: Automated Nomenclature Labeling of the Bronchial Tree in 3D-CT Lung Images. T.Dohi and R.Kikinis (Eds.) MICCAI2002, LNCS2489, pp.1-11, 2002.
3. S. Ema, K. Mori, T. Kitasaka, et al.: An Improved method for automated anatomical labeling of bronchial branches extracted from 3-D CT images, In H.U. Lemke, M.W. Vannier, K. Inamura, A.G. Ferman, K. Doi, J.H.C. Reiber eds., Proceedings of the 18th International Congress and Exhibition on Computer Assisted Radiology and Surgery (CARS) 2004, International Congress Series 1268, p.1358, 2004.
4. P. Rogalla, J. Terwisscha van Scheltinga, and B. Hamm, eds.: Virtual endoscopy and related 3D techniques, Springer, Berlin, 2001.
5. T. Kitasaka, K. Mori, J. Hasegawa, et al: A Method for Extraction of Bronchus Regions from 3D Chest X-ray CT Images by Analyzing Structural Features of the Bronchus, FORMA, 17, pp.321-338, 2002.

Spectral Clustering Algorithms for Ultrasound Image Segmentation

Neculai Archip[1], Robert Rohling[2], Peter Cooperberg[3], Hamid Tahmasebpour[3], and Simon K. Warfield[1]

[1] Computational Radiology Laboratory, Harvard Medical School, Departments of Radiology, Brigham and Women's Hospital, Children's Hospital, Boston, MA, USA
narchip@bwh.harvard.edu

[2] Department of Electrical and Computer Engineering, University of British Columbia, Vancouver, BC, Canada

[3] Department of Radiology, University of British Columbia, Vancouver, BC, Canada

Abstract. Image segmentation algorithms derived from spectral clustering analysis rely on the eigenvectors of the Laplacian of a weighted graph obtained from the image. The NCut criterion was previously used for image segmentation in supervised manner. We derive a new strategy for unsupervised image segmentation. This article describes an initial investigation to determine the suitability of such segmentation techniques for ultrasound images. The extension of the NCut technique to the unsupervised clustering is first described. The novel segmentation algorithm is then performed on simulated ultrasound images. Tests are also performed on abdominal and fetal images with the segmentation results compared to manual segmentation. Comparisons with the classical NCut algorithm are also presented. Finally, segmentation results on other types of medical images are shown.

1 Introduction

Successful segmentation techniques can be used in a variety of clinical applications. In clinical practise, ultrasound images are often segmented manually, but manual techniques can be laborious. More sophisticated techniques are needed. Various methods have been previously proposed. For instance, active contours have been used [1]. Kalman filters are proposed in [2] to improve the segmentation of organ cavities in ultrasound. A statistical shape model is reported for aiding prostate segmentation [3].

However, most of these methods require intensive human interaction. Spectral methods for data clustering have received increasing attention for practical applications in other fields [4]. The spectral methods usually involve taking the top eigenvectors of a matrix constructed from a similarity metric (such as the distance between points) and using them to cluster the various points [5]. Image segmentation can be described as a clustering problem where pixels are the measured data points. For example, Shi and Malik [6] combine spectral clustering and image segmentation. Nevertheless, two important issues need to be

J. Duncan and G. Gerig (Eds.): MICCAI 2005, LNCS 3750, pp. 862–869, 2005.

addressed within this context. First is the determination of the number of clusters to be obtained (supervised vs unsupervised clustering). The second aspect to be considered is execution time. For real images, the matrix for which the eigenvectors should be computed is large ($n^2 \times n^2$ for an image of $n \times n$ pixels). Therefore efficiency is necessary for practical implementations. We focus on the first issue, introducing an unsupervised algorithm. Moreover, using a simple windowing principle, the introduced algorithm has reasonable execution times.

In this paper we show the effectiveness of this novel approach for ultrasound image segmentation. We present validation results on both simulated ultrasound and patient data. Manual segmentation of images by two independent radiologists is the gold standard used to quantify the success of our method. Comparison with a classical related segmentation method - NCut - is also provided. Additionally, we present examples of segmentation results from other imaging modalities.

2 Method

The NCut technique can be applied directly to the ultrasound image, but good results in MRI are reported for a combination of NCut with an anisotropic diffusion filter [7]. Therefore, an anisotropic filter is first applied.

Spectral Clustering and Some Previous Results on Image Segmentation. Spectral methods for image segmentation use the eigenvectors and eigenvalues of a matrix derived from the pairwise affinities of pixels. These eigenvectors induce an embedding of the pixels in a low-dimensional subspace wherein a simple central clustering method can be used to do the final partitioning. Here the partitioning is based on the Normalized Cut (NCut) [6]. Some mathematical notations are first introduced. Let I be the original image of size $N \times N$. The symmetric matrix $S \in R^{N^2 \times N^2}$ denotes the weighted adjacency matrix for a graph $G = (V, E)$ with nodes V representing pixels and edges E whose weights capture the pairwise affinities between pixels. Let A and B represent a bipartition of V, i.e. $A \cup B = V$ and $A \cap B = \emptyset$. Let $cut(A, B)$ denote the sum of the weights between A and B: $cut(A, B) = \sum_{i \in A, j \in B} S_{ij}$. The degree of the ith node is defined as $d_i = \sum_j S_{ij}$. The total connection from nodes in the set A to all nodes in the graph is denoted by $assoc(A, V) = \sum_{i \in A, j \in V} S_{ij}$. The normalized cut between sets A and B is then given by:

$$NCut(A, B) = \frac{cut(A, B)}{assoc(A, V)} + \frac{cut(A, B)}{assoc(B, V)}. \quad (1)$$

The problem is to find A and B such that $NCut(A, B)$ is minimized. Using elements of spectral graph theory, it is shown [6] that an approximate solution may be obtained by thresholding the eigenvector (called the Fiedler vector) corresponding to the second eigenvalue λ_2 of the generalized eigenvalue problem: $(D - S)y = \lambda D y$, where D is a diagonal matrix with entries $D_{ii} = d_i$. Image segmentation is reduced to the problem of partitioning the set V into disjoint sets $V_1,..,V_n$, such that similarity among nodes in V_i is high and similarity across V_i and V_j is low. Here we define the similarity function between two pixels i and j as:

$$S_{ij} = \begin{cases} \frac{1 - \frac{||F(i)-F(j)||_2}{maxF - minF}}{||X(i)-X(j)||_2} & if \ ||X(i) - X(j)||_2 < r \\ 0 & otherwise \end{cases} \tag{2}$$

where $X(i)$ is the spatial location of node i, and $F(i)$ is a feature vector, based on intensity. The values $maxF$ and $minF$ are respectively the maximum and the minimum values of F for the all the pixels in the image. Finally, the similarity matrix S is normalized by $S = S/max(S)$ as proposed by [8]. A requirement of NCut is the number of clusters. Overcoming this problem is a challenging task. Unsupervised clustering, based solely on Fiedler eigenvector is a potential solution. In the unsupervised clustering, the user does not need to explicitly specify the number of clusters. More details follow.

Fiedler Eigenvector for Unsupervised Image Segmentation. Instead of minimizing the NCut function (as suggested by [6]), a property of the Fiedler vector is used. Let each pixel be I_j, $j = 1, ..., N^2$. Given the image pixels $P = (I_1, .., I_{N^2})$ and the Fiedler vector $V = (v_1, .., v_{N^2})$, we consider the permutation $\wp = (i_1, .., i_{N^2})$ that sorts the vector V: $v_{i_1} \leq .. \leq v_{i_{N^2}}$. By applying $\wp$ to the pixel vector P, the vector $(I_{i_1}, .., I_{i_{N^2}})$ is obtained. It satisfies the property that $\exists j_1, .., j_k$ with $\forall p, j_p \leq l \leq j_{p+1} : S(I_l, I_{l-1}) < \epsilon$, where S is the similarity function defined in equation (2). This property provides a way to cluster the original image according to the given similarity metric.

In its new form the vector components are grouped in compact blocks which represent the clusters. It becomes clear that the problem of clustering the initial matrix data is reduced to the problem of determining the sequences of maximum length having similar values in the vector obtained from the Fiedler eigenvector. The pseudocode of the introduced unsupervised segmentation technique is listed in Algorithm 1.

Calculating the eigenvectors for the Laplacian resulting from the whole image is computationally expensive. Therefore a grid is used to divide the whole image into smaller windows. We then apply the clustering algorithm to each of these smaller windows. A global criterion is used to regroup the cluster obtained in every grid cell. There is still no need to know or estimate the number of clusters, K, in advance.

The introduced algorithm requires three parameters to be specified. The first parameter (*DifPixels*) specifies the maximum difference between two pixels to consider them as belonging to the same cluster. This parameter could be determined for specific applications using *a priori* information about the image content. However, for our experiments we used the same value for all examples with good results. The second parameter (*DifClusters*) is the threshold value when two clusters are grouped together during windowing. It can also be customized for a particular application, but is kept constant in the images presented in this paper. Both parameters are present in the majority of the standard segmentation algorithms since one needs to specify when two pixels are similar enough to

Algorithmus 1 Unsupervised clustering of a matrix

Require: image I having the size $N \times N$
Ensure: the number of clusters K and the clusters $C_1, ..., C_K$
Build the similarity matrix S, and the diagonal matrix of node degrees D
$S = S/max(S)$
Solve the generalized eigenvector problem $(D - S)y = \lambda Dy$
Consider λ_2 the second smallest eigenvalue and v_2 its corresponding vector
Consider the permutation $\wp = (i_1, .., i_{N^2})$ sorting v_2
Apply $\wp$ to the image pixels $(I_1, .., I_{N^2})$. Obtain $I' = (I'_1, .., I'_{N^2})$
$K = 1$; $C_K = I'_1$
i=2;
while $i \leq N^2$ **do**
    if I'_i cannot be added to C_K **then**
        $K = K + 1$
    end if
    Add I'_i to C_K
    i=i+1
end while

be grouped in the same region. The third parameter is the window size and is also kept constant. We have also noticed that there are small differences in the clustering results when using different values for the window size. More details follow in the **Results** section.

3 Results

Five simulated ultrasound images of circular objects were created with the Field II program [9]. Various levels of Gaussian additive noise have been used.

Two different metrics are used to compute the error between the boundary of the segmented region and the known object: Hausdorff and the mean error. Although theoretically attractive, the Hausdorff metric is very sensitive to noise in practice.

Abdominal images were also obtained in vivo for patients exhibiting cysts in the liver. The cysts have varying degrees of visibility so are more difficult to segment. Five images were used (see Fig. 1).

The clustering techniques are also used to segment the amniotic fluid present in five images of the fetus. Clinical applications of the segmentation include the diagnosis and quantification of hydramnios or oligohydramnios (see Fig. 2). An example of an ultrasound image segmentation obtained during a prostate brachytherapy procedure is shown in Fig. 3. Finally results of this technique on other imaging modalities, such as CT and microscopic images are illustrated in the Fig. 4. The Hausdorff and mean errors were calculated between the radiologist and NCut, and the radiologist and NCut-Unsupervised.

For the liver images, a second radiologist performed manual segmentation so a comparison can be made between the results with each radiologist. For all tests,

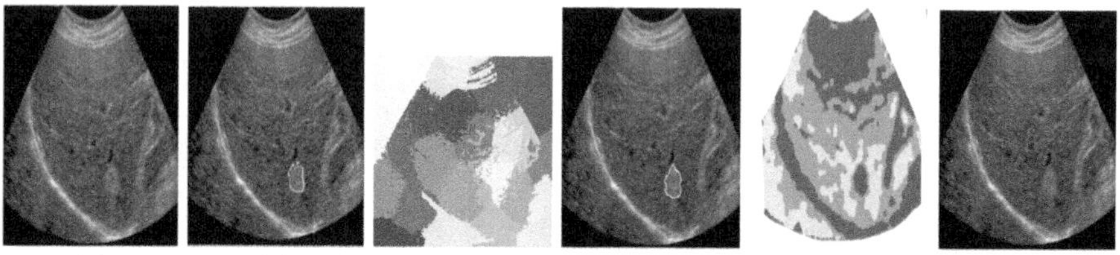

(a) (b) (c) (d) (e) (f)

Fig. 1. Liver cyst image. (a) Original image of a liver with a visible cyst. (b) The manually drawn contour of the cyst. (c) Segmentation using NCUT (9 clusters). (d) The contour of the selected cluster corresponding to the cyst. (e) Segmentation using our unsupervised technique. (f) The contour of the selected cluster corresponding to the cyst.

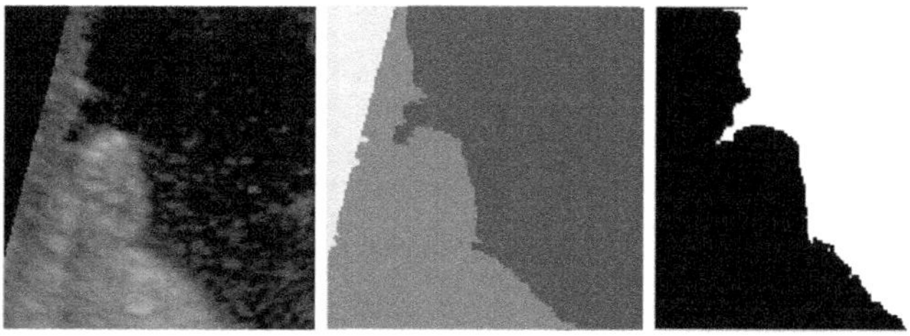

(a) (b) (c)

Fig. 2. Fetus images. (a) An original image of a fetus. (b) Segmentation using NCut. (c) Segmentation using our unsupervised technique. The segmentation closely reflects the underlying anatomy.

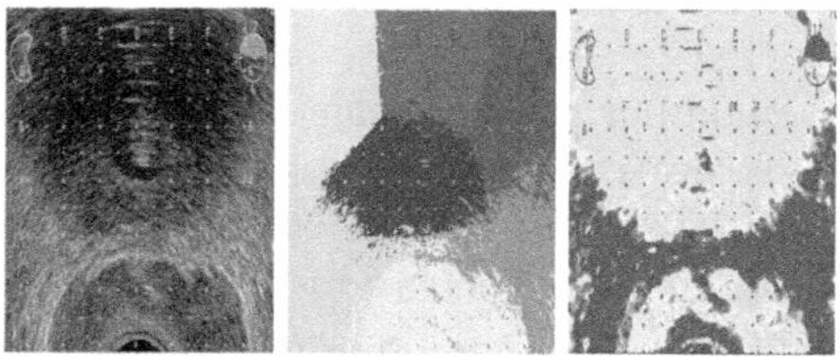

(a) (b) (c)

Fig. 3. Bladder image (a) Original image. (b) Segmentation with NCut. (c) Segmentation with our unsupervised method.

the NCut and NCut-Unsupervised were implemented in Matlab (The Mathworks Inc., Natick, MA, USA). For NCut, the number of clusters was selected manually for each image to get the best segmentation. For NCut-Unsupervised, there was no need to specify the number of clusters. The parameters used for the algorithm had the same values for all the images in the experiments. The values used in the tests are *DifPixels*=5, *DifClusters*=20 and window size=15 pixels. The computation time of the Matlab implementation of both NCut and NCut-Unsupervised is approximately 30 seconds on an image of 150×150. The results in all cases is

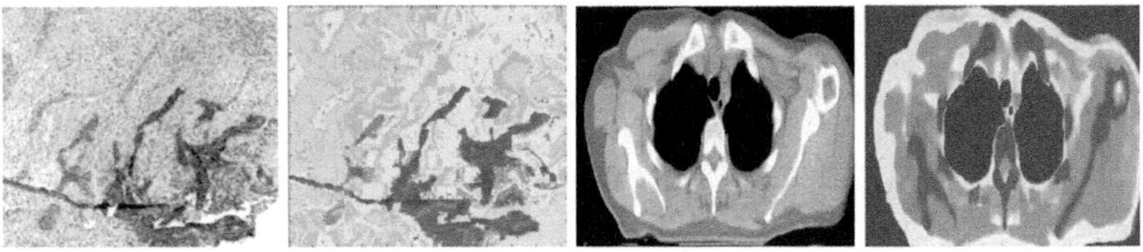

(a) (b) (c) (d)

Fig. 4. (a) Original cancer stain image. (b) Segmentation with our method. (c) CT slice. (d) its segmentation. The segmentation closely reflects the underlying anatomy.

Table 1. Simulated ultrasound images. The errors between the segmented object and the true object are calculated using the Hausdorff metric and the mean differences.

Image	True object vs NCut		True object vs NCut-Unsupervised	
	Hausdorff (mm)	Mean (mm)	Hausdorff (mm)	Mean (mm)
1	3.5	2.2	4.0	2.0
2	3.6	1.3	3.8	1.5
3	3.7	1.2	3.2	1.4
4	3.5	1.4	3.3	1.2
5	2.7	1.9	2.2	1.3
Average	**3.4**	**1.6**	**3.3**	**1.5**

Table 2. Liver cyst images. The errors between NCut-Unsupervised and a manually segmented contour of the cyst are calculated using the Hausdorff metric and the mean differences. The manually segmented contours were drawn by radiologist Rad.1 or Rad.2

Image	Hausdorff Error Rad.1 vs NCut-Uns. (mm)	Mean Error Rad.1 vs NCut-Uns. (mm)	Hausdorff Error Rad.2 vs NCut-Uns. (mm)	Mean Error Rad.2 vs NCut-Uns. (mm)
1	6.5	2.6	6.0	2.4
2	2.3	1.2	2.0	1.1
3	1.7	0.8	2.5	1.1
4	2.5	1.2	2.4	1.0
5	1.2	0.5	1.6	0.7
Average	**2.8**	**1.3**	**2.9**	**1.3**

a partitioning of the image into a set of regions. The clinical user then can select the segmented region of interest and subsequently calculate geometric properties (dimensions, shape, area, volume), build anatomical models, or other types of analysis. For this work, the boundaries of the segmented regions are compared. Numerical results are presented in the Tables 1, 2 and 3. Performance estimates for the segmentation of liver cyst image presented in the Fig. 1 were also obtained using STAPLE [10]. Overall accuracy of the segmentation, summarized as the probability for any voxel that the true segmentation label matched the rater segmentation, was 0.981 (Fig. 1 (b)), 0.965 (Fig. 1 (d)) and 0.989 (Fig. 1 (e)).

Table 3. Fetus images. The errors between NCut, NCut-Unsupervised and a manually segmented contour of the amniotic fluid are calculated using the Hausdorff metric and the mean differences.

Image	Manual vs NCut		Manual vs NCut-Unsupervised	
	Hausdorff	Mean	Hausdorff	Mean
1	6.4	2.8	6.0	2.2
2	5.5	2.9	5.7	3.2
3	5.1	3.2	3.8	3.1
4	5.5	3.0	5.2	2.9
5	4.5	2.2	4.7	1.7
Average	**5.4**	**2.8**	**5.3**	**2.6**

4 Discussion

The simulations show a good match between the spectral clusters and the true object. Small differences along the boundary are likely due to the noise and speckle in the images. There is no significant difference between the NCut and the NCut-Unsupervised techniques (at the 95% confidence level using the paired student t-test). This gives confidence that the changes to the algorithm to make it unsupervised have not caused a drop in accuracy. For the tests on the liver cysts, there was also no significant difference between the following: 1. errors between NCut and manual segmentation and 2. the errors between the two manual segmentations (95% confidence level, using the paired t-test). Nor was there a significant difference between the following: 1. errors between NCut-Unsupervised and manual segmentation and 2. the errors between the two manual segmentations (again with same confidence, 95% using the paired t-test). In other words, the results from either NCut or NCut-unsupervised were within the variation of the two radiologists.

For the tests on the amniotic fluid segmentation, there was also no significant difference between the NCut and theNCut-Unsupervised techniques when compared to the manual segmentation results (95% confidence level, paired t-test). With NCut-Unsupervised, the fluid and the fetus were clearly partitioned into separate clusters. On the other hand, as previously mentioned, the clusters obtained with standard NCut tend to have the same size, so the amniotic fluid was occasionally split in two clusters, and manually combined by clicking both regions.

All of the tests were done without changing the three parameters of the method. The images of the partitioned regions also show the limitations of a spectral clustering approach. Clearly not all separate tissue types are partitioned into separate regions. The objects of interest in this study were partitioned the easiest because they exhibited the most homogeneous properties. For example, the liver cyst forms a single cluster, but the rest of the liver is formed from four more clusters. Some of the liver clusters are also shared with non-liver tissue. Clearly the liver could not be completely segmented with the current partition. So far, the method appears to work well for fluid-filled cavities and vessels.

To perform other segmentation tasks, a more sophisticated similarity criterion may be needed. Additional features, such as texture could be added to the similarity criterion. This may slow the creation of the similarity matrix, but the rest of the algorithm will proceed without change. The main conclusion is that automatic unsupervised spectral clustering on ultrasound images is feasible. The spectral clustering technique is promising, and future research will focus on the development of new similarity criteria, the addition of other *a priori* information, and further improvements to speed.

Acknowledgments

This investigation was supported by NSF ITR 0426558, a research grant from the Whitaker Foundation, a research grant from CIMIT, by NIH grants R21 MH67054, R01 LM007861 and P41 RR13218, by Natural Sciences and Engineering Research Council of Canada and by the Institute of Robotics and Intelligent Systems.

References

1. Ladak, H., Downey, D., Steinman, D., Fenster, A.: Semi-automatic technique for segmentation of the prostate from 2d ultrasound images. In: Proceedings of IEEE BMES/EMBS Conference on Serving Humanity, Advanced Technology. (1999)
2. Abolmaesumi, P., Sirouspour, M.: An interacting multiple model probabilistic data association filter for cavity boundary extraction from ultrasound images. IEEE Transactions on Medical Imaging **23** (2004) 772–784
3. Shen, D., Zhan, Y., Davatzikos, C.: Segmentation of the prostate boundaries from ultrasound images using statistical shape model. IEEE Transactions on Medical Imaging **22** (2003) 539–551
4. Kluger, Y., Basri, R., Chang, J., Gerstein, M.: Spectral biclustering of microarray data: coclustering genes and conditions. Genome Research **13** (2003) 703–716
5. Ng, A.Y., Jordan, M., Weiss, Y.: On spectral clustering: Analysis and an algorithm. In: Advances in Neural Information Processing Systems 14, MIT Press (2002) 849–856
6. Shi, J., Malik, J.: Normalized cuts and image segmentation. IEEE Transactions on Pattern Analysis and Machine Intelligence **22** (2000) 888–905
7. Carballido-Gamio, J., Belongie, S., Majumdar, S.: Normalized cuts in 3-d for spinal mri segmentation. IEEE Transactions on Medical Imaging **23** (2004)
8. Meila, M., Shi, J.: Learning segmentation by random walks. In: Neural Information Processing Systems. (2000) 873–879
9. Jensen, J.: A new calculation procedure for spatial impulse responses in ultrasound. Journal of the Acoustical Society of America **105** (1999) 3266–3274
10. Warfield, S., Zou, K., Wells, W.: Simultaneous truth and performance level estimation (staple): an algorithm for the validation of image segmentation. IEEE Transactions on Medical Imaging **23** (2004) 903–21

Using the Fast Marching Method to Extract Curves with Given Global Properties

Xiaodong Tao[1,*], Christos Davatzikos[2], and Jerry L. Prince[3]

[1] Visualization and Computer Vision Lab, GE Global Research Center,
One Research Circle, KW-C223A, Niskayuna, NY 12309
taox@research.ge.com
[2] SBIA, Department of Radiology,
University of Pennsylvania, Philadelphia, PA 19104
christos@rad.upenn.edu
[3] IACL, Department of Electrical and Computer Engineering,
Johns Hopkins University, Baltimore, MD 21218
prince@jhu.edu

Abstract. Curves are often used as anatomical features to match surfaces that represent biological objects, such as the human brain. Automated and semi-automated methods for extracting these curves usually rely on local properties of the surfaces such as the mean surface curvature without considering the global appearance of the curves themselves. These methods may require additional human intervention, and sometimes produce erroneous results. In this paper, we present an algorithm that is based on the fast marching method (FMM) to extract weighted geodesic curves. Instead of directly using the local image properties as a weight function, we use the surface properties, together with the global properties of the curves, to compute a weight function. This weight function is then used by the FMM to extract curves between given points. The general framework can be used to extract curves with different global properties. The resulting curves are guaranteed to be weighted geodesic curves without cusps usually introduced by intermediate points through which the curves are forced to pass. We show some results on both a simulated image and a highly convoluted human brain cortical surface.

1 Introduction

The problem of finding curve features in an image arises in many computer vision and medical image analysis applications. In particular, curves representing anatomical features can be used to match brain surfaces [1, 2, 3]. The curves of sulcal fundi can be viewed as crestlines [5], sulcal roots [4], or as weighted geodesic curves [3,6], where the weight is usually computed from the local properties (e.g., mean curvature) of the surface [3, 6, 7, 8].

In literature, there have been some methods on how such weighted geodesic curves can be obtained. In [8], finding sulcal fundal curves is formulated as an

* This work was done at Johns Hopkins University.

J. Duncan and G. Gerig (Eds.): MICCAI 2005, LNCS 3750, pp. 870–877, 2005.

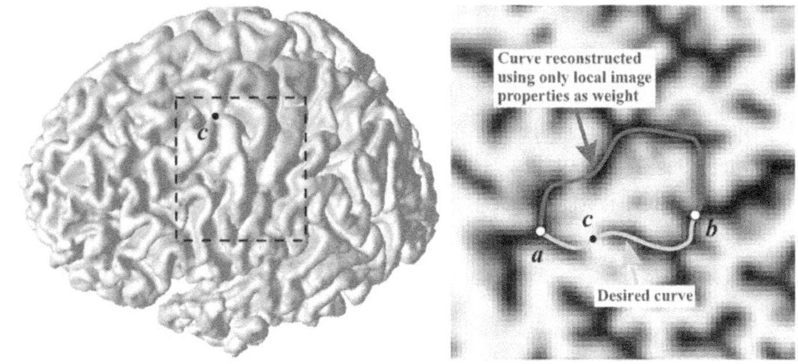

Fig. 1. Left: A human cortical surface. Right: A flattened map [9] of the surface with mean surface curvature of the region around the pre-central sulcus (yellow curve).

optimization problem, which is solved by using a dynamic programming method. The resulting curve is restricted to travel along the edges of the surface, therefore depends on the parameterization of the surface and suffers from metric distortion. More recently, an algorithm based on the FMM has been reported to extract curves of sulcal fundi [3, 6]. In the algorithm, the weight is set to be a function of local "valley-ness". A FMM is used to compute the weighted distance between any points on the surface to a given origin. A weighted geodesic curve can be constructed by following the negative gradient directions. One of the advantages of this algorithm is that it treats the surface as a continuum; therefore, the resulting curves are not restricted to triangle edges and are independent of the surface parameterization.

A problem with both of the above methods is that there is little control over the global properties of the curves. The method may fail in complicated geometries such as the human cortical surface. As an example, consider the situation shown in Fig. 1. When we use a weight function computed from only mean surface curvature to extract the pre-central sulcal curve between **a** and **b**, we will get the upper curve instead. Because the weight function is computed locally, points in the neighborhood of **c** introduce large cost to curves passing them because they have small mean curvature values. Previously, people circumvented this problem by manually picking intermediate points to force the curve to go over the interruption, such as point **c** shown in Fig. 1. This solution, however, is practical only with additional human intervention.

In order to address the above problem, we develop a novel algorithm based on the FMM to extract weighted geodesic curves that have desired global properties. The method uses the desired properties of the curve to compute a weight function, which is then used to extract the curve.

2 Weighted Geodesic Curves

Background. In this section, the problem of finding geodesic curves is stated in 2D Cartesian space, but generalization to surfaces is straightforward with the FMM on triangulated meshes. For a 2D image domain $\Omega = [0,1] \times [0,1]$ and a positive weight function $w(\mathbf{x}) : \Omega \rightarrow \Re^+$, we define the cost for a curve $\mathbf{c}(t) : [0,1] \rightarrow \Omega$ as $\boldsymbol{\Phi}(\mathbf{c}) = \int_0^1 w(\mathbf{c}(t))|\mathbf{c}'(t)|dt$.

If two points $\mathbf{a} = (a_x, a_y), \mathbf{b} = (b_x, b_y) \in \Omega$ are given, the problem of finding the curve connecting $\mathbf{a}$ and $\mathbf{b}$ that minimizes the above cost can be expressed as the following optimization problem:

$$\min \boldsymbol{\Phi}(\mathbf{c}) = \int_0^1 w(\mathbf{c}(t))|\mathbf{c}'(t)|dt, \quad \text{s.t.} \quad \mathbf{c}(0) = \mathbf{a}, \text{ and } \mathbf{c}(1) = \mathbf{b}. \tag{1}$$

By convention, we define $F(\mathbf{x}) = 1/w(\mathbf{x})$ as a *speed function*. The solution to Equation (1) can be obtained by first solving the Eikonal equation for $T(\mathbf{x})$:

$$\|\nabla T(\mathbf{x})\| = F(\mathbf{x}) = 1/w(\mathbf{x}), \text{ with } T(\mathbf{a}) = 0, \text{ for } \mathbf{x} \in \Omega, \tag{2}$$

then following the negative gradient directions of the function $T(\mathbf{x})$ starting from $\mathbf{b}$ until reaching $\mathbf{a}$. The Eikonal equation can be solved efficiently using the fast marching method [10]. If the weight function $w(\mathbf{x}) \equiv 1$, the cost $\boldsymbol{\Phi}(\mathbf{c})$ is the length of the curve. The solution to Equation (1) is a geodesic curve on the surface.

Curves with Global Properties. For the purpose of clarity, the global property is set to be the intensity profile along the curve segment connecting two given points. Generalization to other properties is straightforward.

Given an image $I : \Omega \longrightarrow \mathcal{R}$ and two points, $\mathbf{a}$ and $\mathbf{b}$, we want to find a curve $\mathbf{c}(t) = [x(t), y(t)] \subset \Omega$ with $\mathbf{c}(0) = \mathbf{a}$, $\mathbf{c}(1) = \mathbf{b}$, such that the intensity values of the image along the curve resemble a given function $g(t)$ in the least square sense. This problem can be written as the following optimization problem:

$$\begin{array}{ll} \min \mathcal{E}[x(t), y(t)] = \int_0^1 [I(x(t), y(t)) - g(t)]^2 \sqrt{x'^2(t) + y'^2(t)}dt, \\ \text{s.t.} \qquad x(0) = a_x, y(0) = a_y, x(1) = b_x \text{ and } y(1) = b_y. \end{array} \tag{3}$$

When $g(t)$ is not a constant, the cost function also depends on the parameterization of the curve $\mathbf{c}(t)$, which means that the same curve with different parameterizations will have different costs. One way to circumvent this difficulty is to impose a constant parameterization constraint on the curve $\mathbf{c}(t)$, which can be stated as $|\mathbf{c}'(t)| = L$ with L being the *unknown* length of the curve. Since L is unknown, $|\mathbf{c}'(t)| = L$ cannot be used directly. Instead, we use an equivalent constraint in differential form: $\frac{d}{dt}|\mathbf{c}'(t)| = 0 \Leftrightarrow x'(t)x''(t) + y'(t)y''(t) = 0$.

By doing this, Equation (3) is modified to the following form:

$$\min \mathcal{E}[x(t), y(t)] = \int_0^1 [I(x(t), y(t)) - g(t)]^2 \sqrt{x'^2(t) + y'^2(t)}dt \tag{4}$$

and satisfy the initial and final conditions: $x(0) = a_x$, $y(0) = a_y$, $x(1) = b_x$, and $y(1) = b_y$, and the second order differential equation: $x'(t)x''(t) + y'(t)y''(t) = 0$. This is a Lagrange problem with optimality condition given by Mayer Equations [11], which is a system of nonlinear partial differential equations of order four. Directly solving the problem is difficult. Later, we describe a two-step algorithm to first find a speed function using these global properties, and then extract the weighted geodesic curves using the speed function.

In the above discussion, we assume $g(t)$ is determinant and known. Sometime, we can only estimate the statistical distribution of $g(t)$ from a set of training data. For simplicity, we assume that for fixed t, $g(t)$ follows a Gaussian distribution and for $t_1 \neq t_2$, $g(t_1)$ and $g(t_2)$ are independent. The point-wise mean and variation of $g(t)$ are $\mu_g(t)$ and $\sigma_g^2(t)$. If we want to find a curve $\mathbf{c}(t) = (x(t), y(t))$, such that $I(x(t), y(t))$ has large probability according to the statistical properties of $g(t)$, the problem in Equation (3) can be written as:

$$\begin{array}{ll} \min & \mathcal{E}[x(t), y(t)] = \int_0^1 \left[\frac{I(x(t),y(t))-\mu_g(t)}{\sigma_g(t)}\right]^2 \sqrt{x'^2(t) + y'^2(t)}dt, \\ \text{s.t.} & \mathbf{c}(0) = (a_x, a_y), \mathbf{c}(1) = (b_x, b_y), \text{ and } x'(t)x''(t) + y'(t)y''(t) = 0. \end{array} \quad (5)$$

Again, directly solving the above problem will involve a system of 4th order nonlinear partial differential equations. In the following, we develop an algorithm to find a solution to Equation (5), which we refer to as a *statistical geodesic curve.* We will use speed function $F(\mathbf{x})$ instead of the weight function $w(\mathbf{x})$.

3 Finding Statistical Geodesic Curves

Suppose a curve $\mathbf{c}_0(t)$ is the solution to the problem (5). It minimizes the cost function $\mathcal{E}(\mathbf{c})$ and must be a weighted geodesic curve under a properly chosen speed function. *Since the speed function uniquely determines the curve when the end points are specified, problem (5) is equivalent to finding the proper speed function.* When the speed function is obtained, the curve can be extracted as a weighted geodesic curve using the method described before.

Now, suppose in addition to the point-wise statistics of $g(t)$, we also know that the length of the curve connecting $\mathbf{a}$ and $\mathbf{b}$, ℓ, follows a Gaussian distribution that is independent of $g(t)$. The probability density function is $f_L(\ell) = 1/\sqrt{2\pi}\sigma_L \exp\left\{-(\ell - \mu_L)^2/2\sigma_L^2\right\}$. The probability density function of the intensity value along the curve is $f_G(g;t) = \frac{1}{\sqrt{2\pi\sigma_g^2(t)}} \exp\left\{-\frac{(g-\mu_g(t))^2}{2\sigma_g^2(t)}\right\}$.

We use these probability density functions to find the proper speed function (see Fig. 2 for an illustration). For an image I, on which the end points $\mathbf{a}$ and $\mathbf{b}$ are given, the speed function in the image domain is initialized to be an arbitrary constant. Then an iterative algorithm is applied to successively larger regions surrounding $\mathbf{a}$, until the regions cover the entire image domain. At each iteration, for every point $\mathbf{p}$ [Fig. 2(c)] in the region being processed, a tentative curve, $c_{\mathbf{ap}}(t)$, is reconstructed connecting $\mathbf{a}$ and $\mathbf{p}$ using the current speed function. The length of $c_{\mathbf{ap}}(t)$ and the intensity along $c_{\mathbf{ap}}(t)$ are compared to those of the appropriate segment of the desired curve between $\mathbf{a}$ and $\mathbf{b}$. This step results in a measure of how good $c_{\mathbf{ap}}(t)$ resembles the corresponding part of the desired curve $c_{\mathbf{ab}}(t)$. We use this measure to update the speed value at $\mathbf{p}$.

When we update the weight at $\mathbf{p}$, we *assume* that $\mathbf{p}$ is on the final optimal curve [dotted curve in Fig. 2(c)] and compute the ratio $\tau = \ell_{\mathbf{ap}}/\ell$, where ℓ is the

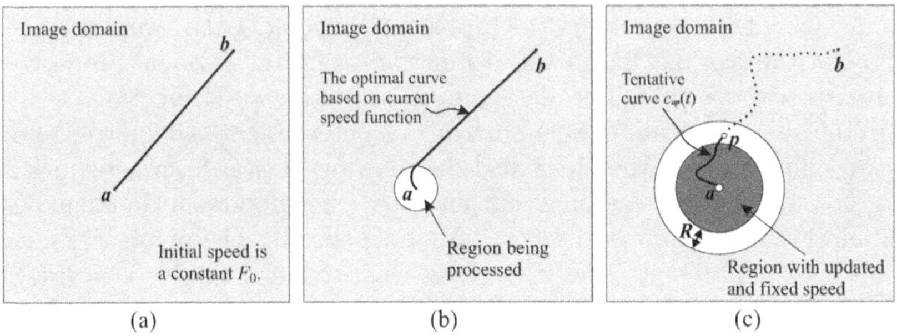

Fig. 2. Demonstration of the iterative algorithm for finding the speed function

curve length of $c_{\mathbf{ab}}(t)$. By assumption, ℓ follows a Gaussian distribution with mean μ_L and variance σ_L^2. The probability distribution of τ is:

$$f_T(\tau|\ell \geq \ell_{\mathbf{ap}}) = \left.\frac{dF_T(\tau|\ell \geq \ell_{\mathbf{ap}})}{d\tau}\right|_{\tau=\tau} = \frac{1}{Z}\frac{\ell_{\mathbf{ap}}}{\tau^2\sqrt{2\pi\sigma_L^2}}\exp\left\{-\frac{(\ell_{\mathbf{ap}}/\tau-\mu_L)^2}{2\sigma_L^2}\right\}, \tag{6}$$

where $Z = \int_{\ell_{\mathbf{ap}}}^{\infty} f_L(s)ds$ is a normalization factor. With the distribution of τ, we compute the distribution of the intensity at $\mathbf{p}$, $f(g) = \int_0^1 f_G(g;\tau)f_T(\tau)d\tau$:

$$f(g) = \frac{\ell_{\mathbf{ap}}}{2\pi Z\sigma_L}\int_0^1 \frac{1}{\tau^2\sigma_g(\tau)}\exp\left\{-\frac{(g-\mu_g(\tau))^2}{2\sigma_g^2(\tau)} - \frac{(\ell_{\mathbf{ap}}/\tau-\mu_L)^2}{2\sigma_L^2}\right\}d\tau. \tag{7}$$

The speed value at $\mathbf{p}$ is updated as:

$$F(\mathbf{p}) = \int_{I(\mathbf{p})-\delta}^{I(\mathbf{p})+\delta} f(g)dg, \tag{8}$$

where $I(\mathbf{p})$ is the image intensity at $\mathbf{p}$ and δ is a parameter. To summarize, the algorithm proceeds as follows.

Step 0. Initialize the speed function to be an arbitrary positive constant F_0;
Step 1. For each point $\mathbf{p} \in \mathcal{N}_k^{\mathbf{a}} = \{\mathbf{p} : \mathbf{p} \in \Omega, (k-1)R \leq \|\mathbf{p}-\mathbf{a}\| < kR\}$, perform steps 2 and 3.
Step 2. Reconstruct a tentative curve $c_{\mathbf{ap}}(t)$ using speed function $F^{(k-1)}(\mathbf{x})$.
Step 3. Update the speed function at point $\mathbf{p}$ using Equations (6)–(8).
Step 4. Increase k by 1 and go to **Step 1.**

The above process proceeds until the speed function at every point $\mathbf{x} \in \Omega$ has been updated. We use the speed function at the final iteration to reconstruct a weighted geodesic curve between $\mathbf{a}$ and $\mathbf{b}$. The image intensity at every point along the resulting curve resembles that presented in the training datasets.

There are two parameters in the algorithm. The first parameter, R, controls the size of the region whose speed function is updated at each iteration. With large R, we need fewer iterations to cover the entire image domain Ω, and therefore need less computation time. But we will also get less accurate results, since at each iteration, the updating of the speed function for two points $\mathbf{p}, \mathbf{q} \in \mathcal{N}_k^{\mathbf{a}}$ may depend not only on the speed function already updated for $\mathcal{N}_j^{\mathbf{a}}$, $j < k$, but also on the speed values of each other. In practice, we choose R to be the pixel size of the image. The parameter δ controls how restrict we are on the intensity at a given point. If δ is large, we allow a point with a wide range of intensity to have relatively large speed value. An extreme is when δ tends to ∞, $F(\mathbf{p}) = 1$, no matter what $I(\mathbf{p})$ is. The resulting curve is a true geodesic curve. If δ is small, we require the resulting curve to have an intensity profile very close to the mean intensity profile presented in the training datasets.

4 Results

In this section, we describe two experimental results of finding the curves connecting two given points with global properties on the intensity profile of the curve. The first experiment is on a simulated image. And the second one is a segment of the pre-central sulcus on a highly convoluted cortical surface.

A simulated example. The simulated image is a gray level image with some bright structures (Fig. 3 left). In the image we specified the end points of the desired curve. If the speed function is set to be the intensity value, the resulting curve will run through regions with high intensity values as much as possible. This is the upper curve in the figure. If instead, the lower curve is desired, without constraints on the global appearance of the curve, we need to specify some intermediate points (circles in the figure). The intensity profile along the desired curve is shown in the right plot of Fig. 3. If we use this intensity as $g(t)$ to solve problem (3), we get the speed function shown in the left image of Fig. 4. By using the FMM with this speed function and the usual curve tracking technique, we get the curve as shown in the right image of Fig. 4.

A curve of sulcal fundi on a cortical surface. In this experiment, we computed the point-wise statistics of the surface mean curvature along a segment of the curve

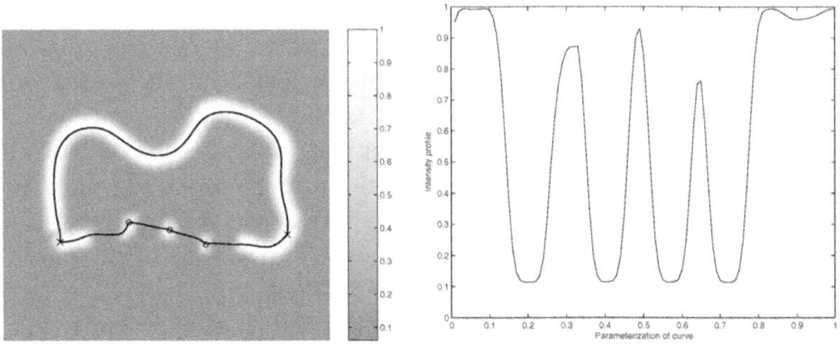

Fig. 3. Left: A simulated image. Right: The intensity profile along the lower curve in the left image.

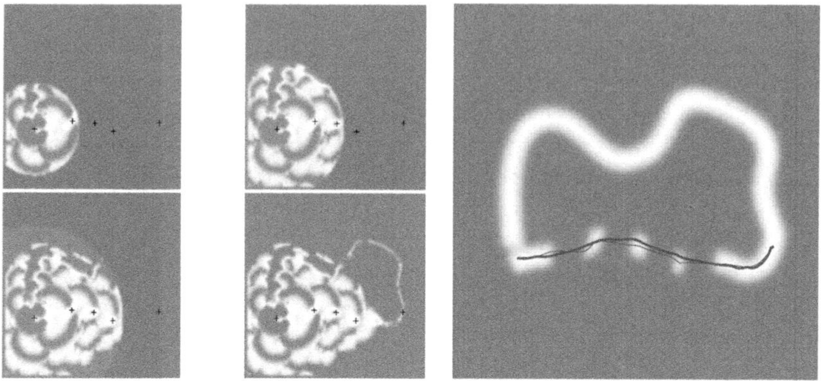

Fig. 4. Left: Speed functions at different iterations. The small crosses are the intermediate points picked in order to get the desired curve. Right: Statistical geodesic curve (thick curve) extracted from two given end points. The thin curve is reconstructed with manually picked intermediate points and the intensity alone as the speed function.

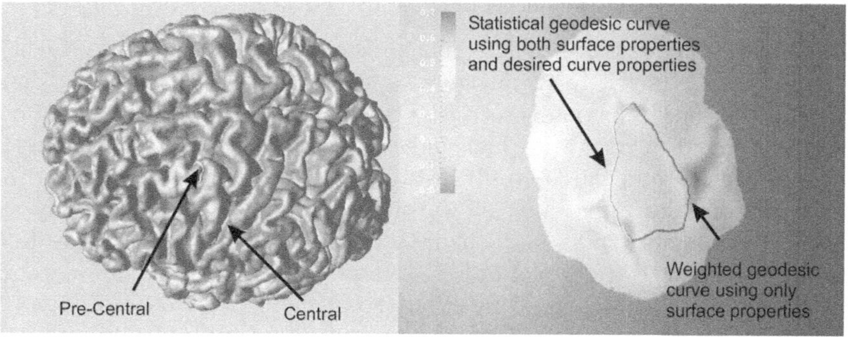

Fig. 5. A statistical geodesic curve on a cortical surface (left), the curve mapped onto the unit sphere with the computed speed function (right, for visualization only)

of pre-central sulcus, and used this information to extract a statistical geodesic curve between two given points on a cortical surface. We used a training set of 30 subjects to estimate the distributions of the length of the sulcal curve and the mean curvature profile along the curve. In the training set, each sulcal curve is extracted using a semi-automatic method with point correspondence built by constant speed parameterization. The results are shown in Fig. 5. When only the mean curvature of the surface is used to extract the curve, we get a segment that connects the pre-central sulcus to the central sulcus (right curve in the figures) because of the structures connecting these two sulci have large local "valley-ness" measure. If we use the statistical information, we are able to get the desired curve representing the part of the pre-central sulcus.

5 Conclusions and Discussion

In this paper, we presented an algorithm to extract curves as weighted geodesics using the FMM. The speed function for FMM is computed using both the surface properties and the global properties of the curves. The algorithm can be easily extended to incorporate different global properties.

There are several advantages of the proposed method. The first advantage is automation. The proposed method allows us to extract the curves from only the most distinctive points, which are relatively easy to be automatically located, while manually picked intermediate points do not necessarily have clear features to facilitate automatic localization. The second advantage is that the entire curve extracted as a statistical geodesic curve is always a weighted geodesic curve under the speed function computed, while curve obtained using manually picked intermediate points consists of pieces of weighted geodesic curve segments, and any intermediate point is a cusp of the curve, where the tangent vector is not continuous.

Future work includes investigation on the optimality of the speed function with given constraints. Although the iterative algorithm presented in this paper solves the problem of finding weighted geodesic curves that satisfies given global constraints, it is not known what the optimal speed is for given properties of the curves. A theoretical understanding of the optimality condition of the speed function, as well as the optimality condition in problem (4) is also needed. Another topic of interest is to use other properties of partically reconstructed curve segments, such as curve shape, as the global properties for curve reconstruction.

References

1. M. Bakircioglu and U. Grenander and N. Khaneja and M. I. Miller, "Curve Matching on Brain Surfaces Using Frenet Distances", *Human Brain Mapping*, 6, 1998.
2. M. Vaillant and A. Davatzikos, "Hierarchical Matching of Cortical Features for Deformable Brain Image Registration", *IPMI*, 1999.
3. X. Tao and X. Han and M. E. Rettmann and J. L. Prince and C. Davatzikos, "Statistical Study on Cortical Sulci of Human Brains", *IPMI*, 2001.
4. D. Riviere, J. F. Mangin, *et al*, "Automatic recognition of cortical sulci of the Human Brain using a congregation of neural networks". MedIA, 6(2), 2002.
5. J.P. Thirion and A. Gourdon, "The 3D Marching Lines Algorithm", *Graphical Models and Image Processing*, 58(6), 1996.
6. A. Bartesaghi and G. Sapiro, "A System for the Generation of Curves on 3D Brain Images", *Human Brain Mapping*, 14(1), 2001.
7. A. M. Lopez and F. Lumbreras and J. Serrat and J. J. Villanueva, "Evaluation of Methods for Ridge and Valley Detection", *IEEE-PAMI*, vol. 21, no. 4, 1999.
8. N. Khaneja, M. I. Miller and U. Grenander, "Dynamic programming generation of curves on brain surfaces", *IEEE-PAMI*, vol. 20, no. 11, 1998.
9. D. Tosun and J. L. Prince, "A Hemispherical Map for the Human Brain Cortex", *Proc. of SPIE Conf. on Medical Imaging,*, 2001.
10. J. A. Sethian, "A fast marching level-set method for monotonically advancing fronts", *Proceedings of the National Academy of Sciences*, vol. 93, 1996.
11. Hans Sagan, "Introduction to the Calculus of Variations", 1992.

Robust Tissue Boundary Detection for Cerebral Cortical Thickness Estimation

Marietta L.J. Scott and Neil A. Thacker

University of Manchester, Manchester, UK
marietta.scott@manchester.ac.uk
http://www.tina-vision.net

Abstract. This paper presents an algorithm for determining regional cerebral grey matter cortical thickness from magnetic resonance scans. In particular, the modification of a gradient-based edge detector into an iso-grey-level boundary detector for reliably determining the low-contrast grey-white matter interface is described and discussed. The reproducibility of the algorithm over 31 gyral regions is assessed using repeat scans of four subjects, and a technique for correcting the misplacement of the grey-white matter boundary is shown to significantly reduce the systematic error on the reproducibility.

1 Introduction

The determination and characterisation of human cerebral cortical grey matter thickness has enormous potential use in the assessment of the severity and progression of pathology and of the processes of normal brain ageing. Grey matter (GM) volume loss is seen throughout adulthood to old age [1] and increased cortical thinning relative to control subjects has been implicated in various degenerative diseases, such as Alzheimer's disease [2], and Multiple Sclerosis [3].

The highly convoluted folding of the cortex provides two challenges to the estimation of thickness. The first is the problem of measuring a thickness of a curved structure, the second is the determination of the boundaries of the GM ribbon, particularly when the opposing banks of two cortical folds are sufficiently close that there is no intervening cerebro-spinal fluid (CSF) or white matter (WM). Assuming that the boundaries of the GM ribbon have been accurately segmented in 3D, there are various measures of distance between the two surfaces that might be employed. First, if an active shape model algorithm using correspondences (eg. [4]) has been used to create the surfaces, the distance between the corresponding points on the two surfaces can be taken. However, anatomical homology within a group of subjects will not be precise. Alternatively, the minimum distance or distance along the surface normal between a given point on one surface to the opposing surface can be used. Of these two methods, the minimum distance will always produce a shorter average cortical thickness than the surface normal method [4].

Segmentation of the GM from the underlying WM and enveloping CSF on MR images requires knowledge of the expected grey-level intensity values for

J. Duncan and G. Gerig (Eds.): MICCAI 2005, LNCS 3750, pp. 878–885, 2005.

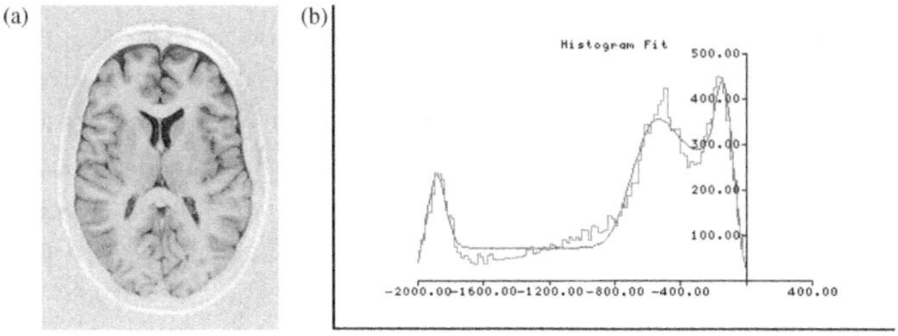

Fig. 1. Example axial inversion-recovery image (a) and corresponding grey-level intensity histogram (b) showing, from left to right, peaks for the CSF, GM and WM

these tissues. The segmentation used must also be able to detect tissue partial voluming and appropriate boundaries should be located under such circumstances. Through-plane magnetic field inhomogeneities should also not be ignored [5]. In addition, the contrast between the tissues needs to be sufficient in order to define their boundaries. Demyelination of WM axons, due to ageing and disease processes will result in the WM appearing more like the non-myelinated GM, making accurate boundary detection less feasible.

The simplest model for boundary determination between two tissues (WM/GM or GM/CSF) is based upon the assumption of a linear image formation process, such that the boundary occurs at the position where the image grey-level intensity is half-way between the two pure tissue values. As can be seen from fig. 1(b) the contrast at the GM/CSF boundary is large and it should be possible to use an edge detector to determine this boundary, whereas the GM/WM contrast is comparable to the noise in the image, so an edge detector could not be used reliably here. The main emphasis of this paper is to describe a modification to the Canny edge detector [6] for the determination of the GM/WM boundary for subsequent use in an original cortical thickness algorithm. The technique allows an assessment of the accuracy of the boundary positioning, and hence a post-processing correction mechanism for the regional thickness estimates. A reproducibility study is presented, showing that the boundary correction can indeed be used to reduce the systematic error on the cortical thickness measurements.

2 Materials and Methods

2.1 Approach Taken to Determine Cortical Thickness

The analysis of the data can be divided into two stages; pre-processing to convert the original volume of data into the required form and the actual cortical thickness estimation. Initially, the mean and standard deviation of the grey-level values of the pure tissues (in this case only GM, WM and CSF are considered) in the image volume are determined for use in future processing steps. Grey-level intensity values from a region (comprising several slices in order to average through-plane inhomogeneities to a certain degree) in the frontal lobe representative of the pure tissue values, are histogrammed (as shown in fig. 1) and a

Bayesian mixture model [7], containing terms for both pure tissues and partial volumes, is fitted to the histogram using simplex to obtain the pure tissue means and standard deviations. To obtain a finer through-plane resolution whilst preserving tissue boundaries, the data is explicitly up-interpolated in the z-direction [8] using a partial volume scheme to constrain the potential tissue boundaries, determined using 3D image gradients, that could pass through a partial volume voxel. The volume of data is then registered to a stereotaxic space (the Talairach atlas [9]) using a linear affine transform. The atlas defines the 31 cortical regions (see table 2 for region names) used later in producing regional histograms of the cortical thickness. Finally, the GM is segmented in the form of the most likely volume estimate in each voxel given the data, based on the defined probability density functions of the image intensity distribution.

The cortical thickness estimation itself proceeds by using a modified edge detection process (see below) to determine the GM/WM boundary. The surface normal to the boundary in 3D at each voxel on the boundary is determined, using a 3D Gaussian smoothed data set (in order to reduce the effects of noise) and a search is performed over 20mm in this direction on the segmented GM map until an edge (see [10] for precise details) is found. The cortical thickness at each boundary voxel is inserted into the appropriate regional histogram according to the registration into stereotaxic space determined earlier. The median of each regional histogram is calculated in order to give a robust estimation of the average cortical thickness for each region.

2.2 Modification to the Canny Edge Detector

The approach to thickness measurement presented here is inherently feature based and the GM/WM boundary is of particular importance. Conventional edge detectors are particularly poor at identifying edge boundaries where the contrast approaches the noise level, such as found at the GM/WM boundary. However, this boundary is expected to have one consistent grey-level value, in the absence of field inhomogeneities and tissue variation, and in this case is defined as the boundary at the average of the two pure tissue (50% transition) values. A simple 'z-score' measure of the consistency of the grey-level of each voxel with this boundary midpoint value is used to construct a likelihood image (which highlights the GM/WM boundary) based on a Gaussian distribution with a standard deviation of ten times the noise in the input image. This is monotonically related to a true hypothesis probability, but has better numerical properties for subsequent processing and sub-voxel peak location. This can be used as the basis for the enhancement process rather than the conventional (summed squares) gradient based measure and subsequent stages of the detection process are applied as normal. The implementation is based upon a version of the Canny edge detector. This new iso-contour Canny (or Iso-Canny) algorithm has the advantage that although noise processes may move the position of the detected boundary, these processes cannot prevent detection of a transition.

The later stages of the standard Canny edge detector perform non-maximal suppression and hysteresis thresholding which results in well localised connected

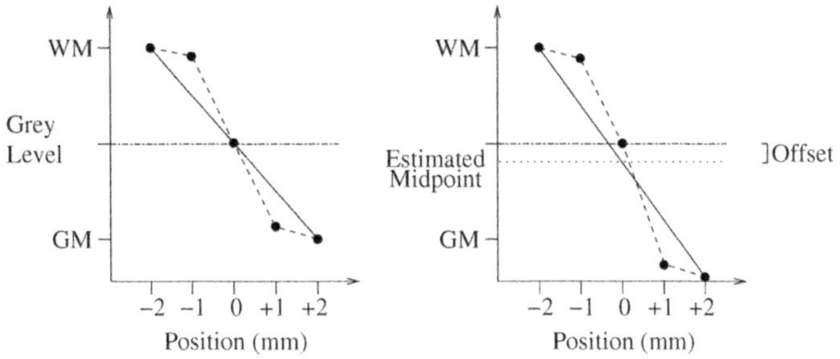

Fig. 2. Diagram illustrating the midpoint offset calculation. The plots show position on the x-axis and grey-level on the y-axis. Marked are the pure tissue grey-level values for GM and WM and the midpoint between them is shown by the dash-dot line. The central position is at the midpoint (edge) and the two positions on each side are in GM and WM. The left-hand plot shows the ideal case, where the linear interpolation (solid line) between the grey-level values of the positions 2mm either side corresponds to the midpoint value. The right-hand plot shows an example of the case where the value of the position in the GM is less than the pure tissue value, so that the interpolated grey-level value at the central position is less by some offset than the midpoint (edge) value.

edge strings which persist into low edge strength regions. Edge locations are computed within each slice of the data to sub-pixel accuracy (to 0.1mm reproducibility) from quadratic fits to the peaks in the edge strength map. This whole process is particularly reliant on the assumption that one accurately determined GM/WM boundary value is applicable in all parts of the image volume. The following section describes the implementation of a quality control process to assess any systematic errors in the analysis, or failures of the calibration process.

2.3 Post-processing to Determine the "Correct" Boundary Position

Use of an incorrect grey-level value for the midpoint of the GM and WM will result in a large systematic error on the regional cortical thickness. Presented here is a technique for monitoring this effect and for correcting for it *post hoc* if required. In order to calibrate such a correction for a given subject, the effect on the median thickness in each region by perturbing the GM/WM grey-level midpoint by -80 to +80 (in increments of 20 grey-levels) was investigated (using in each case the same set of grey-level and probability images). The regression coefficients of median thickness against grey-level perturbation are presented in section 3.2. A method for determining the difference ("offset") between the pre-determined midpoint grey-level value and the value at the actual GM/WM boundary is presented in fig. 2. In order to obtain an average value for each region, the offsets at each tissue boundary location are entered into regional histograms. The position of the peak of each histogram is taken as the offset estimate for that region. This grey-level offset can be used to compute an equivalent median thickness error, using the appropriate regression coefficients (given in table 2) as determined earlier.

2.4 Subjects and Scan Parameters

4 normal volunteers (all male, ages: 34, 40, 40, 46) underwent MR scans on two occasions within 7-21 days apart. All subjects gave informed consent and the study was approved by the Central Manchester LREC. An axial anatomical inversion recovery MR sequence (eg; fig. 1) was acquired (Philips Medical Systems, Best, The Netherlands, 1.5 Tesla, TI/TR/TE=300/6850/18ms, 90° flip angle, echo train length=9, matrix size=256^2, in-plane resolution=0.898^2mm, slice thickness=3.0mm, 51 slices taken covering the whole of the brain). These images were used to determine GM thickness in 31 cortical regions, as described above. Reproducibility of the technique was assessed by comparison of the regional median thicknesses of the two acquisitions from each subject. Images from the subject with the worst reproducibility underwent the correction for the misplacement of the Iso-Canny boundary, and the reproducibility of the modified results was assessed.

3 Results

3.1 Reproducibility Results

Figure 3 shows the 31 regional cortical thickness estimates from the 2nd scan plotted against those of the first, for all four subjects. Table 1 gives the corresponding regression coefficients, and the standard error on their measurement for the 4 subjects. Subjects 2, 3 and 4 have slopes which lie within 5% of the expected value of 1, whereas subject 1 shows a 16% error. The systematic error on the thickness measurements for this group is calculated as the RMS of the differences between the line of equality and the coefficients, scaled by $\sqrt{2}$ because two measurements have been taken, and amounts to 6.2% on the measurement in any given individual. The standard error of the data is indicative of the statistical error due to sampling the thickness distribution on any given region of the data. This can be calculated as the product of the standard error and the $\sqrt{N}$ where N is the number of regions, and amounts to no more than 0.06mm.

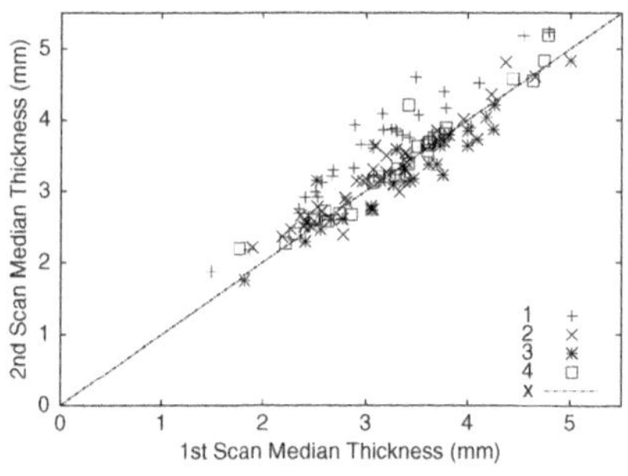

Fig. 3. Scatterplot of 2nd vs 1st scan cortical thickness measurements for 31 regions in each of 4 subjects. The line of equality is also shown.

Table 1. Table of fitted slopes and standard error on the fit for each subject for the data in fig. 2. Note that all regressions are constrained to pass through the origin.

Subject	Slope	Std. Err
1	1.16	0.0148
2	1.04	0.0111
3	0.95	0.0098
4	1.03	0.0088

3.2 Iso-Canny Correction Results

Table 2 gives, for the two scans of subject 1, the regression coefficients of the slopes of median thickness against the extent of GM/WM midpoint perturbation, as well as the estimated offset values by which the boundary was misplaced. In the majority of regions, the slopes are near perfect negative linear correlations of

Table 2. Table of the Talairach regions investigated, values of the slopes of median thickness against Iso-Canny midpoint used and calculated offset values for the two scans of subject 1

Lobe	Region	Slope ($\times 10^{-3}$) (mm/grey-level)		Offset (grey-levels)	
		Scan 1	Scan 2	Scan 1	Scan 2
Frontal	Rectal Gyrus	-4.08	-1.64	8.00	-126.67
	Orbital Gyrus	-1.23	-1.08	-173.33	127.62
	Precentral Gyrus	-4.64	-8.26	-23.33	-50.13
	Inferior Gyrus	-4.37	-6.47	-16.57	-67.88
	Middle Gyrus	-4.50	-6.62	-30.14	-74.17
	Superior Gyrus	-4.96	-7.23	-32.64	-82.07
	Medial Gyrus	-4.33	-7.46	-21.78	-48.68
Limbic	Posterior Cingulate	-1.30	-5.28	-10.26	-45.81
	Anterior Cingulate	-6.32	-7.03	-7.27	-47.69
	Subcallosal Gyrus	-2.12	2.82	-126.67	-60.44
Occipital	Inferior Gyrus	-2.24	-4.28	-3.64	-46.67
	Lingual Gyrus	-2.03	-5.03	-19.39	-95.24
	Middle Gyrus	-2.48	-5.09	5.22	-45.46
	Superior Gyrus	-2.04	-4.82	-55.24	-156.00
	Cuneus	-2.67	-5.61	-20.98	-58.24
Parietal	Insula	-3.15	-2.53	-34.02	-72.94
	Angular Gyrus	-3.93	-4.89	-51.43	-99.26
	Supramarginal Gyrus	-3.43	-6.10	-22.22	-52.08
	Cingulate Gyrus	-3.93	-5.03	-18.58	-54.81
	Inferior Lobule	-4.03	-5.79	-20.39	-88.79
	Superior Lobule	-4.33	-5.80	-37.58	-70.77
	Paracentral Lobule	-3.73	-7.26	-110.30	-108.57
	Postcentral Gyrus	-3.92	-6.85	-34.67	-60.61
	Precuneus	-3.83	-6.48	-34.29	-67.83
Temporal	Transverse Gyrus	-5.58	-9.83	8.48	-20.00
	Uncus	-2.23	-1.37	-42.67	-70.83
	Fusiform Gyrus	-1.93	-4.18	-21.40	-65.78
	Inferior Gyrus	-3.07	-2.88	-41.90	-95.76
	Parahippocampal Gyrus	-1.91	-4.23	-18.63	-76.92
	Middle Gyrus	-2.66	-5.45	-22.48	-54.57
	Superior Gyrus	-3.22	-4.21	2.37	-42.46

thickness with midpoint perturbation. The offset results demonstrate a negative bias (roughly ranging between 0 and -100) which is also seen in a larger cohort (results not shown). This is consistent with the GM grey-levels being lower than expected. The thickness estimation technique assumes that the average of two pure tissue values can be taken as the value at the boundary between these tissues. However, due to the slice thickness of this data, it is likely that there are substantial partial volume effects. GM/CSF partial volumes will result in a more pronounced effect than GM/WM partial volumes, which could explain the peak shift seen in the data If this is the case, the boundary correction may still be used for correcting the systematic error, even though the peak is no longer expected to be at the same grey-level as the assumed tissue boundary.

Applying the Iso-Canny offset correction to the regional cortical thickness measurements from both scans of subject 1 reduces the slope of the regressions from 16% greater than unity to 9.7% and marginally improves the standard error on fitting the regressions from 0.0148 to 0.0133mm.

4 Discussion

This paper has presented some of the difficulties in reliably determining GM cortical thickness from images obtained using MRI. Descriptions of a cortical thickness algorithm and the required pre-processing stages are given. The method is applied to repeat scans of four young normals, and the reproducibility of the *whole* procedure is assessed. The large systematic error, at 6.2%, mainly due to the initial grey-level histogram parameter determination, has implications for the use of this cortical thickness estimation in longitudinal studies. Such an error would be expected to mask any real changes in cortical thickness in an individual over the time scale in which the repeated measurements are likely to be made. However, several steps can be taken in order to achieve greater consistency. Ensuring an identical scanner set-up and subject physiology, as well as fixing the Bayesian prior terms and the ratio of grey-level histogram peaks between scans should reduce variability. Note that natural variation between subjects will be far greater than the effects of the systematic error, such that group-wise comparisons are feasible on tens of subjects. However, the ultimate goal of this work is to provide information suitable for decision support in individual subjects.

The main focus of the paper is a description of a GM/WM boundary detector. The advantage of basing this upon a conventional edge detector is that it provides edge locations computed to sub-pixel accuracy, as is necessary when measuring structures as small as the GM ribbon. In addition, well localised connected edge strings persist even in conventional low edge strength regions. The effect of perturbing the GM/WM midpoint value, in order to determine the effect of modifing the position of the GM/WM edge strings on the regional thickness estimation was used to calibrate a regional correction factor. This was used in conjunction with a technique for determining the inaccuracy in the position of the boundary, for the subject with the greatest systematic error, in order to produce a distance by which the regional thickness was in error. The modified regional estimates were then used to assess any change in reproducibility afforded by the boundary correction technique. The technique improved the systematic error in all 31 regions of subject 1 from 16% to 9%, so the technique appears to be beneficial and implies that through-plane inhomogeneities are partly responsible. However, the error is still greater than that exhibited by the other three subjects, probably for reasons associated with the segmentation. If the tissue value estimations led to inaccuracies in the GM/WM boundary, then the GM/CSF boundary found on the segmented GM maps may also have been inaccurate, although misplacement of the GM/CSF boundary by 50 grey-levels or so will have a much smaller effect on the median thickness than misplacing the GM/WM boundary by the same amount.

Acknowledgements

This work was supported by a grant from the Wellcome Trust. Thanks to Prof. P. Rabbitt for the subject data and Dr. Paul Bromiley for the segmentation code.

References

1. Sowell, E.R., Petersen B.S., Thompson P.M. et al: Mapping cortical change across the human life span. Nature Neuroscience **6** (2003) 309–315
2. Double K.L., Halliday G.M., Krill J.J., Harasty J.A. et al: Topography of brain atrophy during normal aging and Alzheimer's disease. Neurobiol. Aging **17** (1996) 513–521
3. Sailer M., Fischl B., Salat D., Tempelmann C. et al: Focal thinning of the cerebral cortex in multiple sclerosis. Brain **126** (2003) 1734–1744
4. MacDonald D., Kabani N., Avis D., Evans A.C.: Automated 3-D extraction of inner and outer surfaces of cerebral cortex from MRI. NeuroImage **12** (2000) 340–356
5. Jones S.E., Buchbinder B.R., Aharon I.: Three-dimensional mapping of cortical thickness using Laplace's equation. Hum. Br. Map. **11** (2000) 12–32
6. Canny J.F.: A Computational Approach to Edge Detection. Patt. Anal. Mach. Intel. **8** (1986) 679–698
7. Pokrić M., Thacker N.A., Scott M.L.J., Jackson A.: Multi-dimensional medical image segmentation with partial voluming. Proc. MIUA **5** (2001) 77–81
8. McKie S., Thacker N.A.: Step interpolation of MR images with inter-slice gap correction. Tina Memo 2003-010 (2003)
9. Talairach J., Tournoux P.: Co-planar stereotaxic atlas of the human brain. 3-dimensional proportional system: An approach to cerebral imaging. Thieme medical publishers (1988)
10. Scott M.L.J., Thacker N.A.: Cerebral Cortical Thickness Measurements. Tina Memo 2004-007 (2004)

Statistical Analysis of Pharmacokinetic Models in Dynamic Contrast-Enhanced Magnetic Resonance Imaging

Volker J. Schmid[1], Brandon J. Whitcher[2], Guang-Zhong Yang[1], N. Jane Taylor[3], and Anwar R. Padhani[3]

[1] Institute for Biomedical Engineering, Suite 5, Sherfield Building, Imperial College, South Kensington, London SW7 2AZ, United Kingdom
{v.schmid, g.z.yang}@imperial.ac.uk
[2] Translational Medicine & Genetics, GlaxoSmithKline, Greenford Road, Greenford UB6 0HE, Middlesex, United Kingdom
brandon.j.whitcher@gsk.com
[3] Paul Strickland Scanner Centre, Mount Vernon Hospital, Rickmansworth Road, Northwood HA6 2RN, Middlesex, United Kingdom

Abstract. This paper assesses the estimation of kinetic parameters from dynamic contrast-enhanced magnetic resonance imaging (DCE-MRI). Asymptotic results from likelihood-based nonlinear regression are compared with results derived from the posterior distribution using Bayesian estimation, along with the output from an established software package (MRIW). By using the estimated error from kinetic parameters, it is possible to produce more accurate clinical statistics, such as tumor size, for patients with breast tumors. Further analysis has also shown that Bayesian methods are more accurate and do not suffer from convergence problems, but at a higher computational cost.

1 Introduction

The quantitative analysis of dynamic contrast-enhanced magnetic resonance imaging (DCE-MRI) is typically achieved by applying pharmacokinetic (PK) models to the signal intensity, or a nonlinear transformation of it, observed from the scanning process. The contrast agent Gd-DTPA (gadolinium diethylenetriaminepentaacetic acid) is a small molecular weight substance injected after several baseline scans have been acquired. Using T_1-weighted sequences, the reduction in T_1 relaxation time caused by the contrast agent is the dominant enhancement observed [1]. T_1-weighted kinetic curves typically have three phases: the upslope, maximum enhancement, and washout [2]. Quantitative PK parameters are estimated by fitting a nonlinear function, the solution of a system of linear differential equations, to the observations. Each PK parameter has a direct relationship with key biological processes of interest; *e.g.*, volume transfer, leakage space, etc. This is a distinct advantage over the semi-quantitative approach where descriptive statistics of the kinetic curve (onset time, mean rate

J. Duncan and G. Gerig (Eds.): MICCAI 2005, LNCS 3750, pp. 886–893, 2005.

of change, maximum signal intensity, etc.) are estimated, but lack direct tissue or vascular information.

From a statistical point of view this quantitative methods are based on the theory of nonlinear regression [3]. Non-linear models are typically hard to estimate due to optimization problems, but standard software is available. We estimate parameters in pharmacokinetic (PK) models using nonlinear regression in both a likelihood and a Bayesian framework [4] to help alleviate some of the concerns stated above and provide a richer summary of the results, specifically with respect to convergence issues.

Potential clinical applications of DCE-MRI include screening for malignant disease, lesion characterization, monitoring lesion response to treatment, and assessment of residual disease. Newer applications include prognostication, pharmacodynamic assessments of antivascular anticancer drugs, and predicting efficacy of treatment. We propose to look at parameters obtained from the two methods and how they impact clinically relevant statistics such as tumor size.

2 Theory and Methods

2.1 DCE-MRI Data

To evaluate our methods we use a dataset provided by the Paul Strickland Scanner Centre at the Mount Vernon Hospital, Northwood. The data consist of six patients with breast tumors, scanned once at the beginning of treatment and again after six weeks. The scans were acquired with a 1.5 T Siemens MAGNETOM Symphony scanner, TR = 11 ms and TE = 4.7 ms. Each scan consists of three slices of 230×256 voxels. A dose of $D = 0.1$ mmol/kg body weight Gd-DTPA was injected at the start of the fifth acquisition using a power injector.

We use a standard compartmental model [5] to describe the arterial influx of Gd-DTPA into extracellular extravascular space (EES) and its venous efflux. The time series of gadolinium concentration in the tissue is modeled by

$$C_t(t) = K^{\text{trans}} \left[C_p(t) \otimes \exp(-k_{\text{ep}} t) \right], \quad (1)$$

where $C_t(t)$ is the observed Gd-DTPA concentration in the tissue at time t and $C_p(t)$ is the tracer concentration in arterial blood. The parameter K^{trans} represents the transfer from plasma to EES, and k_{ep} is the rate parameter for transport from the EES to plasma. Here, $\otimes$ denotes the convolution operator. The volume of EES per unit volume of tissue (leakage space) is given by

$$v_e = \frac{K^{\text{trans}}}{k_{\text{ep}}}. \quad (2)$$

For the arterial input function $C_p(t)$ we follow the work of Tofts and Kermode [6] and use a bi-exponential function

$$C_p(t) = D \sum_{i=1}^{2} a_i \exp(-m_i t), \quad (3)$$

with the values $a_1 = 3.99\,\text{kg/l}$, $a_2 = 4.78\,\text{kg/l}$, $m_1 = 0.144\,\text{min}^{-1}$ and $m_2 = 0.0111\,\text{min}^{-1}$ and the actual dose per body weight.

To calculate the Gadolinium concentration C_t, the signal intensity was converted to T_1 relaxation time values using T_1-weighted images, proton density weighted images and data from a calibration experiment consisting of phantoms with known T_1 relaxation time. The Gd-DTPA concentration can then be computed via

$$C_t(t) = \frac{1}{r_1}\left[\frac{1}{T_1(t)} - \frac{1}{T_{10}}\right] \tag{4}$$

where T_{10} is the T_1 value without contrast, computed as mean value of the first four images, and $r_1 = 4.24\,\text{l/s/mmol}$ is the longitudinal relativity of protons *in vivo* due to Gd-DTPA.

Regions of interest (ROIs) were drawn manually, on a scan-by-scan basis, using subtraction images from the acquisition of dynamic data. Although the tumor was isolated, in order to save on computation time, enough surrounding tissue was also captured to allow for reasonable contrast between tissue types within the ROI.

2.2 Statistical Models

Likelihood Approach. In each voxel we fitted a nonlinear regression model to the Gd-DTPA concentration time series. By carrying out the convolution in Eqn. 1, the following statistical model can be derived:

$$C_t(t) = D\exp(\theta_1)\sum_{i=1}^{2}\frac{a_i\{\exp(-m_i t) - \exp[-\exp(\theta_2)t]\}}{\exp(\theta_2) - m_i} + \epsilon_t, \tag{5}$$

where ϵ_t is the noise error at time t. We assume the expected value of the error to be zero; i.e. $E(\epsilon) = 0$. Inference is performed by minimizing the sum of squares of the errors $\min \sum \epsilon_t^2$. We use parameters $\exp(\theta_1)$ instead of K^{trans} and $\exp(\theta_2)$ instead of k_{ep} to insure positive values of K^{trans} and k_{ep}. The parameter v_e was computed using Eqn. 2. Estimation of the model was done using the `nls` function of the statistical computing environment R [7]. The function uses a Gauss–Newton algorithm to estimate parameters of interest along with their standard errors.

As comparting models are typically difficult to optimize, we use a multiple search start point approach for the algorithm [8]. To identify the starting values, we follow the ideas of Pinheiro and Bates [9] for first-order compartmental models. Nevertheless, the algorithm still failed to converge in 5% of voxels.

Bayesian Approach. For the Bayesian approach we use the following model

$$C_t(t) = DK^{\text{trans}}\sum_{i=1}^{2}\frac{a_i[\exp(-m_i t) - \exp(-k_{\text{ep}}t)]}{k_{\text{ep}} - m_i} + \epsilon. \tag{6}$$

In the Bayesian framework prior probability density functions (PDFs) have to be specified for all unknown parameters, and hence, we use

$$\begin{aligned}\epsilon &\sim \mathrm{N}(0, \tau_\epsilon^{-1}),\\ \log(K^{\mathrm{trans}}) &\sim \mathrm{N}(0, \tau_{K^{\mathrm{trans}}}^{-1}),\\ \log(k_{\mathrm{ep}}) &\sim \mathrm{N}(0, \tau_{k_{\mathrm{ep}}}^{-1}),\end{aligned}$$

where N denotes the Gaussian (Normal) distribution. The variance parameters for these PDFs are also specified by so-called hyper-priors,

$$\begin{aligned}\tau_\epsilon &\sim \mathrm{Ga}(0.001, 0.001),\\ \tau_{K^{\mathrm{trans}}} &\sim \mathrm{Ga}(0.001, 0.001),\\ \tau_{k_{\mathrm{ep}}} &\sim \mathrm{Ga}(0.001, 0.001),\end{aligned}$$

where Ga denotes the Gamma distribution. So the PDFs of $\epsilon, K^{\mathrm{trans}}$ and k_{ep} have high variance and therefore are very diffuse. This reflects lack of prior information about the parameters of interest. By using a normal prior distribution for $\log(K^{\mathrm{trans}})$ and $\log(k_{\mathrm{ep}})$, we ensure positive values for both parameters as with the likelihood method.

Inference is made by computing the posterior distribution $p(K^{\mathrm{trans}}, k_{\mathrm{ep}} \mid C_t)$ given by Bayes' theorem, so that

$$p(K^{\mathrm{trans}}, k_{\mathrm{ep}} \mid C_t) = \frac{p(K^{\mathrm{trans}}, k_{\mathrm{ep}})\ \ell(C_t \mid K^{\mathrm{trans}}, k_{\mathrm{ep}})}{\int p(K^{\mathrm{trans}*}, k_{\mathrm{ep}*})\ \ell(C_t \mid K^{\mathrm{trans}*}, k_{\mathrm{ep}*})}, \tag{7}$$

where $\ell(C_t \mid K^{\mathrm{trans}}, k_{\mathrm{ep}})$ denotes the likelihood function of $C_t(t)$. Samples from the posterior distribution are obtained via Markov chain Monte Carlo (MCMC) methods [4] implemented in C++. For estimating the parameter and standard errors we use the mean and the empirical standard error of the sample of each parameter, respectively, after a reasonable burn-in phase.

MRIW. Estimation of pharmacokinetic parameters was also performed using MRIW v4.1.6 [10], an established software package for parametric analysis of DCE-MRI data developed at the Institute of Cancer Research, United Kingdom.

3 Results

Both the likelihood and Bayesian methods were applied to six patients, with breast tumor, before and after treatment. Fig. 1 shows the estimated volume transfer constant (K^{trans}), the standard error of $\log(K^{\mathrm{trans}})$ and the leakage space (v_e) from a single slice of patient #2 before therapy. The tumors are clearly visible as a region of high K^{trans}, although the likelihood-based procedure and MRIW failed to converge for approximately 5% of voxels both inside and outside the tumor. Bayesian parameter estimates were available for all voxels. When looking at leakage space the tumor is surrounded by a region of high v_e, making the edges of the tumor difficult to identify.

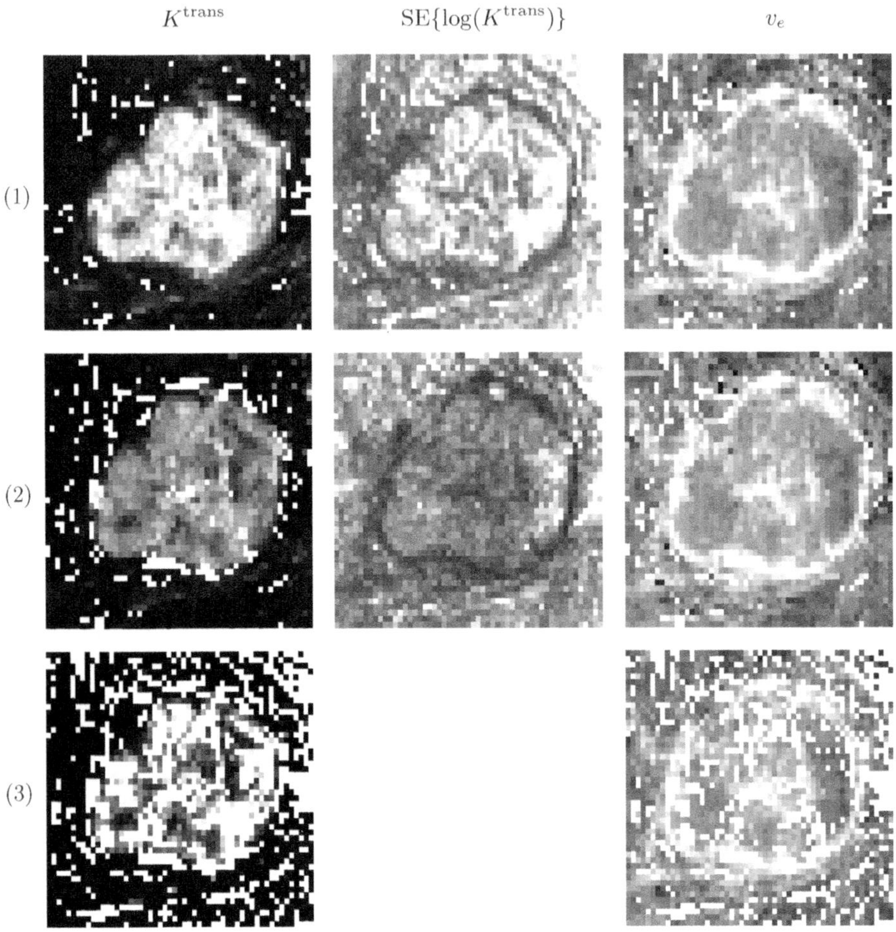

Fig. 1. Parametric maps of kinetic parameters for a region of interest around a breast tumor – from left to right – the volume transfer constant (K^{trans}), the standard error of $\log(K^{\text{trans}})$ and the leakage space (v_e). The rows correspond to three methods likelihood (1), Bayesian (2) and MRIW (3).

To specify the exact region of the tumor, we threshold K^{trans} such that only values exceeding 0.3 remain (Fig. 2, left). This helps to highlight the tumor, but many voxels not associated with the tumor also remain. To produce a better specification, we take advantage of the estimated standard error for K^{trans}. Fig. 1 (right) shows the estimated standard error of $\log(K^{\text{trans}})$ for the likelihood and Bayesian methods (see our model specification in Sec. 2.2). The error is especially high where the estimated value of K^{trans} is high (*e.g.*, in the tumor). Assuming an asymptotic Normal distribution, we can compute the probability of each pixel exceeding the threshold. Fig. 2 (middle) shows this probability map, whereas Fig. 2 (right) shows pixels where the probability of exceeding the threshold (i.e., a pixel being part of the tumor) is greater than or equal to 99%. Utilizing the PDF of K^{trans}, either its asymptotic distribution via the likelihood method or its posterior distribution via the Bayesian method, produces a much better separation between tumor and non-tumor voxels.

We explore the clinical application of these methods by computing the size of the tumor, defined here to be the number of voxels per slice. A tumor mask was created from the estimated K^{trans} for each method (Fig. 3) and the size of the tumor, both pre- and post-treatment, is provided in Tab. 1 for all six patients. There is good agreement between the three methods for most of the scans.

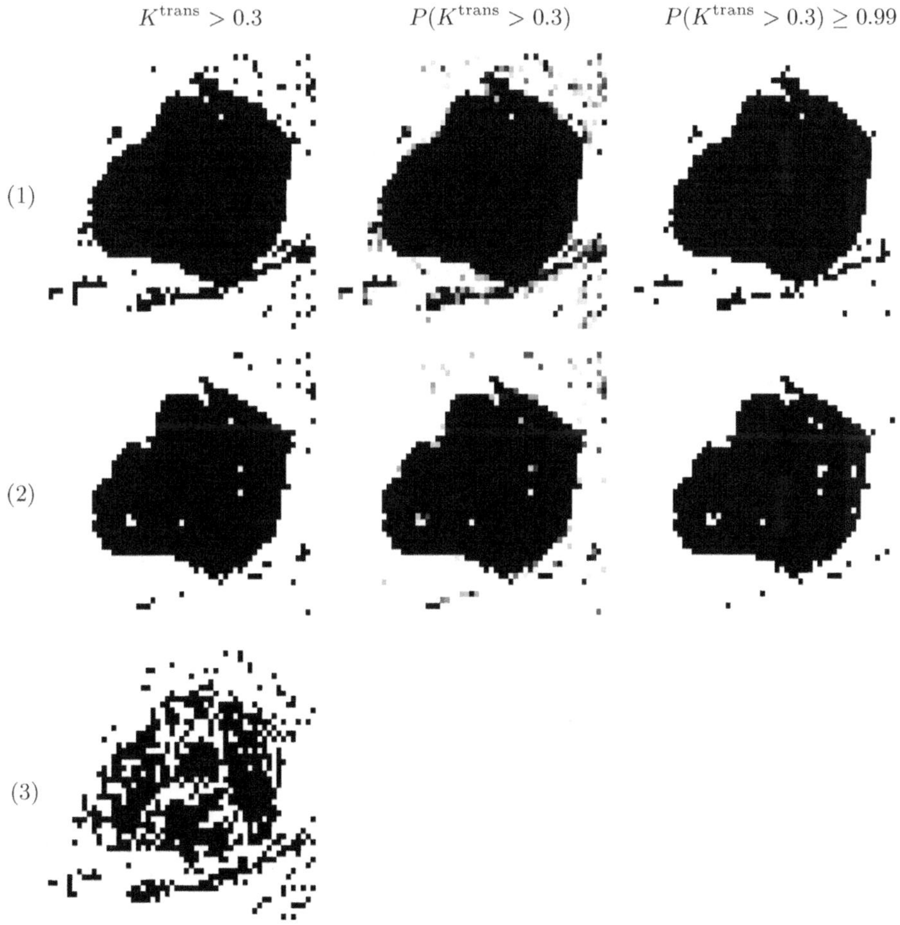

Fig. 2. Threshold maps derived from estimates of K^{trans} of first scan of patient #2 – from left to right – basic thresholding, probability of exceeding the threshold and probability of exceeding the threshold by at least 99%. The rows correspond to three methods – from top to bottom – likelihood (1), Bayesian (2) and MRIW (3).

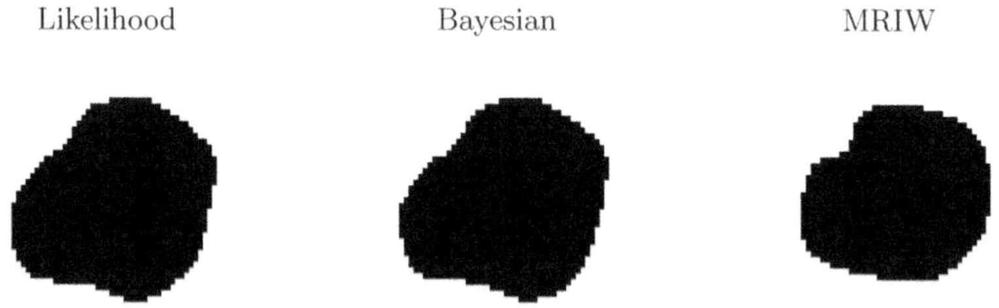

Fig. 3. Mask of the tumor of scan 1 of patient # 2 based on different estimates of K^{trans} – from left to right – likelihood, Bayesian and MRIW

Table 1. Tumor size (number of voxels) derived from K^{trans} for each slice of the six patients, pre- and post-treatment

		Bayes				Likelihood				MRIW			
	Slice	1	2	3	Total	1	2	3	Total	1	2	3	Total
Patient	Treatment												
1	pre	0	557	0	557	0	566	0	566	0	569	0	569
	post	4	32	0	36	5	36	0	41	5	34	0	39
2	pre	663	1068	567	2298	676	1147	582	2405	846	1306	504	2656
	post	0	0	0	0	0	0	0	0	140	0	0	140
3	pre	256	440	192	888	266	429	185	880	289	439	238	966
	post	0	7	0	7	8	0	21	29	0	0	52	52
4	pre	58	292	144	494	57	293	138	488	94	201	261	556
	post	1375	25697	2087	6031	1393	2591	2100	6084	1973	1351	1089	4413
5	pre	450	287	222	959	456	290	207	953	260	227	29	516
	post	1393	1467	1175	4035	1449	1769	1511	4729	445	190	526	1161
6	pre	87	481	114	682	89	503	115	707	104	233	78	415
	post	142	297	0	439	149	301	0	450	134	396	120	450

4 Conclusion

Statistical properties of pharmacokinetic parameters from DCE-MRI have been used to improve clinically relevant quantities of interest. Bayesian techniques allow one to input prior information into the estimation procedure, greatly reducing problems with convergence with the cost of increased computing time. The posterior distribution provides instant access to valuable information about the kinetic parameters without resorting to asymptotic results. We have utilized second-order quantities of the posterior distribution to help discriminate voxels and produce more accurate summaries of clinically meaningful statistics.

With the proposed framework, it is possible to incorporate additional information via the prior distributions including dependence between kinetic parameters and spatial constraints, thus moving towards semi-parametric or non-parametric models in DCE-MRI.

Acknowledgments

Support for Dr. Schmid was financed through a research grant from Glaxo-SmithKline. The clinical data was graciously provided by Dr. A.R. Padhani.

References

1. Parker, G.J.M., Padhani, A.R.: T_1-w DCE-MRI: T_1-weighted dynamic contrast-enhanced MRI. In Tofts, P., ed.: Quantitative MRI of the Brain. Wiley, Chichester, England (2003) 341–364
2. Collins, D.J., Padhani, A.R.: Dynamic magnetic resonance imaging of tumor perfusion. IEEE Engineering in Biology and Medicine Magazine (2004) 65–83
3. Seber, G.A.F., Wild, C.J.: Nonlinear Regression. Wiley, Hoboken, New Jersey (1988)
4. Gilks, W.R., Richardson, S., Spiegelhalter, D.J.: Markov Chain Monte Carlo in Practice. Chapman & Hall, London (1996)
5. Kety, S.: Blood-tissue exchange methods. Theory of blood-tissue exchange and its applications to measurement of blood flow. Methods in Medical Research **8** (1960) 223–227
6. Tofts, P., Kermode, A.: Measurement of the blood-brain barrier permeability and leakage space using dynamic MR imaging–1. Fundamental concepts. Magn Reson Med **17** (1991) 357–36
7. R Development Core Team: R: A language and environment for statistical computing. R Foundation for Statistical Computing, Vienna, Austria. (2003) ISBN 3-900051-00-3.
8. Ahearn, T., Staff, R., Redpath, T., Semple, S.: The use of the Levenberg-Marquardt curve-fitting algorithm in pharmacokinetic modelling of DCE-MRI. Physics in Medicine and Biology **50** (2005) N85–N92
9. Pinheiro, J.C., Bates, D.M.: Mixed-Effects Models in S and S-PLUS. Springer-Verlag, New York (2000)
10. Parker, G., Suckling, J., Tanner, S., Padhani, A., Husband, J., Leach, M.: MRIW: parametric analysis software for contrast-enhanced dynamic mr imaging in cancer. Radiographics **18** (1998) 497–506

Inter-breath-hold Registration for the Production of High Resolution Cardiac MR Volumes

Nicholas M.I. Noble[1,2], Redha Boubertakh[1,2], Reza S. Razavi[2], and Derek L.G. Hill[1]

[1] Centre for Medical Image Computing, University College London, UK
{N.Noble, Derek.Hill}@ucl.ac.uk
[2] Imaging Sciences, Guy's Hospital, Kings College London, UK
{Redha.Boubertakh, Reza.Razavi}@kcl.ac.uk

Abstract. High resolution MRI images of the beating heart permit observation of detailed anatomical features and enable quantification of small changes in metrics of cardiac function. To obtain approximately isotropic sampling with an adequate spatial and temporal resolution, these images need to be acquired in multiple breath-holds. They are, therefore, often affected by through-plane discontinuities due to inconsistent breath-hold positions. This paper presents a method to correct for these discontinuities by performing breath-hold-by-breath-hold registration of high resolution 3D data to radial long axis images. The corrected images appear free of discontinuities, and it was found that they could be delineated more reproducibly than uncorrected images. This reduces the sample size required to detect systematic changes in blood pool volume by 57% at end systole and 78% at end diastole.

1 Introduction

High resolution dynamic 3D volumes of the beating heart are very desirable from both clinical and image processing points of view. Clinically, they permit observation of small anatomical features and enable quantification of small changes in metrics of cardiac function. In addition as we will show, intra-observer variability when delineating such images would appear to be greatly reduced when compared to the repeated delineation of traditional multi-slice cine functional images which have much lower through-plane resolution. From an image analysis perspective, volumetric imaging with isotropic resolution and a sinc point spread function in all directions is desirable because it improves the performance of multi-planar re-formatting and more sophisticated 3D analysis techniques. This should improve the performance of segmentation and model construction techniques, making automatic quantitative image analysis more reliable, and therefore lead to more clinically straightforward imaging protocols.

Currently, clinical MR images used for ventricular function assessment typically feature reconstructed voxel sizes of around 1.5×1.5mm in-plane and $8-10$mm through plane. Two or three slices of this type can be acquired in a single breath-hold, which leads to acquisition times of 4-6 breath-holds for coverage of the entire left ventricle in the short axis. Although these images demonstrate very good contrast, in the z-direction, the resolution is not sufficient to differentiate small features and the point spread function is non-ideal. In this paper, we acquire 3D volumes with reconstructed voxel sizes

J. Duncan and G. Gerig (Eds.): MICCAI 2005, LNCS 3750, pp. 894–901, 2005.

of 1.5×1.5mm in-plane and 1.5mm through plane in chunks of 10 slices during 7-8 breath-holds. During scanning the subject is instructed to hold their breath at the same position, but many patients find this very difficult in practice. Breath-hold inconsistencies result, most clearly visible as jagged structure boundaries in re-formatted long axis images. Translations of up to 23.5mm and rotations of up to 8° due to inconsistent breath-hold positions have been recorded in the literature [1].

Several approaches may be employed to remove through-plane discontinuities. Acquisition approaches include the use of respiratory navigators [2] which when placed through the diaphragm may be used to reject inconsistent breath-holds [3]. However this can greatly increase the scan time as the subject repeatedly attempts to hold their breath within a gating window of 2.5mm. Swingen *et al.* [4] corrected for in-plane translations by fitting a polynomial through the centroids of manually delineated in-slice endocardial contours. Each slice was then translated by the residual error following fitting. Lötjönen *et al.* [5] corrected for 3D translations by registering parallel long axis images and short axis images. Chandler *et al.* [6] corrected for 3D translations and rotations by registering short axis images to 3D volumes. However, these three techniques all seek to correct for breath-hold discontinuities in thick sliced images whose features are somewhat different to those of high resolution near-isotropic images. To date, only Moore *et al.* [7] have attempted to correct for breath-hold inconsistencies in images with high through-plane resolution. They performed successive rigid registrations between each slice and sagital and axial scout slices. This permitted translations in the foot-head and right-left directions to be corrected for. Their images however suffered from very poor SNR. To surmount this, they combined images from multiple subjects (via elastic registration and signal averaging) to form a high resolution atlas.

In this work, to correct for breath-hold discontinuities, 3D translations and rotations are recovered by registration of 2D long axis images acquired with radially oriented slices (figure 1) to high resolution 3D short axis multi-chunk images. Analysis is then performed to determine whether the described technique can be used to reduce the sample size required to detect systematic changes in blood pool volume. Such a reduction is potentially of great importance when performing clinical trials.

2 Data

Following plan scans and identification of the vertical and horizontal long axes, short axis ECG gated steady state free precession 3D volume images with SENSE factor 2 were obtained in 5 healthy male volunteers. Seventy to eighty slices were acquired in 7 or 8 chunks of 10 slices per end-expiration breath-hold. The field of view was adapted for each subject. Imaging parameters were: field of view 330 - 420 mm, acquisition matrix 129×160 with 80% phase encode direction sampling in the in-plane direction, 50% phase encode direction sampling in the through-plane direction, reconstructed to 256×256×70–80 giving a resolution of 1.30×1.30×1.57 mm – 1.64×1.64×1.57 mm, with 8 phases in the cardiac cycle, flip angle 45°, TE 1.5 ms and TR 3.08 - 3.54 ms. An end diastolic ECG gated steady state free precession long axis image containing twelve 2D slices radially oriented about the long axis was then acquired during a single end-expiration breath-hold. The imaging parameters were; slice thickness 8 mm, field of view 400 - 500 mm, acquisition matrix 160×192 with 120% phase encode direction sampling, reconstructed to 256×256 giving a resolution of 1.56×1.56×8 mm – 1.94×1.94×8 mm, flip angle 50°, TE 1.5 ms and TR 3.39 - 3.57 ms. To enable subsequent variability assessment, this procedure was repeated twice during the same scan session for each volunteer.The images were acquired on a Philips Intera 1.5 T with master gradients, using a 5 element cardiac synergy coil and vector ECG.

3 Methods

Before registering the radial long axis and short axis multi-chunk images, transformations must be defined that relate any point in the short axis image to the corresponding point in the radial long axis image. Radial long axis images are stored by stacking radially adjacent images — figure 1.

For each slice (i), locations in voxel coordinates can be related to their position in world coordinates by the following matrix

$$A_{RL(i)} = T_i R_{xi} R_{yi} R_{zi} O_i \tag{1}$$

where R_{xi}, R_{yi} and R_{zi} are 4×4 matrices representing rotations about the respective x, y, and z axes, T_i contains translations in the x, y and z directions and O_i is an orientation matrix with three possible values (corresponding to transverse, sagital and coronal slice orientations). The parameters that make up these matrices were automatically recorded during acquisition and subsequently extracted from the Philips proprietary PAR header file. Likewise, locations in voxel coordinates in the short axis image are related to their position in world coordinates by matrix A_{SA} (composed as per equation 1, but valid for the entire short axis image).

Pseudo radial long axis images were then created from the end diastolic multi-chunk images. For each ten slice chunk, a corresponding short axis 'chunk of interest image' was created. These images were the same as the short axis image, however all voxels that were not acquired during the breath-hold corresponding to that chunk were set to a padding value. The padding value was chosen so that it could not occur elsewhere in the image (-1 in this case). Blank images with the same geometry as the radial long axis image were then created for each chunk of interest image—the pseudo images. For

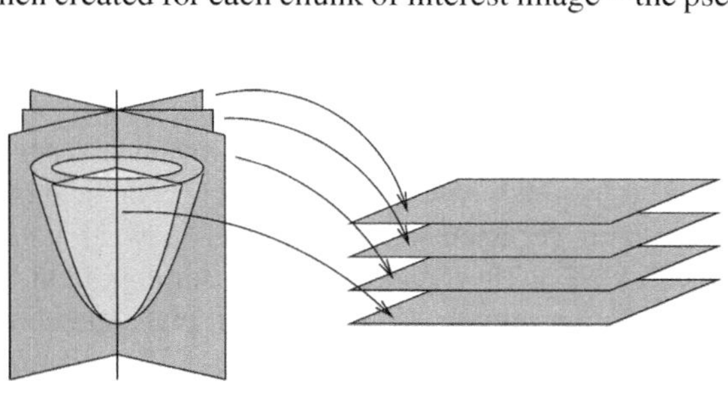

Fig. 1. Illustration of the orientation of radial long axis slice planes with respect to the left ventricle (*left*), and how they are stored in the image (*right*)

each pseudo image, the voxel locations were transformed into world coordinates before being transformed into voxel coordinates in the short axis image.

$$Pos_{SA} = A_{RL(i)} A_{SA}^{-1} Pos_{RL} \tag{2}$$

where Pos_{RL} is a 4×1 matrix representing the voxel location in the radial long axis image and Pos_{SA} represents the corresponding voxel location in the short axis image. These locations were then interpolated using trilinear interpolation to provide the voxel intensity values for the pseudo radial long axis images. Figure 2 shows an example of several slices from pseudo radial long axis images.

To avoid the two stage interpolation associated with transforming the chunk of interest image prior to creating a pseudo radial long axis image, the registration transformation matrix was incorporated into the process of creating the pseudo images. Equation 2 hence becomes

$$Pos_{SA} = A_{RL(i)} T_{REG} A_{SA}^{-1} Pos_{RL} \tag{3}$$

where T_{REG} is a 4×4 matrix which represents a six degree of freedom rigid body transformation.

The correlation coefficient similarity measure between the radial long axis image and each pseudo long axis image was then optimised as a function of the six degrees of freedom of T_{REG} using a simplex search method [8]. Voxels set to the padding value did not contribute to the similarity measure. A two stage optimisation approach was employed; firstly the x, y, and z translations alone were optimised, then all six parameters were optimised. The chunk of interest images were then transformed using trilinear interpolation according to their respective registration matrices. The corrected chunk of interest images were then combined into a single corrected image. Where multiple chunks overlapped, the mean voxel intensity was used. Following correction, small gaps may occur in locations where chunks did not overlap as shown in figure 2. The location of such gaps may be identified by searching for voxels which contain padding values in all of the corrected chunk of interest images. To fill these gaps, for each gap voxel, one dimensional linear interpolation was performed between the nearest non-gap voxels in the inferior and superior z-directions.

For each pair of radial long axis and short axis multi-chunk images, each chunk of the end diastolic multi-chunk image was registered to the radial long axis image. The registration matrices were then used to create corrected short axis image series. The end diastolic and end systolic blood pool volumes were then manually delineated in the original and corrected images by an expert observer using Analyze (Mayo Clinic, Rochester, MN, US).

The reproducibility of manually determined end diastolic and end systolic volume for the original and corrected images was investigated as per [9]. The mean and standard deviation difference between results and the mean and standard deviation percentage variability (defined as the absolute difference of two measurements divided by their mean) were assessed. The correlation coefficient between the first and second set of acquisitions was also calculated. Student's paired t-test was employed to identify any significant differences between the two sets of measurements. The sample sizes (N) required to detect a systematic change (δ) of 1ml with a power (P) of 90% and an α error of 5% were calculated using the following formula

$$N = f(\alpha, P)2\sigma^2/\delta^2 \tag{4}$$

where σ is the standard deviation of the difference as described by Altman [10] and $f(\alpha, P) = 10.5$ for $\alpha = 0.05$ and $P = 90$.

4 Results

Visually, all images registered well. Figure 2 shows example radial long axis views of the corrected images. Note specifically the areas around the right and left ventricular myocardium. The improvements in though-plane continuity can clearly be observed. The uncorrected images can show features that are not present in the corrected images and *vice versa*. This is due to rotations about the z-axis being recovered during registration. The corrected images after filling contain residual intensity fluctuations resulting from the z-axis linear interpolation.

Table 1 shows the reproducibility data. It can be seen that for the corrected images the mean and standard deviation volume differences at both end diastole and end systole are reduced with respect to the uncorrected images. The mean and standard deviation percentage variability for both end diastolic and end systolic volumes of the corrected volumes were also less than for the uncorrected images. For both corrected and uncorrected images the correlation of both end diastolic and end systolic volume between the first and second set of images was very high (correlation coefficient > 0.98). No significant differences between the first and second sets of images were observed ($p < 0.05$).

To detect a change of 1ml in end diastolic and end systolic volume in the uncorrected images requires 83 and 67 subjects respectively. To detect the same change in corrected

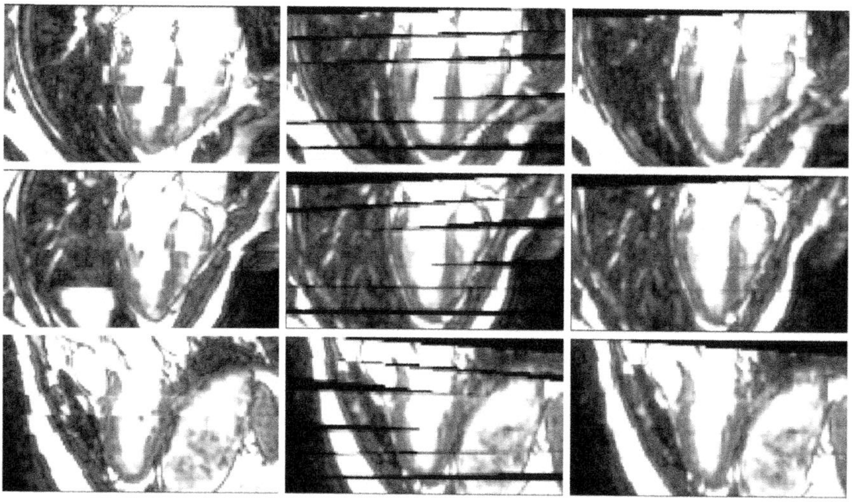

Fig. 2. Pseudo radial long axis images before correction (*left*), following correction (*middle*) and following correction and z-direction interpolation to fill any gaps (*right*)

Table 1. Reproducibility data for uncorrected and corrected images

	Uncorrected		Corrected	
	EDV (ml)	ESV (ml)	EDV (ml)	ESV (ml)
Mean difference $\pm$SD	3.07$\pm$1.99	3.36$\pm$1.79	1.17$\pm$0.92	1.44$\pm$1.18
Correlation coefficient	0.99	0.98	1.00	1.00
t-test *p*	NS	NS	NS	NS
% Variability $\pm$SD	2.25$\pm$1.28	6.94$\pm$3.94	0.97$\pm$0.69	3.55$\pm$2.56

EDV = End Diastolic Volume; ESV = End Systolic Volume; SD = Standard Deviation.

images requires 18 subjects for end diastolic volume and 29 subjects for end systolic volume. In percentage terms, these represent reductions in sample size of 78% and 57% respectively.

It is interesting to note that the standard deviations of differences in end diastolic and systolic volumes in both corrected and uncorrected images are much smaller than when delineating the thick slices exhibited by 2D multislice images —the current gold standard. Standard deviations of 4.3 – 4.7ml at end systole and 2.3 – 3.5ml at end diastole have been reported in the literature when manually delineating 10mm thick slices [9,11]. To put these values in context, this would correspond to sample sizes of 388 – 464 for end systolic volume and 165 – 257 for end diastolic volume to detect a 1ml volume change with $P = 90\%$ and $\alpha = 0.05$. This indicates that the reproducibility of end diastolic and end systolic volumes is much greater for high resolution 3D images.

5 Discussion

We have described a technique for generating high quality dynamic cardiac MR volumes from data acquired using multiple breath-holds. The approach corrects for inconsistent breath-hold positions by registration to a radial stack of long axis slices. We have demonstrated the qualitative benefit of this approach, and also used a power analysis to demonstrate that our technique can provide images that are more sensitive to within- and between-subject changes in cardiac function than the current gold standard technique of multi-slice cine cardiac MRI.

The radial long axis images have a slice thickness of 8mm, whereas the pseudo images are created by sampling high resolution images and have an effective thickness of around 1.5mm. Even at perfect alignment, the radial and pseudo images will appear slightly different because of the disparate slice thicknesses. A possible solution is to simulate thick slices by sampling the chunk of interest images at multiple points normal to the radial long axis slice plane. Weighted combination according to the slice select profile [12] would then produce a simulated thick sliced pseudo radial long axis image, which should better resemble the radial long axis image and may aid registration.

This work has assumed to good effect that misalignment due to inconsistent breath-hold positions can be corrected for by using a rigid transformation model. However, the heart, chest wall and other organs move relative to one another during respiration. In addition, the shape of the heart alters during the respiratory cycle due to changes in the venous return. To further improve registration accuracy, it may be necessary to employ non-rigid registration.

As was seen in figure 2, the corrected images contain residual intensity modulation in the areas of gaps in the data. These intensity modulations could be reduced by using more sophisticated through-slice interpolation (e.g. [13]), or alternatively using the inherent oversampling in each 3D chunk to fill the gaps. The latter approach would require working with the raw data, rather than the exported images, as this oversampled data is discarded prior to image exportation.

6 Conclusion

To conclude, a technique has been described for the correction of breath-hold discontinuities in high resolution short axis images via registration with radial long axis images. Visually, the results are very positive, providing a qualitative indication that the technique has effectively corrected for discontinuities resulting from inconsistent breath-hold positions. Numerical analysis of delineations performed prior to and following correction has shown that correction substantially improves reproducibility. When these results are interpreted in terms of sample size, this improvement corresponds to a reduction of the sample size required to detect systematic changes of 1ml in blood pool volume of between 57% and 78%.

Acknowledgements

This work was funded by the Engineering and Physical Sciences Research Council, grant GT/T11395/01. We are also grateful to Philips Medical Systems Nederland B.V. for research support.

References

1. K. McLeish, D.L.G. Hill, D. Atkinson, J.M. Blackall, and R. Razavi. A Study of the Motion and Deformation of the Heart Due to Respiration. *IEEE Trans. Med. Imaging*, 21(9):1142–1150, 2002.
2. Y. Wang, P.J. Rossman, J.P. Debbins, and R.L. Ehman. 3D Coronary MR-Angiography in Multiple Breath-Holds using a Respiratory Feedback Monitor. *Magn. Reson. Med.*, 34(1):11–16, 1995.
3. R.S. Razavi, D.L.G. Hill, V. Muthurangu, M.E. Miquel, A.M. Taylor, S. Kozerke, and E.J. Baker. Three-Dimensional Magnetic Resonance Imaging of Congenital Cardiac Anomalies. *Cardiol. Young*, 13:461–465, 2003.
4. C. Swingen, R.T. Seethamraju, and M. Jerosch-Herold. An Approach to the Three-Dimensional Display of Left Ventricular Function and Viability using MRI. *Int. J. Comput. Vision*, 19:325–336, 2003.
5. J. Lötjönen, M. Pollari, S. Kivistö, and K. Lauerma. Correction of Movement Artifacts from 4D Cardiac Short- and Long-Axis MR Data. In C. Barillot, D.R. Haynor, and P. Hellier, editors, *Medical Image Computing and Computer-Assisted Intervention—MICCAI 2004*, pages 405–412, 2004.
6. A.G. Chandler, T. Netch, J.A. Schnabel, R. Razavi, D.L.G. Hill, and D.J. Hawkes. Correction of Misaligned Slices in Multi-Slice MR Cardiac Examinations by using Slice-to-Volume Registration. In D. Rueckert, J. Hajnal, and G.-Z. Yang, editors, *Medical Image Understanding and Analysis — MIUA 2004*, pages 33–36, 2004.

7. J. Moore, M. Drangova, M. Wierzbicki, J. Barron, and T. Peters. A High Resolution Dynamic Heart Model Based on Averaged MRI Data. In R. Ellis and T. Peters, editors, *Medical Image Computing and Computer-Assisted Intervention—MICCAI 2003*, pages 549–556, 2003.
8. J.C. Lagarias, J.A. Reeds, M.H. Wright, and P.E. Wright. Convergence Properties of the Nelder-Mead Simplex Method in Low Dimensions. *SIAM Journal of Optimization*, 9(1):112–147, 1998.
9. N.G. Bellenger, L.C. Davies, J.M. Francis, and D.J. Pennell. Reduction in Sample Size for Studies of Remodeling in Heart Failure by the Use of Cardiovascular Magnetic Resonance. *J. Cardio. Magn. Reson.*, 2(4):271–278, 2000.
10. D.G. Altman. *Practical Statistics for Medical Research.* Chapman and Hall, 1991.
11. F. Grothues, G.C. Smith, J.C.C. Moon, N.G. Bellenger, P. Collins, H.U. Klein, and D.J. Pennell. Comparison of Interstudy Reproducibility of Cardiovascular Magnetic Resonance with Two-Dimensional Echocardiography in Normal Subjects and in Patients with Heart Failure or Left Ventricular Hypertrophy. *Am. J. Cardiol.*, 90(1):29–34, 2002.
12. A.G. Chandler. *Improved Slice to Volume Registration using Information-Based Registration and Super-Sampling for Brain MR, Cardiac MR and Lung CT Applications.* PhD thesis, Kings College London, 2005. In Press.
13. G.P. Penney, J.A. Schnabel, D. Rueckert, and M.A. Viergever. Registration-Based Interpolation. *IEEE Trans. Med. Imaging*, 23(7):922–926, 2004.

Consistent Estimation of Cardiac Motions by 4D Image Registration

Dinggang Shen, Hari Sundar, Zhong Xue, Yong Fan, and Harold Litt

Section of Biomedical Image Analysis, Department of Radiology,
University of Pennsylvania, Philadelphia, PA 19104
Dinggang.Shen@uphs.upenn.edu

Abstract. A 4D image registration method is proposed for consistent estimation of cardiac motion from MR image sequences. Under this 4D registration framework, all 3D cardiac images taken at different time-points are registered simultaneously, and motion estimated is enforced to be spatiotemporally smooth, thereby overcoming potential limitations of some methods that typically estimate cardiac deformation sequentially from one frame to another, instead of treating the entire set of images as a 4D volume. To facilitate our image matching process, an attribute vector is designed for each point in the image to include intensity, boundary and geometric moment invariants (GMIs). Hierarchical registration of two image sequences is achieved by using the most distinctive points for initial registration of two sequences and gradually adding less-distinctive points for refinement of registration. Experimental results on real data demonstrate good performance of the proposed method in registering cardiac images and estimating motions from cardiac image sequences.

1 Introduction

Heart attack, stroke and other cardiovascular diseases have been the leading cause of death since 1919 [1]. Importantly, cardiovascular disease kills more Americans than the next seven causes combined, including cancer. Cardiac imaging techniques were developed for providing qualitative and quantitative information about the morphology and function of the heart [2]. In particular, spatiotemporal imaging is a valuable tool for understanding cardiac motion and perfusion, and their relationship with the stages of disease. For assisting the diagnosis and treatment of cardiac diseases, automated methods are needed to analyze a large set of cardiac images and to extract clinically relevant parameters.

Cardiac motion estimation is an important step for quantification of the elasticity and contractility properties of the myocardium, related to the regional function of heart. In the setting of ischemic heart disease, localized regions with abnormal motion are related to the existence of infarcted or hibernating segments, the function of which has been affected by insufficient tissue microcirculation. Extensive research has shown that regional function measures, i.e., wall-thickening, strain, and torsion, may be earlier sub-clinical markers for examining left ventricular dysfunction and myocardial diseases, although ventricular mass, volume, and ejection fraction are considered as a standard for evaluating global function of heart [3].

J. Duncan and G. Gerig (Eds.): MICCAI 2005, LNCS 3750, pp. 902 – 910, 2005.

Many motion estimation methods have been developed for quantification of the deformation of regional myocardial tissue, and they fall into three categories. *The first category* of methods tracks invasive or noninvasive markers in cardiac images. Implanting invasive markers into the myocardium tends to influence the regional motion pattern of the wall muscle. Accordingly, MR tagging was developed to provide noninvasive mathematical markers inside the myocardium, which can deform with myocardial motion [4]. MR imaging and especially tagged MR are currently the reference modalities to estimate dense cardiac displacement fields with high spatial resolution. The deformation fields, as well as the derived motion parameters such as myocardial strain, can be determined with accuracy [5,6]. *The second category* of methods uses segmentation of the myocardial wall, followed by geometrical and mechanical modeling using active contours or surfaces to extract the displacement field and to perform the motion analysis [5,7,8]. For matching two contours or surfaces, curvatures are frequently used to establish initial sparse correspondences, followed by the dense correspondence interpolation in other myocardial positions by regularization or mechanical modeling [5,9]. *The third category* of methods uses energy-based warping or optical flow techniques to compute the displacement of the myocardium [10-12]. There also exists a method taking advantages of *both* the second *and* the third categories, i.e., tracking the cardiac boundaries by image curvatures [13]. Recently, 4D models are also proposed for cardiac registration and segmentation [14,15,16].

We propose a 4D deformable registration method for consistent motion estimation from 3D cardiac image sequences. The main premise of the proposed method is that, if suitable attribute vectors can be designed to serve as morphological signatures for distinctive points in a cardiac image sequence, then by hierarchically matching those attribute vectors along with appropriate regularization we can yield an accurate estimation of cardiac motion. Also, by integrating all temporal cardiac images into a single 4D registration framework, it is possible to estimate temporally consistent cardiac motion, since the constraints of temporal smoothness and consistency can be performed concurrently with the image registration procedure.

2 Method

2.1 Formulating Motion Estimation as Image Registration

Cardiac motion estimation is a problem of finding a transformation to describe how each point $\mathbf{x}$ in the heart moves over the time t. If each point $\mathbf{x}$ in the image at a certain time-point can be related to its corresponding position in the images at other time-points by an image registration method, cardiac motion can be immediately estimated. Thus, for estimating cardiac motion from end-diastole to other times in a periodic sequence of N 3D images, i.e., $I(\mathrm{x},t)=\{I_t, 1\le t\le N\}$ with I_1 as an end-diastolic image, we need only to register end-diastolic image I_1 to images at other time-points.

In order to use a 4D image registration for simultaneously estimating the motion from the end-diastolic image I_1 to all other time-points $\{I_t\}$, we generate a new 4D image, i.e., a new image sequence $T(\mathbf{x},t)=\{I_1,...,I_1\}$, which repeats the end-diastolic image I_1 as images at N different time-points (Fig 1). Thus, by registering the 4D images $I(\mathbf{x},t)$ to $T(\mathbf{x},t)$ via a spatial transformation $h(\mathbf{x},t)$, we can estimate motion for each point $\mathbf{x}$ in the end-diastolic I_1 to all other time-points in a cardiac sequence. Notably, the transformation $h(\mathbf{x},t)$ is restricted to 3D spatial deformations at the same time-point, since no temporal differences exist in the generated image sequence $T(\mathbf{x},t)$ and thus no need to consider temporal variations.

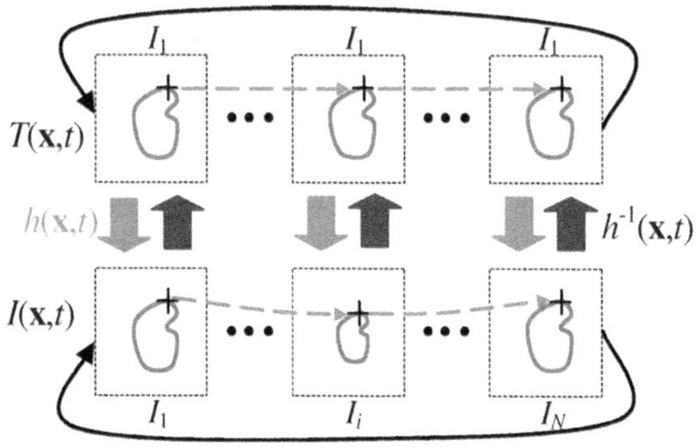

Fig. 1. Formulation of cardiac motion estimation as a 4D image registration problem

2.2 Attribute Vector

In order to register two image sequences accurately, we design for each point a morphological signature, i.e., an attribute vector $\mathbf{a}(\mathbf{x},t)$, for the purpose of minimizing the ambiguity in image matching and correspondence detection during the deformable registration procedure. Each attribute vector includes not only image intensity, but also boundary and Geometric Moment Invariants (GMIs) [17], all of which are computed from the 3D spatial images. For generated image sequence $T(\mathbf{x},t)$, we need only to compute attribute vectors for one 3D image and other identical images just take the same set of attribute vectors. GMIs are computed from different neighborhood sizes, and are concatenated into a long attribute vector. GMIs at a particular scale are calculated by placing a spherical neighborhood around each voxel and calculating a number of parameters that are invariant to rotation. The detailed definitions for attribute vectors and their similarities are the same as in [17].

2.3 Energy Function

The 4D image registration is completed by hierarchically matching attribute vectors in the two image sequences. To make the registration independent of which of the two sequences is treated as the template [18,17], the energy that evaluates the match of two image sequences should be symmetrically designed for two image sequences under registration. That means, both the forward transformation $h(\mathbf{x},t)$ and backward transformation $h^{-1}(\mathbf{x},t)$ should be evaluated in a single energy function, and forced to be consistent with each other.

To allow the registration algorithm to focus on different sets of image points adaptively during different stages of image registration, each point should have its own energy term and the whole energy function should be a weighted summation of all points' energy terms. Therefore, by hierarchically assigning those weights according to the distinctiveness of attribute vectors, i.e., assigning large weights for the energy terms of the points with distinctive attribute vectors (such as points with high curvatures along the left ventricular border) and zero weights for the energy terms of other points, we can focus on the most suitable points to actively drive the image registration. Effectively, this procedure approximates what would be a very high-dimensional (equal to the number of points in the two image sequences) cost function, by a significantly lower-dimensional function of only the active points. This latter function has few local minima, because it is a function of the coordinates of active points, for which relatively unambiguous matches can be found. Therefore, using this strategy, we can speed up the performance of image registration and also reduce the chances of local minima, which in part result from ambiguities in determining the matching pairs of points.

Also, the transformation $h(\mathbf{x},t)$ should be smooth spatially and temporally. Since the image sequences are periodic, i.e., the first image I_1 and the last image I_N are also temporal neighbors as indicated by solid arrows in Fig 1, the temporal smoothness constraint should be applied between the first and the last images in the periodic sequence. In this way, after completing 4D image registration, it is ensured that each point $\mathbf{x}$ moves smoothly along the temporal direction from the end-diastolic image I_1 to other time-points, and importantly moves back to its original position since the first images respectively in the two sequences are identical and transformation between them is thus forced to be exactly zero during the entire registration procedure.

By considering all of above-described requirements, the energy function that our 4D registration algorithm minimizes is defined as follows:

$$E = E_F + E_B + E_C + E_S,$$

where

$$E_F = \sum_{t=1}^{N} \sum_{\mathbf{x}} \omega_T(\mathbf{x},t) \left(\sum_{(\mathbf{z},\tau)\in n(\mathbf{x},t)} d(\mathbf{a}_T(\mathbf{z},\tau), \mathbf{a}_I(h(\mathbf{z},\tau))) \right)$$

$$E_B = \sum_{t=1}^{N} \sum_{\mathbf{x}} \omega_I(\mathbf{x},t) \left(\sum_{(\mathbf{z},\tau)\in n(\mathbf{x},t)} d(\mathbf{a}_T(h^{-1}(\mathbf{z},\tau)), \mathbf{a}_I(\mathbf{z},\tau)) \right)$$

$$E_C = \sum_{t=1}^{N} \sum_{\mathbf{x}} \varepsilon_T(\mathbf{x},t) \left(\sum_{(\mathbf{z},\tau)\in n(\mathbf{x},t),\ t\neq\tau} d(\mathbf{a}_I(h(\mathbf{z},t)), \mathbf{a}_I(h(\mathbf{z},\tau))) \right)$$

$$E_S = \alpha \cdot E_S^{\text{Spatial}} + \beta \cdot E_S^{\text{Temporal}}$$

There are four energy terms in this energy function. The first term E_F is defined on the forward transformation $h(\mathbf{x},t)$, and measures the similarity of attribute vectors between each point in the sequence $T(\mathbf{x},t)$ and its corresponding one in the sequence $I(\mathbf{x},t)$. The second energy term E_B is similar to the first term, while it is defined on the inverse transformation $h^{-1}(\mathbf{x},t)$ to make sure that each point in the sequence $I(\mathbf{x},t)$ also finds its best matching point in the sequence $T(\mathbf{x},t)$. Specifically, in the first energy term, the importance of each point $(\mathbf{x},t)$ in the image registration is determined by its corresponding parameter $\omega_T(\mathbf{x},t)$, which is designed to be proportional to the distinctiveness of this point's attribute vector $\mathbf{a}_T(\mathbf{x},t)$. The match for each point $(\mathbf{x},t)$ is evaluated in its 4D (3D spatial and 1D temporal) neighborhood $n(\mathbf{x},t)$, by integrating all differences between the attribute vector $\mathbf{a}_T(\mathbf{z},\tau)$ of every neighboring point $(\mathbf{z},\tau)$ and the attribute vector $\mathbf{a}_I(h(\mathbf{z},\tau))$ of the corresponding point $h(\mathbf{z},\tau)$ in the sequence $I(\mathbf{x},t)$. The difference of two attribute vectors $d(\cdot,\cdot)$ ranges from 0 to 1 [17]. The size of neighborhood $n(\mathbf{x},t)$ is large initially and decreases gradually with the progress of the deformation, thereby increasing robustness and accuracy of deformable registration.

The third energy term E_C measures the attribute-vector matching of corresponding points in different time-point images of the sequence $I(\mathbf{x},t)$. Notably, for each point $(\mathbf{x},t)$ in the sequence $T(\mathbf{x},t)$, its corresponding point in the sequence $I(\mathbf{x},t)$ is $h(\mathbf{x},t)$. Since the sequence $T(\mathbf{x},t)$ has identical images at different time-points, i.e., same end-diastolic image, points $\{(\mathbf{x},t), 1 \le t \le N\}$ are N corresponding points in the sequence $T(\mathbf{x},t)$; accordingly, N transformed points $\{h(\mathbf{x},t), 1 \le t \le N\}$ are the established correspondences in the sequence $I(\mathbf{x},t)$. In this way, we can require the attribute vector $\mathbf{a}_I(h(\mathbf{x},t))$ of a point $h(\mathbf{x},t)$ in the image $I(\mathbf{x},t)$ be similar to the attribute vector $\mathbf{a}_I(h(\mathbf{x},\tau))$ of its corresponding point $h(\mathbf{x},\tau)$ in the neighboring time-point image $I(\mathbf{x},\tau)$. This requirement is repeated for each position $(\mathbf{z},\tau)$ in a 4D neighborhood $n(\mathbf{x},t)$, and the total attribute-vector difference is weighted by $\varepsilon_T(\mathbf{x},t)$ to reflect the importance of a point $(\mathbf{x},t)$ in the sequence $T(\mathbf{x},t)$. The use of this energy term potentially makes it easier to solve the 4D registration problem, since the registration of cardiac images of neighboring time-points is relatively easier and thus it can provide a good initialization for 4D image registration by initially focusing only on energy terms of E_c and E_S.

The fourth energy term E_S is a smoothness constraint for the transformation $h(\mathbf{x},t)$. For convenience, we separate this smoothness constraint into two components, i.e., a spatial smoothness constraint E_S^{Spatial} and a temporal smoothness constraint E_S^{Temporal}, and these two constraints are linearly combined by their own weighting parameters α and β. For the *spatial* smoothness constraint, we use a Laplacian operator [17] to impose spatial smoothness. Notably, all images in the sequence $T(\mathbf{x},t)$ are identically the end-diastolic image. Thus, for registering two image sequences $T(\mathbf{x},t)$ and $I(\mathbf{x},t)$, we have to register the end-diastolic image with the end-systolic image by a large nonlinear transformation, which might be over-smoothed by the Laplacian operator. To avoid this over-smoothing problem, we use a multi-resolution framework, i.e., multi-level transformations, to implement our registration algorithm. Each resolution will estimate its own level of transformation based on the total transformations estimated from the previous resolutions, and the final transformation used to register two image sequences is the summation of all levels of transformations respectively estimated from all resolutions. Notably, the Laplacian operator is only allowed to smooth the current level of transformation being estimated in the *current resolution*, which effectively avoids smoothing the transformations estimated from the previous resolutions. As for the *temporal* smoothness constraint, we use a Gaussian filter to obtain an average transformation in a 1D temporal neighborhood around each point $(\mathbf{x},t)$, and force the transformation on this point $(\mathbf{x},t)$ to follow its average transformation in temporal neighborhood.

3 Results

The first experiment is designed to show the performance of the proposed method in estimating cardiac motion and deformation fields. There are 33 different time-point images in total, taken from a cardiac cycle of a normal volunteer, with the first time-point at end-diastole. Some selected cardiac images are shown in Fig 2(a). With the transformations established between end-diastolic frame and other frames, we can warp the end-diastolic image to any of the other frames, as shown in Fig 2(b), which becomes very similar to the corresponding frame, partly indicating the accuracy of our registration algorithm. Also, from Fig 2(c) that shows the deformation fields around the left ventricle at end-diastole to other time-points, we can observe that the deformation fields are very smooth in each time-point, and consistent over time.

The accuracy of motion and deformation estimation can also be reflected by the performance of the boundary tracking/labeling results provided by the 4D registration method. For example, if the boundaries of interest have been labeled in the end-diastolic image, we can warp these labeled boundaries to other time-points and obtain the boundary tracking/labeling results at other time-points. Fig 3 shows our semi-automatically labeled boundaries of interest as red contours in two images with black borders, respectively called long-axis and short-axis views at end-diastole. The tracking/labeling results at other time-points are shown by red contours in other images in Figs 3(a) and 3(b). Moreover, we can display the temporal views of short-axis lines to

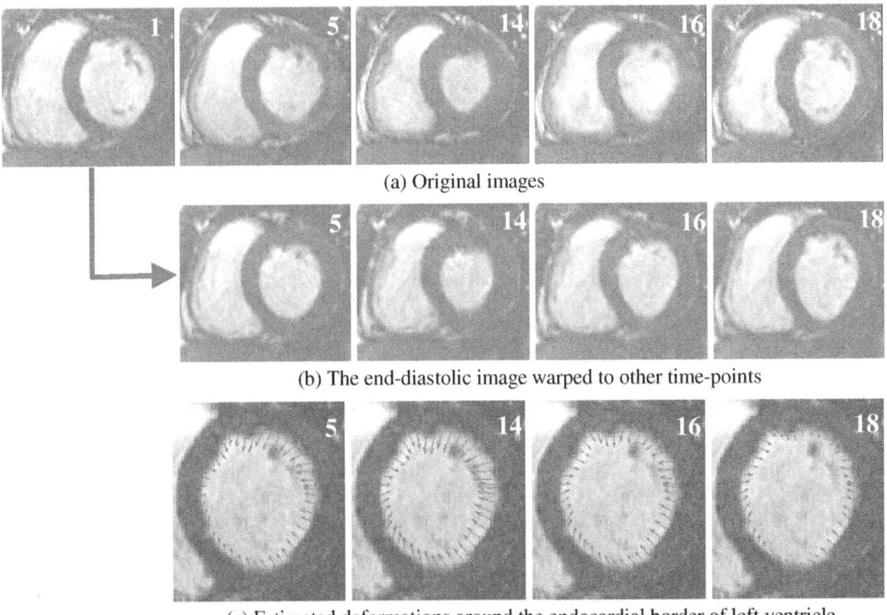

Fig. 2. Estimating deformations from end-diastole to other time-points. (a) 5 selected cardiac images, (b) the results of warping end-diastole to other time-points, (c) deformations around left ventricle, estimated from the end-diastolic image and cropped here for clear display.

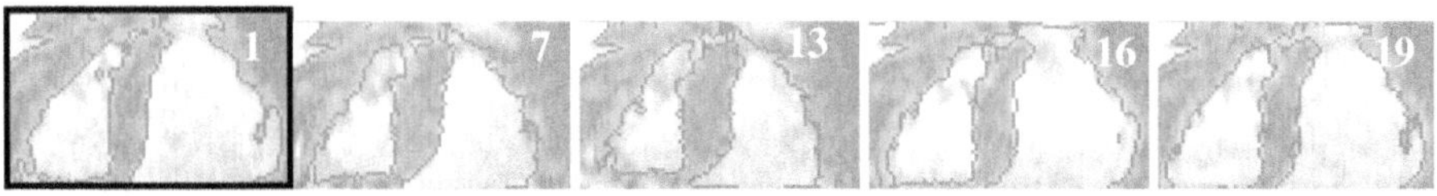

(a) Long-axis view

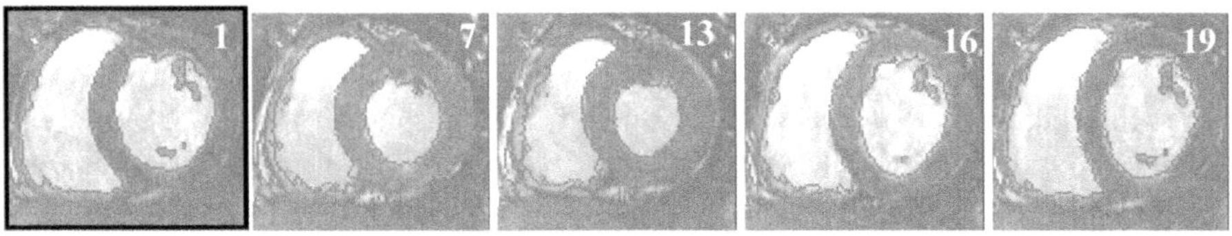

(b) Short-axis view

Fig. 3. Tracking/labeling the boundaries of interest in a cardiac sequence

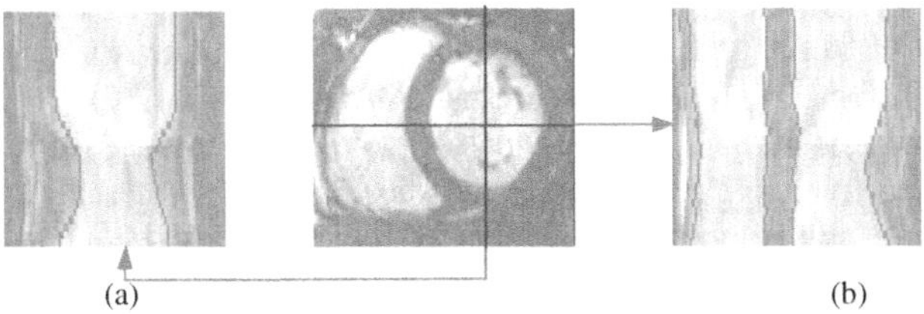

(a) (b)

Fig. 4. Tracking/labeling results in temporal views of two short-axis lines. The red colors indicate the labeling results on the left and right ventricular boundaries.

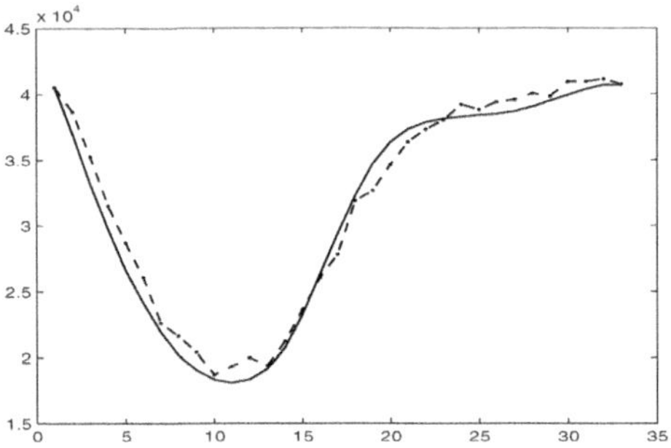

Fig. 5. Left ventricular volume of a selected subject, segmented by our algorithm (solid curve) and by hand (dotted curve) over all frames in a cardiac cycle

show the temporal tracking/labeling results. As shown in Fig 4, the proposed algorithm is able to track/label the two short-axis lines over time.

We also validated our method on a small dataset of 3D cardiac image sequences, by comparing the left-ventricular volumes obtained respectively by manual and automatic segmentations. Average volume error is 3.37%, with standard deviation 2.56%; and average volume overlap error is 7.04%, with standard deviation 3.28%. Correlation coefficient between manual and automatic segmentations is 0.99. Fig 5 shows the comparison on a selected subject over a whole cardiac cycle.

4 Conclusion

We have presented a 4D deformable registration method for estimation of cardiac motions from MR image sequences. The experimental results show consistent motion estimation by our method. This performance is achieved by formulating the cardiac motion estimation as a 4D image registration problem, which simultaneously considers all images of different time-points and further constrains the spatiotemporal smoothness of estimated motion fields concurrently with the image registration procedure. Also, compared to other motion estimation methods that use very simple features such as curvature of the left ventricular border, our method uses a rich set of attributes, including GMIs, to distinguish the corresponding points across different time-points, thereby maximally reducing ambiguity in image matching. Finally, by hierarchically selecting the active points to match, based on the distinctiveness degrees of their attribute vectors, our registration algorithm has more opportunities to produce a global solution for motion estimation.

Our 4D registration method for cardiac applications needs extensive validation in the future, by using both simulated and real data. For simulated data, we will validate the accuracy of our registration algorithm by directly comparing our estimated motions with ground-truth motions that we simulate. For real data, we will compare the algorithm-detected correspondences with the manually placed correspondences in the different frames, in order to validate the motions estimated.

References

1. American Heart Association, 1999. [Online]. Available: http://www.americanheart.org.
2. A.F. Frangi, W.J. Niessen, M.A. Viergever, "Three-Dimensional Modeling for Functional Analysis of Cardiac Images: A Review", *IEEE Trans. Med. Img.*, 20(1): 1-25, Jan 2001.
3. L. Pan, J. A. C. Lima, N.F. Osman, "Fast Tracking of Cardiac Motion Using 3D-HARP", *IPMI'2003*, pp. 611-622.
4. E.A. Zerhouni, D.M. Parish, W.J. Rogers, A. Yang, and E.P. Shapiro, "Human heart: tagging with MR imaging - a method for noninvasive assessment of myocardial motion", *Radiology*, 169(1): 59-63, 1988.
5. P. Shi, A. J. Sinusas, R.T. Constable, and J.S. Duncan, "Volumetric deformation analysis using mechanics-based data fusion: applications in cardiac motion recovery", *International Journal of Computer Vision*, vol. 35, no. 1, pp. 87–107, 1999.
6. J.L. Prince and E.R. McVeigh, "Motion Estimation From Tagged MR Image Sequences", *IEEE Trans. Medical Imaging*, 11(2):238-249, June 1992.
7. X. Papademetris, A.J. Sinusas, D.P. Dione and J.S. Duncan, "Estimation of 3D Left Ventricular Deformation from Echocardiography". *Medical Image Analysis*, 5:17-28, 2001.
8. Y. Wang, Yasheng Chen, and Amir A. Amini, "Fast LV motion estimation using subspace approximation", *IEEE Transactions on Medical Imaging*, Vol. 20, pp. 499-513, 2001.
9. McEachen, II, J.C., Nehorai, A., Duncan, J.S., "Multiframe Temporal Estimation of Cardiac Nonrigid Motion", *IEEE Trans. Image Processing*, 9(4):651-665, April 2000.
10. M.J. Ledesma-Carbayo, J. Kybic, M. Desco, A. Santos, M. Unser, "Cardiac Motion Analysis from Ultrasound Sequences Using Non-Rigid Registration", *MICCAI'01*, pp. 889-896, Utrecht, The Netherlands, October 14-17, 2001.

11. S. Song and R. Leahy, "Computation of 3D velocity fields from 3D cine CT images of a human heart", *IEEE Trans. Med. Imag*, Vol. MI-10, pp 295-306, Sep 1991.
12. R. Chandrashekara, D. Rueckert, R. Mohiaddin, "Cardiac Motion Tracking in Tagged MR Images Using a 4D B-spline Motion Model and Nonrigid Image Registration", *ISBI* 2004: 468-471.
13. N. Lin, X. Papademetris, J.S. Duncan, "Analysis of Left Ventricular Motion Using a General Robust Point Matching Algorithm", *MICCAI*, pp. 556-563, 2003.
14. D. Perperidis, R. Mohiaddin, D. Rueckert, "Spatio-Temporal Free-Form Registration of Cardiac MR Image Sequences", *MICCAI*, pp.911-919, 2004.
15. J. Montagnat, H. Delingette, "4D Deformable Models with temporal constraints: application to 4D cardiac image segmentation", *Med. Image Analysis*, 9(1):87-100, Feb 2005.
16. J. Declerck, J. Feldmar, and N. Ayache, "Definition of a 4D continuous planispheric transformation for the tracking and the analysis of left-ventricle motion," *Medical Image Analysis*, vol. 2, no. 2, pp. 197-213, 1998.
17. D. Shen, C. Davatzikos, "HAMMER: Hierarchical Attribute Matching Mechanism for Elastic Registration", *IEEE Trans. on Medical Imaging*, 21(11):1421-1439, Nov 2002.
18. G.E. Christensen and H.J. Johnson, "Consistent Image Registration", *IEEE TMI*, 20(7), 2001, pp. 568-582.

Multispectral MR to X-Ray Registration of Vertebral Bodies by Generating CT-Like Data

Everine B. van de Kraats[1], Graeme P. Penney[2], Theo van Walsum[3], and Wiro J. Niessen[3]

[1] Image Sciences Institute, University Medical Center Utrecht, The Netherlands
everine@isi.uu.nl
[2] Dept. of Computer Science, University College London
[3] Biomedical Imaging Group, Erasmus MC, University Medical Center Rotterdam

Abstract. A new method for MR to X-ray registration is presented. Based on training data, consisting of registered multispectral MR and CT data, a function is defined that maps multispectral MR data to CT-like data. For new subjects for which multispectral MR data have been acquired, the mapping function is used to generate a corresponding CT-like dataset. The CT-like image is subsequently used for registration to X-ray data, using gradient-based registration. Preliminary experiments indicate that MR to X-ray registration using this method is more accurate and has a larger capture range than gradient-based registration applied directly to MR data.

1 Introduction

In diagnosis and therapy planning, volumetric magnetic resonance (MR) images and computed tomography (CT) datasets are often used. However, in many interventions, intraoperative imaging is limited to 2D; in intravascular procedures and in orthopedic interventions, for example, usually only X-ray projection images are available. In order to relate these images to preoperative data so as to provide 3D insight during the intervention, 2D-3D registration is required.

Several 2D-3D registration methods have been reported in literature. Most algorithms have been designed for CT to X-ray registration. Since both these imaging modalities rely on X-rays, this can be exploited in designing 2D-3D registration methods. MR to X-ray registration is much more challenging, owing to the different underlying contrast mechanism. Several papers have appeared that address registration of magnetic resonance angiography (MRA) to digital subtraction angiography (DSA) images (among others [1, 2, 3]) and little has been done for MR to X-ray registration of bone [4, 5]. Rohlfing [4] compares intensity distributions along all rays to the corresponding pixel intensities of the real projection images by means of a probabilistic extension of histogram-based similarity measures, and Tomaževič [5] optimizes alignment of the gradients in 2D and 3D images. The main difficulty in MR to X-ray registration for bone applications is that bone tissue is not well depicted in MR images. This makes direct application of gradient-based methods, that rely on the bone edge or

J. Duncan and G. Gerig (Eds.): MICCAI 2005, LNCS 3750, pp. 911–918, 2005.

surface, or intensity-based methods, that assume a relation between the image intensities, difficult.

In this paper, a new approach for MR to X-ray registration is proposed. It is investigated whether multispectral MR data can be used to construct a CT-like image, containing sufficient information for registration to X-ray projection images. Hereto, a mapping function is defined, based on training data, which maps multispectral MR data obtained with a standardized acquisition protocol, into a simulated CT dataset. This is not straightforward, as MR imaging is not quantitative and MR intensities are affected by position dependent variations in coil and scanner sensitivity.

In the following, we first introduce the method to construct a CT-like image from multispectral MR data. Next, 2D-3D registration based on the constructed CT-like data is described and the datasets that are acquired for training and evaluation are specified. Subsequently, the experiments are described that were conducted to assess whether in controlled conditions MR intensities can be assumed to be similar across subjects for our purpose, or whether intensity remapping is required. Finally, the 2D-3D registration experiments with the CT-like datasets are detailed and the results are presented and discussed.

2 Method

2.1 Training Multispectral MR to CT Mapping

The general idea is to investigate whether a function can be proposed that maps multispectral MR datasets that are acquired with a standardized protocol to CT-like data. This mapping function can depend on MR image intensities, image features, and spatial information. For a proof of concept, we use a straightforward approach, in which only the image intensities of three different MR scans are used.

In the training stage, registered multispectral MR and CT datasets are used. From these datasets, a look-up table (LUT) is constructed relating MR-value triplets to CT values. Hereto, intensities in each of the MR images are divided in n bins each:

$$\mathrm{BIN_i}(\mathbf{x}) = \left\lfloor \frac{I_i(\mathbf{x}) - \min(I)}{(\max(I) - \min(I))/n} \right\rfloor , \tag{1}$$

where

$$\begin{aligned} I_i(\mathbf{x}) &= \text{intensity of voxel } \mathbf{x} \text{ in MR image } i, \\ \min(I)/\max(I) &= \text{minimum/maximum intensity over all MR images.} \end{aligned}$$

In this preliminary experiment, 64 evenly distributed bins were used. A region of interest is determined containing the specific anatomy that is trained. In our case this is a specific level of the spine (or several spine levels).

The simulated CT value in a certain region corresponding to a specific MR-value triplet, is determined using a mapping function f:

$$\mathrm{LUT}(u, v, w) = f\left(\{\mathrm{CT}(\mathbf{x}) | \mathbf{x} \in S^r_{u,v,w}\}\right) , \tag{2}$$

where

$S^r_{u,v,w}$ = set of voxels $\mathbf{x}$ in region r where
$\text{BIN}_1(\mathbf{x}) = u, \text{BIN}_2(\mathbf{x}) = v$ and $\text{BIN}_3(\mathbf{x}) = w$,
$f : \mathbb{Z}^q \rightarrow \mathbb{R}$ is function that maps the set of CT values corresponding to a certain MR-value triplet into a single estimated CT value.

We chose the median function for f. The mapping functions can easily be extended, *e.g.* by incorporating feature information, information over larger neighborhoods, or spatial information (*e.g.* an atlas). In addition, binning techniques more effective than uniform binning may be useful.

2.2 2D-3D Registration Based on a CT-Like Dataset

For a new subject for which a multispectral MR dataset is available, a trained mapping function as defined in the previous section can be used to generate a CT-like image. This image is subsequently used in 2D-3D registration. Since the CT-like image consists of values that are similar to CT values, intensity-based registration methods as well as feature-based or gradient-based registration methods can be applied.

In this preliminary experiment, we considered a gradient-based 2D-3D registration approach [5], which was previously used for MR to X-ray registration of the spine. Registration to two X-ray images was considered, as one X-ray image is not sufficient to assess the position in three dimensions.

For validation of the 2D-3D registration we applied the framework that was introduced in [6]. Using an accurate reference standard the performance of the method was evaluated by reporting the capture range and final mean TRE (mTRE) of successful registrations within the capture range.

3 Experiments

3.1 Data Acquisition

First, multispectral MR datasets of six healthy subjects (one male and five females with ages ranging from 21 to 54) were acquired using a standardized protocol (see Table 1) with a 1.5-T MR scanner (GyroScan NT, Philips Medical Systems, Best, The Netherlands). Two of the subjects were scanned in two MR scanners, with the same specifications but at different locations, to assess inter-scanner variability. Histograms of all MR images of the same anatomic regions were compared qualitatively, to determine whether intensity remapping of the MR data would be required for training the LUT and applying it to new cases.

Second, multispectral MR (using the same protocol as above), CT, and 3DRX datasets with corresponding X-ray images were acquired from two fresh post-mortem subjects (females aged 102 and 77). CT images were acquired on a clinical multi-slice CT scanner (MX8000, IDT16, Philips Medical Systems). CT and MR datasets were registered using maximization of mutual information.

Table 1. Specifications of the acquired scans

Protocol name	Specifications
Balanced Fast Field Echo (BFFE)	TR 5.29, TE 1.80, NA 8.0, slice thickness 3.0 mm, slice spacing 1.5 mm, pixel spacing 0.5/0.5 mm, flip angle 50°, 512 × 512 × 70
Balanced Fast Field Echo with water selection (BFFE_WS)	TR 6.21, TE 3.10, NA 8.0, slice thickness 3.0 mm, slice spacing 1.5 mm, pixel spacing 0.5/0.5 mm, flip angle 50°, 512 × 512 × 70
Balanced Fast Field Echo with fat selection (BFFE_FS)	TR 6.21, TE 3.10, NA 8.0, slice thickness 3.0 mm, slice spacing 1.5 mm, pixel spacing 0.5/0.5 mm, flip angle 50°, 512 × 512 × 70
CT	$0.35 \times 0.35 \times 0.5\,\text{mm}^3$, slice thickness 1.0 mm
3DRX	$0.43 \times 0.43 \times 0.43\,\text{mm}^3$, 256 × 256 × 256
200 X-ray projections	$0.44 \times 0.44\,\text{mm}^2$, 512 × 512, 25 cm II

These registered datasets were used to train the LUT. 3DRX data and X-ray images were acquired using a 3D C-arm system (Integris BV5000, Philips Medical Systems). Table 1 describes the details of the acquired scans.

The geometrical relation between X-ray images and the 3DRX volume was known, because the 3DRX volume is reconstructed from the X-ray projections. This serves as a reference standard for 3DRX to X-ray registration, as proposed by van de Kraats *et al.* [6]. The CT and MR data were registered to the 3DRX data using maximization of mutual information. As a consequence, the relationship between the X-ray images and the CT and MR data was indirectly derived, which provided the reference standard for MR to X-ray and CT to X-ray registration.

3.2 MR Histogram Inspection

For the six healthy subjects it was investigated whether intensity remapping was required to relate image intensities between subjects. We also qualitatively assessed the relation between MR intensities of healthy subjects and postmortem subjects.

The comparison of MR intensities (across different scans or patients) was performed using the MR intensities that result directly from the Fourier transformed signal intensities, to circumvent the linear transformations that are normally applied in postprocessing steps by MR scanners. We determined regions of interest around the vertebra for each of the subjects and for all the scans. Since the region of interest affects the histogram, it was crucial that similar regions of interest were chosen. In this experiment, a narrow region of interest around vertebral body L3 was taken.

The resulting histograms indicated that the MR intensities were indeed comparable and that age, sex, or scanner did not influence the histograms profoundly. The peaks in the histograms per MR protocol occurred at similar intensities. For the BFFE scan the mean and standard deviation of the position of the peaks was

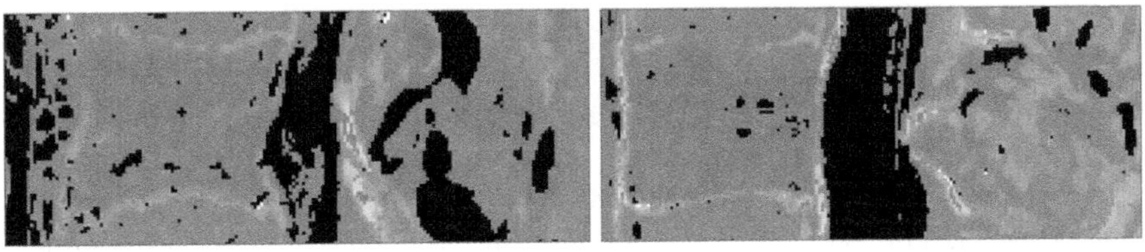

Fig. 1. Sagittal plane through center of vertebra and spinal canal of CT-like images of two healthy subjects constructed using a LUT trained on a postmortem subject (SA-L1)

19.1±3.5, for BFFE_WS this was 47.6±4.9, and for BFFE_FS this was 7.7±1.9. Thus it was expected that application of a LUT trained on any one of these multispectral MR datasets would result in similar CT-like images. A logical step was to verify this by using the trained LUT obtained from the postmortem scans. However, from a similar analysis, it seemed that the histograms of fresh postmortem subjects did not correspond well with healthy subjects. Since the availability of MR, CT, and 3DRX data of the same patient is rare, we had to rely on the (fresh) postmortem data to relate MR and CT intensities. To overcome the intensity correspondence problem, we linearly rescaled the images of the postmortem subjects in such a way that the histogram peaks roughly overlapped with the peaks of the healthy subjects before these were used to train the LUT. This was done in an ad hoc manner; for better histogram overlap more sophisticated techniques can be used. The resulting CT-like images, for which one slice is shown for two subjects in Figure 1, could not be evaluated quantitatively as corresponding CT and 3DRX scans were not acquired of volunteers. The dark areas in the images correspond to locations for which no or insufficient data was present in the training set. These locations can be filled, *e.g.* using gray value dilation or inpainting. The dark areas mainly occur in the spinal canal. This is possibly due to differences between in vivo and in vitro spinal fluid. However, the resulting CT-like images look promising as edges are present at positions where a bone edge is expected.

3.3 2D-3D Registration

Experiments were conducted to determine the performance of 2D-3D registration using the simulated CT-like datasets in the postmortem study. An important aspect was to decide on what dataset and region to train the LUT. Whereas we hypothesize that the LUT will improve with a larger training set, in our first experiments only two datasets were available: a postmortem female aged 102 (SA) and a postmortem female aged 77 (SB). These differred substantially in quality as SA had a very deformed spine with hardly any disc spaces and a high degree of osteoporosis. We therefore did not use this dataset for training, but for evaluation; vertebra L3 (SA-L3) was used for this purpose. To determine the performance as a function of the training data, we trained on SA-L3, SB-L3, SB-L1 and SB-L1,L3.

To assess the performance of 2D-3D registration using the CT-like image in comparison to registrations using 3DRX, CT, and original MR data, we also evaluated the performance of 2D-3D registration using corresponding regions of interest in the 3DRX, CT, resampled CT image ('trans CT', which resembles the resolution of the MR images, $1.5 \times 0.5 \times 0.5\,\mathrm{mm}^3$), and the original MR scan (BFFE). For each of the corresponding vertebra volumes, the same two fluoroscopic images were used for registration. These were approximately at a 90° angle.

For all the datasets, 200 registrations were performed, using the same offsets from the gold standard, which ranged from 0 to 10 mm mTRE with 20 starting positions per 1 mm. The 100 and 90 percent capture ranges, where success was defined as an error smaller than 2 mm mTRE, are reported together with the mean accuracy for successful registrations.

4 Results and Discussion

Figure 2 shows corresponding slices of MR BFFE data, transformed CT data (registered to MR BFFE data), and four generated CT-like datasets (acquired using LUTs trained on different vertebrae) for vertebra L3 of subject A. Whereas it can clearly be seen that when training on the vertebra itself, the generated CT-like image resembles the CT scan best (Figure 2c), in all generated CT-like data edges are present at bone surfaces. There were only a few nontrained MR-intensity triplets (holes in the CT-like datasets), and we thus expect that the unfilled locations have minimal effect on the registration result.

Table 2 lists the 2D-3D registration results. The 100% and 90% capture ranges (where success was defined as a final mTRE less than 2 mm) are reported along with the average error of successful registrations within these ranges. As expected, registration of the 3DRX image to the two X-ray images had the highest 100%/90% capture range (5/6 mm start mTRE) with an mTRE of 0.30 mm, followed by registration of the original CT image to the two X-ray images (4/5 mm

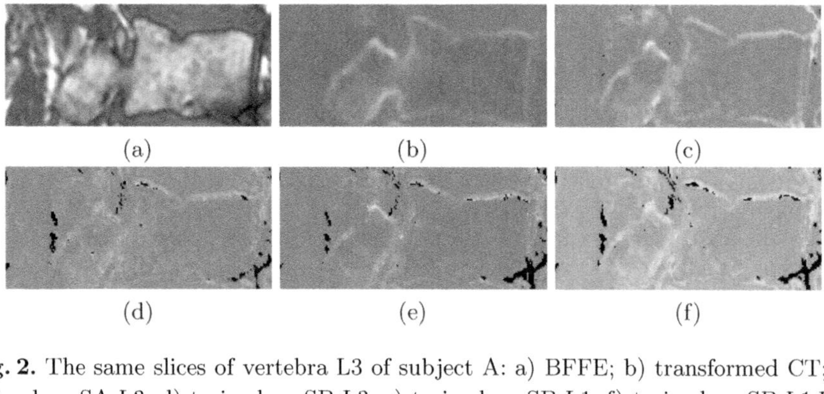

Fig. 2. The same slices of vertebra L3 of subject A: a) BFFE; b) transformed CT; c) trained on SA-L3; d) trained on SB-L3; e) trained on SB-L1; f) trained on SB-L1,L3

Table 2. The 100% and 90% capture ranges and accuracy of successful (< 2 mm mTRE) registrations within the capture range for 2D-3D registration using a gradient-based method on 3DRX data, CT data, transformed/resampled CT data ('trans CT'), and four generated CT-like datasets of vertebra L3 of subject A.

	Gradient-based method		
	100% (mm)	90% (mm)	Err. (mm)
3DRX	5	6	0.30
CT	4	5	0.22
trans CT	3	5	0.34
train SA-L3	3	5	0.46
train SB-L3	2	4	0.55
train SB-L1	3	4	0.45
train SB-L1/L3	3	4	0.61
MR (BFFE)	1	1	0.81

with mTRE of 0.22 mm). Registration of the transformed and resampled CT image, *i.e.* the image used when training the LUT, had a slightly smaller capture range (3/5 mm with mTRE of 0.34 mm). Registration performance for the four generated CT-like datasets (approximately 3/4 mm and mTRE of 0.52 mm) was almost equal to the performance of the transformed CT image. As it can be assumed that the results obtained for the transformed CT image are the best attainable for the CT-like images, since the LUT is trained from the transformed CT image, this indicates the potential of the method. Furthermore, it seemed that the training set used to define the mapping function from multispectral MR intensities to CT values did not have a large influence on the result. The performance of MR to X-ray registration using the CT-like data was much better than when using gradient-based registration directly (after windowing and optimizing parameters for relevant point extraction) on MR data (1/1 mm and mTRE of 0.81 mm) and better than the results reported in literature [5]. This may be explained by numerous points extracted on soft-tissue boundaries in the original MR dataset which introduce boundaries that are not clearly visible in the X-ray images and thus make gradient-based registration applied directly on MR data difficult.

The current study has several limitations. First, we used a limited number of training and evaluation data. Second, the quality of the data was limited, and therefore we should be cautious in generalizing the results. It is subject of further investigation whether the result will be the same when a larger dataset is used and when LUTs are trained and evaluated on more subjects. Moreover, although it is difficult to acquire training data in vivo, this may be required for in vivo application, as we observed considerable differences in the histograms of MR data between healthy subjects and in the postmortem scans.

Furthermore, in our experiment a simple mapping function, *i.e.* the median, was used for generating the LUT. Other mappings of CT intensities can be investigated as well. Possible extensions are to take neighborhood information or other spatial information into account, or using extra features, *e.g.* gradient and texture information or intensity profiles. Another option is to use the variance of the occurring CT values for a specific MR intensity triplet, for example to determine the confidence when generating the CT-like image. It can also be investigated if less than three MR images or other MR protocols can be used to achieve similar results.

Finally, the performance of other types of 2D-3D registration methods, such as feature-based and intensity-based methods, using generated CT-like data should be investigated. By using a CT-like image, intensity-based methods can potentially overcome their current limitation in registering MR data to X-ray images.

5 Conclusions

A method has been presented to simulate CT data from multispectral MR data so as to allow indirect MR to X-ray registration. In preliminary experiments, it was shown that gradient-based registration of the CT-like data to X-ray data yielded results that approximated the accuracy of original transformed CT data to X-ray registration, and that it outperformed registration directly on the MR data.

Acknowledgment. We thank the Netherlands Organization for Scientific Research (NWO) for providing a travel grant.

References

1. Hipwell, J., Penney, G., McLaughlin, R., et al.: Intensity-based 2-D–3-D registration of cerebral angiograms. IEEE Trans. Med. Imag. **22** (2003) 1417–1426
2. Feldmar, J., Malandain, G., Ayache, N., et al.: Matching 3D MR angiography data and 2D X-ray angiograms. In: Proceedings of CVRMed-MRCAS '97. (1997) 129–138
3. Liu, A., Bulitt, E., Pizer, S.: 3D/2D registration via skeletal near projective invariance in tubular objects. In: MICCAI. (1998) 952–963
4. Rohlfing, T., Maurer Jr., C.: A novel image similarity measure for registration of 3-D MR images and X-ray projection images. In: MICCAI, Part 2. (2002) 469–476
5. Tomaževič, D., Likar, B., Slivnik, T., et al.: 3-D/2-D registration of CT and MR to X-ray images. IEEE Trans. Med. Imag. **22** (2003) 1407–1416
6. van de Kraats, E., Penney, G., Tomaževič, D., et al.: Standardized evaluation of 2D-3D registration. In: MICCAI, Part 1. (2004) 574–581

Articulated Rigid Registration for Serial Lower-Limb Mouse Imaging

Xenophon Papademetris[1,2], Donald P. Dione[3], Lawrence W. Dobrucki[3], Lawrence H. Staib[1,2], and Albert J. Sinusas[2,3]

[1] Departments of Biomedical Engineering
[2] Diag. Radiology
[3] Medicine, Yale University New Haven, CT 06520-8042
xenophon.papademetris@yale.edu

Abstract. This paper describes a new piecewise rotational transformation model for capturing the articulation of joints such as the hip and the knee. While a simple piecewise rigid model can be applied, such models suffer from discontinuities at the motion boundary leading to both folding and stretching. Our model avoids both of these problems by constructing a provably continuous transformation along the motion interface. We embed this transformation model within the robust point matching framework and demonstrate its successful application to both synthetic data, and to serial x-ray CT mouse images. In the later case, our model captures the articulation of six joints, namely the left/right hip, the left/right knee and the left/right ankle. In the future such a model could be used to initialize non-rigid registrations of images from different subjects, as well as, be embedded in intensity-based and integrated registration algorithms. It could also be applied to human data in cases where articulated motion is an issue (e.g. image guided prostate radiotherapy, lower extremity CT angiography).

1 Introduction

While non rigid image registration has been extensively applied to brain image analysis [7,2,4,5] (e.g. for comparing shape and function between individuals or groups, developing probabilistic models and atlases, and measuring change within an individual) it has not been extensively applied to other parts of the body to date. Unlike the brain which is a single organ enclosed in the skull with no articulated joints, the abdominal/pelvic cavities and especially regions close to limb joints contain many organs/glands whose relative position/orientation vary substantially from subject to subject. This is of particular importance for non-rigid registration, as the process typically relies on a good initialization often performed by estimating the global linear transformations between the two images. Given the relatively high degrees of freedom (DOF) available in most non-rigid registration methods, the final estimate of the nonlinear transformation is critically dependent on this early step to bring the nonlinear optimization process to a position to enable it to converge to the appropriate local minimum. While the estimation of the initial linear transformation is relatively straightforward in the case of brain images (using both intensity and/or feature methods),

J. Duncan and G. Gerig (Eds.): MICCAI 2005, LNCS 3750, pp. 919–926, 2005.

such simple transformations are inadequate (even for the purpose of initialization) in regions where there are articulated joints. Here the relative orientation of, for example, the proximal and the distal leg is highly dependent on the state of the knee joint and can vary substantially between subjects even when extra care is taken to implement a standardized imaging protocol. This is particularly true in our application of serial hybrid 3-dimensional imaging for the purpose of quantifying the remodeling of existing collateral arteries (arteriogenesis) and increased microvascular density (angiogenesis) associated with peripheral arterial disease of the lower extremities. In this application, x-ray computed tomographic (CT) angiography is used to evaluate lower extremity arteriogenesis, while registered single photon emission computed tomographic (SPECT) images provide a quantitative index of changes in either tissue perfusion or critical radio-labeled molecular markers of the underlying biological process.

While the problem of modeling articulated joints has received extensive interest in computer graphics, it has received little attention to our knowledge, in the medical image analysis literature, the recent early work of Martin-Fernandez et al. [6] being one exception. In their work, the problem of estimating 2D hand motion tracking is modeled using a weighted sum of multiple rigid transformation. While this model is adequate for simple motions, it does not explicitly address the key problem of folding (i.e. ensuring that the resulting transformation remains invertible). A more interesting set of work is the polyrigid/polyaffine model proposed by Arsigny et al. [1], where an elegant method for constructing an invertible transformation as a weighted sum of piecewise rigid/affine transformations is described. The weights are obtained by the solution of an ordinary differential equation. Arsigny et al. present 2D results in the matching of histochemical slices to anatomical data, and they note that this model would also be applicable to articulated registration issues such as the one of concern in this paper. A weakness of their method is the fact that there is no closed form solution to the resulting transformation, rather a numerical solution of the differential equation is needed to generate the final transformation, which makes the model highly computationally intensive.

In this work, we present both a theoretical model with a closed form solution for modeling the piecewise rotational motion of both the hip, the knee, and the ankle joints in mice (and by extension man) in a manner that ensures that the overall map is smooth and invertible and apply this model to the problem of registration of serial CT images acquired from mouse models of angiogenesis. The transformation model is used within the robust point matching registration framework to estimate the piecewise rigid transformation, which can then be used as the initialization to a full nonrigid registration.

2 Methods

2.1 A Model for Non-folding Piecewise Rotations

Our model for computing a non-folding mapping appropriately blends piecewise rotations making the following assumptions: (i) at each joint the motion is a rotation about a rotation axis passing through the joint origin (e.g. the knee). (ii) The two "limbs" linked at the joint can be described without loss of generality as a stationary limb and a moving limb. (iii) A surface can be found which separates the two limbs in the original position (i.e. in the reference image); we label this the joint or motion interface, and (iv) both the joint origin and the axis of rotation are restricted to lie outside the moving limb – this last assumption effectively reduces each joint to having only two degrees of freedom.

Given these assumptions, we now describe our blending piecewise rotation model of articulated joints which provably results in no folding (i.e. the determinant of the Jacobian matrix of the resulting transformations is positive everywhere [2]). Consider the example shown in Figure 1. Here the top part of the cylinder (the moving limb) rotates counter-clockwise, with angle q degrees, with respect to the bottom part of the cylinder (the stationary limb). The axis of rotation shown in yellow (coming out of the paper). If a "naive" piecewise rotation model is used, we observe (Figure 1 middle-top) both folding of the surface where the moving limb moves towards the interface (near point A) and stretching where it moves away from the interface (near point B). Our proposed model (Figure 1 middle-bottom) corrects for both of these problems by appropriately manipulating the angle of rotation. The key to our model is the fact that any complicated 3D rotation can be described as a single rotation about a single axis (the so-called angle-axis representation). Without loss of generality, let the rotation axis pass through the local coordinate origin and be aligned to the $z-$axis. (This can easily be achieved by a global rigid transformation). We next employ a cylindrical polar coordinate system (r, z, θ), where r is the radial distance from the origin and θ the rotational coordinate. In this polar coordinate system, any rotation about the $z-$axis can be expressed as a translation in θ . For example the "naive" piecewise rotation model can be written as:

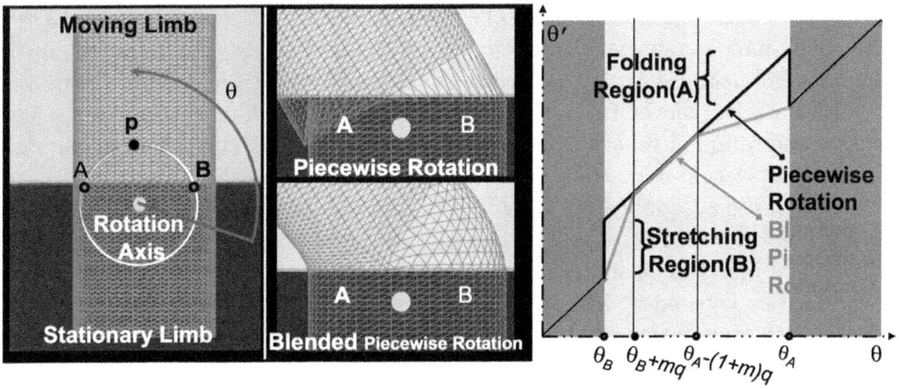

Fig. 1. The blending piecewise model. Left: A simple case of articulated motion where the top part of a cylinder is rotating independently of the bottom part. **Middle Top:** Simple piecewise rotation model exhibiting folding (A) and stretching (B) behavior. **Middle Bottom:** Proposed blending piecewise rotation model which is free from folding and stretching. **Right:** Following transformation to a cylindrical polar coordinate system we plot the original (θ) vs the transformed (θ') polar angle for both the piecewise and the blending models. Note that the blending piecewise rotation model results in an continuous invertible mapping unlike the "naive" piecewise rotation model.

$$\text{Static Limb: } (r, z, \theta) \mapsto (r, z, \theta), \quad \text{Moving Limb: } (r, z, \theta) \mapsto (r, z, \theta + q) \tag{1}$$

$$\text{Static Limb: } \quad \theta' = \theta, \quad \text{Moving Limb: } \theta' = \theta + q \tag{2}$$

where in equation 2 we explicitly reduce this mapping to a one dimensional problem of finding $\theta \mapsto \theta'$, since (r, z) remain constant. Using the same notation, we express our blended piecewise rotation model as:

$$\theta' = \theta + q\phi_{r,z}(\theta) \tag{3}$$

where $\phi_{r,z}(\theta)$ is the to-be constructed continuous function on each circle of constant r, z. Since there is no change in the r, z coordinates, the key to constructing an invertible, continuous mapping is reduced to simply constructing an invertible continuous function $\phi_{r,z}(\theta)$ which is constrained to be close to 0 in the static limb and 1 in the moving limb so as to adhere as much as possible to the overall piecewise rotation. One possible solution to this is demonstrated in figure 1(right) where we plot θ against θ'. For a given circle at constant (r, z), let A and B be the points where the circle intersects the motion interface, with angular coordinates θ_A and θ_B respectively. Our blending model sets $\phi_{r,z} = 0$ in the static limb, and performs all blending in the moving limb – this enables easy hierarchical updating of multi-joint structures such as the leg. Next, in the moving limb, in the region immediately after B (i.e. $\theta_B < \theta < \theta_B + mq$, where $m > 0$ is the dimensionless "extent of blending" parameter typically set to 1) $\phi_{r,z}$ ramps up from zero to one to correct for the stretching problem. In the region $\theta_B + mq < \theta < \theta_A - (1 + m)q$ we have $\phi = 1$ resulting in unconstrained rotation i.e. $\theta' = \theta + q$. Finally as we approach the moving interface $\theta_A - (1+m)q < \theta < \theta_A$ we ramp down the rotation angle back to zero to ensure continuity at the interface point A. This map is both continuous and invertible; a cubic blending method can also be used to make it C^1 continuous if desired. An easily handled special case occurs when the part of the circle that lies in the moving limb is too short (in an angular sense) such that $\theta_A - (1+m)q < \theta_B + mq$. In this case $\phi_{r,z}$ never reaches one and there is no middle portion to the line, rather the ramping functions intersect. We apply folding correction to the right of the intersection and stretching correction to the left.

The practical application of this blending model consists of finding for any given point $p = (r, z, \theta)$, the θ-coordinates of the appropriate intersection points A, B via a bisection search strategy along the circle centered at $(0, z)$. Potential singularities can exist close to the rotation axis $r = 0$; these are avoided by design (see assumption iv above) by ensuring that the rotation axis lies outside the moving limb. A sufficient condition for this is to ensure that the rotation axis lies on a plane (*the local xy-plane*) that is outside the moving limb – this effectively reduces each joint to having only two degrees of freedom.

2.2 Practical Implementation

First, a label image is constructed where each voxel contains a value equal to the index of each limb (i.e. air=-1, main body=0, left hip=1, left knee=2 etc.). Next, for each joint we identify both the position of the joint and a local *xy-plane* that stays completely outside the moving limb on which the rotation axis for the joint is constrained to lie. The joint or motion interface is set to be, for each joint, the bounding surface of the static limb. In the case of the left knee joint, for example, the motion interface is the boundary of the static "limb" which is the union of the main body trunk, the whole right leg, and the left proximal leg, whereas the moving "limb" is the union of the left distal leg and the left foot. The overall transformation model consists in applying a series of transformation in a hierarchical manner, i.e. in the case of a point x in the left foot the overall mapping is:

$$x' = T_{\text{global}} . T_{\text{left-hip}} . T_{\text{left-knee}} . T_{\text{left-ankle}}(x) \tag{4}$$

Here T_{global} is an arbitrary global transformation, whereas $T_{\text{left-hip}}$, $T_{\text{left-knee}}$, $T_{\text{left-ankle}}$ are modeled using our blended piecewise rotation model described above. As an example, the 2-DOF (α, q) transformation $T_{\text{left-ankle}}$ is applied to x as follows:

1. Transform the global coordinate system to the local coordinate system such that the joint origin for the ankle is mapped to the coordinate origin, and the normal of the local *xy-plane* to the local z-axis. (Transformation T_1).
2. Initialize the the rotation axis to be the local x-axis and rotate it by an angle α about the local z-axis to obtain the final rotation axis $\mathbf{l}$.
3. Convert to a cylindrical polar system such that $\mathbf{l}$ maps to the cylindrical polar z-axis. (Transformation T_2).
4. For any point (r, z, θ) compute $\phi_{r,z}(,\theta)$ and map to $(r, z, \theta + q\phi_{r,z}(\theta))$, using the construction discussed in Section 2.1, below equation 3.
5. Transform by $T_1^{-1}.T_2^{-1}$ to get back to the original coordinate system.
6. Consecutively apply $T_{\text{left-knee}}$, $T_{\text{left-hip}}$ and T_{global} in order to get the final transformed point x'.

2.3 Articulated Rigid Robust Point Matching

We embed this new transformation model within the robust point matching (RPM) framework [3]. The registration procedure consists of two alternative steps: (i) the correspondence estimation step – which allows for the handling of outliers both in the reference and target point sets and (ii) the transformation estimation step. The correspondence estimation step is identical to the standard RPM implementation [3] and will not be described here. Given two sets of corresponding points we estimate the $N = 6+2n$ parameters of the articulated model, where n is the number of the articulated joints, by optimizing a functional of the form:

$$G = \underset{g}{\arg\min} \sum_i w_i (g(X_i) - V_i)^2 \tag{5}$$

where g is the articulated rigid transformation, X_i is point i in the reference point set, V_i is its corresponding point in the target data set and the weights w_i are set to give less weight to points termed as outliers by the correspondence process. This functional is optimized using a Conjugate Gradient method.

3 Results

3.1 Synthetic Data

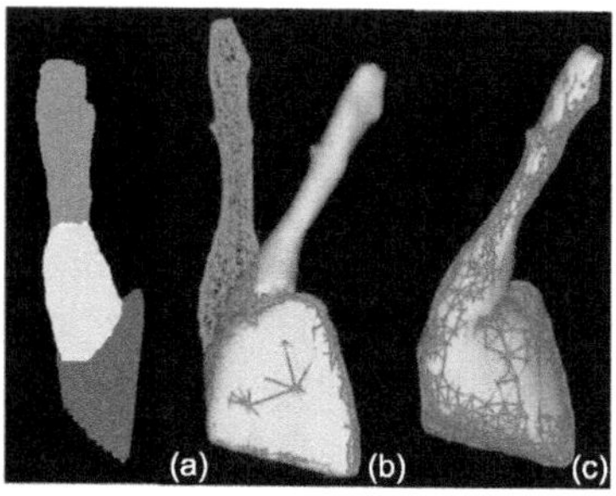

Fig. 2. A Synthetic Mouse Leg Model

To test both the utility of the model as well as the convergence of our registration algorithm, we constructed a three piece (two-joint) synthetic model using the left leg from a real micro-CT mouse image, as shown in Figure 2. The leg is divided into three parts (proximal leg or femur, distal leg and foot) as shown in Figure 2(left) and has two joints (knee,ankle).

A simulated motion of this model using our articulated blended transformation is shown in Figure 2(b) where the original model is shown in red and the transformed model in green. The result of the registration algorithm which consists of the RPM matching strategy and the hierarchical articulated rigid model presented in this paper is shown in Figure 2(c). Note that for this example, the joint rotations where of the order of 25° and the error in the parameter estimates was less than 10% for all parameters.

3.2 Serial Mouse Image Registration

Imaging: We tested the initial utility of our algorithm on three different pairs of mouse micro CT images (resolution $100 \times 100 \times 100\mu m^3$. In two of the pairs the images were acquired 3 weeks apart as part of an angiogenesis imaging protocol, whereas the third case was specially planned to test this algorithm. In this last example, the mouse was positioned in the scanner, imaged and then removed from the scanner. Then the technologist attempted to position the mouse approximately in the same position as in the first acquisition, thereby simulating the actual situation in the case of serial imaging. The images consisted of the lower half of the mouse (roughly from below the lungs to the feet). All figures are based on this last example.

Articulated Model Construction: Prior to registration, the articulated model with six joints was constructed which is shown in Figure 3 (left). The mouse was divided into seven parts namely the main body trunk, the left and right femurs (or proximal legs), the left and right distal legs and the left and right feet, by manually partitioning the image by interactively placing cutting planes to separate the parts. Whereas a single plane was sufficient for the knee and ankle joints, two planes where needed to delineate the boundary between the hips and the main body. In addition, at each joint, the joint origin was located (at the intersection of the bone and the cutting planes) and the local x- and y-axes were defined such that the local x-axis was roughly aligned to the most likely rotation axis. The joint origin was subsequently translated along the local z-axis away from the cutting plane to ensure that the local xy-plane did not intersect the moving limb at each joint, as required by our model.

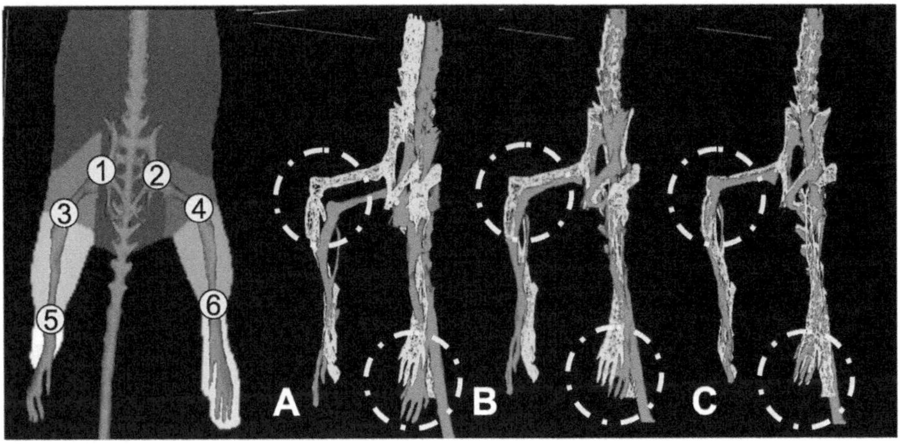

Fig. 3. Left: Schematic of the articulated model with the six joints overlaid on the mouse bony anatomy. (1,2=left/right hip, 3,4=left/right knee and 5,6=left/right ankle) **Right 3 views:** (A) starting position for the registration (red=reference, green=target), (B) result after global rigid alignment, (C) result after articulated rigid alignment. For this result we used points extracted from the bone surfaces of the two images. In particular note the improvement in the registration when using the articulated model at the knee (highlighted by a white circle) and the foot (yellow circle).

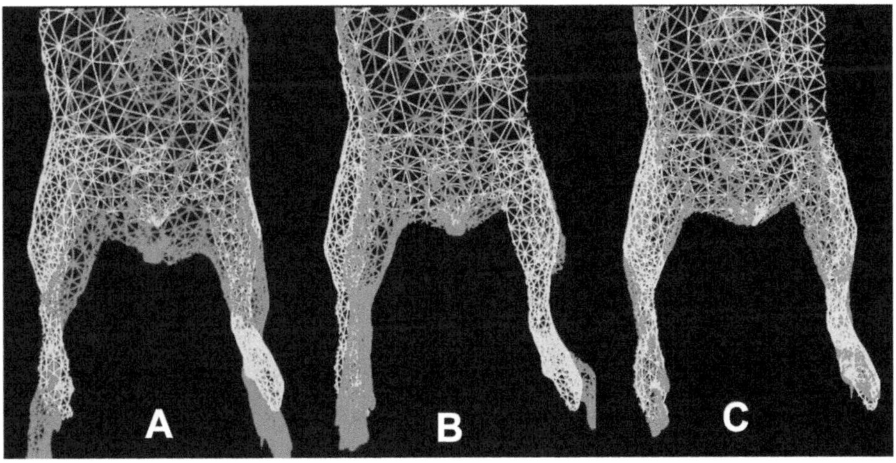

Fig. 4. Surface based registration. In this example, using the same images as in Figure 3 above, we performed the registrations using points sampled from the outer skin surfaces (red=reference, green=target). (A) starting position, (B) after global rigid alignment, (C) after articulated rigid alignment.

Registration: We estimated two different variants of the registration, namely (i) using bone surface points as shown in Figure 3, and (ii) using skin surface points, as shown in Figure 4. While in the case of CT data, the use of the bone surfaces is optimal for estimating the articulation such surfaces are not easily extractable from MRI-data, hence the use of skin surfaces to test for the more general applicability of the method. Visually, at least, our model performs as expected and successfully captured the articulation at the joints, as shown in the figures. In particular, the bone point version of the algorithm was tested on all three datasets and the algorithm successfully recovered joint rotations in the range of 10 to 40°. For this application we represented the bony anatomy with approximately 600 points. RPM was run with a temperature range 10.0 : 2.0 mm and the annealing factor was set to 0.93 [3].

4 Conclusions

In this paper we presented, the first to our knowledge implementation of an articulated rigid registration which embeds a blending piecewise model of the articulated joint that provably results in a continuous and smooth transformation across motion interfaces. The ultimate goal of this work is to use the output of this algorithm to optimally initialize a non-rigid registration algorithm for capturing the deformation of the soft tissue in addition to the overall limb motion, which will in turn provide accurate registrations of both serial intra-mouse images as well as inter-mouse images. This model of articulation is also applicable to human image data, as for example, in the case of the registration of pre-therapy and intra-therapy images in image guided prostate radiotherapy, where there is a significant articulated motion component.

References

1. V. Arsigny, X. Pennec, and N. Ayache. Polyrigid and polyaffine transformations: A new class of diffeomorphisms for locally rigid or affine registration. In Randy E. Ellis and Terry M. Peters, editors, *Proc. of MICCAI'03, Part II*, volume 2879 of *LNCS*, pages 829–837, Montreal, November 2003. Springer Verlag.
2. G. E. Christensen, M. I. Miller, and M. W. Vannier. Individualizing neuroanatomical atlases using a massively parallel computer. *Computer*, pages 32–38, January 1996.
3. H. Chui, L. Win, R. T. Schultz, J. S. Duncan, and A. Rangarajan. A unified non-rigid feature registration method for brain mapping. *Medical Image Analysis*, 7(2):113–130, 2003.
4. D. L. Collins, G. Le Goualher, and A. C. Evans. Non-linear cerebral registration with sulcal constraints. In *Medical Image Computing and Computer Assisted Intervention*, pages 974–984. Springer, Berlin, 1998.
5. C. Davatzikos. Spatial transformation and registration of brain images using elastically deformable models. *Comp. Vision and Image Understanding*, 66(2):207–222, 1997.
6. M. A. Martin-Fernandez, E. Munoz-Moreno, M. Martin-Fernandez, and C. Alberola-Lopez. Articulated registration: Elastic registration based on a wire-model. In *Medical Imaging 2005: Image Processing*, Proceedings of the SPIE 5747.
7. A. W. Toga. *Brain Warping*. Academic Press, San Diego, 1999.

Incorporating Statistical Measures of Anatomical Variability in Atlas-to-Subject Registration for Conformal Brain Radiotherapy

Olivier Commowick[1,2], Radu Stefanescu[1], Pierre Fillard[1], Vincent Arsigny[1], Nicholas Ayache[1], Xavier Pennec[1], and Grégoire Malandain[1]

[1] INRIA Sophia - Epidaure Project, 2004 Route des Lucioles BP 9306902 Sophia Antipolis Cedex, France
Olivier.Commowick@sophia.inria.fr
[2] DOSISoft S.A., 45-47 Avenue Carnot, 94 230 Cachan, France

Abstract. Deforming a digital atlas towards a patient image allows the simultaneous segmentation of several structures. Such an intersubject registration is difficult as the deformations to recover are highly inhomogeneous. A priori information about the local amount of deformation to expect is precious, since it allows to optimally balance the quality of the matching versus the regularity of the deformation. However, intersubject variability makes it hard to heuristically estimate the degree of deformation. Indeed, the sizes and shapes of various structures differ greatly and their relative positions vary in a rather complex manner. In this article, we perform a statistical study of the deformations yielded by the registration of an image database with an anatomical atlas, and we propose methods to re-inject this information into the registration. We show that this provides more accurate segmentations of brain structures.

1 Introduction

Brain radiotherapy must achieve two goals: the complete irradiation of the tumor, and the preservation of certain critical structures (brainstem, eyes, optical tracts, etc.). By customizing the shape of the irradiation beam and modulating the irradiation intensity, conformal radiotherapy allows to optimize the irradiation of the tumor and the critical structures. The planning of conformal radiotherapy requires accurate localizations of the tumor and the critical structures. In existing planning systems, the segmentation of brain structures is manual and each structure has to be delineated in each slice of a 3D image (e.g. MRI). An automatic segmentation algorithm of all the critical structures in a patient image is then an invaluable tool for radiotherapy, and its main requirement is a precise delineation of the structures of interest.

In order to segment all these structures in a specific patient's image, we use an anatomical atlas (described in [1]) containing labels of the structures of the brain. The atlas was manually labeled from an artificial MR image (obtained from the BrainWeb[1]). The first step of the general segmentation method is a rigid

[1] See web site: http://www.bic.mni.mcgill.ca/brainweb/

J. Duncan and G. Gerig (Eds.): MICCAI 2005, LNCS 3750, pp. 927–934, 2005.

matching between the atlas and the patient MRI (usually T1). The recovered transformation is refined using non-rigid registration, and then applied to the atlas labelization in order to obtain a segmentation of the patient image.

Due to its multi-subject nature, the non-rigid registration problem is generally difficult. The topology of the brain, the shape of the ventricles, the number and shape of the sulci vary strongly from one individual to another. Thus, algorithms have to deal with the ambiguity of the structures to match and also to take into account the large variability of the differences between the two brains. The ideal transformation is smooth in some places, and has fine details in others. Registration algorithms based on a uniform regularization lead therefore to local misregistrations as they do not take into account this variability. In the literature, this problem has been explored in the following two ways.

On the one side, some registration algorithms using inhomogeneous regularization [2,3] were recently introduced. They apply a strong regularization where the local deformability is low, and a weak regularization where it is high. However, they use heuristic maps of the deformability. These approaches lead to better results than with uniform regularization, but heuristic models are generally too simple compared to the complexity of the deformability. As a result, the model is not accurate everywhere and there are still local misregistrations.

On the other side, some studies have been conducted on brain asymmetry [4] and on the variability of the cortex surface using a non-rigid registration algorithm [5]. Some studies have also used extrapolation of the variability information on sulci all over the brain [6]. However, to our knowledge, none of them has been used yet to guide in some way a non-rigid registration algorithm.

In this article, we introduce a framework to compute deformability statistics over a database of patient MRI. These statistics are in turn used to guide the regularization of the deformation field. In Section 2, we first introduce an algorithm which is able to take into account scalar or tensor information to guide the regularization. In Section 3, we present the pipeline used to compute the statistics and the two deformability measures we propose. Finally, we present experiments on our image database that demonstrate quantitatively better segmentations with the proposed method, and qualitatively much more consistent from an anatomical point of view.

2 Incorporating Statistics

The registration algorithm proposed in [7] recovers the transformation as an invertible dense displacement field. Given a *target image* I and a *source image* J, the algorithm recovers the deformation field U which makes the deformed source image $J \circ U$ be as similar as possible to the target image. The method consists in the optimization of a three-term criterion:

$$E = Sim(I, J \circ U) + \int_{x \in \Omega} \left\| k(x) \nabla \frac{\partial U}{\partial t}(x) \right\|^2 dx + \int_{x \in \Omega} \| D(x) \nabla U(x) \|^2 \, dx. \quad (1)$$

The first term optimizes the similarity between the target and source image. The second term performs a regularization of the temporal derivative of the displacement field, similar to a fluid regularization of the velocity field in fluid mechanics. By locally weighting this "fluid" regularization with a scalar field k, [8] showed that the algorithm can be rendered robust with respect to potential pathologies in the subject image.

The third term of the criterion performs a regularization of the displacement field, thereby simulating an elastic-like behavior. This "elastic" regularization is weighted by a space-varying field D. If $D(x)$ is scalar, the regularization can model position-dependent deformations: the larger $D(x)$ is, the larger the local deformation can be. If D is a tensor field, the deformability is position-dependent and direction-dependent: the amount of deformation allowed can be separately tuned along spatial directions. Indeed, when one performs a diagonalization of $D(x)$, its eigenvalues model the deformability along the directions represented by the eigenvectors of the tensors (see [7]).

This elastic-like regularization model can very well incorporate deformability statistics: if the deformations are known to be large in some place, $D(x)$ is assigned a low value. Conversely, a high $D(x)$ is assigned if the deformations are known to be locally low. Furthermore, if we also have directional information about the local deformations, D can be a tensor. Its eigenvalues are large if the deformations along the corresponding eigenvectors are small, and vice versa.

3 Computation of Statistical Variability Measures

Our goal here is to build statistical measures of the deformability of the brain, that can be re-introduced as regularization maps $D(x)$ in the algorithm described above. To build the deformability statistics, we need a reference image on which we bring all the images. As choosing one image among the others in the database would introduce a bias in our approach, we use the simulated MRI of the atlas as our reference image. Then, all the images are brought to the atlas geometry using the algorithm described in Section 2 with uniform regularization, meaning that we do not make any assumption about the local deformability of each structure. This pipeline is illustrated on Fig. 1. Once the deformation fields are computed, we need a way to evaluate the mean deformability on the reference image: we now turn to the definition of scalar and tensor measures we propose.

3.1 Scalar Statistics

A good estimator of the local deformation caused by the mapping of the patient's geometry onto the atlas geometry is the Jacobian matrix J of the deformation. Indeed, its determinant $|J(x)|$ indicates whether the region around voxel x locally shrunk ($|J(x)| < 1$) or locally expanded ($|J(x)| > 1$).

Using only the determinant of the Jacobian matrix, it is clear that the contractions and expansions have not a symmetric influence when we compute statistics of the deformability: expansions will have a greater importance than contractions. We therefore propose the following expression based on the determinant:

$$Def_j(x) = \mathrm{abs}(\log(|J_j(x)|)). \qquad (2)$$

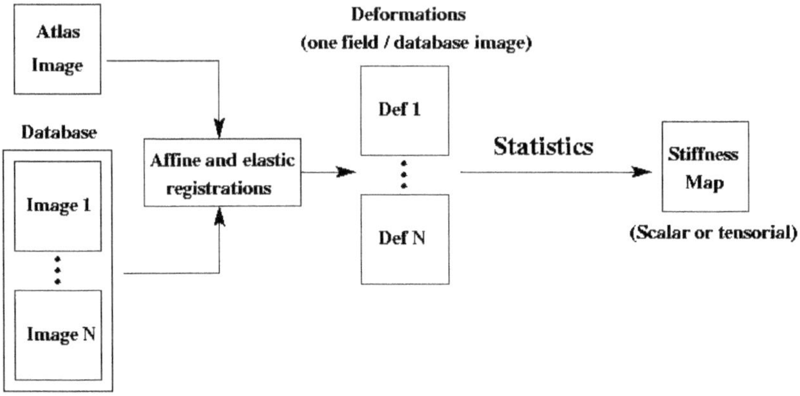

Fig. 1. Schematic view of the pipeline used to compute the deformability statistics. This scheme shows which major steps are done for computing our scalar or tensor stiffness map. (see text)

In this formula, the index j corresponds to the patient while x is the current voxel position. Taking the logarithm symmetrizes the influence of the deformations, thus avoiding to penalize the contractions. The absolute value insures that we have no compensation between contractions and expansions at voxels where both occur in different images. Finally, this distribution can be summarized by its mean value:

$$\overline{Def}(x) = \mathbb{E}\Big(\text{abs}(\log(|J_j(x)|)) \Big). \tag{3}$$

This equation can also be seen as a dispersion measure associated to the median, i.e. a robust version of the standard deviation. However, as we said in Section 2, the quantity of regularization in the algorithm is defined by a stiffness map $D(x)$, where $D(x) \in [0;1]$ is a scalar map. The greater D is, the stronger the regularization is and therefore the less the deformability is. We can see that D is roughly equivalent to the inverse of the measure we defined above. To keep the value of D bounded, we use the following formulation for the stiffness map with $\lambda > 0$: $D(x) = 1/(1 + \lambda\overline{Def}(x))$.

3.2 Tensor Statistics

At this point, we have defined a scalar estimator of the mean deformability of the brain. However, the drawback of a scalar field is that we do not use all the information given by the deformation: we have not taken into account the directional information of the displacements. As the algorithm presented above allows us to perform anisotropic regularization using tensor fields, we would like to have an extension of the preceding formulation to compute tensor statistics of the brain deformability.

The tensor we propose here is based on the Jacobian matrix: $W_j(x) = J_j(x).J_j(x)^T$. This expression can be seen as a measure of the local deformation. A related idea was suggested in [9], but directly on the Jacobian matrix.

However, using the symmetric deformation tensor W allows us to compute simple and efficient (rigid-invariant) statistics.

As for the scalar field, we want to symmetrize the influence of the contractions and the dilatations. We therefore take the matrix logarithm of this expression and the absolute value of the resulting value. Let $W = R.Diag(S_i).R^T$ be a diagonalization of a symmetric matrix (where S_i are the eigenvalues of the matrix). Then, the matrix absolute value is defined by $\text{abs}(W) = R.Diag(\text{abs}(S_i)).R^T$. Finally, we define the measure of deformability by: $\Sigma_j(x) = \text{abs}\Big(\log(W_j(x))\Big)$. And the expression for the mean deformability is simply:

$$\overline{\Sigma}(x) = \mathbb{E}\Big(\text{abs}(\log(W_j(x)))\Big). \tag{4}$$

Similarly to the scalar map, we use the following expression to obtain a bounded stiffness tensor map: $D(x) = \Big(Id + \lambda\overline{\Sigma}(x)\Big)^{-1}$.

4 Experiments and Results

We used in our experiments a database of 36 patients with brain tumors at different grades and positions. For each patient three MRI have been acquired (T1, injected T1 and T2). All these patient images are registered on the atlas MRI following the process in Fig. 1, first by an affine global registration, then using a uniform elastic registration.

Once the deformation fields are obtained, we compute a mask of the region of interest for each image. This allows us to compute our statistical measures only on tissues that are present in both the patient and the atlas images. The problem is similar for tumor and surgical resections. The correspondences are not relevant in these regions as these tissues are not homologous in both images. Then, as we have T1 and T2 images of the patient, we segment the tumor and the surgical resection as in [8] and remove these segmentations from the mask. We are then able to compute deformability statistics on relevant regions using Eqs. (3) and (4). An example of the resulting stiffness maps and fractional anisotropy (FA is an index of the anisotropy of the tensor) for the tensor-based model are given in Fig. 2. As we compute our statistics only on imaged regions of each brain of the database, we do not have any information on some exterior regions of the atlas image, leading to some black regions in the FA map.

As we can see on Fig. 2, the statistical stiffness maps we computed are smoother than the heuristic model used in [7]. We can notice that the heuristic assumptions made in [7] on the deformability of the ventricles are mostly verified. However, in some regions (like the ventricles boundaries), the tensor deformability map is highly anisotropic (see the FA map in Fig. 2). The statistical maps are also very different from the heuristic one in the region in front of the brainstem. This region is attributed a more elastic behavior than in the heuristic map, where it is set to almost 0, resulting in a fluid regularization. However, we can see in Fig. 3 that this assumption can result in relatively bad segmentations

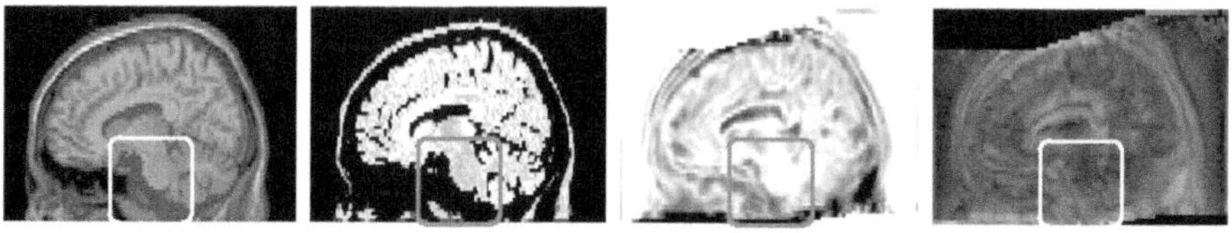

Fig. 2. A slice of the statistical maps obtained in our comparison. The frames show the brainstem and the area in front of it. From left to right: the simulated MRI of the atlas, the heuristic scalar map, the scalar map obtained using Eq. (3), the fractional anisotropy (FA) map obtained using Eq. (4) (see text).

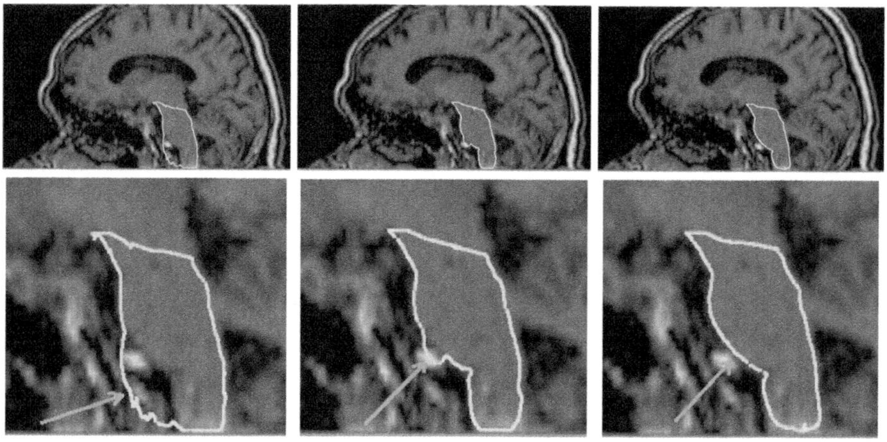

Fig. 3. Comparative results of the atlas-based segmentation. Top: Sagittal slice of the 3D patient image with the segmentation superimposed. Bottom: close-up on the brainstem area. From left to right: registration with the heuristic scalar map, with the statistical scalar map and with the statistical tensor map.

of the brainstem. In this case, the segmented structure often includes the artery just in front of it. This is due to the absence of matter in the atlas image leading to bad correspondences.

Using a fluid registration in this area, as proposed by the heuristic model, leads to non-anatomical deformations. In our scalar stiffness map as well as in its tensor equivalent, the region just in front of the brainstem is assigned to a higher value. Thus, we focus on an example of the automatic segmentation of the brainstem using the image of a patient that was not used to compute the statistics. We can see that the results are improved in this region as shown in Fig. 3. The segmentation is qualitatively more consistent. We can also see that taking into account a directional component in the regularization (tensor map) further improves the results as the artery in front of the brainstem is not anymore included in the segmentation (see arrows in Fig. 3). Finally, the registration process takes about one hour to run in sequential execution on an AMD Opteron 2 GHz, independently of the statistical model used.

Table 1. Statistics obtained using the STAPLE algorithm [10]. Seven expert segmentations for each patient (Sens. stands for Sensitivity, Spec. for Specificity and dist. for the distance to the point (Sens. = 1, Spec. = 1)) (see text).

	Patient 1			Patient 2			Patient 3		
	Sens.	Spec.	Dist.	Sens.	Spec.	Dist.	Sens.	Spec.	Dist.
Heuristic	0.86	0.87	0.19	0.81	0.74	0.32	0.83	0.88	0.21
Scalar	0.84	0.92	0.18	0.82	0.83	0.25	0.81	0.94	0.20
Tensor	0.86	0.91	**0.17**	0.83	0.84	**0.23**	0.82	0.94	**0.18**

At this point, we have seen that our method gives qualitatively better results than the method using a scalar heuristic stiffness map on one example. We also studied in more details the results on three other patient images for which seven experts have manually segmented the brainstem. For each patient image, we compute the ground truth segmentation (see [10]) from the expert segmentations. Then, we use this ground truth to compute the sensitivity and the specificity of each automatic segmentation. We also compute the distance to the best result achievable (Sensitivity = 1, Specificity = 1). The results are reported in Table 1 and confirm our qualitative estimation: the results obtained by the scalar statistics map are slightly better than the ones obtained by the heuristic map. We verify also quantitatively that using an anisotropic regularization map gives better results than using only isotropic information.

5 Conclusion

In this article, we have described a method to incorporate statistics of the deformability of the brain into a non-rigid registration algorithm. We have introduced scalar (isotropic) and tensor-based (anisotropic) models to this end. For each method, we have detailed a symmetric measure of the deformations, on which we can perform consistent statistics. These statistics are also robust since we explicitly exclude the tumor and surgical resection parts of the patients images from the computation of the statistics.

The two ways of re-introducing statistics in the registration result in qualitative and quantitative improvement of the segmentations, the tensor-based model achieving the best results. However, concerning quantitative validation, only three patients were used with only one structure segmented manually by seven experts. We intend to extend this validation to more patients and to more structures in a near future.

The framework we have used has the advantage to be independent of the non-rigid algorithm used to compute the statistics. However, it is sensitive to potential systematic errors in the algorithm used to register images on the atlas image. To compute less biased statistics, it will be interesting to use other non-rigid algorithms (for example parametric algorithms as [11]) or to bring into correspondence manual delineations of structures. Ideally, in order to be as unbiased as possible, we would like to be able to fuse the information provided by several non-rigid registration algorithms into one single statistical map.

Finally, this algorithm can be used on other regions of the body. This approach could bring a way to evaluate the local deformability on regions where it is difficult to have a good idea of the elasticity of the deformation.

Acknowledgments

This work was partially founded by ECIP project MAESTRO and ANRT.
The authors are grateful to Dr. P.-Y. Bondiau for providing the MRI database and the brain atlas used for our experiments.

References

1. PY Bondiau, G Malandain, O Commowick, PY Marcy, S Chanalet, and N Ayache. Atlas-based automatic segmentation of MR images: Validation study on the brainstem in radiotherapy context. In *RSNA*, Chicago, 2004.
2. Hava Lester, Simon R. Arridge, Kalvis M. Jansons, Louis Lemieux, Joseph V. Hajnal, and Anjela Oatridge. Non-linear registration with the variable viscosity fluid algorithm. In *Proc of IPMI;99*, pages 238–251, 1999.
3. R. Stefanescu, X. Pennec, and N. Ayache. Grid powered nonlinear image registration with locally adaptive regularization. *Med. Im. Analysis*, 8(3):325–342, 2004.
4. A.W. Toga and P.M. Thompson. Mapping brain asymmetry. *Nature Reviews Neuroscience*, 4(1):37–48, January 2003.
5. P.M. Thompson, M.S. Mega, K.L. Narr, E.R. Sowell, R.E. Blanton, and A.W. Toga. Brain image analysis and atlas construction. In M. Fitzpatrick and M. Sonka, editors, *Handbook of Medical Image Proc. and Analysis*, chapter 17. SPIE, 2000.
6. P. Fillard, V. Arsigny, X. Pennec, P. Thompson, and N. Ayache. Extrapolation of sparse tensor fields: Application to the modeling of brain variability. In *IPMI'05*, LNCS. Springer, July 2005. To appear.
7. R. Stefanescu. *Parallel nonlinear registration of medical images with a priori information on anatomy and pathology*. PhD thesis, Université de Nice Sophia-Antipolis, March 2005.
8. R. Stefanescu, O. Commowick, G. Malandain, P.-Y. Bondiau, N. Ayache, and X. Pennec. Non-rigid atlas to subject registration with pathologies for conformal brain radiotherapy. In *Proc. of MICCAI'04*, volume 3216 of *LNCS*, pages 704–711. Springer, 2004.
9. R.P. Woods. Characterizing volume and surface deformations in an atlas framework: theory, applications, and implementation. *NeuroImage*, 18(3):769–788, 2003.
10. Simon K Warfield, Kelly H Zou, and William M Wells. Simultaneous truth and performance level estimation (staple): an algorithm for the validation of image segmentation. *IEEE Trans Med Imaging*, 23(7):903–21, July 2004.
11. G.K. Rohde, A. Aldroubi, and B.M. Dawant. The adaptive bases algorithm for intensity based nonrigid image registration. *IEEE TMI*, 22:1470–1479, 2003.

Accurate Image Registration for Quadrature Tomographic Microscopy

Chia-Ling Tsai[1], William Warger II[2], and Charles DiMarzio[2]

[1] National Chung Cheng University, Chiayi 62102, Taiwan
[2] Northeastern University, Boston, MA 02115, U.S.A

Abstract. This paper presents a robust and fully automated registration algorithm for registration of images of Quadrature Tomographic Microscopy (QTM), which is an optical interferometer. The need for registration of such images is to recognize distinguishing features of viable embryos to advance the technique for *In Vitro* Fertilization. QTM images a sample (live embryo) multiple times with different hardware configurations, each in turn producing 4 images taken by 4 CCD cameras simultaneously. Embryo movement is often present between imaging. Our algorithm handles camera calibration[1] of multiple cameras using a variant of ICP, and elimination of embryo movement using a hybrid of feature- and intensity-based methods. The algorithm is tested on 20 live mouse embryos containing various cell numbers between 8 and 26. No failure thus far, and the average alignment error is 0.09 pixels, corresponding to the range of 639 and 675 nanometers.

1 Introduction

With the work pace and stress levels ever increasing, infertility now affects 10% [4] of the population at reproductive age. *In Vitro* Fertilization (IVF) is a method of assisted reproduction in which fertilization takes place in a laboratory dish. Usually, multiple embryos are transferred to the uterus during each cycle to increase the success rate. One cycle of IVF costs an average of $12,400 in the United States. According to the latest statistics, the success rate for IVF is 29.4% live deliveries per egg retrieval, of which about 63% are singletons, 32% are twins, and 5% are triplets or more [4, 1].

To strive for a higher success rate of live deliveries and to reduce multiple births, researchers at Northeastern University, USA, are developing a unique state-of-the-art "fusion microscope" to recognize distinguishing features of viable embryos [6, 11]. This instrument combines 5 imaging modalities for subsurface imaging, including Quadrature Tomographic Microscopy (QTM) and Differential Interference Contrast (DIC) microscopy.

There are two types of registration involved: inter- and intra-modality registration. The work presented in this paper is on intra-modality registration of

[1] In this paper, we define camera calibration as a process that estimates the spatial relationship between the 4 CCD cameras.

J. Duncan and G. Gerig (Eds.): MICCAI 2005, LNCS 3750, pp. 935–942, 2005.

QTM images. Applications for such work include the construction of amplitude and phase images of transparent samples, and cell counting methods involving the combination with DIC images for embryos before the blastocyst stage (less than 30 cells) [7].

2 QTM Images and the Challenges

QTM based on a modified Mach-Zener Interferometer. The laser source is split into two separate beams — signal and reference. The signal beam goes through the sample (embryo) and the reference beam travels the same distance as the signal beam, but is undisturbed. Both are combined later by an unpolarized beamsplitter and their interference is imaged simultaneously by 4 CCD cameras, each having its own coordinate system. An embryo is imaged three times by different hardware configurations (see Fig. 1): (a) mixture, the interference of the reference and signal beams, (b) reference only with the signal beam blocked, and (c) signal only with the reference beam blocked.

Placing all images in the same coordinate system requires calibration between the 4 cameras and registration of images taken at different times. The latter compensates for movement of the embryo. There are two ways to solve the registration problem: (a) for every image pair estimating the transformation directly from features of the embryo, and (b) solving camera calibration first and then eliminating embryo movement. The second method is superior in terms of speed and robustness for the following reasons:

- QTM images of all beam types appear substantially different (see Fig. 2). If registering such an image pair directly, the result is often not accurate

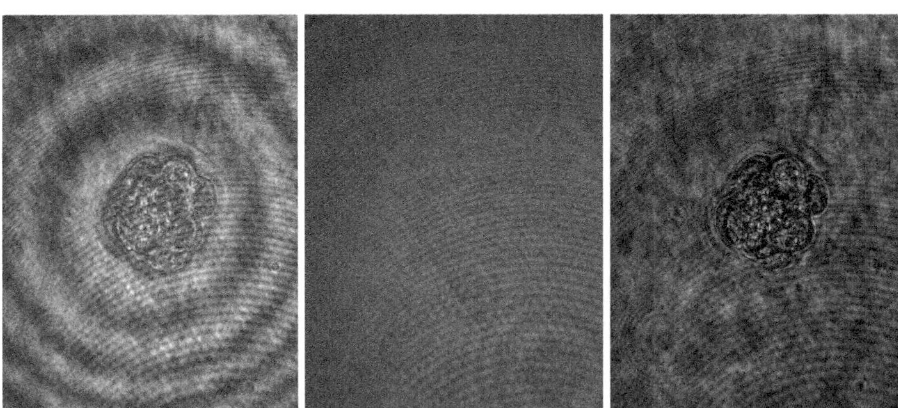

Fig. 1. QTM images of a live embryo taken with different hardware configurations. Accurate registration is required to eliminate the movement of the embryo between imaging. Left: mixture of reference and signal. Middle: reference alone. Right: signal alone.

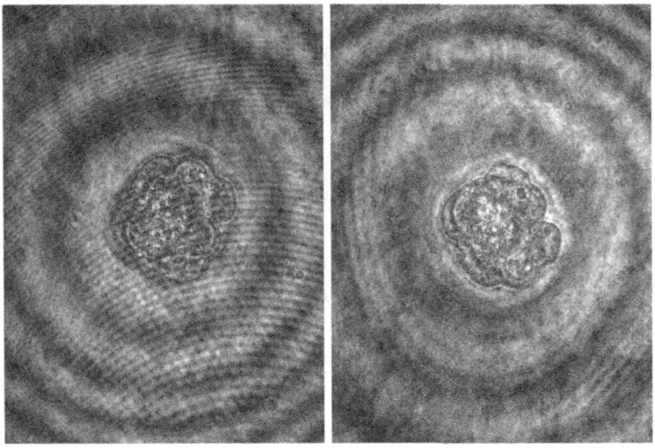

Fig. 2. Two mixture images taken by different cameras. Left: image of x-polarization (first camera). Right: image of y-polarization (second camera).

enough. In addition, it requires a more expensive registration algorithm that exploits the properties of the images. The number of times such an algorithm is applied should be minimized.
- Camera calibration is independent of the object for imaging and performed only when cameras change their relative positions. We can make use of any pattern that allows fast and accurate registration.
- If 4 images of a specific hardware configuration are aligned, we can make use of special optical properties to synthesize images that are similar in appearance. Such images can provide better registration result for elimination of embryo movement between imaging.

3 Camera Calibration

Between two images, the calibration process estimates an affine transformation that allows translation, rotation, reflection, and slight shearing. The image of the

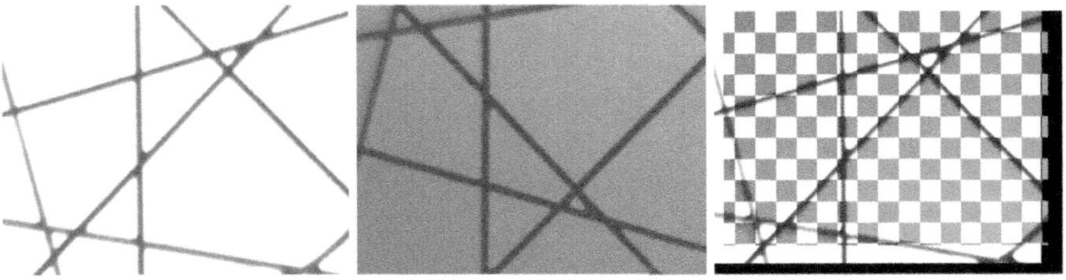

(a) (b) (c)

Fig. 3. The target pattern, imitating a vasculature, designed for automatic calibration of the 4 CCD cameras. (a) The image of the second camera. (b) The image of the fourth camera. (c) The checkerboard mosaic of the registered target images first camera is the anchor (fixed image) for registration. Since camera calibration is independent of the object for imaging, we designed a target pattern that simplifies the registration process. Images of the target are shown in Fig. 3.

The pattern bears strong similarity with a vasculature — both are patterns of lines crossing at random angles. This property allows us to register our target images using feature-based methods in the literature. The features for registration are the centerline points and cross-overs of the dark lines [3, 12]. The transformation model is affine that allows left-right or top-bottom flipping, and significant rotation. We first discuss computation of the transformation Θ that does not involve reflection.

Estimation of Θ follows the method in [9], with some modifications, for full automation. The process consists of 2 steps:

Initialization: To avoid convergence to an incorrect alignment, we need a good initialization scheme to place the transformation in the right domain of convergence. We adopt invariant indexing to automate the process. In particular, for each image, a set of landmark (cross-over) pairs is generated and each pair is associated with a signature vector that is only invariant to similarity transformation, which is the initial transformation model. This is the reason for separation of reflection from the rest of the transformation. The algorithm generates a list of hypothesized correspondence pairs, ordered by the similarity of the invariant features. Each hypothesis provides an initial transformation.

Refinement: The refinement technique is a robust form of ICP (Iterative Closest Points) algorithm which minimizes the sum of point-to-line distances using an M-estimator. It alternates between closest centerline point matching using the current transformation, and transformation estimation using the set of matches. The transformation model for refinement is affine.

The algorithm refines the initial transformations one by one until it reaches one that converges to a good alignment. In practice, we only need to try the very first few.

Special care is needed to register an image pair related by reflection. To do so, the moving image is flipped by Θ_f. Both the flipped and original moving images are registered to the fixed image using the abovementioned procedure, and the best alignment is taken. It does not matter if the moving image is right-left or top-bottom flipped, since rotation of π relates one to the other. This is the major reason for the need of significant rotation. If the flipped is better aligned with the fixed image, the final transformation is the product of Θ and Θ_f.

We validated the algorithm with a small set of target images. Fig. 3(c) contains a checker-board mosaic with sub-pixel accuracy.

4 Elimination of Embryo Movement

The embryo may move between the time two images are acquired with different hardware configurations. In practice, the movement is limited to translation and

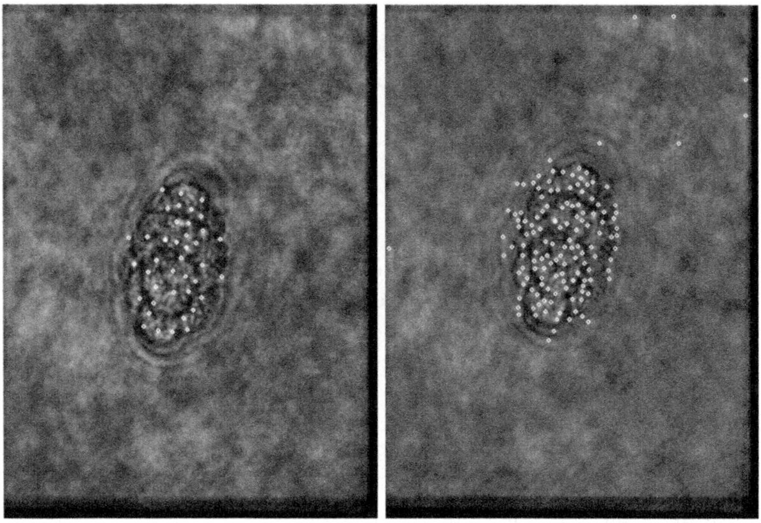

Fig. 4. The synthesized images for registration of signal to mixture images. Features, shown by white dots, are for invariant indexing and refinement. Left: Image I_a, average signal image. Only a subset of features extracted takes part in initialization and refinement. Right: Image I_s, the synthesized signal image. All features are involved in initialization.

rotation. To eliminate the movement, the signal images of the embryo must be aligned with the mixture. Due to the complex optical properties of the QTM, it is hard to directly relate the signal images to the mixture images (see Fig. 1). To overcome this problem, we perform the registration using synthesized images, instead of the original raw images.

Let M_i, be image i of the mixture after camera calibration (i.e. the image mapped to the coordinate system of the first camera). Similarly, R_i is for reference and S_i for signal. The formula for the synthesized image I_s is $\sum_{i=1}^{4}(M_i - R_i)/4$. A very similar image I_a can be generated from S_i using the formula $\sum_{i=1}^{4} S_i/4$.

I_a is registered to I_s, which is in the same space as the first image of the mixture. Fig. 4 shows examples of I_a and I_s from the same set of images. The registration algorithm uses salient features and intensity structure of the images, and consists of 3 steps:

Feature Extraction: Since the background, not the embryo, is already aligned before registration, we want features that concentrate in the embryo to drive the registration out of the local minimum. Edge points are obviously not good candidates, since they are mostly on the fringes in the background. The type of key-point of our choice is harris-corner[5]. We empirically determined the threshold on the corner-like measure to reduce the number of features extracted from the background. Fig. 4 shows a result of the feature extraction.

Initialization: Robust initialization is crucial when the movement of the embryo is significant. Again, we employ invariant indexing. The invariant feature is Lowe's SIFT descriptor [8], a 128-component histogram of normalized gradients. The algorithm generates a list of hypothesized correspondence between two key-points, based on the invariant features. To reduce the number of hypotheses, we only take subset of key-points in I_a. The same set of key-points are used in the refinement stage as well. Each hypothesis provides an initial affine transformation estimate from the location, orientation and scale of each key-point, and is refined separately.

Another common approach is to combine invariant features with RANSAC [2], which examines a number of n correspondences (n is 3 for affine) for the best alignment. We chose invariant indexing over RANSAC for two reasons: (a) invariant indexing can return correct transformation as long as there is one correct match, and (b) SIFT descriptors are distinctive enough for this type of images that invariant indexing can succeed with the first match almost 100% of the time.

Refinement: The refinement algorithm is a variant of ICP that matches key-points based on intensity structure [10]. Unlike initialization, which matches key-points detected in both I_a and I_s, only key-points in I_a are needed.

To generate the corresponding point in I_s, each key-point is associated with a small region R, centering at the location of the key-point p. This region is mapped into the other image (I_s), using the current transformation estimate. Let the transformed location and region be p' and R', respectively. R' is matched against regions centered at pixel locations falling into the

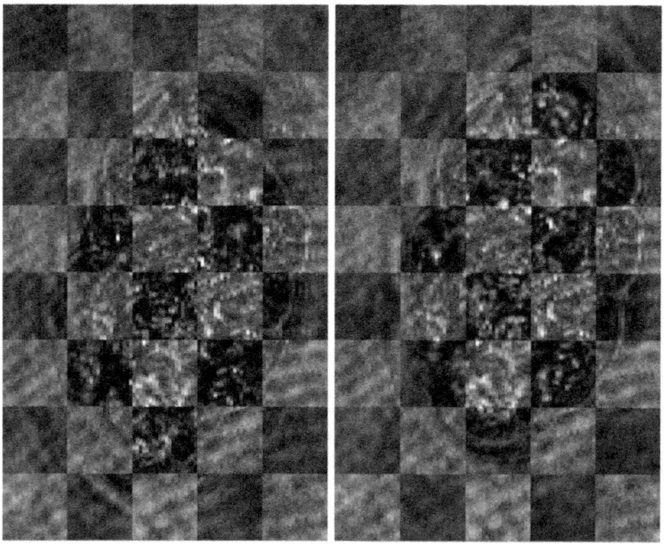

Fig. 5. The registration result, illustrated with cropped checker-board mosaics, of the average to synthesized signal images. Left: before registration. Discontinuity of the border of the embryo manifests the mis-alignment of the images. Right: after registration.

search window of p' in I_s. The width of the window is a multiple of the error scale (uncertainty) of the current transformation; less accurate transformation leads to larger search window for each key-point. The best match has the lowest normalized SSD error measure. The center location of the best matched region defines the new corresponding point to p. Each match is assigned a robust weight which is a product of the distinctiveness of the match and the geometric distance between the corresponding points. The weights are required for robust estimation of the transformation.

We have tested the algorithm on a set of 20 mouse embryos containing various cell numbers between 8 and 26. Some samples were stationary, while others were fairly mobile. The success rate is 100% thus far, with an average alignment accuracy of 0.09 pixel, corresponding to 639 - 675 nanometers. The accuracy is measured in terms of weighted average distance error using the matches generated in the refinement stage. Fig. 5 is the registration result of the two images in Fig. 4. All results were verified manually by visual inspection of the checkerboard mosaics.

We have also attempted registration directly using signal and mixture images of the first camera. The results were not as satisfactory. The set of images in Fig. 1 serves as an example of which signal and mixture images are substantially different. With this set of images, invariant indexing failed with the first 10 hypotheses, which was the threshold. Even if manually initialized by a pair of corresponding points, the final alignment was not as good as our current method.

5 Discussion and Conclusion

We presented a new algorithm for registration of QTM images, and demonstrated its robustness with images of a set of 20 live mouse embryos. The algorithm consists of two parts: camera calibration followed by registration of embryo images taken with different hardware configurations. After registration, all images are aligned with the first camera of mixture. If the embryo movement is present, the images of the embryo are aligned instead. The algorithm is both accurate and efficient — the average alignment error is 639-675 nanometers (0.09 pixel), and it succeeds with the first match almost all the time for both camera calibration and embryo registration.

With registration of QTM images in place, the next step is to apply the technique to synthesis of better amplitude and phase images, which are easily corrupted by embryo movement. Inter-modal registration of QTM phase images with DIC images, for applications such as cell counting, is also simplified by using the registered raw data (mixture and signal images) instead.

References

[1] A. Birmingham. Assisted reproductive technology in the united states: 2000 results generated from the american society for reproductive medicine/society for assisted reproductive technology registry. *Fertility and Sterility*, 81(5), May 2004.

[2] M. Brown and D. Lowe. Recognising panoramas. In *Proc. ICCV*, 2003.
[3] A. Can, H. Shen, J. N. Turner, H. L. Tanenbaum, and B. Roysam. Rapid automated tracing and feature extraction from live high-resolution retinal fundus images using direct exploratory algorithms. *IEEE Trans. on Inf. Tech. in Biomedicine*, 3(2):125–138, 1999.
[4] A. S. for Reproductive Medicine. FACT SHEET: In vitro fertilization (IVF). http://www.asrm.org/Patients/FactSheets/invitro.html.
[5] C. Harris and M. Stephens. A combined corner and edge detector. pages 147–151.
[6] D. Hogenboom, C. DiMarzio, T. Gaudette, A. Devaney, and S. Lindberg. Three-dimensional images generated by quadrature interferometry. *Optics Letters*, 23:783–785, 1998.
[7] W. W. II, J. Newmark, C. Chang, D. Brooks, C. Warner, and C. DiMarzio. Combining optical quadrature and differential interference contrast to facilitate embryonic cell counting with fluorescence imaging for confirmation. In *Proc. SPIE Conference Imaging, Man. Ana. Bio. Cells, Tissue II*, volume 5699, pages 334–341, 2005.
[8] D. G. Lowe. Distinctive image features from scale-invariant keypoints. *IJCV*, 60(2):91–110, November 2004.
[9] C. Stewart, C.-L. Tsai, and B. Roysam. The dual-bootstrap iterative closest point algorithm with application to retinal image registration. *IEEE Trans. Med. Imaging.*, 22(11):1379–1394, 2003.
[10] C. V. Stewart, Y.-L. Lee, and C.-L. Tsai. An uncertainty-driven hybrid of intensity-based and feature-based registration with application to retinal and lung CT images. In *Proc. 7th MICCAI*, Saint-Malo, France, 2004.
[11] D. Townsend, G. L. C. DiMarzio, and M. Rajadhyaksha. Multimodal optical microscope for imaging biological systems. In *Proc. SPIE Conference 3D, Mult. Micro. Image Acqu. Pro. XII*, volume 5701, pages 136–145, 2005.
[12] C.-L. Tsai, C. Stewart, B. Roysam, and H. Tanenbaum. Repeatable vascular landmark extraction from retinal fundus images using local vascular traces. *IEEE Trans. on Inf. Tech. in Biomedicine*, 8(2):122–130, 2004.

Riemannian Elasticity: A Statistical Regularization Framework for Non-linear Registration

X. Pennec, R. Stefanescu, V. Arsigny, P. Fillard, and N. Ayache

INRIA Sophia - Projet Epidaure, 2004 Route des Lucioles BP 93,
06902 Sophia Antipolis Cedex, France
Xavier.Pennec@sophia.inria.fr

Abstract. In inter-subject registration, one often lacks a good model of the transformation variability to choose the optimal regularization. Some works attempt to model the variability in a statistical way, but the re-introduction in a registration algorithm is not easy. In this paper, we interpret the elastic energy as the distance of the Green-St Venant strain tensor to the identity, which reflects the deviation of the local deformation from a rigid transformation. By changing the Euclidean metric for a more suitable Riemannian one, we define a consistent statistical framework to quantify the amount of deformation. In particular, the mean and the covariance matrix of the strain tensor can be consistently and efficiently computed from a population of non-linear transformations. These statistics are then used as parameters in a Mahalanobis distance to measure the statistical deviation from the observed variability, giving a new regularization criterion that we called the statistical Riemannian elasticity. This new criterion is able to handle anisotropic deformations and is inverse-consistent. Preliminary results show that it can be quite easily implemented in a non-rigid registration algorithms.

1 Introduction

Most non-linear image registration algorithms optimize a criterion including an image intensity similarity and a regularization term. In inter-subject registration, the main problem is not really the intensity similarity measure but rather the regularization criterion. Some authors used physical models like elasticity or fluid models [1,2]. For efficiency reasons, other authors proposed to use non-physical but efficient regularization methods like Gaussian filtering [3,4], recently extended to non-stationary but still isotropic diffusion in order to take into account some anatomical information about the tissue types [5,6]. However, since we do not have in general a model of the deformation of organs across subjects, no regularization criterion is obviously more justified than the others. We could think of building a model of the developing organ: inverting the model from the first subject to a sufficiently early stage and growing toward the second subject image would allow to relate the two anatomies. However, such a computational model is out of reach now, and most of the existing work in the literature rather

J. Duncan and G. Gerig (Eds.): MICCAI 2005, LNCS 3750, pp. 943–950, 2005.

try to capture the organ variability from a statistical point of view on a representative population of subjects (see e.g. [7,8,9]). Although the image databases are now large enough to be representative of the organ variability, the problem remains of how to use this information to better guide inter-subject registration.

We propose in this paper an integrated framework to compute the statistics on deformations and reintroduce them in the registration procedure. The basic idea is to interpret the elastic energy as a distance in the space of positive definite symmetric matrices (tensors). By changing the classical Euclidean metric for a more suitable one, we define a natural framework for computing statistics on the strain tensor. Taking them into account in a statistical distance lead to the Riemannian elasticity energy. Notice that we do not enter the fluid vs elastic registration debate as the energy we propose can be used either on the deformation field itself or on its temporal derivative (fluid-like method) [4].

In the sequel, we first recall how to optimize the elastic energy in a registration algorithm. Then, we define in Section 3 the Riemannian elasticity energy as the Mahalanobis distance on the logarithmic strain tensor. To better exemplify its properties, we investigate in Section 4 the isotropic Riemannian Elasticity, which is close to the classical elasticity energy while being inverse-consistent. Preliminary experiments show in Sec. 5 that the Riemannian elasticity framework can be implemented quite effectively and yields promising results.

2 Non-linear Elastic Regularization

Let $\Phi(x)$ be a non-linear space transformation with a positive Jacobian everywhere. We denote by $\partial_\alpha \Phi$ the directional derivatives of the transformation along the spaces axis α (we assume an orthonormal basis). The general registration method is to optimize an energy of the type: $C(\Phi) = Sim(\text{Images}, \Phi) + Reg(\Phi)$. Starting from an initial transformation Φ_0, a first order gradient descent methods computes the gradient of the energy $\nabla C(\Phi)$, and update the transformation using: $\Phi_{t+1} = \Phi_t - \eta \, \nabla C(\Phi_t)$. From a computational points of view, this Lagrangian framework can be advantageously changed into a Eulerian framework to better conserve the diffeomorphic nature of the mappings [6]. In the following, we only focus on the computation of the gradient of the regularization.

2.1 Elastic Deformations

In continuum mechanics [10], one characterizes the deformation of an infinitesimal volume element in the Lagrangian framework using the Cauchy-Green tensor $\Sigma = \nabla\Phi^{\mathrm{T}} \, \nabla\Phi = \sum_\alpha \partial_\alpha \Phi \, \partial_\alpha \Phi^{\mathrm{T}}$. This symmetric matrix is positive definite and measures the local amount of non-rigidity. Let $\nabla\Phi = V \, S \, R^{\mathrm{T}}$ be a singular value decomposition of the transformation Jacobian (R and V are two rotation matrices and S is the diagonal matrix of the positive singular values). The Cauchy-Green tensor $\Sigma = R \, S^2 \, R^{\mathrm{T}}$ is equal to the identity if and only if the transformation is locally a rigid transformation. Eigenvalues between 0 and 1 indicate a local compression of the material along the associated eigenvector, while a value above 1 indicates an expansion. To quantify the deformation, one usually prefers the related Green-St Venant strain tensor $E = \frac{1}{2}(\Sigma - \mathrm{Id})$, whose eigenvalues are null for no deformation. Assuming an isotropic material and a linear Hooks law to relate strain and stress tensors, one can show that the motion equations derive from the *St Venant-Kirchoff elasticity* energy [10]:

$$Reg_{SVKE}(\Phi) = \int \mu \mathrm{Tr}(E^2) + \frac{\lambda}{2}\mathrm{Tr}(E)^2 = \int \frac{\mu}{4}\mathrm{Tr}\left((\Sigma - \mathrm{Id})^2\right) + \frac{\lambda}{8}\mathrm{Tr}(\Sigma - \mathrm{Id})^2$$

where λ, μ are the Lamé coefficients. To minimize this energy in a registration algorithm, we need its gradient. Since $\partial_u \Sigma = \sum_\alpha \left(\partial_\alpha \Phi \, \partial_\alpha u^{\mathrm{T}} + \partial_\alpha u \, \partial_\alpha \Phi^{\mathrm{T}}\right)$, the derivative of the elastic energy in the direction (i.e. displacement field) u is:

$$\begin{aligned} \partial_u Reg_{SVKE}(\Phi) &= \textstyle\int \frac{\mu}{2}\mathrm{Tr}((\Sigma - \mathrm{Id})\, \partial_u \Sigma) + \frac{\lambda}{4}\mathrm{Tr}(\Sigma - \mathrm{Id})\, \mathrm{Tr}(\partial_u \Sigma) \\ &= \textstyle\sum_\alpha \int \langle\, \mu\, (\Sigma - \mathrm{Id})\, \partial_\alpha \Phi \mid \partial_\alpha u \,\rangle + \frac{\lambda}{2}\mathrm{Tr}(\Sigma - \mathrm{Id})\, \langle\, \partial_\alpha \Phi \mid \partial_\alpha u \,\rangle \end{aligned}$$

Using an integration by part with homogeneous Neumann boundary conditions [4], we have $\int \langle\, v \mid \partial_\alpha u \,\rangle = - \int \langle\, \partial_\alpha v \mid u \,\rangle$, so that the gradient is finally:

$$\nabla Reg_{SVKE}(\Phi) = -\textstyle\sum_\alpha \partial_\alpha \big(Z \partial_\alpha \Phi\big) \quad \text{with} \quad Z = \mu(\Sigma - \mathrm{Id}) + \frac{\lambda}{2}\mathrm{Tr}(\Sigma - \mathrm{Id})\,\mathrm{Id} \quad (1)$$

2.2 Practical Implementation

In practice, a simple implementation is the following. First, one computes the image of the gradient of the transformation, for instance using finite differences. This operation is not computationally expensive, but requires to access the value of the transformation field at neighboring points, which can be time consuming due to systematic memory page faults in large images. Then, we process these 3 vectors completely locally to compute 3 new vectors $v_\alpha = Z(\partial_\alpha \Phi)$. This operation is computationally more expensive but is memory efficient as the resulting vectors can replace the old directional derivatives. Finally, the gradient of the criterion $\nabla E = \sum_\alpha \partial_\alpha v_\alpha$ may be computed using finite differences on the resulting image. Once again, this is not computationally expensive, but it requires intensive memory accesses.

3 Riemannian Elasticity

In the standard Elasticity theory, the deviation of the positive definite symmetric matrix Σ (the strain tensor) from the identity (the rigidity) is measured using the Euclidean matrix distance $\mathrm{dist}^2_{Eucl}(\Sigma, \mathrm{Id}) = \mathrm{Tr}((\Sigma - \mathrm{Id})^2)$. However, it has been argued in recent works that the Euclidean metric is not a good metric for the tensor space because positive definite symmetric matrices only constitute a cone in the Euclidean matrix space. Thus, the tensor space is not complete (null or negative eigenvalues are at a finite distance). For instance, an expansion of a factor $\sqrt{2}$ in each direction (leading to $\Sigma = 2\,\mathrm{Id}$) is at the same Euclidean distance from the identity than the "black hole" transformation $\Phi(x) = 0$ (which has a non physical null strain tensor). In non-linear registration, this asymmetry of the regularization leads to different results if we look for the forward or the backward transformation: this is the inverse-consistency problem [11].

3.1 A Log-Euclidean Metric on the Strain Tensor

To solve the problems of the Euclidean tensor computing, affine-invariant Riemannian metrics were recently proposed [12,13,14,15]. Using these metrics, symmetric matrices with null eigenvalues are basically at an infinite distance from any tensor, and the notion of mean value corresponds to a geometric mean, even if it has to be computed iteratively. More recently, [16] proposed the so-called Log-Euclidean metrics, which exhibit the same properties while being much easier to compute. As these metrics simply consist in taking a standard Euclidean metric after a (matrix) logarithm, we rely on this one for the current article. However, the Riemannian Elasticity principle can be generalized to any Riemannian metric on the tensor space without any restriction.

In this framework, the deviation between the tensor Σ and the identity is the tangent vector $\log(\Sigma)$. Interestingly, this tensor is known in continuum mechanics as the logarithmic or Hencky strain tensor and is used for modeling very large deformations. It is considered as the natural strain tensor for many materials, but its use was hampered for a long time because of its computational complexity [17]. For registration, the basic idea is to replace the elastic energy with a regularization that measures the amount of logarithmic strain by taking the Riemannian distance between Σ and Id. This give the *Riemannian elasticity*:

$$Reg_{RE}(\Phi) = \frac{1}{4} \int \operatorname{dist}^2_{Log}(\Sigma, \mathrm{Id}) = \frac{1}{4} \int \|\log(\Sigma) - \log(\mathrm{Id})\|_2^2 = \frac{1}{4} \int \operatorname{Tr}\left(\log(\Sigma)^2\right)$$

It is worth noticing that the logarithmic distance is inverse-consistent, i.e. that $\operatorname{Tr}\left(\log(\Sigma(\Phi(x)))^2\right) = \operatorname{Tr}\left(\log(\Sigma(\Phi^{(-1)}(y)))^2\right)$ if $y = \Phi(x)$. This comes from the fact that $\nabla(\Phi^{(-1)})(y) = (\nabla\Phi(x))^{(-1)}$. In particular, a scaling of a factor 2 is now at the same distance from the identity than a scaling of 0.5, and the "black hole" transformation is at an infinite distance from any acceptable deformation.

3.2 Incorporating Deformation Statistics

To incorporate statistics in this framework, we consider the strain tensor as a random variable in the Riemannian space of tensors. In the context of inter-subject or atlas-to-image registration, this statistical point of view is particularly well adapted since we do not know a priori the deformability of the material. Starting from a population of transformations $\Phi_i(x)$, we define the *a priori* deformability $\bar{\Sigma}(x)$ as the Riemannian mean of deformation tensors $\Sigma_i(x) = \nabla\Phi_i^{\mathrm{T}}\, \nabla\Phi_i$. A related idea was suggested directly on the Jacobian matrix of the transformation $\nabla\Phi$ in [18], but using a general matrix instead of a symmetric one raises important computational and theoretical problems. With the Log-Euclidean metric on strain tensors, the statistics are quite simple since we have a closed form for the mean value:

$$\bar{\Sigma}(x) = \exp(\bar{W}(x)) \quad \text{with} \quad \bar{W}(x) = \frac{1}{N} \sum_i \log(\Sigma_i(x))$$

Going one step further, we can compute the covariance matrix of the random process $\operatorname{Cov}(\Sigma_i(x))$. Let us decompose the symmetric tensor $W = \log(\Sigma)$ into a vector $\mathrm{Vect}(W)^{\mathrm{T}} = (w_{11}, w_{22}, w_{33}, \sqrt{2}w_{12}, \sqrt{2}w_{13}, \sqrt{2}w_{23})$ that gathers all the tensor components in an orthonormal basis. In this coordinate system, we can define the covariance matrix $\mathrm{Cov} = \frac{1}{N}\sum \mathrm{Vect}(W_i - \bar{W})\,\mathrm{Vect}(W_i - \bar{W})^{\mathrm{T}}$.

To take into account these first and second order moments of the random deformation process, a well known and simple tool is the Mahalanobis distance, so that we finally define the *statistical Riemannian elasticity (SRE)* energy as:

$$Reg_{SRE}(\Phi) = \tfrac{1}{4}\int \mu^2_{(\bar{W},Cov)}(\log(\Sigma(x))) = \tfrac{1}{4}\int \mathrm{Vect}(W-\bar{W})\mathrm{Cov}^{(-1)}\mathrm{Vect}(W-\bar{W})^{\mathrm{T}}$$

As we are using a Mahalanobis distance, this least-squares criterion can be seen as the log-likelihood of a Gaussian process on strain tensor fields: we are implicitly modeling the a-priori probability of the deformation. In a registration framework, this point of view is particularly interesting as it opens the way to use Bayesian estimation methods for non-linear registration.

4 Isotropic Riemannian Elasticity

With the general statistical Riemannian elasticity, we can take into account the anisotropic properties of the material, as they could be revealed by the statistics. However, in order to better explain the properties of this new tool, we focus in the following on isotropic covariances matrices. Seen as a quadratic form, the covariance is isotropic if $\mu^2(W) = \mu^2(R\,W\,R^{\mathrm{T}})$ for any rotation R. This means that it only depends on the eigenvalues of W, or equivalently on the matrix invariants $\mathrm{Tr}(W)$, $\mathrm{Tr}(W^2)$ and $\mathrm{Tr}(W^3)$. However, as the form is quadratic in W, we are left only with $\mathrm{Tr}(W)^2$ and $\mathrm{Tr}(W^2)$ that can be weighted arbitrarily, e.g. by μ and $\lambda/2$. Finally, the *isotropic Riemannian elasticity (IRE)* energy has the form:

$$Reg_{IRE}(\Phi) = \int \tfrac{\mu}{4}\mathrm{Tr}\left((\log(\Sigma) - \bar{W})^2\right) + \tfrac{\lambda}{8}\mathrm{Tr}(\log(\Sigma) - \bar{W})^2$$

For a null mean $\bar{W}$, we retrieve the classical form of isotropic elastic energy with Lamé coefficients, but with the logarithmic strain tensor. This form was expected as the St Venant-Kirchoff energy was also derived for isotropic materials.

4.1 Optimizing the Riemannian Elasticity

To use the logarithmic elasticity energy as a regularization criterion in the registration framework we summarized in Section 2, we have to compute its gradient. Let as assume that $\bar{W} = 0$. Thanks to the properties of the differential of the log [19], we have $\mathrm{Tr}(\partial_V \log(\Sigma)) = \mathrm{Tr}(\Sigma^{(-1)}\,V)$ and $\langle\, \partial_V \log(\Sigma) \mid W \,\rangle = \langle\, \partial_W \log(\Sigma) \mid V \,\rangle$. Thus, using $V = \partial_u \Sigma = \sum_\alpha (\partial_\alpha u\,\partial_\alpha \Phi^{\mathrm{T}} + \partial_\alpha \Phi\,\partial_\alpha u^{\mathrm{T}})$ and $W = \log(\Sigma)$, we can write the directional derivative of the criterion:

$$\begin{aligned}
\partial_u Reg_{IRE}(\Phi) &= \int \tfrac{\mu}{2}\,\langle\, W \mid \partial_V \log(\Sigma)\,\rangle + \tfrac{\lambda}{4}\mathrm{Tr}(W)\,\mathrm{Tr}(\partial_V \log(\Sigma))\\
&= \int \tfrac{\mu}{2}\,\langle\, \partial_W \log(\Sigma) \mid V\,\rangle + \tfrac{\lambda}{4}\mathrm{Tr}(W)\,\mathrm{Tr}(\Sigma^{(-1)}\,V)\\
&= \textstyle\sum_\alpha \int \mu\,\langle\, \partial_W \log(\Sigma)\,\partial_\alpha\Phi \mid \partial_\alpha u\rangle + \tfrac{\lambda}{2}\mathrm{Tr}(W)\,\langle\, \Sigma^{(-1)}\,\partial_\alpha \Phi \mid \partial_\alpha u\,\rangle
\end{aligned}$$

Integrating once again by part with homogeneous Neumann boundary conditions, we end up with the gradient:

$$\nabla Reg_{IRE}(\Phi) = -\sum_\alpha \partial_\alpha (Z\, \partial_\alpha \Phi) \quad \text{with} \quad Z = \mu\, \partial_W \log(\Sigma) + \tfrac{\lambda}{2} \mathrm{Tr}(W)\, \Sigma^{(-1)} \qquad (2)$$

Notice the similarity with the gradient of the standard elasticity (eq. 1). For a non null mean deformation $\bar{W}(x)$, we just have to replace W by $W - \bar{W}$ in the above formula. One can even show that the same formula still holds for the general statistical Riemannian elasticity with $Z = \partial_X \log(\Sigma)$ where X is the symmetric matrix defined by $\mathrm{Vect}(X) = \mathrm{Cov}^{(-1)}\, \mathrm{Vect}(\log(\Sigma))$.

4.2 Practical Implementation

Thus, we can optimize the logarithmic elasticity exactly like we did in Section 2.2 for the Euclidean elasticity. The only additional cost is the computation of the tensor Z, which implies the computation of the logarithm $W = \log(\Sigma)$ and its directional derivative $\partial_W \log(\Sigma)$. This cost would probably be prohibitive if we had to rely on numerical approximation methods. Fortunately, we were able to compute an explicit and very simple closed-form expression that only requires the diagonalization $\Sigma = R\, D\, R^{\mathrm{T}}$ [19]:

$$[R^{\mathrm{T}}\, \partial_V \log(\Sigma)\, R]_{ij} = [R^{\mathrm{T}}\, V\, R]_{ij}\, \lambda_{ij} \quad \text{with} \quad \lambda_{ij} = (\log(d_i) - \log(d_j))/(d_i - d_j)$$

Notice that formula is computationally well posed since $\lambda_{ij} = \frac{1}{d}(1 + \frac{1}{12}\varepsilon^2 d^2 + \frac{1}{80}\varepsilon^4 d^4 + O(\varepsilon^6))$ with $d = (d_i + d_j)/2$ and $\varepsilon = d_i - d_j$.

5 Experiments

To evaluate the potential of the Riemannian elasticity as a regularization criterion in non-rigid registration, we implemented the following basic gradient descent algorithm: at each iteration, the algorithm computes the gradient of the similarity criterion (we chose the local correlation coefficient to take image biases into account), and adds the derivative of the Euclidean or the Riemannian elastic energies according Sections 2.1 and 4.1. Then, a fraction η of this gradient is added to the current displacement field. This loop is embedded in a multi-scale pyramid to capture larger deformations. At each pyramid step, iterations are stopped when the evolution of the transformation is too small (typically a hundred iterations by level). The whole algorithm is implemented in C++, and parallelized using Message Passing Interface (MPI) library on a cluster of PCs.

We tested the algorithm on clinical T1 weighted MR images of the brain of Parkinsonian patients (see Fig. 1). The ROI including the full head has 186 x 124 x 216 voxels of size 0.94 x 1.30 x 0.94 mm. Images were first affine registered and intensity corrected. We used a fraction $\eta = 5.10^{-4}$ for the gradient descent and standard values $\mu = \lambda = 0.2$ for both Euclidean and isotropic Riemannian elastic energies. The algorithm took about 1h for the Euclidean elasticity and 3h for the isotropic Riemannian regularization on a cluster of 12 AMD bi-Opteron PC at 2

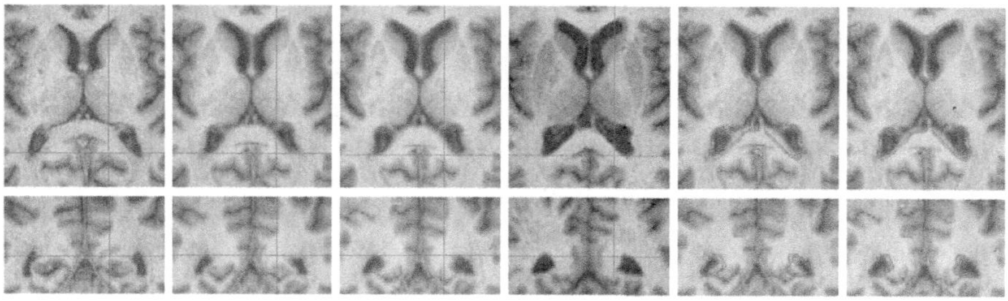

Fig. 1. Experimental comparison of registration with the Euclidean and the Riemannian elasticity regularization. From left to right, we displayed corresponding zoom of axial and coronal slices of: the source image, the elastically deformed source image, the Riemannian elastic result, the target image and the elastic and Riemannian results with the contours of the target image superimposed. Euclidean and Riemannian results are globally equivalent. One can only notice a slightly larger and better deformation of the right ventricle (near the crossing of the axes) with the Riemannian elasticity.

Ghz, connected by a gigabit Ethernet Network. These computations times show that our basic implementation of the Riemannian Elasticity is only 3 times slower than the Euclidean one. The diagonalization of the symmetric matrices being performed using a standard Jacobi method, we could easily design a much more efficient computation in dimensions 2 and 3. In terms of deformation, the results are quite similar for both methods *in the absence of any a priori statistical information.* However, we expect to show in the near future that taking into account statistical information about the expected deformability improves the results both in terms of accuracy and robustness.

6 Conclusion

We proposed in this paper an integrated framework to compute the statistics on deformations and re-introduce them as constraints in non-linear registration algorithms. This framework is based on the interpretation of the elastic energy as a Euclidean distance between the Cauchy-Green strain tensor and the identity (i.e. the local rigidity). By providing the space of tensors with a more suitable Riemannian metric, namely a Log-Euclidean one, we can define proper statistics on deformations, like the mean and the covariance matrix. Taking these measurements into account in a statistical (i.e. a Mahalanobis) distance, we end-up with the statistical Riemannian elasticity regularization criterion. This criterion can also be viewed as the log-likelihood of the deformation probability, which opens the way to Bayesian deformable image registration algorithms.

Riemannian elasticity gives a natural framework to measure statistics on inter-subject deformations. We demonstrate with the isotropic version that it is also an effective regularization criterion for non-linear registration algorithms. There is of course room for a lot of improvements that we plan to tackle in the near future. We are currently computing the deformation statistics (mean and covariance of the logarithmic strain tensor) on a database of brain images to assess their impact on the registration results. We also plan to evaluate carefully how the implementation influences the theoretical inverse-consistency property of the Riemannian elasticity, as this feature may turn out to be very useful for fine measurements of volume changes.

References

1. R. Bajcsy and S. Kovačič. Multiresolution elastic matching. *Computer Vision, Graphics and Image Processing*, 46:1–21, 1989.
2. G. E. Christensen, S. C. Joshi, and M. I. Miller. Volumetric transformation of brain anatomy. *IEEE Trans. Med. Imaging*, 16(6):864–877, 1997.
3. J.-P. Thirion. Image matching as a diffusion process: an analogy with maxwell's demons. *Medical Image Analysis*, 2(3), 1998.
4. Jan Modersitzki. *Numerical Methods for Image Registration.* Numerical Mathematics and Scientific Computations. Oxford University Press, 2004.
5. H. Lester, S.R. Arridge, K.M. Jansons, L. Lemieux, J.V. Hajnal, and A. Oatridge. Non-linear registration with the variable viscosity fluid algorithm. In *Proc of IPMI;99*, pages 238–251, 1999.
6. R. Stefanescu, X. Pennec, and N. Ayache. Grid powered nonlinear image registration with locally adaptive regularization. *Med. Image Anal.*, 8(3):325–342, 2004.
7. P.M. Thompson, M.S. Mega, K.L. Narr, E.R. Sowell, R.E. Blanton, and A.W. Toga. Brain image analysis and atlas construction. In M. Fitzpatrick and M. Sonka, editors, *Handbook of Medical Image Proc. and Analysis*, chapter 17. SPIE, 2000.
8. D. Rueckert, A.F. Frangi, and J.A. Schnabel. Automatic construction of 3D statistical deformation models of the brain using non-rigid registration. *IEEE TMI*, 22:1014–1025, 2003.
9. P. Fillard, V. Arsigny, X. Pennec, P. Thompson, and N. Ayache. Extrapolation of sparse tensor fields: Application to the modeling of brain variability. In *Proc. of IPMI'05*, LNCS, Glenwood springs, CO, USA, July 2005. Springer.
10. P.G. Ciarlet. *Mathematical elasticity Vol. 1: Three-dimensionnal elasticity.* Elsevier Science B.V., 1988.
11. GE Christensen and HJ. Johnson. Consistent image registration. *IEEE Trans Med Imaging*, 20(7):568–82, July 2001.
12. P. Batchelor, M. Moakher, D. Atkinson, F. Calamante, and A. Connelly. A rigorous framework for diffusion tensor calculus. *Mag. Res. in Med.*, 53:221–225, 2005.
13. P.T. Fletcher and S.C. Joshi. Principal geodesic analysis on symmetric spaces: Statistics of diffusion tensors. In *Proc. of CVAMIA and MMBIA Workshops, Prague, Czech Republic, May 15, 2004*, LNCS 3117, pages 87–98. Springer, 2004.
14. Ch. Lenglet, M. Rousson, R. Deriche, and O. Faugeras. Statistics on multivariate normal distributions: A geometric approach and its application to diffusion tensor MRI. Research Report 5242, INRIA, 2004.
15. X. Pennec, P. Fillard, and N. Ayache. A Riemannian framework for tensor computing. *IJCV*, 65(1), October 2005. Also as INRIA Research Report 5255.
16. V. Arsigny, P. Fillard, X. Pennec, and N. Ayache. Fast and simple calculus on tensors in the Log-Euclidean framework. In *Proc. of MICCAI'05*, LNCS, Palm Springs, California, October 2005. Springer Verlag. To Appear.
17. A.D. Freed. Natural strain. *J. of Eng. Materials & Technology*, 117:379–385, 1995.
18. R.P. Woods. Characterizing volume and surface deformations in an atlas framework: theory, applications, and implementation. *NeuroImage*, 18(3):769–788, 2003.
19. V. Arsigny, X. Pennec, P. Fillard, and N. Ayache. Dispositif perfectionné de traitement ou de production d'images de tenseurs. Patent filing 0503483, April 2005.

3D Model-Based Approach to Lung Registration and Prediction of Respiratory Cardiac Motion

Mikhail G. Danilouchkine*, Jos J.M. Westenberg, Hans C. van Assen, Johan H.C. van Reiber, and Boudewijn P.F. Lelieveldt

Division of Image Processing, Dept. Radiology, Leiden University Medical Center, Leiden, The Netherlands

Abstract. This paper presents a new approach for lung registration and cardiac motion prediction, based on a 3D geometric model of the left lung. Feature points, describing a shape of this anatomical object, are automatically extracted from acquired tomographic images. The "goodness-of-fit" measure is assessed at each step in the iterative scheme until spatial alignment between the model and subject's specific data is achieved. We applied the proposed methods to register the 3D lung surfaces of 5 healthy volunteers of thoracic MRI acquired in different respiratory phases. We also utilized this approach to predict the spatial displacement of the human heart due to respiration. The obtained results demonstrate a promising registration performance.

1 Introduction

Over the past decennium image registration has been receiving a significant amount of attention from the medical image processing community. Registration methods aim at establishing a spatial alignment between the tomographic images that were taken at different time points or under different conditions or with different imaging modalities. A vast number of different registration algorithms have been proposed and exhaustively reviewed in literature [1]. Registration algorithms can be split into the following broad categories: intensity- [2,3] and feature-based [4,5] methods or a hybrid of both approaches [6].

The intensity-based methods provide the most accurate way for spatial alignment between two image sets. A registration is performed by transforming one image set with respect to the other and optimizing a measure based on pairs of overlapping voxels. Different similarity measures (i.e. normalized cross correlation, mutual information of pixel intensities etc.) have been adopted to govern the optimization procedure. In spite of the fact that the intensity-based registration algorithms are optimal in terms of accuracy, they remain computationally expensive. The feature-based methods offer a better alternative with respect to numerical efficiency. Commonly two surfaces or point sets, describing the shape

* Partially funded by the Dutch Foundation for Technical Sciences (STW LPG 5651). M.Danilouchkine is now at the Dept. Cardiology, Erasmus Medical Center, Rotterdam, the Netherlands.

J. Duncan and G. Gerig (Eds.): MICCAI 2005, LNCS 3750, pp. 951–959, 2005.

of the same anatomical objects, are aligned with each other, based on a mean squared distance metric. The feature-based registration methods are extremely sensitive to initial mutual alignment of the feature sets.

In this paper, we propose a new model-based registration approach, that combines the best features of the registration algorithms of both categories. We strive to achieve the accuracy comparable with one of the intensity-based registration methods without sacrificing the computational efficiency. Moreover, the model-based approach is much less sensitive to initial misalignment of the feature points with the geometric model.

In this work we adopted the model-driven segmentation method for thoracic MRI images and automated recognition of the organs with the profound air-tissue boundaries proposed in [7]. A new concept of multi-resolution registration is introduced. It significantly improves the computational efficiency and convergence to the globally optimal solution. The energy minimization functional, reflecting a "goodness-of-fit" measure, was adapted to meet the new requirements. This approach is applied to registration of left lung MRI images in extreme respiratory states and to predict the cardiac motion due to respiration.

2 Methods

The components of the model-based registration framework and their interconnections are shown in Fig.1. The basic input data for the registration process are the geometric model of an anatomical organ and the representative set of the feature points describing the same organ. Registration is treated as an optimization problem aimed at finding the spatial mapping that aligns the feature points with the geometric model. The transform component represents the spatial mapping of the features points to the model space. Metric provides a "goodness-of-fit" measure of how well the feature points are brought into alignment with the

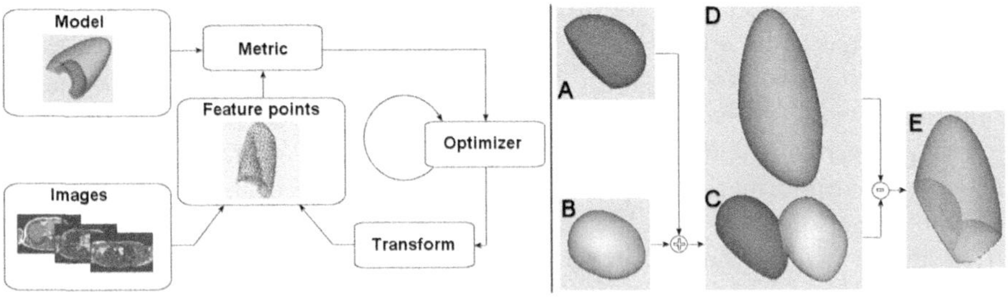

Fig. 1. The main components of the model-based registration framework (left panel). The right panel depicts the 3D geometric model, consisting of the heart (A), spleen (B) and left lung (D) primitives. Those primitives are combined together by means of boolean operators, e.g. *union*-operator for the heart-spleen composite (C) and *difference*-operator for the final model (E), describing the complex shape of the left lung.

model. This measure is the quantitative criterion to be optimized by the optimizer over the search space defined by the transformation parameters.

2.1 3D Geometric Model of Left Lung

Among the vast variety of different modeling paradigms, Implicit Solid Modeling (ISM) [8] allows to describe the shape of an anatomical object in terms of an algebraic implicit function of the spatial coordinates $F(x, y, z)$. The set of points where the function has a predefined cutoff value c describes the surface of the modeled anatomical object. Its interior and exterior are associated with the points where $F(x, y, z) < c$ and $F(x, y, z) > c$, respectively. Different F's can be deduced to describe the analytical template, called primitive, of different anatomical objects. Primitives are organized in a tree-like structure to describe intermediate composites and the final model. The primitives form the leaves of the tree, while the nodes are boolean operators such as differences, unions, etc. The geometric properties of this model are thus expressed in the primitives, while the topological characteristics are stored in the relational tree. Fig. 1 shows the 3D geometric model of the left lung constructed by means of ISM.

2.2 Feature Points

The feature points, describing the shape of the modeled anatomical organ (e. g. left lung), can be extracted automatically from the tomographic images of the examined subject. A cumulative pixel-intensity histogram of scout images typically has a bimodal distribution: one peak corresponds to the pixels with low attenuation or air, contained in the lungs, and the other peak is attributed to tissue or thoracic organs. Expectation-Maximization [9] histogram-based clustering can be utilized to determine the brightness values for air and tissue classes. By fitting a two-component mixture of Gaussian distributions and assigning the class labels according to a maximum *a-posteriori* criterion, the final segmentation of the scout images can be obtained. A set of tuples (x_i, g_i) constitutes the automatically detected feature points, where x_i is a vector of the spatial coordinates of the air-tissue boundaries and g_i is the image gradient at the point x_i.

2.3 Metric and Optimizer

A metric characterizes the fit between the model and feature points. It is defined via the boundary distance field, which was first introduced in [7]. This field represents a mapping $b_\Delta : R^3 \to R$ that computes a value for each point according to the following formula:

$$b_\Delta(x_i) = \begin{cases} |d(x_i)|/\Delta, & |d(x_i)| < \Delta; \\ 1, & |d(x_i)| > \Delta. \end{cases} \tag{1}$$

where $d(x_i) \approx (F(x_i) - c) / \|\overline{\nabla} F(x_i)\|$ is the orthogonal distance from the feature point x_i to the surface of the model; Δ is the effective range of the boundary distance field. The boundary distance value is equal to 0 for the points lying on the model surface, and exhibits approximately linear behavior in the vicinity of the surfaces as the distance to the model surface increases. Outside the effective range, this value is equal to 1.

The energy minimization function to be optimized is given by the formula:

$$E(x_i, g_i) = \sum_{i=1}^{N} w(x_i, g_i) b_{\Delta}^2(x_i) + \rho \cdot \frac{N - \tilde{N}}{N}, \quad \text{where} \tag{2}$$

$$w(x_i, g_i) = \exp\left\{\alpha\left(1 - \arccos\frac{\overline{\nabla} F(x_i) \cdot g_i}{\|\overline{\nabla} F(x_i)\| \cdot \|g_i\|}\right)\right\} \tag{3}$$

The first term in Eq. 2 is a weighted sum of squares of the boundary distance values and quantifies proximity of the feature points to the model. The weighting factor w assures the topological alignment of the feature points. It attains the minimum, when the image gradient lies along the direction of the model gradient, and maximum, when those vectors point in the opposite directions. The second term in Eq. 2 is a penalty factor proportional to the relative number of points lying outside the effective range of the distance field (N - the total number of points and $\tilde{N}$ - the number of points inside the boundary distance field).

The energy minimization function can be optimized by introducing variations in the spatial positioning, scaling and rotation of the feature points. Since the minimization function is the sum of squares, a numerically stable method (e.g. Levenberg-Marquardt [10]) is used in the optimization procedure.

2.4 Multi-resolution Optimization

Multi-resolution approaches are usually employed to improve the computational efficiency and robustness of the registration algorithms. Initially the optimization

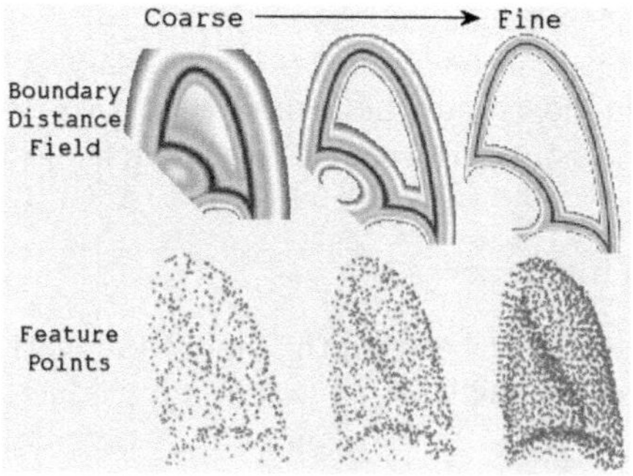

Fig. 2. Multi-resolution approach employed in the model-based registration. The varying effective range of the boundary scalar field (top row) improves robustness of the optimization procedure (boundary distance values are color coded with blue (dark) corresponding to 0 and yellow (light) - to 1), while the variable sparsity factor applied to the feature points (bottom row) increases the computational efficiency.

procedure is solved at the coarsest level. The obtained results are used as a starting guess for finding a solution at the next finer level. The whole procedure iterates until the finest level is reached.

To improve the robustness of the model-based registration, the effective range of the boundary distance field depends on the resolution scale (Fig.2). At the coarsest level, this range is made large. The optimization procedure is primarily governed by the first term of the energy minimization function Eq. 2. The results obtained at a coarser level are subsequently propagated to the next finer level with reduced range of the boundary distance field. At the finer levels both terms in Eq. 2 are equally important. Due to the narrowing effective range, small variations in the spatial positioning, scaling and rotation of the feature points may result in some points moving outside the boundary scalar field, introducing irregularities in the energy minimization function. However, such variations are penalized by the second term, locking the feature points in the vicinity of the global solution and increasing the robustness of the optimization procedure.

The computational efficiency of the model-based registration algorithm is mainly determined by its numerical complexity. The latter can be roughly estimated as $O(MN)$, where N is the number of the feature points and M is the number of primitives constituting the geometric model. While the number of the primitives remains constant, the number of the feature points used at the different resolution scales is made variable. At a coarser level, the optimization procedure is applied to a sparser subset of the extracted feature points, yielding fewer computational costs. At the finer levels the number of the feature points is gradually increased, providing more accurate description of the object of interest and better mutual alignment with the model.

3 Results

In-vivo scout images were obtained from 5 healthy volunteers using a Philips Gyroscan Intera 1.5T MRI scanner. A balanced-FFE protocol (TR 2.32 ms; TE 1.16 ms; flip angle 55°) with prospective VCG was utilized to acquire 60 thoracic images in three standard projections (20 transversal, 20 sagittal, 20 coronal). Two sets of scout images were obtained at full inspiration and expiration for each subject. All volunteers were instructed to withhold from breathing during acquisition. The field of view and slice thickness were equal to 450 mm and 8 mm, respectively. The reconstruction matrix of 256x256 was used, yielding the effective in-plane resolution of 1.75 mm/pixel.

In the first experiment, the model-based registration method was used to identify the anatomically homologous cross-sections of the left lung in extreme respiratory states. The geometric model of this anatomical organ provided the common reference frame for registration. Two sets of the feature points, describing the shape of the left lung of the examined person at full inspiration and expiration, were automatically extracted from the acquired scout images. Both sets were aligned with the model, resulting in two sets of the transformation parameters. A stack of parallel, equidistantly spaced intersecting planes, span-

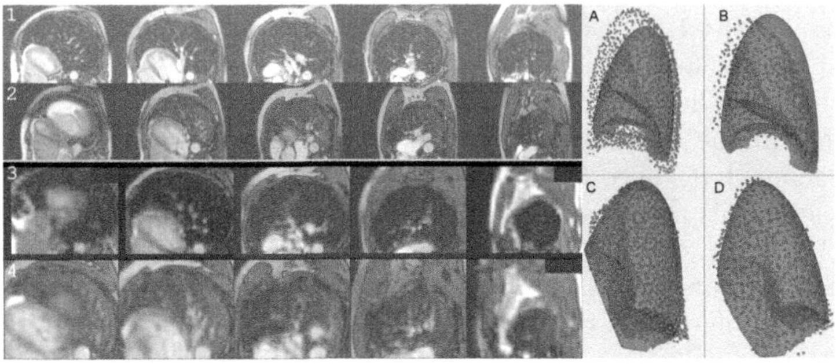

Fig. 3. The results of model-based registration. The spatially homologous cross-sections of the left lung (columns of the first two rows to the left), acquired at full inspiration (1st row) and expiration (2nd rows) show the effect of respiration. The morphologically homologous cross-sections (columns of last two rows to the left), reconstructed after registration, exhibit the anatomical coherence of the left lung appearance. Initial misalignment of the feature points at full inspiration (A) and expiration (B) does not affect the final registration results (C,D).

ning the whole extent of the geometric model in the axial direction, was used to identify the morphologically homologous cross-sections in *in-vivo* imaging data. The geometric parameters of those intersecting planes were projected back from the model into imaging domain by applying the inverse transformation, obtained during registration. The morphologically homologous cross-sections, reconstructed after registration, exhibit the anatomical coherence of the left lung in different slices and are shown in Fig. 3. Before registration, the lung size is generally smaller at full expiration in all slices. Moreover, the cross-section with the liver in the most inferior slice is only visible at full expiration. After registration, the size of the lung is approximately the same in all cross-sections.

Table 1. The results of the quantitative comparison of model- and intensity-based registration approaches (two first columns) using the normalized cross-correlation metric. The assessment of respiratory motion of the heart are summarized in last three columns. The levels of statistical insignificance were found for $^{*} = 0.54$ and for $^{**} = 0.41$.

	NCC*		Heart Displacement (mm)**		
	Intensity-based	Model-based	Actual	Predicted	Abs.Diff.
Normal 1	0.70	0.76	32.76	29.01	3.75
Normal 2	0.92	0.79	26.66	30.62	3.96
Normal 3	0.84	0.82	22.20	26.95	4.75
Normal 4	0.73	0.72	32.35	28.37	3.98
Normal 5	0.77	0.73	28.86	32.55	3.68
Mean	0.79	0.76	28.57	29.50	4.03
StdDev	0.09	0.04	4.36	2.16	0.42

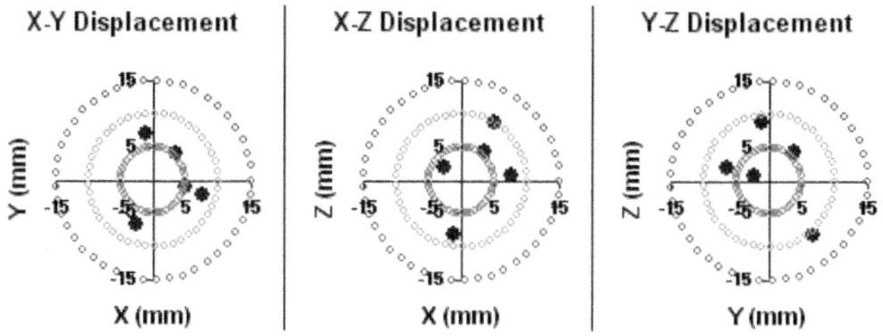

Fig. 4. Difference between actual and predicted heart displacement in projection onto the coordinate planes. The errors are of the same order of magnitude in all projections.

The accuracy of model-based registration was evaluated using the normalized cross-correlation (NCC). The correlation coefficient, normalized by the square root of the autocorrelation, was used to assess the similarity between the morphologically homologous stacks of the left lung at full expiration and inspiration. The NCC results for all subjects as well as the mean and standard deviation are presented in the second column of Tab. 1. For quantitative comparison, the intensity-based registration method was implemented using the Insight Toolkit (ITK) [11]. Prior to registration, the Volume-Of-Interest (VOI) containing the left lung was manually outlined for all subjects and two respiratory states. The affine image registration technique, based on normalized mutual information as a voxel similarity measure and the multi-resolution matching strategy, was employed to align the VOI's at full expiration and inspiration. The quality of intensity-based registration was finally measured using the NCC metric and is shown in the first column of Tab. 1.

In our second experiment, we numerically assessed the displacement of the heart due to respiration. The actual and predicted displacements of the heart were quantitatively compared. The actual displacement was computed by manually delineating the left ventricular (LV) blood pool in all visible cross-sections of the chamber in the scout images, by estimation of the LV center by calculation of the center-of-gravity of the boundary points, and by quantifying the distance between these centers at full expiration and inspiration. The predicted displacement was estimated by back-projection of the center of the LV, comprising the model primitive, from the model to imaging domain using two inverse transformations, obtained during the registration in full exhalation and inhalation. The actual and predicted displacements of the heart along with the absolute difference are shown in last three columns of Tab. 1 and Fig. 4.

4 Discussion and Conclusions

The results show that this new algorithm is a promising tool for left lung registration. The model-based registration with the multi-resolution matching strategy is a fast way of establishing alignment of the left lung in different respiratory states and gives comparable accuracy as the intensity-based registration. The algorithm also produces plausible matches while depending less on correct initial alignment between the feature points and model (Fig. 3). Computational costs for model-based registration amount to 10-12 sec. per match against 60-75 sec. for the intensity-based registration method on a Pentium 2.8 GHz with 1024 MB memory capacity. In particular, the model-based registration is also suitable for the quantitative analysis of respiratory motion of the heart. Our findings are in excellent agreement with those of McLeish [12], obtained with the intensity-based rigid registration of the lungs in extreme respiratory phases.

The proposed model-based registration method was based on two assumptions. Firstly, ISM effectively but coarsely allows to represent the shape of anatomical organs with moderately complex shapes such as lungs and is less suitable to represent highly complex shapes such as cortical sulci or brain ventricles. Secondly, there is a single affine transformation that matches the set of feature points against the model. Although not strictly true, this assumption provides a global but accurate conformal mapping between lungs in extreme respiratory states. That mapping can be beneficial in establishing preliminary correspondence between the major anatomical landmarks of the modeled organ and subsequent intensity-based registration of the lungs in oncological applications [13,14]. Further improvement involves non-rigid transformation that allows to recover local deformation due to the shape changes in the lungs and should be considered as a potential extension of the model-based registration framework.

References

1. Maintz, J.B.A., Viergever, M.A.: A survey of medical image registration. MEDIA **2** (1998) 1–36
2. Wells, W.M., Viola, P., Atsumi, H., Nakajima, S., Kikinis, R.: Multi-modal volume regsitration by maximization of mutual information. MEDIA **1** (1996) 35–51
3. Rueckert, D., Sonoda, L.I., Hayes, C., Hill, D.L.G., Leach, M.O., Hawkes, D.J.: Non-rigid registration using free-form deformations: Application to breast mr images. IEEE TMI **18** (1999) 712–721
4. Besl, P.J., McKay, N.D.: A method for registration of 3d shapes. IEEE PAMI **14** (1992) 239–256
5. Rangarajan, A., Chui, H., Duncan, J.S.: Rigid point feature registration using mutual information. MEDIA **3** (1999) 425–440
6. Stewart, C.V., Lee, Y.L., Tsai, C.L.: An uncertainty-driven hybrid of intensity-based and feature-based registration with application to retinal and lung ct images. In: Proc. MICCAI. LNCS 3216 (2004) 870–877
7. Lelieveldt, B.P.F., Sonka, M., Bolinger, L., Scholz, T.D., van der Geest, H.K.R., Reiber, J.H.C.: Anatomical modeling with fuzzy implicit surface templates: Application to automated localization of the heart and lungs in thoracic mr volumes. CVIU **80** (2000) 1–20
8. Storti, D.W., Ganter, M.A., Nevrinceanu, C.: Tutorial on implicit solid modeling. Mathematica J **2** (1992) 70–78
9. Dempster, A.P., Laird, N.M., Rubin, D.B.: Maximum likelihood from incomplete data via the em algorithm. J Royal Stat Soc(B) **39** (1977) 1–38
10. Press, W.H., Flannery, B.P., Teukolsky, S.A., Vetterling, W.T.: Numerical Recipes in C: The Art of Scientific Computing. Cambridge Univ Press (1992)

11. Ibáñez, L., Ng, L., Gee, J., Aylward, S.: Registration patterns: The generic framework for image registration of the insight toolkit. In: Proc. IEEE Int Symp Biomed Imaging. (2002) 345–348
12. McLeish, K., Hill, D.L.G., Atkinson, D.A., Blackall, J.M., Razavi, R.: A study of the motion and deformation of the heart due to respiration. IEEE TMI **21** (2002) 1142–1150
13. Betke, M., Hong, H., Ko, J.P.: Automatic 3d registration of lung surfaces in computed tomography scans. In: Proc. MICCAI. LNCS 2208 (2001) 725–733
14. Coselmon, M.M., Balter, J.M., McShan, D.L., Kessler, M.L.: Mutual information based ct registration of the lung at exhale and inhale breathing states using thin-plate splines. Med Phys **31** (2004) 2942–2948

Fast DRR Generation for 2D/3D Registration

W. Birkfellner[1], R. Seemann[1], M. Figl[1], J. Hummel[1,2], C. Ede[1], P. Homolka[1], X. Yang[3], P. Niederer[3], and H. Bergmann[1,2]

[1] Center for Biomedical Engineering and Physics, Medical University Vienna, Austria
wolfgang.birkfellner@meduniwien.ac.at
www.bmtp.akh-wien.ac.at/people/birkwo1
[2] Ludwig-Boltzmann Insitute of Nuclear Medicine, Vienna
[3] Department of Biomedical Engineering, Swiss federal institute of Technology, Zurich, Switzerland

Abstract. We present a simple and rapid method for generation of perspective digitally rendered radiographs (DRR) for 2D/3D registration based on splat rendering. Suppression of discretization artefacts by means of computation of Gaussian footprints – which is a considerable computational burden in classical splat rendering – is replaced by stochastic motion of either the voxels in the volume to be rendered, or by simulation of a X-ray tube focal spot of finite size. The result is a simple and fast perspective rendering algorithm using only a small subset of voxels. Our method generates slightly blurred DRRs suitable for registration purposes at framerates of approximately 10 Hz when rendering volume images with a size of 30 MB on a standard PC.

1 Introduction

Generation of simulated X-ray images or digitally rendered radiographs (DRR) is a key technology in 2D/3D registration for image guided therapy (IGT) [1,2,3] and patient alignment in radiation oncology. In general, a DRR is a simulated X-ray image derived from a computed tomography (CT) volume by simulating the attenuation of virtual X-rays. Therefore a DRR is a perspective volume rendering. Raycasting, the computation of line integrals along selected beams emerging from the viewpoint, appears to be the logical rendering algorithm to fulfill this task. From a practical perspective, this approach is barely feasible. In 2D/3D registration patient alignment is achieved by iteratively solving an optimization problem in 6 degrees-of-freedom (dof). During the optimization, the CT-volume undergoes rigid-body transformations where every dof is varied until an optimum match between DRR and X-ray image is achieved. Due to the complexity of the registration task a considerable number of DRRs have to be computed, and the time required for registration is closely related to the efficiency of DRR generation.

Fast perspective volume rendering for DRR generation is therefore a crucial issue for 2D/3D registration. Several alternatives to conventional raycasting such as lightfield- [4] or shear-warp rendering [5] were proposed in the past. In this

J. Duncan and G. Gerig (Eds.): MICCAI 2005, LNCS 3750, pp. 960–967, 2005.

paper, we present a variation of splat rendering [6] – the direct projection of single voxels to the imaging plane – as a fast and simple alternative to these rendering algorithms. The main advantage of splatting lies in the fact that only voxels above a certain threshold are used for DRR generation; this can reduce the number of voxels to be visited during the rendering process significantly. Typically, a DRR of an abdominal CT scan uses less that 10 % of the voxels for splat rendering of bony tissue. Therefore direct projection of voxels easily outperforms methods such as discrete raycasting by a factor of 10 - 20 depending on the minimum Hounsfield density to be rendered. The inherent problem of direct voxel projection is the massive decrease in image quality due to aliasing artefacts. The original splatting algorithm overcomes this problem by calculation of a 3D Gaussian kernel projected onto the image plane providing a discrete point spread function. For orthogonal projection, these so-called footprints can be computed in a preprocessing step. Unfortunately, this is not feasible for perspective splat rendering. As a result of applying antialiasing techniques, time requirements again increase considerable since for each voxel position in the CT volume, the projection of a discrete Gaussian 3D-kernel has to be computed as well. The initial advantage of the splatting algorithm over raycasting – its shorter execution cycle – is actually reversed by this additional task.

In this paper, we present a simple and efficient method for antialiasing of splat - rendered DRRs avoiding the computation of footprints. DRRs from splat rendering and raycasting are compared, and time requirements for DRR - generation were recorded.

2 Materials and Methods

The basic idea of splatting for generating a DRR is simple. Since the exponential weakening of the X-ray beam during body passage – which derives from the general law of linear attenuation [7], p. 59 ff – can be taken into account on the projected image by logarithmization, a perspective summed voxel rendering is an acceptable volume rendering method for this purpose. Thus, every voxel can be projected by an algebraic perspective projection operator P (actually a 4×4 matrix). A setup where the focal spot is located on the z-axis and the imaging plane lies in the x-y plane is, for instance, a good starting point since it shows some favourable symmetry properties for registration [3].

Motion of the CT data set in this coordinate system is given by a 4×4 matrix V which is composed out of a 3×3 rotation matrix and a translation vector. Details on both operators can be found in the literature, e. g. [1,3].

The contribution of each voxel can be computed by applying these operators to every voxel position $\boldsymbol{x}$ in the CT-volume;

$$\boldsymbol{x}_p = PV\boldsymbol{x} \tag{1}$$

resulting in coordinates $\boldsymbol{x}_p$ on the image plane. The HU of the voxel at location $\boldsymbol{x}$ is added to the actual grayscale value of the pixel located closest to $\boldsymbol{x}_p$. After applying eq. 1 to every voxel and integrating the projected density values, a summed voxel rendering of the CT-volume is the result. Discretization artefacts are inevitable when using this technique.

The method of directly projecting single voxel densities onto the projection plane also reveals the inherent advantage of splatting. Since the ordering of voxels relative to each other is of no importance, one can remove all voxels not contributing to the DRR. In the case of 2D/3D registration, this is usually the CT volume content filled with soft tissue and air. After selecting a minimum and maximum threshold for voxels to be rendered, a single preprocessing step allows for reordering the volume.

It should be stated that eq. 1 can easily be generalized to positions of the X-ray tube different to the geometry resulting in the projection operator P. As long as the projection plane remains normal to the central beam of the X-ray tube (for instance in a C-arm), a rigid body transform V^* similar to the matrix V can be used to model motion of the virtual tube focus. The projection operator P is moved to P^* by computing

$$P^* = V^* P \tag{2}$$

As said before the classical splatting technique overcomes the aliasing problem by means of projecting a Gaussian kernel for every voxel position. While the generation of the lookup table containing the splats is simply a preprocessing step in orthogonal projection, this is not the case for perspective projection. On the other hand, projecting such a kernel for every voxel position is a very time-consuming task. The quality of the antialiasing depends on the size of the Gaussian kernel. Taking into account that computation of a $3 \times 3 \times 3$ kernel requires 27 projections for a single footprint, it is evident that rendering times increase considerably, and that kernels with even larger size are definitely out of discussion. As an alternative, we have tested two methods where artefact suppression is achieved by stochastic motion of various parameters in the splatting process. These methods are a.) Gaussian motion of voxels and b.) Gaussian motion of the viewpoint.

The first method resembles a stochastic variant of the original splatting method; in this case, the projected voxel value is not spread on the projection plane by a footprint but by a stochastic Gaussian displacement of voxel positions $\boldsymbol{x}$ in a small range. For each voxel position $\boldsymbol{x}$, a 3×1 Gaussian random vector $\boldsymbol{u}$ with standard deviation σ and mean 0 is computed using the Box-Muller method. Eq. 1 becomes

$$\boldsymbol{x}_p = PV\left(\boldsymbol{x} + \boldsymbol{u}\right) \tag{3}$$

The standard deviation σ of the Gaussian distribution was chosen in such a manner that 3σ approximately equals the voxel size of the volume used.

The second approach is slightly more sophisticated and has the additional appeal of modelling the physics of X-ray generation. To some extent, it resembles methods for rendering of soft shadows in computer graphics. In general, the focal spot of an X-ray tube is not a mathematical point but an area approximately 2.0 mm in diameter [7], p. 42. This behaviour is simulated by stochastic translation of the projector P. parallel to the x-y plane. An additional benefit of this approach is the fact that only two instead of three random numbers have to be computed, as opposed to the first approach. In detail, a 3×1 Gaussian random vector $\boldsymbol{v} = (v_0, v_1, 0)^T$ is computed. Again, mean of the Gaussian distribution is 0 and standard deviation σ is chosen to be $\sigma = \frac{1}{3} D_{fs}$ where D_{fs} is the diameter of the focal spot to be simulated. This displacement is applied to the projection operator P^* (see eq. 2) by computing

$$P' = V^* \begin{pmatrix} 1 & 0 & 0 & v_0 \\ 0 & 1 & 0 & v_1 \\ 0 & 0 & 1 & 0 \\ 0 & 0 & 0 & 1 \end{pmatrix} P \tag{4}$$

Here, the projection operator P is configured in such a manner that it splats the voxels to the x-y plane and the viewpoint is located at the z-axis. Applying P' instead of P or P^* respectively to the volumes voxel positions (eq. 1) results in geometric unsharpness as caused by a focal spot of finite size. We refer to both methods – the Gaussian distortion of voxel positions within the volume and the Gaussian motion of the virtual focal spot of the projector P as 'wobbled splatting' since the antialiasing effect of footprint evaluation as in the classical splatting method is replaced by a random distortion of some splatting parameters.

A small application named SPLATTER for generation of DRRs was written in C++ using the Qt 3.0 graphical user interface toolkit on standard Pentium IV with 2.8 GHz under SuSE Linux 9.0. Additional image processing functionality was implemented using AVW 6.0 library (Biomedical Imaging Resource, Mayo Clinic, Rochester/MN). The Box-Muller method for generation of random numbers with a Gaussian distribution was taken form the GNU scientific library GSL 1.4 (Free Software Foundation, Boston/MA). All illustrations in this paper were generated using SPLATTER. AVW was provided courtesy of Dr. R. A. Robb, Biomedical Imaging Resource, Mayo Clinic, Rochester/MN.

For testing the various antialiasing methods, three CT volume scans were used. First, a clinical pediatric abdominal scan acquired with a Siemens Sensation CT (Siemens AG, Erlangen, Germany) with an original resolution of $512 \times 512 \times 151$ voxels was used. Since all scans were resampled using linear interpolation to $(1\ \text{mm})^3$ voxels, the scan used for rendering had $237 \times 237 \times 302$ voxels and a size of 32.35 MB. It is to be noted that resampling to cubic voxels is performed for the sake of simplying the splatting algorithm, but it is not a necessity [6]. Second, a scan of a pelvis phantom interpolated to $290 \times 205 \times 200$ voxels and a size of 22.67 MB was used. Finally, a clinical scan of mandible ($172 \times 172 \times 72$ voxels, 4.06 MB) was used. The latter two scans were acquired using a Philips Mx 8000 IDT scanner (Philips AG, Best, The Netherlands).

Evaluation was performed by applying various antialiasing techniques on DRRs rendered with an image size of 256×256 pixels and comparison of the outcome. A high-quality rendering using the interpolated raycasting routine from the AVW library was used as a gold standard.

3 Results

Table 1 gives an overview of the visual outcome from the various antialiasing methods. Results from discrete and interpolated raycasting are also included. Voxel wobbling and focus wobbling combined with lowpass-filtering both provide good results. Figs. 1 and 2 show the effects of footprint evaluation and wobbling. The eight DRRs were rendered with a minmum threshold of 0 HU and a maximum threshold of 3072 HU from the pediatric abdomen scan. Fig. 1 shows considerable artefacts, which cannot be fully removed by multiplication with a footprint table generated from $3 \times 3 \times 3$ Gaussian kernels and subsequent lowpass-filtering (fig. 1).

Fig. 2a shows a DRR generated using the same parameters as the DRRs in fig. 1 but rather than performing a footprint-evaluation, the image was generated with voxels being shifted by a Gaussian motion as given in eq. 3 with zero mean and standard deviation $\sigma = 0.4$ mm. Fig. 2c was generated with static voxel positions; antialiasing is introduced by a Gaussian motion of the focal spot (or 'viewpoint') according to eq. 4 with zero mean and $\sigma = \frac{1}{3}$ mm. While discretization artefacts are compensated for, Gaussian noise is clearly visible in both images. 2D lowpass filtering of the DRRs using a Gaussian 3×3 kernel compensate for this flaw (Figs. 2b and 2d).

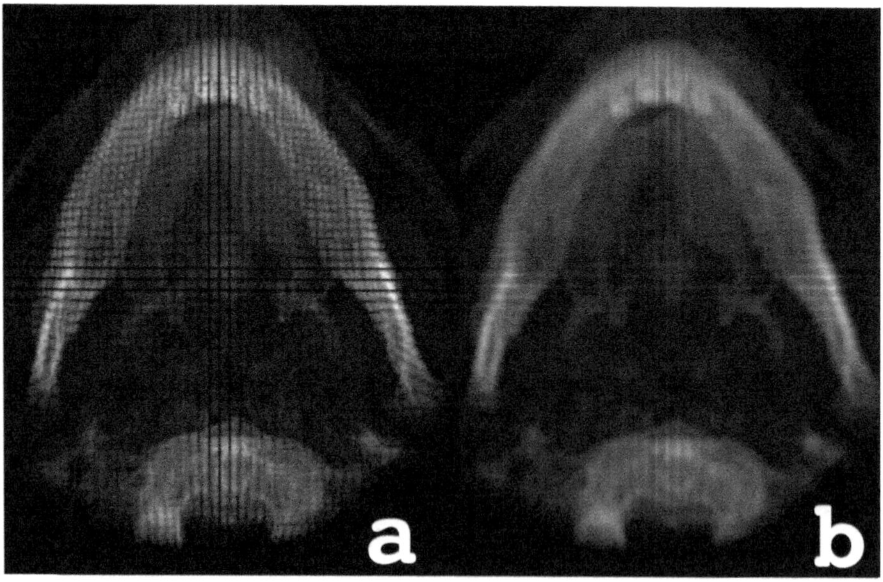

Fig. 1. Results of conventional splatting. The left image shows a direct projection of a mandible CT scan without further antialiasing measures. Discretization artefacts are clearly visible. The right image was splatted using Gaussian 3×3 kernels and lowpass filtering of the resulting DRR with a 3×3 kernel.

Table 2 compares the amount of time required for DRR generation using splatting and raycasting combined with several antialiasing techniques. It is evident that the performance of splat rendering depends on the number of voxels used for DRR generation. Voxel wobbling and focus wobbling combined with subsequent lowpass filtering of the resulting DRR – the antialiasing techniques providing a sufficient result according to table 1 – outperform interpolated raycasting typically by a factor of 20 when using a minimum threshold showing mainly bony tissue. Otherwise, splatting approximately requires the same amount of time as discrete raycasting. It was found that for the DRRs generated for this study, only 5 - 33 % of the voxels had to be used.

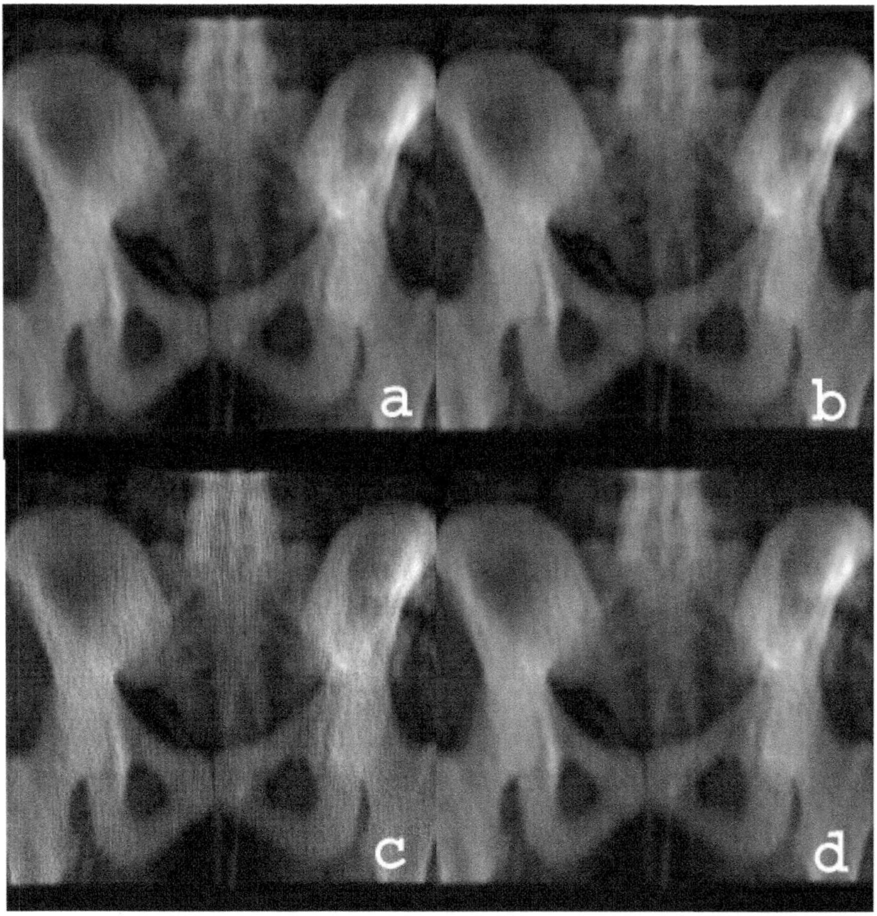

Fig. 2. Results of wobbled splatting. No footprint-table was generated, but either the voxel positions underwent displacement (**a**, voxel wobbling – voxels perform Gaussian movement with mean 0 and standard deviation $\sigma = 0.4$ mm), or the focus position was blurred (**c**, focus wobbling – focal spot performs Gaussian movement with mean 0 and standard deviation $\sigma = 0.33$ mm). **b**) shows **a**) after lowpass-filtering (again with a 3×3 kernel). **d**) shows **c**) after the same filtering procedure.

Table 1. Visual effect of the various combinations of raycasting and antialiasing techniques. Rendering methods are splatting (SPL) and raycasting (RC). Antialiasing measures are lowpass filtering of the DRR using a 3×3 kernel (LP), evaluation of footprints from $3\times3\times3$ Gaussian footprints (GF), voxel wobbling (VW), focus wobbling (FW), and combinations thereof. Outcome was categorized to be heavily stricken with artefacts (−−), aliased (−), fair (...), good (+) and excellent (++).

Renderer/ Anti-aliasing	SPL	SPL/ LP	SPL/ GF	SPL/ VW	SPL/ FW	SPL/ VW, LP	SPL/ FW, LP	SPL/ VW, FW	SPL/ VW, FW,LP	RC	RC/ inter-polation
Visual outcome	−−	−	−	...	...	+	+	...	+	−	++

Table 2. Time required for DRR generation from three different CT scans given in seconds. Splat rendering (SPL) and raycasting (RC) were used as rendering methods. Antialiasing techniques employed for splat rendering were lowpass filtering using a 3×3 Gaussian kernel (LP), prjoection using a footprint (point-spread function) calculated from a $3\times3\times3$ Gaussian kernel (GF), voxel wobbling (VW), focus wobbling (FW), and combiations. Finally, interpolated and discrete raycasting was used as well. Focus and voxel wobbling combined with 2D lowpass filtering – the preferrable antialiasing methods according to table 1 – are printed in boldface.

CT-Volume		Abdomen			Pelvis			Jaw		
		Min. Threshold			*Min. Threshold*			*Min. Threshold*		
Render method	*Anti-aliasing*	-205	0	205	-980	0	350	-1024	0	380
SPL	—	0.92	0.71	0.10	1.41	0.10	0.09	0.19	0.10	0.02
SPL	LP	0.94	0.71	0.10	1.40	0.11	0.12	0.20	0.10	0.02
SPL	GF	43.83	16.87	2.73	33.05	2.52	2.25	4.68	2.20	0.44
SPL	VW	1.24	0.83	0.12	1.65	0.13	0.11	0.23	0.11	0.02
SPL	FW	1.13	0.85	0.12	1.71	0.12	0.12	0.24	0.12	0.02
SPL	**VW, LP**	**1.13**	**0.84**	**0.15**	**1.81**	**0.13**	**0.12**	**0.24**	**0.11**	**0.02**
SPL	**FW, LP**	**1.13**	**0.84**	**0.13**	**1.72**	**0.13**	**0.13**	**0.24**	**0.12**	**0.03**
SPL	VW, FW	1.33	1.00	0.14	2.05	0.15	0.14	0.27	0.13	0.02
SPL	VW, FW, LP	1.40	1.00	0.15	2.03	0.17	0.14	0.28	0.14	0.03
RC	—	1.63	1.68	1.64	1.16	1.07	1.12	0.08	0.09	0.08
RC	interpolation	6.15	2.75	2.33	7.17	1.82	1.77	0.42	0.30	0.13

4 Discussion

A fast DRR algorithm not requiring lengthy preprocessing is definitely desireable for clinical implementations of 2D/3D registration algorithms. For the particular case of iterative DRR generation for registration, splatting has the inherent advantage of its simplicity. The considerable time necessary for generating the footprint tables calls for an alternative solution for the reduction of aliasing artefacts. For this reason, footprint tables generated by Gaussian kernels with a dimension beyond $3\times3\times3$ were not included in this paper. As mentioned before, the reduction of detail due to antialiasing is not considered a severe drawback since measures similar to lowpass filtering have to be undertaken to avoid local minima in the optimization process [1,2]. Aliasing artefacts, on the other hand, cannot be tolerated since small structures with high intensity variations tend to introduce considerable misregistration for a number of 2D/3D cost functions such as minimization of cross-correlation and algorithms based on image gradiente evaluation. The advantage of wobbled splatting compared to anti-aliasing by lowpass-filtering with larger kernels lies in the fact that structure and detail is conserved to some extent. In this paper we have shown that DRRs of bony structures (i. e. DRRs rendered with a minimum threshold above typical soft tissue radioopacity) can be rendered without visible artefacts at framerates of approximately 10 Hz. This amounts to 5 – 7% of the computing time necessary for interpolated raycasting.

While comparing rendering algorithms applied to different volumes remains difficult, it has to be stated that this increase in computational efficiency compares well to the numbers reported in the literature. We conclude that wobbled splatting is comparable to these rendering algorithms in terms of efficiency; it provides an interesting alternative for generation of DRRs in iterative registration applications.

References

1. Lemieux L, Jagoe R, Fish DR, Kitchen ND, Thomas DG: A patient-to-computed-tomography image registration method based on digitally reconstructed radiographs. Med Phys 21(11):1749-1760, (1994)
2. Penney GP, Weese J, Little JA, Desmedt P, Hill DL, Hawkes DJ: A comparison of similarity measures for use in 2-D-3-D medical image registration. IEEE Trans Med Imaging 17(4):586-595, (1998)
3. Birkfellner W, Wirth J, Burgstaller W, Baumann B, Staedele H, Hammer B, Gellrich NC, Jacob AL, Regazzoni P, Messmer P: A faster method for 3D/2D medical image registration–a simulation study. Phys Med Biol 48(16):2665-2679, (2003)
4. LaRose D: "Iterative X-Ray-CT Registration using Accelerated Volume Rendering", PhD thesis, Carnegie Mellon University, (2001)
5. Lacroute P, Levoy M: Fast volume rendering using a shear-warp factorization of the viewing transformation. SIGGRAPH'94:451-458, (1994)
6. Westover L: Footprint evaluation for volume rendering. SIGGRAPH'90:367-376, (1990).
7. Dendy PP, Heaton B: "Physics for Diagnostic Radiology", IOP Medical Science Series, (1999).

Validation of PET Imaging by Alignment to Histology Slices

Philip J. Edwards[1], Ayman D. Nijmeh[2], Mark McGurk[2], Edward Odell[3], Michael R. Fenlon[4], Paul K. Marsden[5], and David J. Hawkes[6]

[1] Department of Surgical Oncology and Technology, ICL, 10th Floor QEQM Wing, St. Mary's Hospital, London W2 1NY, UK
Eddie.Edwards@imperial.ac.uk
[2] Department of Oral and Maxillofacial Surgery, Guy's Hospital, London, UK
[3] Division of Oral Medicine and Pathology, KCL, Guy's Hospital, London, UK
[4] Department of Prosthetic Dentistry, Guy's Hospital, London, UK
[5] Clinical PET Centre, GKT Medical School, St. Thomas' Hospital, London, UK
[6] Centre for Medical Image Computing, University College, London, UK

Abstract. The aim of this project is to verify the accuracy of positron emission tomography (PET) in identifying the tumour boundary and eventually to enable PET-guided resection with removal of significantly smaller margins. We present a novel use of an image-guided surgery system to enable alignment of preoperative PET images to postoperative histology. The oral cancer patients must have a high resolution CT scan as well as undergoing PET imaging. Registration of these images to the patient during surgery is achieved using a device that attaches to the patient's upper or lower teeth. During the procedure markers are placed around the lesion within tissue that is to be resected. These are marked along with any convenient anatomical landmarks using the image guidance system, providing the location of the points in the preoperative images. After the sample has been resected, slices through at least 3 of these points are made and photographed. Registration should be possible using these landmarks, but the accuracy of alignment is much improved by marking the bone surface in the histology image and registering to preoperative CT.

1 Introduction

Histology is generally regarded as the gold standard for identification and labelling of pathological tissues. Imaging techniques can provide a wealth of information about anatomy and physiology in vivo, but its value depends on how closely the image approximates reality. The spatial resolution and level of anatomical or functional detail, however, is much higher in histological slices. Alignment of in vivo images to histology could provide a powerful tool for validation of the imaging process.

Versions of this technique have been used to validate PET. Mega et al registered PET imaging to postmortem brain sections in a patient with Alzheimer's disease [1]. The aim was to compare stained brain sections with a PET scan

J. Duncan and G. Gerig (Eds.): MICCAI 2005, LNCS 3750, pp. 968–975, 2005.

taken 8 hours premortem. A 3D volume was reconstructed from cryosections at 0.5mm intervals and aligned to the PET scan using the method of Woods [2]. The stained sections were also registered to the cryosection data using an outline-based warping algorithm, providing the desired match between stained sections and premortem PET. Humm et al, on the other hand, inserted small rods into a tumour to act as markers for registration of magnetic resonance imaging (MRI) or PET images to histology in rodents [3]. Malandain et al produced a system for alignment of MRI to autoradiographs in tumour bearing mice [4]. Here an initial 3D volume of the autoradiographs is constructed and registered to the MRI image. The alignment for each autoradiographic slice is then refined and a new volume produced, and this process is repeated until a sufficiently good match is achieved.

In all these examples a volume is produced by aligning many histological slices from a postmortem subject. The aim of this project is to examine the accuracy of PET imaging for delineation of tumours in patients, for which we require a means of alignment to the excised tissue. This sample may not be able to provide many parallel slices, so a method that can register a single slice is required.

2 Method

The patient population considered for evaluation had an oral cancer sited in close association with the bone of the upper or lower jaw. A lockable acrylic dental stent (LADS) was made to clamp firmly to the patient's upper or lower teeth.

Fiducial markers can be attached to the LADS which provide accuracy of registration for the head, both in terms of stability and repeatability of positioning, to a tolerance of 1-4mm [5]. Any rotational instability causes greater errors at a distance from the teeth. We would expect accuracy in these cases to be higher, since the lesion is always located very close to the LADS.

2.1 Preoperative Image Acquisition and Processing

Preoperatively, prior to undergoing a PET scan, the LADS and fiducial frame are attached to the patient and the imaging markers filled with 5kBq/ml FDG. This is followed by a CT scan, with the markers filled with iodine solution. Usually there are 8 markers visible in both scans which are used for registration (see Fig. 1).

The position of the fiducials is marked in both sets of images. This provides registration from CT to PET. This was found to be a more accurate and reliable method than automated voxel-based registration [6], since the amount of activity in the PET scan can be quite small unless a significant amount of brain is included and there may be relative movement between the head and the region of interest if the lesion is in the mandible.

The PET scan is segmented using Analyze [7] to remove any activity other than the lesion. A set of surfaces is then produced using marching cubes [8] for

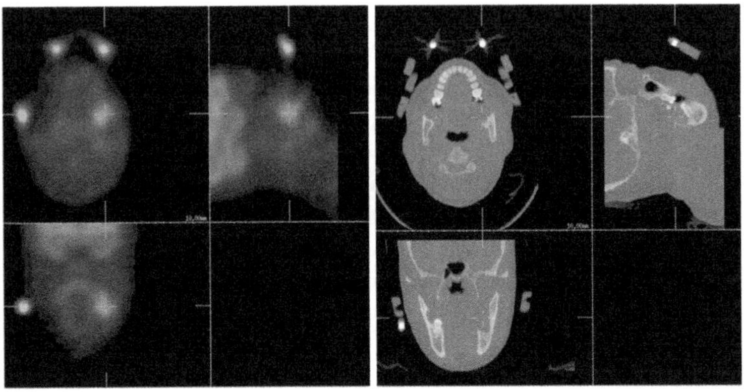

Fig. 1. An example PET scan and CT scan, showing the visibility of the fiducial markers

different thresholds to produce PET models of the lesion. These will be used to produce PET isointensity contours on the resulting histology slice. A bone and teeth surface model is created from the CT scan, also by marching cubes. This is useful for checking registration accuracy and is also required for the outline-based registration step described later.

2.2 Registration to the Physical Space of the Patient

The LADS is designed to carry a tracking frame of 6 infra-red emitting diodes (IREDs). that are located by the Optotrak position sensor from Northern Digital, Inc. Both the tracker and the fiducial frame are attached and the imaging fiducials are replaced by physical markers that dock accurately with a tracked pointer. Marking these points provides their location in the physical coordinate system defined by the IRED tracking frame. Registration to the same points marked in the PET and CT images aligns the preoperative data to the physical space defined by this frame. Now the wings carrying the fiducials can be removed and the intraoperative alignment is performed simply by attaching the LADS to the patient's teeth.

The beauty of using the LADS for this purpose is that the image-to-physical registration process can take place without the patient being present, as long as both the tracking frame and fiducial frame are attached.

It proved instructive to attach the cast of the teeth to the LADS. Then a pointer-based guidance system can be used on the cast to check that the CT is well aligned by marking bone surface points. The lesion can be visualised to check PET alignment (Fig. 2(c)). These planning checks save on operating room time and forewarn of problems with the data.

At surgery only the LADS with the tracking frame is attached to the teeth. The LADS locates and locks onto the teeth with great accuracy [5]. The position of the lesion can now be visualised using pointer-based guidance or augmented reality visualisation (see Fig. 2(d)).

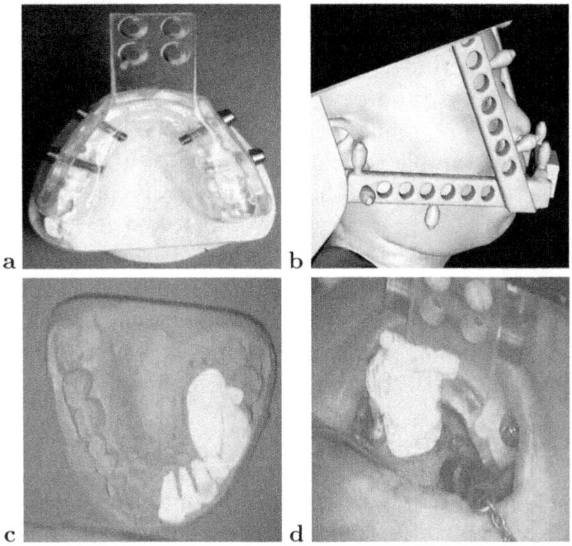

Fig. 2. The LADS registration device, showing attachment to the teeth (a), a rendering of the fiducial frame from CT (b), an overlay on the cast taken when producing the LADS (c) and an overlay during the operation showing that marker pins have been placed around the lesion (d).

2.3 Intraoperative Marker Placement

The surgeon and pathologist decide from the preoperative renderings the position of likely cuts through the lesion for histological assessment of the lesion. We then aim to place markers so that they define this plane, though high accuracy at this stage is not important. At least 3 points are required to define the plane of the cut. If anatomical landmarks are available, such as the cusp of a given tooth, these can be used. Otherwise markers are implanted in the tissue around the lesion. Dental barbed broaches or preferably standard bone screws are used for this purpose.

The screws are then marked with the image-guided surgery system, providing their position in the preoperative images. We use the CT scan as the reference image. The position of all intraoperative markers are recorded.

The surgery then proceeds and the sample containing the lesion and all the markers is removed in one piece to be transferred to the pathology laboratory. It is normal practice for the tumour and a 2cm margin of normal surrounding tissue to be removed.

2.4 Postopertative Histology

The tumour specimen is formalin fixed. With the aid of renderings showing the bone from CT, lesion from PET and the location of the markers, a number of cuts are made through the specimen as close as possible to at least 3 landmarks.

The cuts are made with an Exact 0.3mm thickness diamond grinding band. This part of the process relies on operator skill, but with experience it is possible to produce a cut through the relevant points that is very close to planar. The diamond band should not produce significant distortion of the tissue, especially since we have chosen non-mobile lesions close to the bone.

After each cut the sample is photographed with a Nikon coolpix 900 digital camera set on macro. The plane of the cut is manually placed to be perpendicular to the optical axis of the camera, which is mounted on a camera stand. Two rulers are placed in the same plane as the sample to be used for scaling of the resulting image. The position of the landmarks and the outline of the tumour are identified by the pathologist in the histology image. The landmark positions are released for registration purposes, but the tumour outline is not disclosed until the registration and PET rendering is completed.

2.5 Registration and Refinement

Registration can now be simply performed by point-based alignment of the landmarks from the scaled histology image to the landmark positions in the preoperative images. This process was prone to errors of rotation. The guidance system should be accurate to around 1mm, but the fiducial points are often only a few mm apart. Every effort is made to ensure landmarks are well spread in a triangle, but often this is not possible as the available anatomy at the beginning of surgery may consist of only one tooth. The close proximity of the landmarks can produce significant rotational errors.

To refine the registration the outline of the bone is delineated manually in the histology slice and registered to the bone surface from CT using the iterative closest point (ICP) method [9]. The result of the point-based registration is used as a starting estimate.

2.6 Validation

The technique described here could be used as a validation of PET imaging for tumour localisation, but the method of alignment itself should be validated. Unfortunately there is no easy gold standard registration of PET to histology with which to assess the current method.

It is possible to examine the precision of the registration, however. This is performed for the landmark identification by marking the fiducials intraoperatively six times. For the ICP registration refinement we use multiple random starting estimates within the range of error associated with the landmark registration.

3 Results

An example resulting alignment is shown in figure 3. The outline on the histology slice was provided by the pathologist. Bone from CT and the tumour from PET are overlaid on the histology image using landmark registration (Fig. 3(b)) and after ICP registration (Fig. 3(c)). For landmark registration there is a clear

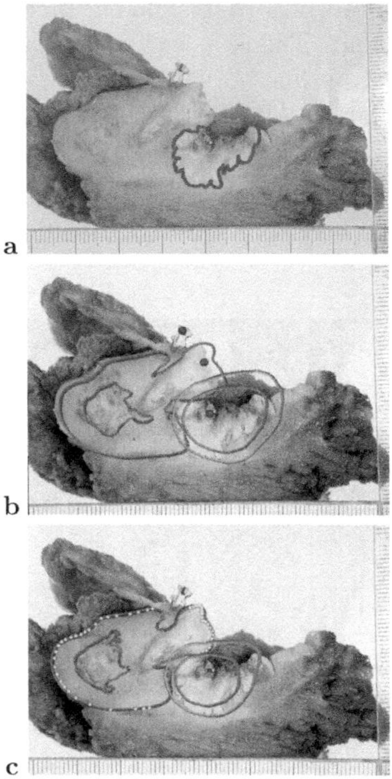

Fig. 3. An example histology slice showing the outline of the lesion (a), an overlay of the bone (brown) and lesion (green) after registration by landmarks (b) and ICP (c). The latter clearly gives a visually better alignment. Two thresholds are used that roughly correspond to the inner and outer boundary of the lesion in PET, demonstrating how we can use this method to help determine how best to use PET for tumour segmentation.

misalignment of the bone surface. After ICP the alignment is visually much improved. Figure 4 shows the position of the histology slice using the two registrations displayed over a rendering of the bone surface from CT and the lesion from PET. The rotational discrepancy between the two registrations is clear.

Repeated marking of the fiducials with the image-guided surgery system gave errors of around 1mm. The RMS residual error on the bone surface points after ICP is 0.34mm. Repeated ICP registrations based on random starting positions were highly consistent, with a mean target registration error (TRE) within the histology slice of 0.54mm. It should be stressed that this is an initial result on one dataset and should not be taken as a true measure of the accuracy of the method.

4 Discussion

We have presented a method for alignment of PET imaging to histology slices. This should enable validation of the ability to delineate a tumour using PET.

An initial result is given in which the alignment precision after ICP registration appears to be around 0.5mm. This is an early result and further experimentation is required. The effect of outline accuracy on precision could be estimated by marking multiple boundaries. Also a true gold standard may be possible with phantom or animal studies. Particularly a series of patients needs to be examined using the system. The initial results do suggest that the use of a guidance system in conjunction with a CT scan to provide the bone surface enables accurate alignment between PET and histology.

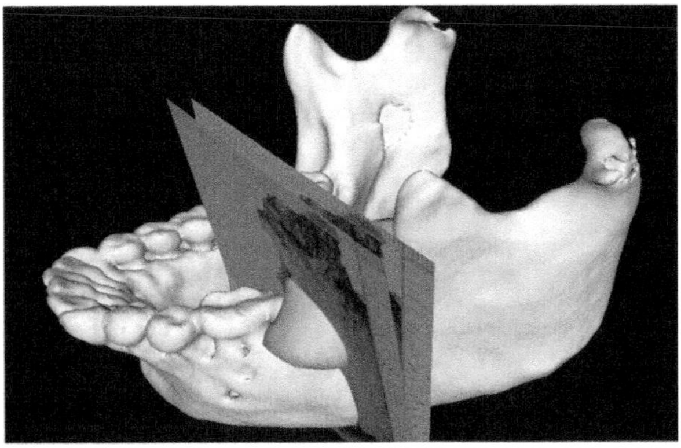

Fig. 4. A rendering of the mandible from CT, lesion from PET and the histology slice, registered using landmarks and ICP. The rotational error between the two registrations can clearly be seen. We believe the ICP result provides accurate alignment.

There are a few caveats when considering this process. Firstly, if the PET scan is taken a significant time before surgery there is the possibility that the lesion may have grown. To minimise this effect scanning was performed 1 week before surgery so as not to allow significant time for tumour growth. In general scanning should take place as near as possible to the time of the operation. Another potential problem is the shrinkage of soft tissue on removal or fixation. By choosing non-mobile lesions that are close to bone, we not only have the advantage of being able to match to the bone surface from CT, but also any deformation of the soft tissue is likely to be minimised. Shrinkage on fixation across the tumour was experimentally assessed to be of the order of 1% linear based on measurement along needles passed through the lesion.

The aim of the project will be to collect a database of PET images aligned to histology slices. This will enable quantitative analysis of the accuracy of PET segmentation techniques for tumour boundary delineation. Once we have confidence in the accuracy of the tumour segmentation we can develop a PET-based image-guided surgery system that will allow complete resection of the lesion with much smaller margins. The current practice is to ensure full resection by taking a significant margin of 1-3cm. Accurate PET-guided tumour resection should result in less-invasive surgery and reduced morbidity for the patient.

This paper presents, to the best knowledge of the authors, the first attempt to use image-guided surgery techniques to perform alignment of PET imaging to histology for verification of tumour boundary segmentation.

References

1. Mega, M.S., Chen, S.S., Thompson, P.M., Woods, R.P., Karaca, T.J., Tiwari, A., Vinters, H.V., Small, G.W., Toga, A.W.: Mapping histology to metabolism: Coregistration of stained whole-brain sections to premortem pet in alzheimer's disease. Neuroimage **5** (1997) 147–153
2. Woods, R.P., Mazziotta, J.C., Cherry, S.R.: MRI-PET registration with automated algorithm. J. Comput. Assist. Tomogr. **17** (1993) 536–546
3. Humm, J.L., Ballon, D., Hu, Y.C., Ruan, S., Chui, C., Tulipano, P.K., Erdi, A., Koutcher, J., Zakian, K., Urano, M., Zanzonico, P., Mattis, C., Dyke, J., Chen, Y., Harrington, P., O'Donoghue, J.A., Ling, C.C.: A stereotactic method for the three-dimensional registration of multi-modality biologic images in animals: NMR, PET, histology, and autoradiography. Med. Phys. **30** (2003) 2303–2314
4. Malandain, G., Bardinet, E., Nelissen, K., Vanduffel, W.: Fusion of autoradiographs with an MR volume using 2-D and 3-D linear transformations. Neuroimage **23** (2004) 111–127
5. Fenlon, M.R., Jusczyzck, A.S., Edwards, P.J., King, A.P.: Locking acrylic resin dental stent for image-guided surgery. J. Prosthet. Dent. **83** (2000) 482–485
6. Studholme, C., Hill, D.L.G., Hawkes, D.J.: Automated 3D registration of MR and CT images of the head. Med. Image Anal. **1** (1996) 163–175
7. Robb, R.A., Hanson, D.P., Karwoski, R.A., Larson, A.G., Workman, E.L., Stacy, M.C.: ANALYZE: a comprehensive, operator-interactive software package for multidimensional medical image display and analysis. Comput. Med. Imaging Graphics **13** (1989) 433–454
8. Lorensen, W.E., Cline, H.E.: Marching cubes: A high resolution 3D surface reconstruction algorithm. Comput. Graph. **21** (1987) 163–169
9. Besl, P.J., McKay, N.D.: A method for registration of 3-D shapes. IEEE Trans. Pattern Anal. Mach. Intell. **14** (1992) 239–256

Adaptive Subdivision for Hierarchical Non-rigid Registration of Multi-modal Images Using Mutual Information

Adrian Andronache, Philippe Cattin, and Gábor Székely

ETH Zurich - Computer Vision Laboratory,
Sternwartstrasse 7, CH - 8092, Zurich
{andronache, cattin, szekely}@vision.ee.ethz.ch

Abstract. In this paper we present an enhanced method for non-rigid registration of volumetric multi-modal images using Mutual Information (MI). Based on a hierarchical subdivision scheme, the non-rigid matching problem is decomposed into numerous rigid registrations of sub-images of decreasing size. A thorough investigation revealed limitations of this approach, caused by a peculiar behavior of MI when applied to regions covering only a limited number of image pixels. We examine and explain the loss of MI's statistical consistency along the hierarchical subdivision. We also propose to use information theoretical measures to identify the problematic regions in order to overcome the MI drawbacks. This does not only improve the accuracy and robustness of the registration, but also can be used as a very efficient stopping criterion for the further subdivision of nodes in the hierarchy, which drastically reduces the computational costs of the entire registration procedure.

1 Introduction

Medical imaging has been developing extremely fast during the last decades, bringing new technologies to improve pre-operative planning and intra-operative navigation. All the related procedures are using a large number of digital images taken at different time intervals or by different radiological modalities. Medical images are usually containing complementary information and their proper integration is often required. The crucial step in this fusion process is the registration procedure to ensure that the images of interest are in a sufficiently good spatial alignment. Several surveys and textbooks (e.g. [1] and references therein) have already been published providing a broad and general overview and analysis of the related problems and techniques proposed in the literature.

Among other, two key elements are to be mentioned in the context of image registration: the measure used to quantify the similarity between the images to be matched, and the spatial transformation that aligns the images. The introduction of MI as a similarity measure [2,3] has especially influenced the development of intensity-based image registration due to its inherent ability to deal with multi-modal matching problems [4]. Because of unavoidable deformations

J. Duncan and G. Gerig (Eds.): MICCAI 2005, LNCS 3750, pp. 976–983, 2005.

of the anatomy between consecutive scanning procedures, classical *rigid, affine* or *projective* registration techniques can only be used in limited special cases. *Non-rigid* registration procedures, capable to deal with more localized spatial changes, are therefore in the focus of current research and development. Likar and Pernuš proposed in [5] a hierarchical subdivision strategy that decomposes the non-rigid matching problem into an elastic interpolation of numerous local rigid registrations of sub-images of decreasing size.

Starting from the original 2D version of the hierarchical strategy, we improved the algorithm presented in [5] and extended it for volumetric data. In this paper, we first present an analysis of difficulties emerging when using this hierarchical registration scheme. Subsequently, solutions to overcome these drawbacks are presented based on a new method to detect noisy patches or regions of homogeneous intensity within an image. Finally, the performance of our method is compared with the original algorithm [5].

2 Method

Even though MI was proven to be a very robust and reliable similarity measure for intensity-based registration of multi-modal images, numerous problems have to be faced if it is applied to small-size images, compromising its usefulness for subdivision schemes. These problems have been identified in connection with either interpolation artifacts or inherent limitations of the MI definition. These difficulties are strongly coupled with the calculation of parameters for the discrete intensity probability distribution estimated by histograms. Therefore, they are increasingly disturbing when the size of the sub-images become smaller with the successive hierarchical subdivision. This effect is, however, less pronounced for 3D data.

The interpolation artifacts have been broadly analyzed in the literature and different solutions have been proposed [6,7].In order to minimize their influence, Likar and Pernuš artificially increased the number of image samples used for histogram generation by incorporating the global joint distribution as a prior. As a consequence, the statistical reliability of MI is increased. For small patch sizes, however, the use of prior information estimated from the entire image may lead to false maxima in the MI goal function. Therefore, we propose to estimate the prior only from a surrounding area relative to the size of the sub-image.

As another consequence of the successive image splitting, patches of low structural content may appear that often lead to morphologically inconsistent local registrations with a low MI response.

Likar and Pernuš suggested to identify such patches by thresholding the MI value and to exclude them from the local adjustment process. However, this way structured sub-images with low MI value, which still can be registered in a morphologically consistent way, will be prevented to become properly adjusted. At the same time, structureless patches may be retained as according to our observations the MI significantly increases when these start to overlap a structure in the reference image.

It is well known in information theory [8], that if two signals are statistically independent then their MI is reaching its minimum possible value, namely zero. Therefore, one would expect that by shifting a structureless noisy patch around its initial position, the similarity measure has a small response. Surprisingly, preliminary experiments clearly demonstrated that even though MI is small, it starts to increase as soon as the structureless patch overlaps a region of higher structural content, leading to wrong local registrations, that a thresholding technique or a regularization procedure may fail to detect or correct. The problem is even more pronounced in the context of multi-modal image registration when not all tissue details can be seen in all modalities, like in the case of CT-MR cross-registration.

The following experiment shows this behavior on a simple one-dimensional case. Let us consider two signals A and B depicted in Fig. 1(a). We generated the reference signal A by adding white noise to a step function. The floating signal B consists of white noise, and is statistically independent of A. Using the basic definition, we can calculate the MI between the two signals as a function of the displacement when the floating signal is translated along the reference signal. The none-zero baseline of the MI, clearly identifiable in Fig. 1(a), can be explained by a combination of two different effects. One is rooted in the difficulty to observe strict independence between signals represented by a finite number of discrete samples. On the other hand, it is well known in the information theory [9] that at the transition from continuous differential entropy to discrete entropy there is systematic bias by an error term depending on the size of the quantization bins used for histogram generation. This theorem does only apply to the marginal entropies $H(A)$ and $H(B)$. We are not aware of any results on deriving a similar relation for the joint entropy $H(A, B)$. Clearly for strictly independent signals A and B the quantization error of the discrete entropy would cancel out. This is, however, not the case if the independency condition is perturbed.

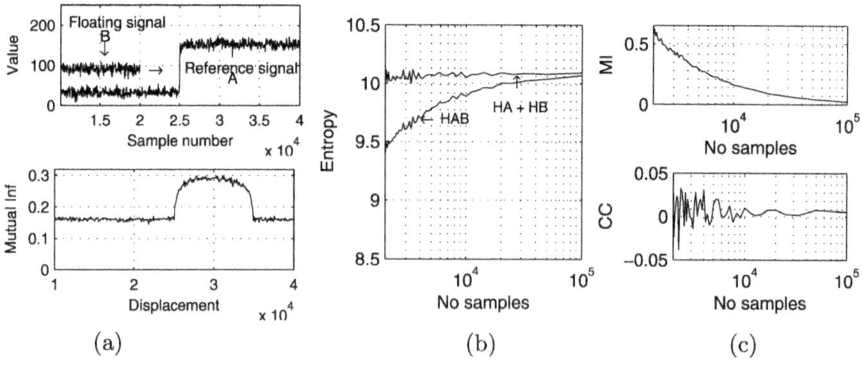

Fig. 1. (a) Experiment, demonstrating the behavior of MI in the presence of noise, showing the original test signals (top) and the response of MI (bottom) when the floating signal B is shifted over the reference signal A. (b) The dependency of the entropies $H(A) + H(B)$ and $H(A, B)$ on the number of samples in the signals. (c) The corresponding dependency of MI and cross-correlation coefficients on the number of samples.

To further investigate the problem, numerical experiments have been carried out showing the dependency of the entropies on the sample size. The results are shown on Fig. 1(b,c). The cross correlation (CC) graph clearly shows, as expected, that the statistical independence of the two finite, discrete random signals improves with the sample length. Figure 1(b), on the other hand, shows a very interesting property of the entropies. While the marginal entropies $H(A)$ and $H(B)$ are only slightly influenced by the sample length and very quickly reach the theoretically predicted value for discrete entropy, the joint entropy $H(A,B)$ requires substantially more samples to show a similarly stable behavior.

Relating this observation to the test signals from Fig. 1(a) it is obvious, that once the floating signal B starts to overlap the step, we get a bi-modal distribution for both $H(A)$ and $H(A,B)$, while $H(B)$ remains constant. The number of available samples needs then to be distributed among two separated distributions for the marginal entropy $H(A)$ and the joint entropy $H(A,B)$. As can be clearly seen from the above graph, the joint entropy $H(A,B)$ decreases much faster than the marginal entropy $H(A)$, necessarily leading to the observed strong increase of the MI. The same behavior has been also noticed when using the normalized mutual information as defined in [10].

As discussed previously, a simple thresholding of the MI during the matching process does not offer a satisfactory solution to the identified problems. Therefore, a new method is necessary, purely relying on the structural content of the single sub-images, allowing to identify structureless nodes in the subdivision scheme. These have to be excluded from both the registration chain and from the further hierarchical splitting process.

Inspired by the point-pattern analysis, where the main goal is to gain information about the spatial pattern or the variation in the data within a region of interest, we propose to use the spatial autocorrelation coefficient to test the consistency of the sub-images. Among different statistical tests proposed in the literature to determine whether the data are randomly or regularly distributed or clustered, the *Moran I* coefficient is favored by most of the analysts because it has highly desirable statistical properties [11]. For a dataset $X = \{x_i, i = 1..N\}$ of mean value $E(X) = \overline{x}$, Moran's I is defined as

$$I = \frac{N}{\sum_{i,j=1}^{N} w_{ij}} \cdot \frac{\sum_{i,j=1}^{N} w_{ij} \cdot (x_i - \overline{x}) \cdot (x_j - \overline{x})}{\sum_{i=1}^{N} (x_i - \overline{x})^2} \tag{1}$$

where $W = \{w_{ij}\}$ is called the contiguity matrix characterizing the amount of interaction between the i and j locations and N is the number of observations.

In order to use Moran's I as an indicator of the structural content in 2D or 3D sub-images, we chose to use a weighting scheme inversely proportional to the Euclidean distance $d(\cdot\,,\,\cdot)$ between the currently inspected pixel at the image coordinates $\boldsymbol{i} = \{i_1, ..i_n\} \in \mathbb{N}^{n=2,3}$ and its neighbors. A maximum interaction distance $\boldsymbol{\mathcal{D}} \in \mathbb{N}^n$ has to be selected according to the minimal size of the structures to be detected in the image. Changing the linearized index notation in (1) to image coordinates, and denoting the vicinity of size $\boldsymbol{\mathcal{D}}$ around $\boldsymbol{i}$ with

$\mathcal{V}_i^{\mathcal{D}} = \{ \boldsymbol{j} \in \mathbb{N}^n, \forall \mid i_k - j_k \mid \leq \mathcal{D}_k \text{ and } k = 1..n \}$, then the contiguity matrix can be expressed as

$$W = \begin{cases} w_{\boldsymbol{ij}} = \frac{1}{d(\boldsymbol{i},\boldsymbol{j})}, & \forall \boldsymbol{j} \in \mathcal{V}_{\boldsymbol{i}}^{\mathcal{D}} \backslash \{\boldsymbol{i}\} \\ 0, & \text{otherwise} \end{cases} \tag{2}$$

Denoting with $a_{\boldsymbol{i}}$ the intensity value of the image voxel located at the spatial position $\boldsymbol{i}$ within an image patch A of size $\boldsymbol{N} \in \mathbb{N}^n$ and mean value $\overline{a}$, the Moran I becomes

$$I = \frac{1}{\sum_{\boldsymbol{j} \in \mathcal{V}_0^{\mathcal{D}}} w_{\boldsymbol{0j}}} \cdot \frac{\sum_{\boldsymbol{i} \in \boldsymbol{N}} \sum_{\boldsymbol{j} \in \mathcal{V}_{\boldsymbol{i}}^{\mathcal{D}}} w_{\boldsymbol{ij}} \cdot (a_{\boldsymbol{i}} - \overline{a}) \cdot (a_{\boldsymbol{j}} - \overline{a})}{\sum_{\boldsymbol{i} \in \boldsymbol{N}} (a_{\boldsymbol{i}} - \overline{a})^2} \tag{3}$$

Moran's I varies in the interval $[-1, 1]$, where the random patterns are characterized by values close to zero. As the associated standard Z value is asymptotically normally distributed [11], a threshold of ± 1.96 corresponding to the 95% confidence interval can be chosen to identify random, i.e. structureless patterns. Figure 3(b-c) shows the result of the analysis at the 5th level of the hierarchy of a 2D neuroradiological MR slice.

We incorporated the enhancements discussed above into the 3D extended version of the hierarchical subdivision scheme described in [5]. The Moran information consistency test is applied to every sub-image in order to pass only the relevant image patches to the succeeding rigid registration stage. For all the sub-images failing this consistency test, the hierarchical splitting is stopped. However, for the 3D version, care has to be given to anisotropic voxel dimensions. In order to avoid discontinuities between neighboring leafs the parameter inheritance from one level to the other, used for the initialization, is done by linearly interpolating the transformations of the parent leaf and its surrounding neighbors. The consistency of the identified individual transformations between neighboring sub-images is ensured by a regularization procedure. It imposes spatial constraints on the centroids of the sub-images by defining a distance range between them. The identified outliers are corrected by assigning them the average transformation of all their surrounding sub-images. Thin-plate splines (TPS) [12] are used to calculate the final deformation field by densely interpolating the regularized local transformations of the sub-images over the whole image domain.

3 Results

For all the experiments, the registration algorithm was using the following parameter settings: (a) the two-dimensional histogram was generated using 256 bins; (b) the prior joint probability was estimated locally only from the direct neighboring sub-windows; (c) the threshold for the magnitude of the standard Z value of Moran's I coefficient used in the information consistency test was set to 1.96; (d) the contiguity matrix was calculated according to a maximum distance of 3 pixels ((7×7) or $(7 \times 7 \times 7)$ for the two- and three-dimensional case respectively), considering also the voxel anisotropy.

We illustrate the performance of our method on a CT-MR cross-registration example. The reference image is a $512 \times 512 \times 46$ CT scan of the head with $0.39 \times 0.39 \times 0.6\text{mm}^3$ voxel dimension and the floating image is a $512 \times 512 \times 28$ MR scan with voxels of the size $0.5 \times 0.5 \times 1.0\text{mm}^3$. Figure 2 visualizes details of our non-rigid registration method in a region where elastic deformation is needed to correct for both MR susceptibility artifacts (e.g. within the left sphenoid sinus) and tissue deformation (e.g. the left ear) between the two acquisitions. In order to better compare the results between a global rigid registration (Fig. 2(c,d)) and after applying the enhanced hierarchical registration process (Fig. 2(e,f)), the outline of the head and of the left sphenoid sinus is extracted from the floating MR volume and overlaid on the reference CT image. The remaining deviations of the two contours are caused by both the spatial constraints imposed by the regularization of the deformation field and the size of the smallest sub-image $(16 \times 16 \times 8)$ given by the number of hierarchical splitting levels.

Figure 3 shows the performance of our enhanced algorithm in comparison with the original method [5] for a two-dimensional registration example. The reference image (Fig. 3(a)) shows one slice from the aforementioned CT scan of the head and the floating image shows the corresponding transversal slice of the rigidly registered MR volume. A comparison between Fig. 3(f) and Fig. 3(g) clearly shows the favorable effect of using Moran's test when the local registration is dealing with structureless sub-images. Depending on the number of structureless sub-images found, the new algorithm can perform significantly faster than the original method (e.g. approximately a factor of two for this experiment). Even more, the Moran's consistency test incorporated into the enhanced algorithm allows us to go further with the hierarchical subdivision down to sub-images of 16×16 pixels, while Likar and Pernuš reported a minimum sub-image size of 95×64 pixels.

To quantify the improvement of the registration, we used an empirical procedure proposed by Ion Pappas et al. [13] to measure the performance of

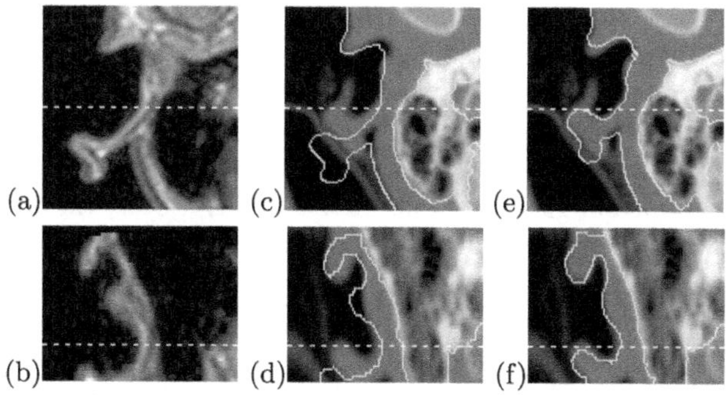

Fig. 2. Result of a CT-MR cross-registration. (a) Transversal and (b) coronal sections of the region of interest in the initial floating MR volume. (c-f) Corresponding sections in the reference CT volume, overlaid with the contours of the head and of the sphenoid sinus after a global rigid (c,d) and after the full hierarchical (e,f) registration. Note: The dashed lines mark the position of the cutting planes.

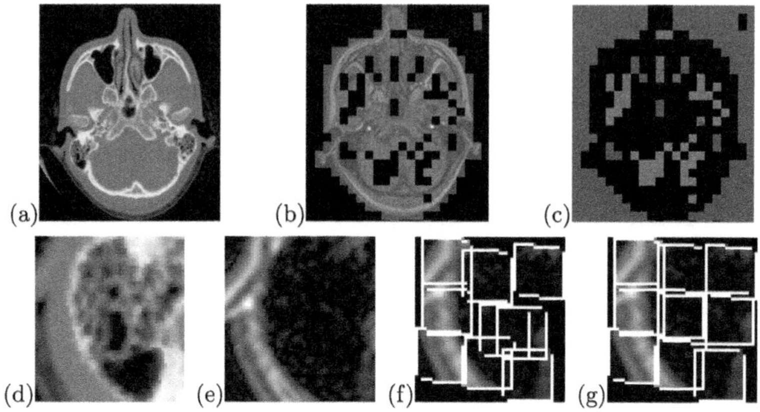

Fig. 3. Registration details of the sphenoid sinus in the left temporal bone at the 5th level of the hierarchy. (a) The reference CT. (b) and (c) The result (cropped images) of Moran's consistency test on the floating MR, divided in 32×32 sub-images of 16×16 pixels. The examined region, ((d) on the CT and (e) on the MR) consists of 3×3 sub-images. (f) Depicts the final position of each image patch after the local rigid registration, while (g) shows the result after applying the local rigid registration only to those MR patches which passed Moran's test. The consistency check clearly prevented the two middle patches from being pulled towards structures in the reference CT.

multimodal registration procedures. Similar to [14], the method estimates the percentage of overlapping volumes segmented from the images of interest. The final score of the registered bony structures using the improved algorithm shows a 2.3% improvement over the original method of Likar et al.

4 Conclusions

In this paper we extended and improved the hierarchical non-rigid registration algorithm relying on the maximization of MI, proposed by Likar and Pernuš. An information consistency test based on Moran's spatial autocorrelation coefficient has been developed and used to detect and eliminate the structureless sub-images from the registration chain, thus avoiding registration errors caused by structurally meaningless extrema of the MI. However, the MI proved to be more robust for the 3D version of the algorithm due to the larger number of available samples. Moran's test results in a very effective stopping criterion for the hierarchical subdivision process allowing to eliminate errors introduced by problematic structureless sub-images and it also speeds up the entire algorithm.

We see several possible directions for future research. Currently, the hierarchical binary splitting is ignoring the image content. An adaptive positioning of the splitting boundaries, enabling better adaptation to the anatomical structures, would not only further reduce the computational load but also improve image registration quality. This adjustment process could also be supported by using

Moran's spatial autocorrelation coefficient. Finally, the regularization method could be significantly improved by adapting the corresponding corrections to the certainty of the estimated transformation parameters, which can be measured by their standard deviation estimated using standard error propagation methods.

Acknowledgments

This work has been supported by the CO-ME/NCCR research network of the Swiss National Science Foundation (http://co-me.ch). We are also grateful to the MEMCenter, University of Bern.

References

1. Hajnal, J.V., Hill, D.L., Hawkes, D.J.: Medical Image Registration. CRC Press (2001)
2. Maes, F., Collignon, A., Vandermeulen, D., Marchal, G., Suetens, P.: Multimodality image registration by maximization of mutual information. Proc IEEE Workshop Mathematical Methods in Biomedical Image Analysis (1996) 14–22
3. Viola, P., W. M. Wells, I.: Alignment by maximization of mutual information. In: ICCV '95: Proceedings of the Fifth International Conference on Computer Vision. ISBN 0-8186-7042-8, IEEE Computer Society (1995) 16
4. Maes, F., Vandermeulen, D., Suetens, P.: Medical image registration using mutual information. Proc IEEE **91** (2003) 1699–1722
5. Likar, B., Pernus, F.: A hierarchical approach to elastic registration based on mutual information. Image and Vision Computing **19** (2001) 33–44
6. Pluim, J.P.W., Maintz, J.A., Viergever, M.A.: Mutual information matching and interpolation artefacts. Proc SPIE Medical Imaging **3661** (1999) 56–65
7. Ji, J.X., Pan, H., Liang, Z.P.: Further analysis of interpolation effects in mutual information-based image registration. IEEE Transactions on Medical Imaging **22** (2003) 1131–1140
8. Shannon, C.E.: A mathematical theory of communication. Technical report, Bell Laboratories (1948)
9. Cover, T., Thomas, J.: Elements of Information Theory. John Wiley & Sons (1991)
10. Studholme, C., Hill, D., Hawkes, D.: An overlap invariant entropy measure of 3d medical image alignment. Pattern Recognition **32** (1999) 71–86
11. Cliff, A., Ord, J.: Spatial Autocorrelation. ISBN 0-85086-036-9. Pion Limited: R.J. Chorley and D.W. Harvey, 207 Brondesbury Park, London NW2 5JN (1973)
12. Bookstein, F.L.: Principal warps: Thin-plate splines and the decomposition of deformations. IEEE Trans Pattern Anal Mach Intell **11** (1989) 567–585
13. Pappas, I.P., Malik, P., Styner, M., Liu, J., Caversaccio, M.: New method to assess the registration of ct-mr images of the head. SPIE Medical Imaging **5370** (2004) 14–19
14. Hellier, P., Barillot, C., Corouge, I., Gibaud, B., Goualher, G.L., Collins, D., Evans, A., Malandain, G., Ayache, N., Christensen, G., Johnson, H.: Retrospective evaluation of intersubject brain registration. Medical Imaging, IEEE Transactions on **22** (2003) 1120– 1130

3-D Diffeomorphic Shape Registration on Hippocampal Data Sets

Hongyu Guo[1], Anand Rangarajan[2], and Sarang C. Joshi[3]

[1] Dept. of CAMS, Texas A&M University-Corpus Christi
[2] Dept. of CISE, University of Florida
[3] Dept. of Radiation Oncology, University of North Carolina at Chapel Hill

Abstract. Matching 3D shapes is important in many medical imaging applications. We show that a joint clustering and diffeomorphism estimation strategy is capable of simultaneously estimating correspondences and a diffeomorphism between unlabeled 3D point-sets. Correspondence is established between the cluster centers and this is coupled with a simultaneous estimation of a 3D diffeomorphism of space. The number of clusters can be estimated by minimizing the Jensen-Shannon divergence on the registered data. We apply our algorithm to both synthetically warped 3D hippocampal shapes as well as real 3D hippocampal shapes from different subjects.

1 Introduction

Shape matching is ubiquitous in medical imaging and in particular, there is a real need for a turnkey non-rigid point feature-based shape matching algorithm [1,2]. This is a very difficult task due to the underlying difficulty of obtaining good feature correspondences when the shapes differ by an unknown deformation. In this paper, we attempt to formulate a precise mathematical model for point feature matching.

Previous work on the landmark matching problem [3,4] ignored the unknown correspondence problem and assumed all the landmarks are labeled. And furthermore, there is a considerable amount of point feature data where the cardinalities in the two shapes are not equal and a point-wise correspondence cannot be assumed. On the other hand, previous work on the correspondence problem [5,6] did not solve the diffeomorphism problem. The deformation model used was splines, like thin-plate splines, Gaussian radial basis functions and B-splines. The principal drawback of using a spline for the spatial mapping or the deformation model is the inability of the spline to guarantee that there are no local folds or reflections in the mapping and that a valid inverse exists.

Here, we are not interested in curve and surface matching because unlike a point-set representation of shapes, which is a universal representation, curve or surface representation of shapes usually require prior knowledge about the topology of the shapes. A point-set representation of shapes is especially useful when feature grouping (into curves and the like) cannot be assumed.

J. Duncan and G. Gerig (Eds.): MICCAI 2005, LNCS 3750, pp. 984–991, 2005.

As far as we know, there is very little previous work on 3D diffeomorphic point matching. Our previous work in [7] deals with 2-D shapes only. The only known competitors are the distance transform-based approach and the recent work of [8]. Due to the indirect approach of transforming point-sets into distance fields, the distance transform method [9] has not seen wide applicability for point-sets.

2 Diffeomorphic Point Matching with the Unknown Correspondence

We use a Gaussian mixture model to describe the data points with a log-likelihood

$$\log p(x|\mathbf{r}, \sigma_T) = \sum_{i=1}^{N_1} \log \sum_{a=1}^{N} \exp(-\frac{1}{2\sigma_T^2}||x_i - r_a||^2), \tag{1}$$

where x is a point in $\mathbf{R}^\mathsf{d}$, $\mathbf{r}$ is the collective notation of a set of cluster centers and σ_T^2 is the variance of each Gaussian distribution. As pointed out by Hathaway [10], the EM algorithm maximizing (1) can be viewed as an alternative minimization of the following objective

$$E(M, \mathbf{r}) = \frac{1}{2\sigma_T^2} \sum_{i=1}^{N_1} \sum_{a=1}^{N} M_{ia}^x ||x_i - r_a||^2 + \sum_{i=1}^{N_1} \sum_{a=1}^{N} M_{ia}^x \log M_{ia}^x \tag{2}$$

with simplex constraints on M. We put together the clustering energy of the two point-sets and the diffeomorphic deformation energy induced in space and our objective function is

$$\begin{aligned} & E(M^x, M^y, \mathbf{r}, \mathbf{s}, v, \phi) \\ &= \sum_{i=1}^{N_1} \sum_{k=1}^{N} M_{ik}^x ||x_i - r_k||^2 + 2\sigma_T^2 \sum_{i=1}^{N_1} \sum_{k=1}^{N} M_{ik}^x \log M_{ik}^x \\ &+ \sum_{j=1}^{N_2} \sum_{k=1}^{N} M_{jk}^y ||y_j - s_k||^2 + 2\sigma_T^2 \sum_{j=1}^{N_2} \sum_{k=1}^{N} M_{jk}^y \log M_{jk}^y \\ &+ \sum_{k=1}^{N} ||s_k - \phi(r_k, 1)||^2 + 2\sigma_T^2 \lambda \int_0^1 \int_\Omega ||Lv(x,t)||^2 dx dt. \end{aligned} \tag{3}$$

Notice we have multiplied each term in the objective function by a constant $2\sigma_T^2$. In the above objective function, the matrix entry M_{ik}^x is the membership of data point x_i in cluster k whose center is at location r_k. The matrix entry M_{jk}^y is the membership of data point y_j in cluster k whose center is at position s_k.

The diffeomorphic deformation energy in Ω is induced by the landmark displacements from r to s, where $x \in \Omega$ and $\phi(x,t)$ is a one parameter diffeomorphism: $\Omega \to \Omega$. The diffeomorphism $\phi(x,t)$ is generated by the flow $v(x,t)$. $\phi(x,t)$ and $v(x,t)$ together satisfy the transport equation $\frac{\partial \phi(x,t)}{\partial t} = v(\phi(x,t), t)$ and the initial condition $\forall x,\ \phi(x,0) = x$ holds. This is in the inexact matching form and the displacement term $\sum_{k=1}^{N} ||s_k - \phi(r_k, 1)||^2$ plays an important role here as the bridge between the two systems. This is also the reason why we prefer the deformation energy in this form because the coupling of the two sets of clusters appear naturally through the inexact matching term and we don't have to introduce external coupling terms as in [7].

3 A Diffeomorphic Point Matching Algorithm

Our joint clustering and diffeomorphism estimation algorithm has two components: i) clustering and ii) diffeomorphism estimation.

For the clustering part, we use the deterministic annealing approach proposed by Rose *et al.* [11] in order to avoid poor local minima. For the diffeomorphism estimation, we expand the flow field in term of the kernel K of the L operator

$$v(x,t) = \sum_{k=1}^{N} \alpha_k(t) K(x, \phi_k(t)) \tag{4}$$

where $\phi_k(t)$ is notational shorthand for $\phi(r_k, t)$ and we also take into consideration the affine part of the mapping when we use thin-plate kernel with matrix entry $K_{ij} = -r_{ij}$ and $r_{ij} = \| x_i - x_j \|$. After discretizing in time t, the objective in (3) is expressed as

$$\begin{aligned} & E(M^x, M^y, \mathbf{r}, \mathbf{s}, \alpha(t), \phi(t)) \\ & = \sum_{i=1}^{N_1} \sum_{k=1}^{N} M^x_{ik} ||x_i - r_k||^2 + T \sum_{i=1}^{N_1} \sum_{k=1}^{N} M^x_{ik} \log M^x_{ik} \\ & + \sum_{j=1}^{N_2} \sum_{k=1}^{N} M^y_{jk} ||y_j - s_k||^2 + T \sum_{j=1}^{N_2} \sum_{k=1}^{N} M^y_{jk} \log M^y_{jk} \\ & + \sum_{k=1}^{N} || s_k - r_k - \sum_{l=1}^{N} \sum_{t=0}^{S} [P(t) d_l(t) + \alpha_l(t) K(\phi_k(t), \phi_l(t))] \, ||^2 \\ & + \lambda T \sum_{k=1}^{N} \sum_{l=1}^{N} \sum_{t=0}^{S} < \alpha_k(t), \alpha_l(t) > K(\phi_k(t), \phi_l(t)) \end{aligned} \tag{5}$$

where $P(t)$ is the homogeneous form of $\phi(t)$. It is easy to find a close form solution for $d(t)$ and $\alpha(t)$ after performing a QR decomposition on P and we use gradient descent to solve for $\phi_k(t)$ when $\alpha_k(t)$ is held fixed.

The clustering of the two point-sets is handled by a deterministic annealing EM algorithm which iteratively estimates the cluster memberships M^x and M^y and the cluster centers r and s. The update of the memberships is the very standard E-step of the EM algorithm [12] and is performed as shown below.

$$M^x_{ik} = \frac{\exp(-\beta \|x_i - r_k\|^2)}{\sum_{l=1}^{N} \exp(-\beta \|x_i - r_l\|^2)}, \forall ik \tag{6}$$

$$M_{jk}^{y} = \frac{\exp(-\beta\|y_j - s_k\|^2)}{\sum_{l=1}^{N}\exp(-\beta\|y_j - s_l\|^2)}, \forall jk\,. \tag{7}$$

The cluster center update is the M-step of the EM algorithm. This step is not the typical M-step. We use a closed-form solution for the cluster centers which is an approximation. From the clustering standpoint, we assume that the change in the diffeomorphism at each iteration is *sufficiently small so that it can be neglected.* After making this approximation, we get

$$r_k = \frac{\sum_{i=1}^{N_1} M_{ik}^{x} x_k + s_k - \sum_{l=1}^{N}\int_0^1 \alpha_l(t)K(\phi_l(t),\phi_k(t))dt}{1+\sum_{i=1}^{N_1} M_{ik}^{x}}, \tag{8}$$

$$s_k = \frac{\sum_{j=1}^{N_2} M_{jk}^{y} y_j + \phi(r_k,1)}{1+\sum_{j=1}^{y} M_{jk}^{y}}, \forall k. \tag{9}$$

The overall algorithm is described below.

- **Initialization:** Initial temperature $T = 0.5(\max_i \|x_i - x_c\|^2 + \max_j \|y_j - y_c\|^2)$ where x_c and y_c are the centroids of X and Y respectively.
- **Begin A:** While $T > T_{\text{final}}$
  - **Step 1**: Clustering
  - Update memberships according to (6), (7).
  - Update cluster centers according to (8), (9).
  - **Step 2:** Diffeomorphism
  - Update (ϕ, v) by minimizing

$$E_{\text{diff}}(\phi, v) = \sum_{k=1}^{C} ||s_k - \phi(r_k,1)||^2 + \lambda T \int_0^1 \int_{\Omega} ||Lv(x,t)||^2 dx dt$$

- **Step 3:** Annealing. $T \leftarrow \gamma T$ where $\gamma < 1$.
- **End**

4 Experiments and Results

4.1 Experiments on Synthetic Data

We selected one hippocampus point-set and warped it with a known diffeomorphism using a Gaussian Radial Basis Function (GRBF) kernel. We choose $\sigma = 60$ for the GRBF because with this larger σ we are able to generate more global warping.

Figure 1 shows the two hippocampal shapes. The set with "+" markers is the original set and the set with point markers is the set after GRBF warping. First, we have no noise added. We used the TPS kernel to recover the diffeomorphism via joint clustering using our algorithm. We experimented with different number of clusters and found the corresponding standard errors. It is easy to see that the standard error goes down as the number of clusters goes up from 100 to 300

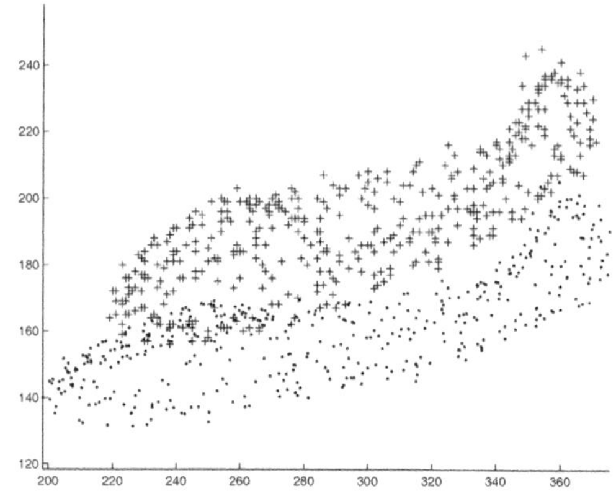

Fig. 1. Hippocampal point-sets

and goes up again when the number of clusters increases further. This is because when we have too few clusters, the points are not well represented by the cluster centers. On the other hand, if we have too many clusters, the variance between the two shapes is too big and the deformation increases dramatically. There is a optimal number of clusters and in this case we find it to be 300.

Next we add noise to the warped data and test the robustness of our algorithm to noise. After GRBF warping we add Gaussian noise to the warped data with different variances σ_N. We experimented with ten trials for each noise level from 0.1 to 1.0 and for each cluster level from 100 to 500. We can see the standard error increase with the increasing noise level but it approximately keeps in the range of the noise. This is easy to see when plotted in Figure 2 with error bars. Figure 2(a) has the errors for 100, 200 and 300 clusters and Figure 2(b) has the errors for 300, 400 and 500 clusters. We can see that at the 300 cluster level we obtain the best matching.

4.2 Experiments on Real Data

We applied the algorithm on different real hippocampal data sets. We have ten 3D point-sets which were extracted from epilepsy patients with left anterior

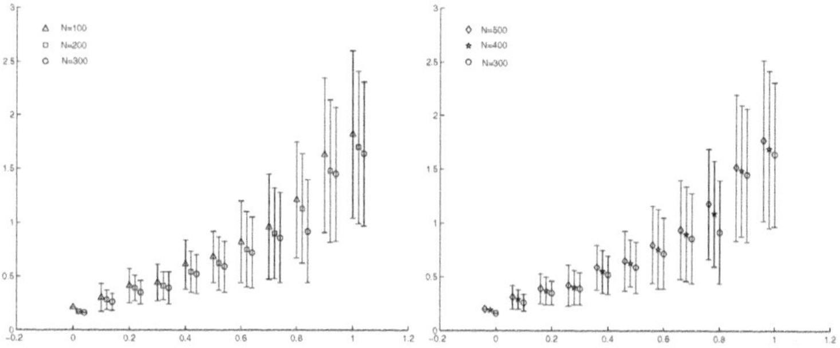

(a) (b)

Fig. 2. Matching results on synthetic data for different number of clusters

Table 1. Matching metrics of various pairs of shapes

	Jensen-Shannon div.					Hausdorff distance					modified Hausdorff				
Trial\No. Clusters	100	200	300	400	500	100	200	300	400	500	100	200	300	400	500
1	0.87	0.31	0.03	0.13	0.21	7.1	7.4	5.7	6.2	7.3	2.8	2.0	1.4	1.2	1.1
2	0.93	0.62	0.47	0.05	0.24	9.3	8.9	7.2	8.3	8.7	3.5	3.1	2.8	2.4	2.3
3	0.76	0.27	0.04	0.16	0.32	7.2	6.1	4.9	5.6	6.4	2.0	1.7	1.4	1.3	1.2
4	0.98	0.52	0.34	0.09	0.45	8.4	7.8	7.2	5.2	6.5	2.7	2.4	2.3	1.7	1.4
5	0.69	0.41	0.14	0.18	0.36	9.6	9.7	8.0	8.4	8.9	3.9	3.6	3.1	2.8	2.7
6	0.57	0.23	0.43	0.78	0.97	9.2	6.3	7.1	7.8	8.6	3.1	2.8	2.5	2.2	2.1
7	0.66	0.21	0.05	0.14	0.30	6.9	5.8	4.4	6.0	7.3	2.4	2.2	2.1	1.7	1.5
8	0.99	0.70	0.25	0.19	0.63	8.9	8.5	7.0	6.4	8.2	3.0	2.6	2.4	2.2	1.9
9	0.85	0.42	0.11	0.68	0.74	9.3	8.0	5.9	7.6	9.1	2.9	2.7	2.3	2.1	1.6
10	0.97	0.62	0.10	0.18	0.55	7.8	7.3	4.7	6.7	8.1	3.2	2.8	2.3	1.8	1.4
11	0.70	0.33	0.06	0.13	0.26	8.7	7.7	5.8	7.4	9.0	2.5	2.1	1.6	1.4	1.2
12	1.02	0.64	0.08	0.44	0.71	9.1	8.3	6.1	7.4	8.6	3.3	3.0	2.5	2.2	2.0
13	0.89	0.54	0.20	0.31	0.65	9.3	8.4	6.5	7.0	8.7	3.6	3.4	3.1	2.4	2.2
14	0.57	0.09	0.15	0.66	0.80	7.4	5.1	5.5	6.8	8.3	3.0	2.7	2.3	2.0	1.8
15	0.88	0.30	0.05	0.29	0.36	8.8	7.1	4.9	6.3	7.8	2.6	2.0	1.5	1.3	1.2
16	0.90	0.75	0.12	0.17	0.44	9.4	9.0	6.1	7.3	8.5	3.2	3.0	2.4	2.1	1.9
17	0.61	0.16	0.28	0.53	0.72	8.6	6.8	7.9	9.0	9.9	3.4	3.5	3.1	2.7	2.4
18	0.91	0.37	0.18	0.40	0.88	9.5	8.2	6.5	7.4	8.0	3.7	3.2	2.9	2.6	2.1
19	1.12	0.80	0.47	0.09	0.28	9.2	7.8	7.2	5.1	6.4	2.8	2.6	2.3	2.2	2.0
20	0.96	0.54	0.33	0.60	0.74	9.6	8.0	7.3	8.7	9.3	3.9	3.5	3.3	3.1	2.7
21	0.65	0.23	0.51	0.78	1.04	8.4	6.1	6.9	7.8	9.5	3.3	3.1	2.8	2.4	2.3
22	0.93	0.46	0.22	0.51	0.68	9.7	8.5	7.0	8.1	9.0	2.9	2.7	2.6	2.3	2.1
23	0.92	0.60	0.28	0.15	0.34	9.6	8.2	7.3	6.5	7.7	2.4	2.1	1.7	1.6	1.5
24	0.80	0.26	0.57	0.69	0.86	7.8	6.6	7.2	8.9	9.6	3.1	2.7	2.5	2.2	1.9
25	1.10	0.62	0.44	0.78	0.97	9.8	7.9	7.6	8.8	9.2	3.8	3.4	3.0	2.8	2.7
26	0.90	0.39	0.05	0.21	0.47	9.0	7.3	5.8	7.0	8.7	2.9	2.4	2.0	1.4	1.2
27	0.58	0.07	0.20	0.56	0.77	7.8	6.0	6.5	7.2	8.3	3.2	2.9	2.5	2.1	1.9
28	0.93	0.51	0.09	0.40	0.63	9.5	8.1	6.1	7.4	8.8	3.0	2.8	2.5	2.1	1.8
29	0.99	0.26	0.18	0.37	0.70	9.7	8.3	6.7	7.0	8.5	3.4	2.7	2.2	1.9	1.7
30	0.60	0.06	0.17	0.54	0.57	7.1	5.6	6.2	7.3	7.8	2.5	2.2	1.8	1.3	1.2
31	0.83	0.19	0.08	0.37	0.76	9.3	6.7	5.8	7.5	8.4	2.7	2.4	2.2	1.6	1.4
32	1.22	0.42	0.57	0.70	0.95	9.9	7.2	7.8	8.5	9.2	3.5	3.0	2.8	2.5	2.3
33	0.80	0.59	0.30	0.86	0.92	8.9	8.0	6.3	7.1	8.7	3.3	3.1	2.6	2.4	2.3
34	0.89	0.76	0.35	0.28	0.67	8.9	8.5	6.7	6.4	7.0	3.0	2.8	2.5	2.2	2.1
35	1.05	0.42	0.37	0.81	1.13	9.6	8.4	7.0	8.1	9.9	3.7	3.4	3.0	2.3	2.0
36	0.92	0.25	0.31	0.60	0.85	8.7	5.9	6.2	7.5	8.4	3.2	2.9	2.5	2.3	2.2
37	0.79	0.35	0.08	0.24	0.40	7.7	6.3	5.4	6.1	7.6	2.4	2.2	1.9	1.6	1.5
38	0.90	0.42	0.16	0.35	0.68	9.5	7.1	5.7	6.6	7.9	2.8	2.4	2.3	2.0	1.8
39	0.86	0.27	0.38	0.50	0.71	9.2	7.3	8.2	8.4	9.0	3.2	3.0	2.7	2.5	2.4
40	0.55	0.04	0.19	0.36	0.67	6.5	5.2	5.8	6.7	7.3	2.0	1.6	1.3	1.1	0.9
41	1.02	0.30	0.47	0.81	0.98	9.4	7.5	7.9	8.6	9.2	3.8	3.2	2.5	2.4	2.3
42	0.43	0.07	0.22	0.56	0.86	7.2	5.8	6.7	7.3	7.9	2.3	1.9	1.6	1.5	1.4
43	0.78	0.56	0.18	0.39	0.61	8.2	7.4	6.0	6.7	7.8	2.9	2.4	2.2	2.0	1.8
44	0.61	0.09	0.25	0.70	0.82	7.1	5.9	6.6	7.5	8.0	2.2	1.9	1.7	1.5	1.4
45	0.44	0.15	0.26	0.53	0.93	7.0	6.5	7.2	7.7	9.1	2.5	2.1	1.9	1.7	1.6

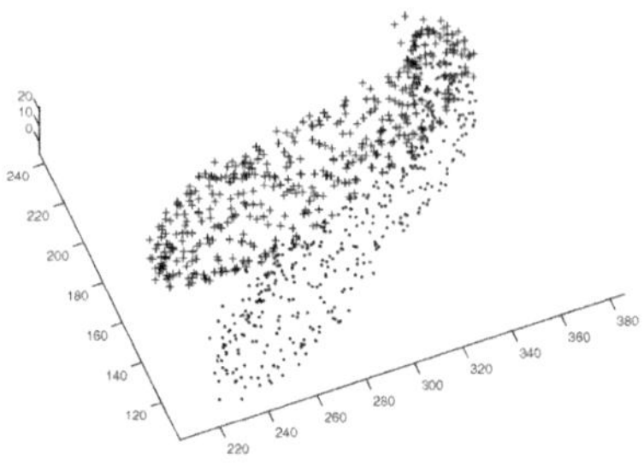

Fig. 3. Two hippocampus shapes

temporal lobe foci identified with EEG. An interactive segmentation tool was used to segment the hippocampus in the 3D anatomical brain MRI of the ten subjects. The shapes vary from point-set to point-set and the number of points in each point-set varies from 310 to 555. Figure 3 shows two hippocampal shapes. We observe when we have 300 clusters, we have a reasonable $\sigma = 1.2$ as the average distance between the nearest neighbors is about 2.65.

We did the matching for all the pairs out of ten hippocampus shapes with totally 45 such pairs. We compare three measures for the matching result with different number of clusters in Table 1. The Jensen-Shannon divergence (a special case with equal weights) [13], Hausdorff distance and modified Hausdorff distance [14]. Notice Jensen-Shannon divergence is highly non-linear. When p and q are completely independent, namely in our matching case, when the two shapes are completely different, D has a maximum of $2\log 2 = 1.39$.

From Table 1 we can see that when we have 300 clusters we have the minimum Jensen-Shannon divergence and Hausdorff distance. However, Hausdorff distance is too sensitive to outliers. We also calculated the modified Hausdorff distance as first introduced in [14]. It is easy to see that when the number of clusters increases, the modified Hausdorff distance decreases.

5 Discussion

The need for a good 3D point feature matching algorithm arises in various application areas of medical image analysis. To our knowledge, this is one of the first attempts at 3D diffeomorphic point matching. We have demonstrated a 3D joint clustering and diffeomorphism algorithm and applied it to hippocampal point-sets. In the process of careful validation, we investigated the role of the different numbers of clusters in the joint clustering and diffeomorphism optimization process. In the current formulation, we still have a free parameter λ whose role has to be determined. The immediate future goal is to further address (theoretically and experimentally), the role of free parameters. The same framework can be used for atlas estimation. Finally, once we have a turnkey 3D diffeomorphic feature matching algorithm, we plan to use it for hippocampal shape classification of epilepsy patients [15].

References

1. Cootes, T., Taylor, C., Cooper, D., Graham, J.: Active Shape Models: Their Training and Application. Computer Vision and Image Understanding **61** (1995) 38–59
2. Duta, N., Jain, A.K., Dubuisson-Jolly, M.: Learning 2D shape models. In: IEEE Conf. on Computer Vision and Pattern Recognition (CVPR). Volume 2. (1999) 8–14
3. Joshi, S., Miller, M.: Landmark matching via large deformation diffeomorphisms. IEEE Trans. Image Processing **9** (2000) 1357–1370
4. Camion, V., Younes, L.: Geodesic interpolating splines. In: Energy Minimization Methods for Computer Vision and Pattern Recognition. Springer, New York (2001) 513–527
5. Chui, H., Rangarajan, A.: Learning an atlas from unlabeled point-sets. In: IEEE Workshop on Mathematical Methods in Biomedical Image Analysis (MMBIA), IEEE Press (2001) 179–186
6. Chui, H., Rangarajan, A.: A new point matching algorithm for non-rigid registration. Computer Vision and Image Understanding **89** (2003) 114–141
7. Guo, H., Rangarajan, A., Joshi, S., Younes, L.: A new joint clustering and diffeomorphism estimation algorithm for non-rigid shape mathcing. IEEE Workshop on Articulated and Non-rigid motion (ANM) (2004)
8. Glaunes, J., Trouve, A., Younes, L.: Diffeomorphic matching of distributions: A new approach for unlabelled point-sets and sub-manifolds matching. In: IEEE Computer Society Conference on Computer Vision and Pattern Recognition (CVPR 04). Volume 2. (2004) 712–718
9. Rosenfeld, A., Plalz, J.L.: Sequential operations in digital picture processing. Journal of ACM **13** (1966) 471–494
10. Hathaway, R.: Another interpretation of the EM algorithm for mixture distributions. Statistics and Probability Letters **4** (1986) 53–56
11. Rose, K., Gurewitz, E., Fox, G.: Statistical mechanics and phase transitions in clustering. Physical Review Letters **65** (1990) 945–948
12. Chui, H., Win, L., Duncan, J., Schultz, R., Rangarajan, A.: A unified non-rigid feature registration method for brain mapping. Medical Image Analysis **7** (2003) 112–130
13. Endres, D.M., Schindelin, J.E.: A new metric for probability distributions. IEEE Transactions on Information Theory **49** (2003) 1858–1860
14. Dubuisson, M.P., Jain, A.K.: A modified Hausdorff distance for object matching. ICPR94 (1994) A:566–568
15. Vohra, N., Vemuri, B.C., Rangarajan, A., Gilmore, R.L., Roper, S.N., Leonard, C.M.: Kernel Fisher for shape based classification in epilepsy. In: Medical Image Computing and Computer-Assisted Intervention (MICCAI02). (2002) 436–443

Two-Stage Registration for Real-Time Deformable Compensation Using an Electromagnetic Tracking Device

Hui Zhang[1], Filip Banovac[1], Neil Glossop[2], and Kevin Cleary[1]

[1] Imaging Science & Information System (ISIS) Center, Department of Radiology, Georgetown University, Washington, DC, USA
{zhang, banovac, cleary}@isis.imac.georgetown.edu
[2] Traxtal, Inc., Bellaire, TX, USA
neil@traxtal.com

Abstract. Electromagnetic tracking systems have the potential to track instruments inside the body because they are not limited by the line of sight constraints that characterize optical tracking systems. To integrate an electromagnetic tracking device into a surgical navigation system, accurate registration is required. We present a two-stage registration mechanism designed to be more accurate than the widely used global fiducial-based registration method. The first stage uses a hybrid Iterative Closest Point (ICP) registration method and the Simulated Annealing (SA) optimization algorithm, to increase the initial registration accuracy. The second stage exploits multiple implanted tracking needles that are used to calculate the affine transform based on the initial transform information, and thereby to compensate for the deformation in real time. Phantom and swine studies have demonstrated the utility of this technique.

1 Introduction

While optical tracking systems are the gold standard for image-guided surgery, recent developments in electromagnetic tracking systems have enabled the development of prototype image-guided systems that can track internal organs. Electromagnetically tracked needles have been constructed that incorporate one or more electromagnetic coils in the needle stylettes. These needles can be as small as 18 gauge, and their stylettes containing the electromagnetic sensor coils can be as small as 19 gauge. Using this technology, our research group has been developing an image-guided system for abdominal interventions such as liver procedures. Liver motion due to respiration is a major concern when trying to precisely target liver lesions. The purpose of this study was to increase the accuracy of the image-guided system using a novel two-stage registration method.

Fiducial and point-based registration is the most widely used registration method for image-guided surgery. In our image-guided system, fiducials are placed on the patient's skin before the pre-operative CT or MR scan. Since the flexibility of the patient's body can cause errors in registration [1], it is essential to place markers in relatively stable locations. In addition, the motion of the liver is not well correlated

J. Duncan and G. Gerig (Eds.): MICCAI 2005, LNCS 3750, pp. 992 – 999, 2005.

with the motion of the skin surface or underlying anatomy. Hence, external tracking of the skin surface may not be sufficient to determine the location of targets within the liver [2].

In a liver biopsy, the needle is inserted percutaneously towards the tumor target. To improve the accuracy of biopsy using our image-guided systems, our algorithm uses multiple points on a needle for registration. According to Fizpatrick [3], formula (1) is used for calculating the target registration error:

$$\langle TRE^2(r)\rangle \approx \frac{\langle FLE^2\rangle}{N}\left(1+\frac{1}{3}\sum_{k=1}^{3}\frac{d_k^2}{f_k^2}\right) \tag{1}$$

where *TRE* is the target registration error in the position r and *FLE* is the fiducial localization error. N indicates the number of fiducials; d_k is the distance of the target from principal axis k; and f_k is the RMS distance of the fiducials. In our algorithm, the fiducial number N is increased by resampling the needle. Also, d_k / f_k is decreased because the principal axis completed from the needle is quite close to the real target. The simulated annealing algorithm and ICP metric are integrated to give the best transformation. This transformation is used as the initial matrix for the second stage: real-time affine transform compensation. The liver and other abdominal organs are not rigid; rather, they are somewhat deformable, so the global transform is not always appropriate due to the intrinsic and extrinsic factors, such as respiration and external forces [4]. In a previous study [5], a tracked reference needle was placed inside the liver to compensate for motion, while still treating the whole model as rigid-body. Compared with the rigid body transform, the affine transform can provide additional scale and shear behavior that can be used to simulate some basic deformation. Our method uses the affine transform, which is computed in real time to reflect the exact internal motion for deformable compensation.

2 Methods

Our method was first tested using a respiratory motion phantom. The phantom includes a rib cage, synthetic skin, and a foam liver model that is mounted on a one degree-of-freedom precision motion platform [6]. The Aurora electromagnetic tracking system from Northern Digital Inc. was the tracking device. Tracked 18-gauge needles (MagTrax Needles, Traxtal Technologies, Bellaire, TX) were placed through the skin and into the liver to define the puncture volume. An image-guided software platform was also developed for the experiment evaluation and clinical research. The overall system implements our own registration algorithm, and also uses ITK for some registration and segmentation, VTK for visualization, and MFC for user interface. The workflow is as follows: DICOM image loading, tracker device initialization, biopsy planning, registration and segmentation, visualization, and motion tracking. The system can be used for biopsy, guide-wire deployment, verterbroplasty, and radio-frequency ablation procedures. The experiment was completed in the interventional suite at Georgetown University Medical Center.

2.1 First Stage: Needle Based Registration

In order to achieve a better registration, three needles are implanted inside the liver and near the tumor target. These three needles bound a volume into which the actual procedure needle will pass through. Multiple points along these needles are used in the registration. The procedure is as follows:

Algorithm 1: Needle-Based Registration

1) Implant three non-parallel needles into the liver;
2) Obtain the pre-operative CT scan;
3) Segment the needles to obtain the image space points;
4) Sample the sensor coils embedded in the stylettes to obtain the corresponding points in tracker space;
5) Process the sampled points to reduce the noise generated by the tracking system;
6) Use ICP as the transformation metric, and integrate the simulated annealing optimization algorithm to get the correct transform.

Usually, the ICP algorithm can efficiently minimize the root mean square (RMS) distance between two feature point sets. However, it may find local minima, especially in noisy feature sets. The ICP algorithm can always reach the local minima, and the simulated annealing algorithm can achieve the global minima position slowly [7, 8]. In our algorithm, we use the ICP algorithm and a Levenberg-Marquardt solver to attain each local minima position. At these local points, the simulated annealing algorithm is applied to the transformation to perturb out and find the global one. The energy function is defined as formula (2), which is the distance between two point sets:

$$E(p_1,\cdots,p_M)=\sum_{i=1}^{N}\left\|RA_i+T-CP(RA_i+T,B)\right\|^2 \tag{2}$$

A and *B* are the source and destination point sets. *R* and *T* are the rotation and translation matrices from point set A to B, respectively. *CP* is the operator that finds the closest point in another data set.

Luck and Penney have described methods that are similar to ours, but the algorithms were implemented differently [8, 9]. Luck used the simulated annealing algorithm to produce "good" starting points for the ICP algorithm. Penny added random Gaussian noise to perturb the positions of the feature set and increase the robustness. Our method applies the simulated annealing algorithm directly to the transformation parameters of each local minimum, as described in formula (3):

$$[P_1,\cdots,P_M]=\min(LM(E(\tilde{p}_1,\cdots,\tilde{p}_M))) \tag{3}$$

$\tilde{p}_i$ represents the disturbed parameters around the last Levenberg-Marquardt solution position, and these parameters are used for optimization. *LM* is the general Levenberg-Marquardt solver.

2.2 Second Stage: Real-Time Affine Transform Compensation

The affine transform aims to simulate the deformation in some sense, and has translation, rotation, scale, and shear operations. The anisotropic scale and shear behavior can be used to simulate the deformable model to some extent [10-12]. A 3D rigid-body transform has three translation factors and three rotation factors. In the affine transform, additional scale factors and other shear factors are incorporated to construct the whole matrix. The computation of the affine transform is described by Horn [13].

The three previously implanted needles are then used for compensation. When the external surgical tool is pushed into the liver body, the pre-calculated global transform will change due to the deformation behavior. Therefore, compensation is required to accurately track the target point. The standard clinical technique uses some external fiducials and internal fiducials, and tracks their positions over several respiratory cycles, trying to find the correlation between the external and internal motion [14]. Clinically, it will use only the external motion to predict the internal movement through the model. The advantage of this method is that it is non-invasive and can be effectively used to synchronize the treatment planning system. However, this method also has several drawbacks. First, it predicts the internal motion from the external motion, whose accuracy greatly depends on the predicting model, without a fixed equation or formula to validate. Second, it treats the whole body as rigid, and then applies the rigid-body compensation to the whole body's motion. Third, the method cannot compensate for the intrusion deformation caused by the surgical tools during the intervention.

The 3D affine transform has 12 defining parameters, and we only use three implanted needles for real-time tracking. Consequently, the orientation information of each needle is used to get three additional points besides three sensor points. Therefore, we have 6 points from three needles for the affine transform registration. These six points are typically chosen as the sensor points and their fixed offset points along the needle direction. The procedure is as follows:

Algorithm 2: Real-Time Affine Transform Compensation

1) At end-expiration period, record the tracking information and generate 6 points in electromagnetic space;
2) Apply the inverse of the transformation calculated in algorithm 1 to get the respective 6 points in the image space. These points are the fixed image points during the tracking;
3) Throughout the whole procedure, record the tracking needles and generate 6 different points in real-time that correspond to the first 6 points due to the deformation;
4) Use point-based registration between these changing tracking points and the fixed image points to update the affine transform in real time;
5) Apply the updated transform to the system, and repeat from step 3.

3 Results

The whole procedure was separated into the two stages explained above. The initial transform calculated from stage one was used for the fixed point set calculation in the second stage. We tested our algorithm with the liver phantom model. In stage one, the final transform matrix and fiducial registration error (FRE) were recorded. Since the target registration error (TRE) is more important for clinical applications, the center point of the triangle defined by the tips of the three needles is considered as the target point. The positions in the image space and in the electromagnetic space were recorded and compared as the TRE.

The intermediate results of the optimization procedure are listed in Table 1 and shown in Fig 1. The final optimization registration result indicates that the FRE is 0.96mm and the TRE is 2.67mm using our registration method. We also computed the registration matrix through the four skin-fiducials in the same case. The result of the skin-fiducial based registration indicates an FRE of 1.49mm and a TRE of 7.54mm. Therefore, the hybrid registration method proposed here is more accurate than the skin fiducial-based registration method.

Fig. 2 shows the point sets before and after the registration method, optimized by ICP and SA algorithms. Fig. 3 shows the needle position validation result after we applied the different matrix to our system. In the left image, we can see the displacement error of the overlaid needle tip compared with the background pre-operative CT image slice. In the right image, the two tips fit together quite well using our registration algorithm.

Table 1. Process for hybrid registration of ICP and SA algorithm

Iteration	FRE (mm)	TRE (mm)	Iteration	FRE (mm)	TRE (mm)
1	60.59	76.42	2	25.67	79.52
3	24.82	80.38	4	24.36	80.34
5	23.91	80.39	6	21.71	5.18
7	15.36	10.75	8	3.20	3.46
9	2.97	3.30	10	2.21	3.20
11	0.96	2.67			

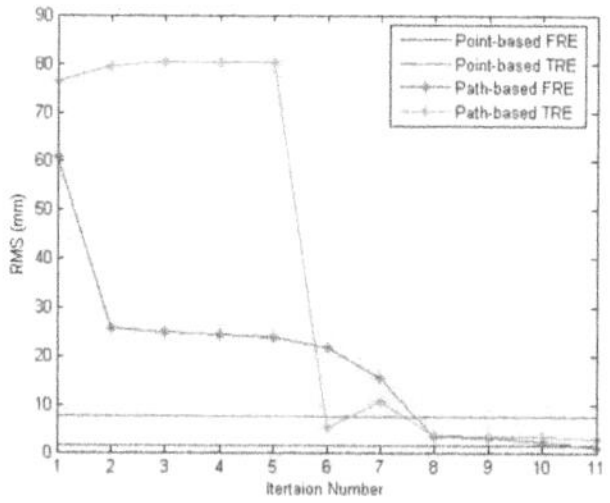

Fig. 1. Optimization process of the hybrid registration. The final registration specification of FRE and TRE is better than the skin fiducial-based registration.

To validate real-time updating of the affine transform, we implanted four needles into the phantom model. Three needles were used in the matrix computation and the fourth needle was used as the target for verification. TRE is calculated by comparing the real position reported by the tracking system and the position generated by the registration transform. Some random deformations of the liver torso by the external force and intrusion were simulated. We also provided the global registration result without affine compensation from the same first-stage transform matrix for

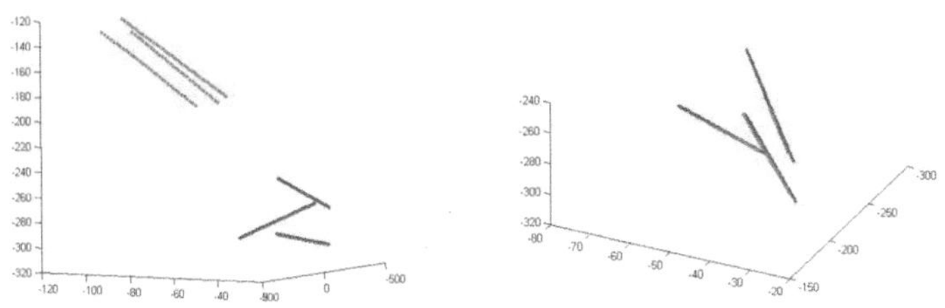

Fig. 2. Point sets before and after registration. Left: The initial position of needles in image space and position sensor space. Right: After the registration. The two point sets agree well and appear as overlaid lines.

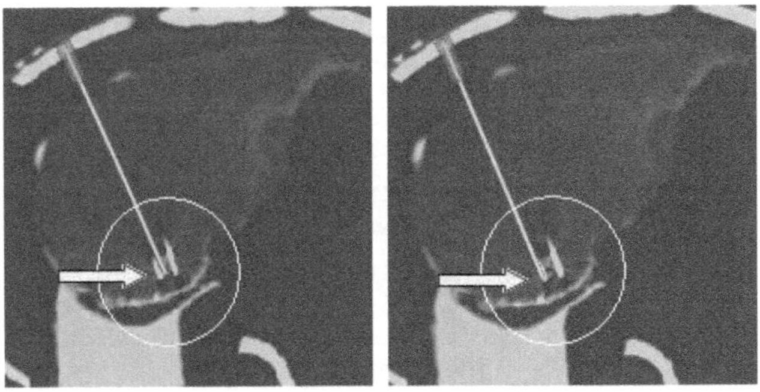

Fig. 3. Needle verification of skin fiducial-based registration and our hybrid registration method. Left: The tip of the needle is a bit off the pre-operative CT image due to the distance between the skin fiducials and target point. Right: The tip is perfectly overlaid with the left band, showing that our needle-based registration algorithm can improve the target registration accuracy.

Table 2. Comparison of the affine compensation with the global registration

	Affine TRE (mm)	Global TRE (mm)	Improvement (%)
Phantom1	2.47±0.03	2.97±0.52	16.74
Phantom2	2.18±0.44	3.40±2.03	36.03
Swine1	3.30±1.16	3.70±1.61	10.84
Swine2	2.07±0.70	2.80±1.45	26.21
Swine3	2.14±0.87	2.82±1.54	24.07

comparison. The results of the phantom simulation and the swine study are given in Table 2, which shows a 10.84% to 36.03% improvement in accuracy, with a standard derivation better than the global one.

A swine study was also completed under an approved protocol, with three needles for real-time affine compensation and the fourth needle for validation. Three 30 second periods, each containing several respiratory cycles, were recorded by the tracking system. The results are shown in Fig. 4. After the registration, the liver target was successfully punctured, guided by our software as shown in Fig. 5.

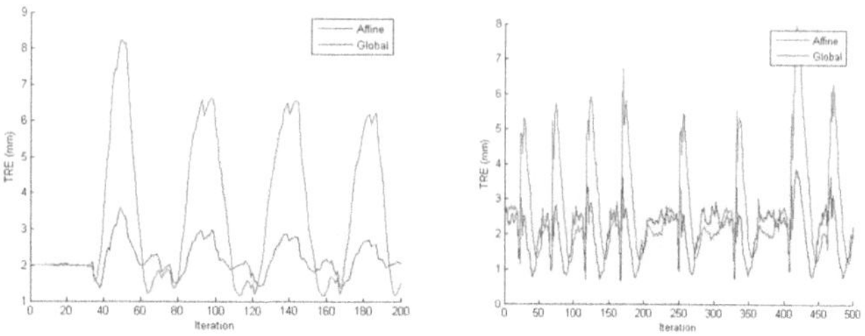

Fig. 4. TRE of affine compensation and global registration. Left: Phantom study with organ deformation. Right: Swine study with respiration deformation.

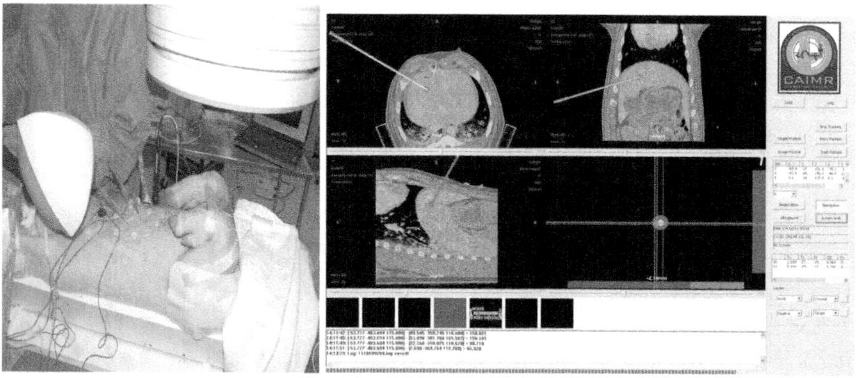

Fig. 5. Left: Image-guided tracking system in swine study. Right: graphical user interface.

4 Discussion

These novel registration methods may be helpful in practical applications. First, we created a hybrid registration method based on the ICP and SA algorithm, which can improve the accuracy of needle insertion. Second, we applied the position information from the tracking needles to update the real-time affine transform and compensate for the basic deformation. Compared with biomechanical model deformation, this method is simple and can be quickly completed. Finally, we proposed a two-stage strategy to combine the different registration methods together. Although we used our registration method in the first stage, any other method can be used in the first stage as the initial transform for the following calculation.

Our needle-based registration method takes advantage of position sensor readings from three reference needles and can provide better accuracy than registration based on skin fiducials. The drawback of this method is that it will take more time to calculate the initial correct transform compared to the real-time computation of point-based registration. However, once the initial transformation matrix is obtained, the affine transform can be updated in real-time to compensate for the deformation.

Acknowledgements. This work was funded by U.S. Army grants DAMD17-99-1-9022 and W81XWH-04-1-0078. The content of this manuscript does not necessarily reflect the position or policy of the U.S. Government.

References

1. Rohlfing T., Maurer, C.R. Jr., O'Dell W.G., and Zhong, J., Modeling Liver Motion and Deformation during the Respiratory Cycle using Intensity-based Nonrigid Registration of Gated MR Images, Medical Physics, 31:427-432, 2004.
2. Achim Schweikard, Greg Glosser, Mohan Bodduluri, Martin Murphy, John R. Adler, Robotic Motion Compensation for Respiratory Movement during Radiosurgery, Computer Aided Surgery, 5(4):263-277, 2000.
3. Fitzpatrick J.M., West J.B., Maurer C.R., Predicting Error in Rigid-Body Point-Based Registration, IEEE Transactions on Medical Imaging, 17(5):694-702, 1998.
4. Julien Jomier, Stephen R. Aylward, Rigid and Deformable Vasculature-to-Image Registration: a Hierarchical Approach, MICCAI 2004, St Malo, France, 2004.
5. Filip Banovac, Neil D. Glossop, David Lindisch, Daigo Tanaka, Elliot Levy, Kevin Cleary: Liver Tumor Biopsy in a Respiring Phantom with the Assistance of a Novel Electromagnetic Navigation Device. MICCAI 2002, 1:200-207, 2002.
6. Kevin Cleary, Filip Banovac, Elliot Levy, Daigo Tanaka, Development of a Liver Respiratory Motion Simulator to Investigate Magnetic Tracking for Abdominal Interventions SPIE Medical Imaging 2002, 4681:25-29, 2002.
7. Zhengyou Zhang. Iterative Point Matching for Registration of Free-Form Curves and Surfaces. International Journal of Computer Vision, 13(2):119-152, 1994.
8. G. P. Penny, P.J. Edwards, A.P.King, J.M. Blackall, P.G.Batchelor, D.J.Hawkes, A Stochastic Iterative Closest Point Algorithm (stochastICP), Medical Image Computing and Computer-Assisted Intervention, MICCAI 2001, 2208: 762-769, 2001.
9. Jason Luck, Charles Little, Willam Hoff, Registration of Range Data Using a Hybrid Simulated Annealing and Iterative Closest Point Algorithm, Proc. of IEEE Int. Conf. on Rob. and Auto., San Francisco, April 24-28, 3739-3744, 2000.
10. GJ Klein, BW Reutter, RH Huesman, 4D Affine Registration Models for Respiratory-Gated PET, IEEE Nuclear Science Symposium, 15:41-45, 2000.
11. J. Feldmar, N. Ayache. Rigid, affine and locally affine registration of free-form surfaces. International Journal of Computer Vision, 18:99–119, 1996.
12. Alain, Pitiot, Gregoire Malandain, Eric Bardinet, Paul M Thompson, Piecewise Affine Registration of Biological Images, WBIR 2003, 91-101, 2003.
13. Berthold K. P. Horn, Closed-form solution of absolute orientation using unit quaternions, Journal of the Optical Society of America A, 4:629-642, 1987.
14. Ritchie CJ, Hsieh J, Gard MF, Godwin JD, Kim Y, Crawford CR., Predictive Respiratory Gating: a new Method to Reduce Motion Artifacts on CT Scans. Radiology, 190:847–852, 1994.

Cadaver Validation of Intensity-Based Ultrasound to CT Registration

Graeme P. Penney[1], Dean C. Barratt[1], Carolyn S.K. Chan[1], Mike Slomczykowski[2], Timothy J. Carter[1], Phillip J. Edwards[3], and David J.Hawkes[1]

[1] Centre for Medical Image Computing (CMIC), University College London, UK
g.penney@cs.ucl.ac.uk
[2] Department of Surgical Oncology and Technology, Imperial College London, UK
[3] i-Orthopaedics, DePuy a Johnson & Johnson Company, Leeds, UK

Abstract. A method is presented for the registration of tracked B-mode ultrasound images to a CT volume of a femur or pelvis. This registration can allow tracked surgical instruments to be aligned with the CT image or an associated preoperative plan. Our method requires no manual segmentation of either the ultrasound images or the CT volume. The CT and US images are processed to produce images where the image intensity represents the probability of the presence of a bone edge. These images are then registered together using normalised cross-correlation as a similarity measure. The parameter which represents the speed of sound through tissue has also been included in the registration optimisation process. Experiments have been carried out on six cadaveric femurs and three cadaveric pelves. Registration results were compared with a "gold standard" registration acquired using bone implanted fiducial markers. Results show the registration method to be accurate, on average, to 1.7mm root-mean-square target registration error.

1 Introduction

Recent years have seen the emergence of image-guidance systems for orthopaedic surgery [1,2,3]. All of these systems require a registration between physical and image space. Most systems achieve this by identifying point landmarks or by delineating surfaces using a tracked pointer. To achieve accurate registrations, bony landmarks, or fiducials attached to bone should be located. Implanting fiducials or exposing additional bone surfaces for registration is invasive and may cause additional pain and risk of infection, whereas limiting surface information to regions exposed in standard procedures may adversely affect registration accuracy. There is a trade off between invasiveness and accuracy of the registration process. The drive to develop less invasive registration methods will increase with the adoption of minimally invasive surgical techniques [4,5], particularly as reduced invasiveness of procedures may be the most powerful argument for the use of computer assisted orthopaedic surgery systems.

J. Duncan and G. Gerig (Eds.): MICCAI 2005, LNCS 3750, pp. 1000–1007, 2005.

Proposals to use B-mode ultrasound (US) for registration to bone in image guided surgery go back approximately a decade [6]. The main application areas have involved registrations on vertebrae [7,8], pelves [9,8,10] and long bones [6,11,12]. The work presented in this paper differs from previously published work in three main ways: firstly, we have used an intensity-based algorithm, therefore no segmentation is required in either the US or CT volume; secondly, our algorithm also optimises the probe calibration parameter which is directly related to the average speed-of-sound through tissue; and thirdly, our validation strategy uses a combination of human cadavers, an independently calculated "gold standard" registration based on bone implanted fiducial markers, and clinically realistic starting positions.

2 Method

2.1 Overview of System

The registration algorithm used in this paper is an extension of an algorithm previously described for registering US images to magnetic resonance images of the liver [13]. An overview of the registration system is given in Figure 1. An optical localiser (Optotrak 3020, Northern Digital Inc., Ontario, Canada) was used to track an US probe and a dynamic reference object (DRO) which is rigidly attached to the bone. Our aim is to calculate the registration transformation, $\mathbf{T}_{reg}$, which transforms physical positions in the coordinate system of the DRO into voxel positions within a preoperative CT volume.

To calculate $\mathbf{T}_{reg}$, 3D freehand US images are acquired of the bone surface. These images are then registered to the preoperative CT volume to obtain transformation, $\mathbf{T}$, which maps pixel positions, $\mathbf{x}_{US}$, in the US images to voxel

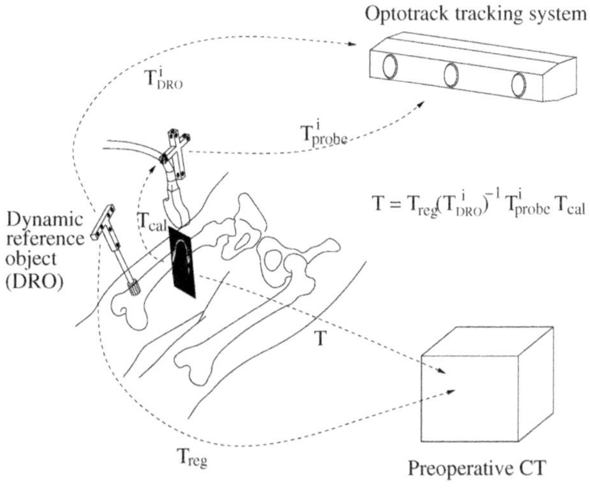

Fig. 1. Overview of system and transformations

positions, $\mathbf{x}_{CT}$, within the CT volume. Transformation $\mathbf{T}$ is computed from four separate transformations:

$$\mathbf{T} = \mathbf{T}_{reg}(\mathbf{T}^{i}_{DRO})^{-1}\mathbf{T}^{i}_{probe}\mathbf{T}_{cal} \quad (1)$$

The calibration matrix, $\mathbf{T}_{cal}$, which transforms positions from the US image to positions relative to the infrared-emitting diodes (IREDs) attached to the probe was calculated using an invariant point method. Transformations $\mathbf{T}_{DRO}$ and $\mathbf{T}_{probe}$ transform positions relative to the IREDs (on the DRO and attached to the US probe respectively) to positions relative to the cameras on the Optotrak localiser.

The algorithm described in this paper calculates the transformation $\mathbf{T}$ by altering the six rigid-body parameters which define transformation $\mathbf{T}_{reg}$ and the probe calibration scaling parameter in the vertical (or y) US image direction, s_y, in order to optimise the value of a similarity measure between the US and CT images. The scaling parameter in the horizontal (or x) US direction, which is not affected by the speed of sound in the imaged medium, was held constant during optimisation. After optimisation $\mathbf{T}_{reg}$ can be used to determine the position and orientation of any tracked and calibrated object (such as a surgical drill) in the CT scan, and so can relate the intraoperative positions of such instruments to a preoperative plan described in the CT image.

The similarity measure for the algorithm is calculated as follows: The current estimate of $\mathbf{T}_{reg}$ and s_y are used to reslice the CT probability image (described in section 2.2) in the plane of each US slice (N.B. therefore, there is no requirement to compound the US slices to produce a 3D volume). The pixel values in these reformatted slices and in the US probability images are then compared using the normalised cross-correlation similarity measure. A three stage hill-climbing optimisation approach is used: low-resolution, high-resolution and then high-resolution which includes s_y optimisation.

2.2 Formation of Probabilistic Images

The US and CT images are converted from intensity images, $I(\mathbf{x})$, into probabilistic images, $P(\mathbf{x})$, where $\mathbf{x}$ represents the image position and $P(\mathbf{x})$ represents the probability of a pixel or voxel containing a bone-to-soft-tissue interface. The probability images, $P(\mathbf{x})$, are calculated using a probability density function (PDF), p, which, given a set of image features, $\mathbf{F}(\mathbf{x})$, returns an estimate of the probability that position $\mathbf{x}$ is a bone-edge, i.e. $P(\mathbf{x}) = p(\mathbf{F}(\mathbf{x}))$.

Converting the CT Volume: The CT PDF, p_{CT}, was based on two image features, so $\mathbf{F}(\mathbf{x})_{CT} = \mathbf{F}(f_{CT1}(\mathbf{x}), f_{CT2}(\mathbf{x}))$. Both CT features were calculated in 2D by applying operators to each CT slice in turn. The first CT feature, $f_{CT1}(\mathbf{x})$, was the intensity of a gradient image calculated using Sobel operators. The second feature, $f_{CT2}(\mathbf{x})$, was set equal to the maximum value under a 3×3 mask centred on pixel $\mathbf{x}$.

A set of training data, comprised of n CT volumes, was used to calculate p_{CT}. Our aim is to identify two sets of voxels in the training data: all of the voxels which lie on a bone-to-soft-tissue boundary, S_{edgeCT}; and all the voxels in the training data, S_{CT}. Therefore, $S_{edgeCT} \subset S_{CT}$, and the PDF is defined as

$$p_{CT}(a,b) = \frac{\text{Number of voxels where } \mathbf{x} \in S_{edgeCT} \text{ with } f_{CT1}(\mathbf{x}) = a \text{ and } f_{CT2}(\mathbf{x}) = b}{\text{Number of voxels where } \mathbf{x} \in S_{CT} \text{ with } f_{CT1}(\mathbf{x}) = a \text{ and } f_{CT2}(\mathbf{x}) = b} \tag{2}$$

Converting the US Slices: The first step is an artifact removal stage. Our method uses simple knowledge of the US image formation process; in particular, that most strong reflections and artifacts cause a loss of signal intensity along the direction of the beam. The algorithm begins at the bottom of each column of pixels in the US image, and moves upwards towards the transducer face. The image is labelled as artifact until a threshold value is reached, see Figure 2(b). A small region (3mm) immediately adjacent to the transducer face is also labelled as artifact to remove artifacts caused by imperfect acoustic coupling at the skin surface boundary. Image regions labelled as artifact were not used in any subsequent image processing.

Two image features, $\mathbf{F}(\mathbf{x})_{US} = \mathbf{F}(f_{US1}(\mathbf{x}), f_{US2}(\mathbf{x}))$, were used for the US PDF, p_{US}. The first US feature, $f_{US1}(\mathbf{x})$, was the intensity of the US image $I_{US}(\mathbf{x})$. The second US feature, $f_{US2}(\mathbf{x})$, was the number of pixels below $\mathbf{x}$ not labelled as artifact. Both of these features are able to highlight bone edges due to the large change in acoustic impedance between soft-tissue and bone. This results in high US intensity values at the boundary (detected by $f_{US1}(\mathbf{x})$) followed by a bone shadow region of very low US intensities (detected by $f_{US2}(\mathbf{x})$). Figure 2 shows an example of an US probability image.

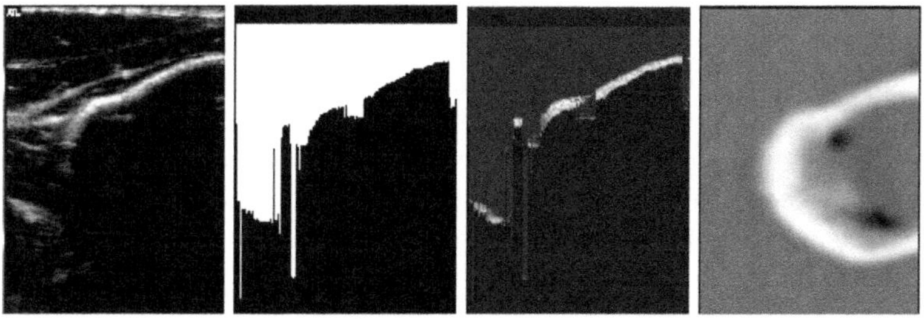

(a) (b) (c) (d)

Fig. 2. Formation of US probability images: (a) sample US slice through femur; (b) mask produced by the artifact removal stage where only pixels in the white region are included for subsequent image processing; (c) probability image; (d) corresponding reformatted slice through the CT volume (calculated using the "gold standard" transformation) included to show the position of bone boundaries. In (c) Some non-bone-boundary pixels can be seen to have been allocated a high value in the probability image and vice-versa. However, it is important to note that our aim is not to produce a perfect segmentation, but to produce probability images of sufficient quality to allow accurate and robust registration.

A set of US slices were used as training data for p_{US}. The bone edge was defined in the training US images as a number of manually selected points connected by straight lines, to give the pixel set, S_{edgeUS}. The pixel set, S_{US}, comprised all the non-artifact US pixels from the training data, and, as before, $S_{edgeUS} \subset S_{US}$. The PDF, p_{US}, is then defined as

$$p_{US}(a,b) = \frac{\text{Number of pixels where } \mathbf{x} \in S_{edgeUS} \text{ with } f_{US1}(\mathbf{x}) = a \text{ and } f_{US2}(\mathbf{x}) = b}{\text{Number of pixels where } \mathbf{x} \in S_{US} \text{ with } f_{US1}(\mathbf{x}) = a \text{ and } f_{US2}(\mathbf{x}) = b} \tag{3}$$

2.3 Experiments

Data Acquisition: for this study was carried out using 3 complete female cadavers. Fiducial markers were implanted into the femur and pelvis of each cadaver (4 in each femur and 5 in each hemi-pelvis) which were used to calculate a "gold standard" registration between image and physical space. A single high-resolution spiral CT scan (Siemens SOMATOM Plus 5) was obtained of the whole pelvis and femurs of each cadaver (voxel dimensions varied between $0.71 \times 0.71 \times 2\text{mm}^3$ and $0.79 \times 0.79 \times 2\text{mm}^3$). Each CT was then reduced into three smaller volumes which contained either a pelvis or femur plus some surrounding anatomy.

Prior to acquiring US images, a dynamic reference object (DRO) was rigidly attached to the bone. All measurements were recorded relative to the co-ordinate system of the DRO. The use of a DRO enabled the position of the cadaver to be changed during US acquisition so that images could be obtained in regions that would otherwise be inaccessible with the cadaver remaining in the supine position. The attachment of DROs [2,3] or external fixators [1] is standard practice for most image-guided orthopaedic surgery systems. Ultrasound images were acquired using a Philips-ATL HDI-5000 scanner and a high frequency probe (5-12 MHz). Between 168 and 565 tracked US images were acquired of each bone using continuous scanning. This took approximately 8 minutes, though we believe that this time could be substantially reduced if an optimal protocol was established. The US images showed no effects of the cadaver preservation process, and so the acquired sets of US images should closely represent clinical data; both in terms of image characteristics, and in terms of in which regions of human femur and pelvis is it possible to obtain clear images of the bone surface using US.

Clinically Realistic Starting Positions: One method for obtaining a starting estimate for the algorithm in a clinical situation is to pick corresponding skin positions in the CT scan and physically using a tracked pointer. We have simulated the above process to obtain 100 starting estimates for each bone. The simulation uses four skin positions on each pelvis, and 3 skin positions and the pivot position for each femur. Our simulation assumes that the skin positions can be selected within a distance of 20mm and the pivot position is accurate to within 10mm.

Training Data for PDF Calculations: For the experiments described in this paper all the CT femur images and between 42 and 100 US images from each femur were used as training data. In order to keep the training data separate from the experimental data the following method was used: All the pelvis experiments used the same US and CT PDFs, which were produced using all the training data. For the femur experiments, separate PDFs were produced for each femur. For a given femur, PDFs were produced using a subset of the training data. This subset comprised all the training data except for the data from the given femur.

3 Results

The results are shown visually using sample overlay images in Figure 3, and numerically in Table 1, where root mean square (RMS) target registration error (TRE) values have been calculated at three stages during the registration process: after the low-resolution optimisation, after the high-resolution optimisation and after the scaling parameter, s_y, is included in the optimisation. The

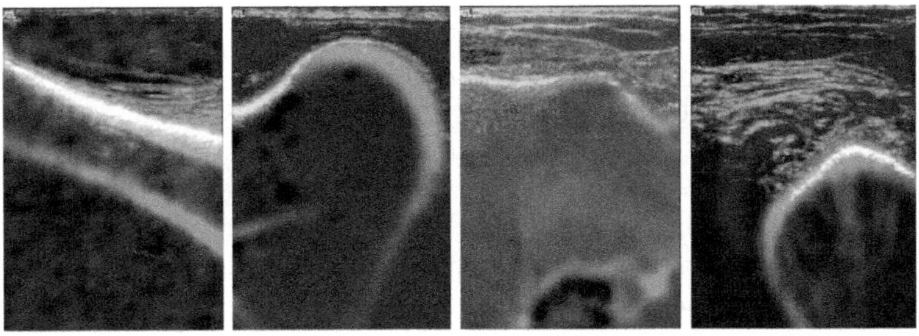

(a) (b) (c) (d)

Fig. 3. Sample overlays of US onto reformatted slices through CT volumes calculated using the intensity-based registration transformation. Images correspond to (a) cadaver 1 pelvis, (b) cadaver 1 L.femur, (c) cadaver 2 L.femur and (d) cadaver 3 R.femur.

Table 1. Registration accuracy, mean RMS TRE, for each bone averaged over all successful registrations. The RMS TRE was calculated over the whole bone surface. A registration was defined to be a failure if its RMS TRE was more than double the mean RMS TRE calculated over all 100 registrations.

Cad	Bone	mean (and s.d.) RMS TRE (mm)				s_y	No. fail	No. US slices
		initial	low-res	high-res 1	inc. scaling			
1	L.Fem	7.3 (2.2)	3.4 (0.6)	2.3 (0.1)	2.2 (0.1)	1.004	0	226
	R.Fem	7.1 (2.3)	4.6 (0.3)	2.2 (0.1)	3.0 (0.1)	1.028	0	168
	Pelvis	11.0 (3.5)	2.2 (0.1)	1.7 (0.1)	1.7 (0.1)	1.001	0	200
2	L.Fem	7.7 (2.5)	4.8 (0.1)	1.3 (0.1)	0.8 (0.1)	0.991	0	247
	R.Fem	7.9 (2.6)	4.9 (0.3)	1.1 (0.0)	1.1 (0.0)	1.000	0	556
	Pelvis	15.1 (7.0)	3.6 (0.2)	1.7 (0.0)	1.0 (0.0)	0.971	1	317
3	L.Fem	7.1 (2.3)	2.6 (0.6)	1.6 (0.4)	1.3 (0.2)	0.965	0	516
	R.Fem	7.3 (2.5)	5.0 (0.3)	2.4 (0.1)	1.4 (0.1)	0.969	0	565
	Pelvis	11.6 (4.0)	5.1 (0.2)	3.0 (0.1)	2.2 (0.1)	0.974	1	331

factor by which s_y has changed, the failure rate and the number of US slices used for each bone registration are also given. The results show that the mean RMS TRE after registration was less than 2.3mm for all the registrations except for the right femur of cadaver 1. The results for this case also show the only instance when the RMS TRE increased when the optimisation included the y scaling parameter; when this parameter was held fixed, the RMS TRE was 2.3mm. These registrations used the smallest number of US images (only 168) compared to over 500 for some of the other femur registrations, and we believe that this may have been a factor in the higher TRE calculated from this case.

4 Discussion and Conclusions

Very basic image processing filters have been used to produce the features on which the probability images are calculated. These have proven sufficient to allow accurate and robust registrations. However, in the future other, more sophisticated filters may be used which are more accurate and robust in their ability to extract bone-to-soft-tissue edges from US and CT images.

The inclusion into the optimisation process of the US image scaling parameter, s_y, improved the TRE values for over half the registrations, once by more than 1mm. Only in one case did the error increase, and this is believed to be due to insufficient numbers of US images.

Future work includes establishing how many US images (and from which anatomical areas) are required for accurate registration. The algorithm speed needs to be improved: current time for registration is between 5 and 22 minutes on a 2.8MHz Intel Pentium 4 processor. We also intend to combine this intensity-based technique with a method which instantiates a shape model [14]. This links in well with the current trend in computer assisted orthopaedic surgery, which is towards the use of CT-free methods.

We have presented an automatic method to register freehand 3D US images to a CT volume of a pelvis or femur. Our method is based on a strategy in which we preprocess images to provide a probability map of corresponding features. This preprocessing step uses information gathered from a set of manually segmented training data. The algorithm also optimises the parameter which defines the speed-of-sound through tissue. Our method had been compared to a "gold-standard" registration based on bone implanted fiducial markers. Registrations have been validated using three cadavers (6 femurs and 3 pelves). Results show that our method is accurate to less than 2.3mm (in all-but-one case), which should be sufficiently accurate for most total hip replacement procedures.

Acknowledgment

We would like to thank the EPSRC (grant number GR/R03525/01) for funding this project. Our thanks also go to Jens Krugman of BrainLab AG, Munich for his assistance in organising the experiments.

References

1. Barger, W., Bauer, A., Borner, M.: Primary and revision total hip replacement using the ROBODOC^r system. Clinic. Orthopaedics and Related Res. (1998) 82–91
2. DiGioia, III, A., Jaramaz, B., Blackwell, M., Simon, D., Morgan, F., Moody, J., Nikou, C., Colgan, B., Aston, C., Labarca, R., Kischell, E., Kanade, T.: Image guided navigation system to measure intraoperatively acetabular implant alignment. Clinic. Orthopaedics and Related Res. (1998) 8–22
3. Nabeyama, R., Matsuda, S., Miura, H., Mawatarim, T., Kawano, T., Iwamoto, Y.: The accuracy of image-guided knee replacement based on computed tomography. J. Bone Joint Surg. (Br) **86-B** (2004) 366–71
4. Berger, R.: Total hip arthroplasty using the minimally invasive two-incision approach. Clinic. Orthopaedics and Related Res. (2003) 232–241
5. DiGioia, III, A., Plakseychuk, A., Levison, T., Jaramaz, B.: Mini-incision technique for total hip arthroplasty with navigation. J. Arthroplasty **18** (2003) 123–128
6. Ault, T., Siegel, M.: Frameless patient registration using ultrasonic imaging. In: Proc. First International Symposium on Medical Robotics and Computer-assisted surgery. Volume 1. (1994) 74–82
7. Brendel, B., Winter, S., Rick, A., Stockheim, M., Ermert, H.: Registration of 3D CT and ultrasound datasets of the spine using bone structures. Comput. Aided Surg. **7** (2002) 146–155
8. Ionescu, G., Lavallée, S., Demongeot, J.: Automated registration of ultrasound with CT images: application to computer assisted prostate radiotherapy and orthopaedics. In Taylor, C., Colchester, A., eds.: Medical Imaging Computing and Computer-Assisted Intervention—MICCAI '99, Springer, Lecture notes in computer science 1679 (1999) 768–777
9. Amin, D., Kanade, T., DiGioia, III, A., Jaramaz, B.: Ultrasound registration of the bone surface for surgical navigation. Comput. Aided Surg. **8** (2003) 1–16
10. Tonetti, J., Carrat, L., Blendea, S., Merloz, P., Troccaz, J., Lavallée, S., Chirossel, J.: Clinical results of percutaneous pelvis surgery. Computer assisted surgery using ultrasound compared to standard fluoroscopy. Comput. Aided Surg. **6** (2001) 204–211
11. Brendel, B., Winter, S., Rick, A., Stockheim, M., Ermert, H.: Bone registration with 3D CT and ultrasound data sets. In: Computer Assisted Radiology and Surgery 2003, Elsevier Sciences B.V. (2003) 426–432
12. Jaramaz, B., Nikou, C., Cavalier, B., Blendea, S., Labarca, R., DiGioia, III, A.: Experimental validation of ultrasound registration of long bones. In Langlotz, F., Davies, B., Bauer, A., eds.: 3rd Annual Meeting of the Int. Soc. for Computer Assisted Orthopaedic Surgery, Steinkopff Darmstadt (2003) 160–161
13. Penney, G., Blackall, J., Hamady, M., Sabharwal, Y., Adam, A., Hawkes, D.: Registration of freehand 3D ultrasound and magnetic resonance liver images. Med. Image Anal. **8** (2004) 81–91
14. Chan, C., Barratt, D., Edwards, P., Penney, G., Slomczykowski, M., Hawkes, D.: Cadaver validation of the use of ultrasound for 3D model instantiation of bony anatomy in image guided orthopaedic surgery. In: Medical Imaging Computing and Computer-Assisted Intervention—MICCAI '04, Springer (2004) 397–404

Author Index

Abolmaesumi, Purang I-83, II-197
Acar, Burak I-213
Adams, J.E. II-733
Adamson, Chris I-294
Admiraal-Behloul, Faiza II-451
Agid, Yves II-385
Agnus, Vincent II-155
Aharon, Shmuel II-773
Aït-Ali, L.S. I-409
Akdemir, U. II-781
Akiyama, Kenta II-543
Alexander, D.C. I-164
Alia-Klein, Nelly I-679
Aljabar, P. II-247
Andronache, Adrian II-976
An, Jung-ha I-286
Anxionnat, R. II-214
Arai, Fumihito I-925
Arbel, Tal II-163
Archip, Neculai II-862
Arridge, Simon R. II-616, II-649
Arsigny, Vincent I-115, II-927, II-943
Ashton, Edward I-451
Atkins, Stella I-868
Audette, Michel I-9
Auvray, Vincent II-352
Avants, Brian B. I-164, II-328
Avila, Ricardo S. I-688
Awad, Mike I-811, II-526
Awate, Suyash P. II-517
Ayache, Nicholas I-115, I-539, I-753, II-295, II-385, II-492, II-927, II-943
Aylward, Elizabeth I-238
Aylward, Stephen R. I-59, I-221, I-523, II-806
Azzabou, Noura I-597

Bach Cuadra, Meritxell I-417
Baegert, Claire II-49
Bajka, M. II-575
Bammer, Roland I-213
Banovac, Filip II-992
Bardinet, Eric II-385, II-492
Bardyn, T. I-474
Barillot, Christian I-409, I-597
Barkovich, J. I-548
Barratt, Dean C. I-605, II-1000
Barta, Patrick I-238
Bauernschmitt, Robert II-287
Bazin, Pierre-Louis II-484
Beg, M. Faisal I-238
Bello, Musodiq I-254
Berezney, Ronald I-876
Berger, M-O. II-214
Bergmann, H. II-960
Bernasconi, A. I-375
Bernasconi, N. I-375
Bertrand, Gilles II-394
Bhagwat, Jui G. I-506
Bhatia, Kanwal K. I-99
Bhattacharjee, Manik II-385
Bhotika, Rahul I-688
Bielen, Didier I-859
Birkfellner, W. II-960
Blackband, Stephen J. I-156
Bland, Peyton H. II-419
Blumenkranz, Steve I-811
Boas, David A. II-649
Bobick, Aaron II-459
Boctor, Emad M. I-621
Boesiger, Peter I-786
Boomsma, Kevin I-786
Borschneck, D.P. I-459
Bos, Clemens I-467
Boubertakh, Redha II-894
Boughner, Derek II-171
Bouix, Sylvain I-515
Boukerroui, Djamal I-262
Boulanger, Jérôme I-893
Bourgeat, Pierrick II-813
Bouthemy, Patrick I-893, II-352
Boyes, R.G. II-247
Bradley, P. I-885
Brandel, Jean-Philippe II-492
Broadbent, Kathy A. I-434
Bryant, J. Tim I-902
Buechel, Christian I-498

Bullitt, Elizabeth I-26, I-59, I-383, II-239
Buonaccorsi, Giovanni A. I-91
Burschka, Darius I-811
Bystrov, Daniel I-467

Cachia, A. II-344
Calcagni, A. II-509
Camara, Oscar I-99
Camara-Rey, Oscar II-616
Campbell, Jennifer S.W. I-123
Cardin, M.A. II-9
Caroli, A. I-392
Carsin, B. I-409
Carson, James I-254
Carter, Timothy J. I-605, II-1000
Cascio, Carissa II-765
Castellanos, Joaquín II-320
Cattin, Philippe II-336, II-976
Chakravarty, M. Mallar II-394
Chan, Carolyn S.K. I-605, II-1000
Chandrashekara, R. I-425
Chang, S. I-442
Chan, Tony F. II-657, II-675
Chapman, Brian E. I-564
Charnoz, Arnaud II-155
Chefd'hotel, Christophe I-662
Chen, Elvis C.S. I-770
Chen, Nan-Kuei I-148
Chen, Yunmei I-278, I-286, II-741
Cheung, Sue I-91
Chiang, Ming-Chang II-666
Chinzei, Kiyoyuki I-9
Chiu, Wah I-254
Choti, Mike I-811, II-526
Christiansen, Claus I-327
Chung, Adrian I-868, I-910
Chung, Albert C.S. I-229
Ciccarelli, O. I-164
Claridge, E. II-509
Clatz, Olivier II-295
Cleary, Kevin II-312, II-992
Clouchoux, C. II-344
Cloutier, Guy I-319
Cocquerez, Jean-Pierre I-262
Cointepas, Y. I-196
Colchester, A.C.F. II-749
Collins, D. Louis I-392, II-163, II-394
Colliot, O. I-375
Commowick, Olivier II-927
Cook, P.A. I-164
Cooperberg, Peter II-862
Cootes, T.F. II-733
Cornu, Philippe II-385
Corouge, Isabelle I-131
Cotin, Stéphane I-43, II-534
Cottone, Lisa I-679
Cotton, S.D. II-509
Coudière, Y. II-607
Coulon, O. II-344
Coupé, Pierrick I-597
Cozzone, Patrick II-492
Cremers, Daniel II-757
Croome, Kris II-57
Crouch, Earl R. III II-591
Crouch, Jessica R. II-591, II-624
Crozier, Stuart II-813
Crum, William R. I-99, II-616
Cuisenaire, Olivier I-417
Cuvillon, Loïc II-551

Dai, Xiangtian (Donald) I-811
Dam, Erik I-327
Danilouchkine, Mikhail G. II-951
Darcourt, Jacques II-369
Darzi, Ara I-360, I-843, II-25, II-114, II-139
Davatzikos, Christos I-1, I-400, II-263, II-500, II-870
Davies, Karen I-91
Davis, B.C. I-442
Davis, Brad II-411
Dawant, Benoit M. II-427
Dawson, Steve I-43, II-534
Deguchi, Daisuke II-543
Deligianni, Fani I-843, I-910, II-139
Delingette, Hervé II-295
de Mathelin, Michel II-551
Descoteaux, Maxime I-9
D'Haese, Pierre-Francois II-427
Diamond, Solomon Gilbert II-649
Dijkers, J.J. I-712
Dikici, Engin II-692
DiMaio, Simon P. I-827
DiMarzio, Charles II-935
Ding, Mingyue II-17
Dione, Donald P. II-919
Dixon, Kat I-335
Dobrucki, Lawrence W. II-684, II-701, II-919

Dold, Christian I-482
Dormont, Didier II-385, II-492
Dornheim, Lars I-335
Downey, Donal II-17
Drisis, Stylianos I-859, II-361
Duchesne, S. I-392
Duncan, James S. I-761, I-778
Dupont, Pierre II-41
Duriez, C. II-534
Dutta, Sandeep I-738

Edan, G. I-409
Ede, C. II-960
Edwards, Phillip J. I-605, II-968, II-1000
Egan, Gary I-294
Eichele, Gregor I-254
El-Baz, Ayman I-34, I-720, II-821
Eldiasty, Tarek I-720, II-821
El-Ghar, Mohamed Abou I-720, II-821
ElHelw, Mohamed A. I-868
Ellis, Randy E. I-75, I-459, I-770, I-902, I-917, II-223
Ema, Sinya II-854
Evelhoch, Jeffrey I-451
Exner, Philipp I-819

Fahmi, Rachid I-531
Fahrig, Rebecca I-631
Falk, Robert I-654
Fan, Yong I-1, II-902
Farag, Aly A. I-34, I-531, I-654, I-720, II-821
Faucheux, Baptiste II-492
Feldman, Michael D. I-729
Feng, Jun II-279
Fenlon, Michael R. II-968
Fenster, Aaron II-17
Ferrarini, Luca II-451
Fetita, Catalin II-830
Feuerstein, Marco II-287
Fevens, Thomas I-670
Fichtinger, Gabor I-621, I-639, II-312
Figl, M. II-960
Fillard, Pierre I-115, II-927, II-943
Finnis, Kirk W. I-835
Firle, Evelyn A. I-482
Fischer, Gregory S. II-73
Fisher, John I-310
Fletcher, P. Thomas I-131
Florie, J. I-712
Florin, Charles I-246
Folkesson, Jenny I-327
Forest, Clément II-155
Forgione, Antonello II-551
Foroughi, Pezhman I-83
Foskey, M. I-442
Foster, Norman L. II-517
Fox, Nick II-616
Franceschini, Maria Angela II-649
Frangi, A.F. II-271
Freiman, M. II-131
Friman, Ola I-107
Fripp, Jurgen II-813
Frisoni, G.B. I-392
Fujiwara, Yasunori II-97
Fukuda, Toshio I-925

Gabrieli, John D. I-205
Galanaud, Damien II-492
Galbraith, Natalie II-57
Gallardo, Greg I-302
Galloway, Graham II-813
Gamper, U. II-336
Gangi, Afshin II-49
Gangloff, Jacques II-551
Gautham, Sardar Mal I-738
Gee, James C. I-164, I-172, II-328, II-725
Geiger, Bernhard I-662
Geiser, Edward I-286
Gerig, Guido I-26, I-131, I-383
Germann, Jurgen II-394
Geroldi, C. I-392
Ghoneim, Mohamed A. II-821
Giddens, Don P. I-490
Gilmore, John H. I-131
Gimel'farb, Georgy I-34, I-720
Gimpel Smith, Rachel II-765
Ginestet, Chantal I-556
Glenn, O. I-548
Glossop, Neil II-992
Goddard, Dorothy A. I-434
Goksel, Orcun I-827
Golby, Alexandra J. II-295
Goldberger, Jacob II-790
Goldberg-Zimring, Daniel I-506
Goldstein, Rita I-679

Golestani, N. I-196
González Ballester, Miguel Ángel I-474, II-369, II-492
Gooding, Mark J. I-434
Gorges, S. II-214
Goshtasby, Ardeshir II-717
Goyal, L. I-442
Grady, Leo I-442, II-773
Grau, Vicente I-589
Greenspan, Hayit II-790
Grenier, Philippe II-830
Grimson, W. Eric L. I-188, 310
Gross, M. II-567
Gu, Xianfeng II-657
Guehring, Jens I-498
Guetter, Christoph II-255
Guiraudon, Gerard II-171
Guo, Hongyu II-984
Guo, Ting I-835

Hadjidemetriou, Stathis I-761
Hager, Gregory D. I-621, I-802, I-811
Haïk, Stéphane II-492
Hajnal, J.V. II-247
Haker, Steven I-188, I-490, I-506, II-147, II-459
Hakozaki, Yoshihide II-97
Harders, M. II-567, II-575
Hasser, Chris I-811
Hassouna, M. Sabry I-654
Hattori, Asaki II-559
Hawkes, David J. I-605, II-968, II-1000
Hayashibe, Mitsuhiro II-559
Hayashi, Kiralee M. II-657
Hayashi, Yuichiro I-696
Hellier, Pierre I-409, I-597
Hendriks, Emile A. II-846
Heng, Pheng-Ann I-572, II-709
Hennig, Jürgen I-482
Hero, Alfred O. III II-271, II-419
Hettleman, Bruce I-67, 704
He, Weijun I-745
He, Y. II-468
Hill, Derek L.G. I-99, I-425, II-607, II-616, II-894
Hill, Nicholas A. II-171
Ho, Hon Pong I-278, II-741
Homolka, P. II-960
Hornegger, Joachim II-255
Huang, Feng I-286
Huang, Heng I-67, I-704
Huang, Ling I-148
Huang, Xiaolei I-745
Huang, Xishi II-171
Hummel, J. II-960
Huppert, Theodore J. II-649
Hushek, Stephen G. I-34

Ianzini, Fiorenza I-302
Ide, Ichiro II-854
Ikeda, Seiichi I-925
Inder, Terrie I-294
Iordachita, Iulian I-621
Iordanova, B. I-548
Ip, Horace H.S. II-279
Irie, Keiko I-925

Jackowski, Marcel II-701, II-717
Jackson, Alan I-91
Jain, Ameet I-639
James, Adam II-25
Janke, Andrew II-813
Jayson, Gordon C. I-91
Jenkinson, Mark I-99
Jiang, T.Z. II-468
Jin, Chao I-670
John, Matthias II-798
Johnston, Leigh I-294
Jolesz, Ferenc A. II-295
Jomier, Julien I-59, I-523, II-806
Jomier, Matthieu II-765
Joshi, Sarang I-131, I-442, II-411, II-984
Joskowicz, L. II-131
Ju, Tao I-254

Kaipio, Jari P. II-649
Kakadiaris, Ioannis A. I-254, I-343
Kalender, Willi A. II-33, II-443
Kameyama, Fumie II-97
Kanade, Takeo II-1
Kao, Chris II-427
Kapoor, Ankur II-89
Karacali, Bilge II-500
Kassim, Ashraf A. I-51, I-270
Katayama, Youichi II-81
Kaufhold, John I-851
Kaur, Manmeen II-205
Kavoussi, L. II-526
Kerrien, E. II-214

Kervrann, Charles I-893
Khamene, Ali II-65
Khan, Ali I-238
Kikinis, Ron I-43, I-310, II-295, II-583
Kim, Jung II-599
Kim, Seyoung I-352
Kiss, Gabriel I-859
Kitasaka, Takayuki I-696, II-543, II-854
Klironomos, D. I-375
Kobayashi, Etsuko II-81
Kolehmainen, Ville II-649
Konrad, Peter E. II-427
Kon, Ryan I-639
Köstler, W. I-474
Kouby, V. El I-196
Koulibaly, Pierre Malick II-369
Koyama, T. II-105
Krasinskas, Alyssa M. I-564
Krishnan, A. II-781
Krissian, Karl I-43
Krzyżak, Adam I-670
Kumar, Rajesh I-811
Kurtcuoglu, Vartan I-786

Laine, Andrew F. II-205
Langan, David I-851
Lanovaz, Joel L. I-770, I-917
Le Bihan, D. I-196
LeDigarcher, Vincent I-59, I-523, II-806
Lee, Su-Lin I-360
Lee, Vivian S. II-205
Lelieveldt, Boudewijn P.F. II-951
Lenoir, J. II-534
Leskovjan, Andreana I-679
Leven, Joshua I-811
Levitt, James J. I-310
Lewis, Emma II-616
Liang, M. II-468
Liénard, Jean II-352
Li, Ming II-89
Li, Shimin II-684
Li, Shuo I-670
Li, Song I-670
Li, X.B. II-468
Likar, Boštjan II-231
Lin, Henry C. I-802
Lin, Mingen I-876
Lin, Ning I-778
Linguraru, Marius George II-492
Litt, Harold II-902
Littmann, Arne I-498
Liu, Huafeng I-278, II-741
Liu, K.-Y. I-885
Liu, Tianming I-148
Liu, Yi-Hwa II-684
Liu, Yuncai II-122
Lo, Benny P.L. II-25
Loeckx, Dirk II-361
Lohmann G. II-749
Lomax, A. II-336
Lorenzen, Peter II-411
Luboz, Vincent I-43
Lucidarme, Olivier II-830
Lui, Lok Ming II-675

Ma, Burton I-75, I-459
Mackey, Michael A. I-302
Madabhushi, Anant I-729
Maddah, Mahnaz I-188
Maeder, Philippe I-417
Maeno, Takashi II-633
Maes, Frederik II-361
Makedon, Fillia I-67, 704
Malandain, Grégoire II-155, II-369, II-385, II-927
Manak, Joseph I-851
Mangin, J.-F. I-196, II-344
Manjeshwar, Ravi I-851
Mansi, T. I-375
Marchal, Guy I-859, II-361
Mareci, Thomas H. I-156
Mareels, Iven I-294
Marohn, Mike I-811
Marquering, Henk A. II-846
Marsden, Paul K. II-968
Martin-Fernandez, Marcos I-515
Maurer, Calvin R. Jr. II-543, II-838
Maurice, Roch L. I-319
Mazilu, D. II-526
McCarley, Robert W. I-515
McGurk, Mark II-968
McShane, Teresa I-451
Meetz, Kirsten I-467
Mekada, Yoshito II-854
Meller, Sebastian II-443
Mellor, Matthew I-434
Mendonça, Paulo R.S. I-688, I-738

Merriam, John C. II-591
Metaxas, Dimitris I-745
Meuli, Reto I-417
Meunier, Jean I-319
Mewes, Andrea U.J. I-188
Meyer, Charles R. II-419
Mian, Asim I-506
Miller, James V. I-688, I-738
Miller, Karol II-583
Miller, Michael I-238
Moallem, Merhdad II-57
Moghari, Mehdi Hedjazi II-197
Mohamed, Ashraf I-400, II-263
Mohiaddin, Raad II-402
Momoi, Y. II-105
Morady, Roya II-57
Moreau-Villéger, V. II-607
Mori, Kensaku I-696, II-543, II-854
Mori, Masaki II-543, II-854
Morimoto, K. II-105
Morris, James I-827
Mortamet, Bénédicte I-383
Mukherjee, Lopamudra I-876
Murase, Hiroshi II-854
Murphy, Todd E. I-802
Mylonas, George P. I-843, II-139

Naessens, V. I-375
Nagai, Noritaka II-633
Nagel, Markus II-33
Naghavi, Morteza I-343
Nain, Delphine II-459
Nakajima, Y. II-105
Nakata, Norio II-559
Natori, Hiroshi II-543, II-854
Navab, Nassir II-287, II-303
Negoro, Makoto I-925
Nelson, Bradley J. I-819
Netsch, Thomas I-467
Neumann, P. II-534
Nicolaou, Marios I-868, II-25
Nicolau, S.A. I-539
Niederer, P. II-960
Niermann, Ken II-427
Niessen, Wiro J. II-911
Nijmeh, Ayman D. II-968
Nio, Y.C. I-712
Nkenke, Emeka II-443
Noble, J. Alison I-589
Noble, Nicholas M.I. II-894
Nolte, L. I-474

Oda, Masahiro I-696
Odell, Edward II-968
O'Donnell, Lauren I-140
O'Donnell, Thomas II-692
Oguz, Ipek II-765
Ohno-Machado, Lucila I-506
Okada, K. II-781
Okamura, Allison M. I-802, II-624
Olofsen, Hans II-451
Olsen, Ole Fogh I-327
O'Malley, Sean M. I-343
Onogi, S. II-105
Otake, Yoshito II-559
Oubel, E. II-271
Ourselin, Sébastien II-813
Özarslan, Evren I-156

Padfield, Dirk R. I-738
Padhani, Anwar R. II-886
Pallavaram, Srivatsan II-427
Papademetris, Xenophon II-701, II-919
Paragios, Nikos I-246
Parker, Geoff J.M. I-91
Park, Hyunjin II-419
Parrent, Andrew G. I-835
Patel, Rajni II-57
Pathak, Chetna II-239
Patriciu, A. II-526
Pearlman, Justin I-67, I-704
Pennec, Xavier I-115, I-539, I-753, II-927, II-943
Penney, Graeme P. I-605, II-911, II-1000
Perchant, Aymeric I-753
Pernuš, Franjo II-231
Perperidis, Dimitrios II-402
Perrimon, N. I-885
Pescatore, J. II-214
Peters, Terry M. I-835, II-171
Pettersen, Paola I-327
Petzold, Ralf II-33
Pham, Dzung L. II-484
Picard, L. II-214
Pichon, Eric I-180
Pidoux, Bernard II-385
Pike, G. Bruce I-123
Pinel, Philippe II-476

Plewes, D.B. II-9
Pohl, Kilian M. I-310
Poline, Jean-Baptiste I-196, II-476
Pollo, Claudio I-417
Poulikakos, Dimos I-786
Poupon, C. I-196
Prastawa, Marcel I-26, I-383
Preece, S.J. II-509
Prêteux, Françoise II-830
Primak, Serguei II-57
Prima, S. I-409
Prince, Jerry L. I-631, II-870

Qian, Xiaoning II-377
Qi, Feihu II-179

Rahn, Norbert II-798
Rajagopalan, Srinivasan I-794
Ramamurthi, Krishnakumar I-631
Ramesh, V. II-781
Rangarajan, Anand II-984
Rayman, Reiza II-57
Razavi, Reza S. I-425, II-607, II-894
Rees, Sandra I-294
Régis, J. II-344
Reiber, Johan H.C. II-451, II-846
Ren, Jing II-171
Reyes, Mauricio II-369
Rhode, K.S. I-425, II-607
Richardson, Theodor II-435
Rit, Simon I-556
Rivaz, Hassan I-613
Rivière, D. I-196, II-344
Robb, Richard A. I-794
Roberts, Caleb I-91
Roberts, M.G. II-733
Rodriguez-Carranza, C. I-548
Rohlfing, T. II-838
Rohling, Robert I-613, I-827, II-862
Rohr, Karl II-320
Röper, Barbara II-303
Rosenman, J. I-442
Rosen, Mark I-729
Ross, James C. I-738, I-851
Rousseau, F. I-548
Rousson, Mikael II-757
Roy Cardinal, Marie-Hélène I-319
Rueckert, Daniel I-99, I-425, II-247, II-402
Ruf, Amit II-790
Rusinek, Henry II-205

Sadikot, Abbas F. II-394
Sakas, Georgios I-482
Sakuma, Ichiro II-81, II-105
Salcudean, Septimiu E. I-827
Saleh, Christian II-385
Samaras, Dimitris I-679
Sánchez Castro, F. Javier I-417
Sanchez-Ortiz, G.I. I-425
Sanderse, Martijn II-846
Sarrut, David I-556
Sauer, Frank II-65, 255
Savadjiev, Peter I-123
Schiwietz, Thomas II-773
Schmidt, Gerd II-33
Schmid, Volker J. II-886
Schnabel, Julia II-616
Schneider, Chad M. II-624
Schreck, Pascal II-49
Schulz, Heinrich I-467
Schutyser, Filip I-368
Schwartzman, David II-1
Schweiger, Martin II-616
Scott, Marietta L.J. II-878
Seemann, R. II-960
Sermesant, M. I-425, II-607
Setser, Randolph II-692
Shafran, Izhak I-802
Shah, Mubarak I-270
Shamir, R. II-131
Shen, Dinggang I-1, II-179, II-263, II-500, II-902
Shen, Li I-67, I-704
Shenton, Martha E. I-310, I-515
Shen, Weijia I-270
Shepherd, Timothy M. I-156
Shi, Fanhuai II-122
Shi, Hongjian I-531, II-821
Shi, Jianbo I-729
Shi, Lin I-572
Shimachi, Shigeyuki II-97
Shi, Pengcheng I-278, II-188, II-741
Shipley, Jacqueline A. I-434
Shoham, M. II-131
Shoshan, Y. II-131
Siddiqi, Kaleem I-9, I-123
Sidler, R. I-474

Sierra, R. II-575
Simpson, A.L. I-459
Singh, M. II-781
Sinusas, Albert J. I-778, II-684, II-701, II-919
Sirohey, Saad A. I-688
Slomczykowski, Mike I-605, II-1000
Smith, Erin J. I-902
Smyth, Padhraic I-352
Soellinger, Michaela I-786
Soler, Luc I-539, II-49, II-155
Solomon, S.B. II-526
Song, Ting II-205
Sonka, Milan I-302
Soulez, Gilles I-319
Speck, Oliver I-482
Spooner, John II-427
Srinivasan, Mandayam A. II-599
Staib, Lawrence H. II-701, II-919
Stefanescu, Radu II-927, II-943
Steinemann, D. II-567
Stern, Hal I-352
Stetten, George I-647
Stiehl, Hans-Siegfried I-498
Stoianovici, D. II-526
Stoll, Jeffrey II-41
Stoyanov, Danail I-843, II-114, II-139
Strobel, Norbert I-631
Studholme, C. I-548
Styles, I.B. II-509
Styner, Martin A. I-474, II-765
Subotic, Vanja II-57
Sudarsky, Sandra I-662
Südkamp, N. I-474
Suenaga, Yasuhito I-696, II-543, II-854
Suetens, Paul I-368, I-859, II-361
Sugano, N. II-105
Sui, M.Q. II-468
Summers, Paul I-786
Sundaram, Tessa A. II-328
Sundar, Hari II-902
Suprijanto, S. I-580
Suzuki, Naoki II-559
Suzuki, Shigeyuki II-559
Suzuki, Takashi II-81
Swennen, Gwen I-368
Szczerba, Dominik II-641
Székely, Gábor II-336, II-567, II-575, II-641, II-976

Tada, Mitsunori II-633
Tagare, Hemant D. II-377
Tahmasebpour, Hamid II-862
Tajine, Mohamed II-155
Takabatake, Hirotsugu II-543, II-854
Takahashi, Ikuo I-925
Talos, Ion-Florin I-506, II-295
Tamura, Y. II-105
Tang, Thomas S.Y. II-223
Tannenbaum, Allen R. I-180, I-490, II-147, II-459
Tao, Xiaodong II-870
Tasdizen, Tolga II-517
Tavakoli, Mahdi II-57
Taylor, N. Jane II-886
Taylor, Russell H. I-811, II-73, II-89, II-312
Teoh, Eam Khwang I-221
Thacker, Neil A. II-878
Thaller, Christina I-254
Thérasse, Éric I-319
Thiran, Jean-Philippe I-417
Thirion, Bertrand II-476
Thompson, A.J. I-164
Thompson, Paul M. II-657, II-666, II-675
Tian, L.X. II-468
Tobon-Gomez, C. II-271
Toews, Matthew II-163
Tolxdorff, Thomas II-320
Tomasi, Dardo I-679
Tomaszeweski, John E. I-729
Tomaževič, Dejan II-231
Tönnies, Klaus D. I-335
Toomre, Derek I-761
Toriwaki, Jun-ichiro I-696
Touhami, Wala I-262
Trousset, Y. II-214
Truyen, R. I-712
Tsai, Chia-Ling II-935
Tsang, Eric C.C. I-572
Tublin, Mitchell E. I-564
Turken, And U. I-205
Turner, Jessica I-352
Turner, Wesley D. I-688

Ungar, Lida I-515

van Assen, Hans C. II-951
van Buchem, Mark A. II-451

Van Cleynenbreugel, Johan I-859
van de Kraats, Everine B. II-911
van der Lugt, Aad II-846
Van Horn, Mark II-239
van Reiber, Johan H.C. II-951
van Vliet, L.J. I-712
van Walsum, Theo II-911
van Wijk, C. I-712
van Wynsberghe, Aimee II-57
Vandermeulen, Dirk II-361
Vavuranakis, Manolis I-343
Vemuri, Baba C. I-17, I-156
Venema, H.W. I-712
Ventikos, Yiannis I-786
Vercauteren, Tom I-753
Vigneron, D. I-548
Villard, Caroline II-49
Villemure, Jean-Guy I-417
Vivert, Christelle I-59
Vogel, M.W. I-580
Volkow, Nora I-679
Vollmers, Karl I-819
von Cramon, D.Y. II-749
von Siebenthal, M. II-336
Vos, F.M. I-580, I-712
Vossepoel, A.M. I-580
Vrooman, H.A. I-580

Wagenknecht, Gudrun II-320
Wainer, Josh II-624
Wang, David I-647
Wang, Defeng I-572
Wang, Fei I-17
Wang, J.X. II-9
Wang, Song II-435
Wang, Yalin II-657, II-666, II-675
Wang, Y.F. II-468
Warfield, Simon K. I-188, I-506, II-295, II-583, II-862
Warger, William II II-935
Warren, Joe I-254
Watson, Yvonne I-91
Weeks, Susan II-239
Wein, Wolfgang II-303
Wei, Zhouping II-17
Wells, William M. III I-310, I-506
Westenberg, Jos J.M. II-951
Westermann, Rüdiger II-773
Westin, Carl-Fredrik I-43, I-107, I-140, I-180
Whitaker, Ross T. II-517
Whitcher, Brandon J. II-886
White, Richard D. II-692
Whitfield-Gabrieli, Susan L. I-205
Wildhirt, Stephen M. II-287
Williams, Jim I-246
Wilson, David I-286, I-851
Wittek, Adam II-583
Wong, Stephen TC I-148, I-885
Wong, Tien-Tsin I-572
Wu, Bing I-647
Wu, Guorong II-179
Wu, Huadong I-564
Wu, Jue I-229
Wu, Xunlei I-43

Xia, Yan I-205
Xie, Jun II-709
Xu, Chenyang II-255
Xu, Jinhui I-876
Xu, Sheng II-312
Xue, Zhong II-500, II-902

Yan, Ping I-778
Yan, Pingkun I-51, 270
Yang, Fuxing I-302
Yang, Guang-Zhong I-360, I-843, I-868, II-25, II-114, II-139, II-886
Yang, X. II-960
Yang, Yan I-490
Yau, Shing-Tung II-657
Yelnik, Jérôme II-385
Yesin, K. Berk I-819
Yeung, Daniel S. I-572
Yeung, Sai Kit II-188
Ying, Xiaoyou I-745
Yonenobu, S. II-105
Yörük, Erdem I-213
Young, Geoffrey I-148
Yuh, David D. I-802
Yuksel, Seniha E. II-821
Yushkevich, Paul A. I-164, I-172, II-725

Zátonyi, J. II-575
Zaitsev, Maxim I-482
Zang, Y.F. II-468
Zehavi, E. II-131

Zeng, Donglin I-383
Zhang, Gary I-811
Zhang, Hui I-164, I-172, II-725, II-992
Zhang, Jing II-122
Zhang, Lei I-679
Zhang, Rong I-67, I-704
Zhao, Zheen I-221
Zhao, Zijian II-122
Zhong, Guang I-910
Zhong, Hua II-1
Zhou, Xiaobo I-885
Zhou, Yu I-639
Zhu, C.Z. II-468
Zhu, Lei I-490, II-147
Zou, Kelly H. I-506

Lecture Notes in Computer Science

For information about Vols. 1–3652

please contact your bookseller or Springer

Vol. 3697: W. Duch, J. Kacprzyk, E. Oja, S. Zadrożny (Eds.), Artificial Neural Networks: Formal Models and Their Applications – ICANN 2005, Part II. XXXII, 1045 pages. 2005.

Vol. 3696: W. Duch, J. Kacprzyk, E. Oja, S. Zadrożny (Eds.), Artificial Neural Networks: Biological Inspirations – ICANN 2005, Part I. XXXI, 703 pages. 2005.

Vol. 3695: M.R. Berthold, R. Glen, K. Diederichs, O. Kohlbacher, I. Fischer (Eds.), Computational Life Sciences. XI, 277 pages. 2005. (Subseries LNBI).

Vol. 3694: M. Malek, E. Nett, N. Suri (Eds.), Service Availability. VIII, 213 pages. 2005.

Vol. 3693: A.G. Cohn, D.M. Mark (Eds.), Spatial Information Theory. XII, 493 pages. 2005.

Vol. 3692: R. Casadio, G. Myers (Eds.), Algorithms in Bioinformatics. X, 436 pages. 2005. (Subseries LNBI).

Vol. 3691: A. Gagalowicz, W. Philips (Eds.), Computer Analysis of Images and Patterns. XIX, 865 pages. 2005.

Vol. 3690: M. Pěchouček, P. Petta, L.Z. Varga (Eds.), Multi-Agent Systems and Applications IV. XVII, 667 pages. 2005. (Subseries LNAI).

Vol. 3689: G.G. Lee, A. Yamada, H. Meng, S.H. Myaeng (Eds.), Information Retrieval Technology. XVII, 735 pages. 2005.

Vol. 3688: R. Winther, B.A. Gran, G. Dahll (Eds.), Computer Safety, Reliability, and Security. XI, 405 pages. 2005.

Vol. 3687: S. Singh, M. Singh, C. Apte, P. Perner (Eds.), Pattern Recognition and Image Analysis, Part II. XXV, 809 pages. 2005.

Vol. 3686: S. Singh, M. Singh, C. Apte, P. Perner (Eds.), Pattern Recognition and Data Mining, Part I. XXVI, 689 pages. 2005.

Vol. 3685: V. Gorodetsky, I. Kotenko, V. Skormin (Eds.), Computer Network Security. XIV, 480 pages. 2005.

Vol. 3684: R. Khosla, R.J. Howlett, L.C. Jain (Eds.), Knowledge-Based Intelligent Information and Engineering Systems, Part IV. LXXIX, 933 pages. 2005. (Subseries LNAI).

Vol. 3683: R. Khosla, R.J. Howlett, L.C. Jain (Eds.), Knowledge-Based Intelligent Information and Engineering Systems, Part III. LXXX, 1397 pages. 2005. (Subseries LNAI).

Vol. 3682: R. Khosla, R.J. Howlett, L.C. Jain (Eds.), Knowledge-Based Intelligent Information and Engineering Systems, Part II. LXXIX, 1371 pages. 2005. (Subseries LNAI).

Vol. 3681: R. Khosla, R.J. Howlett, L.C. Jain (Eds.), Knowledge-Based Intelligent Information and Engineering Systems, Part I. LXXX, 1319 pages. 2005. (Subseries LNAI).

Vol. 3679: S.d.C. di Vimercati, P. Syverson, D. Gollmann (Eds.), Computer Security – ESORICS 2005. XI, 509 pages. 2005.

Vol. 3678: A. McLysaght, D.H. Huson (Eds.), Comparative Genomics. VIII, 167 pages. 2005. (Subseries LNBI).

Vol. 3677: J. Dittmann, S. Katzenbeisser, A. Uhl (Eds.), Communications and Multimedia Security. XIII, 360 pages. 2005.

Vol. 3676: R. Glück, M. Lowry (Eds.), Generative Programming and Component Engineering. XI, 448 pages. 2005.

Vol. 3675: Y. Luo (Ed.), Cooperative Design, Visualization, and Engineering. XI, 264 pages. 2005.

Vol. 3674: W. Jonker, M. Petković (Eds.), Secure Data Management. X, 241 pages. 2005.

Vol. 3673: S. Bandini, S. Manzoni (Eds.), AI*IA 2005: Advances in Artificial Intelligence. XIV, 614 pages. 2005. (Subseries LNAI).

Vol. 3672: C. Hankin, I. Siveroni (Eds.), Static Analysis. X, 369 pages. 2005.

Vol. 3671: S. Bressan, S. Ceri, E. Hunt, Z.G. Ives, Z. Bellahsène, M. Rys, R. Unland (Eds.), Database and XML Technologies. X, 239 pages. 2005.

Vol. 3670: M. Bravetti, L. Kloul, G. Zavattaro (Eds.), Formal Techniques for Computer Systems and Business Processes. XIII, 349 pages. 2005.

Vol. 3669: G.S. Brodal, S. Leonardi (Eds.), Algorithms – ESA 2005. XVIII, 901 pages. 2005.

Vol. 3668: M. Gabbrielli, G. Gupta (Eds.), Logic Programming. XIV, 454 pages. 2005.

Vol. 3666: B.D. Martino, D. Kranzlmüller, J. Dongarra (Eds.), Recent Advances in Parallel Virtual Machine and Message Passing Interface. XVII, 546 pages. 2005.

Vol. 3665: K. S. Candan, A. Celentano (Eds.), Advances in Multimedia Information Systems. X, 221 pages. 2005.

Vol. 3664: C. Türker, M. Agosti, H.-J. Schek (Eds.), Peer-to-Peer, Grid, and Service-Orientation in Digital Library Architectures. X, 261 pages. 2005.

Vol. 3663: W.G. Kropatsch, R. Sablatnig, A. Hanbury (Eds.), Pattern Recognition. XIV, 512 pages. 2005.

Vol. 3662: C. Baral, G. Greco, N. Leone, G. Terracina (Eds.), Logic Programming and Nonmonotonic Reasoning. XIII, 454 pages. 2005. (Subseries LNAI).

Vol. 3661: T. Panayiotopoulos, J. Gratch, R. Aylett, D. Ballin, P. Olivier, T. Rist (Eds.), Intelligent Virtual Agents. XIII, 506 pages. 2005. (Subseries LNAI).

Vol. 3660: M. Beigl, S. Intille, J. Rekimoto, H. Tokuda (Eds.), UbiComp 2005: Ubiquitous Computing. XVII, 394 pages. 2005.

Vol. 3659: J.R. Rao, B. Sunar (Eds.), Cryptographic Hardware and Embedded Systems – CHES 2005. XIV, 458 pages. 2005.

Vol. 3658: V. Matoušek, P. Mautner, T. Pavelka (Eds.), Text, Speech and Dialogue. XV, 460 pages. 2005. (Subseries LNAI).

Vol. 3657: F.S. de Boer, M.M. Bonsangue, S. Graf, W.-P. de Roever (Eds.), Formal Methods for Components and Objects. VIII, 325 pages. 2005.

Vol. 3656: M. Kamel, A. Campilho (Eds.), Image Analysis and Recognition. XXIV, 1279 pages. 2005.

Vol. 3655: A. Aldini, R. Gorrieri, F. Martinelli (Eds.), Foundations of Security Analysis and Design III. VII, 273 pages. 2005.

Vol. 3654: S. Jajodia, D. Wijesekera (Eds.), Data and Applications Security XIX. X, 353 pages. 2005.

Vol. 3653: M. Abadi, L. de Alfaro (Eds.), CONCUR 2005 – Concurrency Theory. XIV, 578 pages. 2005.

GPSR Compliance

The European Union's (EU) General Product Safety Regulation (GPSR) is a set of rules that requires consumer products to be safe and our obligations to ensure this.

If you have any concerns about our products, you can contact us on ProductSafety@springernature.com

In case Publisher is established outside the EU, the EU authorized representative is:

Springer Nature Customer Service Center GmbH
Europaplatz 3
69115 Heidelberg, Germany

Batch number: 10844661

Printed by Printforce, the Netherlands